Sandra Smith's Review for

NCLEX-PN®

EIGHTH EDITION

Sandra F. Smith, RN, MS

JONES AND BARTLETT PUBLISHERS

Sudbury, Massachusetts

BOSTON   TORONTO   LONDON   SINGAPORE

Sandra Smith's Review for

NCLEX-PN®

EIGHTH EDITION

Sandra F. Smith, RN, MS

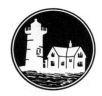

JONES AND BARTLETT PUBLISHERS

Sudbury, Massachusetts

BOSTON   TORONTO   LONDON   SINGAPORE

World Headquarters

Jones and Bartlett Publishers
40 Tall Pine Drive
Sudbury, MA 01776
978-443-5000
info@jbpub.com
www.jbpub.com

Jones and Bartlett Publishers
Canada
6339 Ormindale Way
Mississauga, ON L5V 1J2
CANADA

Jones and Bartlett Publishers
International
Barb House, Barb Mews
London W6 7PA
UK

Jones and Bartlett's books and products are available through most bookstores and online booksellers. To contact Jones and Bartlett Publishers directly, call 800-832-0034, fax 978-443-8000, or visit our website at www.jbpub.com.

Substantial discounts on bulk quantities of Jones and Bartlett's publications are available to corporations, professional associations, and other qualified organizations. For details and specific discount information, contact the special sales department at Jones and Bartlett via the above contact information or send an email to specialsales@jbpub.com.

ISBN-13: 978-0-7637-5676-5

The authors, editor, and publisher have made every effort to provide accurate information. However, they are not responsible for errors, omissions, or for any outcomes related to the use of the contents of this book and take no responsibility for the use of the products and procedures described. Treatments and side effects described in this book may not be applicable to all people; likewise, some people may require a dose or experience a side effect that is not described herein. Drugs and medical devices are discussed that may have limited availability controlled by the Food and Drug Administration (FDA) for use only in a research study or clinical trial. Research, clinical practice, and government regulations often change the accepted standard in this field. When consideration is being given to use of any drug in the clinical setting, the health care provider or reader is responsible for determining FDA status of the drug, reading the package insert, and reviewing prescribing information for the most up-to-date recommendations on dose, precautions, and contraindications, and determining the appropriate usage for the product. This is especially important in the case of drugs that are new or seldom used.

Executive Editor: Kevin Sullivan
Acquisitions Editor: Emily Ekle
Associate Editor: Amy Sibley
Editorial Assistant: Patricia Donnelly
Reprints Coordinator: Amy Browning
Manufacturing and Inventory Control Supervisor: Amy Bacus
Printing and Binding: Malloy, Inc.
Cover Printing: Malloy, Inc.
CD Duplication: New Territories, Inc.

6048

Printed in the United States of America
11 10 09 08 07   10 9 8 7 6 5 4 3 2 1

BRIEF CONTENTS

CONTENTS IN DETAIL

CONTRIBUTING AUTHORS

Marianne Barba, RN, MS
Care New England
Providence, RI

Shirley Chang, RN, MS, PhD
Evergreen College
San Jose, CA

Debra Denham, RN, MS, PhD
Hartnell College
Salinas, CA

Donna Duell, RN, MS, ABD
Consultant-ADN Programs
California

Joseann DeWitt, RN, MSN, BC, CLNC
Legal Nurse Consultant
Vidalia, LA

Marianne Hultgren, RN, MS
Hawaii Pacific University
Honolulu, HI

Susan Yadro, RN, MS
University of Wisconsin
Madison, WI

CONTRIBUTORS TO THE CD-ROM

Audrey Bopp
St. John Fisher College
Rochester, NY

Vera Dauffenbach
University of Wisconsin
Green Bay, WI

Linda Dunaway
Maysville Community College
Maysville, KY

Angie Grabau
University of Nebraska Medical Center
Lincoln, NE

Sammie Justesen
Internet Communications Corporation of America
Logan, UT

Susan Kangas-Packett
Creighton University
Omaha, NE

Kim Kendall
Maysville Community College
Maysville, KY

Sandra Liming
North Seattle Community College
Seattle, WA

Patricia O'Connor
Mariam College
Fond Du Lac, WI

Teresa Shellenbarger
Indiana University of Pennsylvania
Indiana, PA

Jacqueline Thayer
North Seattle Community College
Seattle, WA

CONTRIBUTING AUTHORS

PREVIOUS EDITIONS

Donald Anderson, RN, EdD
Regis College
Weston, MA

Sharon Matusoff Bell, RN, BSN, MA
Columbus Public Schools: Health Occupations
Columbus, OH

Mary Bierly, RN, BSN
Columbus Public Schools: Practical Nursing
Columbus, OH

Lee Brungreber, RN, MS
Cabrillo College
Aptos, CA

Barbara Enderle, RN, BSN
Columbus Public Schools: Practical Nursing
Columbus, OH

Patricia Parr Graves, RN
Columbus Public Schools: Practical Nursing
Columbus, OH

Eva Nunn Gumke, RN, BSN
Hartnell College
Salinas, CA

Judith Hankin, RN, BS, MS
Lively Area Vocational-Technical Center
Tallahassee, FL

Sandra Harper, RN, BSN
Dallas Vocational Nursing Program
Dallas, TX

Susan Tamburro Keiser, RN, BS, EdD
Columbus Public Schools: Practical Nursing
Columbus, OH

Arlene Thorsness Kostoch, RN, PhD
Del Mar College
Corpus Christie, TX

Rhonda R. Martin, RN, MS
University of Tulsa
Tulsa, OK

Patricia Ann Morrissey, RN, MS
Edna McConnell Clark School of Nursing
New York, NY

Doris E. Nay, RN, MA
Boulder Valley Health Occupations
Boulder, CO

Fay Alger O'Brien, RN, MA
De Anza College
Cupertino, CA

Dolores Vaz, RN, MSN, MEd
Bristol Community College
Fall River, MA

REVIEWERS

Brigitte L. Casteel, RN, BSN

John Ficklinger, PhD

Carol J. McFadyen, RN, PhD

Daniel Mobit, RN, BSN

Kathy Peterson-Sweeney, RN, MS, NP

Kathleen A. Pollard, RN, MSN

Carol Sando, RN, DNSc

Linda Wrynn, RN, MS

PREFACE

Passing the National Council Licensure Examination (NCLEX®) is a crucial step in your nursing career. *Sandra Smith's Review for NCLEX-PN,*® written to assist you to prepare for and pass this examination, summarizes in concise outline format the essential nursing content that you must know in order to pass the NCLEX. The content is supplemented by practice questions, providing you the opportunity to test your mastery over nursing theory, principles, and interventions.

The eighth edition of this popular book includes all the material that has been incorporated into prior editions with revisions, updates, deletions, and new, expanded material as appropriate. It also reflects the author's university teaching experience and feedback from many candidates who used earlier editions for NCLEX success.

The first chapter presents useful material on NCLEX background, study and review guidelines, and test-taking strategies.

- The NCLEX description summarizes the current test plan's overall purpose and basic framework. To assist you to understand the test plan, client needs, critical thinking, and the nursing process are reviewed. Cognitive levels are also included, with examples to assist you in identifying the various levels at which questions are written on NCLEX.

- The study and review guidelines suggest how you can design your personal plan for NCLEX preparation, how to use this book effectively, and why testing yourself repeatedly is an important complement to, but not a replacement for, concentrated study of the outline content.

- The test-taking strategies are common sense, but often overlooked, methods of responding to multiple-choice questions. In this edition, priority decision-making strategies, with examples, are included. When taking NCLEX, you must answer each question when it appears on the computer screen. After you confirm an answer selection, you cannot change it or return to an earlier question. Sometimes your best strategy will be an "educated guess in order to move on and not waste valuable time. While the majority of questions are straightforward multiple choice, as of 2003 several variations of questions called "Alternate Item Format Questions" will be included. Examples of the different question formats are in this chapter and in various sections of this edition.

The second chapter covers essential management issues and legal/ethical concerns. This will enable you to understand NCLEX questions that deal with these issues.

The major portion of the book consists of a comprehensive nursing content review organized by clinical area: general nursing concepts, medical/surgical, maternal/newborn, pediatric, and psychiatric nursing. Additional chapters focus on other important subjects, such as pharmacology, laboratory tests, oncology, infection control, nursing through the life cycle, nutrition, management principles, and legal issues. A new chapter, Disaster Nursing—Bioterrorism, has been included.

To assist your review process to be efficient and effective, the nursing content is presented in an outline format. This enables the author to identify and prioritize essential clinical information clearly and concisely. As you progress from subject to subject, you will note that the consistent page design allows you to easily recognize the main topics and their subtopics.

Nursing content in each chapter is organized using the nursing process as the basic framework. The author emphasizes the data collection or assessment and implementation steps, because NCLEX will require you to demonstrate your ability to effectively assess a situation and then implement an appropriate nursing action.

Throughout the text, a special icon (♦) directs your attention to important content for NCLEX preparation. If the icon appears near a major section of content, it means that the entire section is important. Another icon may appear under the same heading indicating especially important material. NCLEX draws upon a test pool containing thousands of questions when selecting the items for your test. Any material in this book could be phrased as a question, so focusing your review exclusively on the icon topics would not be a wise preparation strategy.

Finally, this text is now in its successful eighth edition. Each edition has been revised with the assistance of feedback from candidates who have taken the NCLEX; thus, there is little extraneous or useless information included.

Practice questions are integrated throughout the book to enable you to check your level of understanding of each chapter's contents, or, in the medical/surgical chapter, each section's contents. The answers with rationales are included, along with coding for nursing process, client need, clinical area, and cognitive level.

Review the material, spending a little extra time on the icon areas; answer the practice questions that follow each section or chapter and then review content again if you identify areas of weakness. Finally, take the comprehensive tests at the end of the book. Use the questions on the CD-ROM as a final step in your preparation for NCLEX. All questions are on the CD, so if you prefer to use the computer rather than pencil and paper, you may do so.

The two simulated NCLEX examinations at the back of this book and the additional practice questions on the CD-ROM provide you with substantial opportunity to measure your mastery of the subject matter. The answer rationales throughout the book and on the CD-ROM will reinforce your understanding of the principles that underlie each question. Studying rationales for questions that you answered correctly reinforces your knowledge and understanding. As your understanding increases, so will your confidence.

ACKNOWLEDGMENTS

I wish to thank all of the contributing authors and reviewers who assisted with the development of this and the seven earlier editions. Because of their contributions, this review package will continue to be a valuable resource for PN licensure candidates as they prepare to pass the NCLEX-PN.

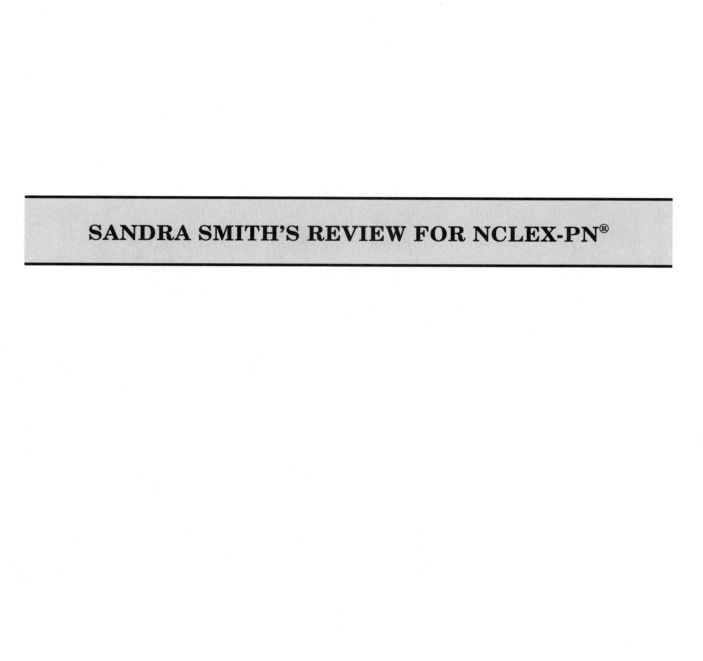

SANDRA SMITH'S REVIEW FOR NCLEX-PN®

The NCLEX-PN® and Test-Taking Strategies

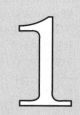

® NCLEX and NCLEX-PN are registered trademarks of
the National Council of State Boards of Nursing, Inc.

INTRODUCTION TO THE NCLEX®

The National Council Licensure Examination for Practical/Vocational Nurses, commonly abbreviated to NCLEX®, measures the licensure candidate's competence to perform safe and effective entry-level nursing practice. This important screening test is designed and administered by the National Council of State Boards of Nursing, Inc., known as the National Council. All 50 states, the District of Columbia, and all U.S. territories are members of the Council and utilize the NCLEX as an integral part of their licensure process. The NCLEX licensure procedures define common entry-level nursing standards throughout the United States while providing health care protection to consumers. Licensed nurses have reciprocity from state to state, an additional benefit provided by a national licensure system.

The NCLEX-PN® Test Plan

In order to plan an effective and efficient study and review program, it is important that you have a general understanding regarding the purpose and framework of the NCLEX. This examination is designed to measure your ability to practice entry-level nursing in a safe, effective manner. The majority of NCLEX questions are presented in the multiple-choice format consisting of the stem of a question followed by four answer choices with only one correct answer. In 2003, the National Council introduced several new alternate item formats. All of the questions are designed to require you to apply your knowledge of nursing care and procedures to specific clinical situations. Your understanding of the overall NCLEX Test Plan and its objectives will assist you in planning what material you should review and how to review it.

Alternate Item Format/Questions

Alternate item format questions have been integrated into the general NCLEX test. These questions use formats different from the multiple-choice items; thus, depending on the format, more than one answer may be required.

Types of Alternate Item Formats
✦ Multiple response questions will offer as many as six possible answers, and the candidate must choose all that apply. The answer must include all that apply to be scored "correct."

> A patient's physician has placed him on a low potassium diet. List the numbers of the following foods that he should avoid because they are high in potassium. The numbers that apply are _____.
>
> 1. Butter.
> 2. Shellfish.
> 3. Milk.
> 4. Frozen vegetables.
> 5. Orange juice.
> 6. Dried dates.
>
> The answers are *3 5 6*. Milk (3), orange juice (5), and dried dates (6) are all high in potassium. The other three foods are high in sodium.

✦ Fill in the blank questions will require the candidate to complete a calculation and type in the correct number, or type in an ordered response where the candidate would put the steps of a skill in proper sequence, for example, *1 4 3 2*.

> The orders are to give warfarin (Coumadin) 12.5 mg. On hand are 5 mg tablets. The nurse would give the patient _____tablet(s).
>
> The answer is 2.5 tablets. This computation can be done using the formula D (dose desired) ÷ H (dose on hand) × Q (quantity of dose on hand). $12.5 \div 5 \times 1 = 2.5$ tablets.
>
> When removing an isolation gown, place in order the steps the nurse would complete to follow infection control protocol:
>
> _____
>
> 1. Remove gloves.   4. Wash hands.
> 2. Untie neck ties.   5. Remove gown.
> 3. Untie front waist strings.
>
> The answer is *3 1 2 5 4*. Untying the waist strings first is appropriate because when they are tied in front, they are considered dirty. The nurse would remove gloves, untie the neck strings (which are considered clean), and then remove the gown. Only if there were no waist strings in front would the nurse remove the gloves first.

✦ Questions may require identification of an area on a line drawing or a graphic; for example, the candidate will use the mouse to point to a spot on a line drawing of the heart.

> Select the location (1–5) at which you would place your stethoscope as you start auscultating breath sounds:

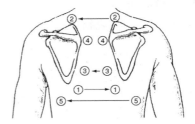

> The answer is that you would place the stethoscope at the top of the back (labeled 2 in the question) as you start auscultating breath sounds. Move down the back according to the numbers (to the fifth position) to complete the procedure.

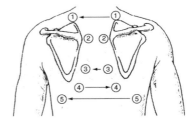

Initially, less than 2% of the questions will be in the alternate item format. This means that in a minimal length exam, the candidate may have only one alternate item format question.

Developing the NCLEX

The National Council contracts with clinical nurses and nurse educators to write questions (referred to as test items) that test your ability to apply your knowledge of nursing. The test questions focus on job tasks normally performed by entry-level PNs during their first six to 12 months on the job. The National Council identifies these tasks by conducting extensive surveys, called practice analyses, about every three years. It is possible that your PN program may have included instruction on certain tasks that are not considered to be entry level by the National Council's job surveys. It is also possible that your PN program may not have provided you with instruction on some of the tasks about which questions have been included in the current test pool.

The practice analysis activities are analyzed by frequency of their performance and their impact on maintaining client safety. The results guide the development of the NCLEX-PN Test Plan framework based upon specific client needs. On a continuing basis, the practice analysis studies are also used to help validate the current test plan and to provide the basis for selecting subjects to be covered by NCLEX.

The Test Plan serves as a guide for examination development and candidate preparation. Each test reflects the knowledge, skills, and abilities necessary for each nurse to safely meet client needs for the promotion, maintenance, and restoration of health.

CLIENT NEEDS

The basic framework for the NCLEX is Client Needs. The health needs of clients are organized into four major categories and 6 subcategories. This section reviews Client Needs so that you can understand how NCLEX is structured and what material you need to master in order to pass this examination. The NCLEX questions are proportional according to a survey conducted every three years by the National Council. Table 1-1 lists the categories and subcategories and provides the percentage of questions for each. You should concentrate your study and review on the categories that are emphasized most by the NCLEX.

Safe and Effective Care Environment

To meet the client's needs for safe, effective care, the nurse must be able to provide nursing care in the following areas:
1. *Coordinated Care*—collaborating with the health care team to facilitate delivery of effective client care.

Table 1-1. CATEGORIES OF CLIENT NEEDS

Categories	Percentage of Test Questions
A. Safe and Effective Care Environment	
• Coordinated Care	11–17%
• Safety and Infection Control	8–14%
B. Health Promotion and Maintenance	7–13%
C. Psychosocial Integrity	8–14%
D. Physiological Integrity	
• Basic Care and Comfort	11–17%
• Pharmacological Therapies	9–15%
• Reduction of Risk Potential	10–16%
• Physiological Adaptation	12–18%

2. *Safety and Infection Control*—protecting clients and health care personnel from environmental hazards.

Health Promotion and Maintenance

To assist in meeting the client's needs for health promotion and maintenance throughout the life cycle, the nurse must be able to provide nursing care in these areas.

Psychosocial Integrity

To assist in meeting the client's needs for psychosocial integrity during periods of illness and common health problems that occur throughout the life cycle, the nurse must be able to provide nursing care in these areas.

Physiological Integrity

To assist in meeting the client's needs for physiological integrity—including acute and/or chronically recurring physiological conditions, as well as potential complications—the nurse must be able to provide nursing care in the following areas:
1. *Basic Care and Comfort*—providing comfort and assistance in the performance of activities of daily living.
2. *Pharmacological Therapies*—providing care related to the administration of medication and parenteral therapies.
3. *Reduction of Risk Potential*—reducing the likelihood that clients will develop complications or health problems related to existing conditions, treatments, or procedures.
4. *Physiological Adaptation*—providing care to clients with acute, chronic, or life-threatening physical health conditions.

Adapted from *Test Plan for the National Council Licensure Examination for Practical/Vocational Nurses,* National Council of State Boards of Nursing, Chicago, 2004.

Integrated Processes

Without specifying as separate Client Needs, several processes are integrated throughout the Client Needs categories and considered fundamental to the practice of nursing. Questions will reflect these processes. They include

- Problem-solving in the Clinical Arena (including nursing process)
- Caring
- Communication and Documentation
- Teaching and Learning

Because the detailed test plan for the NCLEX-PN centers around the categories of Client Needs, you may wish to visit the National Council's web site at *www.ncsbn.org*. This information will help you guide your review process, as it lists specific nursing actions in relation to Client Needs in each of the Nursing Process categories.

NURSING PROCESS

The National Council no longer provides a percentage breakdown of questions according to the individual phases of the Nursing Process. However, the Nursing Process continues to be an integral foundation for nursing education, clinical training, and textbooks. Therefore, it is appropriate for you to understand the concepts and to be able to relate NCLEX questions to the Nursing Process as you apply your knowledge of nursing to select the correct answers.

The four phases of the Nursing Process are Data Collection, Planning, Implementation, and Evaluation. The Nursing Process is a frequently used, but often misunderstood, term. By definition, *process* is a series of actions that lead toward a particular result. When attached to *nursing,* the term *Nursing Process* becomes a general description of a nurse's job: collecting data, planning, implementing, and evaluating. Ideally, this process of decision making results in optimal health care for the clients. While the four steps can be described separately and in logical order, it is obvious that in practice the steps will overlap and events may not always occur in the order listed above, especially when the unexpected happens.

Data Collection

The data collection phase refers to building a data base for a specific client. This phase requires skilled observation and collection of data from the client, family, health team members, and medical records. It also includes a theoretical knowledge base to gather and differentiate data and to document findings. The practical nurse gathers information relevant to the client, assigns meaning to this data, and uses it to participate in the formulation of a nursing diagnosis.

Planning

Based on data collected, the planning phase refers to identifying goals of care. The practical nurse contributes to the nursing care plan, assists in formulating goals, and communicates client needs and nursing measures necessary to achieve goals. This phase of the nursing process also includes nursing measures for the delivery of care. Clients may be involved in this planning phase. A planning question will focus on the development of a plan of care individualized for a specific client.

Implementation

The third phase of the Nursing Process is the implementation or intervention phase. It describes the action component of the Nursing Process. This phase involves initiating and completing those nursing actions necessary to accomplish the identified client goals. Implementation includes performing basic therapeutic and preventive nursing measures, providing a safe and effective environment, recording and reporting specific information, and assisting the client to understand the care plan. Implementation of the plan involves giving direct care to accomplish the specified goal.

Evaluation

The final phase of the Nursing Process is evaluation, or determining the extent to which identified goals were achieved. Evaluation is the examination of the outcome of the nursing interventions. This process is extremely important because without this step, the nursing plan cannot be evaluated and adapted to the client's ongoing needs.

CRITICAL THINKING

All nurses are required to use critical thinking skills. Critical thinking competencies are the cognitive processes that a nurse employs to make clinical judgments, including diagnostic reasoning and decision making. The Nursing Process is the framework for critical thinking competency in nursing:

Data Collection: Obtaining, classifying and organizing data is a principle component of critical thinking.

Planning: Contributing to the care plan by defining realistic goals (both short and long term) and prioritizing these goals also requires critical thinking. The nurse must sort through the available information, evaluate the goals, determine the probable outcomes (which must be time specific), and prioritize them. Nursing Diagnoses are formulated from this step in the critical thinking process.

Implementation: Specifying strategies to achieve positive outcomes is a third key component of critical thinking. Deciding on the appropriate actions (after considering all those possible), and then examining the risks and consequences of each action complete this step in the process.

Evaluation: A critical analysis of each of the patient outcomes is the final step. Was the goal achieved? If not, the plan is revised.

LEVELS OF COGNITIVE ABILITY

Cognitive levels are defined in taxonomy as "the orderly classification of data into appropriate categories on the basis of relationships between them." The practice of nursing requires application of knowledge at various levels of cognitive domain underlying theory, skills and ability. The majority of the NCLEX-PN questions are written at the more advanced levels of application and analysis rather than at the lower levels of knowledge or comprehension. The taxonomy of cognitive levels is as follows:

- **Knowledge:** Recall or recognize theoretical principles or facts of nursing content. Questions ask the nurse to define, identify, recognize, or select the appropriate data.

- **Comprehension:** Understand the information presented. Questions ask the nurse to explain, interpret, predict, or to distinguish data.

- **Application:** Apply or use information in a new or different manner. Questions ask the nurse to problem solve, change or manipulate data, or use the information appropriately.

- **Analysis:** Separate parts of the whole or determine relationships between parts for a new understanding. Questions ask the nurse to analyze, differentiate, evaluate, or interpret data from a variety of sources.

The questions in this book have been coded according to cognitive levels. While all levels are represented, most questions are written at the application and analysis levels. Understanding this component of the test is important because as a licensure candidate, you cannot expect to simply memorize data and recall it for the examination (knowledge level) or interpret data (comprehension level). Rather, most questions will require that you apply your knowledge to clinical problems. This requires application of the data.

Examples of Cognitive Level Questions

Knowledge level

One of the primary developmental tasks of adolescence is

1. Feeling independent.
2. Finding one's identity.
3. Experiencing intimacy.
4. Achieving generativity

Correct answer is (2). Early adolescence has the primary task of finding one's identity and moving out of role diffusion. The task from later adolescence to young adulthood is to experience intimacy (3), not independence and isolation (1). Adults should achieve generativity (4) versus stagnation.

This is a knowledge base question that requires the nurse to recognize or recall knowledge or information learned. (i.e. the developmental tasks of adolescents).

Comprehension level

A mother brings her six-week old infant to the clinic for a well-baby exam. The nurse, when teaching about infant nutrition, would inform the mother that

1. Whole eggs are a good source of iron and can be introduced at six months.
2. Solid foods can be introduced in the sixth week of life.
3. Rice cereal is the least allergenic of the cereals for infants.
4. Only one new food should be introduced per day.

Correct answer is (3). Rice cereal is the least allergenic food. The latest research indicates that solid food (2) should not be given until six months. This may prevent allergies later in life, and the infant's digestive system has had time to mature. Egg yolks, not whole eggs (1), can be introduced because the whites of the egg may cause an allergy. Only one new food should be added each week, not each day (4).

Comprehension involves understanding information (infant nutrition) and being able to explain it effectively in the right context.

Application Level

A patient who is receiving radiation therapy comes to the clinic for a scheduled treatment. The nurse notices that the patient's skin appears wet and weeping. The nursing action is to

1. Not give the treatment and tell the patient to avoid bathing the skin until the weeping has stopped.
2. Give the treatment and make a note on the patient's record concerning the skin condition.
3. Not give the treatment and notify the charge nurse of the patient's skin condition.
4. Give the treatment and instruct the patient to use antibiotic lotion on the lesions.

Correct answer is (3). During the time that the reaction occurs, patients are taken off radiation therapy and instructed to use antibiotic and steroid cream to prevent infection.

Application is the ability to apply knowledge. In this example, understanding that a different intervention, other than the one planned, is necessary based upon new data collection. The nurse is problem solving and applying information appropriately.

Analysis Level

A nurse is assigned to take two patients' vital signs, complete a focus assessment and provide hygienic care, administer meds, and complete a dressing change for a patient with an abdominal wound. Which task will have the highest priority with this assignment?

1. Take the vital signs and provide hygienic care to the first patient.
2. Administer medications to the patients.
3. Complete the dressing change.
4. Take vital signs on the two patients.

The correct answer is (4). Taking vital signs on the two patients would be the priority nursing action to determine if there are any emerging problems. The nurse would next give the meds (2), which can be given within a 30-minute period before or after the ordered time. Because changing the dressing (3) might also involve a pain assessment, this would require more time and should be completed last. Providing hygienic (1) care would take too long at this time.

Analysis requires the nurse to analyze or evaluate data, and then make a determination for nursing action. This example requires the nurse to analyze the situation and then problem solve to a conclusion, or nursing intervention. Taking vital signs first would reveal any problems that require immediate further interventions.

NCLEX APPLICATION PROCEDURES

As a candidate for PN/VN licensure, you will deal with several organizations as you complete your application procedures to take the NCLEX. The key organization is the board of nursing in the state or jurisdiction where you plan to practice. Each state board of nursing sets education and other eligibility requirements for PN licensure. Fortunately, all states and territories accept the NCLEX as the standard licensure examination. Assuming you qualify, the state board will send you an Authorization to Test (ATT). Now you are authorized to contact a Pearson Professional Center of your choice to schedule your test session. The center does not have to be located in the state where you plan to practice. As a first time test taker, you should be able to schedule your test within 30 days of receiving your ATT.

When you receive your ATT from the board of nursing, note its expiration date. You must take the NCLEX before the ATT expires, or you will have to reapply and pay the filing fees again. You should also be aware that the Pearson Professional Centers are highly booked at certain times of the year, especially May through July, so plan your testing date accordingly.

The NCLEX Candidate Bulletin contains a description of computerized adaptive testing and important information regarding NCLEX registration, scheduling and other important procedures. Published by the National Council of State Boards of Nursing, this useful resource is available via the Internet at *www.ncsbn.org*.

Candidates whose applications for licensure have been approved are eligible for an interim permit to practice under the direct supervision of a registered nurse. However, this permit is not renewable and is effect until its expiration date or until the results of NCLEX are mailed to you. These procedures give you strong incentive to pass the NCLEX on your first attempt.

TAKING THE NCLEX

Upon arriving at the Pearson Professional Center, you will present your Authorization to Test and two forms of identification, both signed and one with a photo. A driver's license, school or employee ID, and passport are the most accepted forms. At check-in, you will be photographed and thumbprinted. Before commencing the test questions, you will complete a brief computer tutorial to make certain that you are comfortable with the testing procedures. The National Council advises that no prior computer experience is necessary for CAT. The CD-ROM accompanying this book allows you to practice and become comfortable with CAT procedures.

TESTING PROCEDURES

Two categories of questions appear on NCLEX. The *real* questions test your competency and safety and provide the basis for your pass or fail score. The *tryout* questions are unscored items being field-tested for future NCLEX exams. You have no way of knowing the difference between *real* and *tryout* questions.

The minimum number of questions for each candidate is 85. The National Council maintains that the essential Test Plan categories can be covered by 60 carefully selected questions. The maximum number of questions will be a total of 205 items.

Computer Adaptive Testing does not allow you to skip questions or go back to look at or change questions already answered. Each question has an assigned degree of difficulty. Based on your prior answers—correct or incorrect—the computer selects the next question. Therefore, you must answer each question as it is presented. Because the computer draws from a large pool of questions, each candidate's test is unique. There is no absolute passing score in terms of the number or percentage of questions that you must answer correctly in order to pass.

Although there is no minimum amount of time for your test, the maximum allowable time is five hours, including your computer tutorial and rest breaks. A mandatory rest break of 10 minutes is required after 2 hours of testing and an optional break is available after the next 1½ hours.

Because the number of questions is flexible, from a minimum of 85 to a maximum of 205, there is no optimal amount of time you should spend per question. However, because you won't know how long it will take you to reach the point where the computer stops presenting questions, it is not wise to spend too much time on any one question. If you don't know the answer, guess and move on rather than risk becoming immobilized. When you answer questions correctly, the CAT software presents you with more difficult items. As you answer questions incorrectly, you will receive easier items.

Your test continues until the computer software calculates with a 95 percent degree of confidence that you fall into the safe/competent group or that you do not. The total number of questions answered does not indicate whether you have passed or failed.

GETTING YOUR TEST RESULTS

NCLEX test results are available only from the state board of nursing to which you applied for approval to take the NCLEX. Do not request feedback from the Pearson Professional Center or the National Council. You can expect to receive your results within one month after taking the exam, but often in less time. A failure notice is accompanied by a performance report to help the candidate identify areas of weakness. Most state boards of nursing require that candidates who fail must wait a minimum of 91 days before retaking the exam.

GUIDELINES FOR NCLEX REVIEW

How to Use This Book

Sandra Smith's Review for NCLEX-PN summarizes extensive nursing content to which you have been introduced during your PN education. The material is organized into 17 chapters and presented in outline format for your review.

Nursing theory and practical applications of this theory are included for each major subject area. Nurs-

---

> **NCLEX-PN CAT Quick Reference**
> Test Location: Pearson Professional Centers
> Minimum Number of Questions: 85
> Maximum Number of Questions: 205
> Minimum Testing Time: None
> Maximum Testing Time: 5 hours

---

ing theory includes pathophysiology, signs and symptoms of diseases, diagnosis and treatment of medical conditions, and appropriate nursing care. Tables and appendices are distributed throughout the book to assist you to efficiently review factual material. Familiarize yourself with how the contents are organized in each chapter and how the Nursing Process is integrated throughout the book.

Other features to note for further reference include a detailed index, simulated NCLEX exams at the back of the book, and a CD-ROM attached to the inside of the back cover.

The multiple-choice questions that follow various content review sections are similar in format, subject matter, length, and degree of difficulty to those contained in the NCLEX-PN. The answer and rationale sections provide you with additional learning. If you understand the basic principles of nursing content, you can transfer that knowledge to the clinical situations and questions on the NCLEX.

The questions printed in the book are also presented by chapter on the CD. This provides you with the opportunity to gain computer experience while you assess and review. Also, the CD contains more than 1600 additional questions not printed in the book.

How to Design Your Personal Review Program

Ideally, you will begin your review process several months prior to NCLEX; but if you choose to allocate only a few weeks to prepare for this exam, it is important that you conduct the review process in an efficient manner. The following recommendations are offered to help you achieve maximum results for the amount of time invested.

A. Schedule regular periods for study and review.
   1. Arrange to study when mentally alert. Studying during periods of mental and physical fatigue reduces your efficiency.
   2. Allow short breaks at relatively frequent intervals. Breaks used as rewards for hard study serve as incentives for continued concentrated effort. A 10- to 15-minute break is recommended after each hour of concentrated study.

B. Familiarize yourself with the examination format.
1. Review the NCLEX Test Plan description so that you understand the Client Needs categories. Notice which areas have the greater number of questions and allocate more review time to these topics. Refer to Table 1–1 for the allocation of questions among the subcategories of Client Needs.
2. Study the format used for NCLEX questions. You must know how to read, evaluate, and respond to multiple-choice questions similar to the ones in this book and on the CD-ROM.
C. Identify your strengths and weaknesses.
1. Assess your past performance on classroom tests and written material (clinical pathways or nursing care plans).
2. Learn from your past errors and weaknesses by looking up and studying the appropriate material in this book.
D. Systematically study the material contained in each chapter of this book.
1. First, gain a general impression of the content unit to be reviewed. Skim over the entire section and identify the main ideas.
2. Note the tables, glossaries, and appendices.
3. The special icon (◆) that appears throughout the book's review sections identifies nursing content that is particularly important or involves critical decision-making. If an entire section is marked by an icon, then assume that all this material is important. Do not, however, limit your study to only the icon-marked content; use the icon to help you focus and prioritize. Mark key material that you do not thoroughly understand.
E. Follow up on your priority areas.
1. Set priorities for specific material to be learned or reviewed. Identify the most crucial sections and underline the essential thoughts.
2. Review what you have read. Think of examples that illustrate the main points you have studied.
3. To be sure that you have learned the material, write down the main ideas or explain the major points to another person.
F. Test and retest.
1. Complete the clinical practice questions presented at the conclusion of each chapter. Study the rationale for missed questions so that you understand why you missed them. Refer back to the content outline preceding the questions to study content relating to the topics contained in the questions. Study the rationale for the questions that you answered correctly because this will reinforce your understanding of those topics and increase your confidence about material you firmly understand.
2. After you have worked your way through the clinical questions, take the first simulated NCLEX test at the back of the book. Analyze your results by noting the category of each question missed in terms of nursing process, client needs, and clinical area (*see* Table 1-2). This will help you identify your weaker areas. Refer to the appropriate content for further study and review.
3. Take the second simulated NCLEX test at the back of the book. Repeat the same process of analysis and review. If you studied the content relating to questions you missed, you should see improvement.
4. After you have completed the practice questions and simulated tests in the book, utilize the CD-ROM for additional practice and review. The key to this process is to use the content outline in the various chapters as a learning vehicle to strengthen your grasp of the material. This, in turn, will increase your ability to apply what you know to specific clinical situations tested in the NCLEX.

TEST-TAKING STRATEGIES

The following test-taking strategies will provide you with useful guidelines when answering NCLEX questions. These strategies are neither absolute nor foolproof; they are intended to guide you in choosing the best response for each question.
A. Carefully read each question. Determine what the question is really asking. Some details may not be important. Mentally note important factors; pay attention to key terms and phrases. Read the question as it is presented, not as you would like it to be stated.
B. When answering multiple-choice questions, an effective strategy is to first eliminate the answers that you know are wrong, and then focus on deciding among the remaining answers. If you are not sure about any of the four possible answers, you will have to make an educated guess. Remember, you are not allowed to skip a question, nor will you be able to change any answers that you have selected on previous questions.
C. Your first "hunch" is usually correct. Many candidates have a first impression, choose an answer, and upon reflection, change their mind. Sensing that a particular alternative is correct has some basis. Your brain has made rapid connections. You came to an immediate conclusion based on your knowledge and experience. The fact that you did not go through the logical steps of arriving at the correct solution does not indicate that your choice is incorrect.

Table 1-2. CODING FOR QUESTIONS AND ANSWERS*

Nursing Process:	NP
Data Collection:	D
Planning:	P
Implementation:	I
Evaluation:	E
Client Needs:	**CN**
Safe and Effective Care Environment:	S
Health Promotion and Maintenance:	H
Psychosocial Integrity:	PS
Physiological Integrity:	PH
Content Area: **CA** (will be included only for those questions included in the Comprehensive tests).	
Medical Nursing:	M
Surgical Nursing:	S
Maternity Nursing:	MA
Pediatric Nursing:	P
Psychiatric Nursing:	PS
Cognitive Level:	**CL**
Knowledge:	K
Comprehension:	C
Application:	A
Analysis:	AN

*Each answer will be coded and the reference code will appear at the beginning of each answer section.

D. Be alert for a question that requires you to identify which answer is **not** correct, or a question that asks for a negative response; for example, "Which of the following interventions is inappropriate?"

E. Evaluate the answers in relation to the stem (the question), not to other answers. Choose the answer that best fits the question, rather than an answer that appears to be a correct statement but may not fit the question.

F. The most comprehensive answer is often the best choice. For example, if two alternatives seem reasonable but one answer includes the other (i.e., it is more detailed, extends the first answer, or is more comprehensive), then this answer may be the best choice.

G. Eliminate answers that are obviously different from what is logically right, such as an answer given in grams when other choices are given in milligrams.

H. Do not look for a pattern to the answers. The questions are chosen at random, and the same number may be the correct answer to several consecutive questions.

I. The test administrator will provide you with erasable note boards and a writing implement for your use during the test session. You are not allowed to bring your own notes, scratch paper or writing implements into the test center.

Guidelines for Making Priority Decisions

Priority decision-making is an important test-taking skill. NCLEX places increasingly greater emphasis on requiring candidates to analyze and evaluate information and then to make decisions. The following examples are presented as guidelines to help you recognize and answer priority-based NCLEX questions.

Most Life Threatening

If you are asked which sign or symptom would you respond to first, or which nursing diagnosis would you identify as the priority intervention, you should determine which is the most life threatening. Always choose the critical intervention – airway, breathing, circulation (ABC) – if one is listed as an option.

Example Question

A patient diagnosed with rheumatic heart disease has been admitted to the hospital due to cardiac arrhythmias. The registered nurse, in conjunction with the practical nurse, develops the nursing care plan. The nursing diagnosis to be given the highest priority is

1. Excess fluid volume.
2. Deficient fluid volume.
3. Ineffective tissue perfusion.
4. Ineffective breathing pattern.

Correct answer is (4). Because the atria do not empty fully in atrial fibrillation, the ventricles are not able to pump normal cardiac output. The patient, therefore, may exhibit shortness of breath. Ineffective breathing pattern is the most life threatening condition of the four answer selections. The patient may also show signs of heart failure and decreased cerebral flow, but these symptoms would not be the *most* life threatening.

First Priority Nursing Intervention

When a question focuses on which intervention would you perform *first,* consider which is the most immediate for the well being of the patient. For example, you would suction the patient before administering a routine medication (providing it was not nitroglycerin), because meds can be given up to 30 minutes before or after the ordered time.

Example Question

A patient in the labor room is lying comfortably on her back after receiving an epidural injection 30 minutes earlier. The nurse checks the fetal heart rate and finds the fetal rate is 100 per minute. The first nursing action is to

1. Administer oxygen by mask.
2. Turn the patient onto her left side.
3. Notify the physician immediately.
4. Take the patient's blood pressure.

The correct answer is (2). All of the interventions will be carried out; however, the first action is to turn the patient onto her side to reduce the pressure of the uterus on the vena cava. Oxygen administration should be initiated after turning the patient onto her side. Fetal heart rate should then be checked and rechecked frequently.

Safety Issue

The answer choices that involve a safety issue for the patient will always take priority over other concerns. For example, monitoring the oxygen level in an incubator of a premature infant is a safety issue. If the oxygen level goes above 40% for the premature, it could damage the retinas and lead to blindness. The oxygen level for an adult would not be a serious safety issue unless the client has COPD.

Example Question

After assessing that a blood transfusion allergic reaction has occurred, the first nursing intervention is to

1. Place the patient in high-Fowler's position.
2. Call the physician.
3. Slow the rate of infusion to "keep open" rate.
4. Turn off the transfusion.

The correct answer is (4). If the nurse suspects an allergic reaction, the blood transfusion IV should be turned off immediately. Then, the physician should be notified and the patient placed in a position to facilitate breathing. While in actual practice some nurses advocate slowing the IV rate to "keep open," NCLEX would view this as a safety issue. To be safe, the transfusion should be turned off to prevent a more serious reaction.

Computer Testing Tips

A. When taking the NCLEX, you must answer each question that appears on the computer screen. If you do not recognize a correct answer among the four choices, use your test-taking skills, or if necessary, make your best guess.
B. Be certain of your answer selection before confirming your choice.
C. Take your time and carefully read each question and answer choices.
D. Do not become immobilized by any one question. Spending 5 minutes or more on a question will probably make you more nervous and less attentive as you proceed.
E. Maintain a steady pace of allocating about one minute per question. This strategy will allow you to complete the examination within the required time of five hours should you need to answer 205 questions.

Final Preparation

A. The night before the test.

1. Assemble materials that you will take with you to the test center, such as your ATT, identifications and other items as specified in the *NCLEX Candidate Bulletin*. Do not bring textbooks, notes or any NCLEX study aids to the test center.
2. Get a good night's sleep. Do not stay up all night trying to learn new material.
3. Avoid the use of stimulants or depressants, either of which may affect your ability to think clearly during the test.
4. Approach the test with confidence and the determination to do your best. Think positively and concentrate on all that you do know rather than on what you think you do not know.

B. The day of the test.

1. Eat a high-protein, nonsugar breakfast. Do not rush.
2. Allow ample time to travel to your testing site, including time to park, and to present your Authorization to Test at least 30 minutes before your scheduled testing time.
3. You may wish to take a light, energizing snack and bottled water to have available for your 10-minute break. Secure storage will be provided for your personal items.

The Importance of a Confident Attitude

Anxiety, a forceful deterrent to test-taking success, interferes with your ability to think clearly. Anxiety blocks the search and retrieval process so that you cannot access the knowledge held in your "memory bank." Fear of the unknown is a major source of anxiety. This fear can be overcome by diligent review. As you gain mastery over the nursing content, your self-confidence increases. It is also important to understand test construction and test-taking strategies. This Introduction is designed to reduce many of the unknowns associated with the NCLEX-PN and to provide you with helpful review guidelines and effective test-taking techniques.

These strategies are guidelines, not absolutes. Always use your own judgment, knowledge, and nursing experience. These assets will serve you well.

WEB SITES

For additional information on NCLEX testing procedures and current policies, contact The National Council of State Boards of Nursing at *www.ncsbn.org*.

To register on line to take the NCLEX or to obtain information on Pearson Prefessional Center locations, contact Pearson at *www.vue.com/nclex*.

For information on NCLEX review aids by Sandra F. Smith, RN, MS, contact National Nursing Review at *www.nationalnursingreview.com*.

Management Principles and Legal/Ethical Issues

2

NURSE PRACTICE ACT

Background

A. A series of statutes enacted by each state's legislature to define and regulate the practice of nursing in that state.

B. Establish standards of nursing practice for which the registered nurse and/or the vocational/practical nurse is held legally responsible by a particular state.

C. Provide the framework of statutory law within which the state boards of nursing must function.

D. The Nurse Practice Acts are quite similar throughout the United States, but the professional RN or LVN is held legally responsible for the specific requirements for licensure and regulations of practice as defined by the state in which he or she is working.

Provisions

A. Definition of nursing to include functions, responsibilities, and personal qualifications.

B. Authorization to practice (licensure).

C. Educational requirements and personal qualifications.

D. Implementation and reinforcement of act by State Board of Nursing.

E. Proceedings and penalties for professional misconduct.

Scope of LPN/LVN Functions

A. Administer nursing care, utilizing basic scientific knowledge and understanding, under the direction and supervision of a registered nurse, or licensed physician.
    1. Provide direct and indirect patient care.
    2. Perform and deliver basic health care services.
    3. Implement testing and prevention procedures.

B. Assist the registered nurse or licensed physician with patients who require advanced medical care.
    1. Administer medications and treatments and observe reactions and responses per orders.
    2. Observe and report signs and symptoms of illness.

C. Provide client and family teaching.

D. Act as a client advocate when needed.

E. Document nursing care.

F. Supervise allied nursing personnel.

Legal Issues

A. Legal issues and regulations play a dominant role in nursing practice today.

1. The law provides a framework for establishing nursing actions in the care of patients.
2. Laws determine and set boundaries and maintain a standard of nursing practice.

◆ B. The Nurse Practice Act defines professional nursing.
    ◆1. Recommends those actions that the nurse can take independently.
    ◆2. Recommends those actions that require a physician's order before completion.

C. Each state has the authority to regulate as well as *administrate* health care professionals.
    1. Provisions of Nurse Practice Acts are quite similar from state to state.
    2. The nurse must know the licensing requirements and the grounds for license revocation defined by the state in which he or she works.

◆ D. Legal and ethical standards for nurses are complicated by a myriad of federal and state statutes and the continually changing interpretation of them by the courts of law. Nurses today are faced with the threat of legal action based on negligence, malpractice, invasion of privacy, and other grounds.

E. Legal doctrine holds that an employer may also be liable for negligent acts of employees in the course and scope of employment.
    1. Physicians, hospitals, clinics, and other employers may be held liable for negligent acts of their employees.
    2. This doctrine does not support acts of gross negligence or acts that are outside the scope of employment.

UNUSUAL OCCURRENCE (INCIDENT REPORT)

A. Three purposes.
    1. Help document quality of care.
    2. Identify where in-servcie education is needed.
    3. Record details of an incident for legal reference.

B. Report must include specific details.
    1. Details of the incident.
    2. Patient's reponse.
    3. Nursing action or reaction.
    4. List of personnel who were aware of the incident.
    5. Report forwarded to unit manager, nursing administration, hospital legal department.

C. Useful tool for documenting quality of care.
    1. Identify areas of practice that need improvement (i.e., increase in number of patient falls).
    2. Plan classes or educational seminars to improve deficient areas.

STATE BOARDS OF NURSING

Composition

A. A group invested with authority by a state to administer its Nurse Practice Act.

B. Members of a board are appointed from among the nursing profession and interested public.

Responsibilities

A. Accredits schools of nursing which meet pre-established standards.
1. Withholds accreditation from schools that do not meet standards.
2. Withdraws accreditation from the schools that do not conform to standards.

B. Provides guidelines and minimum standards for nursing curriculum.

C. Governs all aspects of licensing.
1. Administers the nursing licensure examinations.
2. Grants licenses to authorized applicants.
3. Takes necessary legal action required for denial, revocation and suspension of license.

D. Conducts investigations and hearings on violations of established standards, laws, and regulations.

E. Interprets the nurse practice act based on practice, standards of care, and information from all states.

Authorization (Licensure) to Practice Nursing

✦ A. To legally engage in the practice of nursing, an individual must hold an active license issued by the state in which he or she intends to work.

B. The licensing process.
✦ 1. The applicant must pass a licensing examination administered by the state Board of Registered Nursing, or the BRN may grant reciprocity to an applicant who holds a current license in another state.
✦ 2. The applicant for LVN/LPN licensure examination must have attended a state accredited school of nursing, must be a qualified related nursing professional or para-professional, or must meet specified prerequisites if licensed in a foreign country.
3. Boards of Registered Nursing contract with the National Council of State Boards of Nursing, Inc., for use of the National Council Licensure Examination (abbreviated as NCLEX).

C. Licensure is granted to individuals who have met predetermined standards.
1. One reason for licensure is protection of the public from unqualified practitioners.

2. LVN or LPN is responsible to be familiar with the laws of the state in which he or she will practice.

D. Requirements for practice.
1. A license to practice is a mandatory requirement.
   a. Without license, titles of LVN or LPN may not be used.
   b. Without license, compensation for services as LVN or LPN cannot be received.

E. Basis for disciplinary action.
1. Obtaining a license fraudulently.
2. Practicing nursing during period of revocation or suspension of license.
3. Permitting or aiding unlicensed person to perform those nursing activities requiring a license.
4. Performing duties beyond scope of nursing practice.
5. Practicing in a manner that is judged to be incompetent and/or negligent.
6. Practicing when functional ability is impaired by drugs, alcohol, or other disability.
7. Conviction of a felony or crime involving moral turpitude.

VOCATIONAL ETHICS

A. Ethics is a study that deals with issues of good and bad, moral duty, and obligation.

B. Issues are frequently translated into principles of conduct that govern individual or group behavior.

Characteristics of a Set of Principles

A. Principles are generally predetermined and set down by the same group of individuals whose conduct will be guided by them.

B. The group will abide by these principles voluntarily.

C. The moral duties and obligations governing nursing care practice are embodied in the set of guiding principles.

D. The principles clarify desirable attitudes that ought to be basic to a nurse's performance.

NAPNES Code of Ethics

A. The National Association of Practical Nurse Education and Service, Inc. (NAPNES) determines a set code of ethics for the LVN/LPN. This code states that the licensed practical/vocational nurse shall:
1. Consider a basic obligation the conservation of life and the prevention of disease.

2. Promote and protect the physical, mental, emotional, and spiritual health of the patient and his or her family.
3. Fulfill all duties faithfully and efficiently.
4. Function within established legal guidelines.
5. Accept personal responsibility (for his or her acts) and seek to merit the respect and confidence of all members of the health team.
6. Hold in confidence all matters coming to his or her knowledge, in the practice of his or her profession, and in no way and at no time violate this confidence.
7. Give conscientious service, and charge just remuneration.
8. Learn and respect the religious and cultural beliefs of his or her patient and of all people.
9. Meet his or her obligation to patients by keeping abreast of current trends in health care through reading and continuing education.
10. As a citizen of the United States of America, uphold the laws of the land and seek to promote legislation, which shall meet the health needs of its people.
B. The code of ethics provides principles to guide the performance of licensed practical/vocational nurses.

MANAGEMENT PRINCIPLES

LVN Management Duties

A. Responsibilities.
   ✦ 1. Performance, for compensation, of a defined range of health care services, including assessment, planning, implementation, and evaluation of nursing actions as well as teaching and counseling.
   ✦ 3. Supervision of other nursing personnel: The LVN delegates or assigns tasks to unlicensed assistive personnel (UAPs); these are individuals employed in health care settings to augment patient care—persons without licensure under state nurse practice acts.
B. Requirements: specialized skills taught by and acquired at a state accredited nursing school.
✦ C. Standards of competent performance.
   1. A licensed nurse shall be considered competent when he/she consistently demonstrates the ability to transfer knowledge from social, biological, and physical sciences in applying the nursing process.
   2. *Incompetence* means lacking possession of or failure to exercise that degree of learning, skill, care, and experience ordinarily possessed and exercised by a competent licensed nurse.

D. Professional functions of the RN (denoted by state).
   1. Delegates tasks to subordinates based on the legal scope of practice of the subordinate and on the preparation and capability needed in the tasks to be delegated, and effectively supervises nursing care being given by subordinates.
   2. Evaluates the effectiveness of the care plan through observation of the patient's physical condition and behavior, signs and symptoms of illness, reactions to treatment, and through communication with the patient and health team members, modifies the plan as needed.

Risk Management

✦ A. Nurses are responsible to advise hospital authorities of unsafe nursing situations.
✦ B. Nurses are responsible to document unsafe staffing practices in an incident report and internal memo.
   1. Provides legal protection.
   2. These actions may be viewed as mitigating factors if you are sued.
✦ C. The ANA's Code for Nurses states that the nurse is the patient's advocate and must take action if the rights or best interests of the patient are in jeopardy.
D. ANA takes the position that nurses have a professional obligation to refuse assignments that put licenses or patients "in serious jeopardy."

DELEGATION PRINCIPLES

A. Delegation is defined as "transferring to a competent individual the authority to perform a selected nursing task in a selected situation." (*Source:* National Council of State Boards of Nursing.)
B. State licensing laws designate that nurses are legally accountable for quality of care.
✦ C. LVNs must know competency level of unlicensed personnel.
D. Determine which tasks may be delegated.
   1. Some states identify tasks that may *not ever* be delegated (such as a sterile dressing) to unlicensed personnel.
   2. Review individual state rulings regarding tasks that may be legally delegated.
✦ E. LVNs must check with their own states' laws and regulations to determine which activities may *not* be performed by unlicensed personnel. Examples of these tasks follow.
   1. Administration of medications.
   2. Venipuncture or intravenous therapy.

3. Parenteral or tube feedings.
4. Invasive procedures including inserting NG tubes, inserting catheters, or tracheal suctioning.
5. Assessment of the patient's condition.
6. Educating patients and their families concerning health care problems, including post-discharge care.
7. Moderate complexity laboratory tests.

Activity Delegation

✦ A. RN responsibilities that cannot be delegated:
   1. Data entry into patients' charts for all unlicensed personnel to whom tasks are delegated.
   2. Initial health assessments (only by RN).
   3. Care plan objectives—checked by RN if completed by LVN.
   4. Identify parameters for which worker is to notify nurse.
   5. Carry out pain management activities (epidural narcotic analgesia done only by RN).
   6. Organ donation—RN or LVN responsible for carrying out hospital policies.
   7. Complete discharge teaching plan.
✦ B. Determine which tasks may be delegated.
   1. Patient diagnosis.
   2. Legal limits of delegation.
   3. Amount of judgment and experience needed to perform task or skill.
   4. Predictability of outcome of task.
   5. Whether assistant is capable of performing task.
   C. Delegation and responsibility.
   1. The RN is legally responsible for patient care.
      ✦ a. The LVN works with the RN, who initiates the nursing care plan; LVN may update care plan.
      ✦ b. RN completes initial assessment; RN validates assessment changes noted by LVN.
   ✦ 2. RN initiates patient teaching and evaluates the results.
      a. LVNs may *not* initiate patient teaching with exception of using standard care plan.
      b. LVNs may reinforce patient teaching.
   3. Intravenous administration parameters vary by state.
      a. RN may initiate IVs and add medications.
      b. LVNs, depending on each state's standards, may or may not add medications to an IV, do IV push, or administer piggyback solutions.
      c. LVNs may add vitamins and minerals in most states.
      d. LVNs may initiate IV after completing IV course.

Policies and Regulations

A. Many boards of nursing have enacted laws to protect patients in acute care settings.
B. The term UAP refers to health care workers who are not licensed to perform nursing tasks; this group also refers to those workers who are trained and certified, but not licensed.
✦ C. Basic principles of staffing should be based on several criteria.
   1. Patient care needs.
   2. Severity of the patient's condition.
   3. Services needed.
   4. Complexity surrounding these conditions.
D. These policies further state that unlicensed personnel cannot be assigned in lieu of a registered nurse.
✦ E. Unlicensed personnel may not perform functions (even under the direct clinical supervision of an RN) that require a certain amount of scientific knowledge and technical skills.

Unlicensed Assistive Personnel (UAP) or CNA Delegation

A. Value of care extenders (UAPs, PCTs).
   1. Alleviate or lessen nursing workload and stress.
   2. Perform tasks that enable the professional staff to do more complex tasks.
   3. Provide cost-effective, quality patient care.
   4. Provide extra hands to get the work completed in a timely manner.
B. Potential problems in UAP delegation.
   1. Delegating too much responsibility.
   2. Patient welfare in jeopardy as a result of UAP activity.
      a. UAPs are poorly supervised and monitored.
      b. UAPs are unequipped to perform tasks.
   3. UAPs given responsibility beyond the legal limit specified.
   4. Professional staff use UAPs in ways for which they are not prepared—also underutilizing these staff.
   5. Inappropriate delegation leads to unsafe patient situations.
   6. Inability to recognize inappropriate delegation and unsafe patient situations.
   7. Signs are overlooked that indicate the patient's condition is deteriorating and the UAPs do not report it.

Appropriate Delegation to UAPs

✦ A. Use of assistive personnel.
   1. Evaluate specific patient needs.

2. Judge assistant's competence to perform assigned tasks.
3. Communicate expectations.
4. Provide instructions and active monitoring.
5. Monitor progress in patient care through feedback, evaluate outcomes, and follow-up on identified problems.

✦ B. Determining appropriate delegation to an unlicensed health care worker—ask these questions.
1. Can the UAP legally do this procedure according to the Nurse Practic Act in that state?
2. Has the UAP been trained to perform this procedure?
3. Can the UAP demonstrate this procedure safely and consistently?
4. Is the patient status stable, and does this patient require frequent assessment during the procedure?
5. Is the patient response predictable?
6. When performing this task or activity, can the UAP obtain the same or similar results as the LVN?
7. Can the UAP understand the rationale behind each task?

✦ C. Parameters of delegation: many state boards of nursing have identified the parameters of delegation. Examples of these "Rights of Delegation" are:
1. *Right task*—a task that can be legally delegated to a PCT or UAP. Check the state nurse practice act to determine if the caregiver is trained to perform the task. Judge if the UAP is competent to perform the task.
2. *Right circumstance*—the LVN, PCT, or UAP understands the elements of the procedure and the RN is assured that the UAP can perform the procedure safely in an appropriate setting. Caregiver is able to collect the right supplies to perform the procedure.
3. *Right person*—the right person (RN or LVN) delegates the right task (legally can be delegated to a UAP) to the right person (legally can perform the task) on the right patient (stable with predictable outcomes).
4. *Right communication*—person delegating the task (RN or LVN) has described the task clearly including directions, special steps of the task, and the expected outcomes.
5. *Right supervisor*—the RN or LVN delegating the activity answers the UAP's questions and is available to problem solve if necessary (the task cannot be completed or the patient's condition changes). The UAP performing the task reports its completion and the patient response to the nurse who delegated the activity.

Modified from the National Council of State Boards of Nursing.

D. Duties commonly delegated to Unlicensed Assistive Personnel.
1. Take vital signs.
2. Obtain height and weight.
3. Assist a patient to bed.
4. Escort a patient out of the hospital.
5. Bathe and make beds.
6. Daily care activities
7. Personal hygiene activities.
8. Move and turn patients and reposition.
9. Transfer patients.
10. Assigned to patients requiring infection control precautions.
11. Record drainage from an NG tube.
12. Serve a food tray and feed a patient.
13. Provide oral hygiene.
14. Obtain specimens that are nonsterile and noninvasive.
15. Monitor specific gravity.
16. Check urine glucose.
17. Administer disposable enema or tap water enema.
18. Apply elastic hosiery.
19. Perform range-of-motion exercises.
20. Initiate CPR or perform Heimlich maneuver (with CPR certification).
21. Work with a dying patient.
22. Give postmortem care.

THE NURSE AND THE PATIENT

Patient's Rights

A. A violation of a patient's right, or claim to a right, may be established by a court of law.
B. A nurse should be totally familiar with all aspects of a patient's rights when those rights are associated with health care.
C. Basic rights are guaranteed by the United States Constitution.
1. Freedom of expression.
2. Due process of law.
3. Freedom from cruel and inhumane treatment.
4. Equal protection for all citizens.
D. Patients have the right to courteous, individual care without discrimination.
1. Patient's Bill of Rights is a statement of expectations from the institution.
2. The Patient's Bill of Rights is adopted by the American Hospital Association.

Rights and Consent

A. A right or claim may be moral and/or legal.
1. A legal right can be enforced in a court of law.

2. Within the health care system, all patients retain their basic constitutional rights such as freedom of expression, due process of law, freedom from cruel and inhumane punishment, equal protection, and so forth.

B. Patient rights may conflict with nursing functions.
1. Key elements of a patient's rights with which nurses should be thoroughly familiar include consent, confidentiality, and involuntary commitment.
2. The patient's rights may be modified by his or her mental or physical condition as well as his or her social status.

Informed Consent (to Receive Health Services)

A. Consent is the approval by a patient, or those authorized to give consent, to have his or her body touched by health services personnel (such as physician, nurse, or laboratory technician).
B. Two major forms of consent are signed by patients in a health-care facility.
1. The first consent is signed at the time of admission.
   a. Patients sign the form in admissions office or in the emergency department.
   b. This agreement indicates patient will agree to such procedures as medical treatment, x-rays, blood transfusions and injections.
2. The second type of consent is for invasive testing procedures, such as biopsies, surgery, or special studies involving dye injection or other procedures where risk is involved.
C. Factors in consent-giving process.
1. Consent may be implied or expressed in either written or verbal form.
2. Consent must be *informed consent.*
   a. Patient must be fully informed regarding the mode and extent of tests, surgery, and varieties of treatment to be administered.
   b. Patient must understand that intended results may not be accomplished.
   c. Patient must understand that unintended, potentially harmful consequences may result.
   d. Does not mean a patient can insist on having whatever he wants.
   e. The patient has the right to make choices between "acceptable options."
   f. To make decisions, the patient must have the emotional/mental/legal capacity to do so.
3. A prior consent may be rescinded in either verbal or written form.

D. Individuals authorized to give consent for health services.
1. Mentally competent adult patients.
2. Parents or legal guardians of minors.
3. Court-approved individuals responsible for the mentally incompetent patient.
4. Holders of durable power of attorney.
E. Emergency situations requiring immediate life-preserving action require no prior consent.
1. Serious injury and extreme body dysfunction (e.g., cardiac or respiratory arrest).
2. Imminent death from other causes.
F. Liabilities of a nurse regarding consent.
1. Nurse is liable if he or she requests signature of a patient on a consent form when he or she knows (or *should have known*) patient had not been informed by either the physician or authorized hospital staff regarding potential harmful consequences of treatment, procedures, or surgery.
2. Nurse is liable if he or she does not respect rights of a mentally competent adult patient to refuse health care.

The Patient's Bill of Rights

A. The patient has the right to considerate and respectful care.
B. The patient has the right to obtain from his or her physician complete and current information concerning diagnosis, treatment, and prognosis in terms the patient can be reasonably expected to understand.
C. The patient has the right to receive from the physician information necessary to give informed consent prior to the start of any procedure or treatment. Where medically significant alternatives for care or treatment exist, or when the patient requests information concerning medical alternatives, the patient has the right to such information and to know the name of the person responsible for the procedures or treatment.
D. The patient has the right to refuse treatment to the extent permitted by law and to be informed of the medical consequences of his or her action.
E. The patient has the right to every consideration of privacy concerning his or her own medical care program.
F. The patient has the right to expect that all communications and records pertaining to his or her care should be treated as confidential.
G. The patient has the right to expect that within its capacity a hospital must make reasonable response to the request of a patient for services.
H. The patient has the right to obtain information concerning any relationship of the hospital to

other health care and education institutions insofar as his or her care is concerned and any professional relationships among individuals, by name, who are treating him or her.

I. The patient has the right to be advised if the hospital proposes to engage or perform human experimentation affecting his or her care or treatment and has the right to refuse to participate.

J. The patient has the right to expect reasonable continuity of care.

K. The patient has the right to examine and receive an explanation of his or her bill regardless of the source of payment.

L. The patient has the right to know what hospital rules and regulations apply to his or her conduct as a patient.

M. *Inform patient of his/her specific rights.*

Medical Records

A. A medical record is a complete and accurate written account of a patient's medical history, which includes past and present medical conditions, a recording of all tests, surgeries, procedures, medications, and other relevant data.

B. A medical record functions as a tool of communication for health personnel within a hospital, clinic, or physician's office.
1. Documents the history of a patient's medical evaluation and treatment as well as changes in condition.
2. Provides continuity of health care given and to be given to patient.
3. Provides data for purposes of research.
4. Provides data necessary for assessing quality care by hospital obligations.

C. Nurse's legal and ethical obligations.
1. Help to maintain complete and timely records.
2. Sign or countersign only those entries which are accurate and complete.

Patient's Right to Privacy (Confidentiality)

✦ A. Confidential information.
1. Patients are protected by law (invasion of privacy) against unauthorized release of personal clinical data such as symptoms, diagnoses, and treatments.
2. Nurses, as well as other health care professionals and their employers, may be held personally liable for invasion of privacy, as well as other torts, should litigation arise from unauthorized release of patient data.
3. Nurses have a legal and ethical responsibility to become familiar with their employers' policies and procedures regarding protection of patient's information.
4. Confidential information may be released with consent of the patient.
5. Information release is mandatory when ordered by a court or when state statutes require reporting child abuse, communicable diseases, or other incidents.

B. Patient care: nurses have an ethical responsibility to protect the patient's personal privacy during treatment or hospitalization by means of gowns, screens, closed doors, etc.

C. Medical records.
1. As the key written account of patient information such as signs and symptoms, diagnosis, treatment, etc., the medical record fulfills many functions both within the hospital or clinic and with outside parties.
    a. Documents the care given to the patient.
    b. Provides effective means of communication among health care personnel.
    c. Contains important data for insurance and other expense claims.
    d. May be utilized in court in the event of litigation.
2. Nurses have an ethical and legal obligation to maintain complete and timely records, and to sign or countersign only those documents that are accurate and complete.

Health Insurance Portability and Accountability Act (HIPAA)

A. Enacted into law in 1996, phased in gradually.

B. Requires secretary of Health and Human Services (HHS) to devise standards.
1. Improve Medicare and Medicaid programs—efficiency and effectiveness of health care system.
2. Ensures continuing health care insurance if patient has had existing group insurance.
3. Proposed standards for electronic transactions and security signatures.
4. Ensures privacy of individual health information.

C. Privacy rule component became effective April, 2003.
1. Requires health care providrs to protect againt unauthorized disclosures of personal medical information.
2. Requires patient consent for any information disclosed to others.
3. Patients must receive written notice of privacy practices and their rights.
4. Patients may access personal medical records more freely than before.

Advance Directives

✦ A. An advance directive is a document that allows patients to make legal decisions about how they wish to receive future medical treatment. It is written and signed before any such care becomes necessary.
   1. It allows patients to participate in choosing health care providers (physicians and nurses).
   2. It allows patients to choose the type of medical treatments the patient desires.
   3. It allows patients to consent or refuse certain types of medical treatments.
✦ B. Within this document, the patient may indicate the person or persons he or she wishes to make medical decisions in situations in which the patient is unable to do so.
   C. The document needs to be signed and witnessed, and copies should be kept on file in the physician's office and the hospital.
   D. The witness to this document should not be a hospital employee, relative, or heir to the patient's estate.
   E. Advance directives vary among states and, therefore, the nurse must be knowledgeable about the use and type of directives in the state in which he or she practices.

Psychiatric Advance Directives (PAD)

A. PAD is similar to advance directive prepared for end-of-life care.
B. Specific components that may be included in the PAD.
   1. Refusal of specific drugs, surgery, or treatments, i.e., ECT.
   2. Consent for specific psychiatric interventions and conditions under which they may be implemented.
   3. Appointment of a trusted individual who may give consent for the patient.
   4. Willingness to participate in research studies.
C. PADs are not accepted in every state. Popular with mental health providers for providing guidance to family, staff and the courts.

Living Will

✦ A. A living will is a type of advance directive.
✦ B. The document indicates the patient's wishes regarding:
   1. Prolonging life using life support measures.
   2. Refusing or stopping medical interventions.
   3. Making decisions about his or her medical care.
✦ C. Living wills are executed while the patient is competent and able to make sound decisions.

ADVANCE DIRECTIVES

The Patient Self-Determination Act of 1990 (PSDA) is a federal law that imposes on states and providers of health care certain requirements concerning Advance Directives as well as an individual's right under state law to make decisions concerning medical care.

✦ The Omnibus Budget Reconciliation Act (OBRA) of 1990 requires states to provide advance directives as options for patients. This document should be completed and signed before treatment becomes necessary. The nurse should check with the patient's physician to determine that advance directives are on file. Documents include:

- Patient's choice in continuing medical care when the patient is unable to speak or make decisions.
- Living will, power of attorney for health care, or a notarized handwritten document.
- Documents available in patient's medical record.
- Documents witnessed by persons other than medical personnel or relatives of the patient or heirs to the patient's estate.

D. As conditions change, a living will needs to be evaluated for relevance. (States differ in their acceptance of living wills as legal documents.)

Durable Power [of Attorney] for Health Care

A. This is a legal document concerning health care for the patient.
   ✦ 1. This document gives power to make health care decisions to a designated individual in the event that the patient is unable to make competent decisions for him- or herself.
   ✦ 2. It must be prepared and signed while the client is competent.
   ✦ 3. The designated person is obligated to follow the directives outlined in the document.
✦ B. Decisions regarding withdrawing or using life support, organ donation, or consent to treatment or procedures are included in the directives.
   1. As long as the patient is competent, the agent does not have the right to make legal decisions.
   2. The major difference between the Living Will and Power of Attorney is that the latter is more flexible.

Do Not Resuscitate

A. A "Do Not Resuscitate" or DNR order is another type of advance directive.
   1. DNR is a request to *not* have cardiopulmonary resuscitation (CPR) if the patient ceases to breathe or is unable to sustain a heart beat.
   2. This form can be signed at any time before or during hospitalization.

B. When signed, the physician places a DNR notation in the patient's medical chart.

PUBLIC LAW AND THE NURSE

The Law

A. Binding rules and standards of an extended community, which are formally recognized, obeyed, and enforced by authority.
B. The purpose of the law is the preservation of order and the promotion of safety.
C. Obligations of a nurse to the law are no different from that required of other citizens.
   1. An individual is responsible for his or her own behavior unless that individual is mentally incompetent.
   2. An individual is responsible to know the law and its ramifications.
   3. Punitive action may be taken against the individual who fails to abide by the law.

Types of Law

A. Civil. (*See* Table 2-1.)
   1. The harm is against an individual, and guilt requires proof by a preponderance of the evidence.
   2. Civil law covers contracts, labor issues, and, among other areas, tort law (normally involved in malpractice claims). (*See* Table 2-2.)
   3. Punishment is generally the payment of monetary compensation.
B. Criminal.
   1. The harm is against society, and guilt requires proof beyond a reasonable doubt.
   2. Crimes are classified as misdemeanors (lesser) or felonies (serious).
   3. Examples are falsification of narcotics records, withholding life support from terminally ill patients, and administration of drugs that hasten a patient's death.
   4. Punishment may be a payment of compensation and/or imprisonment.

KEY LEGAL TERMS

Liability

✦ A. A nurse has a personal, legal obligation to provide a standard of patient care expected of a reasonably competent professional nurse.
✦ B. Professional nurses are held responsible (liable) for harm resulting from their negligent acts or omission to act.

Table 2-1. NURSING LIABILITY	
Civil Law	**Criminal Law**
Contract	Assault
Unintentional Tort	Battery
Intentional Tort	Murder
Negligence	Manslaughter

Table 2-2. CLASSIFICATIONS OF LAW RELATED TO NURSING	
Classification	**Example**
Constitutional	Patients' rights to equal treatment
Administrative	Licensure and the state BRN
Labor Relations	Union negotiations
Contract	Relationship with employer
Criminal	Handling of narcotics
Tort	
Medical Malpractice	Reasonable and prudent patient care
Product Liability	Warranty on medical equipment

Respondeat Superior

A. Legal doctrine that holds an employer liable for negligent acts of employees in the course and scope of employment.
B. Physicians, hospitals, clinics, and other employers may be held liable for negligent acts of their employees.
C. This doctrine does not support acts of gross negligence or acts that are outside the scope of employment.

Negligence

✦ A. The doctrine of negligence rests on the duty of every person to exercise due care in his or her conduct toward others from which injury may result.
✦ B. *Liability* results from:
   1. A duty to provide on the part of the nurse and a causal relationship between damage or harm to the patient.
   2. An act or an omission to act by the nurse.
C. *Gross negligence* is the intentional failure to perform a duty in reckless disregard of the consequences affecting the patient—a gross lack of care to such a level as to be considered willful and wanton.
✦ D. *Criminal negligence* consists of a duty on the part of the nurse and an act that is the proximate cause of the injury or death of a patient.

PROVING NEGLIGENCE

To prove negligence against a nurse, these 4 elements must be present.
a. Failed a duty to provide a standard of care to the patient.
b. Failed to adhere to the standard of care.
c. Failure to adhere to the standard of care caused injury to the patient.
d. The patient suffered damages as a result of the nurse's negligent action.

Documentation in the patient's chart must show that the nurse met the standard of care.

---

1. Usually defined by statute and punishable as a crime.
2. The act being punished would be a flagrant and reckless disregard for the safety of others and/or a willful disregard to the injury liable to follow.
3. The act is converted to a crime when it results in personal injury or death.

✦ E. One is considered "negligent" if he or she fails to provide a patient with the standard of care that a resonably prudent nurse would exercise under similar circumstances.

Malpractice

✦ A. Any professional misconduct that is an unreasonable lack of skill or fidelity in professional duties.
✦ B. Bad, wrong, or injurious treatment of a patient.
✦ C. Results of treatment may include injury, unnecessary suffering, or death to a patient proceeding from ignorance, carelessness, lack of professional skill, disregard of established rules, protocols, principles or procedures, neglect, or a malicious or criminal intent.
D. It is the nurse's legal duty to provide competent, reasonable care to patients.
  ✦ 1. To ensure that these standards occur, the nurse must know the standards of care, develop patterns of practice that meet these standards, and document these actions.
  ✦ 2. Nursing actions that constitute a breach of standards of care and lead to patient injury can be termed malpractice.

Professional Misconduct

A. Nurses must meet certain standards.
B. Misconduct would be declared for any of the following actions.
  1. Obtaining an LVN/PN license through misrepresentation or fraudulent means.
  2. Giving false information on application for license.

3. Practicing in an incompetent or grossly negligent manner.
4. Practicing when ability to practice is severely impaired.
5. Being habitually drunk or dependent on drugs.
6. Furnishing controlled substances to himself or herself or to another person.
7. Impersonating another certified or licensed practitioner or allowing another person to use his or her license for the purpose of nursing.
8. Being convicted of or committing an act constituting a crime under federal or state law.
9. Refusing to proivde health care services on the grounds of race, color, creed, or national origin.
10. Permitting or aiding an unlicensed person to perform activities requiring a license.
11. Practicing nursing while license is suspended.
12. Practicing medicine without a license.
13. Procuring, aiding, or offering to assist at a criminal abortion.

Nursing Contracts

A. A contract is a binding agreement (usually in printed form) between two or more individuals that gives evidence to specified terms and conditions expected of both parties to the agreement.
B. A contract entered into by a nurse and employer may be in the form of either a written or verbal agreement.
C. Conditions of the agreement.
  1. The nurse is required to perform all nursing duties with skill and knowledge.
  2. Performance is to be in accordance with the standards of care established by the Nurse Practice Act for licensure.
  3. The employer is required to issue fair compensation for services given.
D. Breach of the agreement (contract) occurs when one or more parties to the agreement fail to fulfill the obligations stipulated within it.

LEGAL ISSUES IN DRUG ADMINISTRATION

Definition: In their daily work, most nurses handle a wide variety of drugs. Failure to give the correct medication or improper handling of drugs may result in serious problems for the nurse due to strict federal and state statutes relating to drugs. (*See* Chapter 5 for Drug Administration.)

Regulation

✦ A. The Comprehensive Drug Abuse Prevention Act of 1970 provides the fundamental regulations

LEGAL ASPECTS OF DRUG ADMINISTRATION

✦ A. Nurses must not administer a specific drug unless allowed to do so by the particular state's Nurse Practice Act.
1. Nurses must not administer any drug without a specific physician's order.
2. Nurses must not administer a controlled substance if the physician's order is outdated.
3. LVN/LPNs must be aware of the individual states' Nurse Practice Acts, which state limitations of drug administration (example: some states do not allow LVNs to administer IV push medications).
B. Nurses are to take every safety precaution in whatever action they perform.
C. Nurses are to be certain that the employer's policy allows them to administer a specific drug.
D. A drug may not lawfully be administered unless all the above items are in effect.
E. General rules for drug dispensing:
1. Never leave medicines unattended.
2. Always report errors immediately.
3. Send labeled bottles that are unintelligible back to the pharmacist for relabeling.
4. Store internal and external medicines separately if possible.

(federal) for the compounding, selling, and dispensing of narcotics, stimulants, depressants, and other controlled items.
B. Each state has a similar set of regulations for the same purpose.

Violation

A. Each state's pharmacy act provides standards for dispensing drugs.
B. Noncompliance with federal or state drug regulations can result in liability.
✦ C. Violation of the state drug regulations or licensing laws are grounds for BRN administrative disciplinary action.

LEGAL ISSUES IN PSYCHIATRIC NURSING

Statutes of Protection

A. Laws of certain states protect individuals from themselves.
1. These laws require that such persons be evaluated by competent psychiatric personnel.

2. The laws protect the patient's rights and civil liberties by not allowing psychiatric patients to be hospitalized inappropriately.
B. Laws also protect family members and the general community from persons who are dangerous or severely disturbed.

Admission Procedures

A. There are voluntary and involuntary admissions for psychiatric patients.
B. Voluntary admission occurs when an individual recognizes that he or she needs treatment and signs in to a hospital.
1. After admission, the patient is *not* free to leave before a specified period of time.
2. Such a patient may leave the hospital against the physician's advice if the patient gives notice of such intent at least one or two days prior to leaving.
3. If the physician feels the patient is too ill, he can legally assign the patient to involuntary status.
4. A voluntary patient loses none of his or her civil rights.
C. Involuntary status occurs when the patient is psychiatrically evaluated to be too ill to function outside the hospital.
1. Admission is not initiated by the patient.
2. When a patient is committed, he or she cannot leave the hospital against medical advice.
3. Family members, a physician, a law officer, or a community member can institute commitment proceedings.
4. Patients are permitted to leave only when psychiatric evaluation indicates they are able to care for themselves or are not dangerous to themselves or others.
5. Patient may retain some, all, or none of his or her civil rights. This depends on the individual state laws.
6. The different classifications include emergency admission (time limited), observational (diagnostic evaluation or short term), and indefinite (formal commitment).

PROFESSIONAL ORGANIZATIONS

Purpose

A. Maintain and improve nursing standards.
B. Provide a vehicle for continuing education.
1. Workshops.
2. Publications.
3. National and state conventions.
C. Provide opportunity to share professional interests.
D. Enhance an individual's sense of belonging.

National Associations

A. National Association of Practical Nurse Education and Service, Inc. (NAPNES).
   1. Membership—extended to any individual with an interest in education of practical nurse and/or other aspects of practical nursing.
   2. Publication—*The Journal of Practical Nursing.*
B. National Federation of Licensed Practical Nurses (NFLPN).
   1. Membership—LPNs, LVNs, and practical/vocational nursing students.
   2. Publication—*American Journal of Practical Nursing.*
C. National League for Nursing (NLN).
   1. Membership—extended to any individual with an interest in nursing.
   2. Publications—*Nursing and Health Care, Nursing Research,* and professional directories.
   3. Functions.
      a. Prepare and score selection and achievement tests.
      b. Conduct workshops.
      c. Nationally accredit schools of registered and practical nursing.
D. American Nurses Association (ANA).
   1. Membership—limited to registered nurses, students of registered nursing programs.
   2. Publication—*American Journal of Nursing.*

MANAGEMENT PRINCIPLES AND LEGAL/ETHICAL QUESTIONS

1. A nurse team leader observed another nurse begin an IV without putting on gloves. When confronted, the nurse replied "Oh, I was careful and didn't get any blood on me." The nurse team leader should initially respond

   1. "The regulations state that all of us must wear gloves. If I see you without them, I will place you on report."
   2. "Tell me your understanding of what Standard Precautions for all patients means."
   3. "Well, if you are absolutely sure that you can be careful—but I don't think it is safe nursing practice."
   4. "I think we should clarify this with the charge nurse to see who is right."

2. The LVN is very short staffed because two people did not show up for work. Of the following four patients, which one would the LVN care for first?

   1. A patient just admitted with acute abdominal pain and possible cholecystitis.
   2. A patient with nephrotic syndrome with increasing edema; hourly urine and vital signs.
   3. A confused patient yelling because he is in soft restraints and cannot get out of bed.
   4. A head-injury patient with an IV who was just admitted to the unit.

3. In the presence of the RN, a physician asks the LPN to remove the sutures from the incision before the patient is discharged. The initial response to the physician should be

   1. "LVNs cannot remove the sutures; the RN will do it."
   2. "Please write the order and the sutures will be removed."
   3. "We will remove them right away."
   4. "The LVN will get the suture removal set for you because she/he is not allowed to remove sutures."

4. An LVN has been assigned to work in a subacute nursing unit. The nurse has the help of two UAPs to care for 15 patients. When delegating care, the most important concept for the nurse to keep in mind is

   1. The length of time it takes to care for each patient.
   2. The skill level of the two UAPs.
   3. The length of time each UAP has been on the job.
   4. Which patients the LVN has taken care of before.

5. The LVN observes the nursing assistant (NA) regulating the IV of an oncology patient receiving morphine sulfate for pain. The LVN is responsible for the patient and has assigned the patient to the NA. The appropriate intervention is to

   1. Instruct the NA that this action is not within the realm of responsibility of an NA and reprimand her.
   2. Immediately inform the charge nurse and fill out an incident (unusual occurrence) report.
   3. Call a staff meeting and confront the NA.
   4. Ask the NA to meet with the RN and him/her to discuss the responsibility parameters that are appropriate for the NA.

6. An LPN is assigned three patients when an additional patient, a 90-year-old with COPD, is admitted to the step-down unit. He is short of breath (a CO_2 retainer), and his O_2 stats are 83 percent on 2 L of oxygen. The patient's situation worsens. The supervisor sends a CNA to assist the nurse. Which of the following patients and procedures would the nurse assign the CNA to do?

   1. Carry out pretest procedures and go to the cath lab with a patient.
   2. Vital signs and AM care for a patient with pneumonia and a 2-day postop diabetic patient complaining of pain.
   3. Posttest care for a patient following an arteriogram.
   4. The 90-year-old COPD patient.

7. A male patient admitted himself to the alcoholic treatment unit because he is having blackout spells when he drinks. He is 47 years of age, lives alone, and has a history of early cirrhosis of the liver. In planning for his care, the priority nursing activity is to

   1. Monitor dietary selections and appetite.
   2. Observe for withdrawal symptoms.
   3. Institute 24-hour suicide precautions.
   4. Measure abdominal girth daily.

8. The LVN has a full workload and must reassign some of her patients to the UAP. The most appropriate patient to reassign to the UAP would be a(n)

    1. Patient just returning from the recovery room following colostomy surgery.
    2. Cerebral vascular accident (CVA) patient who has been hospitalized for 2 days.
    3. Oncology patient who is in severe pain controlled by epidural anesthesia.
    4. Newly admitted patient with suspected pancreatitis.

9. The LVN assigns a patient with uremic frost from renal failure to the UAP. The patient is complaining of dry, itchy skin. To alleviate this problem during bathing, the nurse will instruct the UAP to use

    1. Mild soap and water, then lotion.
    2. Bath oil in the water with no soap.
    3. A weak vinegar solution with no soap.
    4. Water only, followed by lotion.

    Clinical Scenario: The nursing unit is very busy. The nurse has five critically ill patients (none are terminal, all are full codes, and have required IV push medications). Seven patients are being discharged and two new patients with chest pain who are on lidocaine drips are being admitted. One of these patients with chest pain had two runs of ventricular tachycardia in the ER. The nurse also has on the unit a comatose terminal patient with a life expectancy of less than 72 hours. This patient has a sump tube, a Foley, and TPN running through a central line, with orders for comfort measures only. **Questions 10–13 relate to this scenario.**

10. Considering the above, the most appropriate person to take care of the critically ill patients is the

    1. RN.
    2. LPN.
    3. CNA.
    4. UAP.

11. The most appropriate person to take care of the terminally ill patient is the

    1. RN.
    2. LPN.
    3. LVN.
    4. UAP.

12. The most appropriate person to take care of the patients being discharged, both of which need teaching to be reinforced, would be the

    1. RN.
    2. LPN.

    3. CNA.
    4. UAP.

13. The patient who is most critical and should be assessed by the RN is the

    1. Diabetic being discharged and requiring patient teaching.
    2. Cardiac patient with a history of ventricular tachycardia.
    3. Patient requiring IV push medication.
    4. Comatose terminally ill patient.

14. Which of the following agencies determine the scope of practice for the LVN?

    1. Individual agency policies employing the LVN.
    2. Joint Commission on Accreditation of Healthcare Organizations.
    3. State Board of Licensed Practical/Vocational Nursing.
    4. American Nurses Association.

15. As the LVN completes charting for a patient, the nurse notices that the information was entered on the wrong patient's chart. The appropriate action is to

    1. Use "white out" and cover all the incorrect information.
    2. Completely block out the information using a black pen.
    3. Draw a single line through the incorrect entry, initial, and write "error."
    4. Discard the notes and ask the staff to rewrite any entries on the page.

16. The nurse's liability in terms of the patient's consent to receive health services is to

    1. Be certain that the physician has prepared the patient.
    2. Ensure that the patient is fully informed before being asked to sign a consent form.
    3. Check that the patient understands the details of the surgery.
    4. The nurse would not be liable—the physician would be.

17. Which of the following might negate liability on the part of the nurse in a negligent action?

    1. The patient consented to the act.
    2. The harm was not reasonably foreseeable.
    3. The nurse had not been taught to do the procedure in nursing school.
    4. Other foreseeable acts occurred that added to the patient's injury.

18. Which of the following statements concerning nursing liability is true?

    1. A physician may assume personal liability for the negligent acts of the nurse.
    2. The nurse is responsible for her own negligent acts.
    3. The doctrine of respondeat superior always protects the nurse.
    4. Malpractice insurance will always cover the damages assessed against the nurse.

19. Patient's rights can be defined as

    1. Rights specifically written into many laws.
    2. A position paper that was developed by the American Hospital Association.
    3. A declaration of the World Health Organization.
    4. Rights not supported by statutory law.

20. A state's Nurse Practice Act would *not* include

    1. A definition of nursing practice.
    2. Qualifications for licensure.
    3. Grounds for revocation of a license.
    4. Difference between RN and LVN functions.

21. The nurse is asked to do a TV commercial for hand lotion. In this commercial, she will wear her nurse's uniform and advocate the use of this lotion by nurses in their work setting. In doing this, the nurse is violating

    1. Consumer fraud laws.
    2. The nurse practice act.
    3. The code of ethics for nurses.
    4. None of the above.

22. For an LVN, which of the following would *not* constitute negligent conduct?

    1. A medication error.
    2. Failure to follow a physician's order.
    3. Failure to challenge a physician's order.
    4. Disagreeing with a physician.

23. The nurse transcribing the physician's order finds it difficult to read. Which of the following people should the nurse consult for clarification of the order?

    1. The head nurse who is familiar with the physician's handwriting.
    2. An RN working with the nurse.
    3. The physician who wrote the order.
    4. The nursing supervisor.

24. If the nurse is involved in a situation in which he or she must countersign the charting of a paraprofessional, which of the following will most aid in decreasing legal liability?

    1. Read the document before it is signed.
    2. Have personal knowledge of the information contained in the document.
    3. Make sure the information is accurate.
    4. Check with a second nurse to see if information is accurate.

25. Which of the following best describes the function and purpose of the unusual occurrence (incident) report?

    1. A legal part of the chart used to furnish data about the incident.
    2. A hospital record used to record the details of the incident for possible legal reference.
    3. A legal hospital business record, which is subject to subpoena and can be used against the hospital personnel.
    4. A hospital record that is entered into the patient's chart if he or she dies.

26. The physician wrote a medication order for a patient. The LVN thought the dosage was incorrect. She questioned the physician who said it was all right. Still questioning, she asked the RN, who said it was all right. The LVN gave the medicine, and the patient died from an overdose. Who is liable?

    1. The physician and the two nurses.
    2. The physician.
    3. The nurse who gave the medication.
    4. Both the physician and the nurse who gave the medication.

27. The decision as to whether or not a nurse can lawfully restrain a patient is made by the

    1. Nurse.
    2. Family.
    3. Hospital administrator.
    4. Physician.

28. One of the elements of negligence is breach of the standard of care. "Standard of care" may be defined as

    1. Nursing competence as defined by the State Nurse Practice Act.
    2. Degree of judgment and skill in nursing care given by a reasonable and prudent professional nurse under similar circumstances.
    3. Health services as prescribed by community ordinances.
    4. Giving care to patients in good faith to the best of one's ability.

29. The primary purpose and criteria of licensure is to

    1. Limit practice.
    2. Define the scope of practice.
    3. Protect the public.
    4. Outline legislative action.

30. The civil rights of a patient would not be jeopardized in which of the following situations?

    1. Trying to forcibly detain a patient who may suffer great harm by leaving the hospital.
    2. Giving emergency medical care to a patient without his or her consent or the consent of the family.
    3. Giving a psychiatric patient's letters addressed to the President of the United States to his physician.
    4. Giving the patient's insurance broker access to his chart.

MANAGEMENT PRINCIPLES AND LEGAL/ETHICAL ISSUES

Answers with Rationales

1. (2)   The best way to determine what the nurse knows and/or understands or believes is to ask this basic question. Once the nurse has baseline data, then teaching about the importance of always using Standard Precautions can be done. When a nurse is inconsistent in the use of these Standard Precautions, patients as well as the other team members are in jeopardy. Universal precautions are to be used for *all* patients when there is a danger of coming into contact with body fluids.

NP:I; CN:S; CA:M; CL:A

2. (4)   Head injury would take the first priority because the danger of increasing intracranial pressure must be assessed and, if it is increasing, or the level of consciousness is changing, these results must be reported immediately. The patient has the most serious and potentially unstable condition; thus, the nursing judgment would be to care for him first. The nephrotic patient (2) is not in critical condition, and the confused patient (3) can also wait; the second priority would be the patient with possible cholecystitis (1) because of the unstable condition.

NP:P; CN:PH; CA:M; CL:AN

3. (2)   LVN/LPNs may remove sutures; however, both nurses must be sure that the physician has written the order to do so.

NP:I; CN:S; CA:S; CL:C

4. (2)   There are two UAPs who probably have different skill levels. It is important to consider their abilities and skill level (as well as the legal parameters for which tasks they can perform) when assigning patients and tasks. The other variables are important, but should be taken into account after the skill level has been evaluated.

NP:P; CN:S; CA:M; CL:C

5. (4)   While regulating or even touching an IV is definitely not within the scope of behaviors that an NA can legally perform, both teaching and clarification of duties are needed in this situation. Before accusing or reprimanding the NA, a nonpunitive environment should be created so that teaching and correction can occur, which will prevent this happening in the future. Unless too much medication was given, an incident report (2) need not be filled out. Confronting the team member in a staff meeting (3) would not be following management principles.

NP:I; CN:S; CA:M; CL:AN

Coding for Questions/Answers Abbreviations: **Nursing Process: NP,** Data Collection: D, Planning: P, Implementation: I, Evaluation: E, **Client Needs: CN,** Safe, Effective Care Environment: S, Health Promotion and Maintenance: H, Psychosocial Integrity: PS, Physiological Integrity: PH, **Clinical Area: CA,** Medical Nursing: M, Surgical Nursing: S, Maternal/Newborn Nursing: MA, Pediatric Nursing: P, Psychiatric Nursing: PS, **Cognitive Level: CL,** Knowledge: K, Comprehension: C, Application: A, Analysis: AN

6. (2) CNAs are trained to provide hygiene and comfort measures for patients. The other patients are either too ill [the patient who had the arteriogram (3) or the COPD patient (4)], and the CNA is not able to carry out pretest procedures for a cardiac cath (1).

   NP:P; CN:S; CA:M; CL:AN

7. (2) The nurse's priority is to observe for symptoms of withdrawal. Although nursing activities may include monitoring diet (1) and measuring abdominal girth (4), there is no need for suicide precautions (3) at this time.

   NP:P; CN:PS; CA:PS; CL:AN

8. (2) The most appropriate patient to assign to the UAP would be the CVA patient. This patient would have been in the hospital for 2 days, so the intial assessment would have been completed. Also, this patient does not require immediate intervention, as does the colostomy patient (1) (assessing for hemorrhage, vital signs, etc.). The oncology patient (3) must be assessed for effectiveness of pain control, and the RN or LVN are the only staff members who can do this. The newly admitted patient with suspected pancreatitis (4) also requires a complete health assessment, and the RN is the only person who can complete this task.

   NP:P; CN:S; CA:M; CL:AN

9. (3) Soaps (1) should be avoided, and bathing daily should be avoided, if possible. Water (4) is drying to the skin. Vinegar solutions may alleviate itching by dissolving crystal deposits in cutaneous layers and leaving an acid layer on the skin. The exact etiology for pruritus in the end-stage renal patient is not known. This is an example of how the LVN has to take responsibility to give the UAP specific instructions for individual patients. The nurse must also receive a report following the care.

   NP:I; CN:PH; CA:M; CL:C

10. (1) An RN is responsible for the continuous assessment of patients. If they are critically ill, they will need continuous assessment. The other patients are not terminal; if they were, they would be able to be cared for by the LPN.

    NP:P; CN:S; CA:M; CL:C

11. (4) This patient is terminal and requires comfort measures only. The RN can assess and maintain the TPN rate via pump, and irrigate the Foley and sump as needed. The UAP can safely provide the care to keep the patient comfortable. Any IV pain medications would be given by the RN.

    NP:P; CN:S; CA:M; CL:C

12. (2) The RNs are needed for the other critically ill patients on the unit. Reinforcement of the teaching can be safely and effectively done by an LPN/LVN.

    NP:P; CN:S; CA:M; CL:C

13. (2) This patient requires constant assessment with the possibility of immediate life support intervention should he have another run of ventricular tachycardia. Given the instability of the patient's situation, the RN should be assessing this patient.

    NP:P; CN:S; CA:M; CL:AN

14. (3) The State Board of Nursing in each state determines the scope of nursing practice by formulating a Nurse Practice Act for the LVN/LPNs within that state. The Nurse Practice Act specifies the rules and regulations for practice and licensure.

    NP:P; CN:S; CA:M; CL:K

15. (3) This is the correct method of indicating an error and the most legally accepted method. The information can be read, if necessary, and it indicates the nurse is not trying to "cover up" a mistake.

    NP:I; CN:S; CA:M; CL:K

16. (2) The patient must be fully informed of potentially harmful effects of the treatment. If this is not done, it could result in the nurse's being personally liable.

    NP:I; CN:S; CA:M; CL:C

17. (2) If basic rules of human conduct are not violated, the elements of liability may not exist. There must be certain elements of liability present; for example, there must exist a causal relationship between harm to the patient and the act by the nurse. There must be some damage or harm sustained by the patient and there must be a legal basis—such as statutory law—for finding liability.

    NP:P; CN:S; CA:M; CL:C

18. (2) The nurse is responsible for her or his own negligent acts; however, legal doctrine holds that an employer is also liable for negligent acts of employees.

    NP:P; CN:S; CA:M; CL:K

19. (1) All but 10 states have some provision for the rights of patients written into a law, and these rights can be enforced by the law.

    NP:D; CN:S; CA:M; CL:K

20. (4) Each state has its own Nurse Practice Act for RNs and LVNs. Separately, they are a series of

statutes enacted by a state to regulate the practice of nursing in that state. It includes all of these plus education.

NP:P; CN:S; CA:M; CL:K

21. (3) The code of ethics is a set of formal guidelines for governing professional action. This situation is not illegal—it is unethical.

NP:P; CN:S; CA:M; CL:C

22. (4) Because the nurse is a licensed professional with an education based on a defined body of knowledge, he or she has the right, indeed the responsibility, to disagree with the physician. This is especially so when the health and welfare of the patient is involved.

NP:I; CN:S; CA:M; CL:K

23. (3) Because the nurse will be responsible (and liable) if she transcribes the order incorrectly, the physician who wrote the order should be consulted.

NP:I; CN:S; CA:M; CL:C

24. (2) To sign a document without having personal knowledge of what occurred would open the possibility of liability.

NP:P; CN:S; CA:M; CL:A

25. (2) The most accurate answer is (2). The other purposes are to help document the quality of care and to identify areas where more inservice education is needed.

NP:P; CN:S; CA:M; CL:C

26. (4) The professional nurse, as well as the physician who wrote the order, are held responsible (liable) for harm resulting from their negligent acts.

NP:E; CN:S; CA:M; CL:A

27. (4) To administer any form of restraint, there must be a physician's order.

NP:P; CN:S; CA:M; CL:K

28. (2) Nursing actions are evaluated against a set of standards referred to as standards of performance.

NP:P; CN:S; CA:M; CL:K

29. (3) The primary purpose of licensing nurses, both RN and LVN, is to safeguard the public by determining that the nurse is a safe and competent practitioner.

NP:P; CN:S; CA:M; CL:K

30. (2) Key elements of a patient's rights are consent, confidentiality, and voluntary commitment.

NP:P; CN:S; CA:M; CL:A

Nursing Through the Life Cycle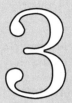

HOMEOSTASIS: STRESS AND ADAPTATION

Homeostasis

✦ *Definition:* The maintenance of a constant state in the internal environment through self-regulatory techniques that preserve the organism's ability to adapt to stresses.

✦ A. Dynamics of homeostasis.
1. Danger or its symbols, whether internal or external, result in the activation of the sympathetic nervous system and the adrenal medulla.
2. The organism prepares for fight or flight (attack–withdrawal).
B. Adaptation factors.
1. Age—adaptation is greatest in youth and young middle life, and least at the extremes of life.
2. Environment—adequate supply of required materials is necessary.
3. Adaptation involves the entire organism.
4. The organism can more easily adapt to stress over a period of time than suddenly.
5. Organism flexibility influences survival.
6. The organism usually uses the adaptation mechanism that is most economical in terms of energy.
7. Illness decreases the organism's capacity to adapt to stress.
8. Adaptation responses may be adequate or deficient.
9. Adaptation may cause stress and illness, i.e., ulcers, arthritis, allergy, asthma, and overwhelming infections.

Stress

✦ A. Definitions of stress.
1. A physical, a chemical, or an emotional factor that causes bodily or mental tension and that may be a factor in disease causation; a state resulting from factors that tend to alter an existing equilibrium.
✦ 2. Selye's definition of stress.
a. The state manifested by a specific syndrome that consists of all the nonspecifically induced changes within the biologic system.
b. The body is the common denominator of all adaptive responses.
c. Stress is manifested by the measurable changes in the body.
d. Stress causes a multiplicity of changes in the body.
B. General aspects of stress.

1. Body responses to stress are a self-preserving mechanism that automatically and immediately becomes activated in times of danger.
a. Caused by physical or psychological stress: disease, injury, anger, or frustration.
b. Caused by changes in internal and/or external environment.
2. There are a limited number of ways an organism can respond to stress (for example, a cornered amoeba cannot fly).

Stress and Disease

A. Stress and individual method of coping are associated with heart disease, cancer and other diseases.
B. Actual physical changes occur with high stress levels.
1. Increased release of adrenalin, cortisol and other hormones lead to increased heart rate, blood pressure and platelet stickiness which may accelerate atherosclerosis and other causes of heart disease.
2. Changes in immune system may interfere with individual ability to recognize and destroy cancer cells.
C. Stress can be both positive and negative. Individual must have adaptive mechanism to cope with stress to increase health and avoid risk for disease.

Selye's Theory of Stress
✦ A. General adaptive syndrome (GAS).
1. Alarm stage (call to arms).
a. Shock: the body translates as sudden injury, and the GAS becomes activated.
b. Countershock: the organism restored to its preinjury condition.
2. Stage of resistance: the organism is adapted to the injuring agent.
3. State of exhaustion: if stress continues, the organism loses its adaptive capability and goes into exhaustion, which is comparable to shock.
✦ B. Local adaptive syndrome (LAS).
1. Selective changes within the organism.
2. Local response elicits general response.
3. Example of LAS: a cut, followed by bleeding, followed by coagulation of blood, etc.
4. Ability of parts of the body to respond to a specific injury is impaired if the whole body is under stress.
C. Whether the organism goes through all the phases of adaptation depends both upon its capacity to adapt and the intensity and continuance of the injuring agent.

1. Organism may return to normal.
2. Organism may overreact; stress decreases.
3. Organism may be unable to adapt or maintain adaptation, a condition that may lead to death.
D. Objective of stress response.
   1. To maintain stability of the organism during stress.
   2. To repair damage.
   3. To restore body to normal composition and activity.

Psychological Stress

✦ *Definition:* All processes that impose a demand or requirement upon the organism, the resolution or accommodation of which necessitates work or activity of the mental apparatus.

Characteristics

A. May involve other structures or systems, but primarily affects mental apparatus.
   1. Anxiety is a primary result of psychological stress.
   2. Causes mental mechanisms to attempt to reduce or relieve psychological discomfort.
     a. Attack/fight.
     b. Withdrawal/flight.
     c. Play dead/immobility.
B. Causes of psychological stress.
   1. Loss of something of value.
   2. Injury/pain.
   3. Frustrations of needs and drives.
   4. Threats to self-concept.
   5. Many illnesses cause stress.
     a. Disfigurement.
     b. Sexually transmitted diseases (STD).
     c. Long-term or chronic diseases.
     d. Cancer.
     e. Heart disease.
   6. Conflicting cultural values, i.e., the American values of competition and assertive vs. the need to be dependent.
   7. Future shock: physiological and psychological stress resulting from an overload of the organism's adaptive systems and decision-making processes brought about by too rapidly changing values and technology.
   8. Cultural shock: stress developing in response to transition of the individual from a familiar environment to an unfamiliar one.
     a. Involves unfamiliarity with communication, technology, customs, attitudes, and beliefs.
     b. Examples: individual moving to new area from foreign country or individual placed in hospital environment.

DANGER SIGNALS OF STRESS*

- Depression, lack of interest in life
- Uncontrolled hyperactive behavior
- Lack of concentration, inability to focus
- Feelings of unreality
- Loss of control, emotional instability
- Pervasive high anxiety level
- Physical manifestations
  Irregular heartbeats
  Tremors, tics
  Gastrointestinal disturbance
  Skin disturbance
  Changes in respiratory patterns
- Insomnia
- Disease
- Increased dependence on alcohol, drugs

*Adapted from Smith, S. F., Duell, D. J. & Martin, B. C. (2004). *Clinical Nursing Skills* (6th ed.). Prentice Hall Health: Upper Saddle River, N.J.

Assessment

✦ A. Assess increased anxiety, anger, helplessness, hopelessness, guilt, shame, disgust, fear, frustration, or depression.
✦ B. Evaluate behaviors resulting from stress.
   1. Apathy, regression, withdrawal.
   2. Crying, demanding.
   3. Physical illness.
   4. Hostility, manipulation.
   5. Senseless violence, acting out.

✦ Implementation

A. Gather information about patient's internal and external environment.
B. Modify external environment so that adaptation responses are within the capacity of patient.
C. Support the efforts of patient to adapt or respond.
D. Provide patient with the materials required to maintain constancy of internal environment.
E. Understand body's mechanisms for accommodating stress.
F. Prevent additional stress.
G. Reduce external stimuli.
H. Reduce or increase physical activity depending on the cause of and response to stress.

GROWTH AND DEVELOPMENT MILESTONES

Birth to Preadolescence

See Pediatric Developmental Chart (Table 3-1) and Erikson's Eight Stages of Personality Development (Table 3-2).

Table 3-1. PEDIATRIC DEVELOPMENTAL CHART

Gross Motor Development	Fine Motor Development	Language Development
1 Month Lifts head slightly from prone Lies awake on back	Follows with eyes to midline Keeps fists clenched Does not grasp objects	Responds to voice Makes throaty noises
2–3 Months Lifts head and chest 45 degrees when prone Turns side to back Rotates head Moves arms vigorously	Grasp becomes voluntary Brings objects to mouth Briefly holds toys	Vocalizes responsively Single vowel sounds Babbles and coos Introduce new sounds
4–5 Months Lifts head and shoulders 90 degrees Moves side to side—tries to roll over Pulls self to sitting position	Follows object 180 degrees Sucks thumb Grasps toy with hand Begins teething Begins hand–eye coordination	Laughs aloud Coos, gurgles Responds to "no"
5–6 Months Sits for short periods alone Rocks and creeps Turns completely over, abdomen to back Weighs twice birth weight	Holds block in each hand Reaches for objects beyond grasp Looks toward objects and sounds Begins hand–eye coordination	Vocalizes vowel sounds Recognizes name Expresses protest
6–12 Months Sits without support (7–8 months) Pulls self to feet Creeps and cruises Stands and walks holding on to objects	Picks up objects fairly well Uses index finger and thumb to grasp Holds own bottle or cup; feeds self Transfers objects hand to hand Follows rapid movements (vision is 20/200)	Speaks one or two words ("Mama," "Dada") Understands several words and commands
12–18 Months Stands and walks alone Climbs stairs with help Throws a ball Weight triples at 12 months Anterior fontanel closes	Fine muscle coordination begins to develop Explores environment Holds a spoon; holds cup with both hands Can release objects at will Does not attempt to change from left to right hand Vision conversion occurs	Uses jargon Understands simple commands Is aware of expressive function of language Has a vocabulary of 10–20 words Makes animal sounds
18 Months–2 Years Walks up and down stairs Climbs on furniture Walks and runs with a stiff gait Kicks a ball in front of self Daytime bladder and bowel control	Uses a spoon without spilling Builds tower of six cubes Fingerpaints Eye accommodation well developed Vision 20/40	Speaks vowels correctly Receptive vocabulary of 300–500 words Begins to use short sentences 100–200 word vocabulary Follows simple directions
2–3 Years Balances on one foot Goes up and down stairs, alternating feet Rides tricycle Swings, climbs, jumps	Copies horizontal and vertical strokes Feeds self; uses fork Pours from pitcher Begins to use scissors Vision is 20/30	Refers to self by pronoun "I" Asks questions about everything Uses "I", "me," "you" speech Has vocabulary of 900 words Can remember and repeat three numbers

Social Development	Play	Toys
1 Month		
May smile	Smile and talk to infant	Music—sing to infant
Alert one out of ten hours	Use touch and cuddle infant	Colorful mobiles
2–3 Months		
Begins social smile	Infant seat	Bright pictures
Differentiates by crying	Bounce infant on bed—let kick	Rattles
Provide social stimulation	Play during feeding	Soft, large animals
4–5 Months		
Knows mother	Increase sensory stimulation	Play music
Demands attention	Give many baths	Soft, colorful toys
Imitates mother		Mirrors, rattles
5–6 Months		
Smiles at familiar people	Holds toys and rattles	Soft, colorful squeeze toys
Shows anticipation	Plays sitting-up games	Toys that don't have removable parts
Begins to recognize strangers	Begins social games (pat-a-cake)	Teething toys
Shows fear and anger		Metal cup and wooden spoon for banging
6–12 Months		
Shows emotions: looks hurt, sad	Protect child from dangerous objects	New objects (blocks)
Is aware of environment: when unfamiliar, may be fearful	Loves to look at pictures	Toys that stimulate senses
Imitates gestures, facial expressions	Allow exploration outdoors	Containers
Entertains self		Bath toys
		Allow security toy
12–18 Months		
Indicates wants	Begins self-directed play rather than adult-directed	Pull and push toys
Likes an audience and will repeat performance	Requires safe environment (medications locked up and harmful items out of reach)	Balls; teddy bears
Shows anxiety about strangers		Pots and pans
Distinguishes self from others	Plays alone but near others (parallel play)	Musical toys
Finds security in a blanket, favorite toy, or thumb sucking	Can identify and play with geometric forms	Telephone
Show affection and encourage child to reciprocate		Sand box and fill toys
		Books and pictures
18 Months–2 Years		
Has fear of parents leaving	Begins peer relationships—needs peers for play	Building blocks
Helps to undress; tries to button	Role-modeling for positive behavior is important	Wagons
Wants to hoard, not share	Self-directed play increases	Pull toys
Begins to have feelings of autonomy		Pounding toys, like a drum
Begins cooperation in toilet training		Books with pictures
2–3 Years		
Knows full name	Pushes and pulls large toys	Manipulative toys for muscle coordination
Displays negativism, temper tantrums	Able to entertain self for short periods	Crayons and paper
Is ritualistic	Engages in associative play	Simple games
Shows poorly developed judgment	Begins imaginative and make-believe play	Climbing apparatus
Wants to please		Tricycle
Begins to share		Record player
Uses toilet by self		

(Continues)

Table 3-1. PEDIATRIC DEVELOPMENTAL CHART (Continued)

Gross Motor Development	Fine Motor Development	Language Development
4–6 Years		
Races up and down steps	Draws man with two to four parts	Asks abundant questions: What? Why? How?
Has good balance	Can button easily	Recites nursery rhymes
Skips, hops, performs stunts	Feeds self	Gives full name
Is agile and graceful	Brushes teeth	Has well-developed vocabulary
Begins to ride two-wheel bicycle	Exhibits small, well-controlled motor movements	Repeats sentence of 10 syllables or more
Runs skillfully	Uses hands as manipulative tools in cutting, pasting, hammering	Talks constantly
Can catch a ball	Begins reading readiness	Defines words by use
Exhibits growth spurt	Vision now 20/20	Learns to read
Is very active, impulsive		Knows number combinations to 10
6–8 Years		
Exhibits better coordination and control	Dresses self	Learns to read
Graceful body movements	Is capable of fine hand movements	Begins to tell time
Speed in movements	Writing improves	Vocabulary increases
Growth spurt	Eyes become fully developed	Defines words by use
		Begins cursive writing
8–10 Years		
Arms grow long in proportion to body	Learns to use script	Increased capacity for logical thought
Good timing and coordination of fine muscles	Demonstrates skill in manual activities because hand–eye coordination is developed	Vocabulary increases
Very active physically		Increased ability to discuss issues
Gains speed and strength	Cares completely for own physical needs	Grasps easy multiplication and division
		Understands money

Preadolescence

A. Physical and motor development.
 1. Begins puberty; physical changes appear in both males and females.
 2. Begins menstruation (females).
 3. May require more sleep due to body changes.
B. Social development.
 1. Participates in community and school affairs.
 2. Tends toward segregation of the sexes.
 3. Likes to be alone occasionally.
 4. Exhibits interest in world affairs.
 5. Comprehends world of possibility and abstraction.
 6. Begins to question parental values.
C. Appropriate games and stimulation.
 1. Provide help in school and sports to channel energy in proper direction.
 2. Provide guidance during dependence/independence conflict.
 3. Set realistic limits.
 4. Give adequate explanation of body changes.
 5. Provide special consideration for child who lags behind in physical development.

Early Adolescence

A. Physical development.
 1. Exhibits further development of secondary sex characteristics.
 2. Shows poor posture.
 3. Exhibits rapid growth and becomes awkward and uncoordinated.
 4. Shows changes in body size and development.
B. Social development.
 1. Needs social approval of peer group.
 2. Strives for independence from family.
 3. Has one or two very close friends in peer group.
 4. Becomes more interested in opposite sex.
 5. Period of upheaval: displays confusion about body image.
 6. Must again learn to control strong feelings (love, aggression).
C. Counseling guidelines.
 1. Provide adult understanding when adolescent deals with social, intellectual, and moral issues.
 2. Allow some financial independence.

Social Development	Play	Toys
4–6 Years		
Shows interest in world about him	Alternate periods of active and quiet play	Books
Sees self as all-important	Explores environment	Puzzles
Begins to share; seeks peer relationships	Enjoys group play in small groups	Drawing
Is less negativistic	Encourage pretending, expressing self and imagination	Utensils
Does simple chores at home	Needs guidance and limits	Puppets
Still requires parental support	Provide exercise to stimulate motor and psychosocial development	Games
Begins to accept authority outside home		Bicycle
6–8 Years		
Is more independent and competitive	Very active	Table games and card games
School is important	Group play is preferred	Magic tricks
Wishes to be like his friends; seeks out clubs and teams	Competitive games	Games that develop physical and mental skill
May have periods of shyness		
8–10 Years		
More self-assured in environment	Likes group projects, clubs	Games of skill
Increased modesty	Through play, learns new concepts: independence, competition, compromise, and cooperation	Competitive games
"Chum" stage occurs; has special friend in whom child confides		Team sports
Needs to be considered important by adults		Books
Questions regarding sex require simple, honest answers		Musical instruments
Lying and stealing may be problem		TV, records
		Organized clubs

3. Provide limits to ensure security.
4. Provide necessary assurance to help adolescent accept changing body image.
5. Show flexibility in adjusting to emotional and erratic mood swings.
6. Be calm and consistent when dealing with an adolescent.

◆ D. Developmental tasks.
  1. Finds identity; moves out of role diffusion.
     a. Integrates childhood identifications with basic drives.
     b. Expands concept of social roles.
  2. Moves toward heterosexuality.
  3. Begins separation from family.
  4. Integrates personality.

Adolescence to Young Adulthood

A. Physical development.
  1. Completes sexual development.
  2. Exhibits signs of slowing down of body growth.
  3. Is capable of reproduction.
  4. Shows more energy after growth spurt tapers off.
  5. Exhibits increased muscular ability and coordination.
  6. Menarche—onset of menstruation—usually occurs between the ages of 11 and 14.

B. Social development.
  1. Less attached to peers.
  2. Shows increased maturity.
  3. Exhibits more interdependence with family members.
  4. Begins romantic love affairs.
  5. Increases mastery over biologic drives.
  6. Develops more mature relationship with parents.
  7. Values fidelity, friendship, cooperation.
  8. Begins vocational development.

C. Counseling guidelines.
  1. Assist adolescent in vocational choice.
  2. Provide safety education, especially regarding driving.
  3. Encourage good attitudes toward health in issues of nutrition, drugs, smoking, and drinking.
  4. Attempt to understand own (parental) difficulties in accepting transition of adolescent to independence and adulthood.

Table 3-2.	**ERIKSON'S EIGHT STAGES OF PERSONALITY DEVELOPMENT**			
Stage	**Approx. Age**	**Psychological Crises**	**Significant Persons**	**Accomplishments**
Infant	0–1 year	Basic trust vs. mistrust	Mother or maternal figure	Tolerates frustration in small doses Recognizes mother as separate from others and self
Toddler	1–3 years	Autonomy vs. shame and doubt	Parents	Begins verbal skills Begins acceptance of reality vs. pleasure principle
Preschool	3–6 years	Initiative vs. guilt	Basic family	Asks many questions Explores own body and environment Differentiates between sexes
School	6–12 years	Industry vs. inferiority	Neighborhood school	Gains attention by accomplishments Explores things Learns to relate to own sex
Puberty and adolescence	12–20 years	Identity vs. role diffusion	Peer groups External groups	Moves toward heterosexuality Begins separation from family Integrates personality (altruism, etc.)
Young adult	18–25 years	Intimacy and solidarity vs. isolation	Partners in friendship, sexual partners	Is able to form lasting relationships with others, committed to work
Adulthood	25–65 years	Generativity vs. stagnation	Partners in friendship, sexual partners	Creative, productive life, caring for others
Late adulthood, elderly	65–death	Ego integrity vs. despair	Partners in friendship, sexual partners	Acceptance of worth and value of one's life

Based on Erikson: *Childhood and Society*

✦ D. Developmental tasks.
　　1. Intimacy and solidarity versus isolation.
　　　　a. Moves from security of self involvement to insecurity of building intimate relationships with others.
　　　　b. Becomes less dependent and more self-sufficient.
　　2. Able to form lasting relationships with others.
　　3. Learns to be productive and creative.
　　4. Handles hormonal changes of developmental period.

Adulthood

Developmental Tasks

✦ A. Achieves goal of generativity versus stagnation or self-absorption.
　　1. Shows concern for establishing and guiding next generation.
　　2. Exhibits productiveness, creativity, and an attitude of looking forward to the future.
　　3. Stagnation results from the refusal to assume power and responsibility of the goals of middle age.
　　　　a. Suffers pervading sense of boredom and impoverishment.
　　　　b. Undergoes but does not resolve midlife crisis.

B. Has relaxed sense of competitiveness.
C. Opens up new interests.
D. Shifts values from physical attractiveness and strength to intellectual abilities.
E. Shows productivity (may be most productive years of one's life).
F. Has more varied and satisfying relationships.
G. Exhibits no significant decline in learning abilities or sexual interests.
H. Shifts sexual interests from physical performance to the individual's total sexuality and need to be loved and touched.
I. Assists next generation to become happy, responsible adults.
J. Achieves mature social and civic responsibility.
K. Accepts and adjusts to physiological changes of middle life.
L. Uses leisure time satisfactorily.
M. Failure to complete developmental tasks may cause the individual to approach old age with resentment and fear.
　　1. Neurotic symptoms may appear.
　　2. Increased psychosomatic disorders may develop.

Values of Adulthood

A. Adult becomes more introspective.
B. Shows less concern as to what others think.
C. Identifies self as successful even though all life goals may not be achieved.

D. Shows less concern for outward manifestations of success.

E. Lives more day-to-day and values life more deeply.

F. Has faced one's finiteness and eventual death.

Parenting in Adulthood

A. Characteristics.
1. Tendency toward smaller families.
2. Career-oriented women who limit family size or who do not want children.
3. Early sexual experimentation, necessitating sexual education, contraceptive information.
4. Tendency toward postponement of children.
   a. To complete education.
   b. Economic factors.
5. High divorce rates.
6. Alternate family designs.
   a. Single parenthood.
   b. Communal family.
B. Family planning.
1. General concepts.
   a. Dealing with individuals with particular ideas regarding contraception.
   b. No perfect method of birth control.
   c. Method must be suited to individual.
   ✦ d. Individuals involved must be thoroughly counseled on all available methods and how they work—including advantages and disadvantages. This includes not only female but also sexual partner (if available).
   e. Once a method is chosen both parties should be thoroughly instructed in its use.
   f. Individuals involved must be motivated to succeed.
2. Effectiveness depends upon:
   a. Method chosen.
   b. Degree to which couple follows prescribed regimen.
   c. Thorough understanding of method.
   d. Motivation on part of individuals concerned.
   See Contraceptive Methods in Chapter 14.

Physiological Changes

Menopause
A. Characteristics.
1. The cessation of menstruation caused by physiologic factors; ovulation no longer occurs.
2. Menopause usually occurs between the ages of 45 and 55.
✦ B. Mechanisms in menopause.
1. Ovaries lose the ability to respond to pituitary stimulation and normal ovarian function ceases.

2. Gradual change due to alteration in hormone production.
   a. Failure to ovulate.
   b. Monthly flow becomes smaller, irregular, and gradually ceases.
3. Menopause is accompanied by changes in reproductive organs—the vagina gradually becomes smaller; uterus, bladder, rectum, and supporting structures lose tone, leading to uterine prolapse, rectocele, and cystocele.
4. Atherosclerosis and osteoporosis are more likely to develop at this time; estrogen replacement decreases rate of bone loss.

Assessment
A. Assess presence of symptoms—varies with individuals and may be mild to severe.
B. Assess feelings of loss as children grow and leave home and aging process continues.
✦ C. Assess presence of physiological symptoms.
1. Hot flashes.
2. Headache.
3. Depression.
4. Insomnia.
5. Weakness.
6. Dizziness.

Implementation
A. Refer patient to physician who can discuss hormonal replacement therapy (HRT) which is now (as a result of the latest studies) considered controversial.
1. Estrogen given on cyclic basis: 1 pill daily except for 5 days during the month when medication is not taken.
2. Progesterone given 10–12 days per month.
B. Various herbs can replace HRT. *See* herbal chart in Pharmacology chapter.

Psychosocial Changes

Midlife Crisis
✦ A. A normal stage in the ongoing life cycle in which the middle-aged person reevaluates his or her total life situation in relation to youthful achievements and actual accomplishments.
1. Struggles to maintain physical attractiveness in relation to younger people.
2. Partner or lover critical to self-definition.
3. Feels he or she has peaked in ability.
4. Blames environment or others for failure to succeed.
5. Displays increased interest in sexuality.
6. Exhibits competitiveness in career plans.
B. Unresolved crisis.
1. May result in stagnation, boredom, and decreased self-esteem and depression.

**MAJOR CAUSES OF
PSYCHOLOGICAL PROBLEMS**

- Fears losing job
- Competition with younger generation
- Loss of job
- Loss of nurturing functions
- Loss of spouse, particularly females
- Realization that person is not going to accomplish some of the things that he or she wanted to do
- Changes in body image
- Illness
- Role change within and outside of family
- Fear of approaching old age
- Physiological changes

---

2. Age for crisis varies.
  a. Women pass through it between 35 and 40 years old.
  b. Men experience the crisis between 40 and 45 years old.

The Aged

Developmental Tasks

✦ A. Maintains ego integrity versus despair.
  1. Integrity results when an individual is satisfied with his or her own actions and lifestyle, feels life is meaningful, remains optimistic, and continues to grow.
  2. Despair results from the feeling that he or she has failed and that it is too late to change.
B. Continues a meaningful life after retirement.
C. Adjusts to income level.
D. Makes satisfactory living arrangements with spouse.
E. Adjusts to loss of spouse. (Forty-five percent of women over 65 are widowed.)
F. Maintains social contact and responsibilities.
G. Faces death realistically.
H. Provides knowledge and wisdom to assist those at other developmental levels to grow and learn.
I. Societal concerns.
  1. In the year 2000, there are approximately 40 million people over the age of 65 in the United States.
  2. More than 5 percent of the aged are currently institutionalized.

Physiological, Psychological, and Socioeconomic Implications

A. Physical changes.
  1. Decrease in physical strength and endurance.
  2. Decrease in muscular coordination.
  3. Tendency to gain weight.
  4. Loss of pigment in hair and skin.
  5. Increased brittleness of the bones.
  6. Greater sensitivity to temperature changes with low tolerance to cold.
  7. Degenerative changes in the cardiovascular system.
  8. Diminution of sensory faculties.
  9. Lowered immune system—decreased resistance to infection, disease, and accidents.
✦ B. Major health problems.
  1. All systems are more vulnerable due to the aging process.
    a. Heart disease (over 250,000 die each year from this condition).
    b. Chronic diseases: diabetes, hypertension, cancer.
    c. Malnutrition; dehydration.
    d. Sensory impairment: blindness and deafness.
    e. Organic brain changes; loss of memory; Parkinson's disease.
    f. Impaired mobility; accidents.
    g. Circulatory impairment.
    h. Osteoporosis.
    i. GI and GU impairment.
  2. Impact of disease on aged.
    a. Diseases may be multiple and chronic (over 40 percent have more than one illness concurrently).
    b. Disability results more readily when an aging person becomes ill.
    c. Response to treatment is diminished.
    d. Resistance is lower due to the aging process so person is more susceptible to disease.
    e. The aged have less resistance to stressors: mental, environmental, and physical.
    f. Changes in the neurological system make the aged person more prone to organic brain changes.
    g. Many elderly take numerous medications and are susceptible to drug reactions and side effects.
C. Developmental process retrogresses.
  1. Increasing dependency.
  2. Concerns focus increasingly on self.
  3. Interests may narrow.
  4. Needs tangible evidence of affection.
D. Major fears of the aged.
  1. Physical and economic dependency.
  2. Chronic illness.
  3. Loneliness.
  4. Boredom resulting from not being needed.
E. Major problems of the aged.
  1. Economic deprivation.
    a. Increased cost of living on a fixed income.
    b. Increased need for costly medical care.
  2. Chronic disease and disability.
  3. Social isolation.

4. Blindness.
5. Organic brain changes.
   a. Not all persons become senile.
   b. Most people have memory impairment.
   c. The change is gradual.
6. Nutritional deprivation.
F. The elderly may provide knowledge and wisdom from their vast experiences, which can assist those at other developmental levels to grow and learn.

DEATH, DYING, AND THE GRIEF PROCESS

The Grief Process

Definition: A process that an individual goes through in response to the loss of a significant or loved person. The grieving process follows certain predictable phases—classic description originally done by Dr. Eric Lindeman. The normal grieving process is described by George Engle, M.D., in "Grief and Grieving," *American Journal of Nursing,* September 1964.

✦ A. First response is *shock and refusal to believe* that the loved one is dead.
1. Displays inability to comprehend the meaning of loss.
2. Attempts to protect self against painful feelings.

✦ B. As *awareness* increases, the bereaved experiences severe anguish.
1. Crying is common in this stage.
2. Anger directed toward those people or circumstances thought to be responsible.

✦ C. *Mourning* is the next stage where the work of *restitution* takes place.
1. Rituals of the funeral help the bereaved accept reality.
2. Support from friends and spiritual guidance comfort the bereaved.

✦ D. *Resolution of the loss* occurs as the mourner begins to deal with the void.

✦ E. *Idealization* of the deceased occurs next where only the pleasant memories are remembered.
1. Characterized by the mourner's taking on certain qualities of the deceased.
2. This process takes many months as preoccupation with the deceased diminishes.

✦ F. Outcome of the grief process takes a year or more.
1. Indications of successful outcome are when the mourner remembers both the pleasant and unpleasant memories.
2. Eventual outcome influenced by:
   a. Importance of the deceased in the life of mourner.
   b. The degree of dependence in the relationship.
   c. The amount of ambivalence toward the deceased.
   d. The more hostile the feelings that exist, the more guilt that interferes with the grieving process.
   e. Age of both mourner and deceased.
   f. Death of a child is more difficult to resolve than that of an aged loved one.
   ✦ g. Number and nature of previous grief experiences—loss is cumulative.
   h. Degree of preparation for the loss.

Counseling Guidelines

✦ A. Recognize that grief is a syndrome with somatic and psychological symptomatology.
1. Weeping, complaints of fatigue, digestive disturbance, and insomnia.
2. Guilt, anger, and irritability.
3. Restless, but unable to initiate meaningful activity.
4. Depression and agitation.
B. Be prepared to support the family as they learn of the death.
1. Know the general response to death by recognizing the stages of the grief process.
2. Understand that the behavior of the mourner may be unstable and disturbed.
✦ C. Use therapeutic communication techniques.
1. Encourage the mourner to express feelings, especially tears.
2. Attempt to meet the needs of the mourner for privacy, information, and support.
3. Show respect for the religious and social customs of the family.

Death and Dying

Impact of Dying Process for Adults

A. Physical symptoms of dying.
1. Cardiovascular collapse.
2. Renal failure.
3. Decreased physical and mental capacity.
4. Gradual loss of consciousness.
✦ B. Stages of dying.
1. The dying process is ably portrayed in *Death and Dying,* by Elisabeth Kübler-Ross, New York, Macmillan Publishing Company, Inc., 1970.
2. *Denial*—individual is stunned at the knowledge he or she is dying and denies it.
3. *Anger* and resentment usually follow as the individual questions, "Why me?"
4. With the beginning of acceptance of impending death comes the *bargaining* stage, that is, bargaining for time to complete some situation in his or her life.

5. Full acknowledgment usually brings *depression;* individual begins to work through feelings and to withdraw from life and relationships.

6. Final stage is full *acceptance* and preparation for death.

7. Throughout the dying process, hope is an important element that should be supported but not reinforced unrealistically.

C. Psychosocial clinical manifestations—behaviors and reactions the nurse may expect to observe in patients who are going through the dying process.

1. Depression and withdrawal.
2. Fear and anxiety.
3. Focus is internal.
4. Agitation and restlessness.

The Concept of Death in the Aging Population

A. In American culture, death is very distasteful.

B. The elderly may see death as an end to suffering and loneliness.

C. Death is not feared if the person has lived a long and fulfilled life, having completed all developmental tasks.

D. Religious beliefs and/or philosophy of life important.

Death and Children

A. Understanding of death for the young child.

✦ 1. Death is viewed as a temporary separation from parents, sometimes viewed synonymously with sleep.

2. Child may express fear of pain and wish to avoid it.

3. Child's awareness is lessened by physical symptoms if death occurs suddenly.

4. Gradual terminal illness may simulate the adult process: depression, withdrawal, fearfulness, and anxiety.

B. Older children's concerns.

1. Death is identified as a "person" to be avoided.

2. Child may ask directly if he or she is going to die.

3. Concerns center around fear of pain, fear of being left alone, and fear of leaving parents and friends.

C. Adolescent concerns.

1. Death is recognized as irreversible and inevitable.

2. Adolescent often avoids talking about impending death, and staff may enter into this "conspiracy of silence."

3. Adolescents have more understanding of death than adults tend to realize.

✦ Nursing Management for Dying Patient

A. Nursing management of the adult.

1. Evaluate pain as the 5th vital sign.
   a. Alleviate patient's pain according to orders —be the patient's advocate for pain relief.
   b. Explore all options (drugs and alternative therapy) for achieving pain relief.

2. Minimize physical discomfort.
   a. Attend to all physical needs.
   b. Make patient as comfortable as possible.

3. Recognize crisis situation.
   a. Observe for changes in patient's condition.
   b. Support patient.

4. Be prepared to give the dying patient the emotional support needed.

5. Encourage communication.
   a. Allow patient to express feelings, to talk, or to cry.
   b. Pick up cues that patient wants to talk, especially about fears.
   c. Be available to form a relationship with patient.
   d. Communicate honestly.

6. Prepare and support the family for their impending loss.

7. Understand the grieving process of patient and family.

B. Nursing management for the dying child.

1. Always elicit the child's understanding of death before discussing it.

2. Before discussing death with child, discuss it with parents.

3. Parental reactions include the continuum of grief process and stages of dying.
   a. Reactions depend on previous experience with loss.
   b. Reactions also depend on relationship with the child and circumstances of illness or injury.
   c. Reactions depend on degree of guilt felt by parents.

4. Assist parents in expressing their fears, concerns, and grief so that they may be more supportive to the child.

5. Assist parents in understanding siblings' possible reactions to a terminally ill child.
   a. Guilt: belief that they caused the problem or illness.
   b. Jealousy: demand for equal attention from the parents.
   c. Anger: feelings of being left behind.

The Hospice Option

A. Hospice care provides treatment, comfort, and support for the terminally ill patient, as well as relief and solace for the family.

B. Hospice neither speeds up nor slows down the dying process—provides a specialized environment where a dying patient may receive medical care in addition to emotional and spiritual support during the dying process.
   1. One of the real advantages of hospice is that the personnel are trained to treat pain aggressively.
   2. The patient should be as pain free as possible, while at the same time remaining as alert as possible.
C. Hospice care includes an interdisciplinary team: a Registered Nurse, a social worker, a home health aide, a chaplain, and trained volunteers.
D. Hospice is reimbursed by Medicare in all states and by Medicaid in 42 states.
E. There are several barriers to hospice care.
   1. The patient's physician must certify that the life expectancy of the patient is six months or less.
   2. Some insurance carriers require patients to waive their rights to medical benefits if they are receiving hospice care.
   3. The largest obstacle may be a problem with communication---between physician and patient, patient and family, and family and patient.
   4. When the finality of dying cannot be discussed, hospice care may not present itself as an option.

HUMAN SEXUALITY

Overview

✦ A. Biological sexuality is determined at conception.
   1. Male sperm contributes an X or a Y chromosome.
   2. Female ovum has an X chromosome.
   3. Fertilization results in either an XX (female) or an XY (male).
B. Preparation for adult sexuality originates in the sexual role development of the child.
   1. Significant differences between male and female infants are observable even at birth.
   2. Biological changes are minimal during childhood, but parenting strongly influences a child's behavior and sexual role development.
   3. Anatomical and physiological changes occur during adolescence which establish biological sexual maturation.
C. Human sexuality pervades the whole of an individual's life.
   1. More than a sum of isolated physical acts.
   2. Functions as a purposeful influence in human nature and behavior.
   3. Observable in everyday life in endless variations.
D. Each society develops a set of normative behaviors, attitudes, and values in respect to sexuality which are considered "right" and "wrong" by individuals.
E. Freud described the bisexual (androgynous) nature of the person.
   1. Each person has components of maleness–femaleness, masculinity–femininity, and heterosexuality–homosexuality.
   2. These components are physiological and psychological in nature.
   3. All components influence an individual's sexuality and sexual behavior.
F. Gender identity (identified at birth) refers to whether a person is male or female.
   1. Cases of "ambiguous genitalia" are rare (1:3000 births), and require special care for the infant and parents.
   2. Ambiguous genitalia is a clinical label similar to slang term *morphodite*, or biological term *hermaphrodite*.
G. Sexual object choice is the selection of a mode of outlet for sexual desire, usually with another person.
   1. Generally occurs during adolescence and beyond.
   2. Includes heterosexuality, homosexuality, bisexuality, celibacy, and narcissism/onanism.
H. Sexual object choice has strong influence on person's lifestyle.
   1. Individual must establish patterns of intimacy and sexual behavior that are acceptable to self, to significant others, and to society to a certain extent.
   2. Psychological demands and expectations throughout life influence an individual's sexual interest, activity, and functional capacity.
   3. Sexual object choice can affect a person's choices in life such as whether to be a parent, where to live, and what career to maintain.

Sexual Behavior

✦ A. Sexual behavior is a composite of developed patterns of intimacy, psychological demands and expectations, and sexual object choice.
   1. Can be genital (sexual intercourse), intimate (holding, hugging), or social (dating, choice of clothing).
   2. Beyond the obvious examples, one never stops "behaving sexually."
   3. Dress, communication, and activity are all expressions of sexuality.
   4. Every person exhibits sexual behavior continually; no one is sexless.

B. *Transvestite* and *transsexual* are two terms that often cause confusion and need definition and differentiation.
  1. Transvestite refers to one who enjoys wearing clothing of the opposite sex; may or may not be homosexual.
  2. Transsexual is a person who chooses sexual reassignment: a complex physical (surgical), psychological, and social process of taking on the gender identity, sex role, sexual object choice, and sexual behavior of the opposite sex.

C. Sexuality, although difficult to define, is pervasive from birth to death, and nurses need to look beyond the framework of reproduction and procreation to understand the influence of sexuality on patients' health and illness.

D. Characteristics.
  1. Difficult to define precisely, human sexuality is considered to be a pervasive life force and includes a person's total feelings, attitudes, and behavior.
  2. It is related to gender identity, sex-role identity, and sexual motivation.
  3. Touching, intimacy, and companionship are factors that have unique meaning for each person's sexuality.
  4. Sex role describes whether a person assumes masculine or feminine behaviors, usually a combination of both.
    a. This role generally considered to be fairly established by age five.
    b. Usually referred to by the concepts boy/girl and man/woman.

Nursing Care Related to Sexual Behavior

✦ A. Assist in providing sex education and counseling.
  1. Patients consider nurses to be experts in sexuality.
  2. Intervention requires knowledge and skill.
  3. Nurses need to know referral sources for interventions beyond their ability.

B. Give patients "permission" or acceptance to maintain sexuality and sexual behavior.

✦ C. Be aware of the effect of medications on patients' sexuality and sexual functioning.
  1. Oral contraceptives are considered by some to have played a major role in creating a sense of sexual freedom in contemporary society.
  2. Drugs that decrease sexual drive or potency may act directly on the physiological mechanisms or may decrease interest through a depressant effect on the central nervous system.
  3. Drugs with an adverse effect on sexual activity include antihypertensive drugs, antidepressants, antihistamines, antispasmodics,

sedatives and tranquilizers, ethyl alcohol, and some hormone preparations and steroids.
  4. Viagra—oral drug therapy (25–100 mg) for erectile dysfunction.
    a. Rapidly absorbed—30–120 minutes, with resulting ability to achieve an erection sufficient for sexual intercourse.
    b. Appropriate for healthy young and elderly males.
    c. Precautions: any male who is at cardiac risk.
  5. Long-term use of any drug or medicine will likely have a negative effect on sexual interest and capability.

D. Be aware of the problems to which nursing personnel should direct themselves in relation to the area of human sexuality.
  ✦ 1. Attitudes.
    a. Nurses should increase their self-awareness of their own attitudes and the effect of these attitudes on the sexual health care of their patients.
    b. Nurses should suppress negative biases and prejudices and/or make appropriate referrals when they cannot give effective or therapeutic sexual health care.
  2. Knowledge.
    a. May have to be actively sought although nursing programs are increasing the sexuality content in their curricula.
    b. Also available through books, journal articles, classes and workshops, and preparation for sexuality therapy on the graduate level.
  3. Skills.
    a. Primary skills needed are interpersonal techniques such as therapeutic communication, interviewing, and teaching.
    b. As with any skill, practice is needed for proficiency in sexual-history taking, education, and counseling.

Sexual Behaviors Related to Health

✦ A. Masturbation.
  1. A common sexual outlet for many people.
  2. For patients requiring long-term care, masturbation may be only means for gratifying sexual needs.
  3. Nurses frequently react negatively to any type of masturbatory activity, especially by male patients.
  4. Patients should be allowed privacy; if nurse walks in on a patient masturbating, he or she should leave with an apology for having intruded on the patient's privacy.
  5. Frequent or inappropriate masturbation may be harmful to the patient's health. Limits

need to be set to protect patient and other patients if behavior is inappropriate.

◆ B. Gender identity issues—homosexuality.

1. Homosexuality is accepted by many as a viable lifestyle.

2. Nurses may have negative attitudes and incorrect knowledge about homosexuality.

◆ 3. A patient's homosexual (gay) lifestyle should be respected. These patients must be treated in an unbiased way without passing judgment on their lifestyle choices.

4. As with any patient, visitors should be encouraged as appropriate for the health/illness status, and these people should not be embarrassed or ridiculed.

5. For chronically ill patients, such as in a nursing home, it is essential that sexuality needs be considered in the total care plan and special efforts be made to have these needs met.

C. Inappropriate sexual behavior.

1. Difficult to precisely define "inappropriate" sexual behavior.

2. Sometimes sexual behavior is in reaction to unintentional "seductive" behavior of the nurses.

◆ 3. Nursing interventions.

   a. Set limits to unacceptable behavior immediately.

   b. Interact without rejecting patient.

   c. Help patient express feelings in an appropriate manner.

   d. Teach alternative behaviors that are acceptable.

   e. Provide acceptable outlets to sexual feelings.

◆ D. Rape.

1. Rape is an act of violence and is only secondarily a sex act.

2. Treatment should consist of both medical and psychological intervention.

3. Sexual assault can have a long-term impact on the victim.

4. Victims may need encouragement and support to report rape occurrences to authorities.

5. Female nurses especially can play a valuable role in giving assistance and support to female rape victims.

6. Many communities have "hot-lines" that offer telephone information and crisis counseling to victims of sexual assault and to professionals.

◆ E. Child sexual abuse.

1. There is only a beginning awareness of this problem area.

2. Most child sexual abuse involves a male adult and female child, but male children can also be victims of female or male sexual abusers.

3. The child may need special protection or temporary placement outside the home, but often the family unit can be maintained.

4. Child sexual abuse or molestation is a form of child abuse, and nurses should know local regulations and procedures for case finding and reporting.

◆ 5. Nursing interventions.

   a. Establish a safe environment for the child.

   b. Allow and encourage child to verbalize or communicate in his or her own way (through drawings or play acting).

   c. Observe for appearance of symptoms over time (withdrawal, depression, phobias).

   d. Encourage ongoing therapy to work through trauma.

◆ F. Sexuality and disability.

1. Physically and developmentally disabled persons are sexual beings also.

2. Developmentally disabled persons should be given sexuality education and counseling in preparation for responsible sexual expression and behavior.

3. After spinal cord injury, the level of the lesion and degree of interruption of nerve impulses influence sexual functioning; adaptation of previous sexual practices may be needed after the injury.

4. Fertility and the ability to bear children are usually not compromised in women with spinal cord injury.

5. Nurses working with disabled patients must make special efforts to include sexuality in total health care and services.

6. Nursing interventions.

   a. Discuss sexual needs openly with patient so he or she will not feel embarrassed to ask questions.

   b. Discuss previous sexual activity and how current needs can be met.

   c. Nurse must maintain a nonjudgmental attitude or relationship will be jeopardized.

   d. Support patient and partner during sexual adjustment period.

   e. Refer to therapy support groups for ongoing support.

G. Contraception.

1. Nurses are considered experts on forms of birth control.

2. Nurses should be familiar with different methods and relative effectiveness of each one.

◆ 3. Patients should be assisted to make their own choices as to whether to use contraception and what method is best for them.

4. More detailed outline of contraception appears in maternity chapter.

H. Therapeutic abortion.
   1. Patients need information about resources for and procedures of therapeutic abortions.
   2. Patients should be given nonjudgmental assistance and support in decision-making process.
   ◆ 3. If nurse cannot in good conscience assist the patient because of conflicting religious or spiritual beliefs, referral should be made to someone who can.
   4. More detailed outline of abortion appears in Chapter 14.

SEXUALLY TRANSMITTED DISEASES (STDs)

Chlamydia

Definition: Caused by *Chlamydia trachomatis;* produces infections in both men and women (fallopian tubes, cervix, urethra) and can develop into PID.

Characteristics

◆ A. Most common sexually transmitted disease (STD) in the United States.
B. 5 million people contract this disease each year.
C. High-risk women: young, nonwhites with multiple sex partners and women not using barrier contraceptives.
D. Chlamydia is not a reportable disease in 50 percent of states.
◆ E. Statistics.
   1. 20 percent of men and 40–50 percent of women with gonorrhea also are infected with chlamydia.
   2. 25–50 percent of pelvic inflammatory diseases (PID) are caused by chlamydia.
   3. 155,000 infants born to mothers with chlamydia are at risk for pneumonia and ophthalmia neonatorium.
   4. Each year 1 billion dollars spent on infection.
F. Chlamydiae are bacteria microorganisms, but have characteristics of both viruses and bacteria.
G. Sensitive to antibiotics (azithromycin or doxycycline).
H. Spread through sexual contact. Incubation period 5–10 days or longer (28 days); gonorrhea is only 2–10 days.
I. Tests for chlamydia include Chlamydiazyme—enzyme immunoassay test and Microtak—direct fluorescent antibody test and amplified DNA assay (BD Probe tec).

Assessment

A. Observe for a discharge—vaginal or urethral.
B. Assess for burning.
C. Check for lower abdominal pain or testicular pain.
D. Assess for bleeding or pain with coitus.
E. Assess for rectal pain or discharge.
F. 33 percent of women report no symptoms.

Implementation

◆ A. Administer antibiotics as ordered.
   1. Doxycycline 100 mg 2x/day for 7 days for non-pregnant women.
      a. Take on an empty stomach.
      b. May cause sensitivity to the sun.
      c. Avoid becoming pregnant.
   2. Erythromycin (base) 500 mg 4x/day for 7 days as second choice (take with meals)—for pregnant women.
   3. Penicillin does not cure chlamydia.
B. Educate men and women about transmission, symptoms, and prevention.
   1. Frequent examinations if people are not monogamous.
   2. If symptoms/signs occur, seek help immediately—teach importance of taking medication as prescribed.
   3. Suggest sexually active people use barrier methods of contraception.
   4. Avoidance of sex until completion of treatment.
C. Provide accurate information about disease, health care, and prevention.

Syphilis

◆ *Definition:* A chronic infectious disease caused by *Treponema pallidum.*

Characteristics

A. Transmission is by intimate physical contact with syphilitic lesions, which are usually found on the skin or the mucous membranes of the mouth and the genitals.
◆ B. Incubation period is 10–90 days following exposure.
◆ C. Primary stage (nonreactive VDRL).
   1. Most infectious stage.
   2. Appearance of chancres, ulcerative lesions.
   3. Usually painless, produced by spirochetes at the point of entry into the body.
◆ D. Secondary stage (reactive VDRL).
   1. Lesions appear about 3 weeks after the primary stage and may occur anywhere on the skin and the mucous membranes.
   2. Highly infectious.
   3. Generalized lymphadenopathy.
◆ E. Tertiary stage.
   1. The spirochetes enter the internal organs and cause permanent damage.
   2. Symptoms may occur 10–30 years following the occurrence of an untreated primary lesion.

3. Invasion of the central nervous system.
   a. Meningitis.
   b. Locomotor ataxia: foot slapping and broad-based gait.
   c. General paresis.
   d. Progressive mental deterioration leading to psychosis.
4. Cardiovascular: most common site of damage is at the aortic valve and the aorta itself.
F. Characteristics relating to pregnancy.
   1. May cause abortion or premature labor.
   2. Infection is passed to the fetus after the fourth month of pregnancy as congenital syphilis.

Assessment
A. Evaluate serum test (STS) for syphilis on first prenatal visit.
B. May repeat just before fourth month, as disease may be acquired after initial visit.

✦ Implementation
A. Educate women to recognize signs of syphilis.
B. Educate women to seek immediate treatment if known exposure occurs.
C. Educate women as to the need for simultaneous treatment of partner as reinfection may occur.
D. Monitor treatment: during pregnancy, 2.4 million units of procaine penicillin G with 2% aluminum monostearate, IM normally in divided doses.
E. Report all cases of syphilis to health authorities for treatment of contacts.

Gonorrhea

✦ *Definition:* An infection caused by *Neisseria gonorrhoeae*, which causes inflammation of the mucous membrane of the genitourinary tract.

Characteristics
A. Transmission is almost completely by sexual intercourse.
B. Incidence is of epidemic proportions in the United States.
✦ C. Signs and symptoms.
   1. Male.
      a. Painful urination.
      b. Pelvic pain and fever.
      c. Epididymitis with pain, tenderness, and swelling.
      d. Mucoid or mucopurulent discharge.
   2. Female (usually asymptomatic).
      a. Vaginal discharge—greenish-yellow.
      b. Urinary frequency and pain.
D. Complications.
   ✦ 1. Female: pelvic inflammatory disease (PID) with abdominal pain, fever, nausea, and vomiting.

2. Male: postgonococcal urethritis and spread of infection to posterior urethra, prostate, and seminal vesicles.
3. PID can lead to sterility.
4. A secondary infection can develop in any organ.
E. Infection may be transmitted to baby's eyes during delivery, causing blindness.

Assessment
A. Obtain culture for gonorrhea (usually done on first prenatal visit).
B. Repeat later as infection may occur during pregnancy.

Implementation
A. Educate women to recognize signs of gonorrhea and to seek immediate treatment.
B. Administer prophylactic medication of a broad-spectrum antibiotic or 1% silver nitrate (not commonly used) to newborn.
C. Monitor treatment: same as for syphilis. Other antibiotics may be used for sensitivity to penicillin.
D. Important to treat sexual partner, as patient may become reinfected.

Herpes Simplex Virus (HSV)

Definition: Herpes infection is caused by the herpes simplex virus (HSV). Forty-five million people in the United States have been diagnosed.

Characteristics
✦ A. HSV type 1 and 2 both present risk to infant.
B. Type 2 most common as genital herpes.
   1. Involves external genitalia, vagina, and cervix.
   2. Development and draining of painful vesicles.
✦ C. Virus may be lethal to fetus if inoculated during vaginal delivery. (Fifty percent of HSV-infected infants die.) Delivery usually by C-section.
D. Safe use of acyclovir has not been established for pregnant women.

Assessment
A. Evaluate for presence of painful, draining vesicles on external genitals, vagina, and cervix.
B. Check for increased temperature and vital signs.

Implementation
A. Educate patient as to dangers to fetus.
B. Encourage patient to report symptoms.
✦ C. Explain to patient about the possibility of a cesarean section should an outbreak occur around the time of delivery. Policy regarding time limit of outbreak in relation to time of delivery varies, but usual policy is an outbreak within 2 weeks.
D. Maintain precautions during vaginal examinations of patient.

E. Maintain isolation precautions during hospitalization if disease is active.
F. Postpartum.
    1. Encourage careful handwashing by patient.
    2. Avoid direct contact with lesions.
    3. Breast-feeding is not contraindicated unless lesions are on breast.

Venereal Warts

✦ *Definition:* A sexually transmitted infection caused by the human papillomavirus (HPV).

Characteristics

✦ A. Almost 1 million Americans develop this condition—major STD of 1990s.
B. The virus affects cervix, urethra, penis, scrotum, and anus.
C. Warts appear 1 or 2 months after exposure, transmitted through intimate sexual contact.

Assessment

✦ A. Assess for small to large wartlike growths on genitals (no symptoms other than lesions).
B. Assess for cervical cell changes—HPV associated with up to 90 percent of cervical malignancies.

Implementation

✦ A. There is no cure for HPV—treatment is cryotherapy, liquid nitrogen, or electrocautery to remove lesions.
B. Key is prevention—similar to any other STD: limit sexual contacts and use condoms.
C. Suggest Pap test every year (cancer risk).

Human Immunodeficiency Virus (HIV)

Definition: A retrovirus that may develop into acquired immunodeficiency syndrome (AIDS). Contracted through exchange of body fluids, it has a long latency period before progressing to AIDS.

✦ Characteristics

A. History of belonging to high-risk group (drug user, prostitution).
B. Pregnancy associated with slight reduction of helper T cells—may increase possibility of opportunistic infections.
C. HIV transmitted to 30 percent of exposed infants—risk increases with low T cell count.

Assessment

A. Assess if HIV infection (mononucleosis-like symptoms) or ARC (pre-AIDS condition).
B. Check for severely compromised immune system (indicates presence of AIDS).
C. Take careful history of risk behaviors.
D. Assess signs and symptoms of STDs and CMV.

Implementation

A. Complete post-test counseling if positive HIV/AIDS results are present.
B. Counsel importance of continued medical care during pregnancy.
C. Maintain body fluid precautions for cell contact with client and teach client precautions.
D. *See* Newborn with AIDS, page 458.

NURSING THROUGH THE LIFE CYCLE QUESTIONS

1. When a person is experiencing severe stress, the nurse would assess for behaviors such as

   1. Restlessness and anxiety.
   2. Crying and upset demeanor.
   3. Laughing and amusement.
   4. Assertiveness and determination.

2. According to Selye's stress theory, when the individual is in the alarm phase of the general adaptive syndrome, the body first responds by

   1. Going into shock and countershock.
   2. Resisting the stressor.
   3. Adapting to the stressor.
   4. Moving to a state of exhaustion.

3. Erik Erikson's theory of personality explains that a child who was never allowed to function autonomously may, in later life, experience the psychological crisis of

   1. Mistrust.
   2. Inferiority.
   3. Guilt.
   4. Shame and doubt.

4. During a routine physical examination, the following reflexes are noted in a 9-month-old child. Which of the following is an abnormal finding and would require further intervention?

   1. Parachute reflex.
   2. Neck righting reflex.
   3. Rooting and sucking reflex.
   4. Moro reflex.

5. The mother of a 1-month-old male infant brings him to a clinic for his well-baby check-up. She asks the nurse when to start solid foods and what to feed him. The *most appropriate* response is to tell her to begin solid food at the age of

   1. 2 months with wheat cereal.
   2. 5 to 6 months with rice cereal.
   3. 4 to 6 months with fruits and vegetables.
   4. 2 to 3 months with bananas and applesauce.

6. A new mother of a 1-month-old infant is concerned because the baby sleeps so much of the day. The best explanation is to tell the mother that infants

   1. Sleep all day and stay awake most of the night until they develop a regular routine.
   2. Should have only one nap during the day.
   3. Need at least 12 hours of sleep during every 24 hours.
   4. Usually sleep about 20 of every 24 hours.

7. When a child is at the toddler stage, what is the most important information to give the mother?

   1. Safety hazards, such as poisons and medicine, must not be within the child's reach.
   2. It is important to help the child master the autonomy stage of development.
   3. It is dangerous for the child to eat dirt.
   4. Beware there is a possibility that the child may show jealousy toward other children.

8. An 8-month-old male child is tentatively diagnosed as being mentally retarded. The parents have come to the hospital for further assessment and counseling. During the nurse's assessment, the observation that will help assess for mental retardation is that the child is unable to

   1. Sit unsupported for brief periods.
   2. Crawl short distances.
   3. Demonstrate a negative Babinski.
   4. Grasp a spoon and bring it to his mouth.

9. Which of the following would be appropriate toys for a 3-month-old infant?

   1. Soft, colorful squeeze toys and teething toys.
   2. Teething toys with small, removable parts.
   3. Push and pull toys and pounding toys.
   4. Balls and toys that stimulate the senses.

10. When caring for a 5-month-old child in the hospital, the *best* toy or object for stimulation would be a

    1. Hanging mobile.
    2. Teddy bear.
    3. Toy that makes noise.
    4. Fabric picture book.

11. At which of the following ages would the nurse first expect a child to sit with no support?

    1. 4 months.
    2. 5 months.
    3. 8 months.
    4. 9 months.

12. The patient is age 4 and while in the hospital, he becomes very bored. The *best* activity to implement for this patient is

    1. Radio and TV.
    2. Puppets.
    3. Books and comics.
    4. Airplane models.

13. A 12 year old can accomplish formal operational thought, according to Paiget. The nurse understands that this statement means that a young person is able to

    1. Ask direct questions.
    2. Use symbols.
    3. Think in concepts.
    4. Understand cause and effect.

14. A teenager has just been told she has herpes simplex 2. When discussing the test results with her, she says, "That's not possible. I've only slept with my boyfriend." The *best* response would be

    1. "Well, then, he has probably slept with someone else who infected him."
    2. "It's all right to tell me the truth. Our conversation is confidential."
    3. "Can you tell me what you know about herpes?"
    4. "How you got it doesn't really matter. What's important is that we treat it now."

15. One of the primary developmental tasks of adolescence is

    1. Feeling independent.
    2. Finding one's identity.
    3. Experiencing intimacy.
    4. Achieving generativity.

16. A patient has just received a diagnosis of breast cancer from her physician. When the nurse asks if she would like to talk about the diagnosis, the patient replies "Oh, no, it's no big deal." The nurse recognizes that this may be a grief response, which probably means that the patient is

    1. Not ready to accept the diagnosis.
    2. In the denial stage of the grief process.
    3. Not comfortable in discussing the diagnosis with the nurse.
    4. Mourning the loss she will have to experience.

17. A nurse who is sensitive to his or her patient's need to talk about dying would recognize which of the following cues as the "need to talk"?

    1. The patient's refusal to talk to anyone.
    2. Constant crying and looking depressed.
    3. The patient's asking the nurse to stay a while.
    4. Constantly asking to be released to go home.

18. The ultimate outcome, when the grieving process is successfully completed, will be when the bereaved

    1. Is able to think of the deceased without emotion.
    2. Remembers only the pleasures of the relationship.
    3. Is no longer emotionally dependent on the deceased.
    4. No longer feels the need to talk about the deceased.

19. A nurse enters the private room of a male patient and realizes he is masturbating. The appropriate response is to

    1. Set limits on his behavior in the hospital.
    2. Apologize for intruding on the patient's privacy.
    3. Tell the patient his behavior is inappropriate.
    4. Ignore the behavior and continue with the intervention planned when entering the room.

20. In the area of human sexuality, nurses may encounter problems in relating to their patients. A major barrier or problem the nurse should be aware of is

    1. Lack of knowledge in human sexuality.
    2. The nurse's personal attitudes toward human sexuality.
    3. Lack of appropriate referrals in this area.
    4. Lack of proficiency in sexual history taking.

NURSING THROUGH THE LIFE CYCLE

Answers with Rationale

1. (2) Crying and being upset is typical behavior experienced when a person is under stress. Restlessness and anxiety (1) might be present, but they are not typical responses. Laughing and humor (3) relieve stress. Assertiveness and determination (4) are not responses to stress.

   NP:D; CN:H; CA:PS; CL:C

2. (1) The first stage is alarm—shock and countershock. The body translates the shock as sudden injury and then is restored to preinjury state (countershock). Resistance (2) is the second stage, and exhaustion (4) is the third stage, according to stress theory.

   NP:P; CN:H; CA:PS; CL:K

3. (4) Erikson's theory explains that at every age the individual has to go through a psychological crisis period of development. In this case, if the toddler is allowed to gain autonomy, he or she will not experience shame and doubt in later life. If the infant develops trust in the maternal figure, he will not mistrust; if the school-age child is industrious, he will not feel inferior later; and, if the preschooler is allowed to show initiative, in later life he or she will not experience guilt.

   NP:P; CN:PS; CA:PS; CL:C

4. (4) The Moro reflex begins to fade at the third or fourth month. Thus, if found in a 9 month old, it would be abnormal. The remaining reflexes would be normal development.

   NP:D; CN:H; CA:P; CL:A

5. (2) Waiting 5 to 6 months to start solid food allows the baby's GI tract to mature. Infants are least allergic to rice cereal, so it is preferable to start feedings with this food.

   NP:I; CN:H; CA:P; CL:A

6. (4) Young infants sleep about 20 hours a day. They are usually awake to eat, gurgle a little, and then go back to sleep. Napping during the day and sleeping only 12 hours a day occurs much later.

   NP:I; CN:H; CA:P; CL:A

7. (1) When there is a choice, safety is always considered first. In this question, safety hazards such as poisons, drugs, or detergents are important to place out of reach or in locked cupboards so they cannot be found by a curious toddler. A toddler is in the stage of autonomy versus shame and doubt according to Erikson (2), but this is not a safety issue. Eating dirt (3) may indicate a nutritional deficiency, but it is not as critical as ensuring home safety.

   NP:P; CN:H; CA:P; CL:A

8. (1) At 6 months of age, a child should be sitting with minimal support. Often, retarded children have flaccid muscles and loose joints, which prevent the attainment of simple developmental milestones. The ability to sit is one of the most important milestones.

   NP:D; CN:PS; CA:P; CL:AN

9. (1) Toys should be visually appealing without small parts that could choke an infant. Exploration through the mouth begins at 3 months. Push and pull toys (3) and balls (4) are appropriate for the mobile, older baby.

   NP:P; CN:H; CA:P; CL:A

10. (1) A mobile is appropriate for a 5 month old, because it provides visual stimulation. A teddy bear (2) is not as interesting or comforting to a 5 month old as it might be to an older child. A toy that makes noise (3) is more appropriate for ages 7 to 9 months, and it requires more motor development than a 5 month old possesses. A 5 month old does

---

Coding for Questions/Answers Abbreviations: **Nursing Process: NP,** Data Collection: D, Planning: P, Implementation: I, Evaluation: E, **Client Needs: CN,** Safe, Effective Care Environment: S, Health Promotion and Maintenance: H, Psychosocial Integrity: PS, Physiological Integrity: PH, **Clinical Area: CA,** Medical Nursing: M, Surgical Nursing: S, Maternal/Newborn Nursing: MA, Pediatric Nursing: P, Psychiatric Nursing: PS, **Cognitive Level: CL,** Knowledge: K, Comprehension: C, Application: A, Analysis: AN

not have the fine motor development required for holding a book (4).

NP:P; CN:H; CA:P; CL:C

11. (3)   Infants begin to sit with support or leaning forward on both hands at 6 months. They sit with minimal or no support between 7 and 8 months. If this milestone does not occur, the infant should be assessed for retardation.

NP:D; CN:H; CA:P; CL:C

12. (2)   Fantasy is very active in this stage of development. Puppets would allow for expression of feelings. Also, this activity is more active than TV (1) or books (3) and involves the nurse with the child, which is a positive way of establishing a relationship.

NP:I; CN:H; CA:P; CL:A

13. (3)   At 12 years plus, a young person is able to think in concepts or conceptualize and do abstract thinking. Before this age, the young person is only able to think concretely. Using symbols (2) and understanding cause/effect (4) occurs at 7 to 12 years. Answer (1) occurs from 4 to 7 years. This is important theoretical information for the nurse to have when the child is in the hospital, because it will give cues as to how much the child or young adult will understand the diagnosis or instructions.

NP:D; CN:H; CA:P; CL:C

14. (3)   This is a good opportunity for patient teaching, and the first thing the nurse must do is assess the patient's level of knowledge.

NP:D; CN:H; CA:M; CL:A

15. (2)   Early adolescence has the primary task of finding one's identity and moving out of role diffusion. Later adolescence to young adulthood's task is to experience intimacy (3), not isolation. Adults should achieve generativity (4) versus stagnation.

NP:D; CN:H; CA:MA; CL:C

16. (2)   The first stage of grief is often denial, along with shock. The patient may also not be ready to accept the diagnosis (1) or wish to discuss it with the nurse (3), but these are not included in the stages of grieving. Mourning (4) is a later stage of the grief process.

NP:D; CN:H; CA:PS; CL:AN

17. (3)   Asking the nurse to stay a while may be a cue that the patient is ready to talk about the difficult subject. The other behaviors do not indicate a willingness to talk.

NP:P; CN:PS; CA:PS; CL:AN

18. (3)   When the grieving process is completed, the bereaved will no longer feel emotionally dependent on the person who died. They will always feel emotion (1) when thinking of the loved one, but they will be able to realistically recall both the good and bad times. There will always be the need to talk about the loved one (4), even when the grief has been resolved.

NP:E; CN:PS; CA:PS; CL:A

19. (2)   The appropriate response is to apologize, leave the room, and return later. Patient's should be allowed privacy, and this is a common sexual outlet for many people. When the behavior is inappropriate, limits should be set (1). The patient's behavior is not necessarily inappropriate for him (3). Continuing with the nurse's intended intervention (4) is also inappropriate because it intrudes on the patient's privacy.

NP:I; CN:H; CA:PS; CL:AN

20. (2)   Negative attitudes, biases, prejudices, or judgments on the part of the nurse can present a major problem for nurses working in the area of sexual health. If these attitudes are negative, the relationship will be compromised. Lack of knowledge (1), referrals (3), or proficiency (4) may all present problems, but do not affect relating to the patient.

NP:P; CN:H; CA:PS; CL:A

General Nursing Concepts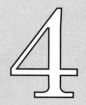

FUNDAMENTAL CONCEPTS

Environment of the Patient

Safety and Comfort
A. Adequate space.
B. Privacy.
C. Comfortable room temperature.
   1. 66°–76°F is normal.
   2. Warmer temperature for very young, old, sedentary, or ill patients.
D. Room humidity 30–60 percent.
E. Adequate lighting.
   1. Natural light if available; avoid glare.
   2. Use of night lights especially with elderly, very young, very ill.
F. Adequate ventilation.
G. Comfortable sound levels.
H. Pleasing, easy-to-clean decor/furniture.
✦ I. Protection from hazards.
   1. Use of handrails, side rails.
   2. Items placed within reach at the bedside.
J. Identification bands/bracelets.
K. Functional call system within patient's reach.

Assessment

Purpose of Assessment
A. Determine person's current health status.
✦ B. Provide baseline for nursing diagnosis and care planning.
   1. First step in the nursing process.
   2. Initial assessment is not the duty of LVN/LPN, but importance of assessment should be understood.
   3. LVN/LPN is responsible for ongoing patient assessments.

Assessment Procedure
A. Collect data by reading chart/care plan.
B. Interview to obtain subjective information/symptoms.
✦ C. Collect cardinal or vital signs.
   1. Temperature: normal range 97°–99.5°F or 36°–37.5°C. Rectal is 1°F higher; ear canal 0.5°F higher.
      a. Electronic—inappropriate for use with infants, after oral surgery, or with patients who are unconscious or receiving oxygen by mask.
      b. Rectal—inappropriate for use with patients who have a rectal disorder or following rectal surgery.
      c. Tympanic or ear canal—used for patients over 3 months old. Takes only 3 seconds to record an accurate temperature and may be used when patient is unconscious.

✦ 2. Pulse: 60–100 beats per minute.
   a. Usually palpated over radial artery.
   b. Apical—used with babies and irregular heart rates.
   c. Pulse deficit—apical rate minus radial rate.
   d. Peripheral—determines the adequacy of perfusion from absent to full and bounding. If peripheral pulse cannot be palpated, a Doppler ultrasound stethoscope is used.
✦ 3. Blood pressure—arterial.
   a. Systolic—the pressure in vessel when heart is contracting. Normal to high normal range is 100–140 mm Hg.
   b. Diastolic—the pressure in vessel when heart is at rest. Normal range is 60–85 mm Hg.
   c. Pulse pressure—the difference between systolic and diastolic.
   d. Blood pressure readings now recorded according to Korotkoff's sounds.
      (1) "K" phase I: first, faint tapping sounds.
      (2) "K" phase II: time during cuff deflation when murmur sounds are heard.
      (3) "K" phase III: sounds are crisper and increase in intensity.
      (4) "K" phase IV: time when distinct muffling of sound is heard.
      (5) "K" phase V: when the last sound is heard.
   e. American Heart Association recommends use of the bell of the stethoscope for blood pressure (Korotkoff's) auscultation.
✦ 4. Respirations: 12–18 breaths per minute.
   a. Quality of respirations is important baseline data.
   b. Breathing pattern, rate and depth.
D. Measure weight and height.
E. Perform a detailed assessment.
   ✦ 1. May be done from the patient's head to toes.
   2. May be done on a system basis.
   3. May be used to determine patient's strengths and weaknesses. (See specific chapters for outlines.)
   4. Phases.
      a. Inspection—overview of patient.
      b. Auscultation—use of stethoscope to listen to heart.
      c. Palpation—use of entire surface of all five fingers.
      d. Percussion—use of middle finger for "tapping."
F. Use data to plan patient care or report the care plan to responsible nurse/team leader for validation, interpretation, or use in planning care.

G. Assist RN to formulate nursing diagnoses.

H. Follow steps of the Nursing Process.

Recording/Charting

✦ **Purpose of Written Records**

A. Method of precise communication between staff members.

B. Legal documentation.

C. Provides for continuity of care and documents progress.

D. Research, statistics, and education.

Types of Charting

A. Computer-assisted—constantly updates information from many sources.

B. Source-oriented.

1. Most common.

2. Organized by sources of information.

3. Types of forms.

a. Order sheets.

b. X-ray reports.

c. Graphs—vital signs.

d. Flow sheets—intake and output.

e. Narrative nurses' notes.

(1) Objective, not interpretive.

(2) Brief and concise.

(3) Use of approved symbols and abbreviations.

(4) Accurate spelling.

(5) Prepared legibly in ink.

(6) Signed with name and status.

C. Problem-oriented—chart is based on a problem list—all the problems, present or potential, associated with the patient.

D. Focus charting—uses the term focus instead of problem.

1. *Subjective:* patient's symptoms and own description of problem (becomes nursing *focus*).

2. *Objective:* factual data, e.g., intake and output, vital signs, drainage, etc.

3. *Assessment:* your conclusions about the problem (nursing *focus*).

4. *Plan:* what you decide to do about the problem.

5. *Implementation:* your nursing interventions.

6. *Evaluation:* how the implementation worked.

7. *Revision:* how you plan to change the PCP if improvement is needed.

Nursing Diagnosis

✦ A. A statement of an actual health problem or a potential one.

1. Derived from the assessment phase of the nursing process.

2. Based on both objective and subjective data.

3. As data base is collected, deviations from normal health patterns are identified.

MASLOW'S HIERARCHY OF NEEDS THEORY

A. Abraham Maslow identified a hierarchy of human needs—the most basic must be met before the next levels can be fulfilled.

B. The most basic needs are bodily drives—hunger, thirst, and physical needs for shelter, sleep, exercise, etc.

C. More general needs follow (also necessary for life) and become the focus after essential physical needs.

1. Feeling safe in the world.

2. Sense of belonging and love.

3. Failure to meet these needs negates fulfillment of even higher needs (respect, self-esteem and self-actualization).

D. Nursing implications: use Maslow hierarchy of needs when you are answering a priority question that involves issues of physiological needs versus needs such as recognitions, belonging, loving. Basic physical needs (such as hunger, pain) must be met first.

✦ B. Specific problem identified is related to a nursing intervention—not a medical one.

C. Major components.

1. Possible risk factors.

2. Possible precipitating factors.

3. Defining characteristics, objective and subjective.

4. Assessment for data base (physical findings, health history, etc.).

5. Formulate nursing diagnosis.

Patient Care Plans

✦ A. The two accepted types are: individualized care plan and standard care plan.

1. Individualized care plans have mutually agreed-upon goals set by the patient, family, and health team members.

2. Specific directions are written to define how these goals can be achieved.

3. The usual care plan format contains patient needs or problems, goals or expected outcomes, a health team action section, with deadline dates, and discharge criteria.

4. Standard care plans provide a guide for patient care.

a. Identify problem relating to all patients having a specific medical condition.

b. Health team actions include routine preventive nursing interventions.

B. The information contained in the care plan must be specific.

C. Care plans become a permanent part of the patient's chart.

1. They must be written in ink.

2. Resolved problems should be crossed out using a colored felt tip pen.

D. Care plans must be updated on a routine basis (generally every 24–48 hours or as the patient's condition changes).

E. Documentation is an essential component of the nurse's role. Importance is based on:
1. Evaluation of planned patient care.
2. Communication to other health care professionals.
3. Patient safety regulations.
4. Reimbursement from the federal government.
5. Legal implications.
6. Joint Commission on Accreditation of Health-Care Organizations (JCAHO).

The Nurse–Patient Relationship

Definition: The nurse–patient relationship is a therapeutic, professional relationship in which interaction occurs between two individuals—the vocational nurse, who possesses the skills, abilities, and resources to relieve another's discomfort; and the patient, who is seeking assistance for alleviation of some existing problem.

Characteristics

A. Create an environment in which the patient has the feeling of being accepted.
1. Accept the patient as having value and worth as an individual.
2. Empathize (feel with the patient) but do not sympathize or use platitudes.
3. Offer emotional involvement but maintain objectivity.
4. Protect and promote patient's self-esteem.

✦ B. Indicate desire to develop mutual trust.
1. Exhibit verbal and nonverbal behavior that is consistent and congruent.
2. Encourage reality orientation.
3. Interact at patient's level of understanding.
4. Understand your own motives and needs.
5. Provide open and honest communication.
6. Communicate with the patient using therapeutic communication techniques.

✦ C. Provide a reality-oriented supportive environment.
1. Focus on the total patient so as to include all physical needs.
2. Set appropriate behavioral limits.
3. Assist patient to identify and cope with feelings.
4. Encourage expression of feelings within a safe limit.
5. Recognize signs of a high anxiety level and seek appropriate help.

✦ Phases of the Relationship

A. Initiating phase.
1. Identify problems.
2. Get to know each other.
3. Test each other's attitudes.
4. Identify expectations.
5. Plan for the conclusion at the beginning of the relationship.

B. Continuing phase.
1. Accept each other.
2. Use specific therapeutic problem-solving techniques.
3. Work actively on problems.
4. Assess and evaluate problem continually.
5. Encourage patient to become more independent and to rely less on the nurse.

C. Terminating phase.
1. Evaluate the initial plan for conclusion.
2. Anticipate problems of termination.
   a. Excessive dependence of patient on nurse, who must encourage independence.
   b. Patient may have feelings of abandonment, rejection, and/or depression about termination.
   c. Discuss patient's feelings about termination.

Communication Techniques

Definition: Communication is the process of sending and receiving messages by means of symbols, words, signs, gestures, or other actions. It is a multilevel process consisting of the content or information of the message, as well as the part that defines the meaning of the message. Messages sent and received define the relationship between individuals.

Characteristics

A. An individual cannot *not* communicate.
B. Communication is a basic human need.
C. It is both verbal and nonverbal expression (also tone, pace, and manner of dress).
D. Effective communication includes:
1. Feedback.
2. Appropriateness.
3. Efficiency.
4. Flexibility.
E. Communication skills are learned as the individual grows and develops.
F. The foundation of the individual's perception of self and the world is based on communicated messages received from significant others.
G. Factors that affect communication.
1. Intrapersonal framework of the individual.
2. Relationship between the participants.
3. Purpose of the sender.
4. Content.
5. Context.
6. Manner in which the message is sent.
7. Effect on the receiver.

Table 4-1. EFFECTIVE COMMUNICATION TECHNIQUES

Listen	→	The act of consciously receiving another person's message. Listen eagerly, actively, responsively, and seriously.
Acknowledge	→	Recognize the person without inserting your own values or judgments. Acknowledgment may be simple and with or without understanding. *Example:* In the response "I hear what you're saying," the person acknowledges a statement without agreeing with it. Acknowledgment may be verbal or nonverbal.
Give feedback	→	The process of the receiver relaying to the sender the effect the message has had. Helps keep the sender on course or alter his course. Involves acknowledging, validating, clarifying, extending, and altering. *Nurse to patient:* "You did that well."
Be congruent (mutual fit)	→	Verbal and nonverbal messages coincide. *Example:* A patient is crying, and the nurse says, "I want to help," and places her hand on the patient's shoulder.
Clarify	→	Checking out or making clear either the intent or hidden meaning of message or determining if the message sent was the message received. *Nurse:* "Are you saying you feel angry now?"
Focus or refocus	→	Pick up on central topic or cue given by the patient. *Nurse:* "You were telling me how hard it was to talk to your mother."
Validate	→	The process of verifying the accuracy of the sender's message by paraphrasing thought. *Nurse:* "Yes, it is confusing with so many people around."
Reflect	→	Echo last few words. This encourages patient to elaborate thought. *Patient:* "I hear voices." *Nurse:* "You hear voices."
Ask open-ended questions	→	Ask questions that cannot be answered "Yes" or "No" or "Maybe" and generally require an answer of several words in order to broaden conversational opportunities and help the patient to communicate. *Nurse:* "What kind of job would you like to do?"
Encourage nonverbally	→	Use body language to indicate interest, understanding, support, caring, and/or listening to extract further information. *Nurse:* Nodding appropriately as patient talks.
Restate	→	Restating what the patient said encourages further communication. *Nurse:* "You said you hate the idea of going home?"
Paraphrase	→	Summarizing or rewording. This enables sender to hear message meaning in another form. *Nurse:* "You mean you're unhappy."
Respond neutrally	→	Show interest and involvement without indicating assent or dissent. *Nurse:* "Yes . . . ." "Uh hmm . . . ."
Use incomplete sentences	→	Encourage the patient to continue. *Nurse:* "Then your life is . . ."
Minimize verbalization	→	Keep your own verbalization at a minimum, and let the patient continue the conversation. *Nurse:* "You feel . . . ?"
Initiate broad statements	→	Open the communication by allowing the patient freedom to talk and focus on himself. *Nurse:* "How have you been feeling?"
Confront with kindness	→	Point out discrepancies in behavior or negative results of behavior. "You say you have no self-confidence, yet you take over every meeting."

✦ **Interviewing Skills**

A. Help the patient feel comfortable so that there is no need to be defensive.

B. Use "I" messages, not "you" messages (e.g., "I feel angry," not "you make me angry").

C. Observe carefully and be alert to cues given by the patient.

D. Participate in planning a goal- and direction-oriented approach.

✦ **Implementation**

A. Encourage the patient to verbalize his or her thoughts and feelings.

B. Assist the patient to clarify or make clear what he or she is saying.

C. Focus on the patient, not on yourself or others.

D. Help the patient understand how he or she affects others.

E. Communicate at the patient's level of understanding.

F. Use "how" questions rather than "why" questions.

G. Focus on the present "here and now" rather than on the past "there and then."

H. Help the patient learn new ways of problem solving.

I. Give constructive feedback so that the patient can self-correct unclear statements.

J. Use nonverbal communication to convey empathy, interest, and encouragement.

K. Send verbal messages that are congruent with your nonverbal messages.

L. Be honest in your answers or statements; say what you mean and mean what you say.

M. Use effective communication techniques (see Table 4-1).

N. Recognize blocks to effective communication (see Table 4-2).

O. Make a sustained effort to give and receive a message.

Table 4-2. BLOCKS TO EFFECTIVE COMMUNICATION	
Make assumptions	→ (Jumping to conclusions.) Suppose or guess meaning of patient's behavior when not validated. The nurse finds the suicidal patient smiling and joking, and tells the staff he's in a cheerful mood.
Give advice	→ Tell the patient what to do, give an opinion, or make a decision that implies patient cannot cope with own self-determination. *Nurse:* "If I were you . . . ."
Change the subject	→ Introduce new topics inappropriately, a pattern that may indicate anxiety. The patient is crying and discussing her fear of surgery when the nurse asks, "How many children do you have?"
Use social response	→ Focus attention on receiver of message rather than sender. *Patient:* "I feel better when the sun is out." *Nurse:* "This sunshine is good for my roses. I have a beautiful rose garden."
Invalidate patient	→ Ignore or deny another's presence, thoughts, or feelings. *Patient:* "Hi, how are you?" *Nurse:* "I can't talk now. I'm on my way to lunch."
Use false reassurance	→ Use cliches, pat answers, cheery words, advice, and comforting statements as an attempt to reassure the patient. Most of what is called "reassurance" is really false reassurance. *Nurse:* "It's going to be all right."
Overload conversation	→ Speak rapidly, change subjects, and give receiver more information than can be absorbed at one time. *Nurse:* "What's your name? I see you are 48 years old and that you like sports. Where do you come from?"
Underload conversation	→ Remain silent and unresponsive, fail to pick up cues, and fail to give feedback. *Patient:* "What's your name?" *Nurse:* Smiles and walks away.
Use incongruent messages	→ Send verbal and nonverbal messages that contradict one another; two or more messages, sent via different levels, seriously do contradict one another. The contradiction may be verbal, nonverbal, and/or content (time, space). This contradiction is a double message. *Patient:* "I like your dress." *Nurse:* Frowns, looks annoyed and disgusted.
Make value judgments	→ Give one's own opinion, moralize or imply one's own values by using words such as "nice," "good," "bad," "right," "wrong," "should," and "ought." *Nurse:* "I think you should leave your husband."

PAIN MANAGEMENT

Characteristics

A. Pain is now considered the 5th vital sign—pain must be assessed regularly (JCAHO) to maintain patient's quality of life.

✦ B. The experience of pain.
1. Pain source—direct causative factor.
2. Stimulation of pain receptor—mechanical, chemical, thermal, electrical, ischemic.
3. Pain pathway.
   a. Sensory pathways through dorsal root, ending on second order neuron in posterior horn.
   b. Afferent fibers cross over to anterolateral pathway, ascend in lateral spinothalamic tract to thalamus.
   c. Fibers then travel to postcentral gyrus in parietal lobe.

Theories of Pain

A. Specificity theory—certain pain receptors are stimulated by a type of sensory stimuli that sends impulses to the brain.
B. Pattern theory—pain originates in spinal cord and results in receptor stimulation coded in CNS and signifies pain.
C. Gate control theory.

1. Pain impulses can be modulated by a transmission blocking action within CNS.
2. Large diameter cutaneous pain fibers can be stimulated (rubbing, scratching) and may inhibit smaller diameter excitatory fibers and prevent transmission of that impulse.
3. Cerebral cortical mechanism that influence perception and interpretation may also inhibit transmission.

D. Endorphins—the brain produces natural brain opioids that fit (lock) into special receptors. Antilocks, called antagonists, keep endorphins from working.

Types of Pain

A. Acute—localized, shorter duration, sharp sensation. Occurs over defined period—6 months or less.
B. Chronic pain—long duration, diffuse, dull aching quality; associated autonomic responses, musculoskeletal tension, nausea. Occurs over 6 month period.
C. Malignant—recurrent, acute episodes; also includes chronic varying in intensity—lasts longer than six months.
D. Psychogenic—due to emotional factors without anatomic or physiological explanation.
E. Pain perception—thalamus/awareness and parietal/integration.

F. Pain interpretation—cerebral cortex; delayed response influenced by previous experiences, culture, existing physical/psychological state.

G. Reactions—psychic and/or physiologic.

Assessment

A. Assess presence of pain.
1. Select a tool based on patient's preferences and cognitive abilities.
2. Examples of Pain Scales—verbal descriptor, numeric rating, FACES®, and pain thermometer.
3. Ask patient to indicate intensity of pain on a scale of zero to ten, zero being no pain and ten being the most pain ever experienced.
4. Use this scale to assess relief of pain after intervention.

✦ B. Assess type of pain.
1. Acute pain: short duration of a few seconds to 6 months.
2. Chronic pain: longer duration of 6 months to years.
3. Intractable pain: severe and constant and resistant to relief measures.

✦ C. Assess location.
1. Ask patient to identify area of the body affected.
2. Superficial or deep.
3. Diffuse or localized.
4. Radiates and where it goes.

✦ D. Assess quality.
1. Stabbing, knifelike.
2. Throbbing.
3. Cramping.
4. Viselike, suffocating.
5. Searing, burning.
6. Other.

E. Assess onset and precipitating factors.
1. How movement affects pain.
2. If coughing affects pain.
3. Impact of emotion on pain, e.g., arguing with spouse or receiving disturbing news.

F. Assess aggravating factors.
1. How position affects pain.
2. Environmental stressors.
3. Fatigue.

G. Assess associated factors.
1. Nausea.
2. Vomiting.
3. Bradycardia/tachycardia.
4. Hypotension/hypertension.
5. Profuse perspiration.
6. Apprehension or anxiety.

H. Assess alleviating factors.
1. Position.
2. Elevation of inflamed extremity.
3. Techniques used at home for pain relief.

I. Assess patient's behavioral responses to pain.
1. Depression, withdrawal, or crying.
2. Stoicism or expressive.

✦ **Implementation**

A. Assess pain before treating.

B. Give reassurance, reduce anxiety and fears.

C. Offer distraction.

D. Give comfort measures as ordered: positioning, rest, elevation, heat/cold applications; protect from painful stimuli.

E. Massage non-surgical area of pain—never massage calf due to danger of emboli.

✦ F. Administer pain medication as ordered: monitor therapeutic or toxic dose, and side effects.
1. Check physician's orders.
2. Use a preventive approach to pain management. Give medication before pain becomes severe. Do *not* withhold medication.
3. Follow steps outlined in assessment to determine the nature, quality, and extent of pain.
4. Start with PO medications. If ineffective or only mildly effective, give IM medications, or combine PO and IM medications.
5. Evaluate result of pain medication. Was it effective? How long did the effect last? What was the extent of relief?
6. Evaluate patient for possible side effects of the medication.
7. Discuss with charge nurse the effects of medication and whether a change of prescription is needed.

G. Monitor alternative methods to control pain.
1. Dorsal column stimulator: stimulation of electrodes at dorsal column of spinal cord by patient-controlled device to inhibit pain.
2. Analgesics: alter perception, threshold, and reaction to pain.
3. Anesthesia: block pain pathway.
4. Local nerve block.
5. Neurosurgical procedures: interrupt sensory pathways; usually also affect pressure and temperature pathways.
   a. Neurectomy: interrupt cranial or peripheral nerves.
   b. Sympathectomy: interrupt afferent pathways (ganglia).
6. Alternative methods of pain control—noninvasive.
   a. Cognitive-behavioral techniques: deep breathing, visualization, imagery.
   b. Physical agents: massage, vibration, biofeedback systems, acupuncture/acupressure.

✦ H. Nurse's role in pain relief.
1. Prevent pain from retarding recovery.

2. Prevent pain from causing nausea and vomiting which could result in fluid and electrolyte imbalance.
3. Prevent pain from causing undue fatigue.
4. Prevent pain from inhibiting moving, ambulating, turning and coughing, and thereby increasing possibilities of secondary problems from inactivity (pneumonia, emboli).
5. Relieve pain or prevent pain from escalating by relaxing muscles (muscle tension increases with pain).
6. Decrease anxiety that present and future pain relief will not be achieved.
7. Bring pain relief to a level acceptable to the patient.

JCAHO Pain Standards (2000–2001)

A. Health care providers must be knowledgeable about pain assessment and management.
B. States that facilities must have policies in place for analgesics and other pain control therapies.
✦ C. JCAHO standards.
  1. Patients have the right to pain assessment.
     a. Facility must provide pain assessment tools.
     b. If facility (i.e., long-term care) cannot treat patient for pain (PCA) patient must be re-referred to facility that can.
     c. Facilities should collect data to monitor effectiveness of pain management.
  2. Patients will be treated for pain and involved in their own pain management.
  3. Health care facilities are expected to comply with these standards for accreditation.
  4. Discharge planning and teaching will include pain management.

CULTURAL SENSITIVITY

A. Demographic shifts influence the direction of health care.
  1. In the United States, 29% of the population is people of color and over 12% are of Hispanic origin.
  2. In 2000, over 20 million foreign-born did not speak English.
  3. These statistics create barriers to health care.
     a. The major barrier is language.
     b. The other barriers are poverty, poor nutrition and poor prevention practices.
  4. Reduced access to health care is a major problem for non-English speaking peoples.
B. It is important for nurses to understand the impact of various cultures on health-care practices.

C. Cultural diversity implications.
  1. Differences in values, beliefs, customs, folklore, traditions, language and patterns of behavior.
  2. Other aspects of differences are personal space related to culture, gender and group behavior.
D. Cultural assessment—important to include in a complete patient assessment.
  1. Cultural background and orientation.
  2. Communication patterns.
  3. Nutritional practices.
     a. Cultural/religious beliefs that do not eliminate whole food groups.
     b. Beliefs that interfere with receiving a healthy, balanced diet (such as a macrobiotic diet).
     c. Food practices that do not allow foods to lose all nutrient value during preparation (overcooking vegetables).
  4. Family relationships.
  5. Beliefs and perceptions related to health, illness, and treatment.
  6. Values related to health.
  7. Education.
  8. Issues affecting health care delivery.

DISEASE PROCESS

Definition: A definite morbid process that affects the body or any of its parts. Symptoms accompany the process; the etiology, course, extent, and prognosis vary.

✦ **Etiology**
A. Mechanical.
  1. Trauma—accidental injury.
  2. Extremes of heat or cold.
  3. Radioactive elements.
  4. Obstruction of normal body passage.
B. Chemical agents.
  1. Caustic substances.
  2. Drugs.
  3. Insect bites.
  4. GI secretions, or blood that is not in GI tract or in vascular system, etc.
  5. Hormones/electrolytes.
C. Genetic/hereditary factors.
D. Infectious agents.
  1. Bacteria.
     a. Cocci—round.
     b. Bacilli—rod-shaped.
     c. Spirochetes—spiral.
  2. Virus—very small, must grow on living cells.
  3. Rickettsias—small, round or rod-shaped microorganisms, transmitted by bites of fleas, lice, ticks.

CULTURAL BELIEFS

Ethnic Group	Cultural Beliefs
Asian/Pacific Islander	→ Extended family has major influence on client.
	Older family members are honored and respected, and their authority is unquestioned.
	Oldest male is decision maker and spokesman.
	Strong emphasis on avoiding conflict and direct confrontation.
	Respect authority and do not disagree with health care recommendations—but they may not follow recommendations.
Chinese	→ Chinese clients will not discuss symptoms of mental illness or depression because they believe this behavior reflects on family; therefore it may produce shame and guilt.
	Use herbalists, spiritual healers, and physicians for care.
Japanese	→ Believe physical contact with blood, skin diseases, and corpses will cause illness.
	They also believe improper care of the body, including poor diet and lack of sleep, causes illness.
	They believe in healers, herbalists and physicians for healing, and energy can be restored with acupuncture, and acupressure.
	They use group decision making for health concerns.
Hindu and Muslim	→ Indians and Pakistanis do not acknowledge a diagnosis of severe emotional illness or mental retardation because it reduces the chance of other family members getting married.
Vietnamese	→ Vietnamese accept mental health counseling and interventions particularly when they have established trust with the health care worker.
Hispanic	→ Older family members are consulted on issues involving health and illness.
	Patriarchal family—men make decisions for family.
	Illness is viewed as God's will or divine punishment resulting from sinful behavior.
	Prefer to use home remedies and consult folk healers known as curanderos rather than traditional Western health care providers.
African-American	→ Family and church oriented.
	Extensive extended family bonds.
	Key family member is consulted for important health-elated decisions.
	Illness is a punishment from God for wrongdoing, or is due to voodoo, spirits, or demons.
	Health prevention is through good diet, herbs, rest, cleanliness, and laxatives to clean the system.
	Wear copper and silver bracelets to prevent illness.
Native American	→ Oriented to the present.
	Value cooperation.
	Value family and spiritual beliefs.
	Strong ties to family and tribe.
	Believe state of health exists when client lives in total harmony with nature.
	Illness is viewed as an imbalance between the ill person and natural or supernatural forces.
	Use medicine man or woman known as a shaman.
	Illness is prevented through elaborate religious rituals.

4. Fungi—yeasts or molds that thrive in a warm, moist place and feed on living plants or animals and decaying organic material.

5. Protozoa—one-celled microscopic organism that belongs to the animal family.

✦ Inflammation

A. Normal body response/homeostatic mechanism.

B. Common local signs/symptoms.
1. Heat.
2. Redness.
3. Swelling.
4. Pain.
5. Loss of motion.

Immunity

A. The body's ability to resist infectious disease.

B. Types.
✦ 1. Natural immunity—"born with"; inborn body characteristic.
✦ 2. Acquired or adaptive immunity.
   a. Develops after exposure to infectious disease or to some form of a particular pathogen or its toxins.
   b. Active—attack of the disease, vaccination, injection of toxoids.
   c. Passive—receive antibodies or antitoxins from mother to unborn fetus or injections of immune serum, gamma globulin, antivenin.

RELIGIOUS DIVERSITY CONSIDERATIONS				
Religious Orientation	**Baptism**	**Death Rituals**	**Health Crisis**	**Diet**
Adventist	Opposed to infant baptism	No last rites	Communion or baptism may be desirable	No alcohol, coffee, tea, or any narcotic
Baptist	Opposed to infant baptism	Clergy supports and counsels	Some believe in healing and laying on of hands Some sects resist medical help	Condemn alcohol Some do not allow coffee and tea
Islam	No baptism	Prescribed procedures by family for washing body and shrouding after death	No faith healing Ritual washing after prayers every day	Prohibit alcohol and pork
Buddhist	Rites are given after child is mature	Send for Buddhist priest Last rite chanting	Family should request priest to be notified	Alcohol and drugs discouraged; some are vegetarian
Christian Scientist	No baptism	No last rites No autopsy	Deny the existence of health crises Many refuse all medical help, blood transfusions, or drugs	Alcohol, coffee, and tobacco viewed as drugs and not allowed
Episcopalian	Infant baptism mandatory	Last rites not essential for all members	Medical treatment acceptable	Some do not eat meat on Fridays
Jehovah's Witness	No infant baptism	No last rites	Opposed to blood transfusions	Do not eat anything to which blood has been added
Judaism	No baptism but ritual circumcision on eighth day after birth	Ritual washing of body after death	All ill people seek medical care Treatment supersedes dietary restrictions	Orthodox observe kosher dietary laws, which prohibit pork, shellfish, and the eating of meat and milk products at the same time
Methodist	Baptism encouraged	No last rites	Medical treatment acceptable	No restrictions
Mormon	Baptism eight years or older	Baptism for the dead can be done by proxy	Do not prohibit medical treatment, although they believe in divine healing	Do not allow alcohol, caffeine, tobacco, tea, and coffee
Roman Catholic	Infant baptism mandatory	Last rites required	Sacrament of the sick	Most ill people are exempt from fasting

Note: There may exist circumstances that require a court order to supervene religious practices (e.g., a blood transfusion to save the life of a child).

C. Antigens.
   1. Substance that causes an immune response.
   2. Examples: pathogen, toxin, foreign protein.
D. Antibodies—substance that protects the body from antigen.

FLUID AND ELECTROLYTES

Fluid Composition of the Body

Body Water
✦ *Definition:*   Total body water represents the largest constituent (45–80 percent) of total body weight, depending on the amount of fat present.
A. Intracellular—represents three-fourths of total body water fluid; contained inside the cell; includes the red blood cells.

B. Extracellular—represents one-fourth of total body water; includes remaining fluid not contained within the cell.
   1. Intravascular (plasma)—liquid in which the blood cells are suspended.
   2. Interstitial—liquid surrounding tissue cells.

Electrolytes
✦ *Definition:*   Electrolytes are compounds that dissolve in a solution to form ions. Each ion carries either a positive or negative electrical charge.
✦ A. Types (see Table 4-3).
   1. Cations—positive charge (Na^+, K^+, Ca^{++}, Mg^{++})
   2. Anions—negative charge (Cl^-, HCO_3^-, HPO_4^-, SO_4^{-})
   3. Equal number of cations and anions (154 each).

Table 4-3. MAJOR ELECTROLYTES			
Cations⁺		**Anions⁻**	
Na^+	Sodium	Cl^-	Chloride
K^+	Potassium	HCO_3^-	Bicarbonate
Ca^{++}	Calcium	HPO_4^{--}	Phosphate
Mg^{++}	Magnesium		

B. Concentration in solution is expressed in mEq/L. Total number of cations (mEq) plus total number of anions (mEq) will be the same in both the intracellular fluid and extracellular fluid, thereby rendering the body's fluid composition electrically neutral.

C. Compartment composition.
1. Extracellular—large quantities of sodium, chloride, and bicarbonate ions.
2. Intracellular—large quantities of potassium, phosphate, and proteins.

Balance of Body Fluid

A. Intake.
1. Ingestion of foodstuff and water (usual intake of fluid is 2000 to 3000 mL/day).
2. Oxidation of foodstuff.

B. Output.
1. Skin and lungs.
   a. Water is lost through vaporization from the skin surface and through expired air from the lungs.
   b. The amount lost increases as metabolism increases.
   c. About 900 mL loss/day.
2. Gastrointestinal tract.
   a. Routes include saliva, gastric secretions, bile, pancreatic juices, and intestinal mucosa.
   b. A volume in excess of seven liters is transferred from the extracellular fluid (ECF) into the gastrointestinal tract, only to be reabsorbed, excepting some 200 mL which is passed with feces.
3. Kidneys.
   a. Carry the heaviest load.
   b. Through glomerular filtration and tubular reabsorption, the kidneys maintain homeostasis.

Fluid Imbalance

◆ Dehydration

A. Extracellular fluid volume deficit.
◆ 1. Possible causes.
   a. Vomiting, diarrhea (GI loss).
   b. Hemorrhage.

DYNAMICS OF INTERCOMPARTMENTAL FLUID TRANSFER

- Osmosis—the movement of water molecules across a semipermeable membrane in a direction that equalizes the concentration of water. The flow of water is into a solution that has a high solute concentration.
- Diffusion—movement of a substance from an area of high concentration to an area of low concentration.
- Active transport—transport of substances across a membrane from an area of low concentration to an area of high concentration.
- Filtration—passage of fluids through a semipermeable membrane as a result of a difference in hydrostatic pressures (pressure exerted by a fluid within a closed system).

   c. Increased urine output.
   d. Excessive loss through respiration or perspiration.
2. The amount of fluid lost increases as metabolism increases.

B. Skin shows initial loss of fluid.
1. Loss of skin turgor (after being pinched and lightly pulled upward, skin very slowly returns to normal).
2. Skin dry and warm.

C. Thirst.

D. Febrile (usually means there is fluid loss through perspiration).

E. Cracked lips.

F. Decreased urinary output (normal output is > 30 mL/hr).

G. Concentrated urine—dark amber color and odorous.

H. Weight loss.

I. Low central venous pressure (CVP).

◆ Circulatory Overload (Extracellular Fluid Volume Excess)

A. Headache.

B. Flushed skin.

C. Tachycardia.

D. Venous distention, particularly neck veins.

E. Increased blood pressure and CVP.

F. Tachypnea (an increase in respiratory rate), coughing, dyspnea (shortness of breath), cyanosis, and pulmonary edema.

◆ Implementation

◆ A. Take central venous pressure to determine fluid balance if CVP catheter is in place. CVP reflects competency of the heart (particularly the right side) to handle the volume of blood returning to it.
1. CVP indicates the comparison of the pumping capacity of the heart and the volume of the circulating blood.
◆ 2. Normal CVP reading: 5–10 cm H_2O.

◆ 3. Increased CVP (> 15 cm H$_2$O) can be indicative of congestive heart failure or circulatory overload.

◆ 4. Decreased CVP (< 5 cm H$_2$O) is indicative of hypovolemia (decreased fluid volume) whether from blood loss or other fluid losses.

◆ B. Monitor patient's condition.
  1. Check condition of skin.
  2. Check body temperature—fever suggests loss of body fluids.
  3. Check for venous distention and increased pulse rate.
  4. Ask patient about unusual related symptoms: headache, shortness of breath.
  5. Monitor fluid intake.
◆ 6. Check urine output at least every 8 hours for maintenance IV therapy or more often for replacement fluid therapy.
  7. Check specific gravity (over 1.025 indicates dehydration; less than 1.010 indicates over-hydration).

Electrolyte Imbalance

◆ **Potassium Imbalance**

Definition: Normal serum or plasma level is 3.5–5.5 mEq/L. Deficiency or excess of potassium in the blood varies from these levels.

◆ **Hyperkalemia (Potassium Excess—greater than 5.5 mEq/L)**
A. Signs and symptoms.
  1. Weakness, flaccid paralysis; irritability.
  2. Hyperreflexia proceeding to paralysis.
  3. Bradycardia.
  4. Ventricular fibrillation.
  5. ECG changes.
  6. Nausea.
  7. Dizziness.
  8. Oliguria.
  9. Apprehension.
  10. Cardiac arrest.
B. Causes of excess potassium levels.
  1. Usually renal disease (cannot excrete potassium).
  2. Burns (due to cellular destruction releasing potassium).
  3. Crushing injuries (due to cellular breakage releasing potassium from cells).
  4. Adrenal insufficiency.
  5. Respiratory or metabolic acidosis.
  6. Excess potassium administration.
C. Treatment of hyperkalemia.
  1. Decrease potassium intake.
  2. IV infusion of sodium chloride, providing kidney function is normal.
  3. Kayexalate enemas.
  4. Dialysis.
  5. Observe ECG tracings.
  6. Measure intake and output.
  7. Withold foods and medication with high potassium content.

◆ **Hypokalemia (Potassium Deficiency—below 3.5 mEq/L)**
A. Signs and symptoms.
  1. Muscle weakness, muscle pain, leg cramps and hyporeflexia.
  2. Hypotension.
  3. Arrhythmias—PVCs particularly.
  4. Nausea, vomiting, diarrhea.
  5. Apathy, drowsiness leading to coma.
  6. ECG changes.
  7. Fatigue.
  8. Weak pulse.
  9. Shortness of breath.
  10. Shallow respirations.
B. Causes of hypokalemia.
  1. Renal loss most common (usually caused by use of diuretics).
  2. Insufficient potassium intake.
  3. Loss from vomiting and diarrhea or from gastrointestinal tract via NG tube placement without replacement of electrolyte solution.
C. Nursing care.
  1. Treatment of hypokalemia—replacement of potassium, orally or parenterally.
  2. Replace no more than 20 mEq of KCl in 1 hour.
  3. Dilute KCL in 30–50 mL IV fluid and administer with IV pump.
  4. Observe ECG monitor if possible.
  5. Observe for adequate urine output.

◆ **Sodium Imbalance**

Definition: Normal serum or plasma level is 135–145 mEq/L. Deficiency or excess of sodium varies from these levels.

◆ **Hypernatremia (Sodium Excess—greater than 145 mEq/L)**
A. Signs and symptoms.
  1. The same as for extracellular fluid excesses.
    a. Pitting edema.
    b. Excessive weight gain.
    c. Increased blood pressure.
    d. Dyspnea.
  2. If hypernatremia is due to dehydration, in which there is a loss of fluid thereby increasing the number of ions, the signs and symptoms include:
    a. Concentrated urine and oliguria.
    b. Dry mucous membranes.
    c. Thirst.

d.   Flushed skin.

e.   Increased temperature.

f.   Tachycardia.

B.   Causes of hypernatremia.

1.   Usually from administration of excessive amount of sodium chloride.

2.   Dehydration from excessive loss of fluids (severe vomiting or diarrhea, fever).

C.   Nursing care.

1.   Monitor administration of NaCl-free IV solutions (dextrose).

2.   Record intake and output.

3.   Restrict sodium in diet.

4.   Weigh daily.

5.   Observe vital signs.

✦ **Hyponatremia (Sodium Deficiency—below 135 mEq/L)**

A.   Signs and symptoms.

1.   The same as those for extracellular fluid deficiency.

a.   Weakness.

b.   Restlessness.

c.   Delirium.

d.   Hyperpnea.

e.   Oliguria.

f.   Increased temperature.

g.   Flushed skin.

h.   Abdominal cramps.

i.   Convulsions.

2.   If sodium is lost but fluid is not, the following signs and symptoms will be present (similar to those of water excess).

a.   Mental confusion.

b.   Headache.

c.   Muscle twitching and weakness.

d.   Coma.

e.   Convulsions.

f.   Oliguria. *(manifestation is polyuria)*

B.   Causes of hyponatremia.

1.   Excessive perspiration.

2.   Use of diuretics.

3.   Gastrointestinal losses.

4.   Lack of sodium in diet.

5.   Renal disease.

6.   Burns.

7.   Diabetes insipidus.

C.   Nursing care.

1.   Monitor IV fluids with sodium (3 percent or 5 percent saline).

2.   Maintain accurate intake and output; restrict water intake.

✦ **Calcium Imbalance**

Definition: Normal serum level is 4.3–5.3 mEq/L., 9–11 mg/dL. Imbalances vary from these levels. Ninety-nine percent of all calcium is found in bones and teeth.

✦ **Hypocalcemia (Calcium Deficiency)**

A.   Signs and symptoms.

1.   Abdominal cramps, muscle cramps.

2.   Tetany, carpopedal spasms.

3.   Circumoral tingling, tingling in fingers.

4.   Convulsions.

5.   Confusion, anxiety and moodiness.

B.   Causes of hypocalcemia.

1.   Vitamin D deficiency.

2.   Magnesium deficiency.

3.   Excessive laxatives.

4.   Malabsorption syndrome.

5.   Acute pancreatitis.

6.   Burns.

7.   Removal of parathyroid glands.

8.   Chronic renal insufficiency.

9.   Massive transfusion (over 2000 mL) blood—requires calcium supplement.

C.   Nursing care

1.   Treatment—reestablish normal plasma level and/or treat underlying cause.

a.   Assess for tetany or convulsions.

b.   If present, notify physician immediately.

✦ 2.   Monitor administration of calcium gluconate IV, followed by oral supplements.

✦ **Hypercalcemia (Calcium Excess)**

A.   Signs and symptoms.

1.   Anorexia, nausea, vomiting.

2.   Lethargy.

3.   Weight loss.

4.   Polydipsia, polyuria, dehydration.

5.   Flank pain, bone pain.

6.   Decreased muscle tone.

B.   Causes of hypercalcemia.

1.   Excessive intake of vitamin D (milk) or calcium supplements.

2.   Hyperparathyroidism, neoplasm of parathyroids, Paget's disease, and specific drugs. (Check for positive Trousseau's or Chvostek's sign.)

3.   Thyrotoxicosis.

4.   Immobilization.

5.   Paget's disease.

C.   Nursing care.

1.   Treatment—treat the underlying cause and/or reestablish normal plasma level of calcium.

2.   Increase fluid intake which decreases tubular reabsorption of calcium.

3.   Promote calcium excretion (sodium salts IV and diuretics).

✦ **Magnesium Imbalance**

Definition: Normal serum or plasma level is 1.3–2.1 mEq/L. Tests for excess or deficit serum levels evaluate kidney function and metabolic disorders.

Hypermagnesemia (Magnesium Excess)

A. Signs and symptoms.
1. Increased level (> 2.5 mEq/L), the higher the level, the more sedative the effect.
2. Loss of deep tendon reflexes.
3. Decrease in respirations.
4. Cardiac arrest.

B. Causes of hypermagnesemia.
1. Severe dehydration.
2. Renal or adrenal insufficiency.
3. Hypothyroidism.
4. Leukemia.
5. Overuse of antacids with Mg (Gelusil).
6. Specific drugs.

C. Nursing care.
1. Increase fluid intake—IV calcium gluconate to promote excretion of excess Mg.
2. Diuretics with possible renal dialysis.

✦ Hypomagnesemia (Magnesium Deficiency)

A. Signs and symptoms.
1. Muscle twitching, hyperactive reflexes, convulsions, tetany indicate neurological signs.
2. Tachycardia, hypotension, ventricular dysrhymia indicage cardiac changes.

B. Causes of hypomagnesemia.
1. Diarrhea, impaired absorption.
2. Acute pancreatitis.
3. Chronic nephritis, diuretic phase of renal failure.
4. Specific drugs (diuretics).
5. Acute alcoholism and cirrhosis.
6. Prolonged IV (3 weeks) without Mg supplementation.
7. Toxemia of pregnancy.

✦ C. Nursing care.
1. Administration of magnesium sulfate IV (10–40 mEq/L in IV fluid) or IM.
   a. Observe for urine output.
   b. Keep antidote (calcium gluconate) available.
2. Promote diet high in Mg (nuts, green vegetables, seafood).
3. Monitor cardiac rhythm.
4. Institute seizure precautions.

✦ Fluid Replacement Therapy

Fluid Replacement Solutions

✦ A. Types of IV solutions.
  ✦ 1. *Hypertonic solution*—a solution with higher osmotic pressure than blood serum.
     a. Solution causes cells to shrink.
     b. Used in severe salt depletion (very rare).
     c. Used in intracranial pressure therapy—reduces edema by rapid movement of fluid out of ventricles into bloodstream.
     d. Common types of solution: normal saline, dextrose 10 percent in saline, dextrose 10 percent in water, and dextrose 5 percent in saline.
     e. Should not be administered faster than 200 mL/hr.
  ✦ 2. *Hypotonic solution*—a solution with lower osmotic pressure than blood serum.
     a. Causes cells to expand or increase in size.
     b. Used to correct diarrhea and dehydration.
     c. Common types of solution: dextrose 5 percent in half strength (0.45 percent) NS, dextrose 5 percent; in one-quarter strength (0.2) NS, and dextrose 5 percent in water.
     d. Should not be administered faster than 400 mL/hr.
  ✦ 3. *Isotonic solution*—a solution with the same osmotic pressure as blood serum.
     a. Cells remain unchanged.
     b. Used for replacement or maintenance (expands extracellular volume); especially used to expand circulating volume.
     c. Common type of solution: lactated Ringer's solution; 5 percent dextrose in NS.

✦ B. Choice of fluid replacement solution—depends on patient's needs.
1. Fluid and electrolyte replacement only.
   a. Saline solution.
   b. Lactated Ringer's solution.
2. Calorie replacement—dextrose solutions.
3. Restriction of dietary intake, such as low sodium.
4. IV medications that are insoluble in certain IV fluids.
5. Rate of administration of IV solution to correct fluid imbalance.
6. Dextrose plays no part in tonicity. It is metabolized off.

C. Purpose of fluid and electrolyte therapy.
1. To replace previous losses.
2. To provide maintenance requirements.
3. To meet current losses.

Implementation

A. Check circulation of immobilized extremity.
B. Check label of solution against physician's order.
C. Check rate of infusion.
D. Observe vein site for signs of swelling.
E. Take vital signs at least every 15 minutes for replacement fluid administration.

✦ Intravenous Calorie Calculation

A. 1000 mL D_5W provides 50 g of dextrose.
B. 50 g of dextrose provides 4 calories per gram (actually 3.4 calories); thus, multiply 50g × 4 Cal.

C. 1000 mL D_5W provides 200 calories.

D. Usual IV total/day is 2000–3000 mL (400–600 calories/day).

✦ Intravenous Regulation ❖ Procedure ❖

A. Check manufacturer's drip rate calibration on administration set package. Macrodrip sets vary from 10–15 gtts per 1 mL.

B Microdrip factor is 60 drops/mL.

C. Y = tubing for blood transfusion is drip factor of 10 drops/mL.

D. Check physician's order for amount of fluid to be delivered per unit of time (e.g., 1 liter q8h, or hourly flow rate such as 100 mL/hr).

E. Calculate flow rate.

1. To find the number of milliliters to be given per hour:

$$\frac{\text{Total solution}}{\text{No. of hours to run}} = \text{mL hour}$$

2. To find drops per minute:

$$\frac{\text{mL/hr x drop factor}}{60 \text{ minutes}} = \text{gtts/minute}$$

Example: Ordered 1000 mL D5W administered over 8-hour period of time.

1. With microdrip, it is easy to remember that the number of drops per minute equals the number of mL to be administered per hour.

Example: $\frac{1000}{8} = 125 \text{ mL/hr}$

Using formula:

$$(8 \times 60) \quad \frac{1000 \times 60}{480} = \frac{60,000}{480} = \frac{125}{\text{gtt/min}}$$

2. With administration set that delivers 10 gtt/mL:

$$\frac{1000 \times 10}{480} = \frac{10,000}{480} = 20.8 \text{ or } 21 \text{ gtt/min}$$

3. With administration set that delivers 15 gtt/mL:

$$\frac{1000 \times 15}{480} = \frac{15,000}{480} = 31 \text{ gtt/min}$$

C. Nursing care with IV therapy.

1. Before infusion, ensure patient is in comfortable position.

2. Carefully check label against physician's orders.

3. Check circulation in the immobilized extremity.

4. Frequently check rate of infusion.

5. Observe for signs of swelling at infusion site.

6. Take vital signs at least every 15 minutes for replacement fluid administration.

ACID–BASE BALANCE

Normal Acid–Base Balance

✦ Principles

A. Acid–base balance is the ratio of acids and bases in the body that are necessary to maintain a chemical balance conducive to life.

B. Acid–base ratio is 20 base to 1 acid.

C. Acid–base balance is measured by arterial blood samples and recorded as blood pH. Range is 7.35–7.45.

D. Acids are hydrogen ion donors. They release hydrogen ions to neutralize or decrease the strength of the base.

E. Bases are hydrogen ion acceptors. They accept hydrogen ions to convert strong acids to weak acids (for example, hydrochloric acid is converted to carbonic acid).

Regulatory Mechanisms

A. The body controls the pH balance by use of:
1. Chemical buffers.
2. Lungs.
3. Cells.
4. Kidneys.

✦ B. The chemical buffer system works fastest, but other regulatory mechanisms provide more reliable protection against acid–base imbalance. The four primary buffer systems are:

1. Carbonic acid—bicarbonate—maintains blood pH at 7.4 with ratio of 20 parts bicarbonate to 1 part carbonic acid.

2. Intracellular and plasma proteins (along with the liver)—vary the amounts of hydrogen ions in the chemical structure of the protein. They can both attract and release hydrogen ions.

3. Hemoglobin—maintains balance by chloride shift. Chloride shifts in and out of red blood cells according to the level of oxygen in blood plasma. Each chloride ion that leaves the cell is replaced by a bicarbonate ion.

4. Phosphate buffer system—composed of sodium and other cations in association with HPO_4^{--} and $H_2PO_4^{-}$; acts like bicarbonate system.

C. Lungs.

1. Next to react are the lungs.

2. It takes 10–30 minutes for lungs to inactivate hydrogen molecules by converting them to water molecules.

3. Lungs can only inactivate the hydrogen ions carried by carbonic acid. The other ions must be excreted by the kidneys.

D. Cells.

1. Cells absorb or release extra hydrogen ions.

2. Cells react in 2–4 hours.

E. Kidneys.
    1. Kidneys are the mainstay of regulatory mechanisms.
    2. Excretion of excessive acid or base is slow. Compensation takes a few hours to several days, but it is the most effective process.
    3. Primary function of kidneys is bicarbonate regulation. Kidneys restore bicarbonate by releasing hydrogen ions and holding bicarbonate ions.

Acid–Base Imbalances

Metabolic Acidosis

Definition: Metabolic acidosis occurs when there is a deficit of bases or an accumulation of fixed acids.

✦ A. Changes in pH and HCO_3.
    1. The pH will become acidic (fall below 7.35).
    2. Bicarbonate, HCO_3, decreased (< 22 mEq/L); normal 22–26 mEq/L.
    3. Note that the serum CO_2 acts as a bicarbonate (HCO_3) determinant. When serum CO_2 is low, HCO_3 is lost and acidosis results.

✦ B. Compensatory mechanisms.
    1. When compensating for metabolic acidosis, the one clinical manifestation usually observed is the "blowing off" of excessive acids. This is manifested by a respiratory rate increase.
    2. The lungs are the fastest mechanism used to compensate for metabolic acidosis.
    3. Renal excretion of acid occurs.

C. Causes of metabolic acidosis (seen particularly in the surgical patient).
    1. Diabetes—diabetic ketoacidosis.
    2. Renal insufficiency—kidneys lose their ability to reabsorb bicarbonate and secrete hydrogen ions.
    3. Diarrhea—excessive amounts of base are lost from the intestines and pancreas, resulting in acidosis.

D. Signs and symptoms.
    1. Headache.
    2. Drowsiness.
    3. Nausea, vomiting, diarrhea.
    4. Stupor, coma.
    5. Twitching, convulsions.
    6. Kussmaul's respiration (increased respiratory rate due to compensation).
    7. Fruity breath (as evidenced in diabetic ketoacidosis as a result of improper fat metabolism).

✦ E. Treatment and nursing care.
    1. These drugs may be given intravenously:
        a. Sodium bicarbonate.
        b. Sodium lactate.
        c. Insulin (in ketoacidosis).
    2. Watch laboratory values closely while treating metabolic acidosis.

3. Watch for signs of hyperkalemia and dehydration in the patient (oliguria, vital sign changes, etc.).
4. Record intake and output.

Metabolic Alkalosis

Definition: Metabolic alkalosis is a malfunction of metabolism that causes an increase in blood base or a reduction of available acids in the serum.

✦ A. Changes in pH and HCO_3.
    1. The pH will become more alkaline (> 7.45).
    2. The CO_2 will increase above 35 mEq/L. Note that this measures the amount of circulating bicarbonate or the base portion of the plasma. (A good way to remember these acid–base values is to recall that as the pH increases, so does the HCO_3. The reverse is true for acidosis.)

✦ B. Compensatory mechanisms.
    1. The lungs will attempt to hold on to the carbonic acid in an effort to neutralize the base state.
    2. As a result, the rate of respiration will decrease.
    3. Renal excretion of bicarbonate occurs.

C. Causes of metabolic alkalosis.
    1. Ingestion of excessive soda bicarbonate (used by individuals for acid indigestion).
    2. Excessive vomiting, which results in the loss of hydrochloric acid and potassium.
    3. Placement of NG tube, which causes a depletion of both hydrochloric acid and potassium.
    4. Use of potent diuretics, particularly by cardiac patients. Not only potassium but also hydrogen and chloride ions are lost, causing an increase in the bicarbonate level of the serum.

D. Signs and symptoms.
    1. Nausea, vomiting.
    2. Diarrhea.
    3. Irritability, agitation, nervousness.
    4. Coma, convulsions.
    5. Restlessness.
    6. Twitching and numbness of extremities.
    7. ECG changes.

✦ E. Treatment and nursing care.
    ✦ 1. Maintain diet of foods high in potassium and chloride (bananas, apricots, dried peaches, Brazil nuts, dried figs, oranges).
    2. Monitor IV solution of added electrolytes.
    3. Give Diamox to promote kidney excretion of bicarbonate.
    4. Administer potassium chloride maintenance doses to patients on long-term diuretics.
    5. Give ammonium chloride to increase the amount of available hydrogen ions, thereby increasing the availability of acids in the blood.
    6. Check laboratory values frequently to watch for electrolyte imbalance.

7. Watch patient for physical signs indicative of hypokalemia or metabolic alkalosis.
8. Keep accurate records of intake and output and vital signs.

Respiratory Acidosis

Definition: Respiratory acidosis refers to increased carbonic acid concentration (accumulated CO_2, which has combined with water) caused by retention of carbon dioxide through hypoventilation. Differs from metabolic acidosis in that it results from altered alveolar ventilation.

✦ A. Changes in pH, PCO_2, and PO_2.
  1. With an increased acidic state, the pH will fall below 7.35.
  2. The PCO_2 will be increased above 45 mm Hg.
  3. The PO_2 is normal (90–100 mm Hg) or it can be decreased as hypoxia increases.
  4. The HCO_3 will be normal (24) if respiratory acidosis is uncompensated.
✦ B. Compensatory mechanisms.
  1. Because the basic problem in respiratory acidosis is a defect in the lungs, the kidneys must be the major compensatory mechanism.
     a. The kidneys work much slower than the lungs.
     b. As a result, compensation may take from hours to days.
  2. The kidneys will retain and return bicarbonate to the extracellular fluid compartment.
C. Causes of respiratory acidosis.
  1. Sedatives.
  2. Oversedation with narcotics in postoperative period.
  3. A chronic pulmonary disorder, such as emphysema, asthma, bronchitis, or pneumonia, leading to
     a. Inability of the lungs to expand and contract adequately—airway obstruction..
     b. Difficulty in the expiratory phase of respiration, which causes retention of carbon dioxide.
  4. Poor gaseous exchange during surgery.
D. Signs and symptoms.
  1. Dyspnea after exertion, tachycardia.
  2. Hyperventilation when at rest.
  3. Cyanosis.
  4. Sensorium changes (drowsiness leading to coma).
  5. Headache, vertigo, tremors, confusion.
  6. Carbon dioxide narcosis.
     a. When body has adjusted to higher carbon dioxide levels, the respiratory center loses its sensitivity to elevated carbon dioxide.
     b. Medulla fails to respond to high levels of carbon dioxide.
     c. Patient is forced to depend on anoxia for respiratory stimulus.
     d. If a high level of oxygen is administered, patient will cease breathing.
✦ E. Treatment and nursing care.
  1. Turn, cough, and hyperventilate patients at least every 2–4 hours postoperatively. Use oropharyngeal suction if necessary. Maintain semi-Fowler's position.
  2. When pulmonary complications present a threat, do postural drainage, percussion, and vibration, followed by suctioning.
  3. Keep patient well hydrated to facilitate removal of secretions. If patient is dehydrated, secretions become thick and more difficult to expectorate.
  4. Monitor vital signs carefully, particularly rate and depth of respirations.
  5. Teach pursed-lip breathing to chronic respiratory patients.
  6. If oxygen is administered, watch carefully for signs of carbon dioxide narcosis (usually start O_2 at 2L).
  7. Place patient on mechanical ventilation if necessary.
  8. Administer aerosol medications.
     a. Bronchodilators (aminophylline)—relieve bronchospasms.
     b. Detergents (Tergemist)—liquefy tenacious mucus.
     c. Antibiotics specific to causative agent.
  9. Drugs that may be given intravenously:
     a. Sodium bicarbonate.
     b. Sodium lactate.
     c. Ringer's lactate—to replace electrolyte loss.
     d. Potassium to maintain serum level.

Respiratory Alkalosis

Definition: Respiratory alkalosis occurs when an excessive amount of carbon dioxide is exhaled, usually caused by hyperventilation. The loss of carbon dioxide results in a decrease in H^+ concentration along with a decrease in PCO_2, and an increase in the ratio of bicarbonate to carbonic acid. The result is an increase in the pH level.

✦ A. Changes in pH, PCO_2, and PO_2.
  1. With an increased alkalotic state, the pH will increase above 7.45, indicating there is a decreased amount of carbonic acide in the serum.
  2. The PCO_2 will be normal to low (< 35 mm Hg), as this measures the acid portion of the acid–base system (30–45 mm Hg).
  3. The PO_2 should be unchanged.
  4. The bicarbonate level (HCO_3 or CO_2 content) should be normal (24) unless the patient is compensating.

Table 4-4. Acid-Base Imbalances			
Metabolic Alkalosis			**Compensation**
pH:	↑	> 7.40	7.40
HCO₃:	↑	> 24	
PCO₂:	normal	40	↑ > 40
Metabolic Acidosis			**Compensation**
pH:	↓	< 7.40	7.40
HCO₃:	↓	< 24	
PCO₂:	normal	40	↓ < 40
Respiratory Alkalosis			**Compensation**
pH:	↑	> 7.40	7.40
PCO₃:	↓	< 40	
HCO₂:	normal	24	↓ < 24
Respiratory Acidosis			**Compensation**
pH:	↓	< 7.40	7.40
PCO₃:	↑	> 40	
HCO₃:	normal	24	↑ > 24

✦ B. Compensatory mechanisms.
   1. Since the basic problem is related to the respiratory system, the kidneys will compensate by excreting more bicarbonate ions and retaining H^+.
   2. This process will return the acid–base balance to a normal ratio.
C. Causes of respiratory alkalosis.
   1. Hysteria—patient hyperventilates and exhales excessive amounts of carbon dioxide.
   2. Hypoxia—stimulates patient to breathe more vigorously.
   3. Following head injuries or intracranial surgery.
   4. Increased temperature.
   5. Salicylate poisoning.
     a. Stimulation of respiration causes alkalosis through hyperventilation.
     b. Acidosis may occur from excessive salicylates in the blood.
D. Signs and symptoms.
   1. Hyperreflexia.
   2. Muscular twitching.
   3. Convulsions.
   4. Gasping for breath.
   5. Lightheadedness, vertigo, tinnitus.
✦ E. Treatment and nursing care.
   1. Eliminate cause of hyperventilation.
   2. Remain with patient and be supportive to reduce anxiety.
   3. Use rebreathing bag to return patient's carbon dioxide to self (paper bag works just as well).
   4. Provide sedation as ordered.
   5. Monitor lab values, especially K and HCO_3.

BLOOD AND BLOOD FACTORS

Blood Grouping

Major Blood Groups
A. ABO blood group (see Table 4-5).
   1. A.
   2. AB.
   3. B.
   4. O.
B. Rh blood group.
   1. Positive (85 percent of the population).
   2. Negative (15 percent of the population).

Antigens and Antibodies
A. Blood type based on type of antigens present in red blood cells as well as type of antibodies in the serum.
✦ B. A and B antigens.
   1. Persons with type A blood have antigen A present; persons with type B blood have antigen B present.
   2. Persons with type AB blood have both A and B antigens present.
   3. Persons with type O blood have no antigens present.
✦ C. Anti-A and anti-B antibodies.
   1. Antibodies develop as a response to exposure. Persons with type A blood have anti-B antibodies. They do not have anti-A antibodies because the blood cells would be destroyed by agglutination.
   2. Persons with type B blood have anti-A antibodies.
   3. Persons with type AB blood have no antibodies.
     a. Considered *universal recipients*.
     b. Cannot destroy donor's red blood cells.
   4. Persons with type O blood have both anti-A and anti-B antibodies.
     a. Considered *universal donors*.
     b. Red blood cells do not contain antigens that could be destroyed by antibodies in recipients' blood.
D. In emergency situations, when time does not allow ABO determination, group 0 red blood cells must be given (whole blood *must* be administered ABO identical).

Transfusion Administration ❖ PROCEDURE ❖

✦ **Procedure**
A. Follow rules for preventing transfusion reaction.
   1. Check physician's orders—type and number of units.
✦ 2. Check carefully for room number, correct name and blood bracelet ID number. Double check blood group donor number (have two persons check information).

Table 4-5. SUMMARY OF ABO BLOOD GROUPING

Blood Type	Antigen in RBCs	Antibodies in Plasma	Incompatible Donor Blood	Compatible Blood Donor
A	A	Anti-B	AB and B	A and O
B	B	Anti-A	A and AB	B and O
AB	A and B	None	None	All blood groups
O	None	Anti-A and anti-B	All blood groups	O

3. Check that patient has signed consent form.

B. Observe blood bag for bubbles, cloudiness, or dark sediment—indicative of contamination.

✦ C. Do not warm blood, as bacteria thrives in this medium. When warming is required in massive transfusions, a blood-warming coil is used.

D. Do not allow blood to be unrefrigerated for more than 30 minutes before administration.

E. Use blood filter to prevent fibrin and other materials from entering the bloodstream.

F. Transfusion will be started with normal saline or another electrolyte solution; blood will agglutinate without the presence of electrolytes.

G. Check blood with another nurse before infusing—sign form according to hospital policy.

✦ **Implementation**

✦ A. Transfusion usually started at 20–25 drops per minute. Closely observe transfusion as reaction usually occurs during the first 15 minutes.

B. Take base line vital signs at beginning and 5, 15, and 30 minutes after beginning transfusion.

✦ C. Transfusion is usually completed in no less than 2 hours and in no more than 4 hours.
1. Usually administered at a rate of 60–80 drops per minute.
2. If patient is hypovolemic, blood can be administered at the rate of 500 mL in 10 minutes by use of a blood pump. Observe for pulmonary edema and hypervolemia.

D. Obtain posttransfusion vital signs.
1. Report a 1°C or 2°F rise in temperature.
2. Increased teperature could indicate transfusion reaction.

Transfusion Reactions

✦ A. Hemolytic or incompatibility reaction.
1. Most severe complication.
2. Caused by mismatched blood.
3. Clinical manifestations.
   a. Increased temperature.
   b. Decreased blood pressure.
   c. Pain across the chest, in kidney region, and at the site of needle insertion.
   d. Chills.
   e. Hematuria.
   f. Backache in the kidney region.
   g. Dyspnea and cyanosis.
   h. Jaundice can occur in severe cases.
4. The reaction is caused by agglutination of the donor's red cells.
   a. The antibodies in the recipient's plasma react with the antigens in the donor's red cells.
   b. The clumping blocks off capillaries and therefore obstructs the flow of blood and oxygen to cells.
5. Nursing care.
   ✦ a. *Stop transfusion immediately* upon appearance of symptoms.
   b. Return remaining blood and the patient's blood sample to the laboratory for type and cross match.
   c. Keep IV patent after changing blood tubing with either normal saline or D_5W.
   d. Take vital signs every 15 minutes.
   e. Insert Foley catheter for a urine sample for red blood cells and an accurate output record.
   f. Check for oliguria.
   g. Administer medications such as vasopressors if indicated.
   h. Administer oxygen as necessary.

✦ B. Bacterial contamination.
1. Check blood for discoloration, cloudiness, and bubbles, which are indicative of contamination.
2. Signs and symptoms.
   a. Sudden increase in temperature.
   b. Sudden chill.
   c. Headache, hypotension.
   d. Peripheral vasodilation.
   e. Malaise.
   f. Lumbar pain.
✦ 3. Nursing care.
   a. Do not use blood that is cloudy or discolored or appears to have bubbles present.
   b. If transfusion has been started, discontinue *immediately*.
   c. Send remaining blood to laboratory for culture and sensitivity. If transfusion has been started, send patient's blood sample as well.

d. Change IV tubing as soon as possible and keep it patent.

e. Check vital signs, including temperature, every 15 minutes; observe for shock.

f. Insert Foley catheter for accurate output and urine specimen as ordered.

g. Control hyperthermia, if present, with antipyretics, cooling blankets, or with sponge baths.

h. Notify physician to obtain order for antibiotic/steroid shock management.

i. Draw blood culture before antibiotic administration.

✦ C. Allergic reactions.
   1. Allergic response to any type of allergen in the donor's blood.
   2. Common reaction, usually mild in nature—urticaria, hives and pruritus.
   3. Signs and symptoms of severe reaction.
      a. Respiratory distress.
      b. Wheezing.
      c. Laryngeal edema.
   ✦ 4. Anaphylactic reaction—shock, loss of consciousness.
   5. Nursing care.
      a. Administer an ordered antihistamine such as Benadryl to control itching and to relieve edema.
      b. If reaction is severe, discontinue the transfusion; otherwise, check with RN for decision to stop or decrease flow rate.
      c. Monitor vital signs and observe for progressive allergic reaction.

COMMON PROCEDURES

General Principles

✦ Nursing Actions Prior to Procedures

A. Most procedures require a physician's order.

B. Review written procedure in your hospital/agency procedure book; seek help from team leader/ head nurse if you do not know method.

C. Explain all procedures to patient; ask patient's cooperation.

D. Wash hands before beginning procedure and maintain medical or surgical asepsis.

E. Provide privacy for patient.

Restraints ❖ Procedure ❖

✦ A. Used as a last resort—legal only to protect patient or others from forseeable harm.
   1. Hospital policy and procedures must be followed when applying restraints.

✦ 2. States and facilities require a physician's order for restraints.
   a. Orders must specify justification for restraint, type of restraint, length of time, and criteria for removal.
   b. Restraints may *not* be ordered PRN; a nurse may legally restrain a patient without an order if essential.

✦ 3. Legal implications for the nurse applying restraints.
   a. A nurse may be charged with assault if restraints are used when not needed.
   b. A nurse may be charged with negligence when patient injury occurs.

B. Types of retraints.
   ✦ 1. Physical restraints—application of a device to restrict movement.
      a. Prevent patient falls.
      b. Discourage patient from disconnecting vital equipment.
      c. Prevent patient from harming self or others.
   ✦ 2. Chemical restraints—sedative or psychotropic medications given to prevent certain behaviors.
      a. Prevent patients from disconnecting vital equipment.
      b. Assist in preventing patient from harming self or others.
      c. Allow staff to care for all patients on a unit.
   3. Seclusion—involuntary confinement in a locked room.

✦ C. Alternatives to restraints.
   1. Encourage family and friends to monitor patient; use sitters to monitor patient.
   2. Use a bed occupancy monitor or similar device to immediately notify nurses when a patient is out of bed.
   3. Provide appropriate and continuing stimulation and monitoring.

✦ D. Restraint guidelines—restraints require a physician's order.
   1. Review hospital policy for the use of restraints.
   2. Use restraints for the patient's protection and to prevent injury, not for the nurse's convenience.
   3. Use the least amount of restraint possible. A torso belt is least restrictive, limb restraint is more restrictive, and chemical (medication) is *most* restrictive.
   4. Allow patients as much freedom of movement as possible. Use slipknots for quick release. Do not use square knots or bows.
   5. Always explain the purpose of the restraint to the patient and family. Afford as much dignity to the patient as possible.

6. Remember that restraints can cause emotional, mental, and physical deterioration and increase the risk of injury if falls occur.
7. Remember that circulation and skin integrity can be affected by restraints.
8. Special precautions should be taken for adult females in restraints to protect breast tissue.
9. Clients must now be observed every 15 minutes; release restraints every 2 hours for 5 minutes to inspect tissues and provide joint range of motion and position change to prevent circulatory impairment. When a patient is combative, release only one restraint at a time.
10. Assess and provide for patient's fluid and elimination needs, pain management, and position change every 2 hours.
11. Pad bony prominences, such as wrists and ankles, beneath a restraint.
12. Attempt to make restraints as inconspicuous as possible for the sake of the patient's relatives and friends, who may be upset by seeing restraints.
13. Clearly document rationale and precautions taken for patient safety.
14. Notify family or significant other if restraints are necessary.

Adapted from Smith, S., Duell, D., & Martin, B. (2004). *Clinical nursing skills* (6th ed.). Upper Saddle River, NJ: Prentice Hall Health.

✦ Catheterization ❖ Procedure ❖

A. Procedure involves putting plastic or rubber tube/catheter in bladder via urethra in order to empty bladder or obtain specimen.
B. It is a sterile procedure—use surgical aseptic technique and avoid contaminating equipment.
C. Position for female patient.
    1. Dorsal recumbent most common.
    2. Sims' or lateral.
D. Make provisions for privacy.
E. Procedure protocol.
    1. Screen, position, and drape patient; wash hands.
    2. Place catheter tray for convenience and open it.
    3. Put on sterile gloves and arrange equipment.
    4. Place sterile drapes (optional).
    5. Lubricate catheter.
    6. Expose urinary meatus (this gloved hand now considered contaminated). Leave hand in position until procedure completed.
    7. Cleanse urinary meatus with provided equipment.
    8. Pick up lubricated catheter (do not contaminate it). Insert catheter into urethra until urine flows.
    9. When urine stops flowing, pinch and withdraw catheter. (If more than 1000 mL

obtained, some facilities suggest clamping catheter for 20 minutes before removing more urine to prevent bladder spasm).
10. Remove gloves.
11. Clean patient and position for comfort.
12. Clean all equipment or discard disposable equipment.
13. Chart time procedure done and amount and character of urine.

✦ F. Retention or Foley catheter (R/C) is inserted in the same manner.
    1. Unless catheter has prefilled balloon, pretest balloon.
        a. Insert tip of prefilled syringe into catheter side arm to inflate balloon.
        b. After testing balloon, pull back on syringe to remove fluid and deflate balloon.
    2. When the catheter is in place, sterile water or sterile air is instilled into a balloonlike structure near the catheter tip. This "balloon" keeps the catheter in the bladder.
    3. The catheter is usually attached to a drainage tube and bag.

✦ Bladder Irrigation ❖ Procedure ❖

A. Surgical aseptic technique used; don clean gloves.
B. Check amount and type of solution ordered.
C. Open method.
    1. Cleanse catheter at connection with drainage tube and separate. Protect drainage tube from contamination with sterile protective cap.
    2. Fill sterile irrigating syringe with sterile solution (30–50 mL) and gently put into catheter.
    3. Remove syringe and allow solution to drain into emesis basin—do not contaminate end of catheter.
    4. Repeat until returns are clear or until ordered amount is used or desired returns are obtained.
    5. Wipe catheter with antiseptic sponge and connect catheter to drainage tube.
D. Closed method—most common.
    1. Place clamp on catheter immediately distal to injection port.
    2. Place 22- or 24-gauge sterile needle on 30-mL sterile syringe. Fill syringe with ordered sterile solution.
    3. Cleanse catheter between side arm and clamp with an alcohol or povidone-iodine swab and insert needle.
    4. Gently and slowly inject solution. When ordered amount injected, withdraw needle and remove clamp.
E. Chart method used, amount and type of solution, description of returns, and patient's reaction.

PREOPERATIVE AND POSTOPERATIVE CARE

✦ Routine Preoperative Care

Psychological Support

A. Reinforce the physician's teaching regarding the surgical procedure.
B. Identify patient's stress level and anxiety; notify physician of extreme anxiety.
C. Listen to patient's verbalization of fears.
D. Provide support to the patient's family (where family can wait during surgery, approximately how long surgery will take, etc.).

✦ Preoperative Teaching

A. Postoperative exercises: leg, coughing, deep breathing, procedures for getting out of bed, etc.
B. Equipment that will be used during postoperative period: ventilator, NG tube to suction, etc.
C. Pain medication and when to ask for it.
D. Explanation of NPO.

Physical Care

A. Observation and recording of patient's overall condition and baseline data.
   1. Nutritional status.
   2. Physical defects, such as loss of limb function, skin breakdown.
   3. Hearing or sight difficulties.
B. Chest x-ray, ECG, and blood and urine samples as ordered.
C. Preoperative history and present physical condition.
D. Determination of any drug allergies.
E. Skin prep when necessary (shaving operative site is no longer recommended); shower with antibacterial soap if ordered.
F. Retention or indwelling catheter, NG tube, or enema if ordered.
G. Have patient void immediately before medicating.
H. Preoperative medications administered.
I. Following preoperative medication, quiet rest with siderails up and curtains drawn.

✦ Nurse's Responsibility

A. Check and report abnormal lab values and vital signs.
✦ B. Check that surgical consent form is signed.
C. Complete preoperative check list.
   1. Remove dentures, nail polish, hairpins, artificial eyes, contact lenses, glasses.
   2. Give preoperative medicines.
D. Complete ordered preoperative nursing interventions.
E. Check ID band, blood bland and allergy bracelet.

✦ F. Complete preoperative teaching.
   1. Postoperative exercises.
   2. Equipment that will be used.
   3. Explanation of NPO.
   4. Pain medication and when to request it.
G. Perform or check skin prep/shave—follow facility guidelines.

Anesthesia

✦ Preoperative Medications

A. Purpose.
   1. Decrease secretions of the mouth and respiratory tract.
   2. Depress vagal reflexes.
   3. Produce drowsiness and relieve anxiety.
   4. Allow anesthesia to be induced more smoothly and in smaller amounts.
✦ B. Types of drugs administered.
   1. Hypnotic or antianxiolytic—given night before surgery.
      a. Decreases anxiety.
      b. Promotes good night's sleep.
   2. Hypnotic or opiate—preoperative medication.
      a. Decreases anxiety.
      b. Allows smooth anesthetic induction.
      c. Provides amnesia for immediate perioperative period.
   3. Anticholinergic—preoperative medication.
      a. Decreases secretions.
      b. Counteracts vagal effects during anesthesia.

General Anesthesia

✦ A. General anesthesia produces a depression of the CNS, amnesia, loss of reflexes, and unconsciousness.
   1. Inhalation agents.
      a. Halothane.
      b. Ether.
      c. Chloroform.
   2. Intravenous anesthesia—thiopental (Pentothal).
   3. Dissociative anesthesia (ketamine HCl and Innovar). Used with nitrous oxide and oxygen for short anesthesia.
B. Stages and planes of general anesthesia.
   1. Stage one: early induction—from beginning of inhalation to loss of consciousness.
   2. Stage two: delirium or excitement.
      a. No surgery is performed at this point—very dangerous stage.
      b. Breathing is irregular.
   3. Stage three: surgical anesthesia.
      a. Begins when patient stops fighting and is breathing regularly.

b. Four planes, based on respiration, pupillary and eyeball movement, and reflex muscular responses.

4. Stage four: medullary paralysis—respiratory arrest.

C. Anesthetic agents.

1. Anesthesia produces insensitivity to pain or sensation.

2. Dangers associated with anesthesia depend on overall condition of patient.

   a. High risk if associated cardiovascular, renal, or respiratory conditions.

   b. High risk for unborn fetus and mother.

   c. High risk if stomach full (chance of vomiting and aspiration).

3. Types of anesthesia.

   a. General—administered IV or by inhalation. Produces loss of consciousness and decreases reflex movement.

   b. Local—applied topically or injected regionally. Patient is alert, but pain and sensation are decreased in surgical area.

D. Reversing anesthetic agents.

1. Anesthesia may affect natural physiologic response for ventilation.

2. Drugs may depress respirations.

3. Thorough assessment necessary to recognize need to reverse these effects.

   a. Naloxone (Narcan) to reverse narcotics.

   b. Atropine or glycopyrrolate (Robinul) with neostigmine to reverse muscle relaxants.

Conscious Sedation

✦ A. Form of IV anesthesia—depressed level of consciousness with the ability to respond to stimuli and verbal commands.

1. Combined sedation and analgesic effect so patient is pain free during procedure.

2. Patient can maintain patent airway.

B. Specfiic drugs used vary with credentials of person administering agents.

1. Versed or Valium IV frequently used.

2. Other drugs used are analgesics (morphine, fentanyl) and reverse agonists (Narcan, Naloxane).

3. Patient must never be left alone and must be closely monitored for respiratory, cardiovascular, or CNS depression.

4. Patient is monitored by ability to maintain airway and respond to verbal demands.

C. Agents may be used alone or in combination with local, regional, or spinal anesthesia.

LEVELS OF SEDATION

- *Minimal:* Patient relaxed and may be awake—understands direction.
- *Moderate:* Patient drowsy—may sleep, but easily awakened.
- *Deep:* Patient sleeps through procedure; has little or no memory; oxygen given because breathing is slowed.

Routine Postoperative Care

✦ Postanesthesic Care Unit (PACU) ❖ PROCEDURE ❖

A. Immediate postoperative care.

✦ 1. Maintain patent airway.

2. Administer humidified oxygen by mask or nasal cannula; monitor oxygen saturation (SaO_2) by pulse oximetry.

3. Check gag reflex.

4. Suction patient as needed.

5. Position patient for adequate ventilation—side-lying is best if not contra-indicated.

6. Observe for adverse signs of general anesthesia or spinal anesthesia.

   a. Level of consciousness.

   b. Movement of limbs.

✦ 7. Monitor vital signs.

   a. Check every 5–15 minutes until stable; then every 30 minutes for 2 hours.

      (1) Pulse—check rate, quality, and rhythm.

      (2) Blood pressure—check pulse pressure and quality as well as systolic and diastolic pressure.

      (3) Respiration—check rate, rhythm, depth, and type of respiration (abdominal breathing, nasal flaring).

   b. Vital signs are sometimes difficult to obtain due to hypothermia.

   c. Movement from operating room table to gurney can alter vital signs significantly, especially with cardiovascular patients.

   d. Maintain temperature (operating room is usually cold)—apply warm blankets.

8. Monitor IV fluids; check IV insertion site.

   a. Verify correct type and amount of solution.

   b. Set appropriate flow rate using IV pump or controller.

   c. Maintain accurate IV intake record.

   d. Monitor blood or blood components.

9. Observe dressings and surgical drains.

   a. Mark any drainage on dressings, and note time by drawing a line around the drainage.

   b. Note color and amount of drainage on dressings and in drainage tubes.

   c. Empty collection device as needed.

d.   Ensure that dressing is secure.

e.   Reinforce dressings as needed.

B.   Overall observations of condition.

1.   Check skin for warmth, color, and moisture.

2.   Check nailbeds and mucous membranes for color (report if cyanotic) and blanching.

3.   Observe for return of reflexes.

C.   Medications—begin routine drugs and administer all STAT drugs; monitor pain level and administer pain medications.

D.   Assessment for return to room—use postanesthesia recovery scoring system in addition to vital signs.

1.   Be sure vital signs are stable and within normal limits; normal skin color.

2.   See if patient is fully awake and reflexes are present (gag and cough reflex).

3.   Take oral airway out (if not out already).

4.   Check ability to cough and deep breathe.

5.   Check blood pressure maintained within 20 mmHg preanesthesia.

6.   Check for movement and sensation in limbs (particularly legs, with spinal anesthesia).

7.   Watch for cyanosis.

8.   Be sure dressings are intact and there is no excessive drainage.

✦ **Phase II Surgical Unit**

A.   Assessment.

1.   Maintain patent airway; administer oxygen as necessary, monitor SaO_2.

2.   Take vital signs—usual orders are VS q 15 minutes until stable; then q 30 minutes × 2, q hour × 4; then q 4 hours for 24–48 hours.

3.   Check IV site and patency frequently.

4.   Observe and record urine output.

5.   Keep accurate records of intake and output.

6.   Observe skin color and moisture.

✦ B.   Nursing care.

1.   Position patient for comfort and maximum airway ventilation.

2.   Turn q 2 hours and PRN—avoid sharply bent knees and hips for good alignment.

3.   Apply elastic stockings and compression device, if ordered.

4.   Encourage coughing and deep breathing every 2 hours.

5.   Keep patient comfortable with pain medications.

6.   Check dressings and drainage tubes q 2–4 hours unless abnormal amount of drainage; then, more frequently.

7.   Give oral hygiene at least q 4 hours; q 2 hours if NG tube, nasal oxygen, or endotracheal tube inserted.

8.   Bathe patient when temperature can be maintained—bathing removes the antiseptic solution and stimulates circulation.

9.   Keep patient warm and avoid chilling, but do not increase temperature above normal.

a.   Increased temperature increases metabolic rate and need for oxygen.

b.   Excessive perspiration causes fluid and electrolyte loss.

10.   Irrigate NG tube q 2 hours and PRN with normal saline to keep patent.

11.   Maintain dietary intake—type of diet depends on type and extent of surgical procedure.

a.   Minor surgical conditions—the patient may drink or eat as soon as he or she is awake and desires food or drink.

b.   Major surgical conditions.

(1)   NPO until bowel sounds return.

(2)   Clear liquid advanced to full liquid as tolerated.

(3)   Soft diet advanced to full diet within 3–5 days (depending on type of surgery and physician's preference).

12.   Place on bedpan 2–4 hours postoperatively if catheter not inserted.

Postoperative Medications

✦ **Narcotic Analgesics**

A.   Pharmacological action—reduces pain and restlessness.

B.   General side effects.

1.   Drowsiness.

2.   Euphoria.

3.   Sleep.

4.   Respiratory depression.

5.   Nausea and vomiting.

C.   Types of analgesics.

1.   Opiates.

a.   Morphine sulfate—potent analgesic.

(1)   Specific side effects: miosis (pinpoint pupils); bradycardia.

(2)   Usual dosage: ¼–⅙ gr IM q 3–4 hours PRN.

b.   Codeine sulfate—mild analgesic.

(1)   Specific side effects: constipation.

(2)   Usual dosage: 30–60 mg q 3–4 hours IM.

c.   Hydromorphone HCl (Dilaudid)—potent analgesic.

(1)   Specific side effects: hypotension, constipation, euphoria.

(2)   Usual dosage: 2–4 mg PO, IM, or IV q 4–6 hours.

d.   Oxymorphone HCl (Numorphan)—potent analgesic.

(1)   Specific side effects: urinary retention, ileus, euphoria.

(2)   Usual dosage: 1–1.5 mg IM q 4–6 hours; 0.5 mg IV q 4–6 hours.

e. Hydrocodone (Vicodin)—potent analgesic.
   (1) Specific side effects: dizziness, drowsiness, sedation, nausea.
   (2) Usual dosage: 10 mg orally every 3–4 hours.
f. Oxycodone HCL (OxyContin) is also Percocet (with acetaminophen) and Percodan (with aspirin).
   (1) Potent opioid analgesic that is very addictive—especially with high, long-term use.
   (2) Usual dosage: 10–80 mg orally.

2. Synthetic opiatelike drugs.
   a. Meperidine HCl (Demerol)—potent analgesic—not commonly used as of 2000.
      (1) Specific side effects: miosis or mydriasis (dilation of pupils); hypotension; tachycardia.
      (2) Usual dosage: 25–100 mg q 3–4 hours IM.
   b. Pentazocine HCl (Talwin)—potent analgesic.
      (1) Specific side effects: gastrointestinal disturbances, vertigo, headache, and euphoria.
      (2) Usual dosage: 50 mg oral tablets q 3–4 hours; 30 mg IM q 3–4 hours PRN.

✦ **Antiemetics**

A. Pharmacological action.
   1. Reduces the hyperactive reflex of the stomach.
   2. Makes the chemoreceptor trigger zone of medulla less sensitive to nerve impulses passing through this center to the vomiting center.
B. General side effects.
   1. Drowsiness.
   2. Dry mouth.
   3. Nervous system effects.
C. Common drugs.
   1. Phenothiazines.
      a. Compazine (prochlorperazine).
         (1) Specific side effects: amenorrhea, hypotension, and vertigo.
         (2) Normal dosage: 5–10 mg q 3–4 hours IM.
      b. Phenergan (promethazine).
         (1) Specific side effects.
            (a) Dryness of mouth.
            (b) Blurred vision.
         (2) Normal dosage: 12.5–50 mg q 4 hours PRN.
   2. Nonphenothiazines.
      a. Dramamine (dimenhydrinate).
         (1) Specific side effects: drowsiness.
         (2) Normal dosage: 50 mg IM q 3 to 4 hours.

b. Tigan (trimethobenzamide).
   (1) Specific side effects (rare).
      (a) Hypotension.
      (b) Skin rashes.
   (2) Normal dosage: 200 mg (2 mL) TID or QID IM.

COMMON POSTOPERATIVE COMPLICATIONS

Respiratory Complications

✦ A. Goal is to maintain pulmonary ventilation so that hypoxemia (deficient oxygen in blood) is prevented.
✦ B. Nursing preventive interventions.
   1. Turn, cough, hyperventilate; encourage deep breathing every 2 hours.
   2. Removal of pooled secretions.
      a. Pharyngeal suctioning required if patient cannot cough up and expectorate secretions.
      b. Endotracheal suctioning usually not required—if ordered, hyperventilate patient with 100% oxygen before and after each suctioning procedure.
C. Mechanical interventions (provide a means of forced-expiration exercise).
   1. Incentive spirometer—promotes lung expansion.
   2. Peak flow measurement.
   3. CPAP/BIPAP—positive pressure application to prevent obstruction of upper airways.
D. Pharmacological therapy (through nebulization or oral route).
   1. Antibiotics—to fight infection by causative organism.
   2. Bronchodilators—to act on smooth muscle to reduce bronchial spasm.
      a. Sympathomimetics (beta$_2$ agonists preferred).
      b. Theophylline (aminophylline).
      c. Anticholinergics (atropine sulfate inhalant).
   3. Adrenocorticosteroids—to reduce inflammation (Prednisone).
   4. Enzymes—to liquefy thick, purulent secretions through digestion.
      a. Dornavac.
      b. Varidase.
   5. Expectorants—to aid in expectoration of secretions.
      a. Mucolytic agents reduce viscosity of secretion (Mucomyst).
      b. Detergents liquefy tenacious mucus (Tergemist, Alevaire).

✦ General Signs and Symptoms

A. Complaint of tightness or fullness in chest.
B. Cough, dyspnea, or shortness of breath.
C. Increased vital signs, particularly temperature and respiratory rate.
D. Restlessness.

✦ Common Respiratory Conditions

A. Pneumonia (see section in respiratory system).
B. Atelectasis, collapse of pulmonary alveoli, caused by mucous plug or by inadequate ventilation.
C. Signs and symptoms.
   1. Asymmetrical chest movement.
   2. Decreased or absent breath sounds over affected area.
   3. Shortness of breath leading to cyanosis.
   4. Painful respirations.
   5. Increased vital signs: temperature, respiration, pulse.
   6. Anxiety and restlessness.

Implementation

A. Encourage coughing and deep breathing exercises; splint incision.
B. Turn frequently and position to facilitate expectoration.
C. Suction as necessary.
D. Instruct in proper use of mechanical measures (blow bottles, etc.).
E. Do clapping, percussion, vibration, postural drainage, every 4 hours.
F. Encourage oral fluid intake to reduce tenacious sputum and to facilitate expectoration.
G. Administer expectorants and other medications as ordered.
H. Place patient in cool room with mist mask or vaporized steam.
I. Administer oxygen if necessary.
J. Mobilize patient as soon as possible.
K. Auscultate breath sounds every 2–4 hours and report unusual occurrences.

Deep Vein Thrombophlebitis (DVT)

Definition: Thrombophlebitis is the formation of a clot in a vein. It occurs most often in deep veins of lower extremities and pelvis.

✦ Etiology

A. Impaired venous flow—stasis.
   1. Dehydration leading to increased cellular components in vessel.
   2. Periods of inactivity such as prolonged bedrest, plane trips, or car rides.
B. Decreased blood flow due to hypothermia and/or decreased metabolic rate during surgery.
C. Injury to vessel during surgery.
D. Malignancy, polycythemia, use of oral contraceptive agents.

✦ Assessment

A. Red, tender, painful calf.
B. Edema of affected leg.
C. Increased temperature in affected area as well as generalized elevation of temperature.
D. Homan's sign not recommended (may mobilize clot) or reliable.

✦ Implementation

A. Maintain strict bedrest—3–4 days.
B. Do not use knee gatch or pillows under knees.
C. Elevate lower extremities 20 degrees; if ordered, raise entire foot of bed.
D. Administer anticoagulants only after checking lab values.
   1. Heparin therapy 7–10 days.
   2. Coumadin for 3 months.
   3. Dose adjusted to keep INR between 2.0–3.0.
E. Check for extension of clot or pulmonary embolism.
   1. Check breath sounds for possible pulmonary emboli.
      a. Cough; rapid, shallow respirations; dyspnea.
      b. Chest pain; tachycardia.
   2. Check extremity involved for extension of signs (tenderness further up leg, etc.), especially in groin.
   3. Check for circulatory difficulties.
F. Position patient to avoid venous stasis, and turn every 2 hours.
G. Take vital signs at least every 4 hours.
H. Use range-of-motion exercises on unaffected limbs only.
I. Do not massage or exercise affected leg unless specified by physician.
J. Apply antiembolic stockings to unaffected leg.
K. Begin exercise gradually with leg-raises to standing briefly every hour, then ambulation.
L. Monitor *intermittent external pneumatic compression* to the legs if applied.

✦ Patient Instruction

A. Avoid standing in one position for any length of time (when exercise program instituted, patients are told to either walk or to lie flat).
B. Avoid wearing constrictive clothing or garments.
C. Keep extremities at consistent, moderate temperature.
D. Wear support hose consistently.
E. Understand correct use of anticoagulants and the necessity for lab tests.
F. Teach prevention—avoid sitting in chair for long periods, elevate foot of bed, do leg and ankle exercises.

Wound Infections

Etiology
A. Usual causative agents.
 1. *Staphylococcus.*
 2. *Pseudomonas aeruginosa.*
 3. *Proteus vulgaris.*
 4. *Escherichia coli.*
B. Usually occur within 3–7 days of surgery.

✦ Assessment
A. Slowly increasing temperature (> 100.4°F) tachypnea and tachycardia.
B. Pain and tenderness surrounding surgical site.
C. Edema and erythema surrounding suture site.
D. Increased warmth around suture site.
E. Purulent drainage.
 1. Yellow if *Staphylococcus.*
 2. Green if *Pseudomonas.*
F. Increased white blood cell count.

✦ Implementation
A. Administer specific antibiotics based on culture for causative agent.
B. For grossly infected wounds, irrigate with solution as ordered (usually normal saline or Ringer's).
C. Keep dressing and skin area dry to prevent skin excoriation and spread of bacteria.
✦ D. Use meticulous handwashing and gloving (standard precautions). CDC is still recommending sterile technique in changing dressings.
E. If excoriation occurs, use karaya powder and drainage bags around area of wound.
✦ F. Changing dressings.
 1. Wet-to-moist—*Purpose:* To maintain a moist environment and prevent damage to granulating tissue.
  a. Cover wound with second moist (normal saline) dressing.
  b. Remove dressing while still damp.
 2. Dressings for pressure ulcers.
  a. Op-Site, Tegaderm or DuoDerm—moist environment to promote autolysis, protect new tissue, and assist with debridement.
  b. Covers ulcer with moisture-retentive dressings—transparent adhesive film or hydrocolloid dressing.
  c. Dressing changed every 5–7 days unless draining.

Wound Dehiscence and Evisceration

✦ *Definition: Dehiscence* is the splitting open of wound edges. *Evisceration* is the extensive loss of clear or serosanguineous fluid (purulent if infection is present) through a wound and the protrusion of a loop of bowel through an open wound. Patient feels as though "everything is pulling apart."

Etiology
A. Usual causes.
 1. General debilitation.
  a. Poor nutrition.
  b. Chronic illness.
  c. Obesity.
 2. Inadequate wound closure (usually during first 3 days).
 3. Wound infection or dehydration.
 4. Severe abdominal stretching (by coughing or vomiting).
✦ B. Occurs about seventh postoperative day.

Implementation
A. Assist patient to lie in supine position.
✦ B. Cover protruding intestine with moist, sterile, normal saline packs; change packs frequently to keep moist.
C. Notify physician.
D. Take vital signs for baseline data and detection of shock.
✦ E. Apply abdominal scultetus binder following dehiscence (preventative measure in obese or debilitated patients).

Pulmonary Embolism

Definition: A clot flowing through the heart into pulmonary circulation where it occludes a pulmonary vessel.

✦ Assessment
✦ A. Sudden sharp stabbing pain in chest.
B. Shortness of breath (dyspnea) most common symptom.
C. Cyanosis.
D. Increased pulse and respirations.
E. Hypotension—symptoms of shock.
F. Distended neck veins caused by congestive heart failure.
G. Decreased breath sounds.
H. Arrhythmias.
I. Anxiety.

✦ Implementation
✦ A. Provide patent airway.
 1. Position in semi- to high-Fowler's position if vital signs allow.
 2. Administer oxygen as needed.
 3. Assist with intubation as needed.
 4. Auscultate breath sounds every 1–2 hours.
 5. Obtain arterial blood gases to ascertain acid–base imbalance.
 6. Check sputum for presence of blood or blood-tinged mucus.
 7. May administer diuretics or cardiotonics.

(Continues on p. 84)

◆ **Table 4-6. POSTOPERATIVE COMPLICATIONS**

Potential Complication	Clients at Risk	Indicative Findings

Atelectasis: collapse of alveoli; may be diffuse and involve a segment, lobe, or entire lung
 	
Potential Onset:
First 48 hours
	All with general anesthesia
	Special risk clients:
	Smokers
	Chronic bronchitis
	Emphysema
	Obesity
	Elderly
	Upper abdominal surgery
	Chest surgery
	Abdominal distention
		Fever to 102°F
		Tachycardia
		Restlessness
		Tachypnea 24–30 minutes
		Altered breath sounds
		    Dullness to percussion
		    Diminished or absent breath sounds
		Crackles
		ABGs: decreased PaO_2

Pneumonia: inflammatory process in which alveoli are filled with exudate
 	
Potential onset:
First 36–48 hours
	Clients with unresolved atelectasis
	Following aspiration
	Smokers
	Elderly
	Chronic bronchitis
	Emphysema
	Heart failure
	Debilitated
	Alcoholic
	Immobile
	Cough suppressant medications
	Respiratory depressant medications
		Client complains of dyspnea; tachycardia; increasing temperature; productive cough, and increasing amount of sputum becoming tenacious, rusty or purulent
		Tactile fremitus
		Dullness to percussion
		Bronchial breath sounds
		Increased crackles or rhonchi
		Voice sounds present
		    Bronchophony
		        Egophony
		            Whispered pectoriloquy
		ABGs: decreased PaO_2

Pulmonary embolism: foreign object has migrated to branch of pulmonary artery *Potential onset:* Seventh to tenth day *Massive embolism:* Pulmonary hypertension, dyspnea, right heart failure, shock, ABGs: decreased PaO_2, increased $PaCO_2$	Superficial vein thrombosis: rare Deep vein thrombosis: 40 to 60 percent Air emboli: intraperitoneal surgery Fat emboli: long bone fracture, split sternum	Only 10% recognized clinically Pain sharp and stabbing, occurs with breathing, localized (right lower lobe most frequent) Marked shortness of breath Increased heart rate—tachycardia Restlessness and other symptoms of hypoxia (severe anxiety)
Pulmonary infarction: necrosis of lung tissue due to occlusion of blood supply (less than 10% develop) *Potential onset:* 2–72 hours after arterial obstruction	Pulmonary embolism	Hemoptysis Cough Fever 101°–102°F Pleural friction rub Pleuritic pain
Thrombophlebitis: inflammation of vein with clot formation *Potential onset:* Seventh to fourteenth day	*Abnormal vein walls:* Varicose veins Previous thrombophlebitis Trauma to vein wall Tight strap on operating room table Surgery on hips or in pelvis Age over 60 years (arteriosclerosis) *Venous stasis:* Immobility, long duration surgery Casts, restrictive dressings Constant Fowler's position Prolonged dependent lower extremities Knee gatch elevated Pillows under knees, calves Obesity Abdominal distention Shock Heart failure *Hypercoagulability:* Surgical stress response Anesthesia Decreased circulation Hypovolemia, dehydration	Superficial vein thrombophlebitis: Pain, redness, tenderness, and induration along course of vein Palpable "cord" corresponding to course of vein History of trauma including IV site *Deep small vein thrombophlebitis:* Increased muscle turgor and tenderness over affected vein Deep muscle tenderness Most frequent site: vessels at calf Affected limb warm to touch with occasional swelling Client complains of tightness or stiffness in affected leg Positive Homan's sign (dorsiflexion of foot leads to calf pain) Fever rarely more than 101°F *Major deep vein thrombophlebitis:* No superficial signs of inflammation Homan's sign unreliable *Femoral vein thrombosis:* Pain and tenderness in distal thigh

Prevention	Intervention	Drug Therapy

Preoperative: Have client practice turning, coughing, and deep breathing
Discuss importance of exercises
Postoperative clients at risk:
   Turn every 30 minutes
   Deep breathe and cough
Other clients:
   Initiate turning and deep breathing exercises every 1–2 hours
Ambulate as soon as possible
Medicate to reduce pain, splinting and resistance to treatment
	Deep breathing and incentive spirometry
	Administer supplemental oxygen as ordered
	Monitor response to treatment
	Monitor for onset of pneumonia
	If entire lobe of lung is involved, prepare for bronchoscopy to remove plug
	Change position q2h
		Analgesics: pain control
		Bronchodilators (nebulized through IPPB); liquefy secretions
		Water or saline (nebulized through IPPB): liquefy secretions

Provide vigorous treatment of atelectasis Prevent aspiration	Turn, cough and deep breathe every 1 hour May need to stimulate cough with nasotracheal suctioning Send sputum for culture and sensitivity Frequent mouth care for comfort Administer oxygen as ordered Increase fluid intake Monitor for response to treatment	Antibiotics: Cephalosporin or ampicillin prophylactically for 48 hours for high risk clients Cephalosporin IV or parenteral for infections Antipyretics: decrease temperature
Provide range of motion Encourage early ambulation Prevent thrombophlebitis Do not massage an area with potential for or suspected thrombus Elastic stockings or leg compression devices	Administer oxygen to relieve hypoxia Reduce anxiety Position client on left side with head dependent to prevent air embolus Prevent recurrent embolization; prepare for fibrinolysis; prepare for anticoagulation Prepare for x-ray, angiography, and/or ventilation/perfusion scan Encourage adequate hydration	Anticoagulation therapy: IV heparin to maintain therapeutic APTT Sodium prophylactically for high risk clients Urokinase, t-PA, streptokinase: thrombolytic effect (24 hours) Analgesics: pleuritic pain control
Prevent thromboembolic pulmonary artery occlusion *See* prevention of thrombophlebitis	Describe indicative findings to physician Institute relaxation techniques to decrease client's anxiety Administer oxygen Support and comfort client	Antibiotics: prevention of infection
Avoid injury to vein wall: Use care when strapping to operating room table Avoid IVs in lower extremities Pad siderails for restless, convulsive, and/or combative client Avoid restraints *Avoid venous stasis:* Encourage early ambulation Provide feet and leg exercises Elastic stockings; sequential-compression devices Increase frequency of exercise for client at risk Prevent client's sitting with legs in dependent position Place pillow between legs while client is lying on side to prevent pressure from upper leg on lower Provide deep breathing exercises Provide active and passive range of motion Increase velocity of blood flow: No standing	*Superficial vein thrombophlebitis:* Treat symptoms Continue ambulation unless accompanied by deep venous involvement Monitor for progression toward saphenafemoral junction (may need ligation) *Deep vein thrombophlebitis:* Provide adequate bedrest Elastic stockings Sequential-compression devices Elevate foot of bed with 6–8-inch blocks Administer warm moist compresses to relieve venospasm and help resolve inflammation Monitor for pulmonary embolism	Streptokinase: thrombolytic effect (24 hours) Heparin IV or sub q: decrease clotting time (short-term) Nonorthopedic surgery—low-dose sub q heparin (or low-molecular-weight heparin) Coumadin PO: decrease clotting time (long-term) Analgesics: pain control Low-molecular-weight dextran IV on operative day and 2 days postoperative Aspirin 1.2 g/day in divided doses

(Continued)

✦ **Table 4-6. POSTOPERATIVE COMPLICATIONS** *(Continued)*

Potential Complication	Clients at Risk	Indicative Findings
Thrombophlebitis *(continued)*	Malignant neoplasms Postpartum Insert rectal tube	and popliteal region Swelling extends to level of knee Oral contraceptives

Ileus: failure of peristalsis
 	
Potential onset:
First 24–36 hours
	All surgical clients
	Stress response to surgical trauma
		No bowel sounds or fewer than
		  5/min (normal: 5–35 clicks or
		  gurgles/min)
		Vomiting
		Abdominal distention

Paralytic ileus: paralysis of
  intestinal peristalsis
 	
Potential onset:
First 3–4 days
	Intraperitoneal surgery
	Peritonitis
	Kidney surgery
	Decreased cardiac output
	Pneumonia
	Electrolyte imbalance
	Wound infection
		No bowel sounds
		Abdominal distention
		No passage of flatus or feces
		Nasogastric drainage green to
		  yellow, 1 to 2 L in 24 hours
		Anorexia, nausea
		Complaints of fullness and diffuse pain

Intestinal obstruction:
  adhesions, trap or kink in
  segment of intestine
Potential onset:
Third to fifth day
The lower the obstruction the
  more gradual the onset
	Abdominal surgery	No postoperative bowel movement
		Abdominal distention
		Client complains of periodic sharp, colicky pains
		Hyperactive, high-pitched, tinkling
		  bowel sounds
		Abdominal tenderness
		Nasogastric drainage: dark brown or black

Urinary tract infection
 	
Potential onset:
Third to fifth day or 48 hours after
  removal of catheter
	Decreased resistance:
	History of bladder distention
	History of urinary retention
	Previous urinary tract infection
	History of prostatic hypertrophy
	History of catheterization
	Diabetic
	Debilitated
	Immobile
		Dysuria
		Frequency
		Urgency
		High fever: up to 104°F with fewer systemic
		  toxic symptoms than would be expected
		Change in urine odor
		Pus in urine
		Sediment
		May be asymptomatic

Wound infection
 	
Potential onset:
Streptococcal: 24–48 hours after
  contamination
Staphylococcus gram-negative rods,
  etc.: 5–7 days postoperatively
	Slow to heal:
	Obese
	Diabetic
	
	Poor nutrition:
	Debilitated
	Elderly
	Ulcerative colitis
	
	Poor circulation:
	Elderly
	Hypovolemic
	Heart failure
	Lack of oxygen to wound:
	Vasoconstriction
	Severe anemia
	Depressed immunity
	Cancer
	Renal failure
	Preoperative steroid therapy
	Prolonged complex surgery (stress
	  response leading to increased ACTH)
	Malnutrition
	Elderly
	At risk for transmission
	Proximity of another client with
	  infection
	Transmission by hands of personnel
		Initial inflammation: 36–48 hours
		Wound tender, swollen, warm,
		  increased redness
		Increasing heart rate
		Increasing temperature (100.4°F or more)
		Increasing or recurring serous drainage;
		  drainage becomes purulent, foul odor
		There may be no local signs if infection
		  is deep
		Elevated WBC
		Malaise

Prevention	Intervention	Drug Therapy

Steady IV flow
Antiembolic stockings (controversial)
Decrease hypercoagulability:
   Provide adequate hydration
   Prevent infections
   Maintain circulation
   Decrease stress/anxiety		

Do not feed until bowel sounds return Offer only sips of water until return of bowel sounds Maintain normal serum potassium level	Monitor for return of normal bowel sounds (enteral feeding following non-GI surgeries will resolve ileus faster) Monitor for distention Monitor for passage of flatus signaling return of peristalsis Monitor signs of hypokalemia	Switch to nonopioid analgesic (opioids slow GI motility), NSAIDs and acetaminophen
Maintain electrolyte balance, especially potassium Maintain cardiac output Prevent pneumonia Provide early ambulation	Treat cause Maintain nasogastric suction until peristalsis returns Monitor for intestinal obstruction	Potassium chloride if serum level is low Dexpanthenol (Ilopan) to stimulate return of peristalsis total parenteral nutrition (TPN) if indicated
None	Identify condition early Report to physician immediately Reduce client anxiety Maintain patent nasogastric tube Prepare for insertion of intestinal tube Prepare for surgery if necessary	Antibiotic therapy: for prevention of infection (optional) Analgesics: pain control Never give laxative or purgative if obstruction is suspected
Maintain sterile technique with catheterization and catheter removal Provide competent indwelling catheter care Encourage early ambulation to decrease retention and stasis	Encourage fluid intake; cranberry juice to decrease urine pH Increase activity to enhance bladder emptying Encourage voiding every 2 hours while awake Send specimen for culture and sensitivity Monitor for residual urine of more than 100 mL	Urinary antiseptics (sulfonamides); bacterial suppression Antibiotics (ampicillin, tetracycline); bacterial suppression Anticholinergics: antispasmodic Topical urinary analgesic: pain relief
Practice meticulous handwashing and gloving Practice aseptic technique in wound care Separate from infected clients Use special caution for a new wound, easily contaminated Maintain nutrition Provide frequent turning Ambulate as soon as possible Maintain PaO_2 Increase attention to prevention for clients with depressed immunity Operative site: clip excess hair and cleanse with povidone-iodine (reduces bacterial counts)	Maintain nutrition Maintain oxygenation Maintain circulation and blood volume Maintain pulmonary toilet Cleanse wound or irrigate as ordered Apply wet-to-moist dressings Monitor for systemic response to infection, fever, malaise, headache, anorexia, nausea Treat symptoms	Administer antibiotics as ordered New cyanoacrylate adhesives (Dermabond, Indermil) close wounds and promote healing Send wound drainage specimen for culture and sensitivity

B. Administer anticoagulants (as ordered) following initial anticoagulation (check lab values each day before administering medication).

C. Take vital signs every 2–4 hours.

D. Turn as directed by physician; do not do percussion or clapping or administer back rubs.

E. Encourage patient to cough and deep breathe every 1–2 hours.

F. Give emotional support.

G. Observe for possible extension of emboli or occurrence of other emboli.

1. Check urine for hematuria or oliguria.

2. Check legs, especially calf.

Fat Embolism

Definition: A type of embolism caused by fat droplets released into the bloodstream.

✦ Etiology

A. Embolism occurs after long bone fractures (particularly from mishandling or incorrect splinting of fractures).

B. Fat droplets are released from the marrow and enter circulation. They usually lodge in the lungs. If they lodge in the brain, the embolism is severe and sometimes fatal.

C. Fat emboli usually occur within the first 24 hours following an injury.

Assessment

✦ A. Classical sign: petechiae across chest, shoulders, and axilla; can also involve conjuctiva.

✦ B. Related pulmonary signs: shortness of breath leading to pallor, cyanosis, and hypoxemia.

C. Diaphoresis.

D. Tachycardia without apparent cause.

E. Change in level of consciousness; shock.

✦ Implementation

A. Position patient in high-Fowler's position to allow for respiratory exchange.

B. Administer oxygen to decrease anoxia and to reduce surface tension of fat globules.

C. Obtain arterial blood gases to maintain sufficient PO_2 levels.

D. Intubate and place on respirator if respirations are severely compromised.

E. Institute preventative treatment to avoid further complications—shock and heart failure.

F. Monitor administration of medications.

1. Alcohol drip.

2. Cortisone therapy to reduce inflammation.

3. Decholin to emulsify fat.

4. Antihyperlipidemic drugs.

ORGAN DONATION

✦ A. Legal aspects of donation.

1. The federal Omnibus Budget Reconciliation Act of 1986 states that all facilities receiving Medicare or Medicaid funding must have policies in place to identify potential organ donors and to inform families about the option to donate.

✦ a. Laws do not require the consent of a family member to retrieve organs if the donor has already declared his wish to donate (must be 18 years of age or older).

✦ b. Choice to donate an organ must be a written document—a donor card, a will, or an advanced directive signed by the patient.

✦ c. Providers are reluctant to act without a family member's permission because of fear of being sued.

✦ d. Some states have limited the family's involvement in the donation process.

2. Legal definition of death.

a. Death is defined legally as cardiac death—total failure of cardiopulmonary system *or*

b. Neurological or brain death—unresponsive to all stimuli, fixed pupils and no brain stem reflexes.

✦ 3. Hospitals are required by law to contact donor team so they may give families the information they need to make an informed decision about organ donation.

4. The Uniform Anatomical Gift Act protects those who are involved in organ procurement from liability, but provider must "act in good faith" and must provide next of kin with complete and accurate information.

✦ B. Allocating organs.

1. United Network for Organ Sharing—patients awaiting transplant (heart or kidney) are assigned priority according to medical need. (Currently there is a waiting list of more than 80,000 for organs.)

2. Ethical question—should more desperately ill receive preference or should priority be given to healthier patients? The answer varies according to facility.

C. Organ donor potential.

1. Review specific facility's death criteria.

2. Generally accepted criteria—brain death.

a. Cause of patient's injury known.

b. Exhibits no brain stem reflexes.

c. No CNS depressants present.

d. Temperature greater than 90°F.

e. Exhibits no spontaneous responses.

f. Unresponsive to noxious stimuli.

REHABILITATIVE NURSING

Definition: The process of restoring a person's ability to live and work in as normal a manner as possible after a disabling injury.

General Principles

Goals

A. Strive for optimal function.
B. Prevent further injury or complications.
C. Restore normal function.
D. Accept philosophy underlying rehabilitative nursing.
  1. Rehabilitation begins with initial contact.
  2. Every illness has intrinsic threat of disability.
  3. Principles of rehabilitation are basic to care of all patients.

✦ Effects of Disability

A. Impact upon the individual's body image.
  1. Physical appearance.
  2. Bodily sensations.
B. Behavior during reaction period.
  1. Appears confused and disorganized.
  2. Denies disability exists.
  3. Overreacts to situations and physical condition.
  4. Assumes false positive attitude.
  5. Becomes self-centered.
  6. Becomes depressed.
  7. Mourns loss of function or body part.
C. Adaptation and adjustment.
  1. Revises body image by modifying former picture of self.
  2. Reorganizes values.
  3. Accepts degree of dependency.
  4. Accepts limitations imposed by disability.
  5. Begins to develop realistic goals.
D. Success in adjusting to a disability depends on:
  1. Individual's prior personality, life experiences, and family relationships.
  2. Person's current behavior and motivation, attitudes, and acceptance.
  3. Comprehensive care from the provider and teamwork.

Duties of the Rehabilitative Nurse

Assessment

A. Specific source of disability or impaired mobility.
B. Presence of accompanying disease state: arthritis, stroke, dementia, diabetes, congestive heart failure (CHF), COPD.
C. Strength and function of limbs and joints.
D. Stability of gait.
E. Presence of pain.
F. Condition of skin.
G. Drug effects—sedation, incontinence, orthostatic hypotension.
H. Motivation for rehabilitation.
I. Nutritional status.
J. History of falls.

Implementation

A. Assist in developing nursing care plan to meet patient's needs.
B. Provide direct nursing care.
C. Establish supportive relationship.
✦ D. Teach activities of daily living (ADLs).
  1. Activities that must be accomplished each day in order for the individual to care for his or her own needs.
  2. Assist in patient evaluation.
    a. Medical condition.
    b. Functional capacity.
    c. Therapeutic goal.
    d. Family background.
    e. Educational background.
  3. Assist in ascertaining best method for completing ADLs for patient.
  4. Demonstrate and encourage individual to practice.
  5. Increase activities as individual progresses and is able to assume activity.
  6. Give positive reinforcement for all effort expended.
E. Record and report nursing observations.
F. Evaluate nursing care plan and alter as necessary.
G. Assist in developing discharge plan.

Prevention of Deformities and Complications

✦ A. Specific nursing actions.
  ✦ 1. Turn and position in good alignment.
    a. Prevent contractures.
    b. Stimulate circulation.
    c. Prevent thrombophlebitis.
    d. Prevent pressure ulcers.
  2. Prevent edema of extremities.
  3. Promote lung expansion.
✦ B. Types of exercises (see Chapter 13, page 402).

Types of Exercise for Rehabilitation

A. Passive.
  1. Carried out by the therapist or nurse without assistance from patient.
  2. Purpose—retain as much joint range of motion as possible, and maintain circulation.
B. Active assistive.
  1. Carried out by the patient with assistance of therapist or nurse.
  2. Purpose—encourage normal muscle function.
C. Active.
  1. Accomplished by the individual without assistance.

2. Purpose—increase muscle strength.
D. Resistive.
   1. Active exercise carried out by the individual working against resistance produced by manual or mechanical means.
   2. Purpose—provide resistance in order to increase muscle power.
E. Isometric or muscle setting.
   1. Performed by the individual without assistance.
   2. Prrpose—maintain strength in a muscle when a joint is immobilized.
F. Range of motion (ROM).
   1. Movement of a joint through its full range in all appropriate planes.
   2. Purpose—maintain joint mobility and increase maximal motion of a joint.
   3. Nursing care.
      a. Assess general condition of patient.
      b. Establish extent of ROM before present condition.
      c. Discontinue ROM at point of pain.
   4. Deterrents to ROM exercises: fear and pain.

✦ **Use of Aids/Devices**
A. Cane.
   1. Purpose.
      a. Provide greater stability and speed when walking.
      b. Relieve pressure on weight-bearing joints.
      c. Provide force to push or pull body forward.
   ✦ 2. Safety factors.
      a. Handle at level of greater trochanter.
      b. Elbow flexed at 25–30-degree angle.
      c. Lightweight material.
      d. Rubber suction tip.
   3. Techniques for walking with cane.
      a. Hold cane close to the body.
      b. Hold in hand on unaffected side.
      c. Move cane at same time as affected leg.
B. Crutches.
   1. Purpose—provide support during ambulating when lower extremities unable to support body weight.
   2. Safety factors.
      ✦ a. Measure 1½ to 2 inches from axillary fold to floor (4 inches in front and 6 inches to side of toes).
      b. Hand piece adjusted to allow 30 degree elbow flexion.
      c. Rubber suction tips on crutches.
      d. Well-fitting shoes with nonslip soles.
   3. *See* gait sequence on page 329.
C. Tilt table.
   1. Board or table that can be tilted gradually from a horizontal to a vertical position.

2. Purpose.
   a. Assist individual to gradually adjust to upright position.
   b. Start weight-bearing activities.
   c. Increase standing tolerance.
   d. Prevent disuse syndrome.
   e. Prevent demineralization of bones.
D. Prosthesis—artificial replacement for a missing body part.
E. Brace—support that protects or supports weakened muscles.

Common Problems from Immobility

Pressure Ulcers

A. Localized areas of necrosis of skin and subcutaneous tissue due to pressure.
✦ B. Cause—pressure exerted on skin and subcutaneous tissue by bony prominences and the object on which the body rests.
C. Predisposing factors.
   1. Malnutrition.
   2. Anemia.
   3. Hypoproteinemia.
   4. Vitamin deficiency.
   5. Edema.
✦ D. Common sites: bony prominences of body such as sacrum, greater trochanter, heels, elbows, etc.
E. Prevention.
   1. Relieve or remove pressure—avoid massaging bony prominences which can lead to deep tissue trama.
      a. Keep bony prominences from direct contact with one another.
      b. Use pillow, foam wedges, elbow pads and heel elevators.
   2. Stimulate circulation—reposition every 2 hours.
   3. Keep skin dry and free of drainage.
   4. Promote adequate diet of protein, calories and nutrients—promote fluid intake.
   5. Place at-risk patients on pressure-reducing devices, i.e., special mattress.
✦ F. Nursing care.
   1. Encourage patient to keep active.
   2. Change position frequently—every 2 hours.
   3. Maintain good skin hygiene—individualize patient's bathing schedule.
   4. Provide for active and/or passive exercises.
   5. Ambulate whenever possible.
   6. Use alternating air pressure mattress, etc., or sheepskin padding.
   7. Inspect skin daily.
   8. Provide for adequate nutritional intake—high protein, calorie and nutrient supplements.

✦ G. Treatment protocol.
1. Stage 1—adhesive film dressing (Op-Site, Bioclusive, or Tegaderm).
2. Stage 2—transparent adhesive film dressing —if wound is draining, irrigate with normal saline and apply hydrocolloid dressing (Duo-Derm).
3. Stage 3—irrigate with normal saline and cover with hydrocolloid dressing.
4. Stage 4—chemical debridement by dressing changes (physician will do surgery or debridement). Wet-to-damp dressing used.

External Rotation of Hip

A. Outward rotation of the hip joint.
B. Cause—lying for long periods of time on back without support to hips or incorrect positioning in bed.
✦ C. Prevention.
1. Trochanter roll extending from crest of ilium to midthigh when positioned on back.
2. Frequent change of position.
3. Proper positioning.

Footdrop

A. A falling or dragging of the foot from tendency to plantar flex—occurs when flexors of the ankle are paralyzed.
B. Causes.
1. Prolonged bedrest.
2. Lack of exercise.
3. Weight of bedclothes forcing toes into plantar flexion.
C. Complications.
1. Individual will walk on his toes without touching heel on ground.
2. Unable to walk.
✦ D. Prevention.
1. Use of special boot, high-top sneakers, or positioning feet against footboard.
2. Use footcradle to keep weight of top linen off toes.
3. Provide range-of-motion exercises.

Contractures

A. Abnormal shortening of muscle, tendon, or ligament so joint cannot function properly.
B. Cause—improper alignment, lack of movement.
✦ C. Prevention.
1. Properly align at all times.
a. Use pillows.
b. Provide supportive splints.
2. Provide for range-of-motion exercises.

Bladder Dysfunction

A. Cause.
1. Disease process.
2. Lack of innervation.
3. Lack of motivation.
✦ B. Bladder training.
1. Purpose.
a. Prevent urinary tract infection and preserve renal function.
b. Keep individual dry and odor free.
c. Help individual maintain social acceptance.
✦ 2. Nursing care. ❖ **PROCEDURE** ❖
a. Set up specific time to empty bladder.
b. Give measured amounts of fluids.
c. Position in normal voiding position.
d. Instruct to Credé bladder.
e. Keep record of amount and time of intake and output.
f. Encourage patient to wear own clothing, particularly underwear.

Bowel Dysfunction

A. Cause.
1. Disease process.
2. Inadequate intake.
3. Poor prior habits.
B. Bowel training.
✦ 1. Purpose.
a. Develop regular bowel habits.
b. Prevent fecal incontinence, impaction, and/or irregularity.
✦ 2. Nursing care. ❖ **PROCEDURE** ❖
a. Establish specific time.
b. Provide for adequate roughage and fluid intake.
c. Use normal posture.
d. Instruct to bear down and contract abdominal muscles.
e. Provide privacy and time.
f. Provide exercise.

Hypostatic Pneumonia

A. Incidence.
1. Very young, very old.
2. Debilitated.
3. Immobile.
B. Cause—stasis of secretions in lungs.
✦ C. Prevention.
1. Assess lung function.
2. Encourage deep breathing, coughing.
3. Turn every 2 hours.
4. Provide for postural drainage, if indicated.
5. Ensure adequate hydration.

GENERAL NURSING CONCEPTS QUESTIONS

1. The nurse understands that it is important to obtain baseline vital signs for her patient preoperatively in order to

   1. Establish a baseline postoperatively.
   2. Inform the anesthetist so he can administer appropriate preanesthesia medication.
   3. Judge the patient's recovery from the effects of surgery and anesthesia when taking postoperative vital signs.
   4. Prevent operative hypotension.

2. A patient has just arrived at the recovery room from surgery. The priority in data collection is to

   1. Assess the patient's need for oxygen.
   2. Check the gag reflex.
   3. Assess vital signs.
   4. Assess airway for patency.

3. Following surgery, a patient has an IV of D_5W to run 50 mL/hr. When the nurse checks his condition for the evening shift, she realizes the IV is 1 hour behind. The first action would be to

   1. Increase the flow rate to make up for the loss within the next 2–3 hours.
   2. Continue IV flow at the same rate.
   3. Increase the flow so that the loss is made up over the remaining hours in the day.
   4. Notify the physician for new orders to decrease the 24-hour total fluid intake.

4. A patient has sustained multiple injuries and fractures in a motor vehicle accident (MVA). During which period would the nurse be most vigilant in observing for the development of a fat embolism?

   1. During the first 24–48 hours after the MVA.
   2. 72–96 hours after the MVA.
   3. During the first week after the MVA.
   4. During the second week after the MVA.

5. One of the duties of the rehabilitative nurse is to teach the activities of daily living (ADLs) to a patient about to be discharged. One of the most important nursing interventions to accomplish these goals is to

   1. Ask if the patient has someone who can help him/her at home.
   2. Determine the best method for the patient to perform the ADLs.
   3. Demonstrate and encourage the patient and then give positive reinforcement.
   4. Record and report the results of the teaching.

6. The nurse responsible for administering a thiazide medication to a patient evaluates his recent lab reports, which are K^+ 3.0 and NA^+ 140. The nurse would

   1. Administer the thiazide drug.
   2. Notify the physician.
   3. Withhold the drug and have the lab repeat the tests.
   4. Withhold the drug and report K^+ level to the physician.

7. The LVN's primary responsibility in monitoring IV therapy is to

   1. Frequently check that the flow of solution is according to the amount ordered.
   2. Check to see that the IV remains open.
   3. Record accurate IV intake for the shift.
   4. Change the IV site every 24 hours to prevent collapse of the vein.

8. While monitoring a patient's blood transfusion, the nurse determines that a hemolysis reaction is occurring. The first nursing intervention is to

   1. Slow down the transfusion.
   2. Administer IV Benadryl.
   3. Stop the transfusion.
   4. Notify the physician.

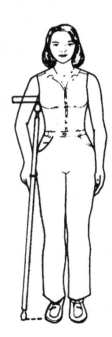

9. When assisting a patient to measure for crutches, you will measure _____ fingerbreadths distance from the axilla to the crutch bar.

10. Following an angry outburst the previous evening, a patient says, "I'm feeling calmer now. I don't know what got into me. You all must think I'm crazy." The best response to this statement would be

    1. "That's all right. We're here to help you."

2. "Why would you think that?"
3. "You think your behavior was crazy?"
4. "How were you feeling last evening?"

11. The patient paces the floor, wringing her hands saying, "Something is going to happen. Help me! Help me!" The nurse says, "You look very upset." The nurse is using the technique of

   1. Giving feedback.
   2. Being reassuring.
   3. Validating a nonverbal observation.
   4. Seeking clarification.

12. The best rationale for the nurse introducing her- or himself to a blind patient and telling him exactly what care will be administered is to

   1. Illustrate the principle of open communication.
   2. Decrease the patient's anxiety and fear of the unknown.
   3. Follow steps for beginning a nurse–patient relationship.
   4. Encourage and utilize clear communication.

13. Assessing the patient following abdominal surgery, the nurse observes pinkish fluid and a loop of bowel through an opening in the incision. The first nursing action is to

   1. Notify the physician.
   2. Notify the operating room for wound closure.
   3. Cover the protruding bowel with a moist, sterile, normal saline dressing.
   4. Apply butterfly tapes to the incision area.

14. Assessing a patient who has developed atelectasis postoperatively, the nurse will be most likely to find

   1. A flushed face.
   2. Dyspnea and pain.
   3. Decreased temperature.
   4. Severe cough with no pain.

15. When completing the preop check list, the patient asks the nurse, "What exactly am I going to have done in surgery?" The appropriate response is

   1. To explain the procedure in nonmedical terms to the patient.
   2. Ask the patient what the physician explained to him.
   3. Check the chart to see what the physician explained and repeat the information to him.
   4. Explain that you don't know and he should ask the physician when he sees him before surgery.

16. The physician tells a patient that he will need exploratory surgery the next day. As the RN and PN determine the preoperative teaching plan, which one of the following interventions is most important?

   1. Answer questions the patient has about his condition or the forthcoming surgery.
   2. Explain the routine preoperative procedures: NPO, shower, medication, shave, etc.
   3. Describe the surgery and what the patient will experience following surgery.
   4. Assure the patient there is nothing to worry about because the physician is very experienced.

17. A patient scheduled for surgery is given a spinal anesthetic. Immediately following the injection, the nurse will position the patient

   1. On his abdomen.
   2. In semi-Fowler's position.
   3. In slight Trendelenburg's position.
   4. On his back or side; head raised.

18. Following spinal anesthesia, a patient is brought into the recovery room. During the initial data collection, which sign or symptom indicates a complication of anesthesia has developed?

   1. Hiccoughs.
   2. Numbness in legs.
   3. Headache.
   4. No urge to void.

19. The nurse is assigned to closely observe a patient for signs of magnesium toxicity following an IV of 4 g magnesium sulfate in 250 mL D_5W. The first indication of this condition is

   1. Decreased urine output.
   2. Peripheral vasodilation.
   3. Extreme thirst.
   4. Change in Babinski reflex.

20. A patient's IV is to run at 125 mL/hr. The IV administration set delivers 20 gtts/mL. At what rate will the nurse adjust the IV?

   1. 21 gtts/min.
   2. 31 gtts/min.
   3. 41 gtts/min.
   4. 125 gtts/min.

21. Pain is now considered the 5th vital sign according to JCAHO. For a patient who is in pain, this change would be important because

   1. The nurse is now responsible for monitoring a patient's pain level.
   2. It helps to maintain the patient's quality of life.

3. As a vital sign it will now be monitored every 15 minutes.
4. The patient's pain level was often ignored by the nursing staff.

22. The most effective method of evaluating a patient's pain level is to

   1. Ask the patient where he feels the pain.
   2. Select a tool to measure pain based on the patient's preferences and cognitive level.
   3. Observe the nonverbal cues to pain level.
   4. Determine if the pain medication ordered is actually taking care of the patient's pain.

23. You are assigned a patient with the diagnosis of intracranial pressure. Physician's orders include an IV of hypertonic solution, dextrose 10% in saline. What is your understanding of the rationale for using this solution?

   1. It reduces edema of the brain.
   2. It provides needed fluid to maintain adequate intake and output balance.

3. This solution causes cells to expand or increase in size.
4. It expands extracellular volume.

24. You are making a home visit to a patient who has the diagnosis of cardiac heart failure and is on daily diuretics. Considering the possibility of potassium deficiency, you will assess for

   1. Pitting edema and excessive weight gain.
   2. Muscle weakness, leg cramps, nausea and fatigue.
   3. Increased blood pressure and dyspnea.
   4. Oliguria, restlessness, weakness and hyperpnea.

25. You are assigned to care for a bedridden patient and one of your nursing goals is to prevent pressure ulcers from developing. The priority nursing action would be to

   1. Massage bony prominences that are reddened.
   2. Provide for active and passive exercises.
   3. Reposition the patient every 2 hours.
   4. Keep the skin moist and supple.

GENERAL NURSING CONCEPTS

Answers and Rationales

1. (3) It is important to have presurgery vital signs so that the patient's progress can be monitored to ensure that his postoperative condition is stable. A baseline (1) is completed presurgery for evaluation postsurgery.

   NP:D; CN:PH; CA:S; CL:C

2. (4) The priority assessment is to determine if the airway is patent. All of the other nursing actions will follow this assessment: need for oxygen, gag reflex, and vital signs.

   NP:D; CN:PH; CA:S; CL:A

3. (3) The loss should be made up over the remaining hours of the day. The nurse would not want to overhydrate the patient by making up the loss too fast.

   NP:I; CN:PH; CA:S; CL:AN

4. (1) Approximately 85 percent of cases of fat embolism occur within 48 hours of injury, making this the most critical time for monitoring the patient for manifestations of this complication.

   NP:D; CN:PH; CA:S; CL:A

5. (3) One of the most important principles of teaching is to demonstrate the activity, encourage the patient to perform, and then give positive reinforcement. It is important that the patient learn to do these activities him- or herself (1). Determining the best method is important (2), but if answer (3) is done, it will encompass this activity and therefore is a more inclusive answer.

   NP:I; CN:H; CA:M; CL:A

6. (4) The appropriate intervention is to withhold the thiazide medication (until the nurse receives further orders) and report the K^+ level to the physician. Normal K^+ is 3.5–5.5 mEq/L. His NA^+ level is normal (range 135–145 mEq/L).

   NP:I; CN:PH; CA:M; CL:AN

7. (1) Frequent checking of the IV flow is the best answer because it would include checking that the IV remains open. Recording (3) is important, but not totally the LVN's responsibility. The IV site is changed (4) every 48–72 hours.

   NP:I; CN:S; CA:M; CL:C

8. (3) The first action would be to stop the transfusion to avoid administering any additional incompatible cells. The incompatible cells can lead to agglutination, oliguric renal failure, pulmonary emboli, and death if administered in large quantities. Some resources state that as little as 50 mL of incompatible blood can lead to severe complications and death.

   NP:I; CN:PH; CA:M; CL:A

9. The answer is 2—two finderbreadths should be between the axilla and the crutch bar. Crutches that do not fit correctly or crutches that are used incorrectly can damage the bracial plexus and cause paralysis.

   NP:I; CN:PS; CA:S; CL:A

10. (4) The patient is encouraged to express his feelings. This may lead to further discussion of the patient's reactions to his own feelings when he feels threatened. Answers (2) and (3) are incorrect and focus on the intellectual aspect of this reaction. Answer (1) is incorrect because it does not encourage the patient to express his feelings and explore his behavior.

    NP:I; CN:PS; CA:PS; CL:A

11. (3) The nurse is sharing her observations and validating that the patient looks and sounds upset, rather than asking for feedback or clarification. This technique may open communication so that the patient can verbalize the fears and be more specific about the kind of help that is needed.

    NP:D; CN:PS; CA:PS; CL:C

Coding for Questions/Answers Abbreviations: **Nursing Process: NP,** Data Collection: D, Planning: P, Implementation: I, Evaluation: E, **Client Needs: CN,** Safe, Effective Care Environment: S, Health Promotion and Maintenance: H, Psychosocial Integrity: PS, Physiological Integrity: PH, **Clinical Area: CA,** Medical Nursing: M, Surgical Nursing: S, Maternal/Newborn Nursing: MA, Pediatric Nursing: P, Psychiatric Nursing: PS, **Cognitive Level: CL,** Knowledge: K, Comprehension: C, Application: A, Analysis: AN

12. (2)   Blind patients become anxious when they hear someone enter the room without talking. The other rationales are not valid for this situation.

NP:P; CN:PS; CA:M; CL:C

13. (3)   The first nursing action, before notifying the physician (1), is to cover the open wound. Evisceration will eventually have to be closed in the operating room (2), but this is a later step. Butterfly tapes would be applied to the wound area (4) to prevent further dehiscence.

NP:I; CN:PH; CA:S; CL:A

14. (2)   Atelectasis is a collapse of the alveoli due to obstruction or hypoventilation. Patients become short of breath, have a high temperature, and usually experience severe pain but do not have a severe cough. The shortness of breath is a result of decreased oxygen–carbon dioxide exchange at the alveolar level.

NP:D; CN:PH; CA:M; CL:C

15. (2)   Find out exactly what the patient has been told. Many times, the patient has been given an explanation and only needs further clarification. If the patient does not have an adequate understanding of the procedure, have the charge nurse notify the physician that he needs to see the patient. The physician has the legal duty to inform the patient about procedures.

NP:I; CN:PS; CA:S; CL:A

16. (1)   It is most important to begin at the patient's level of understanding, so answering questions is more essential than giving explanations (2) until the patient is ready to listen. Describing the surgery (3) is not the nurse's responsibility, and giving false reassurance by assuring the patient there is nothing to worry about (4) is nontherapeutic.

NP:P; CN:PS; CA:S; CL:C

17. (3)   Usually, the patient is positioned on the back following the injection. If a high level of anesthesia is desired, the head and shoulders can be lowered to slight Trendelenburg's. After 20 minutes the anesthetic is set, and the patient can be positioned in any manner.

NP:I; CN:PH; CA:S; CL:A

18. (3)   When spinal fluid is lost through a leak or the patient is dehydrated, a severe headache can occur, which may last several days. Numbness (2) and no urge to void (4) would be expected with spinal anesthesia unless it continues for several hours postop.

The complication of hiccoughs (1) can be associated with abdominal surgery, but is not attributable to spinal anesthesia.

NP:D; CN:PH; CA:S; CL:A

19. (3)   The first sign that the nurse will observe is probably extreme thirst. There will also be a loss of the patellar, not the Babinski (4), reflex. There will also be decreased urine output (1); however, this may be a later sign.

NP:E; CN:PH; CA:MA; CL:A

20. (3)   The general formula to complete this calculation is:

$$\frac{\text{Volume infused} \times \text{drops/mL}}{\text{Time for infusing in minutes}} = \text{Drops/min}$$

$$\frac{125 \times 20}{60} = 41 \text{ Drops/min}$$

NP:I; CN:S; CA:M; CL:C

21. (2)   As a 5th vital sign, pain will be monitored as often as the vital signs which will help to maintain the patient's quality of life. (1) the nurse has always been responsible for monitoring the pain level. Pain does not have to be monitored every 15 minutes (3). A patient's pain level has not been ignored but this additional reminder will assist the nurse to monitor pain more frequently.

NP:P; CH:H; CA:M; CL:A

22. (2)   The most effective way to measure pain is with a scale (either zero to five or zero to ten) that the patient can understand. This allows the evaluation to be consistent over time. Just asking the patient will not yield enough data (1), nor will observing nonverbal cues. This measure will be helpful with a young child or cognitively impaired adult. Just evaluating the pain medication is not an accurate measure for pain control.

NP:E; CH:PH; CA:M; CL:A

23. (1)   Hypertonic solutions are solutions with higher osmotic pressure than blood serum. It is used for intracranial pressure because it reduces edema by rapid movement of fluid out of the ventricles into the bloodstream. Option (2) describes a hypotonic solution which causes cells to expand or increase in size (3). Isotonic solutions expand excellular volume.

NP:P; CN:PH; CA:M; CL:C

24. (2)   Thiazide diuretics are potent anti-hypertensives, but may lead to electrolyte imbalance and

loss of potassium. The symptoms you would assess for are muscle weakness, leg cramps, hypotension and even arrhythmias. Options (1) and (3) are sodium excess symptoms and option (4) is potassium excess.

NP:D; CN:PH; CA:M; CL:A

25. (3) The most important intervention to stimulate circulation and prevent ulcers is to change the patient's position every two hours. It is no longer accepted practice to massage bony prominences because it can lead to deep tissue trauma (1). Option (2) is important, but not the priority intervention. The skin should be kept dry and free of drainage (4).

NP:I; CN:S; CA:M; CL:A

Pharmacology

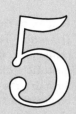

PHARMACOLOGICAL CONCEPTS

Drug Metabolism

Stages of Metabolism

Definition: Drug metabolism in the human body is accomplished in four basic stages—absorption, transportation, biotransformation, and excretion. In order for a drug to be completely metabolized, it must first be given in sufficient concentration to produce the desired effect on body tissues. When this critical drug concentration level is achieved, body tissues change.

A. Absorption.
   1. The first stage of metabolism refers to the route a drug takes from the time it enters the body until it is absorbed in the circulating fluids.
   ✦ 2. Drugs are absorbed by the mucous membranes, the gastrointestinal tract, the respiratory tract, and the skin.
      a. The mucous membranes are one of the most rapid and effective routes of absorption because they are highly vascular.
      b. Drugs are absorbed through these membranes.
   3. Drugs given by mouth are absorbed in the gastrointestinal tract.
      a. Portions of these drugs dissolve and absorb in the stomach.
      b. Drugs are enteric-coated to prevent absorption in the stomach.
      c. The rate of absorption depends on the pH of the stomach's contents, the food content in the stomach at the time of ingestion, and the presence of disease conditions.
      d. Most of the drug concentrate dissolves in the small intestine where the large vascular surface and moderate pH level enhance the process of dissolution.
   4. Methods of administration include intradermal, subcutaneous, intravenous, and intra-arterial injections.
      a. Parenteral methods are the most direct, reliable, and rapid route of absorption.
      b. The actual administration site will depend on type of drug, its action, and the patient.
   5. Another route of administration is inhalation or nebulization through the respiratory system.
      a. This method is not as rapid as parenteral injections but faster than the gastrointestinal tract.
      b. Drugs administered through the respiratory tract must be made up of small particles that can pass through to the alveoli in the lungs.
   6. The final mode of absorption is the skin.
      a. Most drugs, when applied to the skin, produce a local rather than a systemic effect.
      b. The degree of absorption will depend on the strength of the drug as well as where it is applied on the body surface.
✦ B. Distribution.
   1. The second stage of metabolism refers to the way in which a drug is transported from the site of introduction to the site of action.
   2. First, a drug enters or is absorbed by the body.
      a. Drug is transported through circulation to all parts of the body.
      b. If drug binds to plasma protein, it is not effective.
   3. As a drug moves from the circulatory system, it crosses cell membranes and enters the body tissues.
      a. Some of the drug is distributed to and stored in fat and muscle.
      b. Greater masses of tissue (such as fat and muscle) attract the drug.
   4. The amount of drug that is distributed to body tissues depends on the permeability of the membranes and the blood supply to the absorption area.
   5. A drug that first accumulates in the brain may move into fat and muscle tissue and then back to the brain because the drug is still chemically active.
      a. The drug is released in small quantities from the tissues and travels back to the brain.
      b. Equal drug and blood concentration levels in the body are maintained.
✦ C. Metabolism.
   1. The third stage of metabolism takes place as the drug, a foreign substance in the body, is converted by enzymes into a less active and harmless agent that can be easily excreted.
   ✦ 2. Most of this conversion occurs in the liver.
      a. Both synthetic and biochemical reactions take place.
      b. Some conversion does take place in the kidney, plasma, and intestinal mucosa.
   3. Synthetic reactions: liver enzymes conjugate the drug with other substances to make it less harmful for the body.
   4. Biochemical reactions: drugs are oxidized, reduced, hydrolyzed, and synthesized so they become less active and more easily eliminated from the body.
✦ D. Excretion.
   1. The final stage in metabolism takes place when the drug is changed into an inactive form or excreted from the body.

2. The kidneys are the most important route of excretion.

3. The kidneys eliminate both the pure drug and the metabolites of the parent drug.
    a. During excretion these two substances are filtered through the glomeruli.
    b. They are then secreted by the tubules.
    c. Finally, they are reabsorbed through the tubules or directly excreted.

4. Other routes of excretion include the lungs (which exhale gaseous drugs), feces, saliva, tears, and mother's milk.

Factors That Affect Drug Metabolism

A. Personal attributes.
   1. Body weight.
   2. Age.
   3. Sex.
B. Physiological factors.
   1. State of health.
   2. Disease processes.
C. Acid–base and fluid and electrolyte balance.
D. Permeability.
E. Diurnal rhythm.
F. Circulatory capability.
G. Genetic and immunologic factors.
H. Drug tolerance.
I. Cumulation effect of drugs.
J. Other factors.
   1. Psychological.
   2. Emotional.
   3. Environmental.
K. Responses to drugs vary.
   1. Responses depend on the speed with which the drug is absorbed into the blood or tissues.
   2. Responses depend on the effectiveness of the body's circulatory system.

Factors That Affect Drug Absorption

✦ A. Absorption factors.
   1. Solubility of the drug.
   2. Route of administration:oral, sub q, topical, sublingual, or IM.
   3. Patient's sex, age, and health status.
      a. Females absorb IM injections slower than males because they have increased adipose tissue and a smaller blood supply.
      b. Older patients respond more slowly—often related to lower gastric acid in the stomach.
      c. Certain diseases decrease tissue perfusion.
✦ B. Distribution factors.
   1. Cardiac output and circulation influence how the drug reaches the target tissues.
   2. If drug is attached to serum proteins and the protein level is low, there would be more free drug in the bloodstream; this condition

indicates that dosages should be decreased with certain drugs (warfarin, Dilantin, and barbiturates).

3. Drug half-life is the time it takes for a half-dose of the drug to be eliminated from the body.
    a. Four to 5 half-lives are required to reach a steady state of equilibrium in the bloodstream.
    b. For a blood sample to reflect therapeutic action of a drug, there must be a half-life times 4 or 5.

✦ C. Patients with impaired liver function or liver disease may lose much of the therapeutic value of the drug.
   1. Drugs that pass through the liver (called first-pass effect) before being absorbed into the bloodstream may be affected by the liver status.
   2. Certain drugs that go from the GI tract to the portal vein to the liver may need to have their oral dosages adjusted upward to compensate for partial deactivation (lidocaine, morphine, propranolol, verapamil).
D. Kidneys also play a role in drug absorption—depends on tissue perfusion, disease, and urinary pH.
   1. Renal disease interferes with renal clearance, and drugs (potassium chloride or digoxin) can reach toxic levels in the bloodstream.
   2. The more alkaline the urine, the faster certain drugs are excreted (salicylates, barbiturates, and sulfonamides). Sodium bicarbonate will make urine more alkaline.
   3. Some drugs are excreted faster when urine is acidic (amphetamines and ephedrine). Vitamin C will make urine more acidic.

Origin and Naming of Drugs

Common Sources

A. Plant sources.
   1. Roots, bark, sap, leaves, flowers, and seeds from medicinal plants can be used as drug components.
   2. Component substances.
      a. Alkaloid.
         (1) Alkaline (base) in reaction.
         (2) Bitter in taste.
         (3) Physiologically powerful in activity.
      b. Glycoside: a compound containing a carbohydrate molecule.
      c. Resin: soluble in alcohol; insoluble in water.
      d. Gum.
         (1) Mucilaginous (gelatinlike) excretion.
         (2) Used in bulk laxatives; may absorb water.

(3) Used in skin preparations as a soothing effect, e.g., karaya gum.

    e. Oil.

       (1) Fixed oil: does not evaporate on
warming; occurs as a solid, semisolid, or liquid, e.g., castor oil.

       (2) Volatile oil: evaporates readily;
occurs in aromatic plants, e.g., pep-
permint.

B. Animal sources.

  1. Processed from an organ, from organ
secretion, or from organ cells.

  2. Insulin, as an example, is a derivative from
the pancreas of sheep, cattle, or hogs.

C. Mineral sources.

  1. Inorganic elements occurring in nature, but
not of plant or animal origin; may be metallic
or nonmetallic.

  2. Usually form a base or acid salt in food.

  3. Dilute hydrochloric acid (HCl), as an
example, is diluted in water and then taken
through a straw to prevent damage to teeth
by acid.

D. Synthetic sources.

  1. A pure drug made in a laboratory from chemical, not natural, substances.

  2. Many drugs, sulfonamides for example, are
synthetics.

Methods of Naming Drugs

A. Chemical name.

  1. Precise description of chemical constituents
with the exact placement of atom groupings.

  2. "N-methyl-4-carbethoxypiperidine hydrochloride" is an example of a chemical name.

B. Generic name.

  1. Reflects chemical name to which drug
belongs, but is simpler.

  2. It is never changed and used commonly in
medical terminology.

  3. The synthetic narcotic meperidine is an
example of a generic name.

C. Trademark name (brand name, proprietary
name).

  1. Appears in literature with the sign ®, e.g.,
Demerol®.

  2. The sign indicates the name is registered; use
of the name is restricted to the manufacturer
who is the legal owner.

  3. Trademark name is capitalized or shown in
parentheses if generic name stated.

Drug Classification

◆ **Classification by Action**

A. Anti-infectives.

  1. Antiseptics.

    a. Action—inhibit growth of
microorganisms (bacteriostatic).

    b. Purpose—application to wounds and skin
infections, sterilization of equipment,
and hygienic purposes.

  2. Disinfectants.

    a. Action—destroy microorganisms (bacteri-
cidal).

    b. Purpose—destroy bacteria on inanimate
objects (not appropriate for living tissue).

B. Antimicrobials.

  1. Sulfonamides.

    a. Action—inhibit the growth of
microorganisms.

    b. Reduce or prevent infectious process,
especially for urinary tract infections.

  2. Antibiotics (e.g., penicillin).

    a. Action—interfere with microorganism
metabolism.

    b. Usage—reduce or prevent infectious
process.

    c. Specific drug and dosage based on
culture and sensitivity of organism.

C. Metabolic drugs.

  1. Hormones obtained from animal sources,
found naturally in foods and plants.

  2. Synthetic hormones.

D. Diagnostic materials.

  1. Action—dyes and opaque materials ingested
or injected to allow visualization of internal
organs.

  2. Purpose—to analyze organ status and function.

E. Vitamins and minerals.

  1. Action—necessary to obtain healthy body
function.

  2. Found naturally in food or through synthetic
food supplements.

F. Vaccines and serums.

  1. Action—prevent disease or detect presence of
disease.

  2. Types.

    a. Antigenics produce active immunity.

      (1) Vaccines—attenuated suspensions of
microorganisms.

      (2) Toxoids—products of microorganisms.

    b. Antibodies—stimulated by
microorganisms or their products.

      (1) Antitoxins.

      (2) Immune serum globulin.

    c. Allergens—agents for skin immunity
tests.

      (1) Extracts of materials known to be
allergenic.

      (2) Can be used to relieve allergies.

    d. Antivenins—substances which neutralize
venom of certain snakes and spiders.

G. Antifungals—check growth of fungi.

H. Antihistaminics.
1. Action—prevent histamine action.
2. Purpose—relieve symptoms of allergic reaction.
I. Antineoplastics—prevent growth and spread of malignant cells.

Classification by Body Systems

CENTRAL NERVOUS SYSTEM

A. Drugs affect CNS by either inhibiting or promoting the actions of neural pathways centers.
   ✦ 1. Action promoting drug groups (stimulants).
      a. Antidepressants—psychic energizers used to treat depression.
      b. Caffeine—increases mental activity and lessens drowsiness.
      c. Ammonia—used as revival from fainting spell (patient smells cap, not contents of bottle).
   ✦ 2. Action inhibiting drug groups (depressants).
      a. Analgesics—reduce pain by interfering with conduction of nerve impulses.
         (1) Narcotic analgesics—opium derivatives may depress respiratory centers; must be used with caution and respiratory rate above 12.
            (a) A narcotic antagonist drug counteracts depressant drugs.
            (b) Such antagonist drugs are Lorfan, Narcan, and Nalline.
         (2) Nonnarcotic antipyretics—reduce fever and relieve pain.
         (3) Antirheumatics—analgesics given to relieve arthritis pain; may reduce joint inflammation.
      b. Alcohol—stimulates appetite when given in small doses but classified as a depressant.
      c. Hypnotics—sedatives that induce sleep; common form is the barbiturates.
      d. Antispasmodics—relieve skeletal muscle spasms; anticonvulsants prevent muscle spasms or convulsions.
      e. Tranquilizers.
         (1) Relieve tension and anxiety, preoperative and postoperative apprehension, headaches, menstrual tension, chronic alcoholism, skeletal muscle spasticity, and other neuromuscular disorders.
         (2) Tranquilizers and analgesics frequently given together (in reduced dosage); the one drug enhances the action of the other (synergy).
      f. Anesthetics—produce the state of unconsciousness painlessly.

   ✦ B. Precautions to be taken with CNS drugs.
      1. Drugs that act on CNS may potentiate other CNS drugs.
      2. Patient may be receiving other medications; find out drug name and dosage.
      3. Dependence on CNS drugs may occur.

AUTONOMIC NERVOUS SYSTEM

A. This system governs several body functions so that drugs that affect the ANS will at the same time affect other system functions.
B. The ANS is made up of two nerve systems—the sympathetic and parasympathetic.
   1. Parasympathetic is the stabilizing system.
   2 Sympathetic is the protective emergency system.
C. Each system has a separate basic drug group acting on it.
   ✦ 1. Adrenergics—mimic the actions of sympathetic system.
      a. Vasoconstrictors—stimulants such as Adrenalin.
         (1) Action is to constrict peripheral blood vessels, thereby increasing blood pressure.
         (2) Dilate bronchial passages.
         (3) Relax gastrointestinal tract.
      b. Vasodilators—depressants such as nicotinic acid.
         (1) Antagonists of epinephrine and similar drugs.
         (2) Vasodilate blood vessels.
         (3) Increase tone of GI tract.
         (4) Reduce blood pressure.
         (5) Relax smooth muscles.
         (6) *Caution:* If drug is to be stopped, reduce dosage gradually over a period of a week; do not stop it suddenly.
   ✦ 2. Cholinergics—mimic actions of parasympathetic system.
      a. Cholinergic stimulants (e.g., Prostigmin or neostigmine).
         (1) Decrease heart rate.
         (2) Contract smooth muscle.
         (3) Contract pupil in eye.
         (4) Increase peristalsis.
         (5) Increase gland secretions.
      b. Cholinergic inhibitors (anticholinergics).
         (1) Decrease gland secretion.
         (2) Relax smooth muscle.
         (3) Dilate pupil in eye.
         (4) Increase heart action.

GASTROINTESTINAL SYSTEM

A. Drugs affecting GI system act upon muscular and glandular tissues.

✦ B. Antacids—have alkaline base to counteract excess acidity.
  1. Used in the treatment of ulcers.
  2. Neutralize hydrochloric acid in the stomach.
  3. Given frequently (2-hour intervals or more often).
  4. May cause constipation, depending on type of medication.
  5. Baking soda is a systemic antacid which disturbs the pH balance in the body. Most other antacids coat the mucous membrane and neutralize hydrochloric acid.
  6. May contain calcium, but not useful as a calcium supplement because this nutrient is best absorbed in an acidic environment.
C. Emetics—produce vomiting (emesis).
D. Antiemetics—prevent vomiting or nausea but may cause drowsiness.
E. Digestants—relieve enzyme deficiency by replacing secretions in digestive tract.
F. Antidiarrheals—prevent diarrhea.
✦ G. Cathartics—affect intestine and produce defecation.
  1. Provide temporary relief for constipation.
  2. Rid bowel of contents before surgery, and prepare viscera for diagnostic studies.
  3. Counteract edema.
  4. Treat diseases of GI tract.
  5. Contraindicated when abdominal pain is present.
  6. Classifications.
    a. By degree of action.
      (1) Laxative—mild action.
      (2) Cathartic—moderate action.
      (3) Purgative—severe action.
    b. By method of action.
      (1) Increase bulk.
      (2) Lubricate mechanically.
      (3) Irritate chemically.
      (4) Increase or decrease water content with saline.
      (5) Disperse detergent or wetting agent.

RESPIRATORY SYSTEM

A. Drugs act on respiratory tract, tissues, and cough center.
✦ B. Action is to suppress, relax, liquefy, and stimulate.
  1. Respiratory stimulants stimulate depth and rate of respiration.
  ✦ 2. Bronchodilators relax smooth muscle of trachea and bronchi.
    a. Sympathomimetics taken PO or inhaled (fewer side effects); theophylline PO; aminophylline IV.
    b. Beta$_2$ agonists (Albuterol) are preferred drugs.

✦ 3. Anticholinergics (atropine sulfate) given by nebulizer or metered dose inhaler.
✦ 4. Anti-inflammatory agents to reduce bronchospasms: corticosteroids or mast cell inhibitor (cromolyn sodium).
  5. Drug groups that provide cough relief.
    a. Antitussive agents (narcotic, nonnarcotic).
      (1) Sedatives prevent cough.
      (2) Not to be accompanied by water.
    b. Demulcents soothe respiratory tract.
    c. Expectorants liquefy bronchial secretions and increase amount of excretions in respiratory tract.

URINARY SYSTEM

A. Drugs that act on kidneys and urinary tract.
B. Action is to increase urine flow, destroy bacteria, and perform other important body functions.
✦ 1. Diuretics.
    a. Rid body of excess fluid and relieve edema.
    b. Some drugs that act on the GI tract and circulatory system also are diuretic in action.
  2. Urinary antiseptics.
  3. Acidifiers and alkalinizers—certain foods also increase body acids or alkalies.

CIRCULATORY SYSTEM

A. Drugs that act on heart, blood, and blood vessels.
B. Action is to change heart rhythm, rate, and force (altering blood flow), and to dilate or constrict vessels.
✦ 1. Cardiotonics used for heart-strengthening.
    a. Direct heart stimulants that speed heart rate, e.g., caffeine, Adrenalin.
    b. Indirect heart stimulants, e.g., digitalis.
      (1) Stimulate vagus nerve.
      (2) Slow heart rate and strengthen it.
      (3) Improve heart action, thereby improving circulation.
      (4) Do not administer if apical pulse < 60.
✦ 2. Antiarrhythmic drugs used clinically to convert irregularities to a normal sinus rhythm.
    a. Monitor constantly with ECG when administering these drugs.
    b. Quinidine used for its vasodepressor action.
      (1) Slows impulse of sinoauricular node.
      (2) Slows heart rate.
      (3) Side effects include ringing in ears.
✦ 3. Drugs that alter blood flow.
    a. Anticoagulants—inhibit blood clotting action (heparin, Coumadin).
    b. Coagulants—maintain blood fluidity.
    c. Thrombolytic agents (streptokinase, urokinase).

d. Platelet-inhibiting agents (aspirin, dipyridamole).

e. Vasodilators.

4. Blood replacement.

Dosage and Preparation

Solids

A. Extract—obtained by dissolving drug in water or alcohol and allowing solution to evaporate; residue is the extract.

B. Powder—finely ground drugs.

C. Pills—common term for tablet; made by rolling drug and binder into a sphere.

D. Suppository.
   1. Contains drugs mixed with a firm base.
   2. Liquefies at body temperature when inserted into orifice.
   3. Releases drug to produce a local or systemic effect.

E. Ointment—semisolid mixture of drugs with a fatty base.

F. Lozenge—flavored flat tablet that releases drug slowly when held in mouth.

G. Capsule.
   1. Drugs in small, cylindrical gelatin containers that disguise the taste of the drug.
   2. Capsule can be opened and drug mixed with food or jam to mask taste.

H. Tablets.
   1. Dried, powdered drugs that are compressed into a small disk that easily disintegrates in water.
   2. Enteric coated—tablet does not dissolve until reaching intestines, where release of drug occurs.

Liquids

A. Fluid extract.
   1. Concentrated fluid preparation of drugs produced by dissolving crude plant drug in a solvent.
   2. Strength of extract is such that 1 mL (about ¼ teaspoon or 15–16 gtt) represents 1 g of the drug at 100 percent strength.

B. Tincture.
   1. Diluted alcoholic extract of a drug.
   2. Varies in strength from 10–20 percent.

C. Spirit—preparation of volatile (easily vaporized) substances dissolved in alcohol.

D. Syrup—drug contained in a concentrated sugar solution.

E. Elixir—solution of drug made with alcohol, sugar, and some aromatic or pleasant-smelling substance.

F. Suspension.
   1. Undissolved, finely divided particles of drug dispersed in a liquid.
   2. Gels and magma are other forms of suspensions.
   3. Shake all bottles of suspension well before giving.

G. Emulsion—suspension of unmixed oils, fats, or petrolatum in water.

H. Liniment and lotion—liquid suspension of medication applied to the skin.

Packaging Methods and Dispensing

A. Unit dosage package method.
   1. Package contains premeasured amount of drug in proper form for administering.
   2. Pharmacy may deliver to the unit the daily needs for each patient.
   3. Procedures for delivery and storage vary from hospital to hospital.
   4. Nurse administers the medication to the patient.

B. Traditional method.
   1. Nurse prepares medication on the unit.
   2. Supplies come from stock or bulk on the ward or from a multiple dose bottle of patient's.

✦ C. The nurse is responsible for accuracy of the medication given, regardless of the packaging or dispensing method used.

Routes of Administration

Oral Route

A. Ingested (swallowed).

B. Sublingual (under tongue).

C. Buccal (on mucous membrane of cheek or tongue).

Rectal Route

A. Suppository.

B. Liquid (retention enema).

Parenteral Route (Figures 5-1 through 5-5)

✦ A. Intravenous.
   1. The response is fast and immediate.
   2. Over 5 mL medication can be given.
   3. Drug *must* be given slowly and usually in diluted form.
   4. Check medication leaflets to determine if medication route is IM or IV. *Note: Intravenous regulation procedure found in Chapter 4.*

✦ B. Intradermal.
   1. Injected into skin; usual site is inner aspect of forearm or scapular area of back.
   2. A short bevel 26-gauge, 1-cm needle is used.
   3. Needle should be inserted with bevel up.
   4. This route is usually used to inject antigens for skin or tuberculin tests.
   5. Amount injected ranges from 0.01–0.1 mL.

✦ C. Subcutaneous.
   1. A 25-gauge, 1.3- to 1.6-cm needle is used.

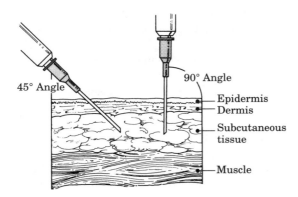

Fig. 5-1 Insert needle at 45- or 90-degree angle for subcutaneous injection. Insert needle at 15-degree angle under the epidermis for intradermal injection.

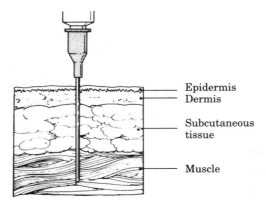

Fig. 5-2 Insert needle at 90-degree angle and deep into muscle tissue for intramuscular injection.

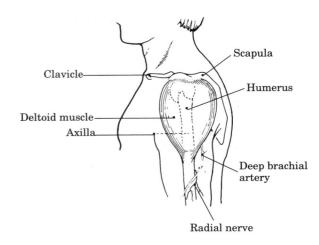

Fig. 5-3 Inject no more than 2 mL solution IM into deltoid muscle.

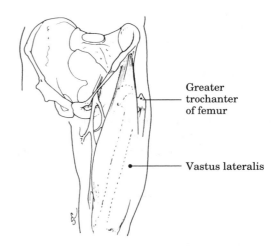

Fig. 5-4 Anatomic frontal view of thigh for intramuscular injection.

2. Injection site is the fatty layer under skin.
    a. Abdomen at navel.
    b. Lateral upper arm or thigh.
3. This route usually used for injecting medication that is to be absorbed slowly with a sustained effect.
4. Amount injected ranges from 0.5–1.5 mL.
5. If repeated doses are necessary, as with insulin for a diabetic person, rotate the injection sites.

✦ D. Intramuscular.
1. Needle gauge and length will vary with site.
    a. Deltoid—located by having patient raise arm.
        (1) A 23- to 25-gauge, 1.6- to 2.5-cm needle is used.
        (2) Administer no more than 2 mL.
    b. Thigh and buttock.
        (1) Needle must be long enough to reach muscle; may vary from 2–8 cm.
        (2) Needle gauge depends on substance of medication.
        (3) Oil bases require 20 gauge; water bases require 22 gauge.
2. Absorption rate of IM medication dependent on circulation of person injected.
3. This route usually used for systemic effect of an irritating drug.
4. Amount of medication must not be over 5 mL, as absorption would be difficult and painful.
5. When giving IM injection, be very sure to avoid sciatic nerve—use ventrogluteal site if possible.
6. Techniques for lessening pain for the patient receiving an IM medication.
    a. Encourage relaxation of area to be injected; request patient to lie on side with flexed knee, or flat on abdomen if giving injection in buttock.
    b. Reduce puncture pain by "darting" needle.

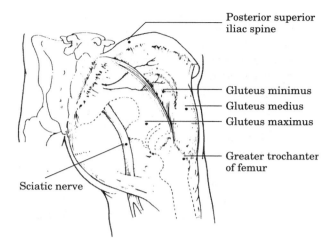

Fig. 5-5 Anatomic view of buttock for intramuscular injection.

c. Prevent antiseptic from clinging to needle during insertion by waiting until skin antiseptic is dry.

d. If medication must be drawn through a rubber stopper, use a new needle for injection.

e. Avoid sensitive or hardened body areas.

f. After needle is under skin, aspirate to be certain that needle is not in a blood vessel.

g. Inject slowly.

h. Maintain grasp of syringe.

i. Withdraw needle quickly after injection.

j. Massage relaxed muscle gently to increase circulation and to distribute medication.

7. Observe for side effects of medication following injection.

Other Routes

A. Inhalation—metered-dose inhaler, nebulizer.

B. Topical route.

Medication Administration

Basic Guidelines for Medication Administration

A. Determine the correct dosage, actions, side effects, and contraindications of any medication before administration.

B. Check with head nurse or RN if medications ordered by the physician do not seem appropriate for patient's condition. This is part of the nurse's professional responsibility.

✦ C. Question the physician about any medication orders that are incomplete, illegible, or inappropriate for the patient's condition.

    1. Remember, the nurse may be liable if a medication error is made.

NURSE PRACTICE ACT GUIDELINES FOR DRUG ADMINISTRATION

- Nurses must not administer a specific drug unless allowed to do so by the particular state's Nurse Practice Act.
- Nurses must not administer any drug without a specific physician order.
- Nurses are to take every safety precaution in whatever they are doing.
- Nurses are to be certain that employer's policy allows them to administer a specific drug.
- Nurses must not administer a controlled substance if the physician's order is outdated.
- A drug may not lawfully be administered unless all of the above items are in effect.
- Nurses are not permitted to fill prescriptions and in most states cannot write prescriptions.
- General rules for drug dispensing:
  Never leave prepared medicines unattended.
  Always report errors immediately.
  Send labeled bottles or packages that are unintelligible back to pharmacist for relabeling.
  Store internal and external medicines separately if possible.

---

2. Report every medication error to the head nurse and/or physician.

3. Complete a medication incident report.

✦ D. Check to determine if the medication ordered is compatible with the patient's condition and with other medications prescribed.

✦ E. Check on what the patient has been eating or drinking before administering a medication.

    1. Determine what effect the patient's diet has on the medication.

    2. Do not administer medication if contraindicated by diet. For example, do not give an MAO inhibitor to a patient who has just ingested cheddar cheese or wine.

F. Check that calculated drug dosage is accurate for young children, elderly people, or for very thin or obese patients. These age and weight groups require smaller or larger dosages.

✦ Narcotic Administration

A. Check medication card or sheet for narcotic orders.

B. Check time frame since last narcotic administered.

C. Open narcotic box or cupboard and find appropriate narcotic container.

D. Count number of pills, ampules, or injectable cartridges in container.

E. Check narcotic sign-out sheet and check that number of narcotics matches number of sign-out sheets.

F. Rectify situation before proceeding with narcotic administration if narcotics and sign-out sheets do not coincide.

G. Sign out for narcotic on narcotic sheets, after taking narcotic out of drawer or cupboard.

H. Lock drawer or cupboard after taking out medication.

I. Sign out narcotics on medication record according to usual procedure.

J. Check narcotics every 8 hours.
1. One off-going and one on-going nurse checks the narcotics.
2. Number of sign-out sheets must match remaining number of narcotics.
3. Each narcotic sheet is checked for accuracy.

K. Return counter (if used) to pharmacy with completed narcotic sign-out sheet when sheet is filled.
1. A new narcotic supply and narcotic check sheet are signed out in pharmacy.
2. The nurse receiving narcotics signs drug record receipt.

Safety Rules—Six Rights

A. The six rights.
1. Right medication.
   a. Compare drug card with drug label three times.
   b. Know general purpose or action, dosage, method of administration.
   c. Know side effects of drug.
2. Right patient: check ID band and room and bed number—ask patient to state name.
3. Right time. Give medication 30 minutes before or after ordered time.
4. Right method or route of administration.
5. Right dose.
   a. Check all calculations of divided dosages with another nurse.
   b. Check heparin and insulin doses with another nurse.
6. Documentation is now considered the sixth right. Document the drug name, dose, route, and time of administration. Patient reaction to the drug may also be documented.

B. The five rights should be practiced each and every time a medication is given.

Documentation of Medications

Medication Orders

✦ A. Medication administered to patient must have a physician's order or prescription before it can be legally administered.

B. Physician's order is a verbal or written order, recorded in a book or file or in patient's chart.

✦ C. If order is given verbally over the telephone, nurse must write a verbal order in patient's chart for the physician to sign at a later date.

D. Written orders are safer—they leave less room for potential misunderstanding or error.

✦ E. Drug order should consist of seven parts.
1. Name of the patient.
2. Date the drug was ordered.
3. Name of the drug.
4. Dosage.
5. Route of administration and any special rules of administration.
6. Time and frequency the drug should be given.
7. Signature of the individual who ordered the drug.

Types of Medication Schedules

A. Routine orders.
✦ 1. Administered according to instructions until it is canceled by another order.
2. Can also be used for PRN drugs.
   a. Administered when patient needs the medication.
   b. Not given on a routine time schedule.
3. Continued validity of any routine order should be assessed—physicians occasionally forget to cancel an order when it is no longer appropriate for patient's condition.

B. One-time orders.
1. Administered as stated, only one time.
2. Given at a specified time or "STAT," which means immediately.

Legal Implications of Medication Errors

✦ A. Nurse who prepares a medication must also give it to patient and chart it.
1. If patient refuses drug, chart that medication was refused—report this information to the physician.
2. When charting medications, use the correct abbreviations and symbols.

✦ B. If error in a drug order is found, it is nurse's responsibility to question the order.
1. If order cannot be understood or read, verify with the physician.
2. Do not guess at the order as this constitutes gross negligence.
3. In many hospitals, it is the pharmacist's responsibility to contact physicians when medication orders are unclear.
   a. Many drugs are now prepared by the pharmacy in unit dose packages.
   b. It remains the nurse's responsibility to know correct drug and dose for the patient.

✦ C. Always report medication errors to the head nurse and/or physician immediately.

1. This action minimizes potential danger to the patient.
2. Measures can be taken immediately to assess and evaluate the patient's status.
3. A plan of action can be implemented to reverse the effects of the medication.

✦ D. Errors in medication are documented in a medication unusual occurrence or incident report and on the patient's record.
   1. This action is necessary for both legal reasons and nursing audits.
   2. Nursing audits are conducted to determine problems in medication administration.
      a. A particular source of problems.
      b. A range of problems that seem to have no connection.

✦ **Legal Issues in Drug Administration**

A. Nurse must not administer a specific drug or use a specific route of administration unless allowed to do so by the particular state's Nurse Practice Act. (Examples are IV push meds and epidural.)
B. Nurse is to take every safety precaution in whatever he or she is doing.
C. Nurse is to be certain that employer's policy allows him or her to administer a specific drug.
D. A drug may not lawfully be administered unless all the above items are in effect.
E. General rules.
   1. Never leave tray with prepared medicines unattended.
   2. Always report errors immediately.
   3. Send labeled bottles that are unintelligible back to pharmacist for relabeling.
   4. Store internal and external medicines separately if possible.

ADMINISTERING MEDICATIONS

Oral Medications

Preparation ❖ Procedure ❖

A. Check medication orders for their completeness and accuracy.
B. Research unfamiliar drugs.
C. Review patient's record for allergies, lab data, etc.
D. Assess patient's physical ability to take medication as ordered.
   1. Swallow reflex present.
   2. State of consciousness.
   3. Signs of nausea and vomiting.
   4. Uncooperative behavior.
E. Check MAR to make sure you have the correct medication for the patient.
F. Assess correct dosage when calculation is needed.
✦ G. Preparing the oral medication.

1. Obtain patient's medication record (MAR). Medication record may be a drug card, medication sheet, or drug Kardex.
2. Compare the MAR with the most *recent* physician's order.
3. Wash your hands.
4. Gather necessary equipment.
5. Retrieve the medication.
6. Compare the label on the bottle or drug package to the MAR.
7. Correctly calculate dosage if necessary and check the dosage to be administered.
8. Pour the medication from the bottle into the lid of the container and then into the medicine cup. With unit dosage, take drug package from medication cart and place in medication cup. Do not remove drug from drug package.
9. Check medication label again to ensure correct drug and dosages if drug is not prepackaged.
10. Place medication cup on a tray, if not using medication cart.
11. Return the multidose vial bottle to the storage area. If medication to be given is a narcotic, sign out the narcotic record sheet with your name.
12. Check medication label for third time before returning bottle to storage.

Implementation

✦ A. Procedure for administering oral medications to adults. ❖ **Procedure** ❖
   1. Take medication tray or cart to patient's room; check room number against medication card or sheet.
   2. Place patient in sitting position, if not contraindicated by his or her condition.
   3. Tell the patient what type of medication you are going to give and explain the actions this medication will produce.
   4. Check the patient's Identaband and ask patient to state name so that you are sure you have correctly identified him or her.
   5. If prepackaged medication is used, read label, take medication out of package, and put into medication cup.
   6. Give the medication cup to the patient.
   7. Offer a fresh glass of water or other liquid to aid swallowing, and give assistance with taking medications.
   8. Make sure the patient swallows the medication.
   9. Discard used medicine cup.
   10. Position patient for comfort.
   11. Record the medication on the appropriate forms.

✦ B. Procedure for administering oral medications to children. ❖ **Procedure** ❖
1. Follow the procedures for the previous intervention, keeping the following guidelines in mind.
   a. Play techniques may help to elicit a young child's cooperation.
   b. Remember, the smaller the quantity of diluent (food or liquid), the greater the ease in eliciting the child's cooperation.
   c. Never use a child's favorite food or drink as an enticement when administering medication because the result may be the child's refusal to eat or drink anything.
   d. Be honest and tell the child that you have medicine, not candy.
2. Assess child for drug action and possible side effects.
3. Explain medication action and side effects to parents.

✦ Patient-Controlled Analgesia (PCA)
❖ **Procedure** ❖

A. Advantages of PCA.
   1. Method provides consistent level of pain control.
   2. Allows patient to self-administer pain medication.
   3. Allows patient to feel in control of pain management.
B. Procedure.
   1. PCA infuser pump is prepared and attached to IV.
   2. Morphine sulfate and hydromorphone (Dilaudid) is delivered in loading dose as ordered and initiates pain management.
   3. Patient is instructed in PCA use and continues to self-administer narcotic.
   4. Dose calculation.
      a. PCA infuser delivers in milliliters.
      b. Maximum rate of administration 20 mL/hour.
      c. Four-hour limit is set for infuser—5- to 30-mL increments.

Narcotic Medications ❖ **Procedure** ❖

A. Check medication sheet for narcotic orders.
B. Check dose and time last narcotic administered.
C. Unlock and open narcotic drawer and find appropriate narcotic container.
D. Count number of pills, ampules, or injectable cartridges in container.
✦ E. Check narcotic sign-out sheet and check that number of narcotics matches number of sign-out sheets.
F. Rectify situation before proceeding with narcotic administration if narcotics and sign-out sheets do not coincide.

G. Sign out for narcotic on narcotic sheets, after taking narcotic out of drawer or cupboard.
H. Lock drawer or cupboard after taking out medication.
I. Sign out narcotics on MAR according to usual procedure.
J. For unit narcotic stock, check narcotics every 8 hours.
   1. One off-going and one on-going nurse check the narcotics.
   2. Number of sign-out sheets must match remaining number of narcotics.
   3. Each narcotic sheet is checked for accuracy.
K. Return empty counter (if used) to pharmacy with completed narcotic sign-out sheet when sheet is filled.
   1. A new narcotic supply and narcotic check sheet are signed out in pharmacy.
   2. The nurse receiving narcotics signs drug record receipt.
L. For automated dispensing system, enter ID code number and user password and continue with dispensing process.

Parenteral Medications

Preparation ❖ **Procedure** ❖

✦ A. Check appropriate method for administration of drug.
   1. *Intradermal (intracutaneous):* injection is made below surface of the skin; inject 0.01 to 0.1 mL.
   2. *Subcutaneous:* small amount of fluid is injected beneath the skin in the loose connective tissues; inject 2 mL.
   3. *Intramuscular:* larger amount of fluid is injected into large muscle masses in the body; inject up to 5 mL.
   4. *Intravenous:* medication is injected or infused directly into a vein—route used when immediate drug effect is desired.
✦ B. Evaluate condition of administration site for presence of lesions, rash, inflammation, lipid dystrophy, ecchymosis, etc.
   1. Ventrogluteal site (patient side-lying).
   2. Dorsogluteal site (patient in prone position).
   3. Vastus lateralis (patient supine with thigh available).
   4. Deltoid site (exposed upper arm).
C. Assess for tissue damage from previous injections.
D. Assess patient's level of consciousness.
   1. For patient in shock: certain methods (subcutaneous) will not be used.
   2. For presence of anxiety: make sure patient is allowed to express his or her fear of injections and offer explanations of ways in which injections will be less frightening.

E. Check patient's written and verbal history for past allergic reactions. Do *not* rely solely on patient's chart.

F. Review patient's chart noting previous injection sites, especially insulin and heparin administration sites.

G. Check label on medication bottle to determine if medication can be administered via route ordered.

✦ H. Preparing the medication.
1. Wash your hands.
2. Obtain equipment for injection: safety needle and syringe, antimicrobial wipes, medication cart (medication container if needed).
3. Select the appropriate-size needle, considering the size of the patient's muscle mass and the viscosity of the medication. Break the seal on the syringe by pulling down on the plunger.
4. Open the antimicrobial wipe and cleanse the top of the vial or break top of ampule.
5. Remove the needle guard.
6. Pull back on barrel of syringe to markings where medication will be inserted.
7. Pick up vial, insert needle into vial, and inject air in an amount equal to the solution to be withdrawn by pushing barrel of syringe down. If using an ampule, break off top at colored line, insert syringe, but do not inject air into ampule as it causes a break in the vacuum and possible loss of medication through leakage.
8. Extract the desired amount of fluid. Remove needle from container and cover needle with guard. Needle should be changed to prevent tracking medication on skin and subcutaneous tissue.
9. Double check drug and dosage against drug card or medication sheet and vial or ampule.
10. Place syringe on tray if tray available.
11. Check label and drug card or medication sheet for accuracy before returning multidose vial to correct storage area.
12. Return multidose vial to correct storage area or discard used vial or ampule.

Implementation

✦ A. Administering intradermal injections.
❖ **Procedure** ❖
1. Take medication to patient's room.
2. Explain the medication's action and the procedure for administration to patient.
3. Check patient's Identaband and ask patient to state name.
4. Wash your hands and don gloves.
5. Select the site of injection.
6. Cleanse the area with an antimicrobial wipe, wiping in circular area from inside to outside.
7. Take off needle guard and place on tray.
8. Grasp patient's forearm from underneath and gently pull the skin taut.

9. Insert the needle at 10- to 15-degree angle with the bevel of needle facing up.
10. Inject medication slowly. Observe for wheals and blanching at the site.
11. Withdraw the needle, wiping the area gently with a dry 2 × 2 bandage to prevent dispersing medication into the subcutaneous tissue.
12. Return the patient to a comfortable position.
13. Activate safety needle and discard supplies in appropriate area.
14. Chart the medication and site used.

✦ B. Administering subcutaneous (sub q) injections.
❖ **Procedure** ❖
1. Take medication to patient's room.
2. Set tray on a clean surface, not the bed.
3. Check patient's Identaband and ask patient to state name.
4. Explain action of medication and procedure of administration.
5. Provide privacy when injection site is other than on the arm.
6. Wash your hands and don gloves.
7. Select site for injection by identifying anatomical landmarks. Remember to alternate sites each time injections are given (see Figure 5-6).
8. Cleanse area with antimicrobial wipe. Using a circular motion cleanse from inside outward.
9. Take off needle guard.
10. Express any air bubbles from syringe.
11. Insert the needle at a 45-degree angle.
12. Pull back on the plunger.

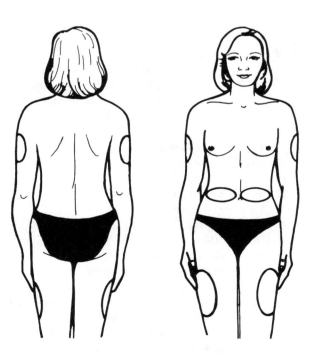

Fig. 5-6 Rotate sites for subcutaneous injections given on a continuing basis.

13. Inject the medication slowly.
14. Withdraw needle quickly and massage area with wipe to aid absorption and lessen bleeding. *Do not* massage area after administering certain drugs such as hep-arin or insulin. Put on Band-Aid if needed.
15. Activate needle safety feature and discard in puncture proof container.
16. Return patient to a position of comfort.
17. Chart the medication and site used.

✦ C. Administering insulin injections.
   ❖ **PROCEDURE** ❖
1. Gather equipment, check medication orders, and injection site. Insulin does not need to be refrigerated.
2. Wash your hands and don gloves.
3. Obtain specific insulin syringe for strength of insulin being administered (U100).
4. Rotate insulin bottle between hands to bring solution into suspension.
5. Wipe top of insulin bottle with antimicrobial swab.
6. Take off needle guard.
7. Pull plunger of syringe down to desired amount of medication and inject that amount of air into the insulin bottle.
8. Draw up ordered amount of insulin into syringe.
9. Expel air from syringe.
10. Replace needle guard.
11. Check medication card, bottle, and syringe with an RN for accuracy. See chart on *Insulin Types and Action* in Medical–Surgical Nursing, Chapter 10, page 314.
12. Take medications to patient's room.
13. Double check site of last injection with patient.
✦ 14. Rotating injection site from one body area to another is no longer recommended due to the variation in insulin absorption and action.
    a. Move injection site 1 inch from previous site.
    b. Absorption is most predictable in the abdomen.
    c. Avoid injecting insulin into an extremity.
15. Provide privacy.
16. Wash your hands.
17. Follow protocol for administration of medications by subcutaneous injections.

✦ D. Administering two insulin solutions.
   ❖ **PROCEDURE** ❖
1. Follow steps 1–6 above.
2. Inject prescribed amount of air into intermediate-acting or long-acting bottle.
3. Pull needle out of insulin bottle and withdraw plunger to prescribed regular insulin dosage.
4. Inject air into regular bottle and withdraw medication. Check dose with another nurse.
5. Expel all air bubbles.

6. Insert needle into second insulin bottle taking care not to push any regular insulin into bottle. This can be avoided by putting pressure on plunger with your small finger when inserting into bottle.
7. Invert bottle and pull back on plunger to obtain prescribed amount of insulin. Remember the total insulin dose will include the amount of regular insulin already drawn up into syringe.
8. Follow steps 9–16 in the previous skill to complete procedure.

✦ E. Insulin pump.
1. This method is a continuous delivery of fixed, small amounts of diluted insulin— mimics release of insulin by the pancreas.
2. Uses regular insulin (50 percent continuous delivery and 50 percent divided into three premeal bolus doses).
3. Amount is calculated by blood glucose monitoring 2–4 times/day.
4. This method is useful for an intelligent, conscientious, active person who can take responsibility.

✦ F. Administering intramuscular (IM) injections.
   ❖ **PROCEDURE** ❖
1. Take medication to patient's room. Check room number against medication card or sheet.
2. Set tray on a clean surface, not the bed.
3. Explain the procedure to patient.
4. Check patient's Identaband and have patient state name.
5. Provide privacy for patient.
6. Wash your hands and don gloves.
7. Select the site of injection by identifying anatomical landmarks. Remember to alternate sites each time injections are given.
8. Cleanse the area with antimicrobial wipe. Using a circular motion, cleanse from inside outward.
9. Hold the syringe; take off needle cover.
10. Express air bubbles from syringe.
11. Insert the needle at 90-degree angle.
12. Pull back on plunger. If blood returns, you know you have entered a blood vessel, textbooks advocate discarding all equipment and medication, but nurses often reposition the needle and aspirate again.
13. Inject the medication slowly.
14. Withdraw the needle and massage the area with a wipe. Put on a Band-Aid, if needed.
15. Activate needle safety feature.
16. Return patient to a comfortable position.
17. Chart the medication and site used.

✦ G. Administering IM injections using Z-track method (Figure 5-7). Used for iron injections.
   ❖ **PROCEDURE** ❖
1. Complete steps 1–7 in the previous skill, Administering IM Injections.

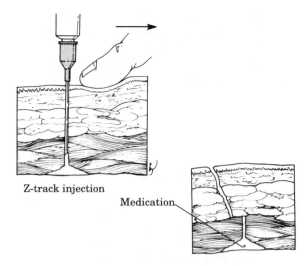

Z-track injection

Medication

Fig. 5-7 Z-track is used to prevent tracking of medications on the skin.

2. Draw up prescribed medication into syringe.
3. Draw up 0.3–0.5 mL of air into syringe.
4. Replace needle with a new 2-inch needle to penetrate deep into muscle.
5. Pull skin 1–1½ inches laterally away from injection site.
6. Cleanse site with alcohol.
7. Insert needle at a 90-degree angle.
8. Inject medication slowly—and wait 10 seconds keeping skin taut.
9. Withdraw needle and then release skin.
10. Apply light pressure with 2″ × 2″ gauze. Do not massage.
11. Discard supplies in appropriate area.
12. Chart medication and site used.

Administering Topical Medications

Preparation
A. Observe skin for open lesions, rashes, or areas of erythema.
B. Check for allergies.

Implementation
A. Obtain patient's medication record.
   ❖ **PROCEDURE** ❖
B. Compare the medication record with the most recent physician's order. Medication record may be a drug card, medication sheet, or drug Kardex, depending on the method of dispensing medications in your facility.
C. Wash your hands.
D. Gather necessary equipment including gloves or tongue blade as needed.
E. Remove the medication from the drug box or tray on medication cart.
F. Compare the label on the medication tube or jar to the medication record.

G. Place medication tube or jar (include a tongue blade with jar) on a tray if not using medication cart.
H. Take medication to patient's room.
I. Wash your hands and don gloves if needed.
J. Provide patient privacy.
K. Squeeze medication from a tube or, using a tongue blade, take ointment out of jar.
L. Spread a small, smooth, thin quantity of medication evenly over patient's skin surface using your gloved fingers or a tongue blade.
M. Protect skin surface with a dressing, if needed, so that medication cannot rub off.
N. Cleanse skin surface with soap and water between medication applications, unless contraindicated by patient's condition.
O. Return medication to appropriate storage area.
P. Check to see that patient is comfortable before leaving room.
Q. Wash your hands.
R. Chart administration.

Administering a Topical Vasodilator

✦ **Implementation**
A. Take medication to patient's room.
   ❖ **PROCEDURE** ❖
B. Wash your hands.
C. Provide patient privacy.
D. Put on gloves to prevent absorbing any medication yourself.
E. Obtain premeasured paper, which accompanies medication tube.
F. Place prescribed medication directly on paper (usually ½- to 1-inch strip).
G. Apply medicated paper to anterior surface of chest.
H. You may apply medicated paper to any area of the body; however, most patients feel the medication works better if applied to the chest surface.
I. Alternate areas of the chest with each dose of medication.
J. Return medication to appropriate storage area.
K. Check to see that patient is comfortable before leaving room.
L. Wash your hands.
M. Chart administration.

HERB-DRUG INTERACTIONS

A. Mixing herbs with traditional medicines may increase or decrease the effects—in some cases this can be dangerous.
   1. Unlike presprescription medicines, herbal products are not regulated by the FDA.
   2. Over 60 million Americans spend 4 billion annually on herbs—over 15 million adults are at risk for potential drug-herb interactions.

B. On the whole, herbal medicine is safe and a gentle form of therapy. However, if the health problem is serious or the person is taking strong orthodox medications, teaching is indicated.

C. Patient teaching with herbs.
   1. When completing a nursing history, ask about taking herbs.
   2. Educate yourself about herbs—check for known side effects, drug interactions and potential risk with certain drugs.
   3. Remind patient to tell his/her physician about any herbs being taken.

Table 5-1. HERB/DRUG INTERACTION CHART

Herb	Action	Side Effects	Drug Interaction	Drugs Affected
Black Cohosh	An herb for females, especially during menopause—maintains healthy levels of luteinizing hormone Decreases menstrual discomfort Sedative, diuretic Lowers blood pressure	Overdose may cause nausea, vomiting, headache, dizziness, tremors and depressed heart rate	Increase effects of drugs—especially synthetic hormones **Congestive heart failure clients and pregnant women should not use this herb**	Hormone replacement therapy (HRT) Contraceptives Heart/Cardiac medications
Echinacea	Immunostimulant Treatment for colds (URIs) and influenza Bladder infections Blood purifier Helps preserve white cells during radiation treatment	Possible, but not common: diarrhea, heartburn, intestinal upset, skin rash	Stimulating immune system may alter effect of certain drugs	Anabolic steroids Amiodarone Methotrexate Ketocanarzole
Ephedra (Ma Huang)	Promotes weight loss and acts as a stimulant (asthma) Considered toxic by FDA	Stimulant, insomnia, headaches, nervousness, seizures, death	Heart attack, seizure or death Additive effect; increased thermogenesis (related to stimulants/coffee) Elevation of BP (related to MAO inhibitors) Reduces drug action—may cause arrhythmias Increased steroid drug clearance/may reduce effectiveness	Decongestants (Actifed, Dristan, Sinutab, Sudafed) Stimulants—caffeine MAO inhibitors Beta blockers Cardiac glycosides Steroids (anti-inflammatories)
Feverfew	Eases pain and nausea of migraine headaches Prevents blood vessel spasms Interferes with action of platelets (which clump together to form clots) Lowers blood pressure	Nervousness, insomnia, and tiredness	Severe bleeding **Pregnant women, children under age two, and people taking drugs as listed should not take this herb**	Warfarin Aspirin NSAIDs (ibuprophen)
Garlic	Contains allicin, natural antibiotic—effective against bacteria and viruses Lowers total cholesterol and increases HDL Reduces blood pressure Reduces blood clot formation (when arteries are narrowed)	Intestinal problems—upset stomach, heartburn	Excessive thinning of blood (bleeding) when used with blood thinners	Warfarin Coumadin

Table 5-1. HERB/DRUG INTERACTION CHART *(Continued)*

Herb	Action	Side Effects	Drug Interaction	Drugs Affected
Ginger	Relieves nausea associated with seasickness, motion sickness or anesthesia Digestive aid; increased secretion of bile Reduces side effects of chemotherapy Reduces congestion and fevers Supports cardiovascular system	Heartburn	Excessive thinning of blood (bleeding) when used with blood thinners Interferes with platelet action Increases gut absorption (may increase drug bioavailability)	Warfarin Take cautiously with all cardiac or diabetic medications; blood pressure therapy
Ginkgo biloba	Improves circulation by thinning blood Enhances flow of oxygen and blood to brain Improves memory and mental function May delay progression of Alzheimer's (jury still out) Asthma	Headache Indigestion Nervousness	Anticoagulant effect and may cause spontaneous or excessive bleeding **Those with blood clotting disorders should not take this drug**	Aspirin Plavix Persantine Ticlid Coumadin Warfarin
Siberian Ginseng	Tonic, boosts energy and stamina Reduces stress Improves sexual performance, regulates hormones Strengthens immune system Raises "good" cholesterol, HDL Protects against heart attacks Preventative for aging	Insomnia, hypertension Low blood glucose Allergy symptoms Increased alcohol clearance Affects insulin level	Increases anticoagulant effect and bleeding Headache, manic behavior Monitoring effect of drug may be difficult—may increase Digoxin levels Stimulates alcohol metabolism **Those who have blood clotting problems, high blood pressure, asthma, emphysema, children and pregnant women should not take this herb** Improves blood sugar and diabetic symptoms (could reduce amount of insulin)	Warfarin Coumadin Aspirin NSAIDs Nardil (MAO inhibitor) Digoxin (Lanoxin) Alcohol Insulin Antidepressants (phenelzine sulfate)
Kava Kava	Sedative effect to treat anxiety	GI problems, liver problems (even failure has been reported) Allergic skin reaction	Sedation, and even coma when taken with certain drugs	Alprazolam Sleeping meds Antipsychotics Alcohol Xanax (antidepressant) Drugs treating Parkinson's disease
Licorice Root	Helps steroid drug withdrawal Helps to heal gastric ulcers Diuretic effect	Raises blood pressure Headache Lethargy Cardiac dysfunction	Potentiates drug levels and offsets effects of NSAIDs Antibiotics reduce herb activity Diuretic effect could result in decreased potassium leading to toxicity	Corticosteroids Thiazides Oral contraceptives Antibiotics

Continues

Table 5-1. HERB/DRUG INTERACTION CHART *(Continued)*

Herb	Action	Side Effects	Drug Interaction	Drugs Affected
Licorice Root *(continued)*			Increased sensitivity to Digoxin or other cardiac glycosides **Pregnant and nursing women, and those with glaucoma, hypertension, stroke and heart disease should not take this herb**	
Saw Palmetto	Supports health of prostate gland Improves urine flow Maintains healthy testosterone metabolism Antiinflammatory	Relatively few: mild nausea, gastro-intestinal disturbance	The safety profile of this herb is very good—no known drug interactions	
Silymarin (Milk Thistle)	Increases liver detox capacity Supports liver function Protects liver from drug damage	Nausea, GI disturbance	Reduces drug toxicity to liver and protects liver from drug damage Reduces toxic side effects of chemotherapy Potentially dangerous for transplant clients—reduces levels of immunosuppressives	Aspirin Alcohol Chemotherapy
St. John's Wort	Relieves mild to moderate depression by countering monamine oxidase (avoid same foods-tyramine-as if taking MAO inhibitor drug) Immune stimulating properties—useful with AIDS because it is antiviral Helps bruises and hemorrhoids	Dry mouth, dizziness, fatigue, digestive problems (fewer side effects than prescription antidepressants) Sensitivity to light	Photosensitivity Decreases level of drugs Decreases immunosuppressant therapy Additive serotonin-like effects—Serotonin syndrome (serious condition: fever, dizziness, sweating, etc.) Could affect action of epilepsy drugs **Patients with hypertension and those on immunosuppressive therapy should not use this herb**	Tetracyclines Cyclosporin Digoxin Oral contraceptives Zoloft and antidepressants Other SSRIs Epilepsy meds
Valerian	Quiets and calms neurological system Promotes sleep Used for headache, anxiety and nervousness	Restlessness, headache, giddiness, nausea, and blurred vision	Use may not be affected by alcohol or barbiturates — use cautiously Not for children under 2 years Effect may be enhanced with sleeping tablets Additive effect—may be used to wean off drugs (diazepam)	Alcohol Barbiturates Sleeping tablets Benzodiazepines

CALCULATIONS AND CONVERSIONS*

Approximate Equivalents
A. The metric system is the universal system of weights and measures.
B. Apothecary and metric do not use same size units; denominations of one system not compatible with the other.
C. Equivalency tables established to list measurement denominations of one system in terms of another. (See Appendix 5-2.)
   1. Conversion from one system to another can be computed, but is not equivalent in absolute terms.
   2. If there is occasion to compute, have computations checked by another licensed nurse.
      a. Do not compute unless allowed to do so by your state's Nurse Practice Act.
      b. Check hospital policy for further guidelines.

Computation
A. Drugs are not always labeled clearly as to number of tablets to administer so computation may be necessary. Always have your computation checked by another licensed nurse.
◆ B. Method.
   1. Both desired (ordered) dose and dose on hand must be in same unit of measurement, e.g., grains, grams, milligrams.
   2. If not same, convert so that unit of measure is the same.
      a. Refer to conversion table (Appendix 5-2).
      b. To convert one measure unit to another, basic equivalencies must be memorized.
   3. After converting, divide desired dose by dose on hand to find amount to administer.

Calculation of Dosages
◆ A. Using equivalent tables to calculate drug dosages.
   1. To make conversions from metric to apothecary or household system, it is necessary to memorize or refer to equivalency tables.
   2. To convert milligrams to grains, use the following formula:

Example: Convert 180 milligrams to grains.

$$\frac{1 \text{ gr}}{\text{mg in gr}} = \frac{\text{dose desired}}{\text{dose on hand}}$$

$$\frac{1}{60} = \frac{x}{180}$$

$$60x = 180$$

$$x = 3 \text{ grains}$$

   3. You may also make this conversion as a ratio:

$$1 \text{ gr} : 60 \text{ mg} :: x \text{ gr} : 180 \text{ mg}$$
$$60x = 180 \quad x = 3 \text{ grains}$$

*Conversion tables are in Appendix 5-2.

4. Check equivalency tables in the drug supplement.
◆ B. Calculating oral dosages of drugs.
   ❖ **PROCEDURE** ❖
   1. To calculate oral dosages, use the following formula:

$$\frac{D}{H} = x$$

where D = dose desired
H = dose on hand
x = dose to be administered

Example: Give 500 mg of ampicillin when the dose on hand is in capsules containing 250 mg.

$$\frac{500 \text{ mg}}{250 \text{ mg}} = 2 \text{ capsules}$$

   2. To calculate oral dosages of liquids, use the following formula:

$$\frac{D}{H} \times Q = x \text{ (quantity to be administered)}$$

where Q = quantity of dosage on hand

Example: Give 375 mg of ampicillin when it is supplied as 250 mg/5 mL.

$$\frac{375 \text{ mg}}{250 \text{ mg}} \times 5$$

$$1.5 \times 5 = 7.5 \text{ mL}$$

You can also set up a direct proportion and following the algebraic principle, cross multiply:

$$\frac{375 \text{ mg}}{x} = \frac{250 \text{ mg}}{5 \text{mL}}$$

$$250x = 1875$$

$$x = 7.5 \text{ mL (of strength 250 mg/5 mL)}$$

C. Calculating parenteral dosages of drugs.
   1. To calculate parenteral dosages, use the following formula:

$$\frac{D}{H} \times Q = x$$

Example: Give patient 40 mg gentamicin. On hand is a multidose vial with a strength of 80 mg/2 mL.

$$\frac{40}{80} \times 2 = 1 \text{ mL}$$

   2. Check your calculations before drawing up medication.
D. Calculating dosages for infants and children.
   1. Calculating dosages for infants and children using BSA:

$$\frac{\text{BSA*}}{1.7} \times \text{adult dose} = \text{pediatric dose}$$

*BSA = body surface area.

2. Calculating dosages for infants and children using Clark's weight rule:

$$\text{Child's dose} = \frac{\text{Child's wt. in lbs.}}{150} \times \text{Adult dose}$$

Check your calculations before drawing up the medications.

✦ Calculation of Solutions

A. Types of solutions.
   1. Volume to volume (v/v): a given volume of solute is added to a given volume solvent.
   2. Weight to weight (w/w): a stated weight of solute is dissolved in a stated weight of solvent.
   3. Weight to volume (w/v): a given weight of solute is dissolved in a given volume of solvent which results in the proper amount of solution.
B. Preparing solutions.
   1. Liquid to drug solutions.
      a. Determine the strength of the solution, the strength of the drug on hand, and the quantity of solution required.
      b. Use this formula for preparing solutions:

$$\frac{D}{H} \times Q = x$$

where D = desired strength
      H = strength on hand
      Q = quantity of solution desired
      x = amount of solute

Example: You have a 100% solution of hydrogen peroxide on hand. You need a liter of 50% solution.

$$\frac{50}{100} \times 1000 \text{ mL} = 500 \text{ mL}$$

If the strength desired and strength on hand are not in like terms, you need to change one of the terms.

Example: You have 1 liter of 50% solution on hand. You need a liter of 1:10 solution. 1:10 solution is the same as 10%.

$$\frac{10\%}{50\%} \times 1000 \text{ mL} = 200 \text{ mL}$$

Add 200 mL of the drug to 800 mL of the solvent to make a liter of 10% solution.
   2. Volume to volume solutions.
      Use the formula:

$$\frac{D}{H} \times Q = x$$

where x = amount of stock solution used

Example: Prepare a liter of 5% solution from a stock solution of 50%.

$$\frac{5\%}{50\%} \times 1000 \text{ mL} = 100 \text{ mL}$$

Add 100 mL to 900 mL of diluent to make 1 liter of 5% solution.
   3. Solutions from tablets.
      a. Use the formula:

$$\frac{D}{H} \times Q = x$$

where x = amount/number of tablets used

Example: Prepare 1 liter of a 1:1000 solution, using 10 grain tablets.

$$\frac{1/1000}{10 \text{ gr}} \times 1000 \text{ mL} = x$$

      b. First convert 10 grains to grams so the numerator and denominator are in the same unit of measure. 1 gm = 15 gr; therefore, 10 gr = 2/3 gm. Now substitute the new numbers in the formula and solve for x.

$$\frac{1/1000}{2/3} \times \frac{1000}{1} \text{ mL} = x$$

$$\frac{3}{2000} \times \frac{1000}{1} = x$$

$x = \frac{3}{2}$ or 1½ tablets

Place 1½ tablets into the 1 liter of solution and dissolve.

GOVERNING LAWS

Federal Food, Drug, and Cosmetic Act of 1938

A. The act is an update of the Food and Drug Act first passed in 1906.
B. It designates *United States Pharmacopeia and National Formulary* as official standard.
C. The federal government has the power to enforce standards.
D. Provisions of the act.
   1. Drug manufacturer must provide adequate evidence of drug's safety.
   2. Correct labeling and packaging of drugs.
E. Amended in 1952 to include control of barbiturates by restricting prescription refills.
F. Amended in 1962 to require substantial investigation of drug and evidence that drug is effective in terms of labeling claims.

Harrison Narcotic Act of 1914

A. Provisions of the act.
   1. Regulates manufacture, importation, and sale of opium, cocaine, and their derivatives.

2. Amendments have added addictive synthetic drugs to the regulated drug listing.

B. Applications of the act.
1. Individuals who produce, sell, dispense (pharmacists), and prescribe (dentists, physicians) these drugs must be licensed and registered; prescriptions must be in triplicate.
2. Hospitals order drugs on special blanks that bear hospital registry number. The following information is recorded for each dose:
   a. Name of drug.
   b. Amount of drug.
   c. Date and time drug obtained.
   d. Name of physician prescribing drug.
   e. Name of patient receiving drug.
   f. Nurse's signature and type of license (RN, LVN, or LPN).

The Controlled Substance Act of 1970

A. Provisions of the act.
✦ 1. Regulates potentially addictive drugs as to prescription, use, and possession.
   a. Regulations refer to use in hospital, office, research, and emergency situations.
   b. Regulations cover narcotics, cocaine, amphetamines, hallucinogens, barbiturates, and other sedatives.
2. Controlled drugs are placed in five different schedules or categorical listings, each governed by different regulations.
   a. The regulations govern manufacture, transport, and storage of the controlled drugs.
   b. The use of the drugs is controlled as to prescription, authorization, mode of dispensation, and administration.
✦ B. Application of the act for use of controlled drugs in hospital.
1. The nurse is to keep the stock supply of controlled drugs under lock and key.
   a. Nurse must sign for each dose (tablet, mL) of drug.
   b. Key is held by the nurse responsible for administration of medication.
   c. At the end of each shift, nurse must account for all controlled drugs in the stock supply.
2. Violations of the Controlled Substance Act.
   a. Violations are punishable by fine, imprisonment, or both.
   b. Nurses, upon conviction of violation, are subject to losing their licenses to practice nursing.

Prescription and Medication Orders

A. Prescription is a written order for dispensation of drugs that can be used only under physician's supervision.

B. Prescriptions outside the hospital.
1. Formula to pharmacist for dispensing drugs to patient.
2. Consists of four parts.
   a. Superscription (symbolized by Rx, meaning "take").
      (1) Patient's name.
      (2) Patient's address (required only for controlled drugs).
      (3) Age (required only if age is factor in dose preparation).
      (4) Date (must always be included).
   b. Inscription.
      (1) Specifies ingredients and their quantities.
      (2) May specify other ingredients necessary to specific drug form.
   c. Subscription—directions to pharmacist as to method of preparation.
   d. Signature—consists of two parts.
      (1) Accurate instructions to patient as to when, how, and in what quantities to take medication; typed on label.
      (2) Physician's signature and refill instructions.

C. Orders inside the hospital.
1. Physician writes medication order in book, file, or patient's chart; if given over phone, nurse writes verbal order which physician later signs.
2. Order consists of six parts.
   a. Name of drug.
   b. Dosage.
   c. Route of administration with time drug was given.
   d. Reason drug required (not always included).
   e. Length of time patient is to receive drug (not always included).
   f. Signature of individual who ordered drug.

Example: Aspirin gr x PO q3h for pain for 3 days.

D. Smith, M.D.

Informational Resources

Official Publications

A. A drug listed in the following publications is designated as official by the Federal Food, Drug, and Cosmetic Act (FDC).
1. *The United States Pharmacopeia* (USP).
2. *National Formulary* (NF).
3. *Homeopathic Pharmacopeia of the United States.*

B. These publications establish standards of purity and other criteria for product acceptability; these standards are binding according to law.

C. Publications contain information on each drug entry.
1. Source.
2. Chemical and physical composition.
3. Method of storage.
4. General type or category.
5. Range of dosage and usual therapeutic dosage.

Other Publications
A. *American Hospital Formulary* is a publication indexed by generic and proprietary names.
B. *Physicians' Desk Reference* (PDR).
1. Annual publication with quarterly supplements.
2. Handy source of information about dosage and drug precautions.

Miscellaneous Resources
A. Package inserts from manufacturers that accompany the product.
B. Pharmacist.
C. Physician.
D. Nursing journals.
E. Pharmaceutical and medical treatment texts.

Appendix 5-1. ABBREVIATIONS AND SYMBOLS

ac	before meals	m	a minim	q3h	every three hours
ad lib	freely, as desired	Mg	magnesium	q4h	every four hours
BID	twice each day	N	nitrogen	R_x	treatment, "take thou"
c̄	with	Na	sodium	s̄	without
C	carbon	NPO	nothing by mouth	ss	one-half (½)
Ca	calcium	oob	out of bed	STAT	immediately
Cl	chlorine	os	mouth	TID	three times a day
dr or ℨ	dram	oz or ℥	ounce	tsp	teaspoon
et	and	pc	after meals	WBC	white blood cell
GI	gastrointestinal	per	by, through	°	degree
gt or gtt	drop(s)	PRN	whenever necessary	−	minus, negative, alkaline reaction
H_2O	water	qd	every day	+	plus, positive, acid reaction
H_2O_2	hydrogen peroxide	qh	every hour	%	percent
IM	intramuscular	QID	four times each day	v	roman numeral five
in	inch	qs	as much as required, quantity sufficient	vii	roman numeral seven
K	potassium			ix	roman numeral nine
lb or #	pound	q2h	every two hours	xiii	roman numeral thirteen

---

Appendix 5-2. CONVERSION TABLES

Table A. HOUSEHOLD EQUIVALENTS (VOLUME)

Metric	Apothecary	Household
0.06 mL	1 minim	1 drop
5(4) mL	1 fluid dram	1 teaspoonful
15 mL	4 fluid drams	1 tablespoonful
30 mL	1 fluid ounce	2 tablespoonfuls
180 mL	6 fluid ounces	1 teacupful
240 mL	8 fluid ounces	1 glassful

Table B. APOTHECARY EQUIVALENTS (VOLUME)

Metric		Apothecary
1	mL	= 15 minims
1	cc	= 15 minims
4	mL	= 1 fluid dram
30	mL	= 1 fluid ounce
500	mL	= 1 pint
1000	mL (1 L)	= 1 quart

Table C. APOTHECARY EQUIVALENTS (WEIGHT)

Metric			Apothecary
1.0 g	or	1000 mg	= gr xv
0.6 g	or	600 mg	= gr x
0.5 g	or	500 mg	= gr viiss
0.3 g	or	300 mg	= gr v
0.2 g	or	200 mg	= gr iii
0.1 g	or	100 mg	= gr 1½
0.06 g	or	60 mg	= gr 1
0.05 g	or	50 mg	= gr ¾
0.03 g	or	30 mg	= gr ½
0.015 g	or	15 mg	= gr ¼
0.010 g	or	10 mg	= gr ⅙
0.008 g	or	8 mg	= gr ⅛
		4 g	= 1 dr
		30 g	= 1 oz
		1 kg	= 2.2 lbs

PHARMACOLOGY QUESTIONS

1. Drug metabolism occurs in four stages. If the drug binds with plasma protein in the blood, it

   1. Is effective.
   2. Is not effective.
   3. Crosses cell membranes.
   4. Is stored in the fat cells.

2. Which of the following actions is *not* accurate when administering a medication using the Z-track method?

   1. Placing 0.3–0.5 mL of air into the syringe.
   2. Using a 2- to 3-inch needle.
   3. Inserting the needle and injecting medication without aspirating.
   4. Pulling skin laterally away from the injection site before inserting the needle.

3. On the images below, identify the 2 areas preferred for insulin injections.

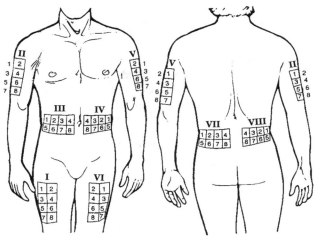

   1. I and II.
   2. II and V.
   3. I and VI.
   4. III and IV.

4. Most drugs are "broken down" in which body area?

   1. Kidney.
   2. Plasma.
   3. Liver.
   4. Intestinal mucosa.

5. Which muscle is preferred for intramuscular injections when possible?

   1. Vastus lateralis.
   2. Gluteus maximus.
   3. Deltoid.
   4. Ventrogluteal.

6. Subcutaneous injections for pain are most commonly injected in which area?

   1. Abdomen.
   2. Buttocks.
   3. Deltoid.
   4. Lateral thigh.

7. The reason for not massaging the site following a heparin injection is to

   1. Prevent rapid absorption of medication.
   2. Maintain heparin in sub q tissue.
   3. Prevent tissue damage.
   4. Prevent tracking medication on skin.

8. A patient with a urinary tract infection is given aminoglycoside (gentamicin) antimicrobial therapy. The nurse understands that this drug is more active when the urine is

   1. Concentrated.
   2. Dilute.
   3. Alkaline.
   4. Acid.

9. The instructions to a patient whose physician recently ordered nitroglycerin are that this medication should be taken

   1. Every 2–3 hours during the day.
   2. Before every meal and at bedtime.
   3. At the first indication of chest pain.
   4. Only when chest pain is not relieved by rest.

10. Which one of the statements is most accurate about the drug cimetidine (Tagamet) and should be discussed with patients who take the medication?

    1. Tagamet should be taken with an antacid to decrease GI distress, a common occurrence with the drug.
    2. Tagamet should be used cautiously with patients on Coumadin because it could inhibit the absorption of the drug.
    3. Tagamet should be taken on an empty stomach for better absorption.
    4. Tagamet is usually prescribed for long-term prevention of gastric ulcers.

11. A 40-year-old patient admitted for a diagnostic workup has orders for Seconal at bedtime. What effect does this drug have on the body?

    1. Tranquilization.
    2. Sedation.
    3. Mood elevation.
    4. Stimulation.

12. Some patients with severely active lupus erythematosus are managed with steroids. A positive response to steroid therapy would be evidenced by

    1. An increase in platelet count.
    2. A normal gamma globulin count.
    3. A decrease in anti-DNA titer.
    4. Negative syphilis serology.

13. A patient has developed agranulocytosis as a result of medications he is taking. In counseling the patient, the nurse knows that one of the most serious consequences of this condition is

    1. The potential danger of excessive bleeding even with minor trauma.
    2. Generalized ecchymosis on exposed areas of the body.
    3. High susceptibility to infection.
    4. Extreme prostration.

14. A patient in liver failure from cirrhosis with ascites is receiving spironolactone. The expected outcome when this drug is given is

    1. Increased urine sodium.
    2. Increased urinary output.
    3. Decreased potassium excretion.
    4. Prevention of metabolic alkalosis.

15. The nurse is assigned to care for a patient preoperatively, whose orders include meperidine 25 mg IM at 7:30 AM. After checking the orders on the chart, the correct nursing action is to

    1. Call the anesthesiologist to double check the dosage, because it is in the lower range of normal.
    2. Use Z-track, not IM, method of injection to protect the injection site.
    3. Follow orders and give the drug as prescribed.
    4. Refuse to administer the medication because the dosage is incorrect.

16. A patient is to receive meperidine (Demerol) 75 mg and atropine 0.2 mg IM. The medications can be mixed together in the same syringe. On hand is Demerol 50 mg per 1 mL and atropine 0.3 mg per 1 mL. What should be the total volume of the two drugs when mixed together into a syringe?

    1. 1.3 mL.
    2. 1.6 mL.
    3. 2.2 mL.
    4. 2.7 mL.

17. The patient's physician orders 20 mEq of KCl. The label on the KCl is 10 mEq/5 mL. The nurse will give the patient

    1. 10 mL.
    2. 2 mL.
    3. 5 mL.
    4. 20 mL.

18. A male patient is currently taking Digitalis 0.25 mg daily, Lasix 100 mg daily, acyclovir 10 mg QID, and Tagamet 300 mg QID. Which one of the following drugs has potential side effects that are the most life threatening?

    1. Digitalis.
    2. Lasix.
    3. Acyclovir.
    4. Tagamet.

19. A 60-year-old male patient with chronic osteoarthritis is severely debilitated. Betamethasone (Celestone) therapy has been ordered for him. The nurse will advise the patient to take a single, daily dose of the drug

    1. At bedtime with a glass of milk.
    2. With orange juice at bedtime.
    3. With milk in the morning.
    4. On an empty stomach in the morning.

20. Teaching a patient about use of the insulin pump in preparation for discharge, the nurse will explain that it uses

    1. A combination of regular and Lente insulin delivered two times each day.
    2. Continuous delivery of small amounts of regular insulin.
    3. A predetermined dose established by a glucose tolerance test.
    4. A combination of NPH and regular insulin with NPH delivered in the morning.

PHARMACOLOGY

Answers with Rationale

1. (1) If a drug binds to plasma protein, it is not effective even though it is transported through the circulatory system to all parts of the body. If it is not bound and travels through the circulatory system, it crosses cell membranes and is stored in the fat.

   NP:P; CN:PH; CA:M; CL:C

2. (3) Pulling back on the plunger, or aspirating, would ensure that the needle had not entered a blood vessel. Therefore, this action would be included in the Z-track method.

   NP:P; CN:S; CA:M; CL:A

3. (4) The area preferred is around the umbilicus in the abdominal area because absorption is quickest and most reliable.

   NP:P; CN:H; CA:M; CL:A

4. (3) Most drugs are broken down in the liver (where they are converted by enzymes into less active and harmless agents), although some conversion does take place in the kidneys (1), plasma (2), and intestinal mucosa (4).

   NP:P; CN:PH; CA:M; CL:C

5. (4) The muscle preferred for an intramuscular injection is the ventrogluteal because it is safer than the dorsogluteal, which is vulnerable to nerve and vascular injury.

   NP:P; CN:S; CA:M; CL:A

6. (3) The deltoid muscle is usually used for injection of a pain medication because blood flow to this area is 7 percent greater than the vastus lateralis and 17 percent greater than the gluteal muscles.

   NP:P; CN:S; CA:M; CL:A

7. (3) Massaging the area after injecting heparin could cause tissue damage. It is also not recommended to massage after injecting insulin. For most other drugs, massaging increases absorption.

   NP:I; CN:S; CA:M; CL:A

8. (3) Aminoglycoside antibiotics are more active when the urine is alkaline, and the patient may receive soda bicarbonate to accomplish creating this environment.

   NP:P; CN:PH; CA:M; CL:A

9. (3) Nitroglycerin should be taken whenever the patient feels a full, pressure feeling or tightness in his chest, not waiting until chest pain is severe. It can also be taken prophylactically before engaging in an activity known to cause angina in order to prevent an anginal attack.

   NP:I; CN:PH; CA:M; CL:A

10. (2) Tagamet can interfere with the absorption of Coumadin and several other drugs such as Dilantin, lidocaine, or Inderal; therefore, the serum levels of the drugs should be monitored closely. Tagamet should not be taken within 1 hour of an antacid, because this will interfere with the absorption. It is best to take the drug with food. Tagamet is usually ordered for short-term treatment of duodenal and active gastric ulcers.

    NP:P; CN:PH; CA:M; CL:A

11. (2) Seconal is a common barbiturate used for sleeplessness. It has a sedative effect on the CNS. Its use should be monitored because of potential addiction or overdose, especially with the elderly.

    NP:P; CN:PH; CA:M; CL:C

12. (3) Anti-DNA antibody levels correlate most specifically with lupus disease activity. A positive response to steroids would show a decrease in these levels. Twenty percent of patients with lupus develop a positive syphilis serology, and

---

Coding for Questions/Answers Abbreviations: **Nursing Process: NP,** Data Collection: D, Planning: P, Implementation: I, Evaluation: E, **Client Needs: CN,** Safe, Effective Care Environment: S, Health Promotion and Maintenance: H, Psychosocial Integrity: PS, Physiological Integrity: PH, **Clinical Area: CA,** Medical Nursing: M, Surgical Nursing: S, Maternal/Newborn Nursing: MA, Pediatric Nursing: P, Psychiatric Nursing: PS, **Cognitive Level: CL,** Knowledge: K, Comprehension: C, Application: A, Analysis: AN

many have hypergammaglobulinemia and a decreased platelet count.

NP:E; CN:PH; CA:M; CL:AN

13. (3) Agranulocytosis is characterized by neutropenia
(decreased number of lymphocytes), which lowers the
body defenses against infection. Granulocytes are
the first barrier to infection in the body.

NP:E; CN:PH; CA:M; CL:A

14. (1) The primary action of spironolactone is to increase urine sodium and thereby cause diuresis. It
is also potassium sparing and helps counteract
metabolic alkalosis by this mechanism.

NP:E; CN:PH; CA:M; CL:AN

15. (3) This is a correct dosage for a preoperative medication, so the nurse would administer the drug as
prescribed. The Z-track method would normally not
be used for this drug, but for injection of iron in
order to protect the tissue.

NP:I; CN:S; CA:M; CL:AN

16. (3) This computation can be done using the formula D (dose desired) divided by H (dose on hand)
multiplied by V (volume). Step I: Compute Demerol
dose: 75 ÷ 50 × 1 = 1.5. Step II: Compute atropine

dose: 0.2 ÷ 0.3 × 1 = 0.66 rounded to 0.7. Step III:
Add Demerol and atropine doses: 1.5 + 0.7 = 2.2 mL.

NP:P; CN:S; CA:M; CL:A

17. (1) 10 mL. To calculate the KCl, use the equation:
20 mEq = x mL; because 10 mEq = 5 mL, calculate
10:20:: 5:x; therefore x = 10 mL.

NP:P; CN:S; CA:M; CL:A

18. (2) Although each of these drugs has significant
side effects, Lasix has the potential for life-threatening cardiac arrhythmias. Potassium is lost as a
result of the drug use. One hundred mg is a large
dose and, thus, a low serum potassium level could
easily occur leading to ventricular arrhythmias.

NP:E; CN:S; CA:M; CL:C

19. (3) A single dose in the morning promotes better
results and less toxicity. It is given with milk to reduce gastrointestinal irritation.

NP:I; CN:PH; CA:M; CL:A

20. (2) The insulin pump mimics the release of insulin
by the pancreas in a continuous delivery of fixed
small amounts of regular insulin. It is capable of
delivering larger doses before meals.

NP:I; CN:PH; CA:M ; CL:A

Nutritional Management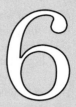

MACRONUTRIENTS

✦ Carbohydrates

A. Chief source of energy.

B. One gram of carbohydrate provides 4 kilocalories.

C. Monosaccharides.
   1. Glucose, fructose, galactose.
   2. Easily digested.

D. Disaccharides: sucrose, lactose, maltose.

E. Polysaccharides.
   1. Starch, dextrin, glycogen, cellulose, hemicellulose.
   2. More complex and harder to digest.

F. Sugar or starch converts to glucose.
   1. Appears in body as blood sugar.
   2. Metabolizes in cells.
   3. Converted in liver to glycogen for storage.

G. The amount and kind of carbohydrates that should be consumed for optimal health are determined by several factors:
   1. Body structure, energy expenditure, basal metabolism and general health status.
   2. The average American diet provides 45% of calories from carbohydrates; experts recommend this be increased to 55–60%.
   3. Simple (refined) sugars should be limited to 10% total calories.

✦ Fats or Lipids

A. Fats or lipids provide energy—each fat gram provides 9 kilocalories.

B. Act as barriers for fat-soluble vitamins, A, D, E, and K.

C. Fatty acids are the basic components of fat and comprise two main groups.
   1. Saturated fatty acids usually come from animal sources.
      a. Saturated fats should be less than 10% of calories.
      b. Cholesterol should be limited to 300 mg/day.
   2. Unsaturated fatty acids primarily come from vegetables, nuts, or seed sources.
      a. This group contains three essential fatty acids.
      b. These acids are called "essential" because they are necessary to prevent a specific deficiency disease.
      c. The body cannot manufacture these acids. They are obtained only from the diet.
      d. These acids are called linoleic acid, arachidonic acid, and linolenic acid.

D. The average American diet provides 35–40% of calories from fat—fats should comprise no more than 25–30% of daily calorie intake.

✦ Proteins

A. Complex organic compounds that contain amino acids.

B. Critical to all aspects of growth and development of body tissues; necessary for the building of muscles, blood, skin, internal organs, hormones, and enzymes.

C. Source of energy—each gram of protein provides 4 kilocalories.
   1. When there is insufficient carbohydrate or fat in the diet, protein is burned.
   2. When protein is spared, it is either used for tissue repair and maintenance or converted by the liver and stored as fat.

D. When digested and broken down, proteins form 20 amino acids.
   1. Amino acids are absorbed from the intestine into the bloodstream.
   2. They are carried to the liver for synthesis into the tissues and organs of the body.

E. Amino acids are the chemical basis for life, and if just one is missing, protein synthesis will decrease or even stop.
   ✦ 1. *All* but nine can be produced by the body; these nine must be obtained from the diet— eight are required by all humans; infants require one more—histidine.
   2. If all nine are present in a particular food, the food is a "complete protein"; foods that lack one or more are called "incomplete proteins."
   3. Most meat and dairy products are complete proteins; most vegetables and fruits are incomplete proteins.
   4. When animal protein is restricted, complementing or combining proteins from plant foods will assure adequate nutrition. For example, the combination of beans and rice is a complete protein food.

F. The National Research Council recommends that 56 g of protein/day for men and 45 g/day for women be consumed. The optimal healthy diet should be 10–12 percent protein (rather than the current 17% consumed by most Americans) or 40–50 g for a person weighing 150 lbs.

✦ Water

A. While not specifically a nutrient, water is essential for survival.
   1. Water is involved in every body process from digestion and absorption to excretion.
   2. It is a major portion of circulation and is the transporter of nutrients throughout the body.

B. Body water performs three major functions.

1. Water gives form to the body, comprising from 50–75 (average is 60) percent of the body mass.
2. It provides the necessary environment for cell metabolism.
3. It maintains a stable body temperature.
C. Almost all foods contain water that is absorbed by the body.
D. The average adult body contains 59 L of water and loses about 3 L a day.
    1. If a person suffers severe water depletion, dehydration and salt depletion can result and will eventually lead to death.
    2. A person can survive longer without food than without water.

MICRONUTRIENTS

✦ Vitamins

A. Vitamins are organic food substances and are essential in small amounts for growth, maintenance, and the functioning of body processes.
B. Vitamins are found only in living things—plants and animals—and usually cannot be synthesized by the human body.
C. Vitamins can be grouped according to the substance in which they are soluble.
D. The fat-soluble group includes vitamins A, D, E, and K.
E. The water-soluble vitamins include B_1, B_2, B_6, B_{12}, niacin, pantothenic acid, folacin, biotin, choline, mesoinositol, para-aminobenzoic acid, and ascorbic acid (vitamin C).
F. Vitamins have no caloric value, but they are as necessary to the body as any other basic nutrient.
    1. Currently, there are about 20 substances identified as vitamins.
    2. Recent research is concerned with identifying even more of these substances since they are so essential to survival.
G. The most commonly used are the listings of the Recommended Dietary Allowances (RDA), based on standards established by the National Academy of Sciences.

✦ Minerals

A. Minerals are inorganic substances, widely prevalent in nature, and essential for metabolic processes.
B. Minerals are grouped according to the amount found in the body.
C. Major minerals include calcium, magnesium, sodium, potassium, phosphorus, sulfur, and chlorine, all of which have a known function in the body.

Table 6-1. FOODS RICH IN FAT- AND WATER-SOLUBLE VITAMINS

Foods Rich in Fat-Soluble Vitamins
Vitamin A—liver, egg yolk, whole milk, butter, fortified margarine, green and yellow vegetables, fruits
Vitamin D—fortified milk and margarine, fish oils
Vitamin K—egg yolk, leafy green vegetables, liver, cheese

Foods Rich in Water-Soluble Vitamins
Vitamin C—citrus fruits, tomatoes, broccoli, cabbage
Thiamine (B_1)—lean meat such as beef, pork, liver; whole-grain cereals and legumes
Riboflavin (B_2)—milk, organ meats, enriched grains
Niacin—meat, beans, peas, peanuts, enriched grains
Pyridoxine (B_6)—yeast, wheat, corn, meats, liver, and kidney
Cobalamin (B_{12})—lean meat, liver, kidney
Folic acid—leafy green vegetables, eggs, liver

D. Trace minerals are iron, copper, iodine, manganese, cobalt, zinc, florine, selenium, and molybdenum and their function in the body remains unclear.
E. There remains another group of trace minerals found in scanty amounts in the body and whose function is also unclear.
F. Minerals form 60–90 percent of all inorganic material in the body, and are found in bones, teeth, soft tissue, muscle, blood, and nerve cells.
G. Minerals act on organs and in metabolic processes.
    1. They serve as catalysts for many reactions such as controlling muscle responses, maintaining the nervous system, and regulating acid–base balance.
    2. They assist in transmitting messages, maintaining cardiac stability, and regulating the metabolism and absorption of other nutrients.
H. Even though they are considered separately, all minerals work synergistically with other minerals, and their actions are interrelated.
    1. A deficiency in one mineral will affect the action of others in the body.
    2. Adequate minerals must be ingested because a mineral deficiency can result in severe illness.
    3. Excessive amounts of minerals can throw the body out of balance and may be toxic.
    4. Additional information can be found in the section on Fluid and Electrolyte Balance.

ASSIMILATION OF NUTRIENTS

Gastrointestinal Tract

A. The main functions of the gastrointestinal system consist of the following.

Table 6-2. ESSENTIAL BODY NUTRIENTS

Carbohydrates
Monosaccharides
    Glucose, fructose, galactose
Disaccharides
    Sucrose, lactose, maltose
Polysaccharides
    Starch, dextrin, glycogen, cellulose, hemicellulose

Fats
Linoleic acid, linolenic acid, arachidonic acid

Proteins
Amino acids
    Phenylalanine, lysine, isoleucine, leucine, methionine,
    valine, tryptophan, threonine, and histidine (for infants)

Vitamins
Fat-soluble
    Vitamins A, D, E, and K
Water-soluble
    Vitamins B_1, B_2, B_6, B_{12}, niacin, pantothenic acid, folacin,
    biotin, choline, mesoinositol, para-aminobenzoic acid, and
    vitamin C

Minerals
Major elements
    Calcium, chlorine, iron, magnesium, phosphorus, potas-
    sium, sodium, sulfur
Trace elements

Water

Table 6-3. MAJOR ENZYMES OF DIGESTION

Enzyme	Source/ Secretion	Substance Acted On
Ptyalin	Oral/Saliva	Starch
Maltose	Oral/Saliva	Maltose
Pepsin	Gastric	Protein
Lipase	Gastric	Fat
Rennin	Gastric	Casein (protein in milk)
Trypsin	Pancreatic	Protein
Steapsin	Pancreatic	Fats
Amylopsin	Pancreatic	Starch
Amylase	Intestinal	Starch
Maltase	Intestinal	Maltose
Lactase	Intestinal	Lactose
Sucrase	Intestinal	Sucrose
Erepsin	Intestinal	Proteins
Enterokinase	Intestinal	Proteins

C. Chemical digestion relies on the action of digestive enzymes and other substances.
   1. *See* Table 6-3.
   2. Hydrochloric acid is secreted by the stomach.
      Aids pepsin in its action on protein.

Gastrointestinal Dysfunctions

A. Dysphagia (difficulty swallowing) occurs in 60% of
   stroke patients and 50% of those with Parkinson's
   disease.
   1. Condition may also occur in cerebral palsy,
      multiple sclerosis, polio, myasthenia gravis.
   2. Most serious complication is aspiration of liq-
      uid or food into lungs.
B. Gastrointestinal hemorrhage may cause a rise in
   serum ammonia which may lead to altered neurologic function.
C. Intestinal obstruction—cessation of peristalsis
   (ileus) results in altered GI movement and
   absorption.

Accessory Organs

A. The accessory organs of the gastrointestinal
   tract play an important role in the utilization of
   nutrients.
✦ B. The liver plays a major role in the metabolism of
   carbohydrates, fats, and proteins.
   1. Liver converts glucose to glycogen and stores
      it. It reconverts glycogen to glucose when the
      body requires higher blood sugar. The
      process of releasing carbohydrates (end prod-
      ucts) into the bloodstream is called
      glycogenolysis.

1. Secretion of enzymes and electrolytes to
   break down raw materials that are ingested.
2. Movement of ingested products through the
   system.
3. Complete digestion of nutrients.
4. Absorption of nutrients into the blood.
5. Storage of nutrients.
6. Excretion of the end products of digestion.
B. Mechanical digestion.
   1. Begins in the mouth with chewing and
      swallowing.
   2. Nutrients are churned, and peristaltic waves
      move the material through the stomach.
   3. At intervals, with relaxation of the pyloric
      sphincter, they move into the duodenum.
   4. Peristaltic waves move the mass through the
      small intestines where some absorption
      occurs.
   5. The large intestine provides for the absorp-
      tion of nutrients and the elimination of waste
      products.
      a. Vitamins K and B_{12}, riboflavin, and thi-
         amine are formed.
      b. Water is absorbed from the fecal mass.

2. Fats are metabolized through the process of oxidation of fatty acids and the formation of acetoacetic acid.
3. Lipoproteins, cholesterol, and phospholipids are formed, and carbohydrates and protein are converted to fats.
4. Proteins are metabolized.
5. The formation of urea and plasma proteins is completed.
6. Bile is secreted.
◆ C. The gallbladder's primary function is to act as a reservoir for bile.
   1. Bile emulsifies fats through constant secretion.
   2. Secretion rate is 500–1000 mL every 24 hours.
◆ D. The pancreas secretes pancreatic juices that contain enzymes for the digestion of carbohydrates, fats, and proteins. These enzymes are activated in the small intestine.

NUTRITIONAL CONCEPTS

Normal and Therapeutic Nutrition

A. Normal nutrition.
   1. A guide for determining adequate nutrition is the U.S. Department of Agriculture recommended daily dietary allowances.
      a. The guide is scientifically designed for the maintenance of healthy people in the United States.
      b. The values of the caloric and nutrient requirements given in the guide are used in assessing nutritional status.
      c. Stress periods in the life cycle, which require alterations in the allowances, should be considered during the planning of menus.
   ◆ 2. The basic four food groups are described in *A Daily Food Guide: The Basic Four* (see Appendix 6-3).
      a. Choices in four food groups are offered to meet the nutrient recommendations during the life cycle. (Caloric requirement is not included.)
      b. Basic nutrients in each food group should be related to dietary needs during the life cycle when menus are planned for each age group.
B. Therapeutic nutrition.
   1. The therapeutic or prescription diet is a modification of the nutritional needs based on the disease condition and/or the excess or deficit nutrition state.
   2. Combination diets, which include alterations in minerals, vitamins, proteins, carbohy-

drates, and fats, as well as fluid and texture, are prescribed in therapeutic nutrition.
   3. Although not all such diets will be included in this review, study of the selected diet concepts will enable you to combine two or more diets when necessary.
C. Normal and therapeutic nutrition considerations.
   1. Cultural, socioeconomic, and psychological influences, as well as physiological requirements, must be considered for effective nutrition.
   2. In any given situation, the nutrition requirements must be considered within the context of the biopsychosocial needs of an individual. *See* Table 6-4.

Diet Related to Heart Disease Risk

A. The lipid hypothesis, introduced in the 1950s, suggested diet and cholesterol (especially saturated fat) presented risk for heart disease.
   1. Total cholesterol over 200 and ratio of high-density lipoproteins (HDL), the "good" cholesterol, to low-density lipoproteins (LDL) or "bad" cholesterol, predict risk.
   2. Goal is to reduce saturated fat in diet.
B. High concentration of homocysteine in blood is also associated with risk for heart disease.

Table 6-4. RECOMMENDED NUTRIENT REQUIREMENTS FOR HEALING*

Total Calories
2800 for tissue repair; 6000 for extensive repair

Protein
50–75 g/day early in postoperative period;
   100–200 g/day if needed for new tissue synthesis

CHO
50–60 percent of calories or sufficient in quantity to meet calorie needs and allow protein to be used for tissue repair

Fat
25–30 percent or not excessive—it leads to poor tissue healing and susceptibility to infection

Vitamins
Vitamin C—up to 1 g/day
Vitamin B—increased above normal
Vitamin K—normal amounts
Vitamin A and beta carotene—stimulates immune response
Vitamin E 400 U—increases O_2 to the tissues
Minerals—normal amount for tissue repair and healing (zinc, selenium, calcium/magnesium)

*Diet will be individualized—depends on assessment of patient's needs.

1. An amino acid forms when diet has a high concentration of meat and dairy products.
2. Excess levels damage artery walls causing the vessel to trap circulating cholesterol.
3. Increasing daily intake of B vitamins (folic acid, pyridoxine and B_{12}) will reduce homocystein levels and risk of heart disease.

Nutritional Problems in the Hospital

A. Nutrition is frequently neglected as an important part of patient care.
B. The nurse must consistently assess the patient to assist in determining needed diet alterations.
   1. Inability to feed self or absence of dentures.
   2. Feelings of depression or fear.
   3. Unpleasant environmental factors prior to meals.
   4. Pain or nausea.
C. Studies conducted at various medical centers claim that as many as 50% of hospitalized patients suffer from malnutrition.

✦ Providing Appropriate Nutrition

A. Verify dietary order.
B. Notify charge nurse and/or physician if patients' needs are not being met.
C. Determine patients' food preferences.
D. Check all diet trays before serving to ensure the diet provided is the one ordered.
E. Ensure that hot food is hot and cold food is cold.
F. Keep food trays attractive. Avoid spilling liquids on tray.
G. Position the patient in a chair or up in bed (unless otherwise ordered) to assist in feeding.
H. Assist the patient with cutting meat and opening milk cartons as needed.
I. Feed the patient if necessary.

✦ Malnutrition Disorders

A. Kwashiorkor—caused by a lack of protein; frequently seen in ages one to three, when high-protein intake is necessary.
B. Nutritional marasmus—a disease caused by a deficiency of food intake. It is a form of starvation.
C. Vitamin A deficiency—night blindness may progress to xerophthalmia and, finally, keratomalacia.
D. Vitamin C deficiency: scurvy—symptoms begin with muscle tenderness as walls of capillaries become fragile. Hemorrhage of vessels results.
E. Vitamin D deficiency: rickets—vitamin D is necessary for adequate calcium absorption by the bones.
F. Thiamine deficiency: beriberi—primarily a disease of rice-eating people; symptoms include numbness in extremities and exhaustion.

G. Niacin deficiency: pellagra—symptoms include dermatitis, diarrhea, dementia, and, finally, death.
H. Iodine deficiency—leads to hyperplasia of the thyroid gland, or goiter.

ENTERAL FEEDING

Nutrients via Tube Feeding

Characteristics

A. Purpose is to maintain adequate food–fluid intake.
B. Reasons for procedure.
   1. Patient is unconscious.
   2. Refusal to take in fluids or solid foods (anorexic).
   3. Trauma to upper GI tract.
   4. Patient is unable to chew or swallow.

Nasogastric Tube Insertion ❖ PROCEDURE ❖

A. Check order for tube feeding.
B. Warm feeding to room temperature.
C. Discuss procedure with the patient.
D. Demonstrate and display items to be used in order to allay the patient's fear and to gain cooperation.
E. Wash your hands and don gloves.
F. Position the patient at 45-degree angle or higher.
G. Examine nostrils and select the most patent nostril by having the patient breathe through each one.
✦ H. Measure from tip of nose to earlobe to xiphoid process of sternum to determine appropriate length for tube insertion. If tube is to go below stomach, a small flex tube is used. Mark point on tube with tape.
I. Lubricate first 10 cm of tube with water-soluble lubricant.
J. Insert tube through nostril to back of throat and ask the patient to swallow. (Instruct patient to flex head forward after tube has passed nasopharynx. Do not have patient hyperextend neck.) Sips of water may aid in advancing tubing past oropharynx.
K. Continue advancing tube until taped mark is reached.
L. Check position of tube.
   1. It is no longer considered safe to place end of NG tube in glass of water and observe for bubbling.
   2. Inject 10 mL of air through nasogastric tube and listen with the stethoscope over stomach for a rush of air. This method cannot be used alone to check tube placement.
   ✦ 3. The most accurate method is to aspirate gastric contents and check pH (sometimes difficult with small-bore tubes). If pH is

acidic—below 3 with litmus paper red—tube is in stomach.

    ✦ 4. Obtain x-ray confirmation. If nasoduodenal or nasojejunal feedings required, patient should have x-ray to confirm correct placement.

    5. Tape tube securely to nose and to cheek.

M. Remain with and talk with the patient until the anxiety level is decreased (tube insertion often raises anxiety).

Tube Feeding Administration ❖ PROCEDURE ❖

A. Obtain order from the physician for appropriate formula (calories and/or amount).

B. Send requisition for formula to diet kitchen.

C. Check early in shift to ensure adequate formula is available.

D. Warm formula to room temperature by setting formula container in basin of hot water—do not use microwave oven.

E. Assemble feeding equipment. If using bag, fill with ordered amount of formula.

F. Explain procedure to the patient and assure privacy.

G. Verify presence of bowel sounds (lack of sounds = no peristalsis).

H. Place the patient on right side in high-Fowler's position.

I. Check position of tube by aspirating stomach contents.

✦ J. Determine amount of residual. Hold feeding if more than one-half amount previously delivered feeding is residual. Return aspirated contents to stomach to prevent electrolyte imbalance.

K. Pinch the tubing to prevent air from entering stomach.

L. Attach barrel of syringe to nasogastric tube and fill syringe with formula. (If using feeding bag, adjust drip rate to infuse over 30 minutes.)

M. Hold syringe no more than 39 cm (18 inches) above patient.

N. Allow formula to infuse slowly (between 20 and 35 minutes) through the tubing.

O. Follow tube feeding with water in amount ordered.

P. Clamp end of the tube.

Q. Wash tray and return it to patient's bedside—change syringe daily.

R. Give water between feedings if tube feeding is the sole source of nutrition.

✦ Nasogastric Tube Irrigation ❖ PROCEDURE ❖

A. Obtain a disposable irrigation set or emesis basin for irrigation solution, a 50-mL syringe, and a normal saline irrigation solution.

B. Wash your hands and don gloves.

C. Place patient in a semi-Fowler's position.

D. Disconnect NG tube from suction, if necessary, and check for nasogastric tube placement by aspirating stomach contents. (*See* Nasogastric Tube Insertion.)

E. Draw up 20–30 mL normal saline into the irrigating syringe.

F. Gently instill the normal saline into the nasogastric tube. Do not force the solution.

G. Withdraw the 20–30 mL irrigation solution and empty into basin.

H. Repeat the procedure twice.

I. Record on I&O sheet the irrigation solution that has not been returned.

✦ Continuous Tube Feedings (Dobhoff, Keofeed Tubes) ❖ PROCEDURE ❖

A. Complete steps A–F from Tube Feeding Administration.

B. Elevate head of bed 30 degrees.

C. Check for bowel sounds.

D. Insert tube (tubes are weighted at the distal end with mercury or tungsten) or check patency of existing tube.

E. Irrigate feeding tube with sterile water or saline at least every 4 hours.

F. Check residual at least every shift.

G. Administer formula at prescribed infusion rate (usually 10 mL/min). Infusion pumps are used to maintain continuous flow.

    1. Avoid keeping formula at room temperature for longer than 4 hours to prevent spoilage and bacterial contamination.

    2. Replace disposable feeding bag and tubing every 24 hours.

H. Routinely assess the abdomen for abdominal distention and bowel sounds.

I. Keep patient in semi-Fowler's position.

J. Turn off flow when placing patient supine.

Gastrostomy Feeding ❖ PROCEDURE ❖

✦ A. Assess gastric contents to determine amount per intermittent feeding.

    1. Hold feeding if more than 50–100 mL.

    2. Return aspirated contents to stomach.

B. Feed slowly through syringe at prescribed rate or adjust rate to infuse over 30 minutes.

C. Observe gastrostomy tube insertion site for signs of dislodging, infection, or skin breakdown.

D. Provide site care; wash area with warm water and soap.

E. Apply skin protective barrier. Cover area with sterile dressing.

Total Nutritional Alimentation (TNA)
❖ PROCEDURE ❖

Assessment

A. Nutritional needs of patients unable to ingest calories normally.

B. Caloric intake necessary to promote positive nitrogen balance, tissue repair, and growth; lipids are included in formula.

C. Ordered additives in each hyperalimentation bottle.

D. Compare label of solution against physician's orders.

E. Check rate of infusion on physician's orders.

F. Ability of patient to understand instructions during procedure.

G. Patency of central venous line following insertion.

H. Observe catheter insertion site for signs of infection, thrombophlebitis, or possible infiltration.

I. Inspect dressing over central line to ensure a dry, noncontaminated dressing.

✦ Implementation

✦ A. Teach the Valsalva's maneuver if patient does not have a cardiac disorder. This maneuver prevents air from entering the catheter during catheter insertion or tubing changes.
  1. Ask patient to take a deep breath and bear down.
  2. Apply gentle pressure to the abdomen.

✦ B. Review physician's order for correct hyperalimentation solution additives.
  1. TNA bottles come directly from the pharmacy and are numbered sequentially.
  2. Each TNA bottle label will include patient's name, room number, additives, IV number, start time, date, and stop time.
  3. Inspect TNA bottle for cracks, turbidity, or precipitates.

C. Assemble IV system with in-line filter and prime IV tubing and filter with ordered solution.

✦ D. Position patient in head-down position with head turned to opposite direction of catheter insertion site. Place a small roll between patient's shoulders to expose insertion site.

E. Cleanse insertion area with Betadine solution.

F. Wash hands and don mask and sterile gloves and assist physician as needed during catheter insertion.

G. Instruct patient in Valsalva's maneuver when stylet is removed from catheter and when IV tubing is connected to catheter.
  1. After tubing is connected, instruct patient to breathe normally.
  2. Tape area between tubing and catheter hub.

H. Turn on IV infusion pump, using normal saline solution at a slow rate of 10 drops/min until x-ray ensures accurate catheter placement. Flush catheter with saline and heparinize with dilute heparin according to agency policy.

✦ I. Confirm catheter placement via x-ray and change IV solution to hyperalimentation solution.
  1. Store hyperalimentation solution in refrigerator until 30 minutes before use. This prevents growth of organisms, but should be warmed to room temperature prior to use.
  2. Change solution every 12 to 24 hours to prevent growth of bacteria.

J. Time tape the bottle after adjusting flow rate. Be prepared to document on IV hourly infusion record.

K. Observe for signs of air embolism, subcutaneous bleeding, pneumothorax, or allergic responses to protein (chills, increased temperature, nausea, headache, urticaria, dyspnea).

L. Apply 4x4 sterile gauze pad over IV site and occlude dressing with micropore or plastic tape.

M. Take vital signs every four hours.

✦ N. Maintain central vein infusion.
  1. Change IV tubing, filter, and infusion pump casette (if used) every 24 hours.
  2. Change extension tubing every 48 hours. Change solution every 12–24 hours (prevents growth of bacteria when using sugar in solution).
  3. Maintain IV flow rate at prescribed rate.
     a. If rate is too rapid, hyperosmolar diuresis occurs (excess sugar will be excreted); if severe enough, intractable seizures, coma, and death can occur.
     b. If rate is too slow, little benefit will be derived from the calories and nitrogen.
     c. Do not correct an overload or deficit in flow, as doing so could result in complications for the patient. Notify physician if this occurs.

O. Check blood sugar via finger-stick every 6 hours. Administer regular insulin according to prescribed "sliding scale."

P. Keep I&O records and weigh daily.

THERAPEUTIC/PRESCRIPTION DIETS

Restricting Dietary Carbohydrates

✦ A. Hypoglycemic diet.
  1. A hypoglycemic diet is utilized to reduce stimulation of excessive insulin by avoiding highly concentrated carbohydrate foods.
     a. Foods prescribed are high protein, moderate complex carbohydrates in 5 or 6 meals/day.
     b. Foods limited are high (noncomplex) carbohydrates, for example, sugar, syrup, candy.

Table 6-5. DIABETIC EXCHANGE DIETS

Food Group	Unit of Exchange	Calories	Foods Allowed
Milk			
Whole	1 cup	170	1 cup whole milk = 1 cup skim milk and 2 fat exchanges
Skim	1 cup	80	
Fruit	Varies according to calories allotted	40	Fresh or canned without sugar or syrup
Vegetables			
A	1 cup	Vary	Green leafy vegetables; tomatoes
B	½ cup	35	Vegetables other than green, leafy
Bread/starch	1 slice	70	Can exchange cereals, starch items, some vegetables
Meat	1 ounce	75	Lean meats, egg, cheese, seafood
Fat	1 teaspoon	45	1 teaspoon butter or mayonnaise = bacon, oil, olives, avocado
Unlimited foods			Coffee, tea, bouillon, spices, flavorings

2. Stevia, a new sugar substitute, is recommended.

✦ B. Diabetic guidelines.
  1. Nutrition is the cornerstone of disease management.
  2. Normal weight must be maintained and may dramatically reduce symptoms.
  3. Diet together with insulin supplement or oral medication and exercise complete the regimen.

C. Goal of dietary therapy is to have a well-balanced diet and stable blood glucose levels by counting carbohydrates (CHO) because CHOs raise blood sugar.
  1. Diabetics do not have to give up their favorite foods; they must learn the amounts that are allowed and substitutions permitted. *See* Table 6-5.
  ✦ 2. General guidelines for nutrient balance:

Carbohydrate   50–60%
(40% from complex CHO)
Fat   20–30%
Saturated fat   10%
(Limit cholesterol to 300 mg)
Protein   10–20%

  ✦ 3. According to the American Dietetic Association, dietary ratio is 5:2:1 carbohydrate to fat to protein.
  4. Also consume 20–35 g. of fiber daily (including soluble and insoluble fiber).

✦ D. Carbohydrate counting is a useful tool to maintain stable blood glucose levels.
  1. Count grams of carbohydrates.
  2. Measure servings or choices.
  3. Use the glycemic index, which describes how much the blood glucose level rises with a specific food when compared with an equivalent amount of glucose. *See* Table 6-6.

Table 6-6. THE GLYCEMIC INDEX OF COMMON FOODS

Low	Moderate
(Recommend in abundance)	(Recommended in moderation)
Green vegetables	Whole-grain breads
Tomatoes	Whole-grain pasta
Beans and peas	Oatmeal
Dried apricots	Sweet potatoes
Berries	Grapes
Grapefruit	Apples
Nuts	Oranges
Rye and barley	Carrots
High	
(Not recommended at all or very sparingly)	
Most sugars	White potatoes
White breads	Corn
Crackers, rice cakes, and chips	Pineapple
Most cold cereals	Raisins
White rice	Ripe bananas

E. Level of activity must be assessed to determine energy requirements.
  1. Increased activity uses more carbohydrates.
  2. Most adults require 30 calories/kg of ideal body weight.

Restructuring Dietary Protein

✦ A. Restricted protein diet.
  1. Utilized for renal impairment: uremia, hepatic coma, and cirrhosis (according to individual requirements).
  2. Purpose of diet: to limit protein intake and the end (breakdown) products of protein

metabolism (nitrogenous waste) which are disturbing the fluid and electrolyte and/or acid–base balance.

3. Diet allowances/requirements.
   a. The number of grams of protein allowed is stated for each diet.
   b. Examples of high-protein foods to be avoided: eggs, meat, milk and milk products.

✦ B. Amino acid metabolism abnormalities diet.
   1. Utilized for phenylketonuria (PKU), galactosemia, and lactose intolerance.
   2. Purpose of diet: to reduce and/or eliminate the offending enzyme in the food intake of protein and utilize substitute nutrient foods.
   3. The main source of enzymes for the three diseases is milk. Milk and milk products must be avoided and substitutes used to meet daily allowances. *See* Table 6-7.

Restricted Dietary Fat

✦ A. Restricted cholesterol diet.
   1. Utilized for cardiovascular diseases, diabetes mellitus, high serum cholesterol levels.
   2. Purpose of diet: to decrease the blood cholesterol level and/or maintain blood cholesterol at a normal level by restricting foods high in cholesterol.
   3. Lipid level goals—cholesterol < 160–200 mg/dL; LDL < 100 mg/dL; HDL > 45 for males and 55 for females.
   4. Restrict total fat to 30% of calories; restrict saturated fat to 10% (or less) of calories.
   5. High-cholesterol foods to be restricted or avoided (primarily originating from animal sources).
      a. Saturated fats.
      b. Examples: egg yolk, shell fish, organ meats, bacon, pork. *See* Table 6-8.
   6. Substitute trans fats and saturated fat with monounsaturated fats (found in plant products); increase essential fatty acids.
   7. Encourage low-cholesterol foods (primarily originating from plant sources).
      a. Polyunsaturated fats.
      b. Examples: vegetable oils, raw or cooked vegetables, fruits, lean meats, fowl.

B. Modified-fat diet.
   1. Utilized according to individual tolerance in malabsorption syndromes, cystic fibrosis, gallbladder disease, obstructive jaundice, and liver diseases.
   2. Purpose of diet: to lower fat content in diet to stop contractions of diseased organs; to reduce fat content where there is inadequate absorption of fat.

Table 6-7. FOODS HIGH IN PROTEIN

Food	Protein (Grams)
Dairy and Eggs	
Cottage cheese, ½ cup	14.0
Milk, 1 cup	8.5
Cheddar cheese, 1 oz.	7.1
Egg, 1 medium	6.1
Ice cream, ½ cup	2.4
Meat and Fish	
Tuna, canned, drained, 4 oz.	32.0
Chicken, 4 oz. cooked	31.2
Hamburger, 4 oz. cooked	30.7
Sirloin steak, 4 oz. cooked	26.7
Grains	
Whole-wheat flour, ½ cup	8.0
Spaghetti, 1 cup cooked	6.0
Cornmeal, ½ cup	5.5
Rice, brown, 1 cup cooked	5.0
Rice, white, 1 cup cooked	4.0
Legumes	
Soybeans, ½ cup cooked	12.0
Peanut butter, 1 oz.	7.1
Lima beans, ½ cup cooked	6.1
Cashews, 1 oz.	4.8

Table 6-8. FOODS HIGH IN CHOLESTEROL

Beef liver	Bacon
Organ meats	Chicken
Eggs	Lobster
Sardines	Turkey
Veal	Ice cream
Lamb	Hot dogs
Beef	White fish
Pork	

a. Foods to be avoided: gravies, fat meat and fish, cream, fried foods, rich pastries.
b. Foods allowed: eggs, lean meat, butter/margarine, cheese.

Restricting Diets for Renal Disease

A. Low-protein—essential amino acid diet.
   1. Utilized for renal failure.
   2. Purpose of diet: to prevent electrolytes and by-products of metabolism from accumulating to a fatal level between artificial kidney treatments.
   3. Foods allowed:
      a. Eggs (1 daily).
      b. Milk (6 ounces).
      c. Low protein bread.

d. Fruit (two to four servings): apples, peaches, pears, cherries, pineapple, strawberries, grapefruit, grapes.

e. Vegetables (two to four servings): usually any vegetable.

f. Free list: for calories—butter, oil, jelly, candy with chocolate; tea, coffee.

4. Foods restricted or not allowed:

a. Meat: chicken, roast beef, fish, lamb, veal.

b. Peanuts; bread other than low-protein bread.

◆ B. Low-calcium diet.

1. Utilized to prevent formation of renal calculi (96 percent of calculi are calcium compounds).

2. Purpose of diet: to decrease the total daily intake of calcium to prevent further stone formation. Total 400 mg calcium instead of normal 800 mg calcium per day.

3. Foods allowed:

a. Milk (one cup daily).

b. Fruit juices, tea, coffee.

c. Eggs (one daily); fats.

d. Fresh fruits; vegetables (except dried).

4. Foods restricted:

a. Rye and whole-grain breads and cereals.

b. Dried fruits and vegetables (peas and beans).

c. Fish, shellfish, dried and cured meats.

d. Cheese, chocolate, nuts. *See* Table 6-9.

◆ C. Low-purine diet.

1. Utilized to prevent uric acid stones; also utilized for gout patients.

2. Purpose of diet: to restrict purine, which is the precursor of uric acid; 4 percent of urinary stones are composed of uric acid.

3. Foods allowed:

a. Carbonated beverages, milk, tea, fruit juices.

b. Breads, cereals.

c. Cheese, eggs, fat.

d. Most vegetables.

4. Foods restricted:

a. Glandular meats, gravies.

b. Fowl, fish, meat (restricted in amount). *See* Table 6-10.

Selected Diets Associated with Mineral Control

◆ A. Restricted sodium diet.

1. Utilized for hypertension, hepatitis, congestive heart failure, renal deficiencies, cirrhosis of liver, adrenal corticoid treatment.

2. Purpose of diet: to correct and/or control the retention of sodium and water in the body by limiting sodium intake. May be done strictly by food restriction or in combination with medications.

Table 6-9. FOODS HIGH IN CALCIUM	
Milk, cream	Shrimp, clams, and oysters
Cottage cheese	Salmon
Mustard greens, turnip greens	Cheese
Kale	Ice cream

Table 6-10. FOODS HIGH IN PURINE	
Meat extracts	Beans, lentils
Shellfish	Peas
Liver and other organ meats	Spinach
Sardines, mussels, anchovies	Cauliflower
Chicken, turkey	Asparagus

Table 6-11. FOODS HIGH IN SODIUM
Table salt and all prepared salts, such as celery salt
Smoked meats and salted meats
Most frozen or canned vegetables with added salt
Butter, margarine, and cheese
Quick-cooking cereals
Shellfish and frozen or salted fish
Seasonings and sauces
Canned soups
Chocolates and cocoa
Beets, celery, and selected greens (spinach)
Foods with salt added, such as potato chips, popcorn

3. Restriction varies from eliminating salt in cooking or at the table to strict food restrictions of any product containing sodium, such as soda bicarbonate.

4. Typical diet provides 4–6 g of sodium/day. *See* Table 6-11.

a. Mild: 2–3 g sodium (no added salt provides 3 g/day).

b. Moderate: 1500 mg sodium.

◆ B. Potassium management in diet.

1. Increased potassium.

a. Utilized for diabetic acidosis, extended use of certain diuretic drugs, burns (after first 48 hours), vomiting, and fevers.

b. Purpose of diet: to replace potassium loss from the body. (Severe potassium loss is managed with intravenous therapy.)

2. Conditions requiring low potassium are glomerulonephritis and dialysis management. *See* Table 6-12.

C. Enhanced calcium diet.

1. Used to prevent or correct post-menopausal osteoporosis and prevent and treat hypertension.

Table 6-12. FOODS HIGH IN POTASSIUM
Fruit juices such as orange, grapefruit, banana, apple
Instant, dry coffee powder
Egg, legumes, whole grains
Fish, especially fresh halibut and codfish
Pork, beef, lamb, veal, chicken
Milk, skim and whole
Dried dates, prunes
Bouillon and meat broths

Table 6-13. FOODS HIGH IN IRON
Organ meats, especially beef liver
Red meat, turkey, chicken
Fish, shellfish
Blackstrap molasses
Egg yolk
Lima beans, legumes
Sunflower seeds
Almonds, pecans, cashews
Dried fruits, apricots, prunes, raisins
Leafy vegetables, broccoli, brussels sprouts
Peas
Kidney beans
Brewer's yeast
Cheese—Swiss, ricotta, roquefort
Wild rice
Yogurt
Wheat germ
Bananas

2. Increase normal adult intake of 1 gm/day to 1.5 gm/day.

3. Lactose intolerant patients take green, leafy vegetables and non-liquid dairy products (cheese, yogurt) to increase calcium intake.

✦ D. High-iron diet.

1. Utilized for anemias (hemorrhagic, nutritional, pernicious), postgastrectomy syndrome, malabsorption syndrome.

2. Purpose of diet: to replace a deficit of iron due to either inadequate intake or chronic blood loss.

3. Foods high in iron content: organ meats (especially liver), meats, egg yolks, whole wheat, seafood, leafy green vegetables, nuts, dried fruit, legumes. See Table 6-13.

4. Diets supplemented with iron and folic acid (for pregnant women) may need to add extra zinc.

Modified Fiber Diets

A. There are 2 types of fiber.

1. Insoluble fibers found in cell wall of plants—do not dissolve in water; speed up elimination of waste products.

2. Soluble fibers (oat bran) dissolve in water. This type decreases cholesterol levels and slows absorption of glucose.

✦ B. High-fiber (roughage) diets.

1. Prescribed for constipation and diverticulosis (prescription varies with physician).

2. Purpose of diet: to mechanically stimulate the gastrointestinal tract.

3. Diet allowances/requirements.

   a. Foods high in residue.

     (1) Any meat or fish that is fried, canned, or smoked; any poultry with skin.

     (2) Cheese.

     (3) Fat in any form.

     (4) Milk and fruit juices.

     (5) Whole-wheat breads, unrefined bran, cereals, shredded wheat.

   b. Foods low in carbohydrates are usually high in residue.

✦ C. Low-fiber (roughage) diets.

1. Utilized for ulcerative colitis, postoperative colon and rectal surgery, diverticulitis (when inflammation decreases diet may revert to high residue), rheumatic fever, diarrhea and enteritis.

2. Purpose of diet: to soothe and be nonirritating residue in the large intestine.

3. Diet allowances/requirements.

   a. Foods low in residue.

     (1) Ground, tender meat; fresh fish; any boiled, roasted, or broiled poultry without skin or fat.

     (2) Hard-boiled egg.

     (3) Creamed cottage cheese and mild cheeses.

     (4) Limited fat, crisp bacon, plain gravies.

     (5) Warm drinks (not iced); no milk.

     (6) Refined, strained, precooked cereals like pablum; enriched white bread; crackers; toast.

   b. Foods low in carbohydrates usually add high residue.

Bland Food Diets

A. These diets are presented in stages, with gradual addition of specific foods.

B. Frequent, small feedings during active stress periods; then regular meals and patterns should be established.

C. May be utilized for duodenal ulcer, gastric ulcers, postoperative stomach surgery.

D. Purpose of diet: to promote the healing of the gastric mucosa by eliminating food sources that are chemically and mechanically irritating.

✦ E. Diet allowances/requirements.
1. Foods allowed.
    a. Milk, butter, eggs (not fried), custard, vanilla ice cream, cottage cheese.
    b. Cooked refined or strained cereal, enriched white bread.
    c. Jello; homemade creamed, pureed soups.
    d. Baked or broiled potatoes.
2. Examples of foods that are eliminated.
    a. Spicy and highly seasoned foods.
    b. Raw foods.
    c. Very hot and very cold foods.
    d. Gas-forming foods (varies with individuals).
    e. Coffee, alcoholic beverages, carbonated drinks.
    f. High fat content (some butter and margarine allowed).

Diets Associated with Surgery

✦ A. Preoperative diet.
1. Purpose of diet.
    a. Maintenance of normal serum protein levels.
    b. Provide adequate carbohydrate to maintain liver glycogen.
    c. Provide adequate amino acids to promote wound healing.
    d. Restore nitrogen balance if protein depleted (burned, elderly, severely debilitated patient).
✦ 2. Recommended nutrient requirements.
    a. 0.8–1.5 g of protein/kg body weight/day.
    b. 25–50 Kcal/kg/day.
        (1) A calorie is a unit of heat measurement defined as the amount of heat required to raise 1 kg of water to 1°C.
        (2) One gram of protein equals 4 kilocalories (Kcal).
3. Recommended diet.
    a. 2500 Kcal.
    b. A high-energy, moderate-protein diet.
    c. High-protein supplements.
✦ 4. Elemental diet.
    a. Low-residue diet.
    b. Contains synthetic mixture of CHO, amino acids, essential fatty acids with added minerals and vitamins.
    c. Bulk free, easily assimilated and absorbed.
    d. Replace clear liquid diet for patients with colon surgery.
    e. Diet products: Vivonex and Precision.

B. Postoperative diet progression.
1. Purpose of diet.
    a. Promote wound healing by adequate protein intake.
    b. Avoid shock from decreased plasma proteins and circulating red blood cells by increasing protein intake.
    c. Prevent edema by adequate protein intake (maintains colloidal osmotic pressure).
    d. Promote bone healing in orthopedic surgery by adequate protein and mineral replacement.
    e. Prevent infection by adequate amino acid replacement (amino acids are involved in body defense mechanisms).
✦ 2. Recommended nutrient requirements.
    a. Total calories: 2800 for tissue repair; 6000 for extensive repair.
    b. Fluid intake.
        (1) Uncomplicated surgery: 2000 to 3000/day.
        (2) Complicated surgery (sepsis, renal damage): 3000 to 4000/day.
        (3) Seriously ill with drainage: 7000/day.
✦ 3. Diet progresses from nothing by mouth (NPO) the day of surgery to a general diet. Phases/steps include:
    a. A clear-liquid diet is 1000 to 1500 mL/day and is comprised of water, tea, broth, Jello, and juices (avoid juices with pulp).
    b. A full-liquid diet lacks many nutrients, so it is used temporarily. Includes clear liquids, milk and milk products, custard, puddings, creamed soups, sherbet, ice cream, and any fruit juice.
    c. A soft diet is full liquid and, in addition, pureed vegetables, eggs (not fried), milk, cheese, fish, fowl, tender beef, veal, potatoes, and cooked fruit.
    d. General diet, taking into consideration specific alterations necessary for patient's health status.

Appendix 6-1. SUMMARY OF DIETARY CONTROL FOR DISORDERS

Malabsorption Syndromes

Cystic fibrosis: high calorie, high protein, with vitamin and mineral supplements; if diet has increased fats (not recommended), add extra enzymes.

Ulcerative colitis: high protein, high calorie, low lactase, low residue.

Crohn's disease: low residue, high protein, and vitamin–mineral supplements.

Diverticulosis: high fiber.

Constipation: high fiber with liquids.

Diarrhea: low residue.

Liver, Biliary, and Pancreatic Problems

Liver involvement: high calorie, high protein, high carbohydrate, low to moderate fat intake.

Gallbladder: low fat and exclude any foods that cause problems (fatty foods, gas-forming vegetables).

Pancreatitis: high protein, high carbohydrate, low fat, and decreased alcohol intake.

Genitourinary Problems

Urinary tract infection: increase acid ash, reduce alkali ash (citrus, milk, vegetables).

Renal failure: high carbohydrate, limited protein, low potassium.

Chronic renal failure: low protein, low salt, restricted fluids.

Renal calculi: acid ash diet for stones formed of exalate or phosphate and alkali ash when stones formed of uric acid or cystine. Force fluids.

Specific Disorders

Gout: restrict foods high in purine, increase fluid intake, high carbohydrate and control of calories.

Hyperthyroidism: high carbohydrate and high protein, restrict caffeine.

Phenylketonuria (PKU): restrict phenylalanine. (Phenylalanine is found in all natural protein foods; meat, milk, etc., are eliminated.)

Obesity: restrict calories but nutritionally sound diet with adequate protein, complex carbhohydrates, and limited fat. (Fat and carbohydrates are retained to ensure protein utilization.)

Appendix 6-2. NUTRITIONAL ASSESSMENT PARAMETERS

Clinical Assessment	Normal	Abnormal
Dietary Data		
Appetite	Remains unchanged	Increased or decreased recently Particular cravings
Nutritional intake	Adequate foods and fluids to supply body nutrients Nonallergic response to major food groups	Elimination of certain food categories that results in limited nutrients Emphasis on some food groups (sugar) to the exclusion of others (vegetables) Allergic response to certain foods
Caloric intake	Average 28 Kcal/Kg/day	Constant use of fad diets to lose weight Use of drugs or chemicals that interfere with appetite or nutrient assimilation
Meal patterns	3–6 home-prepared meals/day Adequate time and calm atmosphere for meals	Fast-food or packaged foods Missed meals, constant snacking, or overeating Eating "on the run" or hurried
General Appearance		
	Alert, responsive healthy appearing eyes and skin	Listless, dull, nonresponsive Skin and eyes appear unhealthy
Physical factors	Adequate chewing and swallowing capability Mouth and gums healthy so food can be ingested Physical exercise adequate for calorie intake	Teeth or gums in poor condition or ill-fitting dentures Swallowing impairs ingestion Inadequate physical exercise to burn calories

Continues

Appendix 6-2. NUTRITIONAL ASSESSMENT PARAMETERS (Continued)

Clinical Assessment	Normal	Abnormal
Presence of disease	No disease process that interferes with nutrient assimilation No congential condition or postsurgery condition that interferes with nutrient assimilation	Disease present that interferes with ingestion, digestion, assimilation, or excretion Congenital condition, rehabilitation phase, or postsurgery that interferes with food assimilation
Elimination schedule	Regular, adequate dlimination of foods Absence of constant flatus, discharge or mucus	Irregular or painful elimination Presence of constant flatus Presence of discharge, blood, or mucus
Anthropometric Measurements		
Height	For bedridden patients, measure arm span —fully extend arms 90° angle to body and measure from tip of one middle finger to the tip of other middle finger for estimated height	Loss of 2–3 inchs in height may indicate osteoporosis
Weight—compared to ideal and usual body weight	Ideal body weight 100 lbs (female); 106 lbs (male) for 5 feet height + 5 lbs for each 1 inch over 5 feet (female) and 6 lbs for each 1 inch over 5 feet (male) Small frame minus 10% Large frame plus 10%	Changed—markedly increased or decreased recently; important indicator of changed nutritional status Loss of more than 10% weight for prior 6 months should be clinically evaluated
Body Mass Index Ratio of weight in kilograms and height in meters	18.5–24.9	Less than 18.5—underweight 25–29—overweight 30–39—obese
Triceps skinfold measurement (mm)	Standard values—male to female 12.5–16.5	If values change over months, may indicate a chronic condition
Circumference of upper arm (cm)	29.3–28.5	
Midarm muscle circumference (cm)	25.3–23.2	Hydration status may influence results
Biochemical Assessments		Examples of possible disease conditions:
Serum albumin	3.5–5.0 g/dL	Decrease signifies lowered nutritional status—protein deficient
Serum transferrin binds iron to plasma and transports to bone marrow	200–430 mg/dL	Reduced levels may indicate chronic diseases and protein deficiency Elevated levels—anemias, liver damage, lead toxicity
Hemoglobin	Male—13.5–17 g/dL Female—12–15 g/dL	Decrease related to iron deficiency (anemias and leukemia)
Prealbumin (PA) serum	20–50 mg/dL	Decreased—protein wasting diseases, malnutrition (< 10.7 indicates severe nutritional deficiency) Elevated—Hodgkin's disease
Blood urea nitrogen/creatinine	10:1–20:1	Nitrogen imbalance, inadequate renal functioning
24-hour urinary nitrogen	Positive balance	Inadequate protein intake

Continues

Appendix 6-2. NUTRITIONAL ASSESSMENT PARAMETERS *(Continued)*

Clinical Assessment	Normal	Abnormal
Sociocultural Data		
Cultural-religious factors	Ability to afford adequate foods in all food categories Cultural beliefs that do not eliminate whole food groups Religious beliefs that do not eliminate whole food groups	Economic position that precludes purchase of adequate food Religious or cultural beliefs that interfere with receiving balanced diet (macrobiotic diets) Inadequate knowledge, experience, or intelligence to prepare healthy meals
Ethnicity	Traditional foods that do not eliminate whole food groups	Beliefs and ethnic preference that eliminate major nutrients from the diet
Lifestyle	Well-balanced meals that include all nutrients Food does not lose all nutrient value in preparation	Fast-paced stressful lifestyle that incorporates fastfood or convenience foods deficient in nutrients or imbalanced (high-fat)

*Laboratory test parameters differ among laboratories. Check the reference range for the specific lab where the patient's blood or urine was tested.

Appendix 6-3 REVISED FOOD PYRAMID (2005)

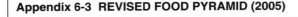

New food pyramid
Pyramid now symbolizes a personalized approach to eating healthy and exercise.

Physical activity
Figure is a reminder on the importance of physical activity. Amount needed:

Minimum: At least 30 minutes most days of the week

To prevent weight gain: 60 minutes

To sustain weight loss: 60 to 90 minutes

Estimating daily calorie needs

Females	Sedentary	Active
9–13 years	1,600	2,200
14–18	1,800	2.400
19–30	2,000	2,400
31–50	1,800	2,200
51+	1,600	2,200
Males		
9–13 years	1,800	2,600
14–18	2,200	3,200
19–30	2,400	3,000
31–50	2,200	3,000
51+	2,000	2,800

Food groups	Grains	Vegetables	Fruits	Oils	Milk	Meat and beans
The five food groups and oils are color-coded for easy identification	At least half should be whole grain	Fresh, frozen, canned, dried, juices	Fresh, frozen, canned, dried, juices	Liquid, not solid	Low- or no-fat, calcium-rich types	Lean meat, poultry, fish; eggs; beans, nuts, seeds; tofu; peanut butter
Daily amount of food from each group by calorie level:						
2,000 calories Moderately active women 26–50	6 oz* (170 g)	2.5 cups	2 cups	6 tsp.	3 cups	5.5 oz.** (720 g)
2,600 calories Moderately active men 26–45	9 oz.* (280 g)	3.5 cups	2 cups	8 tsp.	3 cups	6.5 oz.** (200 g)

Appendix 6-3 REVISED FOOD PYRAMID (2005) *(Continued)*

Milk

Foods Included

- Milk: low or no-fat calcium-rich types

Contribution to Diet: Milk is a leading source of calcium, which is needed for bones and teeth. It also provides a high-quality protein, riboflavin, vitamin A (if milk is whole or fortified), and other nutrients.

Amounts Recommended: Three cups.

Cheese may replace part of the milk. To substitute, figure the amount on the basis of calcium content. Common portions of various kinds of cheese and ice cream and their milk equivalents in calcium are:

2.5-cm cube cheddar-type cheese	= ½ cup milk
½ cup cottage cheese	= ⅓ cup milk
2 tablespoons cream cheese	= 1 tablespoon milk
½ cup ice cream or ice milk	= ⅓ cup milk

Meat and beans

Foods Included:

- Lean meats
- Poultry and eggs
- Fish and shellfish
- Beans, dry peas, lentils, nuts, seeds, tofu, peanut butter

Contribution to Diet: Foods in this group are valued for their protein, which is needed for growth and repair of body tissues, muscle, organs, blood, skin, and hair. These foods also provide iron, thiamine, riboflavin, and niacin.

Amounts Recommended: Choose 5.5 to 6.5 oz. every day. Count as a serving: 62 to 93 g (not including bone weight) cooked lean meat, poultry, or fish. Count as alternates for ½ serving meat or fish: 1 egg, 1/2 cup cooked dry beans, dry peas, or lentils, or 2 tablespoons peanut butter.

Vegetables–Fruits

Foods Included: All vegetables and fruit: Fresh, frozen, canned, dried, juices. This guide emphasizes those that are valuable as sources of vitamin C and vitamin A.

Sources of Vitamin C

Foods included:

Good sources: Grapefruit or grapefruit juice, orange or orange juice, cantaloupe, guava, mango, papaya, raw strawberries, broccoli, brussels sprouts, green pepper, sweet red pepper.

Fair sources: Honeydew melon, lemon, tangerine or tangerine juice, watermelon, asparagus tips, raw cabbage, cauliflower, collards, garden cress, kale, kohlrabi, mustard greens, potatoes and sweet potatoes cooked in the jacket, rutabagas, spinach, tomatoes or tomato juice, turnip greens.

Sources of Vitamin A

Foods included:

Dark-green and deep-yellow vegetables and a few fruits, namely, apricots, broccoli, cantaloupe, carrots, chard, collards, cress, kale, mango, persimmon, pumpkin, spinach, sweet potatoes, turnip greens and other dark-green leaves, winter squash.

Contribution to Diet: Fruits and vegetables are valuable chiefly because of the vitamins and minerals they contain. In this plan, this group is counted on to supply nearly all the vitamin C needed and over half the vitamin A. Vitamin C is needed for healthy gums and body tissues. Vitamin A is needed for growth, normal vision, and healthy condition of skin and other body surfaces.

Amounts Recommended: Choose 2.5 cups vegetables and 2 cups fruit.

Count as one serving: ½ cup of vegetable or fruit; or one medium apple, banana, orange, or potato, half a medium grapefruit, a slice of cantaloupe, or the juice of one lemon.

Grains: at least half should be whole grains.

Foods Included: All breads and cereals that are whole grain, enriched, or restored; check labels to be sure. Specifically, this group includes whole wheat and rye breads, cooked cereal, ready-to-eat whole grain cereal, cornmeal, crackers, , rolled oats, grains (wheat, corn, millet, oats, brown rice), whole-grain or enriched flour.

Contribution to diet: Foods in this group furnish worthwhile amounts of protein, iron, several of the B vitamins, and for energy.

Amounts Recommended: Choose six or more ounces every day. Or, if no cereals are chosen, include an extra serving of whole grain bread or baked goods, which will make at least six ounces from this group daily.

Count as a serving: One slice of bread; 31 g ready-to-eat cereal; ½ to ¾ cup cooked cereal, cornmeal, grits, macaroni, noodles, rice, or spaghetti.

Oils: Liquid, not solid.

Foods Included: Vegetable oils that have no trans fats (olive oil, flax seed oil, cod liver oil, etc.)

Contribution to diet: Major source of vitamine E and polyunsaturated fatty acides including essential fatty acides omega 3 and 6).

Amounts Recommended: 6–8 tsp/day.

NUTRITIONAL MANAGEMENT QUESTIONS

1. A patient has had abdominal surgery and the physician has ordered a bland diet 3 days post-surgery. Which of the following diet trays would have portions removed because it does not adhere to the dietary regimen?

    1. Scrambled eggs, cereal, and white toast.
    2. Baked potato, cottage cheese, and coffee.
    3. Cream soup, Jello, and white toast.
    4. Cooked cereal, boiled egg, and milk.

2. A patient will have a central vein infusion to maintain nutritional status while his gastrointestinal tract is being bypassed. The nurse would expect that the site of catheter insertion for a protein and glucose concentration of 15% would be in the

    1. Jugular vein.
    2. Right subclavian vein.
    3. Right subclavian artery.
    4. Left arm artery access.

3. A patient has injured her eyes with a chemical and must have eye patches in place for several weeks. When her food tray arrives, the most helpful nursing intervention would be to

    1. Feed the patient or assign a nursing assistant to feed her.
    2. Explain that her tray is here and put her hands on it.
    3. Tell her to think of a clock and describe which food is where and put the fork in her hand.
    4. Ask her if she would prefer a liquid diet.

4. A 53-year-old patient with Crohn's disease is placed on total parenteral nutrition (TNA). The fluid in the present TNA bottle should be infused by 8 AM. At 7 AM, the nurse observes that it is empty and another TNA bottle has not yet arrived on the unit. The nursing action is to attach the solution nearest a TNA solution which is a bottle of

    1. D_{25} and water.
    2. D_5 and water.
    3. D_{10} and water.
    4. D_{45} and water.

5. The nurse's discharge teaching for a patient with acute pancreatitis will include advising him to take a dietary supplement of

    1. Vitamin K.
    2. Fat-soluble vitamins.
    3. Vitamin C.
    4. Vitamin B_{12}.

6. The nurse will know that the patient understands presurgical instructions for hemorrhoid surgery if his diet is

    1. Low roughage.
    2. High fiber.
    3. High carbohydrate.
    4. Low fiber.

7. Discharge planning for a patient with a partial colectomy will include which one of the following dietary principles?

    1. High residue, force fluids.
    2. Low residue, no dairy products.
    3. High fiber, no spices.
    4. Regular, no dairy products.

8. The nurse's diet instructions for a patient with a colostomy will be

    1. According to his own individual needs and similar to his preoperative diet.
    2. Low in fiber with a large amount of fluids.
    3. High in fiber with large amounts of fluids and supplemental vitamin K.
    4. Elimination of milk products.

9. Which of the following statements would be correct when counseling a patient about the postoperative diet he would receive following a simple surgical procedure?

    1. A patient undergoing major surgery may have a soft diet the day of surgery.
    2. Approximately 2800 calories are required daily for general tissue repair, so this will be his caloric intake.
    3. Daily fluid intake should be 1500 mL for an uncomplicated surgical procedure.
    4. A mechanical, soft diet should be given the first postoperative day.

10. The nurse will know the patient understands his low-purine diet when he states

1. "I will limit the number of fruit servings each day."
2. "Organ meats must be eliminated from my diet."
3. "I can drink only white wine because red wine is high in purine."
4. "Beef, chicken, and pork are high in purine; therefore, I can have them only once in a while."

11. The nurse will know that the diabetic patient understands his diet when he says that he should obtain the greatest percentage of calories from

    1. Fats.
    2. Complex carbohydrates.
    3. Simple carbohydrates.
    4. Protein.

12. The most appropriate sugar substitute for the type 1 diabetic patient is

    1. Corn sugar.
    2. Honey.
    3. Aspartame.
    4. Fructose.

13. A patient with acute pancreatitis required nasogastric intubation due to persistent vomiting and paralytic ileus. Following NG tube removal, the feeding schedule would start with a diet that is

    1. NPO for 12 hours.
    2. High in protein.
    3. High in carbohydrate.
    4. Clear liquid.

14. A patient with cirrhosis and ascites is placed on a sodium-restricted diet to help control the ascites. In order for this plan to be effective, it is important that the patient also

    1. Restrict his fluid intake.
    2. Increase his potassium intake.
    3. Increase his fluid intake.
    4. Decrease his potassium intake.

15. A patient with a history of pancreatitis should avoid which of the following foods?

    1. Noodles.
    2. Vegetable soup.
    3. Baked fish fillet.
    4. Cheddar cheese sandwiches.

16. The nurse questions the dietary department about the lunch delivered for a patient with the diagnosis of cirrhosis when she finds on his tray

    1. A tuna sandwich.
    2. French fries.
    3. A ham sandwich.
    4. A milkshake.

17. The nurse will know that her teaching has been effective when the patient responds that a low-fiber diet allows the inclusion of

    1. Whole-grain breads, seeds, and legumes.
    2. Fresh fruits and vegetables.
    3. Bran and whole-grain cereals.
    4. Cooked vegetables, fruits, and refined breads.

18. Patients with hepatitis may have a regular diet ordered, unless they become increasingly symptomatic. The diet will then be modified to decrease the amount of

    1. Carbohydrates.
    2. Fats.
    3. Fluids.
    4. Protein.

19. A pregnant patient comes to the clinic, and the nurse is responsible for nutritional counseling. When the patient says that she has eliminated all salt from her diet, the nurse should respond

    1. "That's good. Salt is not healthy."
    2. "What information did you have that led to this decision?"
    3. "At this time we do not advise limiting salt intake."
    4. "You can have all the salt you want."

20. Evaluating the teaching plan for a patient recently placed on a low-sodium diet by her physician, the nurse will know the patient understands the plan when she states

    1. "I will call the dietitian if I can't remember."
    2. "I will look at the list of foods I can have."
    3. "I will read the label on the food product."
    4. "I will cook without adding salt to the food."

NUTRITIONAL MANAGEMENT
Answers with Rationale

1. (2) Coffee is one food eliminated from a bland diet because it is chemically irritating to the stomach. All of the other foods are allowed on a bland diet. Other foods eliminated are raw, spicy, gas-forming, very hot or very cold foods, alcohol, and carbonated drinks.

   NP:I; CN:S; CA:S; CL:AN

2. (2) The most common placement site is the right subclavian vein. The jugular vein (1) might be used as an alternative for high-concentration IV infusions, but it is more difficult to access. The arm (4) is used for insertion of an arterial line for arterial blood gas samples and monitoring.

   NP:P; CN:PH; CA:S; CL:A

3. (3) The most helpful intervention is to assist the patient to help herself, allowing her to be as independent as possible. Feeding her (1) or changing the diet to liquid (4) would not be as therapeutic.

   NP:I; CN:PS; CA:PS; CL:A

4. (3) In order that the patient not experience a sudden drop in blood sugar, the solution nearest most TPN solution concentrations is $D_{10}W$. $D_{25}W$ (1) and $D_{45}W$ (4) could cause osmotic diuresis or fluid overload.

   NP:I; CN:PH; CA:M; CL:A

5. (2) Because the patient will be on a low-fat diet to decrease pancreatic activity, he will need supplements of the fat-soluble vitamins. A well-balanced diet should meet the other vitamin/nutritional needs so a supplement is not required.

   NP:P; CN:PH; CA:M; CL:A

6. (2) A high-fiber diet produces a soft stool without mechanically irritating the hemorrhoidal area. Foods include bran and complex carbohydrates.

   NP:E; CN:PH; CA:S; CL:A

7. (2) The low-residue diet will put less strain on the colon, and eliminating dairy products initially is important because these products cause mucus.

   NP:P; CN:PH; CA:S; CL:C

8. (1) Diets are individualized and patients are generally able to eat the same foods they enjoyed preoperatively. Fresh fruits may cause diarrhea in some, but not all, individuals.

   NP:I; CN:H; CA:S; CL:C

9. (2) A daily intake of 2800 calories is required for usual/general tissue repair, whereas 6000 calories may be required for extensive tissue repair. Fluid intake is 2000 to 3000 mL/day for uncomplicated surgery. Diet progresses from nothing by mouth the day of surgery to a general diet within a few days.

   NP:I; CN:PH; CA:S; CL:C

10. (2) Organ meats, wine, yeast, scallops, and mussels are all high in purine and must be eliminated from the diet of the patient who has gout.

    NP:E; CN:PH; CA:M; CL:A

11. (2) The diabetic's diet should be between 50 and 65 percent carbohydrate calories with only 5 percent of these being simple carbohydrates (sucrose). Fat recommendation is < 30 percent of calories, and protein should be 0.8 mg/kg/day.

    NP:E; CN:PH; CA:M; CL:A

12. (3) Aspartame is the only calorie-free sweetener listed; the others are nutritive, their average caloric value being 20 Kcal per teaspoon. When an equal volume of honey and sugar are compared, honey provides about one and one-third times as many kilocalories as does table sugar.

    NP:P; CN:H; CA:M; CL:K

Coding for Questions/Answers Abbreviations: **Nursing Process: NP,** Data Collection: D, Planning: P, Implementation: I, Evaluation: E, **Client Needs: CN,** Safe, Effective Care Environment: S, Health Promotion and Maintenance: H, Psychosocial Integrity: PS, Physiological Integrity: PH, **Clinical Area: CA,** Medical Nursing: M, Surgical Nursing: S, Maternal/Newborn Nursing: MA, Pediatric Nursing: P, Psychiatric Nursing: PS, **Cognitive Level: CL,** Knowledge: K, Comprehension: C, Application: A, Analysis: AN

13. (3) Foods that are high in carbohydrate are given, because those with high protein or fat content stimulate the pancreas. Alcohol is forbidden. There is no need for the patient to be NPO.

NP:P; CN:PH; CA:M; CL:C

14. (1) It is important that fluids be restricted as well, because unrestricted fluid intake leads to a progressive decrease in serum sodium from dilution. Electrolyte imbalance with potential neurologic complications could result.

NP:P; CN:PH; CA:M; CL:A

15. (4) Patients with this condition must not consume foods high in fat content because there are inadequate pancreatic enzymes to digest the fat. High fat content also causes pain 2 to 4 hours after ingestion. The suggested diet is high in carbohydrates.

NP:P; CN:PH; CA:M; CL:C

16. (3) Ham is high in sodium and can increase fluid retention, leading to edema. Cirrhosis patients are prone to edema as the osmotic pressures change due to a decrease in plasma albumin.

NP:D; CN:PH; CA:M; CL:A

17. (4) Cooked vegetables and fruits as well as refined breads are included in a low-fiber diet. Bran, fresh fruits, and whole grains and seeds are included in a high-fiber diet.

NP:E; CN:PH; CA:M; CL:A

18. (4) With liver cell damage, the liver cannot break down and eliminate protein. Protein needs to be decreased until symptoms dissipate.

NP:I; CN:PH; CA:M; CL:C

19. (3) Research has indicated that pregnant women require a moderate amount of salt, because it is essential in maintaining increased body fluids needed for adequate placental and renal flow as well as tissue requirements. Highly salted foods should still be avoided. Answer (2) is wrong because the patient's information is wrong and needs to be corrected.

NP:I; CN:PH; CA:M; CL:A

20. (3) Patients should be instructed to read labels before purchasing canned, frozen, or processed foods because they are usually very high in sodium. A list of foods will provide guidance, but she should know the sodium content of food. Not adding salt to foods when cooking is also important, but not as critical as answer (3).

NP:E; CN:PH; CA:M; CL:A

Laboratory Tests 7

ROUTINE LAB TESTS

A. Most patients, on admission to the hospital or before, will have several routine lab tests.
   1. These tests are used to determine or verify diagnosis, to establish baseline data, to monitor progress, and to monitor side effects, therapies, and drugs.
   2. These tests are an important component of the patient's general assessment.
B. *See* Routine Blood Chemistry (Table 7-1) and Chem 7.

✦ Chem 7 (SMA 7)

A. Measures serum levels of seven substances: electrolytes (potassium, sodium, and chloride), carbon dioxide, glucose, BUN, and creatinine.
   1. Tests fluid balance and renal function, as well as acid–base status.
   2. When combined with CBC, these tests give a view of how entire body is functioning.
   3. Chem 7 is also part of the preoperative workup.

4. Standard values of Chem 7 (may vary from lab to lab. Check own facility values).
   a. Potassium: 3.5–5.3 mEq/L.
   b. Sodium: 135–145 mEq/L.
   c. Chloride: 98–106 mEq/L.
   d. CO_2: 23–30 mmol/L.
   e. Glucose (fasting): 65–110 mg/dL.
   f. BUN: 7–18 mg/dL.
   g. Creatinine: 0.6–1.3 mg/dL.
✦ B. How these values may be interpreted.
   1. Potassium: an electrolyte that helps maintain acid–base balance.
   2. Sodium: an electrolyte that helps maintain acid–base balance and osmotic pressure.
   3. Chloride: an electrolyte that helps maintain extra electrical neutrality; combines with sodium to form a salt.
   4. CO_2: reflects value of bicarbonate in arterial blood.
   5. Glucose: fasting blood glucose levels may identify diabetes.
   6. BUN: reflects liver's ability to make urea and the kidney's ability to excrete it. With renal disease, the BUN goes up.

Table 7-1. ROUTINE BLOOD CHEMISTRY TESTS

Test	Purpose	Normal Values
Erythrocytes		
Red blood cell count (RBC or Erythrocytes)	Determines actual number of formed blood elements in relation to volume Identifies abnormalities, monitors RBC count	Males: 4.5–6.2 million/mm^3 Females: 4.0–5.5 million/mm^3 Children: 3.2–5.2 million/mm^3
Hematocrit (HCT)	Measures percentage of red blood cells per fluid volume of whole blood	Males: 40–54/100 mL Females: 37–47/100 mL Children: 29–54/100 mL
Hemoglobin (Hgb)	Measures amount of hemoglobin/100 mL blood to determine oxygen-carrying capacity; assists in diagnosing anemia	Males: > 13–18 g/100 mL Females: > 12–16 g/100 mL
Erythrocyte sedimentation rate (ESR)	Measures rate of red blood cells settling from plasma—reflects infections	Wintrobe Method Males: 9 mm/hr Females: 0–15 mm/hr Children: 0–13 mm/hr Westergren Method Males: 0–15 mm/hr Females: 0–20 mm/hr Children: 0–20 mm/hr
Platelet count	Determines number of platelets	Adults: 150,000–450,000/mm^3
Leukocytes		
White blood cell count (WBC or leukocytes)	Establishes quantity and maturity of white blood cell elements	Adults: 4500–11,000/mm^3 Children: 5000–13,000/mm^3 Neutrophils: 3000–7500/mm^3 Band Neutrophils: 150–700/mm^3 Basophils: 25–150/mm^3 Eosinophils: 50–450/mm^3 Lymphocytes: 1500–4500/mm^3 Monocytes: 100–800/mm^3

7. Serum creatinine: more specific test of renal function; elevated levels indicate renal disease.

CARDIAC FUNCTION TESTS

Cardiac Enzyme Studies

A. Enzyme activity evaluation denotes heart muscle damage.
1. When the heart muscle is without oxygen for 30–60 minutes, the cells are damaged which results in necrosis. Intracellular enzymes are released into the bloodstream as the cells die.
✦ 2. Specific enzymes are released into the bloodstream at varying intervals.
   a. Creatine kinase (CK) formerly called creatine phosphokinase or CPK-isoenzymes (CPK-MB)—most valuable measurement. CK-MB is cardiac measurement—level rises within 4 to 6 hours of initial heart muscle damage, peaking at 18 to 24 hours. More than 6 times normal value with damage —returns to normal within 3–4 days.
   b. Compare CK-MB with following two tests (SGOT and LDH) to determine myocardial damage.
   c. Lactate dehydrogenase LDH, LDH$_2$-isoenzymes—level rises in 12–24–48 hours; persists longer; can be as long as 2 weeks.
   d. Serum glutamic oxaloacetic transaminase SGOT+ —not specific to heart disease alone; serial tests helpful.
3. The greater the peak in enzymes and the longer the level remains, the more serious the heart damage.
B. Troponin test.
1. Tested for myocardial injury; when infarction occurs, this substance is released in the bloodstream.
2. Made up of 3 proteins found in striated muscle. Cardiac troponin T rises in 3 to 6 hours and remains up for 14 to 21 days; troponin 1 rises in 7 to 14 hours and remains up 5 to 7 days. Both are accurate assessments for myocardial damage.
3. Normally values are low (troponin T 0.0 to 0.2 ng/mL and troponin 1 less than 0.6 ng/mL); any rise may indicate myocardial cell damage. Serial tests are important.
C. Myoglobin test.
1. Oxygen-binding protein found in cardiac muscle (and skeletal muscle).
2. Level rises shortly after cell dies; peaks in 4 to 6 hours and returns to normal in 24 to 36 hours.

Lipoprotein and Lipid Tests

✦ A. Normal values.
1. Cholesterol— < 200 mg/100 mL (teenager's level should be < 180 mg/100 mL). Levels > 239 mg/100 mL classified as high.
2. Triglycerides—40–150 mg/100 mL.
3. Low-density lipoproteins (LDLs)—60–180 mg/100 mL.
4. Very low-density lipoproteins (VLDLs)—25–50 percent of total cholesterol.
5. High-density lipoproteins (HDLs)—male level, 30–70 mg/100 mL; female level, 30–80 mg/100 mL.
B. Purpose—total cholesterol, lipoproteins, and triglycerides are screening tests to determine risk of atherosclerosis and heart disease.
1. High cholesterol—increased risk of heart disease.
2. High-density lipoprotein—lower risk of heart disease.
3. Low-density lipoprotein—higher risk of heart disease.
4. High triglycerides—higher risk of acute myocardial infarction.
C. Variations.
1. Serum cholesterol increased in: biliary obstruction (cirrhosis), hypothyroidism, pancreatic disease, uncontrolled diabetes, and pregnancy.
2. Serum cholesterol decreased in: liver disease, hyperthyroidism, malnutrition, anemias, malabsorption of cholesterol.
3. Triglycerides increased in: hepatitis, pancreatitis, cirrhosis due to alcoholism, renal failure, acute myocardial infarction.
4. Triglycerides decreased in: hyperparathyroidism, pulmonary disease, malnutrition.

BLOOD STUDIES

Arterial Blood Studies

A. Arterial blood gases.
✦ 1. Assesses respiratory function.
   a. Oxygen (PO$_2$).
      (1) Increased may indicate polycythemia.
      (2) Decreased may indicate COPD, cancer of lung, sickle cell anemia, anemias, cystic fibrosis.
   b. Carbon dioxide (PCO$_2$).
      (1) Increased may indicate COPD, emphysema, bronchitis, asthma attack, pneumonia, cerebral trauma, neuro disorder.
      (2) Decreased may indicate anxiety, hysteria, tetany, increased temperature,

DTs, hyperthyroidism, salicylate
poisoning.

   c. pH—high is alkalotic, low is acidotic.

   d. Oxygen saturation and bicarbonate (HCO_3).

     (1) Oxygen saturation should be viewed
with hemoglobin value.

     (2) Bicarbonate—if low (< 23) or high
(> 27), indicates malfunction of
metabolic process.

2. Determines state of acid–base balance.

3. Reveals adequacy of the lungs to provide oxygen and to remove carbon dioxide.

4. Assesses degree to which kidneys can maintain a normal pH.

◆ B. Normal arterial values.

1. Oxygen saturation—93–98 percent.

2. PaO_2—95 mm Hg.

3. Arterial pH—7.35–7.45 (7.4).

4. PCO_2—35–45 mm Hg (40).

5. HCO_3 content—22–26 mEq/L.

6. Base excess— –3 to +3 (0).

C. Acid–base imbalances.

1. Respiratory acidosis.

   a. pH—7.32.

   b. PCO_2—52 mm Hg.

   c. PO_2—90 mm Hg.

   d. HCO_3—24 mEq/L.

2. Respiratory alkalosis.

   a. pH—7.51.

   b. PCO_2—32 mm Hg.

   c. PO_2—95 mm Hg.

   d. HCO_3—24 mEq/L.

3. Metabolic acidosis.

   a. pH—7.30.

   b. HCO_3—16 mEq/L.

   c. PCO_2—38 mm Hg.

   d. PO_2—95 mm Hg.

   e. Cl—120 mEq/L.

   f. K—5.5 mEq/L.

4. Metabolic alkalosis.

   a. pH—7.50.

   b. HCO_3—38 mEq/L.

   c. PCO_2—38 mm Hg.

   d. PO_2—95 mm Hg.

   e. K—3.0 mEq/L.

   f. Cl—88 mEq/L.

Prostate-Specific Antigen (PSA) Test

A. Values.

1. Normal: 0 to 4–6 ng/mL.

2. Benign prostatic hypertrophy: 4 to 9 ng/mL.

3. Prostate cancer: 10 to 120 ng/mL.

B. Purpose—shows concentration of glycoprotein
from prostate tissue.

1. Increases with benign prostatic hypertrophy
(BPH).

2. Markedly increases with cancer of the prostate.

3. Used to diagnose or to monitor effect of treatment with chemotherapy or radiation.

4. Collect 5 mL of venous blood before rectal or
prostate exam (exam irritates tissue).

Blood Coagulation Studies

A. Clotting takes place in three phases.

1. Phase I—prothrombin activator formed in
response to ruptured vessel or damage to
blood.

2. Phase II—prothrombin activator catalyzes
conversion of prothrombin into thrombin.

3. Phase III—thrombin acts as an enzyme to
convert fibrinogen into fibrin thread.

B. Types of clotting factors.

1. Calcium ions.

   a. Cofactor in coagulation.

   b. Does not enter into reaction.

   c. If absent, neither extrinsic nor intrinsic
system will operate.

2. Phospholipids.

   a. Necessary for formation of final prothrombin activator.

   b. Thromboplastin is phospholipid in extrinsic system.

   c. Platelet factor III is phospholipid for intrinsic system.

3. Plasma protein—all clotting factors from V to
XIII.

◆ C. Coagulation mechanisms.

1. Extrinsic mechanisms.

   a. Extract from damaged tissue is mixed
with blood.

   b. Trauma occurs to tissue or endothelial
surface of vascular wall, releasing thromboplastin.

2. Intrinsic mechanisms.

   a. Blood itself comes into contact with
roughened blood vessel wall.

   b. Platelets adhere to vessel and disinte-
grate, which releases blood factor III containing thromboplastin.

D. Fibrinolytic system.

1. Adequate function is necessary to maintain
hemostasis.

2. Dissolves clots through formation of plasmin.

◆ Prothrombin Time (PT)

A. Normal values—10–13 seconds (some labs use
11–16 seconds).

B. Purpose—prothrombin time provides data on
thrombin generation or how long it takes for a
fibrin clot to form.

1. It is a screening test to detect deficiencies in
the extrinsic clotting mechanism.

2. Useful for control of long-term anticoagulant therapy.
C. Critical values.
   1. If value is above 30 seconds, hemorrhage may occur—observe for bleeding.
   2. Administer vitamin K as ordered.
D. Possible causes of prolonged clotting time.
   1. Inadequate vitamin K in premature and new-born infants or in diet.
   2. Poor fat absorption (obstructive jaundice).
   3. Liver disease (cirrhosis, hepatitis).
   4. Specific drugs (heparin, Coumadin, salicylates).

◆ **Activated Partial Thromboplastin Time (APTT)**
A. Normal values—20–38 seconds with standard technique—different activators will yield different values.
B. Purpose—best single screening test for coagulation disorders.
   1. Test evaluates adequacy of plasma clotting factors—intrinsic clotting mechanism.
   2. Test of choice for monitoring heparin therapy.
   3. Used for patients with hemophilia.
C. Arterial values—if APTT is very prolonged (100 seconds), assess for spontaneous bleeding coagulant disorder.
D. Possible causes of prolonged clotting time.
   1. Vitamin K deficiency.
   2. Liver disease.
   3. Hemophilia.
   4. Specific drugs (heparin, warfarin, Coumadin, salicylates).
E. When APTT is prolonged, physician may order protamine sulfate (or, in severe cases, whole blood or plasma transfusion).

◆ **International Normalized Ratio (INR)**
A. Designed to standardize values and improve monitoring process. Test provides a more accurate assessment of patient's anticoagulant; a uniform value where PT is expressed as a ratio.
B. Standardizes PT ratio by allowing all thromboplastin reagents to be compared to an international standard thromboplastin (sensitivity index) provided by WHO.
   1. INR is a mathematical correction to prothrombin time ratio (PTR).
   2. Value is calculated using patient's PT divided by the mean of normal PT; target range is 2.5 to 3.5.
   3. INR is calculated by raising the observed PT ratio to the power of the sensitivity index, depending on the reagent used.
C. The INR is the best lab value for monitoring anticoagulation therapy; improves the effectiveness of the medication.

D. Should only be used after patient has been stabilized on warfarin (which takes at least 1 week).

RENAL FUNCTION TESTS

A. Phenolsulfonphthalein (PSP) test indicates the functional ability of the kidney to:
   1. Excrete waste products.
   2. Concentrate and dilute urine.
   3. Carry on absorption and excretion activities.
   4. Maintain body fluids and electrolytes.
B. Renal concentration tests.
   1. Evaluate the ability of the kidney to concentrate urine.
   2. As kidney disease progresses, renal function decreases. Concentration tests evaluate this process.
   3. Renal concentration is measured by specific gravity readings.
◆ C. Specific gravity.
   1. Normal value—range is 1.003–1.030, usually 1.010–1.025.
   2. If specific gravity is 1.018 or greater, it may be assumed that the kidney is functioning within normal limits.
   3. Specific gravity that stabilizes at 1.010 indicates kidney has lost ability to concentrate or dilute urine.
◆ D. Blood urea nitrogen (BUN).
   1. Normal value—10–20 mg/100 mL.
   2. Purpose—tests for impaired kidney function by testing the body's urea production and urine flow.
   3. BUN level affected by protein intake and tissue breakdown.
◆ E. Serum creatinine.
   1. Normal value—male: 0.8–1.2 mg/dL; female: 0.6–0.9 mg/dL. If normal value doubles, overall renal function and glomerular filtration rate (GFR) has decreased by half.
      a. When elevated, suggests hypertension or drugs such as steroids.
      b. Decreased indicates mild to severe renal impairment, muscular dystrophy, or use of certain drugs.
   2. Purpose—tests renal function by evaluating the balance between production and filtration of glomeruli.
   3. This is the most sensitive of renal function tests.
◆ F. Concentration and dilution tests.
   1. Fishberg concentration test—high protein dinner with 200 mL fluid is ordered. Next AM on arising, patient voids q 1/hr. One specimen should have specific gravity more than 1.025.

2. Dilution test—NPO after dinner. Morning voiding discarded. Patient drinks 1000 mL in 30 to 45 minutes. Four specimens at 1 hour intervals are collected. One specimen will fall below 1.003.

3. Specific gravity—urine 1.010 to 1.025. Increased solutes cause increased specific gravity.

◆ G. Glomerular filtration rate (GFR) or endogenous creatinine clearance.
   1. Normal value—125 mL/min (male) and 110 mL/min (female).
   2. Purpose—kidney function is assessed by clearing a substance from the blood such as inulin, a polysaccharide found in plants (filtration in the glomerulus).
   3. Common test is the amount of blood cleared of urea per minute.
   4. Test done on 12-hour or 24-hour urine specimen.

H. Electrolyte tests.
   1. Kidney function is essential to maintain fluid and electrolyte balance.
   2. Tests for electrolytes (sodium, potassium, chloride, and bicarbonate) measure the ability of the kidney to filter, reabsorb, or excrete these substances.
   3. Impaired filtration leads to retention, and impaired reabsorption leads to loss of electrolytes.
   4. Tests are performed on blood serum, so venous blood is required.

◆ Urine Analysis

A. Normal values.
   1. Specific gravity—1.010–1.025.
   2. Urine pH—4.5–8.0.
   3. Color—straw.
   4. Odor—aromatic.
   5. Appearance—clear.
   6. Protein—negative or zero.
   7. Glucose—negative or zero.
   8. Ketones—negative or zero.
   9. Red blood cells—0–3.
   10. White blood cells—0–4.
   11. Casts—none; occasional.
   12. Crystals—negative.
   13. Yeast cells—none.
   14. Parasites—none.

B. Urinalysis is a critical test for total evaluation of the renal system and for indication of renal disease.

◆ C. Specific gravity shows the degree of concentration in urine.
   1. Normal value—1.010–1.025.
   2. Indicates the ability of the kidney to concentrate or dilute urine.

3. Change from normal range.
   a. Elevated (> 1.030) indicates diabetes mellitus, dehydration, vomiting/diarrhea, contrast media (1–2 days).
   b. Low (< 1.010) indicates diabetes insipidus, overhydration, renal disease.

4. Renal failure—specific gravity constant at 1.010.

◆ D. Analysis of urine pH.
   1. pH is the symbol for the logarithm of the reciprocal of the hydrogen ion concentration.
   2. A measurement of hydrogen ion concentration is taken—the lower the number, the higher the acidity of urine.
      a. Normal value range—4.5 to 8.0 (normal pH is 6 to 7).
      b. Lower than 6 is acidic urine, and higher than 7 is alkaline urine.
   3. Regulation of urine pH is important for treatment of certain conditions.
      a. Alkaline pH suggests urinary tract infection, metabolic or respiratory alkalosis, drug influence, or a highly alkaline or vegetarian diet.
      b. Acidic pH may reflect renal TB, PKU, pyrexia, acidosis.
      c. Acid urine may be desired when treating blood infections or phosphate stones.

◆ E. Chemical analysis of urine.
   1. Protein or albumin—zero is normal for a 24-hour specimen.
      a. Presence may indicate renal disease, such as nephritis or nephrosis.
      b. Inflammatory processes any place in the body may result in proteinuria.
      c. Toxemia of pregnancy yields a finding of proteinuria.
      d. Renal calculi indicate positive test results.
      e. Appearance in urine may be due to dehydration, strenuous exercise, high protein diet.

   ◆ 2. Glucose—normal range is zero.
      a. Presence of glucose may indicate head injury, diabetes, Cushing's, hyperthyroidism.
      b. Test is usually done by test strips or tablets; change in color indicates presence of glucose (done occasionally in the home).
      c. Urine testing for glucose has been replaced by testing for blood glucose.

   ◆ 3. Ketone bodies—normal range is zero.
      a. Ketonuria primarily indicates diabetic acidosis but is also present with starvation and pernicious vomiting.
      b. Test is usually done by strip or powder mixed with urine; purple color indicates positive test.

4. Bilirubin—normal range is zero.
   a. Presence in urine may indicate liver disease and may appear before the clinical symptom of jaundice.
   b. Detected in the urine by qualitative methods, such as inspection of color.
5. Blood—normal range is zero.
   a. If red blood cells present, may indicate disease of kidney or urinary tract, and the source of hemorrhage must be determined.
   b. Specific diagnosis is made by complete urine analysis for casts and epithelial cells.

F. Microscopic examination of urine.
   1. Evaluation of urinary sediment is important for diagnostic purposes.
   2. Test for cellular elements (epithelial cells, white and red blood cells).
   3. Test for casts, fat bodies, and crystals.

G. Levels of albuminuria.
   30 mg/100 mL = 1+
   100 mg/100 mL = 2+
   300 mg/100 mL = 3+
   1000 mg/100 mL = 4+

H. Schilling urine test.
   1. Determines absorption of vitamin B_{12} necessary for erythropoiesis—definitive test for pernicious anemia and intestinal malabsorption syndrome.
   2. 7% excretion of radioactive B_{12} in urine within 24 hours—when less is excreted it confirms diagnosis.

GASTROINTESTINAL TESTS

Analysis of GI Secretions

A. Contents of the GI tract may be examined for the presence or absence of digestive juices, bacteria, parasites, and malignant cells.
B. Stomach contents may be aspirated and analyzed for volume and free and total acid.

✦ Gastric Analysis

A. Performed by means of a nasogastric tube.
   1. Maintain NPO 6–8 hours prior to the test.
   2. Pass nasogastric tube; verify its presence in the stomach; tape to patient's nose.
B. Collect fasting specimens.
   1. Administer agents, such as alcohol, caffeine, histamine (0.2 mg subcutaneous), as ordered, to stimulate the flow of gastric acid.
      a. Watch for side effects of histamine, including flushing, headache, and hypotension.
      b. Do not give drug to patients with a history of asthma or other allergic conditions.
   2. Collect specimens as ordered, usually at 10- to 20-minute intervals.
   3. Label specimens and send to laboratory.
   4. Withdraw nasogastric tube; offer oral hygiene; make patient comfortable.
   5. Gastric acid is high in the presence of duodenal ulcers, and is low in pernicious anemia.

✦ C. Tubeless gastric analysis.
   1. Enables the determination of acidity or its absence.
   2. Have patient fast for 6–8 hours prior to the examination.
   3. Administer gastric stimulant followed by Azuresin or Diagnex Blue, as ordered.
   4. Acid in the stomach displaces the dye, which is then released, absorbed by the bowel mucosa, and excreted in the urine.
   5. The bladder is emptied; the specimen saved. One hour after taking dye resin, patient is instructed to void again. Urine is analyzed, and an estimation is made of the amount of free acid in the stomach.

✦ D. Gastric washings for acid-fast bacilli.
   1. Instruct patient to fast 6–8 hours prior to the procedure.
   2. Insert nasogastric tube and secure gastric washings.
   3. Send specimens to the laboratory to determine the presence of acid-fast bacilli.
   4. Wash your hands carefully and protect yourself from direct contact with specimens.
   5. This procedure is performed on suspected cases of active pulmonary tuberculosis when it is difficult to secure sputum for analysis.

Stool Analysis

A. Stool specimens are examined for amount, consistency, color, shape, blood, fecal urobilinogen, fat, nitrogen, parasites, food residue, and other substances.
   1. Stool cultures are also done for bacteria and viruses.
   2. Some foods and medicines can affect stool color—spinach, green; cocoa, dark red; senna, yellow; iron, black; upper GI bleeding, tarry black; lower GI bleeding, bright red.

✦ B. Stool abnormalities.
   1. Steatorrhea—bulky, greasy and foamy, foul odor.
   2. Biliary obstruction—light gray or clay-colored.
   3. Ulcerative colitis—loose stools, with copious amounts of mucus or pus.
   4. Constipation or obstruction—small, hard masses.

✦ C. Specimen collection.
   1. Specimens for detection of parasites should be sent to the laboratory while the stool is still warm and fresh.
   2. Examinations for blood are performed on small samples. A tongue blade may be used to place a small amount of stool in a disposable waxed container, or place a drop on a commercial card, which will turn color if blood is present in the stool.
   3. Stools for chemical analysis are usually examined for the total quantity expelled, so the complete stool is sent to the laboratory.

Liver Function Tests

Pigment Studies
✦ A. Serum bilirubin—abnormal in biliary and liver disease causing jaundice.
   1. Direct (conjugated)—normal: 0.2 mg/100 mL, soluble in H_2O.
   2. Indirect (unconjugated)—normal: 0.8–1.0 mg/100 mL, insoluble in H_2O.
   3. Total serum bilirubin—normal: 1.0 mg/100 mL.
   B. Urine bilirubin—normally none is found.
   C. Urine urobilinogen—0–4 mg/24 hours.
   D. Fecal urobilinogen—40–280 mg/24 hours.
✦ E. Serum cholesterol—150–250 mg/100 mL.

✦ Protein Studies
   A. Total protein—6–8 g/100 mL.
   B. Serum albumin—3.5–5.0 mg/100 mL.
   C. Serum globulin—1.5–3.0 mg/100 mL.
   D. Prothrombin time—11–16 sec.
   E. Cephalin—0–1+.
   F. In liver damage, fewer plasma proteins are synthesized; thus, albumin synthesis is reduced.
   1. Serum globulins produced by the plasma cells are increased.
   2. PT is reduced in liver cell damage.

Fat and Carbohydrate Metabolism
   A. Fat metabolism—serum lipase 1.5 units.
   B. Carbohydrate metabolism—glucose tolerance levels should return to normal in 1–2 hours.

Liver Detoxification
   A. Bromsulphalein excretion (BSP).
   B. Less than 5 percent dye retention after 1 hour.
   1. Dye is injected intravenously and removed by the liver cells, conjugated, and excreted.
   2. Blood specimen is obtained at 30-minute and 1-hour intervals after injection.
   3. Increased retention occurs in hepatic disorders.

✦ Enzyme (Transaminase) Indicators
   A. Elevations reflect organ damage.

B. Levels.
   1. AST (formerly SGOT)—10–40 units/mL.
   2. ALT (formerly SGPT)—5–35 units/mL.
   3. LDH—100–200 u/L.
   4. GGT—10–48 units/mL.

✦ Alkaline Phosphatase
   A. 2–5 units (varies with method used).
   B. Elevated in obstructive jaundice and in liver metastasis.

✦ Blood Ammonia
   A. 20–120 µg/dL. Range varies with method used.
   B. Ammonia level rises in liver failure because liver converts ammonia to urea.
   C. Metabolic alkalosis increases the toxicity of NH_3.

THYROID FUNCTION TESTS

✦ Radioactive Iodine (RAI) Uptake (Radioiodine ^{131}I)
   A. Normal values—5–35 percent in 24 hours (recently lowered values in United States due to increased ingestion of iodine).
   1. Elevated values indicate—hyperthyroidism, thyrotoxicosis, hypofunctioning goiter, iodine lack, excessive hormonal losses.
   2. Depressed values indicate—low T_4, antithyroid drugs, thyroiditis, myxedema, or hypothyroidism.
   B. Purpose—measures the absorption of the iodine isotope to determine how the thyroid gland is functioning.
   C. Principles.
   1. The use of ^{123}I rather than ^{131}I is now preferred because of its lower radiation hazard. (^{123}I can be used on pregnant women; ^{131}I is contraindicated.)
   2. The amount of radioactivity is measured 2, 6, and 24 hours after ingestion of the capsule.
   3. ^{131}I evaluates the storage of iodine and gives a distribution pattern, as does ^{123}I.

✦ TSH Ultrasensitive Assay
   A. Normal values—0.5–5.0 µU/mL.
   1. Increased values: > 20 µU/mL indicates hyperthyroidism, Addison's disease, goiter, and toxicity from certain drugs.
   2. Decreased values: first-degree hypothyroidism is < 0.3 µU/mL, and second- to third-degree hypothyroidism is < 0.1 µU/mL.
   B. Test is an ultrasensitive indicator that has mostly replaced all other thyroid tests.
   1. If assay is normal, no other test is indicated.
   2. If test is abnormal, it should be validated by a T_4 assay.

✦ T$_3$ and T$_4$ Resin Uptake Tests

A. Normal values.
    1. T$_4$—3.8–11.4 percent.
    2. T$_3$—25–35 percent.
    3. T$_4$.
        a. Elevated—hyperthyroidism, early hepatitis, exogenous T$_4$.
        b. Decreased—hypothyroidism, abnormal binding, exogenous T$_4$.
    4. T$_3$.
        a. Elevated—hyperthyroidism, T$_3$ toxicosis.
        b. Decreased—advancing age.
B. Purpose—both of these in vitro tests are used as screening tests for diagnosis in thyroid disorders. T$_4$ is 90 percent accurate in diagnosing hyperthyroidism and hypothyroidism.
C. Principles.
    1. Levels of T$_3$ and T$_4$ in the blood regulate thyroid stimulating hormone (TSH).
    2. These levels alter according to a balancing system of negative feedback.
    3. Venous blood sample is obtained to directly measure concentration of unsaturated thyroxine-binding globulin in the serum.
    4. Thyroid function tests should be interpreted according to the clinical situation.

✦ Thyroid Stimulating Hormone

A. Normal values less than 10 µU/mL (may vary with laboratory).
    1. Increased values indicate primary hypothyroidism.
    2. Decreased values indicate Hashimoto's thyroiditis, hyperthyroidism, large doses of glucocorticoids, secondary hypothyroidism.
B. Purpose—differentiates primary from secondary hypothyroidism and assesses level of thyroid gland activity.
C. Principles.
    1. Administration of IM TSH (thyrotropin) measures the responsiveness of the thyroid gland.
    2. Blood samples are obtained at intervals.

BLOOD GLUCOSE STUDIES

Glucose Tolerance Test

A. Normal values are between 70 and 105 mg fasting and no sugar in the urine.
    ✦ 1. > 126 mg/dL fasting and 200 mg/dL 2-hour postprandial are diagnostic of diabetes.
    2. The oral glucose tolerance test and IV glucose are no longer recommended for routine clinical use.

B. Purpose—primary aim is to diagnose or rule out diabetes, but also important for unexplained hypoglycemia and malabsorption syndrome.
C. Principles.
    1. This test determines rate of removal of a concentrated dose of glucose from the bloodstream.
    2. Test is indicated when there is sugar in the urine or when fasting blood sugar is elevated.
    3. This is a timed test done in the morning after fasting for at least 12 hours. Blood and urine samples are taken at intervals up to 3 hours.
    4. This test is contraindicated for recent surgical patients or patients with history of myocardial infarctions.

✦ Fasting Plasma Glucose (FPG)

A. > 126 mg/dL can signify diabetes or is required to diagnose diabetes.
    1. Normal fasting level is 8—100 mg/dL. In November, 2003, the lower cutoff level was changed from 110 to 100 mg/dL.
    2. Fasting is defined as no calorie intake for 8 hours.
B. FPG is also used to diagnose hypoglycemia.

✦ Random (Casual) Plasma Glucose Levels

A. Levels of > 200 mg/dL on more than one occasion are diagnostic of diabetes.
B. Casual is any time of day without regard to when the last meal was eaten.

IMMUNODIAGNOSTIC TESTS

✦ HIV-1 Antibody Test

A. The ELISA (enzyme-linked immunosorbent assay) test was developed to screen national donor blood.
    ✦ 1. This test does not test for AIDS, but the antibodies to the HIV virus.
    2. Once exposed to a virus, it takes the body time to produce antibodies. A person may already be infected and if the body has not yet produced antibodies, the ELISA test will be negative.
    3. Test is also imperfect in that it may produce a false positive or false negative.
B. All positive results must be retested.
C. The Western blot test is given for final confirmation—used to confirm seropositive blood as identified by ELISA.
D. The indirect immunofluorescence assay (IFA) is used by some physicians rather than the Western blot to confirm positive for HIV.

✦ Coombs' Test

A. Normal values—negative.
B. Purpose—test to discover presence of antibodies present in Rh negative mother's blood.
   1. Test also will confirm diagnosis of hemolytic disease in the newborn.
   2. Titration determines extent to which antibodies are present.
C. Types of test for Rh incompatibility.
   1. Indirect Coombs'—mother's blood reveals antibodies as result of previous transfusion or pregnancy.
   2. Direct Coombs'—tests newborn's cord blood—determines presence of maternal antibodies attached to baby's cells.

✦ Venereal Disease Research Laboratory Test (VDRL)

A. Normal values—serum is nonreactive.
B. Purpose—to screen for primary or secondary syphilis.
C. Differential diagnosis.
   1. Biological false positive tests may occur with hepatitis, mononucleosis, leprosy, malaria, rheumatoid arthritis, lupus erythematosus.
   2. A nonreactive result does not rule out syphilis, as it takes up to 4 weeks after infection to cause an immunologic response.
D. The Rapid Plasma Reagin Circle Card test (RPR-CT) is also used to screen for diabetes.

Epstein–Barr Virus Antibodies (EBV)

A. Normal values—negative (antibodies appear within first 3 weeks, then decline rapidly).
B. Purpose—to diagnose infectious mononucleosis or to determine the antibody status of EBV infected people.
C. Test—serum is tested for heterophile antibodies (Monospot test).
D. Differential diagnosis.
   1. Positive results may occur with infectious mononucleosis, hepatitis A and B, cancer of the pancreas.
   2. A negative Monospot does not always rule out acute or past EBV.

✦ Serologic Tests for Hepatitis A, B

A. Normal values—negative for hepatitis A, B, C, and D.
B. Purpose—serologic tests diagnose and differentiate different forms of hepatitis.

C. Test variations.
   ✦ 1. Hepatitis A (HAV).
      a. Anti-HAV IgM presence confirms recent infection of hepatitis A—detectable for 3 to 12 weeks.
      b. Anti-HAV IgG indicates previous exposure to HAV, recovery and immunity. Appears after acute infection and is detectable for life.
   ✦ 2. Hepatitis B (HBV).
      a. Hepatitis B surface antigen—appears in 27–41 days and is the earliest indicator of HBV.
      b. Antibody to hepatitis B surface antigen indicates clinical recovery with subsequent immunity.
   ✦ 3. Hepatitis C has no serologic or laboratory test to establish diagnosis—usually made by excluding other causes of hepatitis.
   4. Hepatitis D or Delta is associated with hepatitis B and depends on HBV for replication. It is found in the serum 7–14 days during acute infection.

✦ Rubella Viral Serologic Test

A. Normal values.
   1. Negative titer of < 1.8 or 1.10 (depending on test)—no antibody detected, therefore, not immune.
   2. Positive titer of > 1.10—antibody detected, therefore immune.
B. Purpose—exposure to rubella is important to detect because exposure to this virus—if a woman is in the first trimester of pregnancy—may result in congenital abnormalities, abortion, or stillbirth.

✦ Papanicolaou Smear

A. Diagnosis to identify preinvasive and invasive cervical cancer.
B. Vaginal secretions and secretions from posterior fornix are swabbed and smeared on a glass slide.
✦ C. Pathological classifications. Early cellular changes may be detected before disease becomes clinically observable.
   1. Class I—no abnormal or atypical cells present.
   2. Class II—atypical or abnormal cells present but no malignancy found; repeat Pap smear and follow-up if necessary.
   3. Class III—cytology, suggestive of malignancy; additional procedures indicated (biopsy, D & C).
   4. Class IV—cytology, strongly suggestive of malignancy; additional procedures indicated (biopsy, D & C).
   5. Class V—cytology results conclusive of malignancy.

LABORATORY TESTS QUESTIONS

1. The nurse should explain to a patient who takes Lasix and has a potassium of 3.2 mEq/L that he should

   1. Avoid apple juice, orange juice, and instant coffee.
   2. Eat three servings daily of fruits and meat or fish.
   3. Maintain a fluid intake of 2 liters per day.
   4. Avoid driving or operating electrical equipment.

2. The premenstrual hemoglobin of a 24-year-old patient with no history of trauma, recent surgery, or hemorrhage is 9.8 g/dL. The nurse interprets that this value is due to

   1. Iron-deficiency anemia.
   2. Hypovolemia.
   3. Dehydration.
   4. Cardiogenic shock.

3. A patient is scheduled for a carotid endarterectomy in 3 days. Which of the following preadmission lab test results must be immediately reported to the physician?

   1. Sodium of 151 mEq/L.
   2. Chloride of 105 mEq/L.
   3. Potassium of 3.8 mEq/L.
   4. Bicarbonate of 23 mEq/L.

4. At the physician's office, a patient has a random plasma glucose test. The results were 250 mg/dL. The patient asked the office nurse why the doctor told him to come back the next day to repeat the test. The best answer is

   1. "The doctor always repeats this test."
   2. "You may have diabetes and the doctor wants to be sure."
   3. "This test requires that it be done at least twice for accurate results."
   4. "It was a little high, so the doctor wants to check the results."

5. A patient comes to the clinic complaining of a variety of symptoms including pain. The patient has a gastric analysis done and results show that gastric acid is high. This test result would indicate to the nurse that the patient may receive the diagnosis of

   1. Pernicious anemia.
   2. Peptic ulcer.
   3. Tuberculosis.
   4. Duodenal ulcer.

6. A TSH ultrasensitive assay has been ordered for a patient, and she asks the nurse the purpose of this test. The most appropriate reply is to say

   1. "This test is a screening test to diagnose thyroid disorders."
   2. "The doctor is testing whether you have Hashimoto's disease."
   3. "This test measures the absorption of iodine and how it relates to the thyroid gland."
   4. "The test indicates whether your thyroid gland is over- or underactive."

7. A 60-year-old patient is admitted to the surgery unit for removal of fibroid tumors. When the nurse checks the lab results for routine blood chemistry, she notes that the sedimentation rate is 29 mm/dL. The appropriate intervention is to

   1. Ask the patient if she has been sick and has had a fever.
   2. Do nothing—the value is normal.
   3. Notify the physician.
   4. Ask the lab to repeat the test.

8. A patient is admitted to the hospital for evaluation. His physician writes in the chart "rule out liver cancer" and schedules a liver biopsy. Before the procedure, the nurse reviews the PT results just returned from the lab: 24—INR, 4.0. The nurse also notes that this patient is not on an anticoagulant. The nursing intervention is to

   1. Do nothing—the results of the PT are normal.
   2. Notify the head nurse or physician before the biopsy procedure.
   3. Ask the lab to repeat the test tomorrow and notify the physician.
   4. Ask the patient if he has been eating foods high in vitamin K.

9. A patient with coronary artery disease has an LDL cholesterol level of 140 mg/dL. His physician has recommended that he start on Mevacor to lower the level and slow the progression of atherosclerosis. While reinforcing discharge teaching, the nurse should emphasize

   1. Taking this medication with niacin to lower the LDL level.
   2. Notifying the physician if the patient's gums begin to bleed.

3. Reporting a rash, myalgia, or blurred vision.

4. The drug causes sensitivity to the sun, hence the need for sunscreen and protective clothing.

10. A patient with suspected HIV will receive which test(s) to verify the diagnosis?

   1. Home Access HIV-1 Test System.
   2. Enzyme-linked immunosorbent assay (ELISA) and Western blot assay.
   3. Indirect immunofluorescence assay (IFA).
   4. ELISA and DNA.

11. As part of an annual physical exam, a 60-year-old man has had lab work done. Which of the following serum creatinine levels would indicate that the patient has a mild degree of renal insufficiency?

   1. 4.0 mg/dL.
   2. 3.3 mg/dL.
   3. 1.7 mg/dL.
   4. 0.8 mg/dL.

12. A patient who has sustained head trauma in a motor vehicle accident has been diagnosed and treated for having the syndrome of inappropriate antidiuretic hormone (SIADH) secretion. Which of the following urine specific gravity values would indicate that the situation had not resolved?

   1. 1.005.
   2. 1.018.
   3. 1.025.
   4. 1.035.

13. A patient with damaged or impaired lungs cannot remove all of the CO_2 from the body. When the excess CO_2 combines with H_2O, it will form

   1. H_2CO_3.
   2. HCO_3.
   3. H^+.
   4. CO_2.

14. A patient has been advised to take a bile acid sequestrant (Colestid) to lower his LDL. It comes in powder form or tablets. The nurse should inform the patient that if he chooses tablet form, he should

   1. Take milk with the medication.
   2. Take up to 30 tablets per day for the medication to be effective.
   3. Take the tablet every 6 hours.
   4. Not take the medication with citric acid (orange juice).

15. A 60-year-old woman has a tentative diagnosis of myocardial infarction (MI). Which of the following laboratory values is the *best* indicator of an MI?

   1. CK-MB.
   2. LDH_1.
   3. SGOT.
   4. WBC.

16. An 80-year-old patient has been admitted to the hospital with influenza and dehydration. Which of the following blood urea nitrogen (BUN) levels would indicate to the nurse that the patient has received adequate fluid volume replacement?

   1. 40 mg/dL.
   2. 29 mg/dL.
   3. 17 mg/dL.
   4. 3 mg/dL.

17. A person who is infected with HIV will be diagnosed with AIDS when the CD4 lymphocyte count falls below

   1. 75.
   2. 200.
   3. 350.
   4. 500.

18. A patient with symptoms of nausea and vomiting is admitted to the emergency department. He states that before he came to the hospital, when he tried to lie down, his abdominal pain got worse and was not relieved by antacids. When questioned, he states that he had consumed a large meal and two glasses of wine. The tentative diagnosis is acute pancreatitis. The physician orders lab work. With this complaint picture and diagnosis, the nurse would expect lab results to indicate

   1. Decreased white blood cell count.
   2. Elevated serum amylase and lipase.
   3. No change in serum bilirubin level.
   4. Elevated alkaline phosphatase.

19. A male patient has advanced cirrhosis. His blood test results have been returned and indicate a prothrombin time of 30 seconds. The nurse would expect the physician to order

   1. Vitamin K.
   2. Heparin.
   3. Coumadin.
   4. Ferrous sulfate.

20. Which group of cells is the first line of defense against bacterial infection working primarily through phagocytosis?

   1. Monocytes.
   2. Platelets.
   3. Neutrophils.
   4. Basophils.

LABORATORY TESTS

Answers with Rationale

1. (2)   The normal potassium level is 3.5–5.0 mEq/L. The patient's potassium level is low, and he needs to replenish what has been lost as a result of taking the Lasix. In addition to taking potassium supplements, the patient should be given a list of the appropriate foods that have an average of 7 mEq potassium per serving. (1) is wrong because these foods contain potassium. Answers (3) and (4) do not relate to this question. Fruit, meat, fish, instant coffee, and milk are high in potassium.

   NP:P; CN:PH; CA:M; CL:A

2. (1)   The normal Hgb for a female is > 12–16 g/dL. With the data given, the nurse would suspect anemia. Hypovolemia (2) will alter Hgb if the loss of blood volume was due to hemorrhage. Dehydration (3) may increase the level by hemoconcentration. Cardiogenic shock (4) may increase the Hgb because of the need for increased oxygen carrying capacity.

   NP:D; CN:PH; CA:M; CL:C

3. (1)   The normal electrolyte values for an adult are as follows: sodium of 135–145 mEq/L, chloride of 100–106 mEq/L, potassium of 3.5–5.0 mEq/L, and bicarbonate of 22–29 mEq/L. The serum sodium is the only abnormal value.

   NP:D; CN:S; CA:M; CL:AN

4. (3)   The best answer is to be truthful, but not to frighten the patient by telling him that he may have diabetes (2) (this is the domain of the physician). Levels of > 200 mg/dL on more than one occasion would, however, be diagnostic of diabetes, so the doctor would order at least two tests.

   NP:I; CN:PH; CA:M; CL:A

5. (4)   High gastric acid levels may indicate a duodenal ulcer. Pernicious anemia (1) would yield low results. TB (3) may be diagnosed by gastric washings for acid-fast bacilli, especially if sputum analysis is difficult to procure.

   NP:P; CN:PH; CA:M; CL:C

6. (4)   The clearest and best reply is a general description of the test, but not specific enough to frighten the patient (1, 2). Answer (3) is inaccurate because this answer refers to the radioactive iodine uptake test.

   NP:I; CN:PS; CA:S; CL:A

7. (2)   This is a normal sed rate for a female over age 60. Under age 50, normal is 20 mm/hr. If it were increased, it would indicate presence of infection or inflammation, and surgery might have to be postponed.

   NP:I; CN:PH; CA:M; CL:AN

8. (2)   Because the patient is not on anticoagulant therapy, the results are abnormal (normal PT is 11–15 seconds). It is important to notify the head nurse or physician before the biopsy; bleeding could be life threatening. The patient will probably be given vitamin K therapy and when the PT results return to the normal range, the procedure can be done. Liver disease likely caused the prolonged PT.

   NP:I; CN:S; CA:M; CL:AN

9. (4)   Sensitivity to the sun or photosensitization is a risk for patients taking HMG-COA reductase inhibitors (Mevacor). (1) Niacin is usually given with bile acid sequestrants because they work synergistically. (2) Bleeding from the gums or rectum is a sign of vitamin K deficiency from bile acid sequestrants (Questran). (3) These common adverse effects are from fibric acid derivatives, which are not very effective in lowering LDL.

   NP:I; CN:PH; CA:M; CL:A

10. (2)   ELISA is the first test used to confirm the presence of the antibody to HIV and indicates the

---

Coding for Questions/Answers Abbreviations: **Nursing Process: NP,** Data Collection: D, Planning: P, Implementation: I, Evaluation: E, **Client Needs: CN,** Safe, Effective Care Environment: S, Health Promotion and Maintenance: H, Psychosocial Integrity: PS, Physiological Integrity: PH, **Clinical Area: CA,** Medical Nursing: M, Surgical Nursing: S, Maternal/Newborn Nursing: MA, Pediatric Nursing: P, Psychiatric Nursing: PS, **Cognitive Level: CL,** Knowledge: K, Comprehension: C, Application: A, Analysis: AN

person has been exposed to or infected by HIV. The Western blot assay is used to confirm seropositivity as identified by ELISA. The Home Access Kit (1) has been approved by the FDA, but false-positive test results are possible and must be verified. The IFA (3) is an indirect test and must be confirmed by the Western blot. DNA (4) may be used to track HIV.

NP:P; CN:H; CA:M; CL:K

11. (3) The normal serum creatinine level for a male is 0.6–0.9 mg/dL. A patient with a mild degree of renal insufficiency would have a slightly elevated level, which in this case would be 1.7. Levels of 3.3 (2) and 4.0 (1) may be associated with acute or chronic renal failure.

NP:D; CN:PH; CA:M; CL:C

12. (4) This value is above normal limits (the normal range of a urine specific gravity is 1.010–1.025). Answer (1) may be seen when the patient is in the diuretic phase of a head injury or insult. Answers (2) and (3) are within normal limits, but (3) is indicative of concentrated urine.

NP:D; CN:PH; CA:M; CL:A

13. (1) Excess CO_2 in the blood, when combined with H_2O, forms H_2CO_3, carbonic acid. Depending on the amount of acid in the blood, the lungs will increase or decrease ventilation to remove excess CO_2 (4). The kidneys can excrete or retain H^+ (3) and HCO_3 (2); thus, the equation representing homeostasis is:

$$CO_2 + H_2O = H_2CO_3 = H^+ + HCO_3.$$
$$\text{(Lungs)} \qquad \text{(Kidney)}$$

NP:P; CN:PH; CA:M; CL:C

14. (2) If the patient chooses to take the tablets rather than the powder, he will have to take up to 30 tablets a day. The powder can be taken with a beverage or cereal.

NP:I; CN:PH; CA:M; CL:A

15. (1) All of these laboratory studies provide information about the condition, but the CK-MB is the most valuable measurement. The level rises within 6 hours of myocardial cell death and remains elevated for about 3 days.

NP:P; CN:PH; CA:M; CL:K

16. (3) The normal BUN is 10–20 mg/dL. Answers (1) and (2) indicate unresolved dehydration. Answer (4) is significantly lower than normal and may indicate fluid overload.

NP:D; CN:PH; CA:M; CL:A

17. (2) Criteria for a diagnosis of AIDS in an HIV-infected person includes a CD4 lymphocyte count of < 200.

NP:D; CN:H; CA:M; CL:K

18. (2) These elevated serum levels (amylase and lipase) are the hallmark of acute pancreatitis. Increased white blood cell count and serum bilirubin level is also seen with acute pancreatitis. Elevated alkaline phosphatase (4) is found in chronic pancreatitis.

NP:P; CN:PH; CA:M; CL:C

19. (1) A prothrombin time of 30 seconds indicates the clotting time is prolonged and bleeding could occur (15 seconds is maximum normal reading). A vitamin K injection will increase the synthesis of prothrombin by the liver.

NP:P; CN:PH; CA:M; CL:C

20. (3) Neutrophils are the first line of defense against infection. They live in the circulation for about 6 hours after bacteria are ingested. The cells die and become the main component of pus. Monocytes (1) are the second group to defend the body. Platelets (2) are blood components that go to the site of injury and stem blood loss. Basophils (4) release heparin and histamine in areas that are invaded by antigens.

NP:P; CN:S; CA:M ; CL:K

Infection Control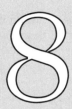

INFECTION

The Infectious Process

A. For an infection to occur, a process involving six links or steps must be present.
   1. If any links are missing, the infection will not occur.
   2. Infection control measures can interrupt the process by eliminating one or more of the steps.
✦ B. Six links form the chain of infection.
   1. Infectious agent (microorganism): bacteria, virus, fungi, etc.
      a. Capability of producing an infection depends on:
         (1) Virulence and number of organisms present.
         (2) Susceptibility of host.
         (3) Existence of portal of entry.
         (4) Affinity of host to harbor microorganism.
      b. The circumstances above must be present to produce an infection.
   2. Reservoir: people, equipment, water, etc., provide survival for organism.
      a. Appropriate environment for growth and multiplication of microorganism must be present.
      b. Reservoirs include respiratory, gastrointestinal, reproductive and urinary tracts, and the blood.
   3. Portal of exit: allows the microorganism to move from reservoir to host (includes excretions, secretions, skin, droplets).
   4. Route of transmission of microorganisms: five routes. Three primary (contact, droplet and airborne); two lesser routes (vehicle and vector).
      a. Contact—most frequent source of nosocomial infection.
         (1) Direct contact—transmission body-to-body and physical transmission (sexual intercourse, kissing or touch).
         (2) Indirect contact—contact with contaminated intermediate object (needle, dressing, dirty hands).
      b. Droplet—transmission of large particle droplets (larger than 5 microns); diphtheria, pertussis, pneumonia, etc.
      c. Airborne—transmission of small particle droplets or residue of 5 microns (measles, varicella, TB).
      d. Two lesser routes.
         (1) Common vehicle: transmission by contaminated items such as food, water, devices.
         (2) Vector-borne: mosquitoes, fleas, rats, etc.
   5. Portal of entry: mucous membrane, gastrointestinal (GI) tract, genitourinary (GU) tract, respiratory tract, and nonintact skin.
   6. Susceptible host: a host who is immunosuppressed, fatigued, malnourished, weakened by other diseases, elderly, stressed, or hospitalized with wounds, IVs, and catheters are at high risk.

Barriers to Infection

✦ A. The primary barrier to infection is the individual's general health and immunologic system (defense mechanisms).
B. Factors that contribute to infection susceptibility.
   1. Disease states.
   2. Altered nutritional status.
   3. Stress and fatigue.
   4. Metabolic function.
   5. Age.
   6. Medications.
✦ C. The body's protection against infection.
   1. The immune process.
      a. Natural immunity is inherited.
      b. Acquired immunity comes from disease exposure or vaccinations.
   2. Anatomic barriers (skin and mucous membranes).
      a. Integrity of the skin and mucous membrane—when integrity is broken, bacteria can enter the body.
      b. How quickly a wound heals depends on the degree of vascularization in the injured area.
   3. The inflammatory process.
✦ D. Conditions predisposing patient to infection.
   1. Surgical wounds.
   2. Alterations in the respiratory or genitourinary tracts (most common site for nosocomial infections).
   3. Invasive devices or venipuncture sites.
   4. Implanted prosthetic devices—cardiac valves, grafts, shunts, or orthopedic joints or pins.

CDC GUIDELINES

Principles of Precautions

✦ A. Risk reduction.
   1. Standard Precautions—handwashing primary method.
   2. Follow procedures to recognize and reduce risks.
B. The CDC guidelines, revised in 1994, contain two tiers of precautions.

◆ C. First-tier *Standard Precautions* blends the major features of universal precautions (blood and body fluids precautions) and body substance isolation into a single set of precautions.
 1. Used for the care of all patients in hospitals regardless of diagnosis or infection status.
 2. Applies to blood, all body fluids, secretions, and excretions, whether or not they contain visible blood; nonintact skin; and mucous membranes.
 3. Precautions designed to reduce the risk of transmission of both recognized and unrecognized sources of infection in hospitals.
 4. As a result of the new category of Standard Precautions, diseases or conditions that previously required category-specific or disease-specific precautions are now covered under this category and do not require additional precautions.

◆ D. The second tier, *Transmission-Based Precautions,* are designed only for the care of specified patients. It reduces the disease-specific precautions into three sets of precautions based on routes of transmission.
 1. Categories are designed for patients documented or suspected to be infected or colonized with highly transmissible or epidemiologically important pathogens which require additional precautions to interrupt transmission to others in the same environment/facility.
 ◆ 2. Three types of transmission-based precautions include airborne precautions, droplet precautions, and contact precautions.
  a. *Airborne precautions* reduce the risk of airborne transmission of infectious agents, such as measles, varicella, and tuberculosis.
  b. *Droplet precautions* are used to prevent the transmission of diseases, such as meningitis, pneumonia, scarlet fever, diphtheria, rubella, and pertussis.
  c. *Contact precautions* are used for patients known or suspected to have serious illnesses easily transmitted by direct contact, such as herpes simplex, staphylococcal infections, hepatitis A, respiratory syncytial virus, and wound or skin infections.
 3. All three types of precautions may be used at one time when multiple routes of transmission are suspected. These precautions are always used in conjunction with Standard Precautions.

 E. Transmission-based precautions used (in addition to Standard Precautions) when a patient is infected with microorganisms or communicable disease.

◆ 1. Airborne precautions.
 a. Implemented when infections can spread through the air (TB, chickenpox, rubeola).
 b. Pathogens can be suspended in air for long periods and are transmitted when a person inhales particles that contain the pathogen.
 c. Health care workers should wear HEPA (high-efficiency particulate air) filter respirator when working with tuberculosis (TB).

◆ 2. Droplet precautions.
 a. This system used when caring for patients who have infections that spread by large-particle droplets containing microorganisms (includes rubella, diphtheria, mumps, pertussis, influenza).
 ◆ b. Patients with this type of infection should be in a private room or with another patient with same disease.
 c. Health care workers should wear a surgical mask for protection when coming within 3 feet of the patient.

◆ 3. Contact precautions.
 a. These precautions used when caring for patients infected or colonized by microorganisms that spread by direct contact (skin to skin) or indirect contact (touch) with a contaminated object.
 ◆ b. Patient requires private room or room with another patient with same illness.
 c. Wear gloves when entering room and change gloves as needed during care. Remove gloves and wash hands when leaving patient's room.
 d. Wear gown if clothing may come into contact with patients, environmental surfaces, or items in room, if patient has diarrhea, wound drainage, or GI surgery.
 e. Use dedicated equipment when a patient has multiple-resistant microorganisms.

◆ F. Transmission guidelines.
 1. Infections and conditions fall into two categories because microorganisms are transmitted in more than one way.
 a. Chickenpox and zoster can spread through both airborne and contact routes.
 b. Adenovirus infection can spread through droplet and contact.
 2. If patient's infection spreads through two transmission routes, institute both precautions and hang both signs on door.

◆ G. Transmission-based precautions and patient transfer.
 1. When patient is transferred to another unit or area for testing, patient must wear a mask and impervious dressing.

2. Transporter takes necessary precautions and wears appropriate barriers.

3. Staff in receiving area have been notified and understand precautions.

✦ H. Methods of infection prevention.
   1. Vaccinations.
      a. Currently more than 25 vaccines licensed in United States.
      b. Preventative vaccines: smallpox, measles, mumps, rubella, polio, diphtheria, pertussis, and tetanus.
      c. Goal of vaccines—prevent specific infectious diseases in a specific population.
   2. Education.

Standard Precautions

✦ A. The term *Standard Precautions* incorporates universal blood and body fluid precautions.

✦ B. Apply Standard Precautions to all patients regardless of diagnosis or infection status.

✦ C. The following guidelines are recommended by the Centers for Disease Control and Prevention (CDC) for use with all patients (whether identified as infectious or not), to prevent transmission of infections. Please follow these guidelines when caring for all patients.

   ✦ 1. Wash hands thoroughly with soap and water or alcohol-based handrub or gel before and after all contact. Wash hands and change gloves between contact with patients.

   2. Wear gloves if there is a possibility of direct contact with blood or bodily secretions (pus, sputum, urine, feces, blood, saliva, etc.).
      ✦ a. This includes a neonate before first bath.
      b. Wash as soon as possible if unanticipated contact with these body substances occurs.

   3. Gloves should be worn when in contact with items or surfaces soiled with blood or body fluids.

   4. In 2003, the CDC stated that healthcare workers in contact with patients must remove all false fingernails.

   5. Protect clothing with gowns or plastic aprons if there is a possibility of being splashed or direct contact with contaminated material.

   6. Wear masks and/or goggles or face shields to avoid being splashed; especially during suctioning, irrigations, and deliveries.

   7. Do not break needles into receptacles; rather, discard them intact and uncapped into containers.

   8. Handle laboratory specimens with care. All specimens are potentially infected.

   9. Place soiled linen in a laundry bag, then in a plastic bag to prevent leakage. Check hospital policy for double-bagging procedure.

   10. Clean spills quickly with 1:1000 solution of bleach if spill occurs in an HIV/AIDS patient's room.

   11. Incineration is preferred method of disposal of infectious waste and should be used whenever possible.

   12. Place patients at risk for contaminating the environment in a private room or with another patient with the same infectious organism.

ACQUIRED HOSPITAL INFECTIONS

Risks of Hospitalization

✦ A. Major risk—nosocomial infections—leading cause of death in United States.
   1. More than 88,000 deaths/year as direct or indirect result of infections (CDC).
   2. These infections begin in hospital or health care facility—each year 2 million patients in the United States acquire infections in these settings (CDC).
   3. Major source of nosocomials: health care workers and patients are reservoirs.
   4. One-third of all nosocomials could be prevented with effective infection control programs in health care facilities.
   5. CDC states these figures can be reduced with education and strict adherence to infection control practices.
   6. A CDC study in 2000 showed that infections contracted in hospitals by patients hospitalized for other health reasons cost 5 billion dollars/year.

✦ B. Most common sites for infection.
   1. Urinary tract infections most common (80% related to catheterization).
   2. Pneumonia second most common nosocomial.
      a. Affects 40 percent of all critically ill or immunocompromised patients.
      b. Causes 15 percent of all in-hospital deaths.
   3. Surgical wound infections—account for 60 percent of additional hospital days.

✦ C. Intravascular devices present increased risk.
   1. Risk of infection related to device itself, site of insertion, and technique of insertion.
   2. *Staphylococcus* is usual cause of infection and bacteremia.

D. Drug-resistant strains of pathogens are increasing nosocomials.
   ✦ 1. Vancomycin-resistant enterococcus (VRE) was a serious development in the 1990s.
      a. *Enterococcus faecium* (called a supergerm) frequently invades surgical wounds, heart valve replacements, and abdominal and urinary tracts.

   b. Enterococcal infections are often impervious to antibiotics—25 percent of these infections in intensive care patients were untreatable.

✦ 2. Methicillin-resistant *Staphylococcus aureus* (MRSA).

   3. Resistant strain of *Mycobacterium tuberculosis.*

E. In 2000, the FDA approved a new super antibiotic called Zyvox, which is a new weapon against drug-resistant infections.

   1. The first entirely new type of antibiotic in 35 years.

   2. Drug should be reserved to fight life-threatening infections that are resistant to other antibiotics.

Basic Infection Control Measures

A. Washing hands.

✦ 1. Many nurses believe wearing gloves eliminates the need to wash hands—not so!

   a. Donning gloves with unclean hands can transfer microorganisms to outside of glove (people carry between 10,000 and 10 million bacteria on each hand).

   b. Important to wash hands between patient contact *and* before and after using gloves.

✦ 2. Proper method of washing hands.

   a. Wet hands with warm running water.

   b. Apply soap or antimicrobial agent.

   c. Rub hands together vigorously for at least 10 to 15 seconds—include all surfaces of fingers and hands.

   d. Rinse hands thoroughly under running water to remove all soap.

   e. Dry hands with paper towels removed one at a time from dispenser.

   f. Use paper towel to turn off faucet if there is no foot pedal.

   3. Washing with waterless agents.

   a. Apply small amount on palm of hand.

   b. Use only if hands are free of dirt.

   c. Rub hands together vigorously covering all surfaces of hands and fingers.

   d. Rub until dry.

✦ B. Gloving: basic infection control measure.

   1. The Occupational Safety and Health Administration (OSHA) stipulates that gloves in all sizes are to be available for health care workers.

   2. Gloves necessary for any task or procedure that may result in blood or body fluid exposure to hands.

   3. Important to change gloves *and* wash hands between patients.

   4. Latex allergy to gloves.

   a. Affects 8 to 12 percent of health care workers.

   b. Classified as immediate immunological reaction caused by latex proteins.

   c. Reaction may progress to anaphylaxis.

   d. Know symptoms of latex allergy: contact dermatitis, local swelling, itching, hives, redness.

   e. Assess allergy to avocados, bananas, kiwi fruit, or chestnuts. Patients or staff may have cross-sensitivity to latex.

   f. If health care worker thinks he or she has latex allergy, they should switch to latex-free gloves *immediately*.

✦ C. Items needed as protective barriers.

   1. Gloves most common barrier protection: protects health workers from mucous membranes, wounds, or infectious body substances.

   2. Face mask: prevents airborne infection—change mask every 30 minutes, or sooner if it becomes damp.

   3. Face shield or goggles: reduces risk of contamination of mucous membranes of eyes. Wear when there is risk of being sprayed or splashed with contaminated body fluids.

   4. Gown: protects clothing from splashed blood or body fluids.

✦ D. Removing protective garb.

   1. Untie ties of gown if tied in front (ties are contaminated).

   2. Remove gloves.

   a. Do not touch outer surface to skin.

   b. Pull first glove down, turning inside out as you pull it off.

   c. Insert two fingers of ungloved hand inside glove edge and pull downward.

   d. Discard gloves in paper receptacle.

   3. Remove gown: unfasten waist ties (if tied in back), then neck ties. Pull gown off shoulders and over arms, turning gown inside out as it is removed, and discard.

   4. Remove face shield or goggles (do not touch face) and discard.

   5. Remove mask: untie lower string first, then upper strings, and discard.

   6. Complete procedure by washing hands.

✦ E. Isolation protocol.

   1. Prepare for isolation.

   a. Check physician's orders.

   b. Obtain isolation cart.

   c. Place isolation cart at patient's door.

   d. Place linen hamper and trash cans conveniently.

   2. Follow dressing procedure when entering or leaving room.

   a. Gown or wear plastic apron.

REMOVING BIOHAZARD WASTE

- Biohazard waste is any solid or liquid waste that presents a threat of infection.
  a. Separate at point of origin or before it leaves patient's room—reduces risk of exposure.
  b. Use impermeable red plastic bag labeled "biohazard." Close securely and double bag.
  c. Red bags cannot be placed with other waste—could contaminate all waste.
- Storage of biohazard material.
  a. Appropriately sealed. May be stored for 30 days.
  b. Waste must be restricted, locked up or stored separately.
  c. Waste must be labeled correctly so tracking may be done.

---

    b.   Use a mask (HEPA filter recommended).
    c.   Use eyeshield or goggles if appropriate.
  3. Remove items from isolation room by double-bagging (using red biohazard bags).
F. Governmental regulatory agencies.
  ✦ 1. CDC goal is disease reduction.
  ✦ 2. OSHA goal is to reduce risk exposure.
  3. OSHA requires that health care facilities have educational protocols in place for prevention of blood-borne pathogens and hepatitis B control.

Nosocomial Infections

Definition: Infections acquired while the client is in the hospital—infections that were not present or incubating at the time of admission.
A. Affect more than 2 million and estimated to cause or contribute to more than 90,000 deaths annually in the U.S.
B. Many of these infections are caused by pathogens transmitted from one to another by healthcare workers.
C. Usually caused by poor or no handwashing technique between patients.

Nosocomial Infectious Diarrhea

✦ A. Most common cause *Clostridium* (C.) *difficile*–associated diarrhea (CDAD)—infectious diarrhea.
  1. Anaerobic, gram-positive bacillus—20–40 percent of hospitalized patients become colonized within a few days of entering hospital.
  2. Spores and microbes found on hospital toilets, bedpans, floors, and health care workers' hands.
✦ B. Recognizing signs and symptoms of CDAD.
  1. Diarrhea occurring after antibiotics.
  2. Abdominal pain—crampy pain and abdominal tenderness.

  3. Fever—above 102.2°F (39°C).
  4. Leukocytosis—WBCs can go as high as 50,000/mm3 (average is 4500 to 11,000).
  5. Lab tests will confirm CDAD with positive stool assay for toxin A or B and autotoxin neutralization test.
✦ C. Preventive methods.
  1. Wash hands before and after patient contact *and* after removing gloves with antiseptic soap.
  2. In addition to Standard Precautions, institute contact isolation precautions—includes placing patient in a private room and always wearing gloves and gown when in direct contact with patient.
  3. After removing gloves and gown, do not touch any potentially contaminated surface.
  4. Use dedicated equipment such as stethoscope and BP cuff—*never* use electronic thermometer because of the potential for spreading bacteria.
  5. Dispose of all contaminated items (bed linens, towel) in proper receptacles.
  6. Instruct family and friends to use infection precautions.
D. Treatment.
  1. Antibiotics for a mild case.
  2. For more severe cases, the physician may discontinue the antibiotic and start antimicrobial therapy (metronidazole is drug of choice).
  3. CDC has recently advised against using vancomycin to treat CDAD because of vancomycin-resistant enterococcus (VRE).

✦ Nosocomial Bloodstream Infections

A. Types of infection.
  1. Presence of bacteria in bloodstream.
  2. Fungemia—infection in bloodstream caused by a fungal organism.
✦ B. Two categories of infection.
  1. Primary infection means host has no preexisting infection but there is direct introduction of microorganisms into bloodstream and host becomes infected via external (catheter) or internal means (internal tubing during manipulation).
  2. Secondary infection occurs when host has another site of infection (urinary tract) that enters bloodstream.
✦ C. Preventive measures.
  1. IV therapy increases risk of invasion of harmful microorganisms (invasive devices and venipuncture sites provide route for infection to occur).
  2. Use of impeccable Standard Precaution methods will reduce risk.

Nosocomial Pneumonia

✦ A. Second most common infection—affects 40 percent of all critically ill or immunosuppressed patients.
  1. Aspiration of gram-negative bacteria are typically acquired in the hospital.
  2. Gram-positive strain (*Staphylococcus aureus*) is leading cause of condition—develops into methicillin resistant condition (MRSA).
    a. Vancomycin, drug of choice to treat MRSA, is rapidly losing its effectiveness.
    b. May occur when food, fluid, or gastric contents enter lung via aspiration.
    c. May also occur when airborne particles are inhaled through respirations or anesthesia equipment.
  3. Viral pneumonia (causes 20 percent of all nosocomials). Most common are adenoviruses, influenza, and respiratory syncytial viruses (RSV).
  4. Fungal pneumonia *Aspergillus* through contact with unfiltered air system, food, or plants.
✦ B. Preventative measures.
  1. Change ventilator tubing frequently—every 48 hours.
  2. Use closed suction system.
  3. Remove pooled secretions above cuff when endotracheal (ET) tube is repositioned.
  4. Provide frequent mouth care.
  5. Provide 100 percent relative humidity at body temperature with all ventilation systems (will help patient fight off pneumonia infection).
  6. Recognizing signs and symptoms.
    a. Onset 72 hours after hospital admission.
    b. Crackles in lung and dullness on percussion.
    c. Purulent sputum.
    d. Positive bacterial or fungal culture.
    e. In elderly patient, may be confusion and fatigue with no fever.
  C. Treatment.
  1. Administer antibiotics as prescribed.
  2. Observe for dyspnea, respiratory rate, and administer O_2 (as prescribed) to maintain PaO_2 at 80 mm Hg plus.
  3. Position patient at 45-degree angle.
  4. Encourage fluid intake—good nutrition.
  5. Encourage incentive spirometry.

Nosocomial Tuberculosis

✦ A. Tuberculosis is an infectious disease caused by the tubercle bacillus *Mycobacterium tuberculosis*.
  1. Currently 100 million afflicted—30–40 million will die and 1/3 may be resistant.
  2. Main reservoir for the organism is respiratory tract.
  3. Transmission occurs between individuals through respiratory contact via droplets transmitted through productive coughing.
✦ B. Symptoms.
  1. Occur 4–12 weeks after exposure.
  2. Active disease and symptoms of cough, weight loss, and fever usually occur within first 2 years after infection.
  3. Latent infections (asymptomatic) are not infectious and may last a lifetime.
  4. Without treatment, tuberculosis progresses.
✦ C. Multidrug-resistant tuberculosis (MDR-TB).
  1. Disease can progress from diagnosis to death in 4–15 weeks.
  2. Patients develop resistance to standard drug regimen as a result of noncompliance and/or inappropriate drug therapy.
✦ D. Effective tuberculosis control requirements: early identification, isolation, and treatment of persons with active tuberculosis.
  1. Purified protein derivative (PPD) skin test used to quickly identify infection in the absence of clinical symptoms.
  ✦ 2. Sputum specimens for acid-fast bacilli (AFB), culture, sensitivity, and chest x-rays.
    a. PPD skin test is read 48–72 hours after the injection.
    b. Positive skin test is indicated by an induration of 10 mm or more at site of injection.
    c. HIV or immunosuppressed—5 mm or more is considered positive. If positive, chest x-ray will rule out active TB.
  ✦ 3. CDC recommendation for tuberculosis isolation—directional air-flow, negative-pressure ventilation system in room.
    a. Anyone entering the patient's room should wear a mask that forms a tight-fitting seal against particulates 1–5 μ.
    b. Disposable particulate respirators are suggested by the CDC when adequate ventilation is not available in the room.

Nosocomial Infected Wounds

✦ A. The longer a person is hospitalized prior to the surgical procedure, the greater risk of postsurgical infection.
  B. Factors that influence infection rates.
  1. Duration of time in the operating room.
  2. Time surgery is done (between midnight and 8 am is period of greatest risk).
  3. Whether patient has postsurgical drains in place.
  4. If the surgery enters a colonized or infected part of the body.

EMERGING VIRUSES AND INFECTIOUS DISEASES

Biology of Diseases

A.   Various forms of flora help protect the human from invasion of pathogens, usually microorganisms that can cause disease.

B.   Host defenses determine whether infection will occur.
1.   Natural barriers: skin and mucous membranes.
2.   Nonspecific immune responses: white cells.
3.   Specific immune responses: antibodies.

C.   Pathogeneses of infection.
1.   Toxins: protein molecules that cause development of disease (diphtheria, cholera, tetanus, etc.).
2.   Virulence factors: assist pathogens in invasion and resistance of host defense mechanism (different forms of *H. influenza).*
3.   Microbial adherence: ability to adhere to surfaces to invade tissue (*Escherichia coli* attaching to human cells in GI tract).
4.   Antimicrobial resistance: agents that can exert selective pressures on microbial populations allowing bacteria to develop resistance to an antimicrobial agent (MRSA).

Marburg and Ebola Virus

Definition: Acute infection (perhaps related to exposure to monkeys in Africa or the Philippines) that produces severe illness.

Characteristics

A.   Vector is unknown, human to human.
B.   Transmission occurs via skin and mucous membrane contact with an infected person.
C.   Incubation period is 5–10 days.
D.   Mortality rate is 25–90%.

Assessment

A.   Fever with myalgia and headache with upper respiratory symptoms.
B.   Hemorrhagic symptoms begin within a few days.

Implementation

A.   Mask–gown–glove precautions.
B.   There is no vaccine or effective antiviral therapy.

Hanta Virus

Definition: Acute infection caused by the hantavirus transmitted to humans from rodents.

Characteristics

A.   Transmission is through inhalation of infectious aerosols from rodent excreta.

B.   Characterized by acute renal failure or acute pulmonary edema.
C.   Incubation period 7–36 days.

Assessment

A.   Sudden onset with high fever, headache, backache and abdominal pain.
B.   Hemorrhages appear; severe neurological symptoms occur in 1%; severe cases are 10–15%.

Implementation

A.   Treatment is ribavirin IV and supportive care.
B.   Overall fatality is 6–15%.

Lassa Fever

Definition: Systemic arenavirus infection that involves visceral organs; spares the CNS.

Characteristics

A.   Most human cases result from contamination of food with rodent urine; human-to-human transmission can occur.
B.   Mortality rate 16–45%.
C.   Incubation period 1–24 days.

Assessment

A.   Initial symptoms are sore throat, fever, headache, myalgia and malaise.
B.   Onset of severe symptoms take several days; severity correlates with amount of virus absorbed and degree of fever.

Implementation

A.   Standard precautions, airborne isolation including high-efficiency mask and negative pressure room.
B.   Ribavirin used to reduce mortality rate, given within 6 days of onset.
C.   Supportive care including fluid and electrolyte balance critical.

Dengue Fever

Definition: Acute febrile disease caused by flavivirus, transmitted by bite of *Aedes* mosquito.

Characteristics

A.   Occurs mostly in children living when Dengue is endemic (Southeast Asia, China and Cuba); endemic in tropics and subtropics, including Puerto Rico, U.S. Virgin Islands and Tahiti.
B.   Incubation period is 3–15 days.

Assessment

A.   Abrupt onset with chills, headache, aching joints with rapid rise in temperature (104°) followed by afebrile period for 24 hours.
B.   Second rise in temperature follows with rash covering entire body.

Implementation

A. Dengue prophylaxis requires eradication of mosquito vector.

B. Treatment is symptomatic—complete bed rest and acetaminophen (avoid aspirin).

Severe Acute Respiratory Syndrome (SARS)

Definition: A respiratory illness of unknown etiology; the first severe and readily transmittable viral disease of the 21st century.

Characteristics

A. First detected in November, 2002, in China; in March, 2003, the World Health Organization (WHO) announced a global alert. SARS proceeded to be reported in 30 countreis.

B. SARS is belived to be caused by a new variety of the coronavirus (the common cold).

C. Transmission of SARS.
   1. Spread by person-to-person contact.
   2. Possibly spread by contact with objects that have been contaminated with infectious droplets.
   3. Disease may be airborne spread, but this is still undetermined.

D. Incubation period is 2 to 7 days (or possibly as long as 10 days).

Assessment

A. SARS begins with elevated temperature (> 100.4°F or > 38°C).
   1. Fever may be associated with chills, headache or malaise.
   2. During this prodromal period, patient may develop mild respiratory symptoms.

B. After 3 to 7 days, lower respiratory symptoms develop.
   1. Dry, nonproductive cough and dyspnea.
   2. Hypoxemia may develop, as well as respiratory distress syndrome.

C. The last stage of SARS is classified as atypical pneumonia.

D. No definitive diagnostic test for SARS; CDC has serum tests to detect antibodies to the virus but specificity is still being evaluated.

E. Epidemiological criteria: travel (through an airport) within 10 days of onset of symptoms; close contact with a person known or suspected to have SARS.

Implementation

A. Implement immediate infection control measures with a suspected case of SARS.
   1. Use standard hand hygiene (soap and water or alcohol-based gel).
   2. Use contact protection (gloves, gown, and eye shield).
   3. Use airborne protection: N95 disposable respirators; place patient in a negative pressure isolation room.

B. No accepted medical treatment.
   1. A viral drug, Ribavirin (a drug used to treat AIDS patients) may be useful for those under age 40.
   2. Elderly patients do not react well to this drug.

C. Give supportive care; in some cases mechanical ventilation is started when normal functioning of the lungs is compromised.

D. Complementary physicians are recommending the herb, echinacea, because it boosts immune responses and aids in fighting the virus.

West Nile Virus

Definition: A mosquito borne viral disease that has been detected in 43 states. It is a single-stranded RNA virus of the family of encephalitis-causing viruses.

Characteristics

A. First cases were identified in New York City in 1999, introduced by an infected host (bird or human) or vector (mosquito).

B. Transmission occurs in summer and early fall when mosquitos are active.

Assessment

A. Infection occurs in 3 to 14 days after infected mosquito bites; symptoms last 3–6 days.
   1. 80% of infections are mild, without symptoms.
   2. 20% develop flu symptoms, lasting less than 1 week.
   3. Less than 1% develop a severe illness: encephalitis or meningitis.

B. Assess for symptoms of severe neurologic disease.
   1. Fever, headache, stiff neck, and mental confusion.
   2. Tremors, muscle weakness and convulsions in about 15% (of the 1%).

C. Symptoms may be confused with (or misdiagnosed as) Guillain-Barré.

D. MAC-ELISA is the best diagnostic test to detect antibody in serum or cerebro-spinal fluid (collected with 8 days of illness onset).

Implementation

A. No treatment is needed for asymptomatic West Nile virus.

B. Patients with symptoms of encephalitis or meningitis require hospitalization.
   1. No specific therapy is available; give supportive therapy.

2. Airway management, respiratory support (mechanical ventilation) may be ordered to control cerebral edema.
3. Fluid management.

C. Use Standard Precautions to protect health care workers.

D. Teach patients preventive methods.
   1. Avoid mosquito bites.
   2. Use the chemical insect repellent, DEET, which will offer protection. (Studies show DEET lasts 5 hours after application.)

IMMUNOSUPPRESSION

The Immunosuppressed Patient

✦ *Definition:* An acquired immune deficiency characterized by a defect in natural immunity against disease. With loss of the immune system, the individual is susceptible to a variety of "opportunistic infections."

Characteristics

A. The immune system—how it functions.
   1. A complex system of organs and cells that work to distinguish foreign invaders from natural components in the body.
      a. The body's skin and mucous membranes provide the *first line of defense* against invading organisms.
      b. When a foreign organism enters the body, it may be destroyed by circulating white blood cells, macrophages and neutrophils—the *second line of defense.*
   ✦ 2. The immune system is triggered when an antigen has not been stopped or destroyed by the body's first and second defense system.
      a. Lymphocytes then mobilize to defend the body against invaders or antigens.
      b. Lymphocytes fall into two classes.
         (1) B cells (30 percent of blood lymphocytes) develop in the bone marrow.
         (2) T cells (70 percent of blood lymphocytes) originate in the bone marrow but complete development in the thymus gland.
✦ B. Etiology of immunosuppression.
   1. Drug treatment protocols.
      a. Cancer chemotherapeutic agents.
      b. Antibiotics such as tetracycline, chloramphenicol, streptomycin, gentamicin inhibit cellular immunity.
      c. Mafenide and silver sulfadiazine inhibit neutrophil movement to the area of inflammation.
      d. Steroids cause temporary lymphocytopenia, increase in neutrophils, decrease in monocyte and eosinophils.
         (1) Chronic use leads to nonresponsive immune system.
         (2) Anergy may lead to susceptibility to opportunistic infections.
   2. Age—the older a patient's chronologic age, the more susceptible to infections.
   3. Acute and chronic diseases.
      a. Acquired immune deficiency syndrome (AIDS).
      b. Cancer.
      c. Inflammatory bowel disease.
      d. Diabetes.
      e. Chemical sensitivity.
      f. Chronic fatigue syndrome.
   4. Poor nutritional status.
      a. Protein and calorie depletion lead to lymphocyte suppression.
      b. Iron deficiency causes atrophy of the liver, spleen, bone marrow, and lymphoid tissue.
      c. Zinc deficiency affects thymus gland.
   5. Surgery and anesthesia.
   6. Stress, both specific and generalized.
      a. Environmental stress such as pollution, high-intensity sound or noise may create stress that results in immunosuppression.
      b. Stressful life events, such as loss of job, marriage, or death, decrease immune function.
   7. Psychiatric illness, especially major illness such as schizophrenia, depression, or manic episode.
   8. Lesions of the central nervous system, especially the hypothalamus, produce changes in the immune response.

Assessment

✦ A. Observe for possible sites of infection.
   1. IV sites and invasive devices (prosthetic devices).
   2. Catheter sites.
   3. Surgical wounds.
   4. All body crevices.
   5. Respiratory tract (lungs) and genitourinary tract.
✦ B. Observe for signs of inflammation or systemic infection.
   1. Changes in temperature—fever may be only sign, since signs of inflammation may not appear due to diminished neutrophils.
   2. Changes in white blood cell count and differential count.
   3. Signs of inflammation: pain, redness, swelling and heat.
C. Assess lungs for adventitious sounds.
D. Assess nutritional status.

1. Calorie and protein intake to build immune system.
2. Adequate vitamins (including vitamins A and C) and minerals (iron and zinc).

Implementation

✦ A. Prevention and early detection of infection.
  ✦ 1. Handwashing and gloving are essential for prevention.
     a. Wash hands frequently during the care, and wash thoroughly before and after any contact with an immunosuppressed patient. Use antiseptic, not bar soap or waterless antiseptic.
     b. Wear gloves for any contact where there is possibility of contact with blood, body secretions, or contaminated surface.
  ✦ 2. Use of aseptic technique when caring for all possible entrance sites for infection: catheters, central lines, endotracheal tubes, pressure-monitoring lines and peripheral IV lines.
  ✦ 3. Be aware of possibility of cross contamination—deliver care first to the immunosuppressed patient.
  ✦ 4. Assign patient to private room, if possible.
     a. Keep door closed to prevent transmission of airborne organisms.
     b. Keep room well ventilated.
  5. Use masks for all persons with the slightest evidence of upper respiratory or other type of infection.
  6. Damp dust with a disinfectant solution when cleaning room or objects used in care.
  7. Use a humidifier to reduce microorganisms that may thrive in an arid environment.
  8. Do not allow water to collect and stagnate; change every 24 hours to prevent breeding of organisms.
  ✦ 9. Prevent contamination of suctioning equipment.
     a. Use two-glove technique to prevent spread of organisms.
     b. Complete thorough handwashing before and after suctioning.
     c. Clean connecting tubes with germicide solution.
     d. Change tubes every 8 hours.
  ✦ 10. Use strict aseptic technique for every dressing change.
✦ B. Complete impeccable skin care for the immunosuppressed patient.
  1. Observe all pressure areas for signs of breakdown.
  2. Turn frequently, every hour if patient is immobile.
  3. Complete passive or active range of motion when indicated.
  4. Change any wet clothing or dressing immediately; wetness will break down skin.
  5. Lubricate and massage skin to prevent cracks and stimulate blood circulation to potential areas of breakdown.
✦ C. Perform pulmonary toilet.
  1. Assess pulmonary function frequently for lung sounds, coughing, drainage, and ability to breathe.
  2. Perform toilet every 2–4 hours.
D. Monitor nutritional status.
  1. Provide high-calorie, high-protein diet; without adequate nutrients, patient cannot produce enough lymphocytes to fight infection.
  2. Malnutrition impairs the immune response.
  3. Administer enteral feedings for patients with normal GI functions.
  4. Administer total parenteral nutrition (TPN) if GI tract is not functioning. This achieves high-density caloric support.
E. Assist client to handle stressful conditions.
F. Present realistic optimism when caring for patient—a no-hope attitude on the part of the nurse will be conveyed.

Acquired Immune Deficiency Syndrome (AIDS)

Definition: Aquired immune deficiency diseases linked to HIV. A retrovirus, it primarily affects the helper T cells, causing the immune system to collapse.

Characteristics

A. Specific etiology is unknown.
  1. HIV virus attaches to protein on surface of helper T cells.
  2. Helper T cells are unable to activate B cells and killer T cells.
  3. Immune system collapses when many helper T cells have been destroyed.
B. Risk factors.
  1. IVdrug abusers.
  2. Homosexual males with multiple sexual partners or bisexual men.
  3. The above 2 groups make up 85 percent of all AIDS cases.
C. Incubation period may be as long as 8 to 10 years.
D. Individuals may have antibodies and be carriers but not exhibit AIDS.
E. Some individuals exhibit a mild version of immune system depression.
F. Transmission of virus is known to be through body fluids such as semen and blood products.
G. Disease is known to be lethal in a high proportion of persons, especially those with *Kaposi's sarcoma*.

H. HIV statistics.
   1. 800,000 to 900,000 Americans are living with HIV—40,000 new cases occur each year.
   2. WHO estimates that in 2010 75 million HIV cases in 5 industrial nations will be infected with HIV.

Assessment

A. HIV-1 antibody test—tests for antibodies to HIV virus.
   1. The ELISA test was developed to screen national donor blood.
   2. Test may produce false positive or negative.
   3. All positive results must be retested via ELISA.
B. Initial symptoms indicative of syndrome onset.
   1. Weight loss, anorexia.
   2. Elevated temperature.
   3. Lymphadenopathy.
   4. Malnutrition.
   5. Diarrhea.
   6. Chronic fatigue, malaise.
   7. Dry, productive cough.
   8. Acute onset presents with overwhelming infection.
C. Lungs exhibit adventitious sounds (*Pneumocystis carinii*), a parasitic infection of the lungs.
D. Purple lesions on skin (*Kaposi's sarcoma*), a type of cancer.
E. Mucous membranes of mouth have fungus from *Candida albicans* and ulcerating infections.

Implementation

A. Treatment is oriented toward aggressive antiviral therapy.
   1. HAART (highly active antiretroviral therapy).
   2. One protease inhibitor and two nonnucleoside reverse transcriptase inhibitors is recommended.
   3. This combination "cocktail" is now standard of care.
B. Maintain nutritional status of patient.
   1. Dietary supplements.
   2. Fluids 1500 to 2000 mL/day.
   3. Antiemetics to minimize anorexia and nausea.
C. Provide good skin care to prevent breakdown.
D. Provide respiratory care: turn, cough and deep breathe.
E. Place on secretion precaution.
F. Provide pain control and comfort measures for fatigue.
G. Provide supportive care for patient who develops Pneumocystosis (an acute pneumonia caused by *Pneumocystis carinii*).
   1. Disease occurs in about 60 percent of AIDS patients and is a major cause of death.

   2. There is an abrupt onset with fever, tachycardia, severe hypoxemia, and uncompensated respiratory alkalosis.

Psychosocial Care for the AIDS Patient

✦ A. Identify problem area.
   1. Fear of contagion.
      a. Family and friends fear contagion because of lack of knowledge about AIDS transmission.
      b. The person with AIDS is actually the most vulnerable to contagion.
   2. Fear of rejection.
      a. Disclosing AIDS, especially if one is a homosexual, to family or friends leads to fear of rejection.
      b. Guilt and shame accompany a diagnosis of AIDS.
   3. Planning for terminal care.
      a. Resources and funds may be depleted when terminal care is needed.
      b. Long-term total care is often needed for physical as well as mental debilitation.
B. Provide milieu of individual acceptance.
   1. Use of nonjudgmental attitudes.
   2. Encourage open, honest communication from staff to patient.
✦ C. Assist patient to clarify fears and concerns of rejection.
   1. Encourage verbalization of fears and feelings but only if patient is ready to verbalize.
   2. Encourage honesty when telling others of diagnosis, concerns, and needs.
D. Mediate between patient, parents, and loved ones.
   1. Clarify role patient wishes friends, partner, and family to take during illness.
   2. Assist patient to clarify decisions regarding treatment, finances, and caregiving.
E. Assist patient to go through grieving process caused by loss (of self-image, independence, identity, and worthiness).
F. Support parents and loved ones who are bereaved at loss of partner or child.

Hepatitis

See Hepatitis A, B, C, D in Chapter 10.

Health Care Workers' Exposure to HIV

A. In 1997, the Public Health Service updated recommendations for management of health care workers' exposure to HIV. The decision to recommend HIV postexposure prophylaxis (PEP) takes into account:
   1. The nature of the exposure.

2. The amount of blood or body fluid involved in the exposure.

✦ B. Health care facilities should have the protocols available and mandate prompt reporting and postexposure care.
1. Health care workers must be educated to report occupational exposures immediately after they occur.
2. PEP is most likely to be effective if implemented as soon after the exposure as possible.
3. Exposure is defined as a percutaneous injury, contact of mucous membrane or nonintact skin, or contact with intact skin when the duration of contact is prolonged.
4. Risk assessment is performed on all health care workers who have been exposed to potentially HIV-infected blood or body fluids.
5. Goal is to balance risk for infection against potential toxicity of the PEP drugs.

C. Recommendations for PEP:
1. A basic 4-week regimen of two drugs (zidovudine and lamivudine) for most HIV exposures.
2. Expanded regimen that includes the addition of a protease inhibitor (indinavir or nelfinavir) is recommended for increased risk for transmission of HIV exposures.

HIV–HBV Health Care Worker Alert

A. Accidental contact with blood or body fluids.
✦ 1. Any percutaneous or mucocutaneous exposure should receive immediate first aid.
   a. Percutaneous exposure—a break in the skin caused by contaminated needle or sharp instrument, broken glass container holding blood or body fluids, or human bite.
   b. Mucocutaneous exposure—body fluid contact to open wounds, nonintact skin

(eczema), or body fluid splash to mucous membranes (mouth, eyes).
✦ 2. Apply immediate first aid to site.
   a. Needlestick or puncture wound; scrub area vigorously with soap and water for 5 minutes.
   b. Oral mucous membrane exposure: rinse area several times with water.
   c. Ocular exposure: irrigate immediately with water or normal saline solution.
   d. Human bite: cleanse wound with povidone–iodine (Betadine) and sterile water.
3. Report unusual occurrence to the charge nurse or supervisor.
4. Complete an unusual occurrence form and follow reporting requirements mandated by OSHA.

B. Health Care Worker Protection Act.
1. The Health Care Worker Protection Act was passed to reduce number of health care workers who are accidentally exposed to potentially contaminated, infected blood via a needlestick.
   a. Between 600,000 and 800,000 needlesticks and injuries are reported yearly.
   b. Most common cause of exposure to bloodborne pathogens is needlestick injuries.
2. This act makes the use of safe needle devices a requirement if facility receives Medicare funding.
✦ 3. More than 20 pathogens can be transmitted through small amounts of blood.
   a. Hepatitis B is the most common infectious disease transmitted through work-related exposure to blood and needlesticks.
   b. In addition to HIV and hepatitis B, syphilis, varicella-zoster, and hepatitis C can be transmitted via this route.

INFECTION CONTROL QUESTIONS

1. The single major risk a patient faces when entering a hospital in the United States for any reason is

    1. Resistant strain of *Staphylococcus*.
    2. Vancomycin-resistant enterococcus.
    3. Nosocomial infection.
    4. Death.

2. Considering the most basic infection control measures, which of the following statements is correct?

    1. Wearing gloves eliminates the need to wash hands between patients.
    2. Donning gloves, even with unclean hands, will protect the patient.
    3. It is important to wash hands between patients and before and after using gloves.
    4. OSHA stipulates that gloves must be worn for all patient contact.

3. The nurse has instituted contact precautions on a patient with herpes infection. These precautions would *not* include

    1. Special particulate (HEPA) filter mask.
    2. Private room or double room with a patient with the same illness.
    3. Gloves when providing patient care and changing gloves following contact procedures.
    4. Gown if clothing will come in contact with the patient, environmental surfaces, or items in the room.

4. For an infection to occur, six links or steps must be present. Which of the following is *not* considered a link?

    1. Infectious agent.
    2. Reservoir.
    3. Portal of entry.
    4. Droplet transmission.

5. The most common nosocomial infection is

    1. Urinary tract infection.
    2. Infectious diarrhea (*C. difficile*).
    3. Pneumonia (gram-negative bacteria).
    4. Bloodstream infection.

6. A patient returns to the unit following neurosurgery for removal of a meningioma. The patient has been in intensive care for 2 days and now is assigned to a step-down unit. When completing an assessment, the nurse notes that the patient has a fever of 102°F and is complaining of cramps and pain in the stomach. The appropriate intervention is to

    1. Repeat the assessment in 12 hours.
    2. Check what the patient has eaten in the last meal.
    3. Do nothing—these symptoms are expected with this condition.
    4. Report the symptoms and request a stool assay for toxin A or B.

7. A nurse accidentally has had a needlestick in her hand as she pulled an IM needle from the muscle. The first action is to

    1. Report the accident to the charge nurse.
    2. Scrub the area vigorously with soap and water for 5 minutes.
    3. Cleanse area with povidone–iodine (Betadine).
    4. Irrigate the wound with sterile water.

8. All staff must wear disposable particulate respirators (HEPA filter) when

    1. Working with a patient in isolation.
    2. There is inadequate room ventilation.
    3. Working with a patient with tuberculosis.
    4. There are suspected colonized microorganisms.

9. A nurse is assigned to take two patients' vital signs, complete a focus assessment and provide hygienic care, administer meds, and complete a dressing change for a patient with an abdominal wound. Which task will have priority with this assignment?

    1. Complete a focus assessment and provide hygienic care on the first patient.
    2. Administer medications to the patient.
    3. Complete the dressing change.
    4. Take vital signs on the two patients.

10. CDC guidelines are specific for patients with tuberculosis. The major differences in providing care for the patient with TB versus other patients requiring barrier nursing are the

    1. Staff must wear gowns, mask, and gloves.
    2. Patient should be in a private room with a special ventilation system.

3. Patient may be placed in a room with other patients requiring barrier nursing protocol.
4. Protocol of donning and removing isolation garb before entering or leaving the patient's room is different.

11. The nurse is assigned to care for two patients. One patient has just returned from surgery for an abdominal resection. The second patient is hospitalized with an acute case of tuberculosis. What special precautions should the nurse take when providing care for these two patients?

1. Proper handwashing between patients and use of specific isolation garb.
2. Provide care to the patient with tuberculosis before the patient with abdominal surgery.
3. Strictly adhere to barrier nursing principles.
4. Thorough handwashing and gloving is sufficient in this situation.

12. A nurse is just exiting an isolation room. Considering infection control protocol, which action would the nurse take first?

1. Bag equipment and double-bag it out at the door.
2. Remove protective gear.
3. Dispose of equipment appropriately inside the room.
4. Wash hands.

13. The LVN team leader will assign a healthcare worker to provide basic hygiene care for a patient in isolation. Which team member would be appropriate for this assignment in terms of legal and Nurse Practice Act restrictions?

1. LVN/LPN only.
2. LVN/LPN, CNA.
3. LVN/LPN, UAP.
4. LVN/LPN, CNA, UAP.

14. Protective eyewear should be worn at all times when the nurse is

1. Giving personal care to an AIDS patient.
2. Bathing a neonate for the first time.
3. Drawing cord blood.
4. Taking a specimen to the laboratory.

15. Gloves are an important component of infection control protocol. Which of the following situations would not require that gloves be worn?

1. When the nurse is in contact with urine.

2. Suctioning a patient who does not have an infectious disease.
3. Changing an ostomy pouch.
4. Delivering a food tray to a patient with AIDS.

16. A nurse is assigned to provide care for a patient with AIDS. Infection control guidelines specify that a gown should be worn when the nurse

1. Enters the room to provide patient care.
2. Administers IV medications.
3. Completes a dressing change.
4. Administers an IM injection.

17. When removing an isolation gown, steps the nurse should take would be to

1. Untie the neck strings, remove gloves, and untie waist strings.
2. Untie front waist strings, remove gloves, and untie neck ties.
3. Remove gloves, untie waist strings, and wash hands.
4. Remove gloves, untie neck strings, and wash hands.

18. Two major factors that influence whether an infection occurs in an individual are

1. Age and general health status.
2. Underlying disease status and exposure to infectious agent.
3. Inherent health and immunologic status.
4. Type of organism and age.

19. Which of the following is a type of transmission-based precaution?

1. Droplet.
2. Respiratory.
3. Blood.
4. Body fluids.

20. The census on the unit is 90 percent and there are no private rooms available. An elderly patient with influenza is admitted. Which of the following rooms would it be appropriate to assign this patient?

1. A double room with another patient who has the same diagnosis.
2. A four-bed room with three patients who have had orthopedic surgery.
3. A double room with an elderly patient with a diagnosis of chickenpox.
4. A double room with a patient admitted for impetigo.

INFECTION CONTROL

Answers with Rationale

1. (3) The major risk for any hospitalized patient for any reason is developing a nosocomial infection. There are 2 million infections per year acquired in hospitals, with 88,000 deaths as a direct or indirect result of infections (CDC stats). Option (1) and (2) are two of the possible infections that can be contracted. The end result of any infection could be death.

   NP:D; CN:S; CA:M; CL:K

2. (3) The only totally correct statement is to wash hands between patients as well as before and after using gloves. Wearing gloves does *not* eliminate the need to wash hands (1) and microorganisms can be transmitted (when the hands are unclean) even if gloves are worn (2). Gloves are not necessary for all patient contact (4)—just contact that may result in blood or body fluid exposure to the hands.

   NP:P; CN:S; CA:M ; CL:C

3. (1) A HEPA filter mask would work for droplet precautions for a patient with tuberculosis or any disease that is spread via droplet (such as diphtheria or pertussis) rather than contact (skin to skin).

   NP:P; CN:S; CA:M; CL:A

4. (4) Droplet transmission is not considered a link in the six-step process of infection. Droplet is one of the three precautions (the other two are contact and airborne) based on the route of transmission. The additional three links needed for an infection to occur are route of transmission, portal of exit, and susceptible host.

   NP:D; CN:S; CA:M; CL:C

5. (2) The most common cause of nosocomial infections is *C. difficile* diarrhea. Twenty to 40 percent of hospital patients become colonized within a few days. The second most common cause is pneumonia—gram negative, gram positive, and viral.

   NP:P; CN:S; CA:M; CL:K

6. (4) The symptoms suggest infectious diarrhea. Up to 40 percent of hospitalized patients contract this infection within days of entering the hospital. A stool assay is indicated so that antibiotics or antimicrobial medication can be initiated immediately. The cramps and stomach pain do not relate to what the patient ate (2).

   NP:I; CN:PH; CA:M; CL:AN

7. (2) Immediate first aid is to scrub the area vigorously. The nurse would then report and write up the accidental needlestick (1). Cleansing the area with Betadine (3) would be appropriate for a human bite. Irrigating with sterile water (4) is appropriate first aid for ocular exposure to blood or body fluid.

   NP:I; CN:S; CA:M; CL:A

8. (2) Staff must wear disposable respirators when there is inadequate room ventilation. If the room has a directional negative-pressure ventilation system, the staff would not be required to wear a HEPA filter mask, even if the patient had TB. These masks are required for droplet transmission–based conditions.

   NP:P; CN:H; CA:M; CL:A

9. (4) Taking vital signs on the two patients would be the priority nursing action to determine if there are any emergent problems. Next, the nurse would give the meds (2) that need to be given within a certain time frame. Third, the nurse would complete the focus assessment (reporting the results to the RN) and if possible, assign the hygienic care to a CNA. Because changing the dressing (3) might also involve a pain assessment, this would take more time and should probably be done last.

   NP:P; CN:S; CA:M; CL:AN

10. (2) Patients with tuberculosis are placed in private rooms with directional air-flow, negative-pressure

Coding for Questions/Answers Abbreviations: **Nursing Process: NP,** Data Collection: D, Planning: P, Implementation: I, Evaluation: E, **Client Needs: CN,** Safe, Effective Care Environment: S, Health Promotion and Maintenance: H, Psychosocial Integrity: PS, Physiological Integrity: PH, **Clinical Area: CA,** Medical Nursing: M, Surgical Nursing: S, Maternal/Newborn Nursing: MA, Pediatric Nursing: P, Psychiatric Nursing: PS, **Cognitive Level: CL,** Knowledge: K, Comprehension: C, Application: A, Analysis: AN

ventilation systems. Negative pressure pulls air away from the hallway and exhausts it out of the room to areas away from the intake vents. The other elements are the same for any patient requiring barrier nursing precautions or isolation protocols.

NP:P; CN:S; CA:M; CL:A

11. (3) There are no special precautions; however, the nurse must strictly adhere to barrier nursing principles and the two patients must be treated separately. Providing care to the abdominal surgery patient before the TB patient would be appropriate. Proper handwashing is essential (1), but isolation garb is needed only for the TB patient.

NP:I; CN:S; CA:M; CL:AN

12. (3) The first action would be to dispose of "dirty" equipment in a garbage bag before removing protective gear. Then, the nurse would remove gear beginning with the gown (2) and place it in a garbage bag (1). Finally, the nurse would wash hands (4) and dispose of all "double–bagged" equipment in the dirty utility room and wash hands again.

NP:I; CN:S; CA:M; CL:A

13. (4) All members of the team, even unlicensed personnel, can legally perform some activities of care for a patient in isolation.

NP:P; CN:S; CA:M; CL:AN

14. (3) Protective eyewear should be worn when drawing cord blood, because the blood could easily splash into the nurse's eyes. Gloves should be worn when giving personal care to an AIDS patient or bathing a neonate for the first time, but eyewear is not required protocol.

NP:P; CN:S; CA:M; CL:A

15. (4) Delivering a food tray to an AIDS patient would not require the nurse to don gloves. However, correct protocol would require that the nurse wash hands before delivering another tray. The other interventions would absolutely require gloving because the nurse is in contact with body fluids.

NP:I; CN:S; CA:M; CL:A

16. (3) Whenever a dressing is changed, the nurse could come in contact with body fluids; thus, a gown should always be worn. Entering a room (1) and administering IV meds (2) or an IM injection (4) are interventions that do not necessarily require gowning.

NP:P; CN:S; CA:M; CL:A

17. (2) Removing the waist strings first is appropriate because when they are tied in front, they are considered dirty. The nurse would remove gloves, untie the neck strings (which are considered clean), and then remove the gown. Only if there were no waist strings in front would the nurse remove the gloves first.

NP:P; CN:S; CA:M; CL:K

18. (3) Inherent health and the health of one's immune system are the two major factors that determine whether an infection will occur. Other factors that have an impact are general health status (1) and underlying disease status (2) (which would weaken the immune system). Neither age nor exposure time to the infectious agent is a major factor.

NP:P; CN:S; CA:M; CL:C

19. (1) Droplet is a type of transmission-based precaution. The other two types are contact and airborne. The remaining answers are not considered types of precautions.

NP:E; CN:S; CA:M; CL:K

20. (1) If a private room is not available, the patient should be placed with another patient with the same diagnosis where droplet precautions would already be in place. The staff and visitors should be told to stay at least 3 feet away without a mask because large-particle droplets travel only about 3 feet before falling from the air. The orthopedic patients (2) should not be exposed to the flu or chickenpox (3) (which require airborne precautions). Impetigo (1) requires contact precautions, so this patient should not be exposed to the flu or vice versa.

NP:I; CN:S; CA:M; CL:AN

Disaster Nursing—Bioterrorism*

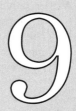

*This is a very inclusive chapter because there is so little information available in the nursing textbooks.

INTRODUCTION TO DISASTER NURSING

A. Preparedness for a terrorist-caused disaster is critical for containment and protection of the population.

B. The Centers for Disease Control (CDC) has developed a strategic plan based on five focus areas.
   1. Preparedness and prevention.
   2. Detection and surveillance.
   3. Diagnosis and characterization of biological and chemical agents.
   4. Response.
   5. Communication.

✦ C. Disaster is defined as an event of such magnitude that essential services are disrupted and current resources are overwhelmed.
   1. Disasters may be natural (caused by an earthquake, hurricane, tornado, blizzard, flood, etc.).
   2. Disasters may be caused by human actions such as civil disturbance, a hazardous material incident, or act of terrorism.
   3. Disasters have several characteristics in common.
      a. They are unexpected with little or no warning.
      b. Lives, public health, and the environment are endangered.
      c. Emergency services and personnel must be called to action.

D. Public policy in relation to mass casualties.
   ✦ 1. Hospitals are the last link in community response to a mass casualty incident and will receive most seriously injured and ill casualties.
   2. Hospitals must follow federal legislation known as EMTALA (for the Emergency Medical Treatment and Labor Act).
      a. By federal law, a hospital is not allowed to turn away patients. .
      b. EMTALA ensures that all individuals must be screened, evaluated, and stabilized before being transferred.
   3. The Public Health Security and Bioterrorism Response Act of 2002 authorizes 4.3 billion dollars to combat terrorism through detection, treatment, and containment.

E. Disaster impact on the infrastructure will affect transportation, electrical systems, telephone, water, and fuel supplies.

F. JCAHO has focused on security management and has a developed plan.
   1. Provides for designation of personnel to report and investigate security incidents.
   2. Provides identification for participants.
   3. Controls access and egress to sensitive areas.
   4. Provides an education program and performance standards for a mass casualty event.

WEAPONS OF MASS DESTRUCTION

✦ A. Biological agents.
   1. Biological terrorism is the use of specific agents to cause harm or kill people, and includes the use of organisms such as bacteria, viruses and toxins.
   2. Agents possess unique characteristics.
      a. Easily disseminated or transmitted person-to-person and can be dispersed over a wide geographical area.
      b. Cause high mortality with the potential for major public health impact.
      c. Require specific actions in order that public health preparedness is secured.

✦ B. Chemical agents.
   1. Chemical terrorism is the deployment of chemical weapons with the intention of causing death.
   2. Chemical weapons can be pulmonary agents (phosgene, chlorine), cyanide agents (hydrogen cyanide), vesicant agents (mustard, oxime), nerve agents (tabun, sarin, VX), or incapacitating agents (agent 15, BZ).
      a. The most dangerous of these agents are nerve gases (sarin, tabun, VX), extremely toxic and easy to disseminate in the air.
      b. Nerve agents are designed to kill people by binding up a compound known as acetylcholinesterase, which is the body's "off" switch.

✦ C. Radiation.
   1. Radioactive substances emit radiation in the form of rays (waves) or extremely small particles.
      a. *Waveforms* are x-ray and gamma rays. *Particle forms* are alpha, beta, and neutron.
      b. Ionizing radiation is radiation that has enough energy to cause atoms to lose electrons and become ions.
      c. Charged particles are emitted from ionizing radiation, the most likely to be dispersed following a terrorist attack.
   2. A cell that has been exposed to any type of radiation is damaged and may die.
   3. A critical point of discrimination is whether a victim is exposed to, or contaminated by, radiation.
      a. If exposed, the victim is *not* a hazard to others. Radiation is absorbed by or passes through the body, but does not result in radioactive contamination.
      b. Radioactive contamination as radioactive particulate material is a major cause for concern. The source of contamination, resulting from spillage, leakage, deliberate dispersal, or attached to dust particles in the air, can be passed on to health care workers.

✦ 4. Measuring radiation.
   a. RAD (radiation absorbed dose) is a unit of measure for radiation exposure; 1 rad results in absorption of 100 ergs of energy/gram of tissue exposed.
   b. The international system now measures the unit of exposure by Gray (Gy). 1 Gy equals 100 rads.
   c. Radiation dose is a specific calculated measurement of the amount of energy deposited in the body.
   d. The unit of dose is called REM, which takes into account the type of radiation.
   e. A survey instrument measures radiation levels.
      (1) The readout is in units of R (either rad or rem), which is exposure or dose.
      (2) An instrument reading of 50R/hr tells the healthcare worker that if he stays in the exposed area for 1 hour, he will receive a 50 rad exposure.
      (3) A radiation detection device (film badge) should be worn by personnel who come in contact with the exposed area or victims.
✦ 5. Health effects of radiation.
   a. A victim contaminated by radiation is at risk. How much risk is dependent on how much radiation is absorbed.
   b. Victims who absorb less that 0.75 Gy will not experience symptoms of exposure.
   c. Those who absorb 8 Gy could die. Between 0.75 and 8 Gy, the victim could develop acute radiation syndrome (ARS).
   d. Background radiation is derived from natural sources such as radiation from outer space, industrial, academic, military or radiation used in medicine.
   e. All these sources combine to give us a background radiation dose of 0.360 rem per person per year.

BIOLOGICAL AGENTS AND ANTIDOTES

Assessment

A. Identify epidemiologic features.
   1. Rapidly increasing incidence of specific signs and symptoms.
   2. Unusual number of patients seeking care, especially with flu-like symptoms, fever, respiratory complaints.
   3. An endemic disease that rapidly emerges.
   4. Clusters of patients from one area.
   5. Large numbers of fatalities.

B. Identify mode of dissemination and incubation period.
C. Assess the appropriate therapy/antidotes necessary to treat victims of a bioterrorist attack.
D. Assess need for collecting a clinical specimen to identify a specific bioterrorism agent.

✦ Anthrax

Definition: An acute infectious disease caused by *Bacillus anthracis,* a spore forming gram-positive bacillus. Human anthrax occurs in three forms: cutaneous, gastrointestinal or inhalation, the form most dangerous.

Characteristics

A. Clinical features.
   1. Inhalation or pulmonary form.
      a. Early signs and symptoms: developing within days, nonspecific flu-like illness with malaise, dry cough, mild fever, and headache.
      b. Delayed signs and symptoms: severe respiratory distress, hemodynamic collapse—victim may die, even with antibiotic treatment.
   2. Cutaneous form.
      a. Early signs and symptoms: local skin involvement with intense itching; painless, papular lesions (commonly seen on head, forearms or hands).
      b. Delayed signs and symptoms: papular lesion turned vesicular, developing into black eschar with edema.
   3. Gastrointestinal form (from contaminated meat).
      a. Early signs and symptoms: abdominal pain, nausea and vomiting, severe diarrhea.
      b. Delayed signs and symptoms: gastrointestinal bleeding and fever; usually fatal after progression to toxemia and sepsis.
B. Mode of dissemination and incubation period.
   1. Inhalation of spores: aerosol—no person-to-person transmission. Incubation: 2 to 60 days (usually 48 hours).
   2. Cutaneous: direct contact with skin lesions.
   3. Gastrointestinal ingestion of contaminated food: no person-to-person transmission; incubation: 1 to 7 days.

Implementation

A. Manage decontamination.
   1. Remove contaminated clothing.
   2. Instruct patients to shower thoroughly with soap and water.
   3. Instruct personnel to use Standard Precautions.

4. Decontaminate environment with 0.5% bleach (1 part to 9 parts water), or EPA approved germicidal agent.
B. Institute isolation precautions.
1. Inhalation—Standard Precautions, wash victim thoroughly (use 0.5% diluted bleach for visible contamination); store clothing in sealed plastic bag with biohazard label.
2. Cutaneous—contact precautions (gown and gloves).
3. Gastrointestinal—Standard Precautions.
C. Assign patient placement.
1. Private room placement *not* necessary.
2. Airborne transmission does *not* occur.
3. Skin lesions may be transmitted by direct skin contact only.
D. Implement therapy for anthrax infection.
1. Ciprofloxacin 400 mg IV q8–12 hrs; 500 mg PO q12 hrs;
   Doxycycline 200 mg IV (1 dose); 100 mg IV q8–12 hrs; or
   100 mg PO q12 hrs, or
   Amoxicillin may also be ordered.
2. Continue treatment for 60 days.

✦ Plague

Definition: Acute, severe bacterial infection, caused by gram-negative bacillus. Seen in bubonic or pneumonic form; caused by *bacillus yersinia pestis*. A bioterrorism outbreak could be airborne, causing pneumonic plague.

Characteristics
A. Clinical features.
1. Bubonic form.
   a. Swollen, tender lymph nodes (femoral or inguinal commonly most involved).
   b. High temp (39.5 to 41° C), chills.
   c. Pulse rapid, hypotension.
   d. Extreme exhaustion.
2. Pneumonic form.
   a. High fever, chills, tachycardia, headache.
   b. Cough with foamy hemoptysis.
   c. Tachypnea and dyspnea.
B. Know mode of dissemination and incubation period.
1. Transmitted from rodents to humans by infected fleas; incubation 2–8 days.
2. Human-to-human transmission occurs by inhaling droplets through cough.
3. Bioterrorism-related through dispersion of aerosol. Incubation: 1–3 days.

Implementation
A. Manage decontamination—procedure should be done in a room designed for this purpose or at a special site outside the hospital.
1. Instruct patients to remove clothing and store in closed plastic biohazard bags.

2. Instruct patients to shower thoroughly with soap and water—include all crevices.
3. Home decontamination: employ Standard Precautions (gloves, gown, face shield, when necessary).
4. Use 0.5% diluted bleach or EPA-approved germicidal agent.
B. Institute isolation precautions.
1. Bubonic form—routine aseptic (Standard) Precautions.
2. Pneumonic form—add droplet precautions to Standard Precautions (eye protection and surgical mask when within 3 feet of patient) until 72 hours of antimicrobial therapy.
C. Assign patient placement.
1. Bubonic form—private isolation room or cohort with patients with similar symptoms.
2. Maintain at least 3 feet between patients when cohorting is not possible.
3. Do not place patient with immunosuppressed patient.
D. Implement therapy.
1. Doxycycline 100 mg 2 x daily.
2. Ciprofloxacin 500 mg 2 x daily.

✦ Botulism

Definition: A muscle-paralyzing disease caused by an anaerobic gram-positive bacillus that produces a potent neurotoxin. Foodborne botulism is the most common form; inhalational botulism is most likely to occur through a bioterrorist release of aerosol.

Characteristics
A. Recognize clinical features.
1. Foodborne botulism.
   a. Gastrointestinal symptoms: nausea, vomiting, diarrhea.
   b. Leads to symptoms of inhalational botulism.
2. Inhalational botulism.
   a. No fever—patient is responsive.
   b. Symetric cranial nerve paralysis: drooping eyelids, blurred vision, diplopia, difficulty swallowing, dry mouth.
   c. Symptoms progress to paralysis of arms, respiratory muscles, and legs.
   d. Symptoms may be confused with Guillain-Barré syndrome.
B. Know mode of dissemination and incubation period.
1. Food borne botulism: generally transmitted through toxin-contaminated food; incubation is 12–36 hours after ingestion.
2. Inhalational botulism: transmitted through aerosolization of the toxin. Incubation is 24–72 hours post-exposure.

Implementation

A. Manage decontamination.
　　1. Patient does not require decontamination.
　　2. Contaminated clothing washed with commercial soap.
B. Institute isolation precautions.
　　1. No evidence of person-to-person transmission.
　　2. Standard Precautions for patients.
C. Assign patient placement: patient room selection and care according to facility policy. Patient-to-patient transmission does not occur.
D. Implement therapy.
　　1. Early recognition of botulism important for administration of antitoxin that may stop or reduce paralysis.
　　2. Administer trivalent botulinum antitoxin (per CDC orders); requires skin testing due to 95% hypersensitivity reactions.
　　3. Monitor patient for respiratory failure and provide supportive care.

Typhoidal Tularemia

Definition: A disease caused by *firaneisella tularensis* bacterium. Extremely infectious and can be transmitted via aerosol or contaminated water or food.

Characteristics

A. Clinical features.
　　1. Early symptoms: headache, cough, fever, and chills, malaise.
　　2. Delayed symptoms: pharyngeal ulcers, pleuritic chest pain, pneumonia, pericarditis—may progress to respiratory failure.
B. Mode of dissemination and incubation period.
　　1. Bioterrorism mode is aerosol.
　　2. This disease may not be recognized unless a bioterrorism attack is suspected.
　　3. Incubation period: 2–12 days (average 3–5 days) after exposure.

Implementation

A. Manage decontamination: general decontamination measures for clothing of infected person—shower with soap or use 0.5% bleach. Because there is no transmission person-to-person, no other measures are necessary.
B. Institute isolation precautions.
　　1. This disease is not transmitted person-to-person, so isolation measures are not required.
　　2. Standard Precautions recommended.
C. Assign patient placement: cohort patients and do not place with immunosuppressed patients.
D. Implement therapy: Ciprofloxacin 250 mg. PO q12 hrs x 14 days. Streptomycin 15 mg/Kg BID IM x 10–14 days or Gentamycin 1.5 mg/Kg q8 hrs IV x 10–14 days.

Viral Hemorrhagic Fever (VHF)

Definition: An infection caused by agents such as Ebola, Marburg, Larsa, Argentine, Yellow and Dengue fevers. These viruses could be life-threatening (moderately-high lethalitiy) and could be delivered by aerosol in a biological attack.

Characteristics

A. Clinical features.
　　1. Each illness has unique clinical manifestations; however, some features are similar.
　　2. Characterized by abrupt onset of fever, myalgia, headache, prostration.
　　3. Other signs and symptoms are nausea and vomiting, diarrhea, pain in abdomen and chest, cough, and pharyngitis.
　　4. A maculopapular rash, prominent on the trunk, develops in most patients 5 days after onset of illness.
　　5. Bleeding manifestations may occur as the disease progresses. Even though it is rare for this life-threatening condition to occur, bleeding (intracranial hemorrhage), could result; hence, the term, hemorrhagic fever.
B. Mode of dissemination and incubation period.
　　1. Viruses are zoonotic (animal-borne), but can be spread person-to-person.
　　2. All viruses (except Dengue fever) could be spread by aerosol in a biological attack.
　　3. Incubation period: usually 5–10 days, with a range of 2–21 days.

Implementation

A. Manage decontamination: the virus is transmitted person-to-person; decontamination with overt attack: victim undresses, showers with soap or 0.5% diluted bleach.
B. Institute isolation procedures.
　　1. Communicable person-to-person; risk is highest after infection has progressed. Isolation precautions (including airborne and contact), including respirators, face shields, gowns, gloves, shoe and head covers.
　　2. Negative-pressure ventilated rooms with an anteroom.
C. Assign patient placement.
　　1. Patients should be under strict isolation precautions, including a negative-pressure room with anteroom.
　　2. Only patients with the same form of hemorrhagic infection should be cohorted.
D. Implement therapy.
　　1. Primarily supportive.
　　2. Ribavirin, 30 mg/Kg IV x 1 dose; 15 mg/Kg IV q6 hrs x 4 days.

Q Fever

Definition: A rickettsial organism (*coxiella gurnetti*), naturally found in sheep, cattle, and goats. Bioterrorism mode of dissemination will be aerosol or food supply sabotage.

Characteristics
A. Clinical features.
    1. Early signs and symptoms: headache, fever, chills, malaise, diaphoresis, anorexia; insidious onset with nonspecific flu-like symptoms.
    2. Delayed signs and symptoms: double vision, sore throat, cough, chest pain, nuchal rigidity, encephalitis, hallucinations, weight loss.
    3. Differential diagnosis: atypical pneumonias.
B. Mode of dissemination and incubation period.
    1. Aerosol or food supply.
    2. Incubation period: 10–40 days (average 10–14 days).

Implementation
A. Manage decontamination.
    1. Have victim undress and shower thoroughly with soap. May use 0.5% diluted bleach.
    2. Clean environment with 0.5% diluted bleach.
B. Institute isolation precautions: none required. Rarely transmitted person-to-person. Use Standard Precautions.
C. Assign patient placement: transmissibility rare, so patients can be cohorted.
D. Implement therapy.
    1. Tetracycline 500 mg PO q6 hrs x 5–7 days; Doxycycline 100 mg PO q12 hrs x 5–7 days.
    2. Continue treatment for 2 days post-febrile condition.

✦ Ricin Toxin

Definition: Produced from the castor bean plant and secreted in castor seeds; *Ricinus communis* is a cytotoxin that blocks protein synthesis, killing the cell.

Characteristics
A. Clinical features.
    1. Signs and symptoms depend on route of exposure. Diagnosis is difficult. ELISA test of blood will identify Ricin.
        a. Ingestion: nausea, vomiting, diarrhea, and severe abdominal cramps occur before vascular collapse (GI bleeding) leading to death on 3rd day.
        b. Aerosol—inhalation: cough, fever, hypothermia and hypotension (usually nonspecific symptoms); cardiovascular collapse leads to death in 36 to 48 hours.
    2. This biotoxin has been used by assassins to cause death; in 2003 ricin was found in a ter-

---

THE DANGER OF BIOLOGICALLY TOXIC AGENTS
- Biological incidents will be the most difficult of all attacks for the community to recognize and actively coordinate a response.
- Most viruses are useful as bioterror agents—they cause unique signs and symptoms that require intervention and isolation of the victims to prevent spread.
- Specific incapacitating viral or bacterial agents slowly produce signs and symptoms.
    a. Signs and symptoms are nonspecific and difficult to recognize; onset of incident may remain unknown for days before symptoms appear.
    b. It may be necessary to identify "clusters" of illness—many victims become sick within a short period of time in one location.
- If agents are detected early most can be treated with antibiotics or antivirals.
- The most common form of agents that could be used in a bioterror attack are bacteria.

rorist cell in England—potential use unknown.
B. Mode of dissemination and incubation period.
    1. Ricin can be delivered via the castor bean through a chemical process (ingested) or through inhalation method.
    2. Incubation period is within hours to days (ingestion: 3 days; inhalation 3–4 days).

Implementation
A. Manage decontamination.
    1. Ingested biotoxin does not require decontamination.
    2. Aerosol exposure—victim should shower with soap or use 0.5% diluted bleach.
B. Institute isolation precautions. This toxin is not transmitted to others, but Standard Precautions should be implemented.
C. Assign patient placement. There is no communicability person to person or transport through the skin, so placement is planned to protect patient's immune system.
D. Implement therapy. There is no approved antitoxin treatment or prophylaxis (vaccination) at this time.
    1. Therapy is supportive; give oxygen and hydration.
    2. If there is ingestion, GI decontamination would be implemented.

SMALLPOX—AGENT OF TERROR

✦ Smallpox Disease

Definition: An acute viral disease caused by the *variola virus*. It was eradicated in 1977, and in the early

1980s routine vaccinations were discontinued. Because there is a large nonimmune populaton, authorities fear it could be a bioterrorism weapon, transmitted via the airborne route as aerosol.

Characteristics

A. Recognize clinical features.
1. Initially, symptoms resemble an acute viral illness like influenza with fever, myalgia, headache, and backache.
2. Rash appears, progressing from macules to papules (in 1 week) to vesicles, and scabs over in 1–2 weeks.
3. Distinguishing rash from varicella (chicken pox): smallpox has a synchronous onset on face and extremities, rather than arising in 'bunches," starting on the trunk.
B. Mode of dissemination and incubation period.
1. Smallpox is transmitted by large and small respiratory droplets; thus, both respiratory and oral secretions spread the disease, as well as lesion drainage.
2. Patients are considered more infectious if they are coughing or have a hemorrhagic form of the disease.
3. Vaccination effective if given within 4 days.
4. Incubation: 7–17 days; average is 12 days.

Assessment

A. Determine patients who could be in a high-risk group for smallpox vaccination.
B. Assess need for smallpox vaccination.
C. Observe post-vaccination reactions and compare with adverse reactions.
D. Assess patient's understanding of post-vaccination evaluation.

Implementation

A. Manage decontamination.
1. Decontamination of patients is not indicated with smallpox.
2. Careful management using contact precautions of potentially contaminated equipment and environmental surfaces—clean, disinfect, and sterilize when possible.
3. Dedicated or disposable equipment for each patient should be used.
B. Institute strict isolation precautions *immediately*.
1. Airborne and contact precautions in addition to Standard Precautions; includes gloves, gown, eye shields, shoe covers and correctly fitted masks (very important).
2. Airborne precautions: Microrganisms transmitted by airborne droplet nuclei (particles 5 microns or smaller).
   a. Respiratory protection when entering patient's room (particulate respirators, N95); must meet N10SH standards for particulate respirators.
   b. Isolate in room under negative pressure with high-efficiency particle air filtration.
3. Contact precautions: Patients known to be infected or colonized with organisms that can be transmitted by direct contact or indirect contact with contaminated surfaces.
   a. Wash hands using antimicrobial agent when entering and leaving room.
   b. Don gloves when entering room.
   c. Wear gown for all patient contact or contact with patient's environment.
   d. Wear gown when entering room and remove before leaving isolation area.
C. Assign patient placement.
1. Rooms must meet ventilation and engineering requirements for airborne precautions.
   a. Monitored negative air pressure with 6–12 air exchanges/hour.
   b. Appropriate discharge of air to outdoors, or high-efficiency filtration of air.
2. Door to room must remain closed; private room is preferred. Patients with same diagnosis may be cohorted.
3. Limit transport of patients; use appropriate mask if unavoidable.
D. Implement therapy.
1. Post-exposure immunization (*vaccinea virus*) is available.
   a. Vaccination alone if given within 3 days of exposure.
   b. Passive immunization (VIG) if greater than 3 days port-exposure.
   c. VIG given at 0.6 mL/kg IM. Check with CDC for up-to-date recommendations.
2. Prophylactic care with precautions.
E. Identify patients exposed to the smallpox virus.
1. Persons who were exposed to initial release of the virus.
2. Persons who had face-to-face, household or close-proximity contact (< 2 meters = 6.5 feet) with a confirmed or suspected smallpox patient after patient developed fever and until all scabs have separated (no longer infectious).
F. Identify health care workers exposed to the virus—must be evaluated for possible vaccination.
1. Personnel involved in evaluation, care, or transportation of confirmed, probable, or suspected smallpox patients.
2. Laboratory personnel involved in collection or processing of clinical specimens.
3. Other persons with increased likelihood of contact with infectious materials from a smallpox patient (laundry or medical waste handlers).

4. Other persons or staff who have a reasonable probability of contact with smallpox patient or infectious materials (e.g., selected law enforcement, emergency response, or military personnel).

5. Because of potential for greater spread of smallpox in a hospital setting due to aerosolization of the virus from a severely ill patient, all individuals in the hospital may be vaccinated.

✦ G. Determine contraindications for vaccination of noncontacts.
1. Certain medical conditions have a higher risk of developing severe complications following vaccination.
2. Diseases or conditions which cause immunodeficiency (HIV, AIDS, leukemia, lymphoma, generalized malignancy, agammaglobulinemia).
4. Serious, life-threatening allergies to the antibiotics.
5. Persons who have ever been diagnosed with eczema or other acute or chronic skin conditions such as atopic dermatitis, burns, impetigo or varicella zoster (shingles).
6. Women who are pregnant.

✦ Administering Smallpox Vaccine

Implementation
A. Prepare the vaccine.
1. Identify patient(s) to be vaccinated according to public health protocol.
2. Reconstitute *vaccina* vaccine.
   a. Bring vaccine vial to room temperature.
   b. Don gloves.
   c. Use prefilled syringe of diluent and inject into vaccine vial.
   d. Allow vial to stand for 3–5 minutes.
   e. Record date and time of reconstitution.
   f. Dispose of equipment in biohazard bag.
3. Gather equipment.
4. Wash hands.
B. Administer the smallpox vaccine.
1. Remove aluminum seal and rubber stopper from vaccine vial and place in sterile container.
2. Choose site of vaccination—one that is easily accessible for vaccination and later evaluation of site. (The outer aspect of the upper right arm over the insertion of the deltoid muscle is the standard vaccination site.)
3. Clean vaccination site only if grossly contaminated. Let dry thoroughly.
4. Dip point of a sterile bifurcated needle into vial of reconstituted vaccine and withdraw needle perpendicular to the floor.
5. Do not redip needle into vaccine vial if needle has touched skin. This contaminates the vial.

6. Hold needle at a 90° angle (perpendicular) to skin and apply 15 up-and-down (perpendicular) strokes rapidly within a 5mm diameter area. This number of strokes will deliver specified dose to patient.
7. Examine for a trace of blood at vaccination site which will indicate successful vaccine delivery.
8. Cover vaccination site with gauze bandage and tape.
9. Dispose of bifurcated needle in a puncture-resistant medical waste sharps container.
10. Instruct patient to keep site dry.
11. Recap vial with sterile rubber stopper and store capped vial at 2 to 8° C.
12. Remove gloves, dispose in appropriate receptacle, and wash hands.
✦ C. Assess post-vaccination reactions.
1. Identify persons who should be revaccinated. If the vaccination did not take, the individual will remain vulnerable to the smallpox virus.
   a. They will have delayed type of skin sensitivity consisting of *erythema only* within 24 to 48 hours.
   b. This represents a response to inert protein in a previously sensitized person and can occur in a highly immunized person or in individuals with little or no immunity; it is indistinguishable from the immediate or immune reaction.
2. Confirm successful vaccination.
   a. Presence of a pustular lesion in previously unvaccinated persons.
   b. Pustular lesion or an area of definite induration or congestion surrounding a central lesion 7 days following revaccination in a previously vaccinated person.
   c. Vaccinees who do not exhibit a "major" reaction at vaccination site on day 7 should be revaccinated.
3. Recognize adverse reactions.
   a. The overall risk of serious complications following vaccination with vaccinia vaccine is low.
   b. Complications occur more frequently in persons receiving their first dose of vaccine, and among young children (< 5 years of age).
   c. The *most frequent* complications of vaccination are inadvertent inoculation, generalized vaccinia, eczema vaccination, progressive vaccinia, and postvaccination encephalitis.
D. Instruct patient in post-vaccination evaluation.
1. Successful vaccination is associated with tenderness, redness, swelling, and a lesion at the vaccination site.

2. May also be associated with fever for a few days, malaise, and enlarged, tender lymph nodes in the axilla of the vaccinated arm.

3. Inoculation site becomes reddened and pruritic 3–4 days after vaccination.

4. A vesicle surrounded by a red areola, enlarges, becomes umbilicated, and then pustular by the 7th to 11th day after vaccination.

5. The pustule begins to dry, redness subsides, and lesion becomes crusted between 2nd and 3rd week.

6. By the end of the 3rd week, scab falls off, leaving a permanent scar that at first is pink in color, but eventually becomes flesh-colored.

E. Identify indications for vaccinia immune globulin (VIG) administration.

1. Identify post-vaccination complications for which VIG may be indicated.
   a. Eczema vaccinatum.
   b. Progressive vaccinia (vaccinia necrosum).
   c. Severe generalized vaccinia if client has a toxic condition or serious underlying illness.
   d. Inadvertent inoculation of eye or eyelid without vaccinial keratitis.

2. Check physician's orders for VIG treatment of complications due to *vaccinia* vaccination.

3. Administer VIG intramuscularly (IM) as early as possible after onset of symptoms.

4. Give VIG in divided doses over a 24 to 36 hour period. Doses may be repeated at 2–3 day intervals until no new lesions appear.

Collecting and Transporting Specimens

Implementation

A. Acquire and follow specific recommendations for diagnostic sampling of the specific agent.

1. Perform all sampling according to Standard Precautions.

2. Check that laboratory has capacity and equipment to handle specific sample.

✦ B. Wear protective gear when entering environment where potential for exposure exists.

C. Collect specimen and place in appropriate container (zip-closure plastic bag, sealed).

1. Remove original gloves handling specimen, and place in biohazard container.

2. Don new pair of gloves.

3. Place specimen bag in second zip-closure bag and seal, or if specimen is large, in trash bag.

D. Remove protective gear and place in biohazard bags.

E. Wash hands.

F. Label specimen with appropriate label outside of bag: date, person collecting specimen, location, and contact person.

G. Collect an acute phase serum sample, as well as a later convalescent serum sample for comparison.

H. Transport specimens.

1. Coordinate with local and state health departments and the FBI.

2. Include a chain of custody form with specimen information from moment of collection, completed each time specimen is transferred to another party.

✦ CHEMICAL AGENT EXPOSURE

Assessment

✦ A. Pulmonary agents (chlorine, chloropicrin or phosgene): when inhaled produce pulmonary edema with little damage to other pulmonary tissues (with resulting hypoxemia) and hypovolemia.

1. Immediate symptoms are irritation of eyes, nose and upper airways—often not distinctive enough to be recognized as chemical agent exposure.

2. Two to 24 hours later, victim develops chest tightness, shortness of breath with exertion (later, at rest).

3. Cough produces clear, frothy sputum, fluid that leaked into lungs.

4. If symptoms begin soon after exposure, death may occur within hours.

✦ B. Cyanide agents (gases or solids, such as hydrogen cyanide or cyanogens chloride): with high concentrations death occurs in 6 to 8 minutes.

1. Initial symptoms are burning irritation of eyes, nose and airways, and smell of bitter almonds.

2. Victim's skin may be acyanotic, cherry-red (oxygenated venous blood) or normal.

3. Large amount of gas inhaled: hyperventilation, convulsions, cessation of breathing (3 to 5 minutes) and no heartbeat (6 to 10 minutes).

✦ C. Vesicant agents: cause vesicles or blisters; common agents are sulfur mustard and lewisite. More lethal than pulmonary agents and cyanide.

1. Mustard—initial symptoms not observable; effects begin hours after exposure: erythema, burning and itching with blisters; burning of eyes; airway pain, sore throat, nonproductive cough.

2. Lewisite—oily liquid that results in topical damage; vapor causes immediate pain, burning and irritation of eyes, skin and upper airways.

3. Cellular damage occurs that can result in hypovolemic shock.

✦ D. Nerve agents (Sarin, tabon, Soman, GF and VX): liquids or vapors that are the most toxic of all chemical agents.

1. Nerve agents block the enzyme acetylcholinesterase, so activity in organs, glands,

---

**TRIAGE IN THE HOT ZONE FOLLOWING A
CHEMICAL AGENT TERRORIST ATTACK**

- First responders will probably not be able to identify the
  exact agent.
- Early intervention is critical for nerve agents and cyanide.
- Pulmonary agent exposure will be treated later.
- Intervention in the hot zone generally has to do with airway, breathing and circulation (ABCs); add antidotes for
  nerve agents.

---

muscles, smooth muscles and central nervous system cannot turn off; body systems
wear out.

2. Effects of nerve agent depends on route
   (vapor or droplet) of exposure and amount; it
   is felt within seconds.
   a. Felt first on face: eyes, nose, mouth and
      lower airways—watery eyes, runny nose,
      increased salivation and constriction of
      airways, shortness of breath.
   b. The most common signs of nerve vapor
      exposure is constricted pupils (miosis)
      with reddened, watery eyes.
   c. Large concentration of vapor: loss of con-
      sciousness, convulsions, no breathing.

✦ **Implementation**
   A. Pulmonary agents: patient with pulmonary
      edema must be on immediate bedrest with no ex-
      ertion and receive oxygen.
   B. Cyanide agents: administer antidotes.
      1. Patient inhales amyl nitrite, or is given
         sodium nitrite IV (10 mL; 300 mg); frees
         bound cyanide from hemoglobin to allow O_2
         transport.
      2. Sulflur thiosulfate IV (50 mL; 12.5 gm); sul-
         fur converts cyanide to form a nontoxic sub-
         stance.
      3. Give antidotes sequentially and slowly,
         titrated to monitor effects; ventilate with oxy-
         gen, and correct acidosis.
   C. Vesicant agents.
      1. Mustard: immediate decontamination (within
         1 minute) will minimize damage; longer will
         be too late. Irrigate affected skin areas and
         eyes frequently and apply antibiotics to skin 3
         to 4 times/day.
      2. Lewisite: similar to mustard; Immediate de-
         contamination is important. An antidote for
         systemic lewisite is British-Anti-Lewisite
         (BAL), a drug given IV for heavy metal poi-
         soning.
   D. Nerve agents.
      1. Personal protection equipment is necessary
         when decontaminating victims.

Decontamination must take place first, before
management begins.

2. Antidotes.
   a. *Atropine* 2 to 6 mg (average dose 2 to 4
      mg) IM. 2 mg more may be administered
      in 5 to 10 minutes if no improvement. A
      high initial dose is necessary to block ex-
      cess neurotransmitter, especially if vic-
      tim is unconscious.
   b. *Protopam,* an oxime, 600 mg given slowly
      IV to counteract nerve agent by removing
      agent from the enzyme.
   c. *Valium* might be used for prolonged con-
      vulsions.

3. The military has a device (Mark I Auto-
   Injection Kit) that holds 2 spring-powered injectors containing two antidotes, Atropine
   and Protopam, that can be used effectively
   and quickly to administer antidotes.

ACUTE RADIATION SYNDROME

Characteristics
✦ A. An acute illness characterized by manifestations
     of cellular deficiencies caused by the body's reac-
     tion to ionizing radiation (radiation that has the
     energy to cause atoms to lose electrons and be-
     come ions).
   1. Prodromal period: loss of appetite, nausea,
      vomiting, fatigue and   diarrhea.
   2. Latent period: symptoms disappear for a pe-
      riod of time.
   3. Overt illness follows the latent period—infec-
      tion, electrolyte imbalance, diarrhea, bleeding.
   4. The final phase is a period of recovery or
      death.
  B. The higher the radiation dose, the greater the sever-
     ity of early effects and possibility of late effects.

Assessment
✦ A. Attempt to identify dose exposure of patient.
     (Treatment is according to dose exposure. A RAD,
     radiation absorbed dose, is the unit of measure for
     radiation exposure; dose is now measured in
     terms of Gray or Gy—1Gy=100 RAD.)
   1. Dose less than 2 Gy (200 rads) is usually not
      severe; nausea and vomiting seldom experi-
      enced at 0.75 to 1 Gy (75–100 rads) of pene-
      trating gamma rays.
      a. Hospitalization unnecessary at less than
         2 Gy, thus outpatient care indicated.
      b. Closely monitor and administer frequent
         CBC with differential blood tests.
   2. Dose greater than 2 Gy (200 rads). Signs and
      symptoms become increasingly severe with
      increased dose.

✦ ACUTE RADIATION SYNDROMES

- Hematopoietic syndrome
  a. Characterized by deficiencies of RBC, lymphocytes and platelets, with immunodeficiency.
  b. Increased infectious complications, including bleeding, anemia, and impaired wound healing.
- Gastrointestinal syndrome
  a. Characterized by loss of cells lining intestine and alterations in intestinal motility.
  b. Fluid and electrolyte loss with vomiting and diarrhea.
  c. Loss of normal intestinal bacteria, sepsis, and damage to the intestinal microcirculation, along with the hematopoietic syndrome.
- Cerebrovascular–central nervous system
  a. Primarily associated with effects on the vasculature and resultant fluid shifts.
  b. Signs and symptoms include vomiting and diarrhea within minutes of exposure, confusion, disorientation, cerebral edema, hypotension, and hyperpyrexia.
  c. Fatal in short time.
- Skin syndrome
  a. Can occur with other syndrome.
  b. Characterized by loss of epidermis (and possibly dermis) with "radiation burns."

B. Identify if radiation dose includes radioactive iodine—uptake of this isotope could destroy thyroid tissue.

Implementation

A. Give supportive care—treat gastric distress with H_2 receptor antagonists (Tagamet, Pepcid, etc.).

B. Prevent and treat infections—monitor viral prophylaxis.

C. Consult with hematologist and radiation experts.

D. Observe for erythema, hair loss, skin injury, mucositis, weight loss and fever.

✦ E. Administer potassium iodide before exposure, if possible, or as soon as available (within 4 hours).
  1. Blocks uptake of specific damaging isotope.
  2. Protects thyroid tissue.

PERSONAL PROTECTION EQUIPMENT

Assessment

A. Identify patients who present risk to healthcare professionals.

B. Assess need for special equipment (biohazard bags, specimen bags, etc.).

C. Determine type of protection equipment required according to biohazard that is identified (biological, chemical or radiological).

D. Assess need for decontaminating victims prior to triage.

E. Assess strategy for decontamination at site of incident.

F. Assess need for mass casualty decontamination.

Implementation

✦ A. Protective equipment for biological exposure.
  1. Respirators—type selected according to hazard identified and its airborne concentration.
    a. High level of protection: Self-contained breathing apparatus (SCBA) with full facepiece. Provides highest level of protection against airborne hazards when used correctly—reduces exposure to hazard by a factor of 10,000.
    b. Minimal level of protection: Half-mask or full facepiece air-purifying respirator with particulate filters like N95 (used for TB) or P100 (used for hantavirus).
  2. Protective clothing includes gloves and shoe covers—necessary for full protection.
    a. Level A Protective Suit used when a suspected biological incident occurs and type, dissemination method, and concentration is unknown.
    b. Level B Protective Suit used when biological aerosol is no longer present.
    c. Full facepiece respirator (P100 or HEPA filters) used if agent was *not* aerosoled or dissemination was by letter or package that could be bagged.

✦ B. Protective equipment for chemical exposure.
  1. Cover all skin surfaces with protective clothing impervious to chemicals—necessary for protection until exact chemical agent is identified.
    a. Use Mission Oriented Protective Posture (MOPP) suit, if available (chemical protection suit).
    b. Use fire department chemical suits as alternative.
  2. Don masks with filtered respirator. (HEPA filter respirator—N100 with full facepiece—and fit-tested N95 meet CDC performance criteria for chemical exposure.)
  3. Wear boots or boot covers to prevent tracking contaminant.
  4. Initiate decontamination procedures with trained personnel.
    a. Decontaminate at site, if possible.
    b. Otherwise, decontaminate outside of facility.
  5. Use chemical detection devices, if available, to validate presence or absence of agent.

✦ C. Protective equipment for a radiological attack.
  1. Don protective clothing: basic gear will stop alpha and some beta particles, not gamma rays.
    a. Scrub suit.

    b. Gown and cap.

    c. Mask.

    d. Eye shield.

    e. Double gloves—one pair under cuff of gown and taped to close all entry; second pair can be removed and/or replaced.

    f. Masking tape, 2" wide.

    g. Shoe cover with all seams taped.

    h. Radiation detection device: able to detect energy emitted from a radiation source. Several detectors available: Geiger counters, dosimeters, etc.

    i. Film badge.

2. If radiation incident is suspected, self-contained breathing apparatus (SCBA) and flash suits are indicated to reduce potential exposure of healthcare providers.

3. If SCBA suits not available:

    a. Use surgical attire or disposable garments (such as those made of Tyvek).

    b. Use eye protection and double gloves.

    c. Use masks with respirators.

✦ 4. Triage patient's medical condition first, regardless of radiation exposure—first priority is delivery of emergency medical services, including transport.

    a. Administer emergency medical treatment to radiation-exposed patients.

    b. Decontaminate patients who have been contaminated on the scene before transport.

5. Complete decontamination of victims.

6. Implement isolation techniques for contaminated victims to confine contamination and protect personnel.

7. Recheck radiation levels at each stage of treatment until reduced to background levels.

8. Dispose of used protective gear appropriately.

DECONTAMINATION

Characteristics

A. Utilize Standard Precautions for all patients admitted to or arriving at the hospital.

B. Follow routing patient placement for normal number of admissions.

1. Isolate suspicious cases.

2. Group similar cases.

C. Utilize alternative placement for large numbers of patients.

1. Co-group patients with similar syndromes in a designated area.

2. Establish designated unit, floor, or area in advance.

3. Place patients based on patterns of airflow and ventilation with respirator problems, smallpox, or plague.

4. Place patients after consultation with engineering staff.

D. Control entry to patient designated areas.

E. Transport bioterrorism patients as little as possible—limit to essential movement.

F. Clean, disinfect, and sterilize equipment according to principles of Standard Precautions.

1. Use procedures facility has in place for routine cleaning and disinfection.

2. Have available approved germicidal cleaning solutions.

3. Contaminated waste should be sorted and disposed of in accordance with biohazard waste regulations.

4. For patients with bioterrorism-related infections, use Standard Precautions for cleaning unless infecting organism indicated special cleaning.

Decontamination Procedures

A. Decontaminate at scene of incident (hot zone) to prevent hospital system from absorbing contaminated victims and protect health care providers and uncontaminated casualties.

✦ B. Familiarize emergency personnel with stages of decontamination.

1. Gross decontamination.

    a. Decontaminate those who require assistance.

    b. Remove and dispose of exposed victim's clothing. (This will remove 70–80 percent of contaminant.)

✦   c. Perform a thorough head-to-toe tepid water rinse. (Cold water can cause hypothermia and hot water can result in vasodilation, speeding distribution of the contaminants.)

✦ 2. Secondary decontamination.

    a. Perform a full-body rinse with clean tepid water. (Water is an effective decontaminant because of rapidity of application.)

    b. Wash rapidly from head to toe with cleaning solution (HTH chlorine is effective) and rinse with water. (HTH chlorine can decontaminate both chemical and biological contaminants.) Note: Undiluted household bleach is 5.0% sodium hypochlorite.

3. Definitive decontamination.

    a. Perform thorough head-to-toe wash and rinse.

    b. Dry victim and don clean clothes.

C. Initial decontamination may be accomplished by the fire department with hoses spraying water at reduced pressure. (This will remove a high percentage of contaminant at an early stage.)

SETTING UP A SITE FOR DECONTAMINATION

- Establish upwind from contamination area.
- Set up site on a downhill slope, if possible, or on flat ground (so that runoff can be captured).
- Have water source available and, if possible, decontamination solution.
- Have decontamination equipment available, if possible.
- Supply personal protection equipment for health care personnel.
- Notify health care facilities nearby to be available, if possible.
- Maintain security and privacy for site.
- Institute post-decontamination monitoring and checks.

✦ D. Decontaminate salvageable patients first. (This allows those in need of medical intervention to be treated.)
  1. Non-symptomatic and ambulatory victims have lowest priority for decontamination. (The goal is to decontaminate victims who have been exposed, yet are salvageable.)
  2. Patients who are dead or unsalvageable have lowest priority for decontamination.
E. Reduce extent of contamination in facility by decontaminating patients prior to receiving in health care facility—to ensure safety of patients and staff.
  1. Establish decontamination site outside facility using a decontamination tent prior to needing it.
  2. Set up procedures for decontamination, depending on infectious agent.

Specific Decontamination Steps

Implementation
✦ A. Following a biological terrorist event.
  1. Identify dermal exposure, if possible.
  2. Remove victim's clothing as soon as possible and place in biohazard bags.
  3. Cleanse exposed areas using soap and tepid water (large amounts) or diluted sodium hypochlorite (0.5%).
  4. Adhere strictly to Standard Precautions for emergency personnel to prevent secondary contamination of personnel.
  5. Send victims home, if possible, to continue decontamination procedure.
    a. Instruct to wash thoroughly with soap and water.
    b. Instruct victims to monitor for signs and symptoms of agent.
✦ B. Following a chemical terrorist event.
  1. Know general principles to guide actions following a chemical agent incident.

    a. Expect a 5:1 ratio of unaffected to affected casualties.
    b. Decontaminate immediately (ASAP).
    c. Disrobing is decontamination, head-to-toe; the more removal, the better.
    d. Large volume water flush is best decontamination method.
    e. Following exposure, first-responders must decontaminate immediately to avoid serious effects.
  2. Practice triage guidelines for Mass Casualty Decontamination. (Chemical exposure can be deadly, so early decontamination is critical.) Prioritize casualties by identifying those:
    a. Closest to point of release.
    b. Reporting exposure to vapor or aerosol.
    c. With liquid deposits on clothing or skin.
    d. With serious medical conditions.
    e. With conventional injuries.
  3. Decontaminate victims as early as possible. (Requirements differ according to type of chemical agent used: sarin dissipates quickly in the air; VX remains lethal for hours.)
    a. Nerve agents may be absorbed on all body surfaces must be removed quickly to be effective.
    b. Vesicant (blister) agents are not always identified due to latent effects.
  4. Treat eyes and mucous membranes with special protocol.
    a. Flush with copious amounts of water.
    b. If available, isotonic bicarbonate (1.26%) or saline (0.9%) may be used as a flushing agent.
  5. Monitor victim for remains of agent or contaminate using chemical agent monitor (CAM) or M-8 paper for chemical agents.
✦ C. Following radiation exposure.
  1. Determine cause of incident to identify radiation exposure or contamination. (Exposure does not necessarily indicate need for decontamination.)
    a. First responders may be told by those requesting assistance that there has been a radiation-exposure event.
    b. First responders may recognize radiation exposure from observation at incident site.
  2. Understand difference between exposure and contamination.
    a. Exposed victim: presents no hazard; requires no special handling; and presents no radiological threat to personnel.
    b. Externally-contaminated victim: may mean individual has come in contact with unconfined radioactive material.
  3. Decontaminate all victims; remove all clothing and complete a full body wash.

4. Institute isolation techniques to confine contamination and protect others.
5. Decontaminate equipment touched by patient.
    a. Gurney used to transfer patient.
    b. Equipment used in patient care, e.g., BP cuff, stethoscope, etc.
    c. Ambulance.
6. Decontaminate care providers who touched or moved patient (protective clothing may be contaminated).
7. Examine surrounding area (walls, floor that patient may have touched).
8. Control victims' entry and exit to/from area. (Radioactive particles adhere to dust, may become airborne, and can contaminate other patients and personnel.)

TRIAGE

Characteristics
✦ A. Triage, a French word (trier) meaning to sort, is a medical process of prioritizing treatment urgency.
   1. The triage system can quickly assess large numbers of people with multiple problems.
   2. Rapid identification determines which patients require immediate treatment and which can safely wait.
✦ B. Categorizing triage.
   1. **Emergent** triage refers to a life-threatening or potentially life-threatening condition that requires immediate treatment.
   2. **Immediate,** or Urgent, triage is not life-threatening or acute, but refers to patients who need treatment as soon as possible (within 2 hours). These patients have stable vital signs and require no immediate intervention.
   3. **Nonemergent,** or Nonurgent, includes patients who have a condition that would not be affected by a delay in treatment.
C. A second way of implementing the strategy of triage:
   1. **Immediate (I)**—the victim has a life-threatening injury (airway, bleeding or shock) that demands immediate attention (the same as Emergent);
   2. **Delayed (D)**—an injury that does not jeopardize the victim's life if definitive treatment is delayed; and finally,
   3. **Dead (DEAD)**—no respiration after 2 attempts to open airway. (CPR is not performed in a disaster environment because it demands extensive resources, including personnel time.)
D. The goal of triage is to do the greatest good for the greatest number.

E. From triage, victims are taken to a designated medical treatment area (Immediate Care, Delayed Care, or Morgue), and from there, transported out of the disaster area (see flow chart on the next page).

Assessment
A. Assess need to establish triage treatment areas.
B. Validate that public health parameters are established.
C. Observe that steps of triage are followed.
D. Assess that victim is not in immediate danger, or conversely, requires immediate intervention.
E. Assess vital signs of victims.
F. Assess the treatment steps necessary to treat life-threatening conditions
   1. Observe for signs of respiratory distress.
   2. Assess need for establishing an airway.
   3. Observe for amount and source of bleeding and need for intervention.
   4. Recognize shock state and need for intervention.
G. Assess victims post-triage and observe for any signs or symptoms that indicate major injury.
H. Identify victims having a severe psychological reaction to bioterrorism event.
I. Assess possibility of post-traumatic stress syndrome developing.

✦ Implementation
A. Assign roles to personnel in treatment areas.
B. Select a site as soon as possible–advance planning is essential.
   1. Select safe area, free of hazards and debris.
   2. Position site upwind of hazard zone.
   3. Determine site is accessible to transportation vehicles (ambulances, trucks, helicopters).
   4. Be sure site is able to expand.
   5. Survey entire scene, including area above you, for threats to your safety before beginning triage or team work.
C. Protect treatment area and delineate area using tarps, covers, etc.
D. Set up signs to identify subdivisions of area.
        I = Immediate care.
        D = Delayed care.
        Dead = Dead for morgue.
   1. Establish I and D areas close together in order to facilitate verbal communication between workers; this also allows them to share medical supplies and transfer victims quickly when status changes.
   2. Position victims in head-to-toe configuration, with 2 to 3 feet between victims, facilitating effective use of space and personnel.
   3. Establish morgue site secure and away (and not visible) from medical treatment areas.

TRIAGE CATEGORIES

Field Triage

Red	=	Emergent (hyperacute–1st priority)
Yellow	=	Immediate (serious–2nd priority)
Green	=	Urgent (injured–3rd priority)
Blue	=	First-Aid
Black	=	Dead or dying

Catastrophic Triage (First Option)

I	=	Immediate (life threatening)
D	=	Delayed (may delay treatment without death)
Dead	=	Dead

Catastrophic Triage (Second Option)

Red Tag	=	Potential to survive
No other victims tagged.		

START Categories

Color Tag			Decontamination Priority
Red Tag	=	Immediate	1. Serious signs/symptoms Known agent contamination
Yellow Tag	=	Delayed	2. Moderate-to-minimal signs/symptoms Known agent or aerosol contamination Close to point of release
Green Tag	=	Minor	3. Minimal signs/symptoms No known exposure to agent
Black Tag	=	Deceased/ Expectant	4. Very serious signs/symptoms Grossly contaminated Unresponsive

E. Establish public health parameters.
  1. Assign personnel to monitor public health concerns where disaster victims are sheltered.
  2. Have available search and rescue safety equipment.
  3. Maintain proper hygiene by washing hands and using gloves.
     a. Wash hands with soap and water if dirty or antibacterial gel between victims.
     b. Wear gloves at all times.
     c. Change gloves between victims if possible. If not, clean them between victims in a bleach and water solution (1 part bleach to 10 parts water).
  4. Wear a mask and goggles.
  5. Avoid direct contact with body fluids.
  6. Maintain sanitation.
     a. Mark and have available specific biohazard waste disposal containers where bacterial sources (gloves, dressings, etc.) are discarded.
     b. Place waste products in plastic bags and bury them in designated area.
     c. Bury human waste.

  7. Purify water for drinking, cooking, medical use, if potable water is not available.
     a. Boil water at rolling boil for 10 minutes.
     b. Use water purification tablets.
     c. Use unscented liquid bleach (16 drops per gallon of water or 1 teaspoon per 5 gallons; mix and let stand for 30 minutes).
F. Steps of trauma assessment applied to triage.
  1. Perform a rapid systematic assessment. (Trauma is a multisystem condition so all systems must be assessed.)
  2. Complete a primary trauma assessment. (To identify victim's primary and critical problem.)
     a. Airway.
     b. Breathing capability.
     c. Shock—circulation and bleeding.
     d. Neurological—level of consciousness, mental status.
     e. Exposure to contaminate.
     f. Disability.
     g. Evacuation necessity.
  3. Complete a secondary assessment (post-triage) that includes a focus assessment.

DISASTER MANAGEMENT— COMMUNICATION

Characteristics

A. Communication systems are likely to be overwhelmed in a disaster.
   1. Establishing backup and redundant communication systems is essential.
   2. Communication coordination is an important component in the infrastructure system.
B. There must be communication amongst the triage team (out-of-hospital) establishing victim care priorities, the hospital or treatment staff (in-hospital), and state and federal agencies.
✦ C. Hospitals must have an ongoing, open channel of communication with emergency response teams, who will have been notified first of a mass casualty incident.
   1. A community-wide network, all using the same channel of communication, is necessary.
      a. A single communication site for obtaining victim and locator information should be established.
      b. A clear and open information system, using both telecommunication and a position-to-position cascade in the event of the primary system being overloaded, is necessary.
   2. Adequate equipment, such as cell phones, walkie-talkies, even runners, must be available if current phone land lines are overwhelmed.

Implementation

A. Understand lines of communication. (When lines of communication are compromised, effective triage and intervention cannot take place.)
   1. Mass casualty incident occurs.
   2. Local public health official notifies FBI—lead agency for crisis plan.
   3. FBI notifies HHS and CDC and FEMA.
   4. State health agency requests CDC to deploy response teams if needed.
B. Understand the network of communication that will be activated in response to a suspected or actual bioterrorism event.
   1. Emergency response team.
      • Local and state public health officials.
      • Infection control personnel in notified facilities.
      • FBI field offices.
      • CDC.
      • Local emergency medical services (EMS).
      • Local police and fire departments.
   2. In turn, the Federal Response Plan will be activated.
C. Activate Federal Response Plan. (When the local area cannot cope with the disaster, federal assistance is available.)
   • Department of Health and Human Services (HHS) is primary agency.
   • Office of Emergency Preparedness is action agency.
   • Emergency Support Function N8 coordinates federal assistance to supplement state and local resources (directed by HHS).
   • Implemented when state requests assistance and FEMA agrees.
D. Establish a viable communication system.

TREATING LIFE-THREATENING CONDITIONS

Implementation

A. Implement Simple Triage and Rapid Treatment (START), the first step for treating multiple casualties in a disaster.
B. Gather all equipment needed for interventions.
✦ C. Begin triage interventions according to protocols.
   1. Check breathing immediately.
      a. Open airway. (If airway is obstructed, victim cannot get oxygen.)
      b. Move fast—time is critical. (Heart function will be affected within minutes, and brain damage is possible after 4 minutes.)
      c. Check if tongue is obstructing airway. (This is the most   common airway obstruction, especially when victim is positioned on back).
   2. Use head-tilt/chin-lift method if victim is not breathing and airway is not obstructed.
      a. Touch victim and shout "CAN YOU HEAR ME?"
      b. If victim does not respond, place one hand on forehead, 2 fingers of other hand under chin, and tilt jaw upward and head back slightly.
      c. Look for chest to rise, listen for air exchange, and feel for abdominal movement.
      d. If no response (victim does not start breathing) repeat procedure. (If AED is available, may apply to victim.)
      e. If victim does not respond after 2nd attempt, move on to next victim. (Goal of disaster intervention is to do the greatest good for the greatest number of victims.)
      f. If the victim begins breathing–maintain airway (hopefully with a volunteer holding airway open) or place soft object under victim's shoulders to elevate them, keeping airway open.
   3. Control bleeding. If bleeding is not controlled within a short period of time, victim will go into shock—loss of 1 liter of blood, out of a total of 5 in the human body, will result in risk of death.

4. Identify type of bleeding.
   a. Arterial bleeding (spurting blood).
   b. Venous bleeding (flowing blood).
   c. Capillary bleeding (oozing blood).
5. Choose appropriate method to control bleeding.
   a. Direct local pressure–place direct pressure over wound (using clean or sterile pad) and press firmly. (95% of bleeding can be controlled by direct pressure with elevation.)
   b. Maintain compression by wrapping wound firmly with pressure bandage.
   c. Elevate wound above level of heart.
   d. Use pressure point to slow blood flow to wound, brachial point for arm, femoral point for leg.
6. Use tourniquet if bleeding cannot be controlled by other methods (consider this a last resort, as tourniquets can pose serious risks to affected limbs.)
   a. Incorrect material or application can cause more damage and bleeding; if too tight, nerves, blood vessels or muscles may be damaged.
   b. If tourniquet is left in place too long, limb may be lost.
   c. If tourniquet is applied, leave in plain sight and affix label to victim's forehead, stating time tourniquet was applied.
   d. Notify physician to remove tourniquet.
7. Recognize and treat shock.
   a. Body will initially compensate for blood loss, so signs of shock may not be observable.
   b. Continually evaluate victim's condition.
8. Observe for signs/symptoms of shock.
   a. Rapid, shallow breathing (> 30/minute).
   b. Cold, pale skin (capillary refill > 2/second).
   c. Failure to respond to simple commands.
9. Administer treatment for shock.
   a. Position victim supine with feet elevated 6–10 inches.
   b. Maintain open airway.
   c. Maintain body temperature (cover ground and victim).
   d. Avoid rough or excessive handling, and do not allow victim to eat or drink.

POST-TRIAGE INTERVENTIONS

Assessment

A. Perform head-to-toe assessment, always in the same order. This will enable you to complete it more quickly and accurately: head, neck, shoulders, chest, arms, abdomen, pelvis, legs, back.

B. Complete assessment before beginning any treatment; to prioritize treatment interventions, a complete assessment must be done.
C. Observe for any sign/symptom that indicates major injury.
   1. Assess how person received injury (mechanism of injury).
   2. Airway obstruction.
   3. Signs of shock.
   4. Labored or difficult breathing.
   5. Excessive bleeding.
   6. Swelling/bruising.
   7. Severe pain.

Implementation

A. Provide immediate treatment. Reclassify victim during treatment, if necessary.
B. Evaluate that victim is not in immediate danger.
   1. If available staff, continue to assess for signs of head, neck, and spinal injury.
      a. Change in level of consciousness (unconscious, confused).
      b. Unable to move body part.
      c. Severe pain in head, neck, back.
      d. Tingling or numbness in extremities.
   2. Continue to assess other signs and symptoms.
      a. Difficulty breathing or seeing.
      b. Heavy bleeding/blood in eyes or nose.
      c. Seizures.
      d. Nausea, vomiting.
C. Immobilize head, neck or spine by keeping spine in straight line, putting cervical collar on neck, or placing victim on board–if equipment is available.
D. Document person's identity and relevant medical information.
E. Care for those who died.
   1. Victims pronounced DOA (dead on arrival) must be tagged.
      a. Add special tag "not to remove personal effects."
      b. Incorporate special instructions for people performing autopsies, preparing bodies for burial or transportation.
   2. Place bodies in cordoned off area for field triage. (Decontamination may have to be completed before transport.)
   3. Notify those performing post-mortem care of victim's diagnosis to protect staff handling post-mortem care.
      a. Autopsies performed carefully using all personal protective equipment and Standard Precautions, including use of masks and eye protection.
      b. Incorporate any special instructions about biological–chemical–radiological agent present.

4. Complete a record for all bodies including identification, name of person declaring death, diagnosis, if known, name of agency removing body, etc.

F. Care for patients with psychological reactions.
   1. Expect major psychological reactions of fear, panic, anger, horror, paranoia, etc., following a bioterrorism event.
   2. Plan prior to such an event for professional and educated volunteers to be on site.
   3. Minimize fear and panic in staff.
      a. Provide educational materials that include risks to healthcare workers, accurate information of bioterrorism facts, plans for protecting workers, and how to use personal protection equipment.
      b. Encourage team participation in disaster drills to experience in handling a disaster will build confidence and allay anxiety.
   4. Cope with psychological reactions of fear and anxiety.
      a. Minimize panic by clearly explaining care given with explanations.
      b. Offer rapid evaluation and treatment and avoid isolation, if possible.
   5. Treat major anxiety reactions in unexposed persons with factual information, reassurance and medication, if indicated. (Anxiety is communicable; prompt intervention will allay group anxiety. "Worried well" persons could overwhelm hospitals if they leave area and go to closest health care facility.)
   6. Prevent post-terrorism trauma.
      a. Gather victims into a group with a skilled therapist soon after event (within 24 hours) to prevent a major post-trauma reaction.
         (1) Early opportunity for catharsis will help prevent suppression of traumatic event emotions.
         (2) Group victims according to age and experience.
      b. Follow initial group meeting with subsequent meeting within one week to discuss feelings about event. (Research has found that group meetings following traumatic event has eliminated 80% post-traumatic stress disorder.)

◆ G. Identifying post-traumatic stress disorder.
   1. Recognize possibility of existing condition.
      a. Traumatic event occurs and is re-experienced as flashbacks, dreams, or memory state.
      b. Abreaction occurs: vivid recall of painful experience with original emotions.
      c. Individual cannot adjust to event.
   2. Assess signs and symptoms of anxiety and depression
      a. Emotional instability, withdrawal and isolation.
      b. Nightmares, difficulty sleeping.
      c. Feelings of detachment or guilt.
   3. Assess aggressive or acting-out behavior; may be explosive or impulsive behavior.
   4. Assist patient to go through recovery process.
      a. Recovery—reassure patient that he is safe following experience of the traumatic event.
      b. Avoidance—patient will avoid thinking about traumatic event; support client.
      c. Reconsideration—patient deals with event by confronting it, talking about it, and working through feelings.
      d. Adjustment—patient rehabilitates and adjusts to environment following event; patient functions well and is able to view future positively.

DISASTER NURSING—BIOTERRORISM QUESTIONS

1. You are assigned to participate in mass casualty decontamination. You understand that triage guidelines dictate that the group who will be decontaminated last are the casualties

    1. Closest to the point of release of the toxin.
    2. Who do not have serious medical conditions.
    3. With liquid deposits on their skin.
    4. With conventional injuries.

2. If a disaster occurs, one example of how the disaster will impact the infrastructure of a city is by the effect it will have on the

    1. People who live in the city.
    2. Houses and land of the city.
    3. Water supply of a city.
    4. First responders.

3. A preparedness plan for a community-wide communication network has the local emergency response system activated. The individual person or agency who is notified *first* would be the

    1. Local health officer commander.
    2. FBI field office.
    3. Health and Human Services.
    4. Centers for Disease Control (CDC).

4. Health care workers' exposure to radiation is measured by an instrument readout in units of RAD (R). 50 R tells the worker that if he stays in the exposed area 1 hour, he will receive a RAD exposure of

    1. 50 RAD.
    2. 5 RAD.
    3. 0.75 RAD.
    4. 100 RAD.

5. When you are assigned to decontaminate patients, the primary decontamination material that is used as a first step in the process of decontamination is

    1. Bleach
    2. Hydrogen peroxide.
    3. Tepid water.
    4. Hot water.

6. Which piece of equipment is *not* necessary when implementing standard precautions?

    1. Soap or waterless antiseptic.
    2. Gloves.

    3. Gown.
    4. Shoe covers.

7. Contraindications for administering the smallpox vaccination would include persons with all of the following conditions *EXCEPT* those

    1. With immunodeficiency, such as HIV, AIDS.
    2. Who have life-threatening allergies to antibiotics.
    3. With flu, cold, or bronchitis.
    4. Who have been diagnosed with eczema.

8. When establishing a triage site following a major disaster, the area that will *not* be included is

    1. Immediate care.
    2. Intermediate care.
    3. Delayed care.
    4. The Morgue or other designated area for the deceased.

9. The precautions healthcare professionals will plan to take for an attack of anthrax are

    1. Strict isolation.
    2. Isolation.
    3. Droplet Precautions.
    4. Standard Precautions.

10. The precaution protocol necessary to implement for the biohazard of Pneumonic Plague is

    1. Standard Precautions plus Droplet.
    2. Strict isolation with Standard Precautions.
    3. Droplet Precautions.
    4. Contact Precautions.

11. Which of the following groups would be considered high-risk for smallpox vaccinations?

    1. Health care workers over 50 years of age.
    2. Laboratory personnel.
    3. Persons with non-active eczema.
    4. Persons with a cold or flu.

12. The best rationale for informing patients about the smallpox vaccination process is to

    1. Avoid a later lawsuit.
    2. Meet government expectations.
    3. Provide safety information.
    4. Make the patient comfortable in signing the permission form.

13. The most toxic of all chemical agents is/are

    1. Cyanide.
    2. Vesicant.
    3. Pulmonary.
    4. Nerve.

14. The rationale for setting up a decontamination unit for radiological exposure prior to victims entering the hospital is

    1. That it is closer to medical care than a unit in the field.
    2. To prevent contamination of patients and health care workers.

    3. That it is preferable to decontamination at the site.
    4. Protection for health care workers is better closer to the hospital.

15. If a mass casualty incident occurs and the first responders do not know what type of personal protection gear is needed, the action the team should take is to

    1. Wait until the type of equipment needed is known.
    2. Decontaminate victims before intervening.
    3. Choose the highest level of equipment available—full Level A protection.
    4. Wear a radiation and biological device before entering the area.

DISASTER NURSING—BIOTERRORISM
Answers with Rationale

1. (2) When triaging casualties, you will first triage serious medical conditions, then those close to the point of release with liquid on their skin or those who report exposure to the agent. You will then treat those with conventional injuries. Last, treat those who do not have a serious medical condition.
NP:P; CN:S; CA:M; CL:C

2. (3) The infrastructure of a city includes transportation, electrical equipment, telephone connections, fuel supplies, and water. People and housing are not part of the infrastructure. Water could be affected by disruption of service, inadequate supply to fight a fire, and increased risk to public health if the supply is not pure.
NP:E; CN:H; CA:M; CL:C

3. (1) Once the local emergency response system is activated, the local health officer commander (who has been pre-chosen) is notified first, and he/she in turn notifies the FBI field office, HHS, and the CDC.
NP:P; CN:S; CA:M; CL:K

4. (1) One hour is equal to an exposure of 50 RADs. Gray is also a unit of exposure; so the worker should know that if he receives less than 0.75 Gray (when 1 Gray equals 100 RADs), his exposure will be in the safe range.
NP:E; CN:S; CA:M; CL:C

5. (3) The primary decontamination material used is tepid water. Water is an effective decontaminant because of the rapidity of application. Water should be tepid because cold water can cause hypothermia and hot water will cause vasodilation, speeding distribution of the contaminants.
NP:P; CN:S; CA:M; CL:A

6. (4) Shoe covers are not considered standard equipment for precautions, but a mask and eye or face shield are included.
NP:P; CN:S; CA:M; CL:A

7. (3) Persons who have a cold, flu, or bronchitis are not excluded from having a smallpox vaccination. Other categories of conditions that are excluded (in addition to the ones mentioned in the question) are cardiac conditions, leukemia, lymphoma, pregnant women or burns.
NP:P; CN:S; CA:M; CL:C

8. (2) Triage sites will be set up in three areas. The area that is not included is Intermediate Care. Following a disaster, the area sites are simple and straight forward—those who need immediate care, delayed care or no cure (dead).
NP:P; CN:S; CA:M; CL:A

9. (4) An attack of anthrax would require Standard Precautions. Isolation is not necessary because anthrax is not transmitted via droplet or person to person.
NP:P; CN:S; CA:M; CL:A

10. (1) Precautions include Standard plus Droplet (eye protection and surgical mask)—until 48–72 hours after antibiotic treatment. Isolation and contact are not necessary because this disease is not spread via this method.
NP:I; CN:S; CA:M; CL:A

11. (3) Persons with eczema, even if it is non-active, as well as other skin diseases, such as dermatitis, shingles, etc., are considered in the high risk group. General personnel are not at risk, even if they have a cold or flu.
NP:E; CN:S; CA:M; CL:C

12. (3) The best rationale for providing information is the safety element, so the patient will know how to recognize side effects, care for the blister, and not contaminate others. Regulations state that patients cannot sue following a vaccination. The government has specific regulations about this being voluntary, not a government expectation. A permission form must be

Coding for Questions/Answers Abbreviations: **Nursing Process: NP,** Data Collection: D, Planning: P, Implementation: I, Evaluation: E, **Client Needs: CN,** Safe, Effective Care Environment: S, Health Promotion and Maintenance: H, Psychosocial Integrity: PS, Physiological Integrity: PH, **Clinical Area: CA,** Medical Nursing: M, Surgical Nursing: S, Maternal/Newborn Nursing: MA, Pediatric Nursing: P, Psychiatric Nursing: PS, **Cognitive Level: CL,** Knowledge: K, Comprehension: C, Application: A, Analysis: AN

signed and adequate information would make the patient more comfortable, but it is not a safety issue.

NP:P; CN:H; CA:M; CL:C

13. (4) The most toxic chemical agents are nerve agents, such as Sarin, tabon, Soman, GF and VX. These agents block acetycholinesterase, which regulates activity in organs, glands, muscles, and the CNS. With no ability to "turn off," the body wears out and death occurs within a short time.

NP:D; CN:H; CA:M; CL:C

14. (2) It is preferable to decontaminate at the site of radiological exposure, but if it cannot be done, the next choice is to decontaminate prior to entering the hospital to prevent contamination of the patients and workers.

NP:P; CN:S; CA:M; CL:A

15. (3) Because it is critical that the response team be fully protected, they must wear the highest level of equipment; this includes SCBA full protection suit, shoe covers, double gloves and biological detection device, if available. Wearing a radiation or biological device alone is not sufficient protection. Waiting or decontaminating victims will not provide enough safety.

NP:P; CN:S; CA:M; CL:A

Medical-Surgical Nursing

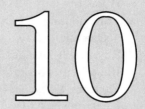

NEUROLOGIC SYSTEM

The nervous system (together with the endocrine system) provides the control functions for the body. It handles thousands of bits of information and stimuli from the sensory organs. This system of nerves and nerve centers coordinates and regulates all of this data and determines the responses of the body.

ANATOMY AND PHYSIOLOGY OF THE NERVOUS SYSTEM

Structure and Function

Neuron

A. Structure.
    1. Cell body (gray matter).
    2. Processes—dendrites (to cell body) and axon (from cell body).
    3. Synapse—chemical transmission of impulses from axon to dendrites.
    4. Nerve fiber—axon and its myelin sheath (white matter).
        a. Myelin sheath insulates; correlates with function and speed of conduction.
        b. Produced by neurolemma cells in peripheral nerve fibers and neuroglia cells in CNS fibers.

B. Classification by function.
    1. Sensory (afferent)—conduct impulses from end organ to CNS.
    2. Motor (efferent)—conduct impulses from CNS to muscles, glands.
    3. Internuncial (connector)—conducts impulses from sensory to motor neurons.
    4. Somatic—innervate body wall.
    5. Visceral—innervate the viscera.

C. Regeneration of destroyed nerve fibers.
    1. Peripheral nerve—can regenerate, possibly due to neurolemma.
    2. CNS—cannot regenerate as it lacks neurolemma.

D. Reflex arc—basic unit of function.
    1. Involuntary stereotyped response to stimulus.
    2. Components—sensory receptor, sensory neuron, internuncial neuron, motor neuron, and effector.
    3. Classification of reflexes—three types: superficial (cutaneous), deep (tendon), pathological.

Central Nervous System—Brain and Spinal Cord

A. Forebrain.
  ✦ 1. Cerebrum—highest level of functioning.
        a. Governs all sensory and motor activity, thought, and learning.
        b. Analyzes, associates, integrates, and stores information.
    ✦ c. Cerebral cortex (outer gray layer) divided into four major lobes.
           (1) Frontal.
               (a) Motor function.
               (b) Motor speech area.
               (c) Prefrontal lobe—controls morals, values, emotions, judgment.
           (2) Parietal.
               (a) Integrates general sensation.
               (b) Interprets pain, touch, temperature, and pressure.
               (c) Governs discrimination.
           (3) Temporal.
               (a) Auditory center.
               (b) Sensory speech center.
           (4) Occipital—visual area.
    2. Basal ganglia.
        a. Part of extrapyramidal tract.
        b. Controls associated motor movements.
    3. Internal capsule—contains projection fibers connecting cortical areas with other parts of the CNS.

B. Brain stem.
    1. Diencephalon.
        a. Thalamus.
            (1) Screens and relays sensory impulses to cortex.
            (2) Lowest level of crude conscious awareness.
     ✦ b. Hypothalamus—regulates autonomic nervous system, stress response, sleep, appetite, body temperature, water balance, emotion.
    2. Midbrain—motor coordination, conjugate eye movements.
    3. Pons.
        a. Contains projection tracts between spinal cord, medulla, and brain.
        b. Controls the involuntary respiratory reflexes.
    4. Medulla oblongata.
        a. Contains all afferent and efferent tracts.
        b. Contains cardiac, respiratory, vomiting, and vasomotor centers.

C. Cerebellum.
    1. Connected by afferent/efferent pathways to all other parts of CNS.
  ✦ 2. Coordinates muscle movement, posture, equilibrium, and muscle tone.

D. Pyramidal tract.
  1. Initiates skilled voluntary movements.
  2. Originates with cell bodies in motor cortex; fibers form projection tracts that pass through internal capsule and medulla where most decussate; fibers from corticospinal tracts, which terminate at anterior horn.
E. Extrapyramidal (outside of pyramidal tract).
  1. Inhibitory or facilitory effect on motor function.
  2. Includes basal ganglia, cerebellum, reticular formation, cortex, and spinal cord.
✦ F. Spinal cord—conveys messages between brain and periphery.
  1. Structure.
    a. Extends from foramen magnum to second lumbar vertebra.
    b. Inner column of H-shaped gray matter which contains the two anterior and two posterior horns.
    c. Posterior horns—contain cell bodies that connect with afferent (sensory) nerve fibers from posterior root ganglia.
    d. Anterior horns—contain cell bodies giving rise to efferent (motor) nerve fibers.
    e. Lateral horns—present in thoracic segments; origin of autonomic fibers of sympathetic nervous system.
  2. Ascending tracts (sensory pathways).
  3. Descending tracts (motor pathways).
✦ G. Protection for CNS.
  1. Skull—rigid chamber with opening at the base (foramen magnum).
  2. Meninges.
    a. Dura mater—tough, outermost, fibrous membrane.
    b. Arachnoid membrane—delicate membrane that contains subarachnoid fluid.
    c. Pia mater—vascular membrane.
  3. Cerebrospinal fluid.
    a. Protective cushion; aids exchange of nutrients, wastes.
    b. Secreted from choroid plexuses in the four ventricles.
    c. Volume is 80–200 mL; average is 130 mL.
    d. Circulates within interconnecting ventricles and subarachnoid space.
  4. Blood–brain barrier.
    a. Prevents damaging substances from entering CSF.
    b. Brain parenchyma.
  5. Blood supply—conductor of oxygen vitally needed by nervous system.
    a. Internal carotids.
    b. Vertebral arteries.
    c. Circle of Willis.

Peripheral Nervous System
A. Carries voluntary and involuntary impulses.
✦ B. Cranial nerves (12 pairs).
  1. *Olfactory*—sensory; nasal cavity
  2. *Optic*—conducts sensory information from the retina.
  3. *Oculomotor*—motor nerve that controls four of the six extraocular muscles. Raises the eyelid and controls the constrictor pupillae and ciliary muscles of the eyeball.
  4. *Trochlear*—a motor nerve that controls the superior oblique eye muscle.
  5. *Trigeminal nerve*—a mixed nerve with three sensory branches and one motor branch. Corneal reflex is supplied by the ophthalmic branch.
  6. *Abducens*—controls the lateral rectus muscle of the eye.
  7. *Facial*—a mixed nerve. The anterior tongue receives sensory supply. Motor supply to glands of nose, palate, lacrimal, submaxillary, and sublingual. The motor branch supplies hyoid levators and muscles of expression and closes eyelid.
  8. *Acoustic*—a sensory nerve with two divisions: hearing and semicircular canals.
  9. *Glossopharyngeal*—a mixed nerve. Motor innervates parotid gland and sensory innervates auditory tube and posterior portion of taste buds.
  10. *Vagus*—a mixed nerve with motor branches to the pharyngeal and laryngeal muscles and to the viscera of the thorax and abdomen. Sensory portion supplies the pinna of the ear, thoracic and abdominal viscera.
  11. *Accessory nerve*—a motor nerve innervating the sternocleidomastoid and trapezius muscles.
  12. *Hypoglossal*—a motor nerve controlling tongue muscles.
✦ C. Dysfunction of cranial nerves.
  1. Eye deviation from midline or unusual movements.
    a. Unilateral pupil dilation: compression of the third cranial nerve (controls pupillary constriction).
    b. Fixed pupils, often unequal: midbrain injury.
    c. Pinpoint, fixed pupils, often unequal: pontine damage.
  2. Reflexes present with dysfunction.
    a. Babinski: dorsiflexion ankle and great toe with fanning of other toes; indicates disruption of pyramidal tract.
    b. Corneal: loss of blink reflex indicates dysfunction of fifth cranial nerve (danger of corneal injuries).

c. Gag: loss of gag reflex indicates dysfunction on the ninth and tenth cranial nerves (danger of aspiration).

✦ D. Spinal nerves (31 pairs).
1. All mixed nerve fibers formed by joining of anterior motor and posterior sensory roots.
2. Anterior root—efferent nerve fibers to glands and voluntary and involuntary muscles.
3. Posterior root—afferent nerve fibers from sensory receptors. Contains posterior ganglion (cell body of sensory neuron).

Autonomic Nervous System

A. Structure and function.
1. Part of peripheral nervous system controlling smooth muscle, cardiac muscle, and glands.
2. The ANS is divided into 2 components: sympathetic and parasympathetic.
3. Two divisions make involuntary adjustments for integrated balance (homeostasis).
B. Sympathetic nervous system—thoracolumbar division.
1. Fight, flight, or freeze; diffuse response.
2. May cause variation in heart rate, blood pressure.
3. Dilates pupils, bronchi.
4. Problem with nerve trunk can cause decreased peristalsis and bowel paralysis.
C. Parasympathetic nervous system—craniosacral division.
1. Repair, repose; discrete response.
2. Decreases heart rate, blood pressure.
3. Constricts pupils, bronchi.

Basic Neurologic Assessment

✦ Signs and Symptoms

A. Numbness, weakness.
B. Dizziness, fainting, loss of consciousness.
C. Headache, pain.
D. Speech disturbances.
E. Visual disturbances.
F. Disturbances in memory, thinking, personality.
G. Nausea, vomiting.

Level of Consciousness

✦ A. Most sensitive, reliable index of cerebral function.
✦ B. Assessment of consciousness.
1. Orientation of patient as to place, purpose, time.
2. Response to verbal and tactile stimuli or simple commands.
3. Response to painful stimuli.
C. Describe behaviors indicating levels of consciousness: clouding, confusion, delirium, stupor, coma.

Pupillary Signs

✦ A. Light reflex—most important sign differentiating structural from metabolic coma.
✦ B. Pupil assessment.
1. Size—measure in millimeters—compare each eye.
2. Equality—equal, unequal, fluctuations.
3. Reactions to light—brisk, slow, fixed.
4. Unusual eye movements or deviations from midline.
C. Pupillary abnormalities—deviation from midline.
1. Unilateral dilation.
2. Mid-position, fixed (often unequal).
3. Pinpoint, fixed.

Motor Function

A. Pattern of motor dysfunction gives information about anatomic location of lesions, independent of level of consciousness.
B. Assessment of face, upper and lower extremities.
1. Muscle tone, strength, equality.
2. Voluntary movement.
3. Involuntary movements.
✦ 4. Reflex response 0–4; absence is 0, hyperreflexia is 4.
   a. Babinski—dorsiflexion ankle and great toe with fanning of other toes.
   b. Corneal—blink reflex.
   c. Gag—gag and vomiting reflex.
C. Patterns of motor function.
1. Appropriate—spontaneous movement to stimulus or command.
2. Absent—hemiplegia, paraplegia, quadriplegia.
3. Inappropriate (nonpurposeful).
   a. Posturing in response to stimuli.
   b. Involuntary: choreiform (jerky, quick); athetoid (twisting, slow); tremors; spasms; or convulsions.
✦ D. Posturing in response to stimuli.
1. Decorticate—nonfunctioning cortex, flexion of upper extremity.
2. Decerebrate—brain stem lesion, total extension.

Sensory Function

A. Assess general sensory function in all extremities: touch, pressure, pain.
B. If no motor response to command, may elicit response by sensory stimuli such as supraorbital pressure.
C. Use minimal amount of stimulus necessary to evoke a response.

Vital Signs

A. Monitor for trends—changes often unreliable and occur late with increasing intracranial pressure.

SIGNS OF MENINGEAL IRRITATION

- Brudzinski's sign—flexion of head causes flexion of both thighs at the hips and flexion of the knees.
- Kernig's sign—in supine position, thigh and knee flexed to right angles; extension of leg causes spasm of hamstring, resistance, and pain.
- Nuchal rigidity.
- Irritability.
- Increased temperature.

B. Blood pressure and pulse—changes may indicate increasing intracranial pressure.
   1. Rise in blood pressure and widening pulse pressure.
   2. Reflex slowing of pulse.
✦ C. Respiration.
   1. Rate, depth, and rhythm more sensitive indication of intracranial pressure than blood pressure and pulse—especially periods of apnea.
   2. Cheyne–Stokes—respiratory increase and decrease in rate and depth, rhythmically alternating with periods of apnea.
   3. Neurogenic hyperventilation—sustained regular, rapid, and deep.
   4. Ataxic—totally irregular, random rhythm and depth.
✦ D. Temperature (rectal or electronic).
   1. Early rise may indicate damage to hypothalamus or brain stem.
   2. Slow rise may indicate infection.
   3. Elevated temperature increases brain's metabolic rate.

DIAGNOSTIC PROCEDURES

Radiologic Procedures

A. Skull series.
   1. Procedure—x-rays of head from different angles.
   2. Purpose—to visualize configuration, density and vascular markings.
   3. Tomograms—layered vertical or horizontal x-ray exposures.
B. Myelography.
   1. Procedure—injection of dye or air into lumbar or cisternal subarachnoid space followed by x-rays of the spinal column.
✦   2. Purpose—to visualize spinal subarachnoid space for distortions caused by lesions.
   3. Potential complications.
     a. Same as for lumbar puncture.
     b. Cerebral meningeal irritation from dye.
   4. Nursing care.
     a. Same as for lumbar puncture.

✦   b. If dye is used, elevate head and observe for meningeal irritation.
     c. If air is used, keep head lower than trunk.
C. Cerebral angiography.
   1. Procedure—injection of radiopaque dye into carotid and/or vertebral arteries followed by serial x-rays.
   2. Purpose—to visualize cerebral vessels and localize lesions such as aneurysms, occlusions, angiomas, tumors, or abscesses.
   3. Potential complications.
     a. Anaphylactic reaction to dye.
     b. Local hemorrhage.
     c. Vasospasm.
     d. Adverse intracranial pressure.
   4. Nursing care.
     a. Prior to procedure.
       (1) Check allergies.
       (2) Take baseline assessment.
       (3) Measure neck circumference.
✦   b. During and after procedure.
       (1) Have emergency equipment available.
       (2) Monitor neurological and vital signs for shock, level of consciousness, hemiparesis, hemiplegia, and aphasia.
       (3) Monitor for swelling of neck, difficulty in swallowing or breathing.
       (4) Apply ice collar.

Magnetic Resonance Imaging (MRI)

A. Procedure—visualization of distribution of hydrogen molecules in the body in three dimensions.
B. Technique has revolutionized diagnostic medicine and is surpassing more conventional methods—yields greater contrast in images of soft-tissue structues than CT scan.
   1. Procedure is noninvasive.
   2. Does not use harmful ionizing radiation.
   3. Superior imaging of body's soft tissue.
✦ C. Purpose—to differentiate types of tissues, including those in normal and abnormal states. Includes brain, both tumors and vascular abnormalities; cardiac and respiratory conditions; blood vessels; liver disease, renal abnormalities, gallbladder, and tumors.
✦ D. Safety measures.
   1. Patients with pacemakers are excluded from MRI.
   2. Metal objects must be removed from patients.
   3. Patients with metal implants (hip prostheses, vascular clips, artificial valves, etc.) are prohibited from MRI imaging.
   4. Closely monitor patients with potential respiratory or cardiac collapse.
E. Nursing implementation.
   1. Maintain safety measures with MRI use.

2. Explain procedure and machine to allay anxiety.
3. Provide patient and family teaching.

Tomography

A. Procedure—intravenous injection of radioactive isotope substance followed by anterior-posterior and lateral scanning. Concentration of substance is greatest in pathological areas.
B. Purpose—to localize tumors with high degree of accuracy. Accuracy is increased if scanning is combined with arteriography or encephalography.
C. Type of brain scan that relies on tissue density—EMI scanner (CT scan).
D. Xenon computed tomography—quantitative cerebral blood flow test.
 1. Measures blood flow to various areas of the brain—defines degree of ischemia in an acute neurologic condition.
 2. Enables clinicians to identify irreversible brain damage.
 3. Test used to:
  a. Select patients for thrombolytic therapy.
  b. Diagnose brain death.
  c. Determine degree of hyperventilation in head trama patients with ICP.
  d. Evaluate interventions to increase cerebral perfusion.
 4. Xenon gas is eliminated from body in 20 minutes.

Positron Emission Tomography (PET)

A. Used to determine regional metabolism of the brain.
B. Noninvasive means of determining biochemical processes that occur in the brain.

Electroencephalography (EEG)

A. Procedure—graphic recording of brain's electrical activity by electrodes placed on the scalp.
✦ B. Purpose—to detect intracranial lesion and abnormal electrical activity (epilepsy); now used to detect and indicate "brain death."
C. Nursing care.
 1. Wash hair.
 2. Withhold sedatives or stimulants.
 3. Administer fluids as ordered.

Electromyography (EMG)

A. Procedure—recording of muscle action potential by surface or needle electrodes.
B. Purpose—to diagnose or localize neuromuscular disease.

Lumbar Puncture (LP)

A. Procedure—insertion of spinal needle through L3–L4 or L4–L5 interspace into lumbar subarachnoid space.
B. Purpose.
 1. To obtain cerebrospinal fluid (CSF).
 2. To measure intracranial pressure.
 3. To instill air, dye, or medications.
✦ C. Potential complications—headache, backache, and herniation with brain stem compression (especially if intracranial pressure is high).
✦ D. Nursing care.
 1. Have patient empty bowel and bladder.
 2. Assist with specimens and pressure measurement.
 3. Maintain strict asepsis.
 4. Monitor vital signs.
 5. Maintain patient in horizontal position.
 6. Encourage fluids if not contraindicated.
 7. Inspect puncture site.
✦ E. Queckenstedt–Stookey test.
 1. Normal pressure is 60–150 mm H_2O when patient is in lateral recumbent position. Pressure increases with jugular compression and drops to normal 10 to 30 seconds after release of compression.
 2. Partial block if slow rise and return to normal.
 3. Complete block if no rise.

CONDITIONS OF THE NEUROLOGIC SYSTEM

The Unconscious Patient

Definition: Unconsciousness is the state of depressed cerebral function with altered sensory and motor function.

Assessment
See Basic Neurologic Assessment, p. 203.

Glasgow Coma Scale

A. Comatose state based on three areas associated with level of consciousness.
B. Scoring system.
 1. Based on a scale of 1 to 15 points.
 2. Any score below 8 indicates coma is present.
C. Eye opening is the most important indicator.

Treatment and Implementation
✦ A. Maintain open airway and adequate ventilation.
 1. Airway obstruction.
 2. Breath sounds.
 3. Positioning.
  a. Semiprone (to prevent tongue from occluding airway and secretions from pooling in pharynx).
  b. Frequent change of position.
 4. Bronchial toilet.
  a. Include deep breathing and coughing when possible.

GLASGOW COMA SCALE ❖ Procedure ❖

- **Motor response**   Points
  - Obeys a simple command   6
  - Localizes painful stimuli   5
  - Withdrawn—moves purposelessly in response
    to pain   4
  - Abnormal flexion—decorticate position   3
  - Extensor response—decerebrate position   2
  - Nil—no motor response to pain   1
- **Verbal response**   Points
  - Oriented to time, place, and person   5
  - Confused conversation; disorientated   4
  - Inappropriate words   3
  - Incomprehensible sounds   2
  - Nonverbal responses/nil (record T if endotracheal
    or tracheostomy tube is in place)   1
- **Eye opening**   Points
  - Spontaneous when person approaches   4
  - In response to speech   3
  - Only in response to pain   2
  - Do not open, even to painful stimuli (record C
    if eyes closed by swelling)   1

    b.   Suctioning of secretions as necessary.

5.   Assisted ventilation.

6.   Have emergency equipment available.

✦ B. Maintain adequate circulation.

    1.   Positioning to encourage circulation.

       a.   Avoid Trendelenburg's position with head or neck injuries.

       b.   Change position frequently, from horizontal to sitting or standing, as soon as possible.

       c.   Passive, active ROM.

    2.   Caution against Valsalva's maneuver (technique of clearing or testing patency of the eustachian tubes).

    3.   Monitor blood pressure (for increased intracranial pressure), pulse, and heart sounds (may be premature ventricular contractions).

✦ C. Maintain optimal positioning and movement.

    1.   Prevent further trauma.

       a.   Maintain body alignment, support head and limbs when turning, logroll.

       b.   Do not flex or twist spine or hyperextend neck if spinal cord injury suspected.

    2.   Positioning.

       a.   Semi-prone or side-lying position.

       b.   Maintain and support joints and limbs in most functional anatomic position.

       c.   Avoid improper use of knee gatch or pillows under knee.

       d.   Use footboard or high-top sneaker to prevent footdrop—remove sneakers daily and inspect feet.

    3.   Avoid complete immobility.

       a.   Perform ROM (against resistance if able), weight bearing; provide tilt table.

       b.   Encourage self-help.

D. Maintain integrity of the skin.

  ✦ 1.   High risk of pressure ulcers.

       a.   Loss of vasomotor tone.

       b.   Impaired peripheral circulation.

       c.   Paralysis, immobility, and loss of muscle assistance to blood flow.

       d.   Hypoproteinemia.

    2.   Loss of sensation of pressure, pain, or temperature—decreased awareness of developing pressure ulcers or burns.

    3.   Skin care.

       a.   Clean and dry skin; avoid powder because it may cake.

       b.   Smooth on lotion around and toward bony prominences if not reddened areas—massage could cause further trauma.

       c.   Turn patient every 2 hours; position with pillows to protect bony prominences.

       d.   Use air fluidized therapy bed or eggcrate mattress.

       e.   Keep linen from wrinkling; avoid mechanical friction against linen.

✦ E. Institute safety precautions.

    1.   Use siderails at all times.

    2.   Remove dentures or bridges and contact lenses.

F. Maintain personal hygiene.

    1.   Eye—loss of corneal reflex may contribute to corneal irritation, keratitis, blindness.

       a.   Observe for signs of irritation.

       b.   Instill artificial tears or apply moistened pads to protect cornea.

  ✦ 2.   Nose—trauma or infection in nose or nasopharynx may cause meningitis.

       a.   Observe for drainage of CSF.

       b.   Clean and lubricate nares; do not clean inside nostrils.

       c.   Change nasogastric tube per policy and PRN.

    3.   Mouth—mouth breathing contributes to drying and crusting excoriation of mucous membranes, which may lead to aspiration and respiratory tract infections.

       a.   Examine the mouth daily with a good light.

       b.   Clean teeth, gums, mucous membranes, tongue, and uvula to prevent crusting and infection; lubricate lips.

       c.   Inspect for retained food in the mouth of patients who have facial paralysis.

  ✦ 4.   Ear—drainage of CSF from the ear indicates damage to the base of the brain and a danger of meningitis.

a. Inspect ear for drainage of CSF. If clear drainage tests positive for glucose (using a Labstix) drainage is CSF.

b. Loosely cover ear with sterile, dry dressing.

G. Promote adequate nutrition, fluid and electrolyte balance.

1. Intravenous fluids.
   a. Electrolyte solutions, hyperalimentation.
   ✦ b. Caution with IV rates if intracranial pressure is elevated.
✦ 2. Tube feedings—high in proteins and calories.
   a. Position patient in semi-Fowler's position, slightly turned to right side.
   b. Check position of tube; aspirate and measure gastric contents; usually if > 100 mL, return and subtract that amount from feeding.
   c. Give feeding by gravity flow; flush tubing with water; prevent air from entering stomach via tubing.
   d. Monitor intake and output, and daily weight.
3. Oral feedings.
   a. Check swallowing with ice chips.
   b. Put patient in semi-Fowler's position.
   c. Have suction equipment available.
   d. Give semiliquid, soft, or blended foods.

H. Promote elimination.
   ✦ 1. Catheter (Foley)—strict asepsis, catheter care.
   2. Cathartic—enema on a regular schedule.
   3. Bowel/bladder retraining if necessary.

I. Provide psychosocial support for patient and family.
   ✦ 1. Assume that an unconscious patient can hear; frequently reassure and explain procedures to the patient.
   2. Encourage family interaction.

J. Observe signs and symptoms for potential complications.

1. Neurological (*See* Basic Neurologic Assessment, p. 203).
2. Respiratory function.
   a. Color, chest expansion, deformities.
   b. Rate, depth, and rhythm of respirations.
   c. Movement of air at nose/mouth or intratracheal tube.
   d. Breath sounds.
   e. Accumulation of secretions or blood in the mouth.
   f. Signs of respiratory distress, failure, hypoxemia, hypercapnia, infection, atelectasis.
3. Cardiovascular function.
   a. Blood pressure, pulses.
   b. Skin color, temperature, edema, leg pain.
   c. Heart sounds, arrhythmias.
   d. Signs of shock, hypertension, orthostatic hypotension.

4. Condition of skin.
   a. Inspect entire body, especially susceptible pressure points (heels, malleoli, trochanteric areas, ischium, sacrum).
   b. Note redness, pallor, edema, excoriation, or skin breakdown.
5. Bladder/bowel function.
   a. Bladder distention—urinary stasis, incontinence.
   b. Urinary tract infection.
   c. Urinary calculi—stasis, infection, alkalinity, decreased volume of urine and citric acid.
   d. Abdominal distention—paralytic ileus, constipation, impaction, diarrhea, trauma.
6. Nutrition, fluid and electrolyte balance.
   a. Intake—NPO while unconscious; tube feedings, IV, observe for dehydration, fluid overload.
   b. Output—urinary, feces; check emesis, nasogastric.
   c. Electrolytes, acid–base.
   d. Thirst, loss of sensation of thirst.
   e. Check for swallowing, gag reflex.
7. Musculoskeletal function.
   a. Muscle strength—weakness, paralysis.
   b. Muscle tone or resistance to passive movement—flaccid, atrophied, spastic.
   c. Limitation of function—deformities, contractures.
   d. Osteoporosis.
8. Process of psychological adaptation—patient/family.
   a. Changes in body image; social and family roles.
   b. Sensory deprivation.
   c. Emotional/physiological stress.
   d. Adaptation to loss—anxiety, fear, denial, depression, dependency.

Increased Intracranial Pressure

Definition: An increase in intracranial bulk due to blood, CSF, or brain tissue, leading to an increase in pressure.

Characteristics
A. Etiology: trauma, hemorrhage, tumors, abscess, hydrocephalus, edema, or inflammation.
B. Pathology.
   1. Cranial cavity is a solid compartment with relatively little room for expansion.
   2. Increased intracranial bulk from blood, CSF, or brain tissue will increase intracranial pressure.
   3. Increased pressure impedes cerebral circulation, absorption of CSF, and function of the nerve cells.

4. Increasing pressure if transmitted downward toward the brain stem can lead to eventual tentorial herniation, brain stem compression, and death.

✦ Assessment

A. *See* Basic Neurologic Assessment, p. 203.

✦ B. Level of consciousness (most sensitive indicator of increasing intracranial pressure) changes from restlessness to confusion to declining level of consciousness and coma.

C. Headache—tension, displacement of brain.

D. Vomiting—may be projectile.

✦ E. Pupillary changes.
1. Unilateral dilation of pupil: slow reaction to light (light reflex is most important sign differentiating structural from metabolic coma).
2. Unilatral fixed dilated pupil is ominous sign requiring immediate action—may indicate herniation of the brain.

F. Motor function—weakness, hemiplegia, positive Babinski, decerebrate, seizure activity.

✦ G. Vital signs—rise in blood pressure; widening pulse pressure; reflex slowing of pulse; abnormalities in respiration, especially periods of apnea; temperature elevation.
1. Cushing reflex—when systolic pressure rises and pulse slows, but is more forceful, ICP is rising but body is coping.
2. When systolic pressure drops (< 50 mm Hg), and pulse becomes irregular, thready, and rapid, body is not coping—danger.

Implementation

✦ A. Elevate head of bed 30 to 40 degrees as ordered; avoid Trendelenburg's.

✦ B. Limit fluid intake (1200 mL/day).

✦ C. Administer medications as ordered: steroids, osmotic diuretics.
1. Steroids (Decadron) decrease cerebral edema by their anti-inflammatory effect.
   a. Decrease capillary permeability in inflammatory processes, thus decreasing leakage of fluid into tissue.
   b. Histamine blocker (Zantac) given with steroids to counter excess gastric acid.
2. Mannitol decreases cerebral edema; provides diuretic action by carrying out large volume of water through nephrons.
3. Hypertonic IV solution administered because it is impermeable to blood–brain barrier; reduces edema by rapid movement of water out of ventricles into bloodstream.

D. Maintain patent airway and administer mechanical ventilation if ordered.

E. Prevent further complications.
1. Monitor neurological dysfunction versus cardiovascular shock.
2. Prevent hypoxia: avoid morphine which masks signs of increased ICP and decreases respirations.
3. Monitor fluids: electrolyte and acid–base balance.

F. Decrease environmental stimuli—dim lights, speak softly, limit visitors, avoid routine procedures if possible.

G. Surgical management (chronic phase).
1. Ventriculoperitoneal shunt systems (most common). Designed to shunt cerebrospinal fluid from the lateral ventricles into the peritoneum.
2. Postoperative care.
   a. Monitor closely for signs and symptoms of increasing intracranial pressure due to shunt failure.
   b. Check for infection (a common and serious complication). If present, removal of the shunt system is indicated in addition to appropriate chemotherapy.
   c. Position patient supine and turn from back to unoperative side.

Spinal Cord Injury

Definition: May include cervical injury leading to quadriplegia or respiratory failure, thoracic injury leading to flaccid/spastic paraplegia, or lumbar injury leading to flaccid paraplegia.

Pathophysiology

✦ A. Neurological signs generally due to edema, concussion, compression, hemorrhage, partial or complete transection of cord, and disruption of sensory and motor pathways.

B. Spinal shock—initial flaccid paralysis, loss of sensation and reflexes, urinary and bowel retention, disturbed nerve supply to blood vessels, and hypotension.

✦ C. Autonomic dysfunction—absence of sweating; decreased blood pressure and temperature in affected areas; poor response to reflex stimuli; paralytic ileus often occurs.

D. After spinal shock recedes—spastic paralysis and hyperreflexia; bowel and bladder control may be retained.

E. Lumbar injury (cauda equina)—persisting flaccid paralysis of lower extremities, bladder, and rectum; muscle atrophy.

Classification of Cord Involvement

✦ A. Functional deficiencies.
1. Quadriplegia (tetraplegia)—all four extremities functionally involved—cervical injuries (C1–C8).

2. Paraplegia—both lower extremities functionally involved—thoracic–lumbar region (T1–L4).

✦ B. Trauma usually related to vertebra fracture—most common cause of cord damage.
   1. Common traumas from auto and motorcycle accidents, sports injuries, falls, stab wounds, and bullets.
   2. Most common cause of abnormal cord movement is acceleration and deceleration.

C. Transection of the cord.
   1. Complete cord transection.
      a. All voluntary motor activity below injury is permanently lost.
      b. All sensation dependent on ascending pathway of segment is lost.
      c. Reflexes may return if blood supply to cord below injury is intact.
   2. Incomplete injuries.
      a. Motor and sensory loss varies and is dependent on degree of incompleteness.
      b. Extent of reflex dysfunction dependent on location of neurological deficit.
   3. Central cord syndrome—leg function returns, arm function does not, as damage has occurred to peripheral cord, which innervates arms.
      a. More common in older adults.
      b. Frequently a result of hyperextension of osteoarthritis spine.
   4. Brown–Séquard's syndrome—one side of cord damaged, resulting in paralysis on one side of body and loss of sensation on the other side.
      a. Transection or lesion of half of spinal cord.
      b. Usually caused by penetrating injuries (gunshot or stabbing).

✦ D. Autonomic hyperreflexia (also called autonomic dysreflexia); most common cause is distended bladder or impacted rectum.
   1. Occurs in patients with lesions above T6, most often those with cervical injuries, after spinal shock has resolved.
   2. Acute emergency—result of exaggerated autonomic responses to stimuli (most often distended bladder or impacted rectum)—treat immediately to prevent stroke.
   3. Symptoms include severe headache, profuse diaphoresis, nausea, bradycardia, and hypertension.
   4. Interventions focused on reducing blood pressure and eliminating stimulus.
      a. Immediately elevate head to decrease blood pressure and monitor vital signs every 15 minutes.
      b. Eliminate stimulus—relieve bladder distention by catheterizing or remove fecal mass.

5. If severe hypertension does not resolve with removal of stimulus, an antihypertensive drug (Apresoline) will be ordered IV.

Implementation

A. Direct efforts toward primary nursing goals: prevent further injury or complications and maintain optimal body functioning while patient is immobilized. (*See* The Unconscious Patient, p. 205.)

B. Maintain open airway and adequate ventilation—high cervical injuries can cause complete paralysis of muscles for breathing; observe for any signs of respiratory failure.

✦ C. Immobilize patient as ordered (stabilize cervical spine), to allow fracture healing and prevent further injury.
   1. Stryker frame permits change of position between prone and supine.
      a. Maintain optimal body alignment.
      b. Place patient in center of frame without flexing or twisting.
      c. Position armboards, footboards, canvas.
      d. Turn; reassure patient while turning.
      e. Free all tubings; secure bolts and straps.
   2. Regular hospital beds used in many rehabilitation centers—Roto beds commonly used.
   3. Halo traction with body cast allows early mobilization.
   4. Soft and hard collars and back braces used about 6 weeks postinjury.
   5. Maintain skeletal traction if part of treatment.
      ✦ a. Cervical tongs for hyperextension (Crutchfield, Gardner–Wells, Vinke).
         (1) Traction is applied to vertebral column by attaching weights to pair of tongs.
         (2) Tongs are inserted into outer layer of parietal area of skull.
      b. Facilitates moving and turning of patient while maintaining spine immobilization.
      c. Observe site of insertion for redness or drainage, alignment, and position.

✦ D. Monitor for potential complications. Neurologic assessment should include watching for changes in muscle tone, motor movement, sensation, bladder/bowel function, presence/absence of sweating, and temperature.

E. Maintain optimal positioning.
   ✦ 1. If turning permitted, logroll with firm support to head, neck, spine, and limbs.
   2. Maintain good body alignment with 10-degree flexion of knees, heels off mattress or canvas, and feet in firm dorsiflexion.
   3. Convalescence—cervical collar, tilt table, wheelchair, braces, parallel bars.

✦ F.   Maintain integrity of the skin.
  ✦ 1.   Turn patient every 2 hours and check skin.
  ✦ 2.   Do not administer IM medication below level of the lesion due to impaired circulation and potential skin breakdown.
    3.   Provide elastic stockings to improve circulation in legs.
✦ G.   Promote adequate nutrition, fluid and electrolyte balance.
    1.   Provide diet high in protein, vitamins, calories, and bulk.
    2.   Avoid all citrus juices, which alkalize the urine and contribute to infection and renal calculi.
    3.   Avoid gas-forming foods and foods with high residue.
    4.   Monitor calcium, electrolyte, and hemoglobin levels.
    5.   Encourage fluids to 3000 mL/day unless patient is on intermittent catheterization when fluids will be restricted.
  H.   Establish optimal bladder function.
    1.   During spinal shock—bladder is atonic with urinary retention; danger of overdistention, stretching.
    2.   Possible reactions:
      a.   Hypotonic—retention with overflow.
      b.   Hypertonic—sudden reflex voiding.
    3.   Check for bladder distention, voiding, incontinence.
    4.   Provide aseptic catheter care.
    5.   Prevent urinary tract infection, calculi.
    6.   Initiate bladder retraining.
      a.   Hypertonic—sensation of full bladder, trigger areas, regulation of fluid intake.
    ✦ b.   Hypotonic—the manual expression of urine (Credé).
  ✦ 7.   Administer medications to treat incontinence.
      a.   Hypertonic—propantheline bromide, diazepam.
      b.   Hypotonic—bethanechol chloride.
  I.   Establish optimal bowel function.
  ✦ 1.   Incontinence and paralytic ileus occur with spinal shock; later, incontinence, constipation, impaction.
  ✦ 2.   For severe distention, administer neostigmine methylsulfate and insert rectal tube, which decompresses intestinal tract.
    3.   Initiate bowel retraining.   ❖ **PROCEDURE** ❖
      a.   Record bowel habits before and after injury.
      b.   Provide well-balanced diet with bulky foods.
      c.   Encourage fluid intake.
      d.   Encourage development of muscle tone, ability to sit in chair.
      e.   Administer suppository as ordered.
      f.   Emphasize importance of a regular, consistent routine.

✦ J.   Major medications used in treatment.
    1.   Corticosteroids—given IV within 8 hours of injury to prevent secondary cord damage from edema and ischemia.
    2.   Vasopressors—used to treat bradycardia and hypotension.
    3.   Antispasmodics—used to treat spasms.
    4.   Analgesics.
  K.   Provide psychological support to patient and family.
    1.   Adjustment to paralysis may be very difficult as patient is usually young; may be inclined toward suicide.
    2.   Provide nonjudgmental atmosphere, security, sensory input.
    3.   Provide diversionary activities, socialization, independence, explanations, support.
    4.   Give encouragement and reassurance but never false hope.
  L.   Encourage optimal physical activity as tolerated by patient.
    1.   Physical therapy exercises.
    2.   Independent activity within limitations.
    3.   Extensive program of rehabilitation and self-care.

Head Injury

Definition: Trauma to the skull by means of compression, tension, and/or shearing force resulting in varying degrees of injury to the brain.

Types of Injury

A.   Brain concussion—violent jarring of brain within skull; temporary loss of consciousness.
B.   Brain contusion—bruising, injury of brain.
C.   Skull fracture—linear, depressed, compound, or comminuted.
✦ D.   Hemorrhage.
    1.   Epidural hematoma—most serious; hematoma between dura and skull from tear in meningeal artery; forms rapidly.
    2.   Subdural hematoma—under dura due to tears in veins crossing subdural space; forms slowly.
    3.   Subarachnoid hematoma—bleeding into subarachnoid space, brain, or ventricles.
    4.   Intracerebral hematoma—usually multiple hemorrhages around contused area, frontal and temporal lobes.

Assessment

A.   Impaired level of consciousness, unconsciousness, confusion.
B.   Headache, nausea, vomiting.
C.   Pupillary changes.
D.   Changes in vital signs, reflecting increased intracranial pressure or shock.

E. Rhinorrhea, otorrhea, nuchal rigidity.

F. Overt scalp/skull trauma.

✦ G. Positive Babinski sign (dorsiflexion of toes when bottom of foot is stroked).

Implementation

A. Direct efforts toward primary nursing goals: recognize, prevent, and treat complications. (*See* The Unconscious Patient, p. 205, for measures to maintain optimal body functioning.)

B. Maintain open airway and adequate ventilation.

✦ C. Awaken the patient as completely as possible to assess level of consciousness.
 1. Complete neurologic assessment every 15 minutes initially, then every hour until stable.
 2. Maintain slight head elevation to reduce venous pressure.

D. Assess and treat convulsions. (*See* Convulsions, p. 215.)

✦ E. Control pain and restlessness.
 1. Avoid morphine, a respiratory depressant, which will increase intracranial pressure.
 2. Use codeine or other milder analgesic (use sparingly).

F. Prevent infection.
 1. High risk of developing meningitis, abscess, osteomyelitis, particularly in the presence of rhinorrhea, otorrhea.
 2. Maintain strict asepsis.

G. Assess and treat other complications.
 1. Shock—significant cause of death.
 2. Cranial nerve paralysis.
 ✦ 3. Rhinorrhea (fracture ethmoid bone) and otorrhea (temporal).
  a. Check discharge—bloody spot surrounded by pale ring; positive test tape reaction for sugar.
  b. Do not attempt to clean nose or ears.
  c. Do not suction nose.
  d. Instruct patient not to blow nose.
 4. Ear—drainage of CSF from the ear indicates damage to the base of the brain and a danger of meningitis.
  a. Inspect ear for drainage of CSF.
  b. Loosely cover ear with sterile, dry dressing.

H. Prevent complications of immobility.
 1. Prevent contractures.
 2. Continue range-of-motion activities.

Encephalitis

Definition: Severe inflammation of the brain caused by arboviruses or enteroviruses. Can be fatal; diagnosed by MRI, PET scan and spinal fluid culture.

Assessment

A. Fever, headache, vomiting.

B. Signs of meningeal irritation.

C. Neuronal damage, drowsiness, coma, paralysis, ataxia.

D. Symptoms resemble meningitis, but have a more gradual onset.

Implementation

A. Monitor vital signs frequently.

B. Monitor neurologic signs for alterations in condition.

✦ C. Administer medications.
 1. Anticonvulsant medications as ordered: phenytoin.
 2. Glucocorticoids as ordered: reduces cerebral edema.
 3. Sedatives as ordered: relieves restlessness.

D. Manage fluid and electrolyte balance to prevent fluid overload and dehydration.

✦ E. Position to maintain patent airway and prevent contractures. Provide passive or active range-of-motion exercises.

F. Promote adequate nutrition through tube feedings, and parenteral hyperalimentation if necessary.

G. Provide hygienic care, i.e., skin care, oral care, and perineal care.

H. Provide safety measures if patient is confused.

Postpolio Syndrome (PPS)

✦ *Definition:* A neurologic condition caused by the poliovirus that invaded the central nervous system decades earlier.

Characteristics

A. Risk of developing PPS.
 1. Risk manifests as people reach age 45 to 60 (35 years from the original polio infection).
 2. Progresses over time, but becomes a major risk if acute health problem develops.
 3. Patients who had nonparalytic or "mild" polio are also at risk for developing PPS.

B. For original polio infection, see Chapter 15, p. 497.

C. Cause of PPS appears to be neuromuscular failure—chronic overuse of polio-damaged nerves and muscles together with normal aging process.

D. If no medical records are available, electromyographic testing will confirm diagnosis of PPS.

Assessment

A. Clinical manifestations of PPS.
 1. Excessive fatigue.
 2. Muscle weakness (in both muscles involved in original infection and those that were not).
 3. Joint pain.
 4. Breathing problems.
 5. Impaired swallowing.
 6. Intolerance to cold.
 7. Inability to carry out activities of daily living.

B. Onset usually insidious, but any sudden change in health status (severe illness or general anesthesia for surgery), onset may be sudden.

Implementation

A. Monitor respiratory function.
   1. Position for maximum chest excursion.
   2. Monitor oxygen.
   3. Muscle-relaxing medications and narcotic analgesics may be life threatening if respirations are depressed.
B. Surgery presents special risks.
   1. General anesthesia not tolerated well—regional anesthesia is a better option.
   2. Patients should not undergo nonessential surgical procedures.
C. Maintain blood volume and fluid and electrolyte balance (especially K+, important to replace after surgery).
D. Cold intolerance may present a special challenge for patient undergoing surgery.

Creutzfeldt–Jakob Disease (CJD)

✦ *Definition:*   Central nervous system disorder caused by proteinaceous infectious particle found in brains of patients. There appear to be varying forms of this disease, now labeled variant CJD or vCJD.

Characteristics

A. Etiology.
   1. May be inherited (10%).
   2. Patients who received human growth hormone prior to more stringent purification methods instituted after 1978.
   3. Corneal transplants or cadaver dural grafts.
   4. Incubation ranges from 4–20 years.
B. Creutzfeldt–Jakob-like disease (also called mad cow disease) recently appeared in Great Britain.
   1. Caused by bovine spongiform encephalopathy from people who eat beef fed with scrapie (infected sheep parts).
   2. Early onset followed by slow progression and a longer course of illness.

Assessment

A. Onset gradual with first symptom usually memory loss.
   1. Assess for memory loss progressing to global dementia.
   2. Death may occur after a few months.
B. History—inquire if patient has been living in Great Britain for more than 6 months.

Implementation

A. Prevention centers around caution in handling body fluids (blood) and other material from pa-

tients with this diagnosis and, for mad cow disease, not eating contaminated beef.
B. The U.S. Blood Bank has implemented guidelines that refuse blood from anyone who has lived in Great Britain for more than 6 months.

Brain Attack/Cerebrovascular Accident (CVA or Stroke)

✦ *Definition:*   Impaired blood supply in the brain caused by a hemorrhage or occlusion that results in a sudden focal neurologic deficit. It is the most common cause of brain disturbance.

Pathophysiology

A. Causes.
   1. Thrombosis.
   2. Embolism.
   3. Hemorrhage.
   4. Compression or spasm.
B. Risk factors.
   1. Circulatory—atherosclerosis, hypertension, anticoagulation therapy, cardiac valvular disease, synthetic valve and organ replacement, atrial arrhythmias.
   2. Diabetes.
   3. Sickle cell disease.
   4. Substance abuse.
   5. Sedentary lifestyle.
   6. High lipids.
C. Cerebral anoxia longer than 10 minutes to a localized area of brain causes cerebral infarction (irreversible changes).
D. Surrounding edema and congestion cause further dysfunction.
E. Lesion in cerebral hemisphere results in manifestations on the opposite side of the body.
F. Permanent disability unknown until edema subsides. Order in which function may return: facial, swallowing, lower limbs, speech, arms.

Transient Ischemic Attack (TIA)

✦ A. A precursor symptom or warning of impending CVA.
   1. Rapid onset and short duration (30 minutes to 24 hours); by definition, must be resolved within this time period.
   2. Following resolution, no permanent neurologic deficit.
   3. Most common symptoms: vision loss, diplopia, contralateral hemiparesis, aphasia, confusion, slurred speech, and vertigo.
✦ B. Carotid endarterectomy is surgical procedure for carotid stenosis—often done following TIA or presence of bruit indicating stenosis.
   1. Procedure removes atherosclerotic plaque from arterial wall.

2. Monitor closely first 24 hours for cerebral ischemia or thrombosis or intolerance from carotid clamping.

Assessment

A. Condition status depends on site and size of involved area.
   1. Appears suddenly with embolism.
   2. More gradually with hemorrhage and thrombosis.
✦ B. Generalized symptoms—headache; hypertension; changes in level of consciousness, convulsions; vomiting, nuchal rigidity, slow bounding pulse, Cheyne–Stokes respirations.
C. Focal—hemiparesis, hemiplegia, central facial paralysis, language disorders, cranial dysfunction, conjugate deviation of eyes toward lesion, flaccid hyporeflexia (later, spastic hyperreflexia).
D. Residual manifestations.
   ✦ 1. Lesion left hemisphere.
      a. Right hemiplegia; aphasia, expressive and/or receptive.
      b. Behavior is slow, cautious, disorganized.
   ✦ 2. Lesion right hemisphere.
      a. Left hemiplegia.
      b. Behavior is impulsive, quick; unaware of deficits; poor judge of abilities, limitations; neglect of paralyzed side.
   3. General.
      a. Memory deficits; reduced memory span; emotional lability.
      b. Visual deficits; loss of half of each visual field.
      c. Apraxia (can move but unable to use body part for specific purpose).

Implementation

A. Strive for initial nursing goal: support life and prevent complications; long-term goal is rehabilitation.
B. Bedrest as ordered.
✦ C. Maintain patent airway and ventilation.
   1. Elevate head of bed 20 to 30 degrees unless patient is in shock.
   2. Give oxygen as needed. Begin at 3 L/min.
   3. Recent studies indicate the sooner oxygen is administered, the faster the recovery.
D. Monitor clinical status to prevent complications.
   1. Neurologic.
      a. Include assessment of recurrent CVA, increased intracranial pressure, bulbar involvement, hyperthermia.
      b. Continued coma is a negative prognostic sign.
   2. Cardiovascular—shock and arrhythmias, hypertension.

3. Apply elastic stockings or pneumatic compression stockings as ordered to reduce risk of deep vein thrombosis.
   4. Lungs—pulmonary emboli.
✦ E. Maintain optimal positioning—prevent contractures.
   1. Siderails up and use safety straps if necessary.
   2. During acute stages, quiet environment and minimal handling may be necessary to prevent further bleeding.
   3. Upper motor lesion—spastic paralysis, flexion deformities, external rotation of hip.
   4. Positioning schedule—2 hours on unaffected side; 20 minutes on affected side; 30 minutes prone, BID–TID.
   5. Complications common with hemiplegia—frozen shoulder, footdrop; use footboard, active or passive range-of-motion exercises.
✦ F. Maintain skin integrity; turn and provide skin care every 2 hours.
G. Maintain personal hygiene—encourage self-help.
H. Promote adequate nutrition, fluid and electrolyte balance.
   1. Encourage self-feeding if swallow and gag reflex present.
   2. Food should be placed in unparalyzed side of mouth.
I. Promote elimination.
   1. Bladder control may be regained within 3–5 days.
   2. Retention catheter may not be part of treatment regimen.
   3. Offer urinal or bedpan every 2 hours day and night.
J. Provide emotional support.
   1. Behavior changes as consciousness is regained—loss of memory, emotional lability, confusion, language disorders.
   2. Reorient, reassure, and establish means of communication.
K. Promote rehabilitation to maximal functioning.
   1. Comprehensive program—begin during acute phase and follow through convalescence.
   ✦ 2. Guidelines to assist patient with *left hemisphere lesion*.
      a. Do not underestimate ability to learn.
      b. Assess ability to understand speech.
      c. Act out, pantomime communication; use patient's terms to communicate; speak in normal tone of voice.
      d. Divide tasks into simple steps; give frequent feedback.
   ✦ 3. Guidelines to assist patient with *right hemisphere lesion*.
      a. Do not overestimate abilities.
      b. Use verbal cues as demonstrations; pantomimes may confuse.

c. Use slow, minimal movements and avoid clutter.

d. Divide tasks into simple steps; elicit return demonstration of skills.

e. Promote awareness of body and environment on affected side.

Cerebral Aneurysm

Definition: A dilation of the walls of a weakened cerebral artery leading to rupture from arteriosclerosis or trauma.

Assessment

✦ A. Diplopia, eye pain, blurred vision, or ptosis.
B. Hemiparesis, nuchal rigidity.
C. Headache, tinnitus, nausea.
D. Irritability, seizure activity.

Implementation

A. Establish and maintain a patent airway.
✦ B. Administer oxygen at 3 L/min unless patient has COPD.
✦ C. Place patient on bedrest in semi-Fowler's or side-lying position.
D. Turn, cough, and deep breathe patient every 2 hours.
E. Suction only with specific order.
F. Provide darkened room without stimulation, i.e., limit visitors and lengthy discussions.
G. Avoid strenuous activity; provide range-of-motion exercises.
H. Provide diet low in stimulants such as caffeine.
I. Restrict fluid intake to prevent increased intracranial pressure.
J. Monitor intake and output.
✦ K. Monitor vital signs for hypertension or cardiac irregularities. *Do not take rectal temperature due to vagal stimulation leading to cardiac arrest.*
L. Observe for complications indicating rebleeding, clot formation, or increased size of aneurysm.

Hyperthermia

Definition: Increased temperature that has reached 41°C (106°F); associated with increased cerebral metabolism, which may increase risk of hypoxia.

Assessment

A. Shivering.
B. Respiratory function—ventilation and patent airway.
C. Cardiac function—pulse and rhythm; arrhythmias.
D. Urinary function—color, specific gravity, and amount.
E. Nausea and vomiting.
F. Seizures with very high temperature.
G. Signs of dehydration.

Treatment and Implementation

A. Methods for inducing hypothermia, the primary focus of treatment for a patient with hyperthermia.
✦ 1. External—cool bath, fans, ice bags, hypothermic blanket (most common).
✦ 2. Drugs.
   a. Chlorpromazine—reduces peripheral vasoconstriction, muscle tone, shivering.
   b. Meperidine—relaxes smooth muscle, reduces shivering.
   c. Promethazine—dilates coronary arteries, reduces laryngeal and bronchial irritation.
3. Effect of treatment protocols used.
   a. Reduces cerebral metabolism and demand for oxygen.
   b. Decreases cerebral and systemic blood flow.
   c. Reduces CSF pressure.
   d. Decreases endocrine, liver, and kidney function.
   e. Decreases pulse, blood pressure, and respiration; may affect cardiac pacemaker.
✦ B. Continually monitor patient who is experiencing induced hypothermia.
1. Temperature.
   a. Continuous probe or rectal thermometer.
   b. Read and record every 15 minutes.
✦ 2. Prevent shivering.
   a. Shivering increases CSF pressure and oxygen consumption.
   b. Treatment: chlorpromazine or meperidine.
✦ 3. Prevent trauma to skin and tissue.
   a. Frostbite—crystallization of tissues with white or blue discoloration, hardening of tissue, burning, numbness.
   b. Fat necrosis—solidification of subcutaneous fat creating hard tissue masses.
   c. Initially give complete bath and oil the skin; during procedure, massage skin frequently with lotion or oil to maintain integrity of the skin.
4. Prevent respiratory complications.
   a. Hypothermia may mask infection and cause respiratory arrest.
   b. Institute measures to maintain open airway and adequate ventilation.
5. Prevent cardiac complications.
   a. Monitor cardiac status; hypothermia can cause arrhythmias and cardiac arrest.
   b. Have emergency equipment available.
6. Monitor renal function.
   a. Insert Foley catheter.
   b. Monitor urinary output, BUN; may monitor specific gravity.
7. Prevent vomiting and possible aspiration; patient may have loss of gag reflex and reduced peristalsis.

8. Monitor changes in neurological function during hypothermia.

Convulsions

Definition: Forceful involuntary contractions of voluntary muscles; may be one component of a seizure.

Etiology
Cerebral trauma, congenital defects, epilepsy, infection, tumor, circulatory defect, anoxia, metabolic abnormalities, excessive hydration.

Classification
◆ A. Tonic convulsion—sustained contraction of muscles.
◆ B. Clonic convulsion—alternating contraction/relaxation of opposing muscle group.
   C. Epileptoid—any convulsion with loss of consciousness.

Assessment
A. Presence of aura.
B. Type of motor activity.
C. Pattern of seizure activity.
D. Length of seizure activity.
E. Loss of bowel or bladder control.
F. Loss of consciousness.
G. Signs of respiratory distress.
H. Characteristics during the postictal state.

Implementation
◆ A. Protecting patient from further injury is primary goal.
   1. Maintain patent airway.
   ◆ 2. Keep padded tongue blade at bedside; use only with physician's orders. Do not force between teeth if they are already clenched.
   ◆ 3. Be sure siderails are padded and there is padding around head.
   4. Avoid use of any restraints.
   5. Remove any objects from environment that may cause injury.
   6. Remain with patient.
   7. If patient is standing, guide to floor and protect head and body from hard floor.
   8. Be prepared to suction patient if in hospital.
B. Observe and record characteristics of seizure activity.
   1. Level of consciousness.
   2. Description of aura, if present.
   3. Description of body position and initial activity.
   4. Monitor activity—initial body part involved, character of movements (tonic/clonic), progression of movement, duration, biting of the tongue.
   5. Respiration, color.
   6. Pupillary changes, eye movements.
   7. Incontinence, vomiting.
   8. Total duration of seizure.
   9. Postictal state—loss of consciousness; sleepiness; impaired speech, motor, or thinking; headache; injuries.
   10. Postconvulsion, neurologic and vital signs.
   11. Frequency and number of convulsions.
C. Care after the seizure.
   1. Maintain open airway—positioning, suction.
   2. Reorient to environment; give reassurance and support.
   3. Monitor clinical status.
   4. Administer anticonvulsants.
   5. Maintain quiet environment.

Epilepsy

Definition: A combination of several disorders characterized by chronic seizure activity; a symptom of brain or CNS irritation. A seizure is an abnormal, sudden, excessive neuronal discharge of electrical activity within the brain.

Characteristics
A. Incidence in United States may be as low as 1 million or as high as 2.5 million.
B. Major problems may be an electrical disturbance (dysrhythmia) in nerve cells in one section of the brain.
C. Seizures are associated with changes in behavior, mentation, and motor or sensory activity.
D. Causes may be genetic, trauma, brain tumor, circulatory or metabolic disorder, toxicity, or infection.
E. Diagnostic tests include CT to determine underlying CNS changes, EEG for a distinctive pattern, MRI, blood studies, lumbar puncture, etc.

Seizures—Four Types
◆ A. Tonic–clonic seizures, traditionally known as "grand mal."
   1. May begin with an aura, then a tonic phase—symmetrical stiffening or rigidity of muscles, particularly arms and legs, usually lasts for 10 to 20 seconds.
   2. Clonic phase follows—hyperventilation with rhythmic jerking of all extremities; usually lasts for 30–40 seconds.
   3. Loss of consciousness occurs; may be incontinent of urine or feces; may bite tongue.
   4. Full recovery may take several hours.
◆ B. Absence seizures, formerly "petit mal."
   1. Brief, often just seconds, loss of consciousness; almost no loss or change in muscle tone.
   2. May occur 100 times/day. More common in children; may appear to be "daydreaming."
◆ C. Myoclonic seizure.
   1. Characterized by a brief, generalized jerking or stiffening of the extremities.

2. May occur singly or in groups; may throw person to the floor.

♦ D. Atonic or akinetic seizures, also called "drop attacks."
   1. Characterized by sudden, momentary loss of muscle tone.
   2. Usually causes person to fall to the ground; injuries from falling are common.

Assessment

♦ A. Assess for partial seizures (focal seizures).
   1. Simple partial seizure.
      a. Localized (confined to a specific area) *motor symptoms,* accompanied by *sensory symptoms.*
      b. Patient remains conscious throughout episode and may report an aura before seizure takes place.
   2. Complex partial (psychomotor) seizure; may progress to generalized tonic–clonic.
      a. Area of brain most involved is temporal lobe (thus, this type of seizure is called *psychomotor*).
      b. Characterized by period of altered behavior and automatism (patient is not aware of behavior); evidenced by such mannerisms as lip smacking, chewing, picking at clothes, etc.
      c. Patient loses consciousness for a few seconds.

B. Idiopathic or unclassified seizures.
   1. This type of seizure accounts for half of all seizure activity.
   2. Occurs for no known reason and fits into no generalized or partial classification.

C. Assess for specific phases of seizure activity.
   1. Occurs without warning or following an *aura* (peculiar sensation that warns of an impending seizure—dizziness, visual or auditory sensation).
   2. Behavior at onset of seizure.

Implementation

A. Protect patient from injury or complication during seizure. (*See* Convulsions, p. 215.)

B. Eliminate precipitating factors of seizure.
   1. Accurate observation and recording of seizures.
   2. Possible factors: drugs, alcohol, sleep, nutrition, loud noises, music, flickering lights, hyperventilation.
   3. Treatment of underlying cause—tumor, infection.

♦ C. Promote physical and mental health.
   1. Establish regular routines for activities of daily living.

a. Diet, sleep, physical activity (activity tends to inhibit seizure activity).
b. Provide appropriate safeguards during exercise and sports.

2. Avoid alcohol, stress, exhaustion.

3. Foster self-esteem and confidence; avoid overprotection of patient.

4. Provide patient and family with facts regarding epilepsy.
   a. Control of the disorder.
   b. Recognition of impending seizure and care during seizure.
   c. Importance of carrying identification card in case of emergency.
   d. Organizations that provide services, such as the National Epilepsy League and the National Association to Control Epilepsy.

♦ D. Administer and monitor effects of medications.
   1. Medication regimen may require periods of adjustment and/or a combination of drugs.
   2. Reinforce necessity for taking medication regularly as prescribed; observe response, any side effects or seizure activity.
      a. Medications given continuously and throughout life of patient.
      b. Usually used in combination—decreased dosage lessens side effects.
   ♦ 3. Phenytoin (Dilantin).
      a. Prevents seizures through depression of the motor areas of the brain.
      b. Side effects include GI symptoms, rash, and bleeding gums.
      c. Check CBC and calcium levels.
      d. Give PO drug with meals; supplement with vitamin D and folic acid.
      e. Caution against alcohol—deactivates medication.
   4. Diazepam (Valium).
      a. For relief of restlessness.
      b. To decrease seizure activity.
   5. Phenobarbital (Luminal).
      a. Reduces responsiveness of normal neurons to impulses arising in the focal site.
      b. Side effects are drowsiness, ataxia, nystagmus, respiratory depression.
      c. Toxic effects produce rash but usually no nausea and vomiting.
   ♦ 6. Carbamazepine (Tegretol).
      a. Inhibits nerve impulses by limiting influx of sodium ions across cell membranes.
      b. Give with meals; monitor for side effects—diplopia, blurred vision, ataxia, vomiting, leukopenia.
   ♦ 7. Clonazepam (Klonopin).
      a. Decreases frequency, duration, and spread of discharge in minor motor

seizures (absence, akinetic, myoclonic seizures).

 b. Side effects: lethargy, ataxia, vertigo thrombocytopenia—monitor CBC.

8. Gabapentin (Neurontin).

 a. Do not take 1 hour before or less than 2 hours after antacids.

 b. Liver function studies regularly, as ordered, to detect early signs of hepatitis or liver problems.

9. Monitor toxic side effects of drugs: drowsiness, skin rash, nervousness, nausea, ataxia, gum hyperplasia, blood dyscrasias.

10. Avoid sudden withdrawal of drugs—may precipitate status epilepticus.

11. Monitor other drugs patient is taking (aspirin, certain antibiotics, Diamonx, folic acid, narcotics, oral contraceptives, etc.) because of interaction with anti-convulsants.

✦ E. *Status epilepticus*—a dangerous complication.

1. Successive major convulsions without regaining consciousness between attacks are considered a medical emergency, which may cause death.

2. Most frequent cause is sudden withdrawal of anticonvulsants; other factors include insulin, electroshock, acute infections, trauma, and metabolic disorders.

3. Management of complications.

 a. Maintain open airway.

 b. Terminate seizure with IV medications: phenobarbital, Dilantin, diazepam, paraldehyde.

 c. Monitor patient's condition frequently for complications: cardiac, respiratory, and neurologic status; arterial blood gases, glucose, calcium, electrolytes, renal and liver function.

F. Surgical treatment used (excision of tissue involved in seizure activity) when attempts to control seizure activity fail.

Multiple Sclerosis (MS)

Definition: Chronic, slowly progressive, noncontagious, degenerative disease of the CNS.

✦ Etiology

A. Definite cause unknown; autoimmunity or virus likely cause.

B. Incidence is greater in colder climate, equal in the sexes, and usually occurs between ages 20 and 40 years.

Pathophysiology

✦ A. Demyelination of nerve fibers within long conducting pathways of spinal cord and brain.

B. Lesions (plaques) are irregularly scattered—disseminated.

C. Destruction of myelin sheath creates patches of sclerotic tissue, degeneration of the nerve fiber, and disturbance in conduction of sensory and motor impulses.

D. Initially, the disease is characterized by periods of remission with exacerbation and variable manifestations but is followed by irreversible dysfunction.

E. Clinical course may extend over 10 to 20 years.

Assessment

A. Highly variable, depending on area of involvement: sensory fibers, motor fibers, brain stem, cerebellum, internal capsule.

B. Weakness, paralysis, incoordination, ataxia, intention tremor, spasticity, numbness, tingling, loss of position sense.

C. Bladder/bowel retention or incontinence.

D. Impaired vision (diplopia, nystagmus).

E. Dysphagia, impaired speech.

F. Emotional instability, impaired judgment.

G. Charcot's triad—nystagmus, intention tremor, and scanning speech.

Implementation

✦ A. Prevent precipitation of exacerbations.

1. Avoid fatigue, stress, infection, overheating, chilling.

2. Establish regular program of exercise and rest.

3. Provide a balanced diet.

✦ B. Administer and assess effects of medications.

1. Steroids hasten remission. Prednisone is used for short-term therapy.

2. Chlordiazepoxide for mood swings.

3. Baclofen or dantrolene for spasticity.

4. Bethanechol or oxybutynin to relieve urinary retention.

5. Antibiotics, vitamin B, essential fatty acids.

6. Tegretol to treat paresthesia.

7. Symmetrel or Cylert to treat fatigue.

8. Inderal or an anticonvulsant to treat ataxia.

✦ C. Promote optimal activity.

1. Moderation in activity with rest periods.

2. Physical and speech therapy.

3. Diversionary activities, hobbies.

4. During exacerbation, patient is usually put on bedrest.

✦ D. Promote safety.

1. Sensory loss—regulate bath water; use caution with heating pads; inspect skin for lesions.

2. Motor loss—avoid waxed floors, throw rugs; provide rails and walker.

3. Diplopia—apply eye patch.

E. Encourage regular elimination—bladder/ bowel training programs.
F. Provide education and emotional support to patient and family.
  1. Encourage independence and realistic goals; assess personality and behavior changes; observe for signs of depression.
  2. Provide instruction and assistive devices; provide information about services of the National Multiple Sclerosis Society.
G. Assess and prevent potential complications.
  1. Most common: urinary tract infection, calculi, pressure ulcers.
  2. Contracture pain due to spasticity, metabolic or nutritional disorders, regurgitation, depression.
  3. Common cause of death: respiratory tract infection, urinary tract infection.

✦ Myasthenia Gravis

Definition: Neuromuscular disease characterized by marked weakness and abnormal fatigue of voluntary muscles.

Etiology
A. Unknown; question autoimmune reaction.
B. Patients with myasthenia have a high incidence of thymus abnormalities and frequently have systemic lupus erythematosus.

Pathophysiology
A. Basic pathology is a defect in transmission of nerve impulse at the myoneural junction, the junction of motor neuron with muscle.
B. Normally, acetylcholine is stored in synaptic vesicle of motor neurons to skeletal muscles.
C. Defect may be due to:
  1. Deficiency in acetylcholine/excess acetylcholinesterase.
  2. Defective motor-end plate and/or nerve terminals.
  3. Decreased sensitivity to acetylcholine.
D. Generally, there is no muscle atrophy or degeneration; there may be periods of exacerbations and remissions.

Assessment
A. Symptoms are related to progressive weakness and fatigue of muscles when used; muscles generally are strongest in the morning.
B. Eyes are affected first: ptosis, diplopia, and eye squint.
C. Impaired speech; dysphagia; drooping facies; difficulty chewing, closing mouth, or smiling; breathing difficulty and hoarse voice.
D. Respiratory paralysis and failure.

E. Diagnosis confirmed with Tensilon test.
  1. Positive for myasthenia—improvement in muscle strength.
  2. Negative—no improvement or even deterioration.

Implementation
A. Primary goals are to improve neuromuscular transmission and prevent complications.
✦ B. Administer and assess effects of medications.
  1. Anticholinesterase drugs increase levels of acetylcholine at myoneural junction.
    a. Neostigmine, pyridostigmine, ambenonium—main difference is duration of effect.
  ✦ b. Edrophonium (Tensilon)—is a rapid, brief-acting anticholinesterase used for testing purposes.
    c. Side effects.
      (1) Related to effects of increased acetylcholine in parasympathetic nervous system: sweating, excessive salivation, nausea, diarrhea, abdominal cramps; possibly bradycardia or hypotension.
      (2) Excessive doses lead to cholinergic crisis—atropine given as cholinergic blocker.
    d. Nursing measures.
      (1) Give medications exactly on time, 30 minutes before meals.
      (2) Give medication with milk and crackers to reduce GI upset.
      (3) Observe therapeutic or any toxic effects; monitor and record muscle strength and vital capacity.
  2. Steroids.
    a. Suppress immune response.
    b. Usually the last resort after anticholinesterase and thymectomy.
  ✦ 3. The following drugs must be avoided.
    a. Streptomycin, kanamycin, neomycin, gentamicin are drugs that block neuromuscular transmission.
    b. Ether, quinidine, morphine, curare, procainamide, Innovar, sedatives—aggravate weakness of myasthenia.
C. Monitor patient's condition for complications.
  1. Vital signs.
  2. Respirations—depth, rate, vital capacity, ability to deep breathe and cough.
  3. Swallowing—ability to eat and handle secretions.
  3. Muscle strength.
  4. Speech—provide method of communication if patient unable to talk.
  5. Bowel and bladder function.
  7. Psychological status.

D. Encourage optimal activity.
1. Plan short periods of activity and long periods of rest.
2. Time activity to coincide with maximal muscle strength.
3. Encourage normal activities of daily living.
4. Encourage diversionary activities.
E. Provide instruction and emotional support.
1. Instruct patient about medications and treatment regimen and importance of adhering to medication schedule.
2. Instruct patient to avoid infection, stress, fatigue, and over-the-counter drugs.
3. Instruct patient to wear identification medal and carry emergency card.
4. Provide information about services of Myasthenia Gravis Foundation.

✦ **Myasthenic or Cholinergic Crisis**
✦ A. Myasthenic crisis.
1. Acute exacerbation of disease may be due to rapid, unrecognized progression of disease; failure of medication; infection; or fatigue or stress.
2. Myasthenic symptoms—weakness, dyspnea, dysphagia, restlessness, difficulty speaking.
✦ B. Cholinergic crisis.
1. Cholinergic paralysis with sustained depolarization of motor-end plates is due to overmedication with anticholinesterase.
2. Symptoms similar to myasthenic state; restlessness, weakness, speaking difficulty, dysphagia, dyspnea.
3. Cholinergic symptoms—fasciculations, abdominal cramps, diarrhea, nausea, vomiting, salivation, sweating, increased bronchial secretion.

✦ **Tensilon Test**
A. Test used to differentiate crises, as symptoms are similar.
✦ 1. Tensilon is given and if strength improves, it is symptomatic of myasthenic crisis and the patient needs more medication; more severe weakness is symptomatic of cholinergic crisis and overdose has occurred.
✦ 2. Be prepared for emergency with atropine, suction, and other emergency equipment for respiratory arrest.
B. Crisis with respiratory insufficiency; patient cannot swallow secretions and may aspirate.
1. Bedrest maintained.
2. Endotracheal or tracheostomy tube to assist with ventilation may be required.
3. Atropine given and anticholinesterase (cholinergic) may be held.
4. Anticholinesterase (myasthenic) begun.

Parkinson's Disease

Definition: Degenerative disease of the brain resulting in dysfunction of the extrapyramidal system.

Etiology
A. Idiopathic.
B. Other possible causes: atherosclerosis, drug induction, postencephalitis.

Pathophysiology
A. Degeneration of basal ganglia due to depleted concentration of dopamine.
B. Depletion of dopamine correlated with degeneration of substantia nigra (midbrain structures that are closely related functionally to basal ganglia).
C. Loss in inhibitory modulation of dopamine to counterbalance cholinergic system and interruption of balance-coordinating extrapyramidal system.
D. Slowly progressive disease with high incidence of crippling disability; mental deterioration occurs very late.

Assessment
A. Appears in five stages: unilateral, bilateral, impaired balance, fully developed severe disease, and confinement to bed or wheelchair.
✦ B. Symptoms.
1. Tremor at rest—especially in hands and fingers (pill-rolling).
   a. Increases when stressed or fatigued.
   b. May decrease with purposeful activity or sleep.
2. Rigidity—blank facial expression (masklike).
   a. Drooling, difficulty with swallowing or speaking.
   b. Short, shuffling steps with stooped posture.
   c. Propulsive gait.
   d. Immobility of muscles in flexed position, creating jerky cogwheel motions.
   e. Loss of coordinated and associated automatic movement and balance.
3. Akinesia—difficulty initiating voluntary movement.
4. Autonomic dysfunction—lacrimation, incontinence, decreased sexual function, constipation.

Implementation
A. Strive for primary goals: reduce muscle tremor and rigidity and prevent complications.
✦ B. Administer and assess effects of medications.
1. Amantadine (Symmetrel): used to treat patients with mild symptoms but no disability; side effect uncommon with usual dose.
2. Anticholinergic drugs: most effective is ethopropazine (Parsidol); used to treat tremors and rigidity, and inhibit action of acetylcholine; side effects include dry mouth, dry

skin, blurring vision, urinary retention, and tachycardia.

✦ 3. Levodopa (Larodopa, Dopar); converted in body to dopamine.
   a. Reduces akinesia, tremor, and rigidity.
   b. Passes through blood–brain barrier.
   c. Effectiveness may decline after 2 to 3 years.
   d. Side effects.
      (1) Anorexia, nausea, and vomiting (administer drug with meals or snack; avoid coffee, which seems to increase nausea).
      (2) Postural hypotension, dizziness, tachycardia, and arrhythmias (monitor vital signs; caution patient to sit up or stand up slowly; have patient wear support stockings).
   e. Contraindicated in patients with closed-angle glaucoma, psychotic illness, and peptic ulcer disease.
✦ 4. Sinemet—combination of carbidopa and levodopa; has fewer side effects than levodopa.
   5. Antihistamines: reduce tremor and anxiety; side effect is drowsiness.
   6. Antispasmodics (Artane, Kemadrin): improve rigidity but not tremor.
   7. Bromocriptine (Parlodel); drug often used to replace levodopa when it loses effectiveness.
      a. Acts on dopamine receptors.
      b. Side effects: anorexia, nausea, vomiting, constipation, postural hypotension, cardiac arrhythmias, headache.
      c. Contraindicated in patients with mental illness, myocardial infarction, peptic ulcers, peripheral vascular disease.
✦ 8. Avoid the following drugs:
      a. Phenothiazines, reserpine, pyridoxine (vitamin B_6)—block desired action of levodopa.
      b. Monamine oxidase inhibitors—precipitate hypertensive crisis.
      c. Methyldopa—potentiates parkinsonian effects.
C. Provide appropriate nursing care following surgery.
   1. Stereotactic surgery (pallidotomy or thalamotomy) to reduce tremor.
   2. Implantation of electrodes through burr holes into target area of brain; creation of lesion with high frequency of coagulation probe.
      a. Performed under local anesthesia.
      b. Effective in relieving symptoms—interrupts nerve pathways to alleviate tremors or rigidity.
D. Maintain regular patterns of elimination.
   1. Constipation is often a problem due to side effects of medications, reduced physical activity, and muscle weakness.

   2. Provide stool softeners, suppositories, mild cathartics.
✦ E. Promote physical therapy and rehabilitation.
   1. Provide preventive, corrective, and postural exercises.
   2. Institute massage and stretching exercises, stressing extension of limbs.
   3. Encourage daily ambulation; have patient lift feet up when walking and avoid prolonged sitting.
   4. Facilitate adaptation for activities of daily living and self-care; encourage rhythmic patterns to attain timing; foster independence; utilize special aids and devices.
   5. Remove hazards that might cause falls.
F. Provide education and emotional support to patient and family.
   1. Remember, intellect is usually not impaired.
   2. Assess changes in self-consciousness, body image, sexuality, moods.
   3. Instruct patient to avoid emotional stress and fatigue, which aggravate symptoms.
   4. Instruct patient to avoid foods high in vitamin B_6 and monamine oxidase.

Meningitis

Definition: Acute infection of the pia-arachnoid membrane. Caused by infection of meningococcus, staphylococcus, streptococcus, pneumococcus, *Haemophilus influenzae,* tuberculous, or a virus.

✦ **Assessment**
A. Inflammation, infection, ICP cause cardinal signs and symptoms.
B. Meningeal irritation.
   ✦ 1. *Kernig's sign* (supine position, thigh and knee flexed to right angles. Extension of leg causes spasm of hamstring, resistance, and pain).
   ✦ 2. *Brudzinski's sign* (flexion of head causes flexion of both hips and knee flexion).
   3. *Nuchal rigidity*—painful, stiff neck.
C. Symptoms are progressive.
   1. Headache, high fever, and changes in mental status are first indications.
   2. Nausea, vomiting, disorientation, muscle aches, and Kernig's sign follow.
D. Severe headache, photophobia.
E. As illness progresses, lethargy, irritability, stupor, coma.
F. Diagnosis made by testing CSF obtained from lumbar puncture.

✦ **Implementation**
A. Maintain open airway—oxygen as needed.
B. Treat the infective organism—antimicrobic therapy, intravenously for 2 weeks.

C. Droplet isolation for 24 hours after antibiotic therapy initiated.
D. Assess and treat increased intracranial pressure or seizures (Mannitol may be given for cerebral edema).
E. Control body temperature.
F. Provide adequate fluid and electrolyte balance.
G. Maintain bedrest and a quiet environment.

CRANIAL NERVE DISORDERS

Trigeminal Neuralgia (Tic Douloureux)

✦ *Definition:*   Sensory disorder of the fifth cranial nerve, resulting in severe, recurrent paroxysms of sharp facial pain along the distribution of the trigeminal nerve. Etiology and pathology are unknown; incidence is higher in older women.

Assessment
A. Trigger points on the lips, gums, nose, or cheek.
B. May be stimulated by a cold breeze, washing, chewing, food/fluids of extreme temperatures.
C. Pain—limited to areas innervated by branches from fifth nerve.

Treatment and Implementation
A. Observe characteristics of attack and ways patient protects face from stimulus.
B. Avoid extremes of heat or cold; give small feedings of semiliquid or soft food.
✦ C. Medical treatment.
   1. Massive doses of B_{12}.
   2. Inhalation: 10–15 drops of trichloroethylene on cotton.
   3. Anticonvulsants: Dilantin and Tegretol.
   4. Alcohol injections to produce anesthesia of the nerve for pain relief.
   5. Glycerol injection to the nerve.
D. Surgical treatment.
   1. Peripheral—avulsion of supraorbital, infraorbital or mandibular division.
   2. Intracranial.
     a. Division of the sensory nerve root for permanent anesthesia.
     b. Patient may experience numbness, stiffness, or burning after surgery.
     c. Microsurgery allows for selective sectioning of the fifth nerve.
     d. Pain and temperature fibers are destroyed, and sensation of touch and corneal reflex are preserved.
E. Assess and treat complications after surgery.
   1. Facial paralysis.
   2. Irritation or ulceration of cornea due to loss of sensation.
   3. Local trauma to inside of mouth.

Bell's Palsy (Facial Paralysis)

Definition: Lower motor neuron lesion of the seventh cranial nerve, resulting in paralysis of one side of the face. Diagnosis made by exclusion—no definitive test.

Assessment
A. Flaccid muscles.
B. Shallow nasolabial fold.
C. Inability to raise eyebrows, frown, smile, close eyelids, or puff out cheeks.
D. Upward movement of eye when attempting to close eyelid.
E. Loss of taste in anterior tongue.

Implementation
✦ A. Palliative (most patients recover in a few weeks without residual effects); moist heat, massage.
B. Analgesics, steroids, physiotherapy, support of facial muscles, protection of cornea.
C. Promote active facial exercises to prevent loss of muscle tone.
D. Instruct patient to chew food on unaffected side.
E. Present attractive, easy-to-eat foods to prevent anorexia and weight loss.
F. Provide special eye care to prevent keratitis; dark glasses, artificial tears.
G. Reassure and support.

Ménière's Disease

Definition: Dilatation of the endolymphatic system causing degeneration of the vestibular and cochlear hair cells.

Etiology
A. Etiology is unknown.
B. Possible causes may include allergies, toxicity, localized ischemia, hemorrhage, viral infection, and edema.

Treatment and Implementation
A. Direct care toward alleviating obstruction and reducing the pressure.
B. Surgical procedures.
   1. Surgical division of vestibular portion of the nerve or destruction of the labyrinth may be necessary for severe cases.
   2. Endolymphatic shunt.
   3. Vestibular section.
   4. Labyrinthotomy and labyrinthectomy.
C. Maintain bedrest during acute attack.
   1. Prevent injury during attack.
   2. Provide siderails if necessary.
   3. Keep room dark when photophobia present.
D. Provide drug therapy.
   1. Vasodilators (nicotinic acid).
   2. Diuretics, antihistamines (Benadryl).
   3. Sedatives.

E. Monitor diet therapy.
   1. Low sodium.
   2. Lipoflavonoid vitamin supplement.
   3. Restricted fluid intake.
F. Assist with ambulation if necessary.

Guillain–Barré Syndrome

✦ *Definition:*   An acute rapidly progressive and potentially fatal form of polyneuritis. Immune system overreacts to an infection, destroying the myelin sheath.

Characteristics
A. Etiology is unknown.
B. Occurs at any age but increased incidence between 30 and 50 years of age.
C. Both sexes equally affected.
D. Recovery is a slow process, taking 2 months to 2 years.
E. Diagnostic test results: CSF contains high protein, abnormal EEG.

Assessment
A. First report may be of a mild upper respiratory infection or gastroenteritis.
B. Initial symptom of weakness of lower extremities with ascending paralysis/paresthesia.
✦ C. Gradual progressive weakness of upper extremities and facial muscles (24 to 72 hours); paresthesias may precede weakness.
D. Respiratory failure may occur.
E. Sensory changes—usually minor, but in some cases severe impairment of sensory information occurs.
F. Cardiac arrhythmias.

Implementation
✦ A. No specific treatment available; supportive treatment includes monitoring for complications (respiratory, circulatory).
B. Carefully observe for respiratory paralysis and inability to handle secretions.
C. Provide chest physiotherapy and pulmonary toilet.
D. Maintain cardiovascular function.
   1. Monitor vital signs and cardiac rhythm.
   2. Vasopressors and volume replacement.
E. Prevent complications of immobility.
   1. Turn frequently.
   2. Provide skin care.
F. Provide appropriate diversion.
G. Reassure patient, especially during paralysis period.
H. Previous treatment included corticosteroids; this is now considered controversial.

Amyotrophic Lateral Sclerosis (Lou Gehrig's Disease)

✦ *Definition:*   The most common motor neuron disease of muscular atrophy. It is a rapidly fatal, upper and lower motor neuron deficit affecting the limbs.

Characteristics
A. May result from several causes.
   1. Nutritional deficiency related to disturbance in enzyme metabolism.
   2. Vitamin E deficiency resulting in damage to cell membranes.
   3. Metabolic interference in nucleic acid production by nerve fibers.
   4. Autoimmune disorders.
B. Inherited in 10 percent of the cases.
C. Occurs after age 40; most common in men.
D. Is fatal within 3 to 10 years after onset. Riluzole slows progression of disease.
E. Diagnostic tests: EMG and muscle biopsy; increased protein in CSF.

Assessment
A. Atrophy and weakness of upper extremities.
B. Difficulty swallowing and chewing.
C. Respiratory excursion and breathing patterns.
D. Impaired speech.
E. Secondary depression.

Implementation
A. Assist with rehabilitation program to promote independence.
✦ B. Monitor for complications.
   1. Prevent skin breakdown: reposition regularly, provide back care, and utilize pressure-relieving devices.
   2. Prevent aspiration of food or fluids: offer soft foods and keep patient in upright position during meals.
   3. Promote bowel and bladder function.
C. Provide emotional support.

INTRACRANIAL SURGERY

Preoperative and Postoperative Care

Preoperative Care
A. Observe and record neurological symptoms.
   1. Paralysis.
   2. Seizure foci.
   3. Pupillary response.
✦ B. Prepare patient physically and psychologically for surgery.
   1. Prep and shave cranial hair (save hair).
   2. Apply scrub solution to scalp, as ordered.

3. Avoid using enemas unless specifically ordered; the strain of defecation can lead to increased intracranial pressure.

4. Explain postoperative routine orders such as neurologic checks and headaches.

5. Administer steroids or mercurial diuretics, as ordered, to decrease cerebral edema.

6. Insert NG tube and/or Foley catheter as ordered.

General Postoperative Care

A. Observe neurologic signs.
- ✦ 1. Evaluate level of consciousness.
    - a. Orientation to time and place.
    - b. Response to painful stimuli.
    - c. Ability to follow verbal command.
- ✦ 2. Evaluate pupil size and reactions to light.
    - a. Are pupils equal, not constricted or dilated?
    - b. Do pupils react to light?
    - c. Do pupils react sluggishly or are they fixed?
  3. Evaluate strength and motion of extremities.
    - a. Are handgrips present and equal?
    - b. Are handgrips strong or weak?
    - c. Can patient move all extremities on command?
    - d. Are movements purposeful or involuntary?
    - e. Do the extremities have twitching, flaccid, or spastic movements (indicative of a neurological problem)?
- ✦ 4. Observe vital signs (TPR and BP).
    - a. Keep patient normothermic to decrease metabolic needs of the brain.
    - b. Observe respirations for depth and rate to prevent respiratory acidosis from anoxia.
    - c. Observe blood pressure and pulse for signs of shock or increased intracranial pressure.
- ✦ 5. Evaluate reflexes.
    - a. *Babinski*—positive Babinski is elicited by stroking the lateral aspect of the sole of the foot, backward flexion of the great toe, or spreading of other toes (Figure 10-1).
    - ✦ b. *Romberg*—when patient stands with feet close together, he or she falls off balance. This sway is positive; may have cerebellar, proprioceptive, or vestibular difficulties.
    - ✦ c. *Kernig*—patient is lying down with thigh flexed at a right angle; extension of the leg upward results in spasm of hamstring muscle, pain, and resistance to additional extension of leg at the knee (indicative of meningitis).
  6. Watch for headache, double vision, nausea, or vomiting.

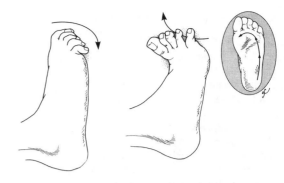

Negative Babinski   Positive Babinski

Fig.10-1

B. Provide for special needs.
- ✦ 1. Maintain patent airway—oxygen deprivation and an increase of carbon dioxide may produce cerebral hypoxia and cause cerebral edema.
    - a. Intubate if values indicate to be necessary (as ordered).
    - b. PO_2 below 80 mmHg or PCO_2 above 50 mmHg.
  2. Suction as necessary, but not through nose without specific order.
- ✦ 3. Maintain adequate oxygenation and humidification.
  4. Place patient in semi-prone or semi-Fowler's position (or totally on side). Turn every 2 hours, side to side unless contraindicated by surgical procedure.
  5. Maintain fluid and electrolytes.
    - a. Do not give fluid by mouth to semiconscious or unconscious patient.
    - b. Weigh to determine fluid loss.
    - c. Monitor IV fluids; overhydration leads to cerebral edema.
  6. Record accurate intake and output.
  7. Take seizure precautions.
  8. Provide hygienic care, including oral hygiene.
  9. Observe dressing for unusual drainage (bleeding, cerebrospinal fluid).
  10. Prevent straining with bowel movements.

✦ Medications

A. Steroids.
  1. Decrease cerebral edema by their anti-inflammatory effect.
  2. Decrease capillary permeability in inflammatory process, thus decreasing leakage of fluid into tissue.
- ✦ B. Mannitol.
  1. Decreases cerebral edema.
  2. Diuretic action by carrying out large volume of water through the nephron.

PRECAUTIONS FOR CARE OF NEUROSURGICAL PATIENT

- Do not lower head in Trendelenburg's position or place in supine position.
- Do not suction through nose without specific order.
- Be careful when administering sedative drugs and narcotics.
  a. Cannot evaluate neurologic status.
  b. May cause respiratory embarrassment.
- Do not give oral fluids unless patient is fully conscious.
- Do not administer enemas or cathartics (may cause straining, therefore increasing intracranial pressure).
- Do not place on operative side if large tumor or bone removed.

♦ C. Dilantin.
  1. Prevents seizures through depression of the motor areas of the brain.
  2. Side effects include gastrointestinal symptoms and rash.
  D. Valium.
  1. Relieves restlessness.
  2. Decreases seizure activity.
  E. Phenobarbital.
  1. Reduces responsiveness of normal neurons to the nervous impulses arising in the focal site.
  2. Side effects are drowsiness, ataxia, nystagmus.
  3. Toxic effects produce rash but usually no nausea and vomiting.

Neurosurgical Postoperative Complications

Increased Intracranial Pressure

♦ A. Signs and symptoms.
  1. Brain becomes compressed as intracranial pressure increases.
  2. Change in level of consciousness.
  3. Lethargy, slurring speech, and slow responses.
  4. Changes in condition (often rapid).
     a. Patient becomes restless.
     b. Patient becomes confused.
     c. Increased drowsiness.
     d. Stupor to coma.
  ♦ 5. Changes in vital signs.
     a. Pulse changes—may decrease to 60 or occasionally increase above 100.
     b. Respiratory irregularities—progresses to Cheyne–Stokes and apnea can result.
     c. Blood pressure increases with wide pulse pressure (difference between systolic and diastolic).
     d. Moderately elevated temperature.
  6. Headache.
  7. Vomiting.

  8. Pupil changes—increasing pressure or an expanding clot can displace the brain against the oculomotor or optic nerve.
♦ B. Nursing care.
  1. Inform physician of any vital sign changes or sensorium changes.
  2. Observe intake and output for possible fluid overload leading to cerebral edema.
  3. Observe surgical incision site for signs of edema.
  4. Administer diuretics or steroids to decrease edema as ordered.
  5. Administer anticonvulsant drugs as ordered.
  6. Have spinal or ventricular puncture tray available to drain off cerebrospinal fluid as necessary.
  7. Observe for level of consciousness—lethargy, slurred speech, slowed responses.
  8. *See* Precautions for Care of Neurosurgical Patient (above).

Seizures

A. Signs and symptoms—tonic–clonic seizures (grand mal, *see* p. 215).
B. Nursing care.
  1. Administer drugs as ordered (Dilantin, phenobarbital, and other related drugs).
  ♦ 2. Provide safe environment.
     a. Pad siderails.
     b. Do not restrain during seizure.
     c. Only use tongue blade to prevent tongue from falling back into throat prior to seizure onset.
  3. Observe and record.
     a. Activities preceding the seizure (aura, movements, etc.).
     b. Type of movements and area of body involved.
     c. Incontinence.
     d. Presence of unconsciousness during seizure.
     e. Length of seizure.
     f. Conditions following seizure.
        (1) Somnolent.
        (2) Continuation of previous activities.
        (3) Awareness of seizure activity.
  4. Provide privacy during seizure.

Brain Abscess or Wound Infection

A. Signs and symptoms.
  1. Increased temperature unless abscess walled off, in which case temperature can be subnormal.
  2. Headache.
  3. Neurologic deficits relative to area involved (focal seizures, blurred vision, etc.).
  4. Increased intracranial pressure.

Table 10-1. POSITIONS FOR NEUROLOGIC CONDITIONS

Condition	Position
Cerebral edema	Elevate head to promote venous return from brain to heart
Stroke with increased intracranial pressure	Head elevated—avoid neck flexion or severe head rotation; prone position impedes venous outflow from brain
CSF fistula, right- or left-sided dependent posturing	Head-up position to promote drainage and lower CSF pressure
Cerebrovascular accident (CVA)	Encourage flat in bed except for ADLs; prevent hip flexion deformities with padded splint at night, trochanter roll and footboard
Rupture of intracranial aneurysm with subarachnoid hematoma	30- to 40-degree elevation, low-Fowler's to facilitate drainage from brain; bedrest
Subdural hematoma	Avoid sudden change in position; promote rest
Brain/head injury	Low position at all times; semi-prone or lateral recumbent prevents aspiration and increases gaseous exchange; turn side to side to prevent stasis of secretions and skin excoriation
Cerebral aneurysm	Elevate head of bed; bedrest
Cerebral concussion and contusion	
Unconscious patient	Semi-prone position; prevent tongue from obstructing airway; encourage drainage of secretion and increased gaseous exchange
Intracranial surgery	
Supratentorial surgery (above the cerebellum)	Head of bed elevated 45 degrees with pillow under head and shoulders; lessens possibility of hemorrhage and improves circulation of CSF
Infratentorial surgery	Bed flat, small pillow under nape of neck and patient turned to either side; avoid flexion of neck causing brain stem compression and coughing and vomiting, because these increase ICP

B. Nursing care.
  1. Observe neurologic signs.
  2. Decrease temperature: sponge bath, antipyretic drugs (Tylenol), cooling blanket.
  3. Administer appropriate antibiotics for causative agent.

EYE CONDITIONS AND SURGERY

Cataracts

Definition: Clouding or opacity of the lens that leads to blurring vision.

✦ **Characteristics**
A. Opacity is due to chemical changes of the fibers or chemical changes in protein of the lens—most often caused by the slow degenerative changes of age.
B. Surgical procedure is usually based on individual needs: that is, how much the patient can see out of the other eye.
  1. If any inflammation is present, surgery is not performed.
  2. Cataracts are usually removed under local or topical anesthesia.
  3. Some simple cataracts are removed by use of alpha-chymotrypsin, which loosens the zonular fibers that hold the lens in position.
  4. Surgery is performed on one eye at a time.

✦ C. Types of surgical extraction.
  1. Extracapsular—the lens is lifted out without removing the posterior lens capsule.
  2. Phacoemulsification (ultrasonic)—the lens is broken up by ultrasonic vibrations and extracted via extracapsular.
  3. Intracapsular—the lens is removed within its capsule (rarely done today).
D. Intraocular lens implant at time of surgery is a common alternative to sight correction with glasses.

Implementation
✦ A. Check that patient understands preoperative instructions.
  1. Patient must be transported to and from hospital.
  2. Patient must have someone at home following surgery.
  3. Patient should be NPO and shampoo hair before surgery.
  4. Review instructions to decrease intraocular pressure. (Do not bend, cough, strain, or lift.)
✦ B. Administer prescribed preoperative medications.
  1. Mydriatics (atropine sulfate) and cycloplegics to paralyze ciliary muscle—note whether pupil dilates following drug instillation.
  2. Topical antibiotics—prevention of infection.
  3. Hyperosmotic agents (oral: glycerol, or IV: mannitol).

✦ C.   Provide postoperative care. Most procedures are done on outpatient basis.
   1.   Instruct patient in postoperative drugs.
       a.   Mydriatics (atropine sulfate)—2–6 weeks after surgery.
       b.   Steroids (prednisolone suspension).
       c.   Analgesics.
   2.   Instruct in ways to alleviate symptoms that could result in complications.
       a.   Nausea and vomiting.
       b.   Restlessness.
       c.   Coughing or sneezing.

Retinal Detachment

Definition: The retina is the part of the eye that perceives light; it coordinates and transmits impulses from its seeing nerve cells to the optic nerve. As the detachment extends and becomes complete, blindness occurs.

✦ **Assessment**
A.   Opacity of the eyes.
B.   Flashes of light.
C.   Floating spots—blood and retinal cells that are freed at the time of the tear and that cast shadows on the retina as they drift about the eye.
D.   Progressive constriction of vision in one area.
   1.   The area of visual loss depends on the location of detachment.
   2.   When the detachment is extensive and rapid, the patient feels as if a curtain has been pulled over his eyes.
   3.   Painless.

Preoperative Implementation
A.   Keep patient on bedrest.
B.   Cover both eyes with patches to prevent further detachment.
C.   Position patient's head so the retinal hole is in the lowest part of the eye.

Surgical Procedure
A.   Immediate surgery with drainage of fluid from subretinal space so that retina returns to normal position.
✦ B.   Retinal breaks are sealed by various methods that produce inflammatory reactions (chorioretinitis).
   1.   Cryosurgery—cold probe applied to sclera causes chorioretinal scar—most common procedure.
   2.   Laser beam seals small retinal tears—can also be used to produce the chorioretinitis.
   3.   Diathermy—causes retina to adhere to choroid.

Postoperative Implementation
✦ A.   Maintain safe environment.
   1.   Keep siderails up.

   2.   Feed patient.
   3.   Maintain bedrest for 1 or 2 days.
   4.   Keep bed flat or in low-Fowler's position.
   5.   Give patient call bell and answer immediately.
✦ B.   Prevent complications.
   1.   Observe for hemorrhage, which is a common complication. Notify head nurse immediately of any sudden, sharp eye pain, restlessness.
   2.   Cover both eyes; keep lights dim.
   3.   Position so area of detachment is in dependent position. (If air bubble is present, position on abdomen.)
   4.   Prevent clinical manifestations which can cause hemorrhage.
       a.   Nausea and vomiting.
       b.   Restlessness.
   5.   Encourage patient to do deep breathing but to avoid coughing.
   6.   Administer good skin care to prevent breakdown.
   7.   Avoid external eye pressure.
C.   Provide emotional support.
   1.   Provide audible stimulation.
   2.   Warn patient as you enter the room and always speak before touching.
   3.   Orient to surroundings.
✦ D.   Provide patient instruction.
   1.   During convalescent period.
       a.   Wear patch at night to prevent rubbing of eyes.
       b.   Wear dark glasses.
       c.   Avoid squinting.
   2.   During postconvalescent period.
       a.   Avoid straining and constipation.
       b.   Avoid lifting heavy objects for 6–8 weeks.
       c.   Avoid bending from the waist.
       d.   Avoid reading for 3 weeks.
       e.   May return to more active life in 6–8 weeks.

Glaucoma

Definition: An eye disorder in which intraocular pressure is too high for the health of the eye—causes atrophy of the optic nerve.

Characteristics
✦ A.   Open-angle (chronic) glaucoma.
   1.   Results from an overproduction or obstruction to the outflow of aqueous humor.
   2.   Sixty to seventy percent of all glaucoma cases are of this type.
✦ B.   Closed-angle (narrow-angle—acute) glaucoma follows an untreated attack of acute closed-angle glaucoma.

1. Results from an obstruction to the outflow of aqueous humor.
2. Caused by trauma, drugs, or inflammation.

C. Risk conditions.
1. Over 40 years of age.
2. Diabetic.
3. Black patient.
4. Hypertensive.
5. Familial history of glaucoma.
6. "Large-eyed" children.
7. History of eye injury.

Assessment

✦ A. Schiotz or Goldmann's Applanation Tonometer Test (7–21 mmHg is normal).

B. Primary open-angle.
1. Slow loss of peripheral vision.
2. Eventual loss of central vision.

C. Primary closed-angle glaucoma (accounts for 10 percent of all glaucomas).
1. Unilateral inflammation.
2. Pain.
3. Pressure over eye. (Increased pressure 24–32 mmHg to much higher). One-sixth of patients with glaucoma have pressures within normal range.
4. Moderate pupil dilation, nonreactive to light.
5. Cloudy cornea.
6. Blurring and decreased visual acuity.
7. Photophobia.
8. Halos around light.
9. Nausea and vomiting.

Treatment and Implementation

✦ A. For primary open-angle glaucoma.
1. Aqueous humor production decreased through beta blockers or prostaglandins.
2. Treated first with medication; new drugs include a_2-selective adrenergic agonists, prostaglandin analogs, etc.
3. When medication no longer controls intraocular pressure, patient prepared for surgery—trabeculoplasty or trabeculectomy, photocoagulation using argon laser or cyclocryotherapy for freezing tissue.

✦ B. For acute closed-angle glaucoma.
1. Treated as an emergency problem.
2. Drugs administered to lower intraocular pressure—B-blockers, IV or oral, carbonic anhydrase inhibitors, topical adrenergic agonists.
✦ 3. Patient prepared for laser peripheral iridectomy.
   a. Part of iris is excised to reestablish aqueous humor outflow.
   b. Acetazolamide, mannitol administered.
   c. Pilocarpine given to constrict pupil and force iris away from trabecular, allowing fluid to escape.

✦ C. For chronic closed-angle glaucoma.
1. Pilocarpine administered.
2. Patient is prepared for bilateral peripheral iridectomy.

✦ D. Postoperative care.
1. Cycloplegic eyedrops to affected eye to relax the ciliary muscle and decrease inflammation.
2. Observe unaffected eye for symptoms of acute closed-angle glaucoma if cycloplegic drops are given by mistake.
3. Instruct patient to limit activities that increase intraocular pressure—straining, coughing, stooping, or lifting.

Age-Related Macular Degeneration (ARMD)

✦ *Definition:* Macula cells fail to function and cell regeneration lessens, which causes loss of central vision.

Characteristics

A. The leading cause of vision loss in Americans over 52 years.
1. Most cases are age-related.
2. More common in white than black people.
3. New procedures are now in clincial trials to reverse ARMD.

B. There are two types.
1. Dry (atrophic)—photoreceptors in the macula of the retina fail to function and are not replaced due to age.
2. Wet (exudative)—less common form; retinal tissue degenerates allowing fluid to leak into the subretinal space.

Assessment

✦ A. Painless loss of central vision in one or both eyes.
1. Blurred vision.
2. Distortion of straight lines.
3. Dark spot in the central vision area.

B. Decreased ability to distinguish colors.

C. Check if patient has difficulty with everyday activities—reading, driving, watching television, recognizing faces.

Implementation

A. Assist patient to learn to compensate for visual deficit in the home.

B. Discuss patient's fear of blindness.

C. Discuss optical aids available, closed-circuit television, telescopic lenses.

D. Refer patient to a low-vision support group.

E. If patient is hospitalized with this condition, orient to room, remove clutter, assist with meals, and always identify self when entering room.

F. Vitamin and nutrient supplements (lutein, lycopene, and beta-carotene) provide alternative therapy and prevention.

◆ **Instilling Eye Drops** ❖ Procedure ❖

A. Take medication to patient's room and check room number against medication card or sheet.
B. Check patient's Identaband and ask patient to state name.
C. Wash your hands.
D. Explain procedure to patient.
E. Tilt patient's head slightly backward.
F. Squeeze the prescribed amount of medication into eye dropper. Hold dropper with bulb in uppermost position.
G. Give tissue to patient for wiping off excess medication.
H. Expose lower conjunctival sac.
I. Drop prescribed medication into center of sac. (Do not place medication directly on cornea, because medication can cause injury to cornea.)
J. Ask patient to close eyelids and move eyes to distribute solution over conjunctival surface and anterior eyeball.
K. Remove excess medication from surrounding tissue.

◆ **Removal of Foreign Body from Eye** ❖ Procedure ❖

A. Have patient look upward.
B. Expose and evert lower lid to expose conjunctival sac.
C. Wet cotton applicator with sterile normal saline and gently twist swab over particle and remove it.
D. If particle cannot be found, have patient look downward. Place cotton applicator horizontally on outer surface of upper lid.
E. Grasp eyelashes with fingers and pull upper lid outward and upward over cotton stick.
F. With twisting motion upward, loosen particle and remove.

◆ **Ophthalmic Drugs**

◆ A. Miotics: pilocarpine HCl 1–6 percent solution; carbamylcholine 1.5–3 percent solution; cholinergic agonists.
   1. Action is contraction of ciliary muscle, which increases flow of aqueous humor.
   2. Treatment for glaucoma and certain types of lens implants.
   3. Side effects: headache, conjunctival irritation, and inflammation.
◆ B. Mydriatics: atropine sulfate 0.25–2 percent solution; epinephrine HCl 0.1 percent solution; cyclopentolate HCl 0.5–1 percent.
   1. Action is to block sphincter muscle response—dilates pupil.
   2. Treatment for ocular surgery and used in eye examinations.
   3. Side effects: headache, dizziness, dry mouth, flushing, and hyperemia.

◆ C. Beta blockers: timolol maleate; betaxolol, levobunolol.
   1. Action is to reduce intraocular pressure by decreasing formation of aqueous humor or may facilitate outflow of aqueous humor.
   2. Treatment for glaucoma.
   3. Side effects: eye irritation.
◆ D. Carbonic anhydrase inhibitors: acetazolamide, dichlorphenamide.
   1. Action is to restrict action of the enzyme necessary to produce aqueous humor—mild diuretic action.
   2. Treatment for glaucoma.
   3. Side effects: CNS disturbance, GI irritation, acidosis, hypokalemia.
◆ E. Hyperosmotic agents: glycerol (oral) or mannitol.
   1. Action is to increase blood osmolarity—reduce intraocular pressure.
   2. Treatment for cataract surgery as preoperative medication.
   3. Side effects: CNS—headache, confusion, blurred vision; GI irritability; nausea; dehydration.
F. Nonselective adrenergic agonists—epinephrine, dipivefrin.
   1. Action is to increase aqueous outflow and decrease aqueous production.
   2. Topical treatment for glaucoma.

EAR SURGERY—STAPEDECTOMY

Definition: Surgery performed to correct otosclerosis; otosclerosis is a condition in which the normal bone of the middle ear is replaced by abnormal osseous tissue.

◆ **Surgical Procedure**

A. An incision is made deep within the ear canal, close to the eardrum, so that the drum can be turned back and the middle ear exposed.
B. The surgeon frees and removes the stapes and the attached footplate, leaving an opening in the oval window.
C. The patient can usually hear as soon as this procedure has been completed.
D. The opening in the oval window is closed with a plug of fat or Gelfoam, which the body eventually replaces with mucous membrane cells.
E. A steel wire or a Teflon piston is inserted to replace the stapes.
   1. The wire is attached to the incus at one end and to the graft or plug at the other end.
   2. The wire transmits sound to the inner ear.

Implementation

✦ A. Keep patient in low-Fowler's position on unoperated side, or as ordered by physician.

B. Do not turn the patient.

C. Put siderails up.

D. Have patient deep breathe every 2 hours until ambulatory, but do not allow coughing.

E. Check for drainage; report excessive bleeding.

F. Prevent vomiting.

G. Give antibiotics as ordered.

H. Patient may have vertigo when ambulatory; stay with the patient and avoid quick movements.

I. Advise patient not to smoke.

✦ **Irrigation of External Auditory Canal**

❖ **PROCEDURE** ❖

A. Remove any discharge on outer ear.

B. Place emesis basin under ear.

C. Gently pull outer ear upward and backward for adult, or downward and backward for child.

D. Place tip of syringe or irrigating catheter at opening of ear.

E. Gently irrigate with solution at 95°–105°F, directing flow toward the sides of the canal.

F. Dry external ear.

G. If irrigation does not dislodge wax, instillation of drops will need to be carried out.

CARDIOVASCULAR SYSTEM

The heart and the circulatory system, both systemic and pulmonary, comprise one of the most essential parts of the body. Failure of the heart to function results in death of the organism. Blood, composed of cells and plasma, circulates through the body and is the means by which (1) oxygen and nutritive materials are transported to the tissues and (2) carbon dioxide and metabolic end products are removed from the tissues for excretion.

CARDIOVASCULAR ANATOMY

Gross Structure of the Heart

A. Four chambered muscular organ that functions as a pump.
B. Separated by a septum into a right, or venous, chamber and into a left, or arterial, chamber. Each half is divided into upper and lower chambers—upper chambers are called atria and lower chambers called ventricles.

Layers
A. Pericardium.
   1. Fibrous pericardium—fibrous sac.
   2. Serous pericardium—allows for free cardiac motion.
B. Epicardium—covers surface of heart, extends onto great vessels, and becomes continuous with the inner lining of the pericardium.
C. Myocardium—muscular portion of heart.
D. Endocardium—thin, delicate inner layer of tissue, which lines cardiac chambers and covers surface of heart valves.

✦ Chambers of the Heart
A. Right chambers.
   1. Right atrium (RA)—thin-walled, distensible, low-pressure collecting chamber for systemic venous return (receives deoxygenated blood from superior vena cava, inferior vena cava, and coronary sinus and sends it to the right ventricle).
   2. Right ventricle (RV)—thin-walled, low-pressure receiving chamber for blood from right atrium (pumps blood into low-resistance pulmonary system).
B. Left chambers.
   1. Left atrium (LA)—thin-walled, low-pressure collecting chamber that receives oxygenated blood from the pulmonary venous system (receives oxygenated blood via the four pulmonary veins).
   2. Left ventricle (LV)—thick-walled, high-pressure chamber that propels blood into the high-resistance systemic circuit (pumps oxygenated blood via aorta to all body tissues).

Valves
A. Strong membranous openings that operate to permit flow of blood only in one direction.
B. Classifications of valves.
   1. Atrioventricular valves, located as heart-guard openings between atria and ventricles, prevent backflow of blood from ventricles to atria during systole.
      a. Tricuspid—right heart valve.
         (1) Three cusps, or leaflets.
         (2) Free edges anchored to papillary muscles in right ventricle by chordae tendineae, which contract when the ventricular walls contract.
      b. Mitral—left heart valve (systole).
         (1) Two cusps, or leaflets.
         (2) Free edges anchored to papillary muscles in left ventricle by chordae tendineae, which contract when the ventricular walls contract (systole).
   2. Semilunar valves, located at blood's exit points inside pulmonary artery and aorta, prevent backflow from the aorta and pulmonary artery into the ventricles during diastole.
      a. Pulmonic—three cusps, or leaflets.
      b. Aortic—three cusps, or leaflets.

Coronary Blood Supply
A. Arteries.
   1. Two arteries provide the myocardium with its own blood supply.
      a. Right coronary artery supplies mainly the right ventricle but also part of the left ventricle.
      b. Left coronary artery divides into two branches (left anterior descending artery and circumflex artery) and supplies mainly the left ventricle.
   2. Coronary blood flow is regulated by oxygen needs of the myocardium.
   3. Aortic pressure determines perfusion of myocardium.
B. Veins.
   1. Principle coronary veins empty into coronary sinus.
   2. Coronary sinus veins drain into right atrium.

Conduction System

A. Composed of specialized tissue that initiates rapid transmission of electrical impulses for orderly sequence of cardiac contraction.

✦ B. Sinoatrial (SA) node.
  1. Main pacemaker of heart in which normal, rhythmic, self-excitatory impulse is generated.
  2. Normal heart elicits 60–100 electrical impulses/minute.
  3. External control is through autonomic nervous system.
    a. Sympathetic—increases rate and increases force of contraction.
    b. Parasympathetic—slows rate and decreases force of contraction; has predominant control.

C. Internodal tracts—transmits electrical impulses through atria from sinoatrial node to atrioventricular node.

D. Atrioventricular (AV) node—contains delay tissue to allow atrial contraction to eject blood into ventricle before ventricular contraction.

E. Bundle of His—conducts the electrical impulse from AV node into ventricles.

F. Left and right bundles to Purkinje fibers—conduct impulses to all parts of the ventricles.

Gross Structure of Vasculature

Arteries

A. Arteries are elastic, muscular tubes that transport blood from the heart to the capillaries in the body tissue.

B. Strong, muscular walls of the arteries force blood onward to all parts of the body.

C. Blood flows rapidly to the tissues.

✦ D. Factors influencing arterial flow.
  1. An adequate volume of blood (cardiac output).
  2. A closed system of unobstructive tubes.
  3. Set of heart valves to ensure flow of blood in one direction only.
  4. Resistance to flow, i.e., an increased thickness of blood causes slowing of blood flow.

Capillaries

A. Capillaries are minute passageways in which the exchange of blood, metabolic waste products and fluid take place.

B. Capillary walls are thin and permeable to fluid and small substances.

C. Blood flow varies depending on type of tissue.

D. Capillaries permit rapid exchange of water and solutes.

Veins

A. Veins are thin-walled tubes that transport blood from tissues back to the heart.

✦ B. Venous system.
  1. Pressure is low.
  2. Walls able to contract or expand, which permits storing of small or large amounts of blood.
  3. Many veins, particularly in the extremities, have valves, which help to prevent backflow of blood.

✦ C. Factors influencing venous return.
  1. Decrease in volume of circulating blood decreases venous return.
  2. Resistance in the venous system (such as occurs in CHF) decreases venous return.
  3. Muscle contraction (walking, leg exercises) increases venous return.
  4. Gravity (elevating legs).
  5. Respiration.
    a. Inspiration increases venous return.
    b. Expiration decreases venous return.
  6. Ability of right heart to handle venous return (CVP).

CARDIOVASCULAR PHYSIOLOGY

Function of Heart and Vessels

A. Heart supplies sufficient amounts of blood to meet the metabolic demands of body tissues.

B. Vessels provide the means of transporting blood to every part and organ of the body.

Regulation of Cardiac Activity

A. Properties of cardiac cells.
  1. Automaticity—ability to initiate an electrical impulse without external stimuli. Conduction of the impulse: SA node → AV node → bundle of His → Purkinje system.
  2. Conductivity—ability to transmit electrical impulses.
  3. Contractility—ability of muscle to shorten with electrical stimulation.
  4. Excitability—ability to be stimulated.

✦ B. Cardiac cycle—cycle is one complete heart beat.
  1. Contraction (systole).
    a. Atria contract, AV valves close, ventricles pump out blood.
    b. "Lub" sound heard through stethoscope.
  2. Relaxation (diastole).
    a. Closure of semilunar valves, relaxation of atria and ventricles (volume of blood is constant in chambers).
    b. "Dub" sound heard through stethoscope.

✦ C. Cardiac output (CO)—the amount of blood pumped out by the heart in 1 minute.
  1. Stroke volume (SV) is the volume of blood ejected from each ventricle with each contraction.

2. Calculation of cardiac output: stroke volume × heart rate = cardiac output.

Example: Stroke volume (SV) = 90 mL
Heart rate (HR) = 60 beats/min
Then, 90 mL (SV) × 60 (HR) = 5400 mL (CO)

3. Factors affecting cardiac output.
   a. Heart rate.
   b. Stroke volume.
      (1) Preload—volume of blood in the ventricles before contraction.
      (2) Afterload—peripheral vascular resistance that the left ventricle must pump against.

D. Cardiac reserve—ability of the heart to respond to increased demands by increasing cardiac output.

Cardiac Muscle Principles

A. Frank–Starling law states that, within physiological limits, the more the heart muscle is stretched by blood flow, the greater is the force of contraction.
   1. The heart can pump a large or a small amount of blood depending on the amount that flows into it from the veins.
   2. The heart can adapt to whatever the required load may be within the physiological limits of the total amount the heart can pump.

B. All or none principle states that cardiac muscle either contracts or does not contract when stimulated.

Compensatory Cardiac Mechanisms

A. Cardiac reserve—the difference between actual work being done and the maximum effort of which the heart is capable; a normal heart can increase its output four to six times.

B. Alterations in heart rate—a normal heart will increase its rate in response to increased oxygen need.

C. Dilatation—an increase in the length of the muscle fibers of the heart.
   1. Characterized by an increase in the *volume* of the heart chambers.
   2. There are physiological limits to dilatation.

D. Hypertrophy—an increase in the *diameter* of the muscle fibers of the heart.
   1. Characterized by *thickening* of the walls of the heart chambers.
   2. There are physiological limits to hypertrophy.

Pulse

A. Rhythmic dilation of an artery caused by contraction of the heart.
B. Palpated over any large surface artery.
✦ C. Pulse deficit—difference between apical and radial pulse, which is due to weakened or ineffective contraction of the heart.

Blood Pressure

A. *Definition:* a measure of pressure exerted on walls of arterial system.
B. Pulse pressure—difference between systolic and diastolic pressure.
✦ C. Factors influencing blood pressure.
   1. Force of heart contractions.
   2. Volume of blood (hemorrhage, for example, will cause decrease in blood pressure).
   3. Diameter and elasticity of blood vessels (arteriosclerosis, for example, will increase blood pressure).
   4. Viscosity of blood (polycythemia vera, for example, will increase blood pressure).

Nervous System Control

A. Control of the heart—impulses from the autonomic nervous system can modify the rate and strength of cardiac contractions.
   1. Sympathetic nervous system (adrenergic).
      a. Secretes epinephrine and norepinephrine.
      b. Increases heart rate.
      c. Increases force of contraction.
   2. Parasympathetic nervous system (cholinergic).
      a. Secretes acetylcholine.
      b. Exerts constant control as the "brake of heart."
      c. Slows heart rate.
      d. Decreases force of contraction.

B. Control of blood vessels.
   1. Sympathetic nervous system.
      a. Causes vasoconstriction of blood vessels.
      b. Causes vasodilation of coronary arteries.
   2. Parasympathetic nervous system.
      a. Causes vasodilation.
      b. Has little direct effect on coronary arteries.

Blood Components

A. Plasma.
   1. Accounts for 55 percent of the total volume of blood.
   2. Plasma composition.
      a. Consists of 92 percent water and 7 percent proteins (proteins include serum, fibrinogen, albumin, gamma globulin).
      b. Less than 1 percent organic salts, dissolved gases, hormones, antibodies, and enzymes.

B. Solid particles (blood cells and platelets).
   1. Comprise 45 percent of the total blood volume.
✦ 2. Blood cells.
   ✦ a. Erythrocytes (red blood cells).
      (1) Normal count in an adult male is 4.6 million–6.2 million cells, adult female is 4.2 million–5.4 million cells/mm^3 of blood.

(2) Contain hemoglobin, which carries oxygen to cells and carbon dioxide from cells to lungs.

(3) Originate in bone marrow and are stored in the spleen.

(4) Average life span is 10–120 days.

✦ b. Leukocytes (white blood cells).

(1) Normal count in an adult is 4500–11,000 cells/mm³ of blood.

(2) Primary defense against infection.

(3) Leukocyte types.

(a) Neutrophils play an active role in the acute inflamma-tory process and are phago-cytic (able to destroy bacteria).

(b) Lymphocytes play an important role in immunologic responses.

(c) Monocytes are the largest of the leukocytes.

✦ c. Platelets (thrombocytes).

(1) Normal count in an adult is 150,000–400,000/mm³ of blood.

(2) Necessary for normal blood coagulation.

(3) Decreased platelet count leads to bleeding problems.

Spleen

A. Glandlike organ located in the left upper quadrant of the abdominal cavity.

B. Functions.

1. Stores blood.
2. Purifies blood by removing waste and infectious organisms.
3. Provides the primary source of antibodies in infants and children.
4. Produces lymphocytes, plasma cells, and antibodies in adults.
5. Produces erythrocytes in fetus.
6. Destroys erythrocytes when they reach the end of their life span.

Cardiovascular System Assessment

Patient History

A. Consider geriatric status.

1. Valves—thicker and stiffer.
2. SA node—decreased number of pacemaker cells.
3. Sympathetic nervous system diminished.
   a. Decreased response to physical and psychological stress.
   b. Less sensitive to beta adrenergic agonist drugs.
4. Arterial blood vessels—thicker with decreased elasticity, resulting in elevated blood pressure.

B. Check for relevant signs and symptoms.

1. Pain.
   a. Character.
   b. Location.
   c. Duration.
   d. Intensity.
   e. Precipitating, aggravating factors.
   f. Relieving factors.

✦ 2. Respiratory problems.
   a. Dyspnea—shortness of breath, feeling of inability to get enough air.
      (1) Exertional dyspnea (DOE)—occurs while exercising.
      (2) Paroxysmal nocturnal dyspnea (PND)—has sudden onset and interrupts patient's sleep.
   b. Orthopnea—occurs while in recumbent position.

3. Fatigue—result of less cardiac output.
4. Palpitations (heart feels like it is pounding).

✦ 5. Cerebral anoxia.
   a. Irritability.
   b. Restlessness.
   c. Confusion.
   d. Apprehension.
   e. Syncope.

6. Hemoptysis—coughing and spitting up of blood.

✦ 7. Edema—collection of fluid in interstitial spaces.
   a. Rales present in lungs.
   b. Ascites (abdominal cavity).
   c. Dependent (pedal).

8. Condition of extremities.
   a. Color.
   b. Temperature.
   c. Skin integrity.
   d. Presence of petechiae.

✦ 9. Syncope—transient loss of consciousness due to inadequate cerebral blood flow.

10. Neck vein distention.
11. Peripheral pulses.
    a. Presence or absence; character; rate.
    b. Grade peripheral pulses.
       (1) 0 = absent.
       (2) 1+ = weak/thready.
       (3) 2+ = normal.
       (4) 3+ = bounding/full.
12. Pulse deficit.
13. Blood pressure—lying, sitting, and standing.
14. Lung sounds.
    a. Crackles (rales): fine, medium, coarse.
    b. Rhonchi: sibilant, sonorous.

C. Check for predisposing factors.

1. Hypertension.
2. Obesity.
3. Diabetes mellitus.
4. Hypercholesterolemia.

5. Smoking.
6. Sedentary lifestyle.
7. Emotional stress.
D. Assess heart sounds by auscultation.
    1. Auscultatory areas.
        a. Aortic: Second intercostal space right of sternum.
        b. Pulmonic: Second intercostal space left of sternum.
        c. Tricuspid: Fifth intercostal space left, close to sternum.
        d. Mitral: Fifth intercostals space mid-clavicular.
        e. PMI: Point of maximal impulse.
    ✦ 2. Heart sounds—frequency, pitch, intensity, duration.
        a. S_1—("Lub") closure of mitral and tricuspid valve.
        b. S_2—("Dub") closure of aortic and pulmonic valve.
        a. S_3 and S_4—diastolic filling sounds.
            (1) S_3—rapid filling of ventricle in early diastole; heard after S_2; sign of heart failure in patient over age 40.
            (2) S_4—coincides with atrial contraction due to poorly compliant ventricle.

DIAGNOSTIC PROCEDURES

Electrocardiogram

✦ A. ECG is a record of the heart's electrical activity as reflected by changes in electrical potential at skin level.
B. Purpose is to determine types and extent of heart damage, cardiac irregularities, and electrolyte imbalance.
    1. Noninvasive and nonpainful, but procedure should be explained to patient.
    2. Requires relaxation so as to reduce electrical interference from muscle movement.
C. 12-lead ECG essential for diagnosing cardiac abnormalities.
D. ECG interpretation (Figures 10-2 through 10-6).
    1. Normal cardiac cycle.
        a. P wave—atrial muscle depolarization.
        b. P-R interval—atrial depolarization.
        c. QRS wave—ventricular muscle depolarization.
        d. ST segment—early ventricular repolarization.
        e. T wave—ventricular muscle repolarization and ventricular diastole.
    2. Determining heart rate.
        a. Calculate atrial rate (P-P interval) and ventricular rate (R-R interval). Normal pulse 60–100.
        b. Determine regularity of rhythm (atrial and ventricular).
    3. Etiology of arrhythmias.
        a. Heart failure, electrolyte imbalance, acidosis or alkalosis, hypoxemia, drugs, hypotension, emotional stress.
        b. Precipitating or contributing diseases—infection, hypovolemia, anemia, thyroid disorders.

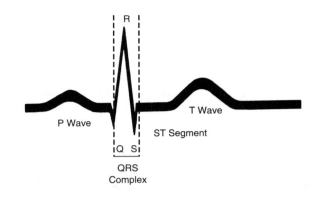

Fig. 10-2 ECG Pattern.

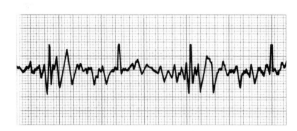

Fig. 10-3 ECG pattern showing artifact.

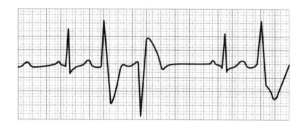

Fig. 10-4 Multifocal PVCs.

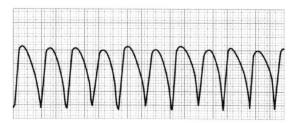

Fig. 10-5 Ventricular tachycardia.

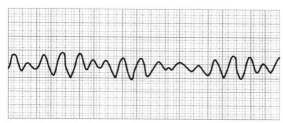

Fig. 10-6 Ventricular fibrillation.

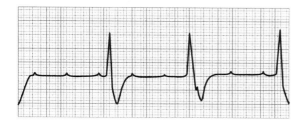

Fig. 10-7 Third-degree heart block.

Exercise Electrocardiography (Stress Test)

A. An electrocardiogram that is taken while the patient is exercising on a stationary bike or treadmill.

B. Purpose is to determine possible cardiac irregularities that may occur during exercise.

C. Test is monitored by physician.

D. Test is discontinued if electrocardiogram records change, if blood pressure increases, or if patient complains of angina.

Cardiac Catheterization/Coronary Angiography

A. Invasive angiography procedure—insertion of a catheter into the heart and vessels surrounding the heart to examine one or both sides of the heart.

✦ B. Purpose is to collect data such as pressure measurements of various chambers, blood oxygen measurement, cardiac output determination, and confirmation of the presence of coronary vessel disease.

C. Catheter may be passed through arterial system into left side of the heart or through venous system into the right side of heart.

✦ D. Possible complications/consequences.
   1. Fatigue, backache.
   2. Pain, bleeding, ecchymosis, swelling at insertion site.
   3. Thrombosis at insertion site.
      a. Numbness, tingling, or coldness of extremity.
      b. Loss of peripheral pulse—notify physician.
   4. Arrhythmias with passage of catheters through ventricles, especially premature ventricular contraction and ventricular fibrillation.
   5. Respiratory complications—hypoventilation, hypoxia, pulmonary edema.
   6. Decreased urine production.

✦ E. Nursing care.
   1. Prior to procedure.
      a. Obtain history of allergy, especially to shellfish, iodine or drugs.
      b. Serum BUN and creatinine for renal function.
      c. Check coagulation studies.
      d. Give no food and fluids (for 6 hours) as ordered.
      e. Establish vital sign baseline.
      f. Prep skin in areas of insertion site.
      g. Have patient rest quietly for 3 or more hours.
      h. Inform patient that there will be little or no pain, but that a fluttery sensation may be felt around heart as catheter is passed through vessels into heart.
   ✦ 2. After the procedure.
      a. Provide bedrest as ordered.
      b. Take vital signs same as for any postop patient. Report blood pressure decreases of more than 10 percent or pulse increases of 10 percent.
      ✦ c. Check peripheral pulses distal to catheter insertion site (radial or pedal).
      d. Observe insertion sites for bleeding, swelling, infection, or thrombosis (pressure dressing may be in place).
      e. Elevate extremity if bleeding occurs.
      f. Instruct patient not to bend limb used for insertion site.
      g. Force fluids to flush system (contrast dye is nephrotoxic) if not contraindicated.
      h. Observe for and report arrhythmias.

Hemodynamic Monitoring

✦ A. Pulmonary artery catheter measures several parameters.
   1. Central venous pressure (CVP): 5–10 cm H_2O.
   2. Right atrial pressure (RAP): normal is 5 mm Hg.
   3. Pulmonary artery pressure (PAP): normal is 20/10 mm Hg with mean of 15 mm Hg.
   4. Pulmonary artery wedge pressure (PAWP): mean pressure 4.5 to 13 (mean of 10) mm Hg.

B. Pulmonary artery catheter has four to five lumens.
   1. Two lumens used to measure CVP, cardiac output, and inject selected solutions.
   2. Distal lumen used to measure PAWP.
   3. Third lumen used for balloon inflation.
   4. Fourth lumen used to measure cardiac output.

C. Prepare for insertion.
   1. Prepare patient and bring emergency cart to patient's room.
   2. Prepare solution bag with heparin.

✦ 3. Calibrate and balance transducer.
   a. Transducer must be at level of patient's right atrium (fourth intercostal space) to ensure accurate reading.
   b. Continuously monitor patient's ECG.
4. Assist physician to insert catheter.

✦ D. Obtain pressure readings.
   1 Expose distal port for PAWP.
   2. Inject air into balloon port and leave in no longer than 5–10 seconds.
   3. Observe waveform change—wedge pressure "A" depicts left atrial contraction and left ventricular relaxation, and "V" left atrial relaxation and left ventricular contraction.

Central Venous Pressure (CVP) Monitoring

✦ A. CVP is pressure within right atrium and reflects right ventricular function—indicates the right side of the heart's ability to manage fluid load.
   1. CVP is a guide for fluid replacement.
   2. Measure of circulating blood volume.

✦ B. Changes in CVP correlate with patient's clinical status.
   1. Elevated CVP can be late sign of left ventricular failure.
   2. Lowered CVP indicates hypovolemia.

✦ C. CVP measured by height of column of water in a manometer.
   1. Measuring CVP is done by using zero mark on manometer as standard reference point.
   2. Transducer placed at phlebostatic axis.
   3. Normal CVP is 5–10 cm H_2O.

D. Monitor for infection and air embolism—most common complications.

Nuclear Cardiology Tests

✦ A. Technetium-99m pyrophosphate scan.
   1. Special camera scans heart to identify areas of increased uptake of radioisotope (hot spots).
   2. Radioisotope accumulates in damaged areas of the heart and will evidence a recent MI.
   3. Hot spots appear within 12 hours, seen most clearly in 48–72 hours and disappear within 7 days.

✦ B. Thallium-201 scan. A radioactive isotope (^{201}TI) is injected into the antecubital vein to evaluate blood flow through vessels and scanning is done within 4–10 minutes.
   1. Necrotic or ischemic tissue will not reflect radioisotope as will tissue with normal blood supply and healthy cells.
   2. Detects myocardial scarring and perfusion, an acute or chronic MI, or evaluation of prior cardiac surgery.

✦ C. Thallium scan with exercise.
   1. Test involves exercise; takes 1 hour and 15 minutes and 3 hours later, a 30-minute resting scan is performed.
   2. Imaging with exercise may demonstrate perfusion problems not apparent when patient is at rest.

D. Gated cardiac blood pool scan.
   1. After an intravenous injection of a red blood cell tagging agent, the computer is synchronized with the ECG reading.
   2. This test evaluates left ventricular function.

E. Positron emission tomography (PET).
   1. Scan that provides information about myocardial perfusion and metabolism.
   2. Radioisotopes administered are measured by PET camera—provides detailed specific information.

Other Cardiac Tests

A. Routine chest films—for observation of silhouette of heart, chambers, and great vessels.
B. Fluoroscopy—examination of heart, lungs, and vessel movement as viewed on fluorescent screen in darkened room.
C. Coronary artery angiography—taking pictures of coronary circulation after injection of radiopaque dye.
D. Phonocardiogram—record produced by registering sounds produced by action of heart; sounds translated into electrical energy by a microphone.

✦ E. Tests for serum enzymes levels.
   1. Elevated following myocardial damage.
   2. Serum enzyme studies include serum glutamic pyruvic transaminase (SGPT), lactate dehydrogenase (LDH), creatine kinase (CK-m8), troponin, and myoglobin protein enzyme tests. (*See* Laboratory tests.)

F. Echocardiography—records high-frequency sound vibrations; assists in evaluating structures of the heart, dimensions of the chambers, and thickness of septum and walls.
G. Holter monitor—tape-recorded ambulatory electrocardiogram. Monitors cardiac cycle for 24 hours.

HEART DISORDERS

Coronary Artery Disease (CAD)

Definition: Occurs as the result of accumulation of fatty materials (lipids, cholesterol being primary one), which narrows the lumen of coronary arteries. Clinical manifestations of disease reflect ischemia to myocardium, resulting from inadequate blood supply to meet metabolic demands.

✦ **Risk Factors**

A. Diet—increased intake of cholesterol and saturated fats.

B. Hypertension—aggravates atherosclerotic process.

C. Cigarette smoking.

D. Diabetes mellitus—accelerates atherosclerotic process.

E. Lack of exercise; sedentary living.

F. Psychosocial tensions (stress)—may precipitate acute events.

G. Obesity—susceptibility to hypertension, diabetes mellitus, hyperlipidemia.

H. Male sex—three times greater incidence.

Assessment

✦ A. Chest pain.
1. Angina, burning, squeezing, crushing tightness substernally or over precordial area.
2. May radiate down arms.

B. Nausea, vomiting.

C. Increased perspiration and cool extremities.

Treatment and Implementation

A. Monitor vital signs, particularly blood pressure and pulse.

B. Assist with ECG.

✦ C. Administer nitrates if chest pain present (as ordered).

D. Evaluate if chest pain—type, duration, is relieved with medication.

E. Monitor breath sounds and signs of peripheral edema to detect early complications.

F. Lipid-lowering agents.

G. Revascularizaiton.
1. Percutaneious transluminal coronary angioplasty (PTCA).
2. Stent placement.
3. Atherectomy.
4. Laser angioplasty.

✦ H. Lifestyle modification.
1. Regular aerobic exercise.
2. If overweight, reduce calorie intake.
3. Diet of 20 percent fat, < 300 mg cholesterol, 8–10 percent saturated fats.
4. Refrain from smoking.
5. Stress reduction.

Stable Angina Pectoris

Definition: Intermittent chest pain or discomfort due to temporary inability of coronary arteries to meet metabolic needs of myocardium. Pathophysiology involves narrowing of lumen of coronary artery, usually by atherosclerotic process. There is an interference with supply of oxygen to the heart.

Precipitating Factors

A. Physical exertion and effort.

B. Emotional upsets.

C. Tachyarrhythmias.

D. Extremes of temperature, especially cold.

E. Smoking, consumption of heavy meals.

F. Sexual activity.

Assessment

✦ A. Pain.
1. Location—precordial, substernal.
2. Character—compressing, choking, burning, squeezing, crushing, and heaviness.
3. Radiation—arm, jaw, neck, back.
4. Duration—usually 5–15 minutes; relieved by rest or nitroglycerin.

✦ B. Dyspnea.

C. ECG changes; may not be evident at rest.

D. There are no physical signs 90 percent of the time.

Implementation

✦ A. Instruct patient how to reduce frequency of attacks.
1. Learn to live with moderation; physical activity should be sufficient to maintain general physical state, but short of causing angina.
2. Avoid stress and emotional upset.
3. Reduce caloric intake if overweight.
4. Refrain from smoking.
5. Decrease use of stimulants, e.g., coffee, tea, cola.
6. Avoid heavy meals.
7. Avoid extremes of temperature, especially cold, and high altitudes.

✦ B. Primary medication—nitroglycerin.
1. Drug action.
    a. Dilates coronary arteries that are not atherosclerotic.
    b. Enhances blood flow to myocardium without increasing oxygen consumption.
2. Use of drug is to relieve pain from myocardia ischemia.
3. Side effects—hypotension, headache, tachycardia.
✦ 4. Important considerations.
    a. Nitroglycerin effective sublingually or metered dose spray.
    b. Dosage of 1–2 tablets may be repeated at 5-minute intervals, up to 3 doses.
    c. Physician should be called if no relief in 15 minutes—may call 911.
    d. No limit to number that may be taken in 24-hour period.
    e. Is not addictive.
    f. May be used prophylactically before engaging in activity known to precipitate angina.

g. Avoid alcohol consumption with drug.

h. Must be stored in closed, dark glass container to avoid light, heat, and moisture. Has 3–6-month shelf-life.

i. Patient should wear Medic-Alert band.

C. Alternatively—instruct patient in use of nitroglycerin ointment/transdermal patch.

❖ PROCEDURE ❖

1. Apply directly to skin.
2. Wash off remaining ointment before new application.
3. Change skin placement with each application.
4. Wear patch 12 hours/day to prevent tolerance.

D. Other medications used.

1. Long-acting nitrites (Isordil, Cardilate).
2. Beta blockers: propranolol (Inderal).
3. Calcium-blocking agents (Calan, Cardizem).
4. Platelet-inhibiting agents (aspirin or clopidogrel).
5. Morphine sulfate as analgesic and sedative—reduces preload and myocardial O_2 consumption.

E. If medications ineffective, may require coronary artery bypass surgery, percutaneous transluminal coronary angioplasty (PTCA), stent placement, artherectomy or laser angioplasty.

Unstable Angina

✦ *Definition:*   Also called preinfarction angina—previously stable angina has now onset while at rest and is less responsive to medication. Condition signifies dynamic change in the vessels.

Assessment

A. Assess for pain that differs from previous attacks, attacks that increase in frequency and duration. Unstable angina leads to myocardial infarction (MI).

B. Changes in the ECG.

C. Serial cardiac enzyme changes.

Implementation

✦ A. Monitor unstable status that could progress to an MI or may heal and return to stable status.

B. Immediate hospital admission with bedrest and hemodynamic monitoring.

C. Monitor medications.

1. Heparin infusion.
2. Platelet-inhibiting agents (ASA, clopidogrel).
3. Narcotic pain management (morphine sulfate).
4. Nitroglycerin infusion (Tridil) titrated for pain relief (requires continuous blood pressure monitoring for hypotension).
5. Beta blockers.

D. Oxygen administration (2–4 L/min).

Myocardial Infarction

Definition: The process by which cardiac muscle is destroyed due to interruption of or insufficient blood supply for a prolonged period, resulting in sustained oxygen deprivation.

Etiology and Risk Factors

A. Atherosclerotic heart disease.

B. Coronary artery embolism.

C. Decreased blood flow with shock and/or hemorrhage.

D. Direct trauma.

E. Risk factors.

1. Smoking.
2. Obesity.
3. High cholesterol/low density.
4. High stress.
5. Poor diet (high fat, low fiber).
6. Sedentary lifestyle.

Assessment

A. Take a complete history—precipitating factors, interventions leading to relief, and associated symptoms.

✦ B. Assess pain that is similar to angina but is usually more intense and has longer duration (30 minutes or longer).

1. Location—left precordial, substernal.
2. Character—crushing, viselike, tightening, and burning.
3. Radiation—jaw, back, arms.

C. Feeling of apprehension or doom.

D. Dyspnea or orthopnea; nausea and vomiting.

E. Diaphoresis.

F. Pallor or cyanosis.

G. Arrhythmias.

H. Signs of congestive heart failure.

✦ Diagnosis

A. History (very important) of ischemic type chest discomfort.

B. ECG changes—ST segment elevated with acute injury.

✦ C. Laboratory studies—serum enzymes (SGPT, LDH, CK) released with death of tissue.

1. Creatine kinase MB (CK-MB)—isoenzymes, level rises in 3–6 hours—most valuable measurement.
2. LDH—LDH_2, level rises in 6–8 hours.
3. Myoglobin—protein found in cardiac and skeletal muscle—sensitive and early indicator—occurs 1–2 hours following injury.
4. Troponin—myocardial muscle protein released after injury.
   a. Troponin T—peaks in 12 hours—high specificity at 3–6 hours.

   b.   Troponin I—rises in 4–6 hours—remains elevated 6 days.
D.   Increase of white cell count.
E.   Increased sedimentation rate.
F.   Isotope scanning of myocardium.

Treatment and Implementation

✦ A.   Death-producing arrhythmias treated immediately with lidocaine.
B.   IV or IM narcotic analgesics (morphine sulfate), as ordered, to relieve pain and anxiety.
C.   Cardiac rhythm monitored continuously.
D.   Lidocaine drip for frequent and complex PVCs.
E.   Oxygen via cannula.
F.   Monitored closely for signs of CHF (seen within first 24 hours).
G.   IV nitroglycerin drip.
H.   Swan–Ganz catheter with PAWP and cardiac output (CO) readings.
I.   Beta blocker therapy to reduce reinfarction rate and sudden death.
J.   Nursing care.
   1.   Administer narcotic analgesics to relieve pain and anxiety.
   2.   Administer oxygen with cannula.
   3.   Observe for arrhythmias.
   4.   Monitor vital signs, urine output.
   5.   Observe for signs of congestive heart failure.
   6.   Monitor for use of thrombolytic agents to reduce infarction size—streptokinase, tissue-type plasminogen activator, anistreplase.
      a.   Must be administered within 6 hours.
      b.   Monitor for complications: systemic bleeding (streptokinase), allergic reaction, dysrhythmias.
   7.   Provide physical rest and emotional support.
      a.   Sedation, graduated activity.
      b.   Use of commode and self-feed.
   8.   Maintain patient on stool softeners and, after liquid diet for 24 hours, soft diet to prevent increased workload on heart and prevent Valsalva maneuver.
   9.   Provide low-fat, low-cholesterol, low-sodium diet.
   10. Rehabilitate patient to enable him to return to physical level according to cardiac capability.
      a.   Plan exercise program.
      b.   Provide psychological support.
      c.   Avoid stressful environment.
      d.   Consider possible change of lifestyle.
J.   Rehabilitation: encourage patient to participate in organized cardiac rehabilitation program. Program usually consists of:
   1.   Monitored exercise program based on METs.
   2.   Stress reduction classes.
   3.   Alterations in nutrition.
   4.   Sex counseling.

Complications

A.   Arrhythmias.
B.   Congestive heart failure.
C.   Cardiogenic shock.
D.   Thrombophlebitis.
E.   Pericarditis.
F.   Ventricular aneurysm or rupture (late complication) due to weakened area of myocardium as result of myocardial infarction.

Heart Valve Stenosis

Definition: A progressive scarring and calcification of the valve cusps that results in the narrowing of the lumen of the valve opening.

Assessment

A.   Predisposing factors.
   1.   History of congenital heart disease.
   2.   Rheumatic heart disease.
   3.   Arteriosclerosis.
B.   May be asymptomatic.
C.   May evidence mild symptoms.
   1.   Decreased cardiac output—tired and lethargic.
   2.   Dizziness and syncope.
   3.   Angina.

Implementation

A.   Treat heart failure and arrhythmias.
B.   Decrease cardiac workload.
C.   Prevent and/or treat infections.
D.   Monitor administration of anticoagulants for treatment and/or prevention of thrombi.
E.   Provide emotional support.
F.   Prepare patient for valvotomy if no calcification of valve or for surgical replacement of the valve.
G.   Complications.
   1.   Atrial fibrillation.
   2.   Subacute bacterial endocarditis.
   3.   Thrombi formation.
   4.   Heart failure.

Heart Failure

✦ *Definition:*   A group of symptoms, not a disease, which results from decreased pumping effectiveness of the heart. Circulatory congestion occurs in response to the decreased or inadequate cardiac output (forward failure) and venous congestion (backward failure). Also known as *cardiac decompensation* or *cardiac insufficiency*.

✦ Types of Heart Failure

A.   Differentiate heart failure types: Left or right-sided failure, systolic or diastolic, high-output failure or acute versus chronic.
B.   High output failure is caused by hypermetabolic states (infection, hyperthyroidism) that require increased blood flow to meet O_2 demands.

C. Acute versus chronic failure is abrupt onset (MI) versus progressive deterioration (cardiomyopathy, CHD).
D. Left vs. right-sided failure.
   1. Left heart failure—congestion occurs mainly in the lungs due to inadequate ejection of the blood into the systemic circulation.
   2. Right heart failure—congestion occurs systemically due to inadequate pumping of the blood from the systemic circulation into the lungs.
✦ E. Differentiate systolic from diastolic dysfunction—heart failure is manifest by systolic and diastolic dysfunction, or both.
   ✦ 1. Systolic dysfunction.
      a. Primarily a problem of ventricular contractile dysfunction—inadequate ventricular emptying leads to increased preload, diastolic volume, and pressure (the tissues do not receive adequate circulatory output).
      b. Most common causes are coronary artery disease, hypertension, and cardiomyopathy with viruses and toxic substances such as alcohol and medications being a possible cause.
      c. Conventional therapy includes diuretics (loop diuretics preferred), digitalis, ACE inhibitors, and beta blockers to improve performance of left ventricle.
      d. The above regimens may be inappropriate for diastolic dysfunction; avoid digitalis and vasodilators.
   ✦ 2. Diastolic dysfunction.
      a. Results when heart cannot completely relax during diastole as a consequence of reduced ventricular compliance.
      b. Manifestations include shortness of breath, tachypnea and respiratory crackles for left ventricle involvement; enlarged liver, neck vein distension, anorexia and nausea for right ventricle involvement.
      c. Patients cannot tolerate reduced blood pressure or plasma volume, so diuretics, ACE inhibitors, and vasodilators are usually contraindicated. Digoxin is also contraindicated.
      d. May respond to calcium channel blockers and beta blockers (to slow the heart rate).
      e. Nitrates may be used to decrease preload.

Pathophysiology
✦ A. Left heart failure.
   1. Damage to myocardium of the left ventricle.
   2. Left ventricle unable to pump adequate amount of blood; pressure increases in pulmonary vessels.
   3. Backflow of blood into the lungs causes pulmonary congestion and increased pressures in the pulmonary system.
   4. Symptoms are pulmonic in nature (pulmonary edema) dyspnea, shortness of breath and cough.
✦ B. Right heart failure.
   1. Increased pulmonary pressure.
   2. Right ventricle unable to effectively pump blood to lungs.
   3. Right side of heart becomes congested with blood.
   4. Venous blood returning to right heart cannot be pumped quickly and efficiently.
   5. Congestion of blood develops in the large veins leading to the right heart and, eventually, in the organs and tissues of the body.
   6. Symptoms are systemic in nature: congested abdominal organs and peripheral edema.

✦ Assessment of Left Heart Failure
A. Fatigue and weakness.
B. Dyspnea—labored breathing (early symptom).
C. Orthopnea (difficulty breathing when lying flat).
D. Anxiety, apprehension, irritability, confusion, restlessness.
E. Moist, hacking cough—may be associated with blood-tinged, frothy sputum.
F. Bibasilar crackles.
G. Cyanosis or pallor.
H. Arrhythmias.
I. Diaphoresis, palpitations.

✦ Assessment of Right Heart Failure
A. Peripheral edema results from elevation in venous pressure (pitting type) in dependent parts—feet and legs, sacrum, back, buttocks.
B. Ascites, which can lead to pulmonary distress.
C. Nausea, vomiting, anorexia due to congestion in liver and gut.
D. Weight gain.
E. Hepatomegaly, liver congestion.
F. Oliguria during day; polyuria at night.
G. Arrhythmias.
H. Increased central venous pressure.
I. Jugular vein distention.

Implementation
✦ A. Goal is to reduce workload on the heart, reduce fluid, and increase efficiency of contractions.
✦ B. Reduce pain and anxiety.
   1. Morphine sulfate.
   2. Physical and emotional rest.
✦ C. Administer oxygen therapy as ordered; use cannula rather than mask because patient already feels he or she cannot breathe.
   1. Administer 2 L/min for COPD patients.

2. IPPB decreases venous return.

✦ D. Reduce fluid and sodium retention.
   1. Diuretics.
   2. Restrict fluid intake.
   3. Moderate sodium restriction—1.5–2 g.
   4. Bedrest in Fowler's position.
   5. Intake and output measure.
   6. Weigh daily.
   7. Special skin care to edematous areas.

✦ E. Reduce preload (the volume of blood present in the heart with each contraction).
   1. Preload drugs—vasodilators, diuretics, digitalis.
   2. Drugs decrease venous blood return to heart and exert force on ventricles to contract.
   3. Administer nitrates that cause generalized vasodilation.
   4. Monitor diuretics; prevent fluid retention by restricting fluid and sodium.
   5. Rotating tourniquets to decrease venous return (no longer commonly used).
      a. Previously used for pulmonary edema—mechanically reduced volume of blood returning to the heart.
      b. New drugs with increased ability to monitor fluid volume status are replacing rotating tourniquets. Multilumen pulmonary artery catheters now used.
   6. Fowler's position to facilitate breathing.
   7. Record intake and output; weigh daily.

✦ F. Reduce *afterload* (resistance against which the ventricles must pump to empty their blood supply).
   1. Afterload drugs—vasodilators: calcium channel blockers and hydralazine (Apresoline).
   2. Drugs increase left ventricle stroke volume and cardiac output; decrease peripheral vascular resistance, pulmonary, and peripheral venous pressure.

✦ G. Monitor medications.
   1. Administer digitalis—increases strength of contraction and decreases rate—for systolic dysfunction.
   2. Drug not used in diastolic dysfunction.
   3. Loading dose given for acute condition.
   4. Digitalis has a cumulative effect—important to monitor for toxic symptoms.
   H. Observe for arrhythmias.
   I. Provide emotional support.
   J. Instruct patient in principles of care.

Complications

✦ A. Digitalis toxicity.
   1. Most common predisposing factor for toxicity is hypokalemia, which potentiates effect of digitalis.
   2. Low potassium levels (from diuretics) lead to excitable heart and dysrhythmias.
   3. Potassium levels requiring intervention—below normal: 4.0–5.4 mEq/L.
   B. Electrolyte imbalance from diuretics, especially decreased potassium.
   C. Oxygen toxicity, especially with COPD.
   D. Myocardial failure.
   E. Cardiac dysrhythmia.
   F. Pulmonary infarction; emboli, pneumonia from bedrest—circulatory stasis.

Acute Pulmonary Edema

✦ *Definition:* An excessive quantity of fluid in the pulmonary interstitial spaces or in the alveoli usually following severe left ventricular decompensation.

Characteristics

✦ A. The most common cause is greatly elevated capillary pressure resulting from failure of left heart and damming of blood in lungs.
   B. Alveoli filled with fluid and bronchioles congested.
   C. Retention of fluid resulting from reduced renal function. May be associated with barbiturate or opiate poisoning.

Assessment

✦ A. Moist rales and pink, frothy sputum—primary symptoms.
✦ B. Severe anxiety, feelings of impending doom, and restlessness.
   C. Marked dyspnea.
   D. Stertorous breathing.
   E. Marked cyanosis.
   F. Profuse diaphoresis—cold and clammy.
   G. Blood pressure and pulse changes.
   H. Heart symptoms.
      1. Tachyarrhythmias.
      2. Gallop rhythm (S3).
   I. Increase in wedge pressure and CVP.

✦ Implementation

   A. Place in high-Fowler's position.
   B. Administer oxygen at 6 L/min if patient does not have COPD.
   C. Administer medications (diuretics and digitalis, morphine, and nitroglycerin) to improve myocardial contractility and reduce pulmonary and systemic blood volume.
   D. Instruct patient in deep breathing and coughing exercises.
   E. Monitor fluid intake and output, weigh daily.
   F. Monitor vital signs.
   G. Provide sedation with ordered medication. Observe respiratory rate and depth.
   H. Administer drug therapy for preload or afterload as ordered: nitroglycerin, nitroprusside, hydralazine.

I. Assist with rotating tourniquets on patient's extremities if ordered.
1. Now, this procedure is *not* commonly used; used only in emergencies.
2. Purpose.
   a. Reduce venous return to heart.
   b. Pool blood temporarily in extremities.
   c. Treatment for pulmonary edema.

Cardiomyopathy

✦ *Definition:* Heart muscle disease of unknown origin that manifests as three types: dilated congestive, hypertrophic, and restrictive cardiomyopathy.

Characteristics

A. The most common type, dilated congestive cardiomyopathy, is diffuse coronary artery disease.
B. Hypertrophic type is asymmetrical ventricular hypertrophy which results in impaired ventricular filling and decreased cardiac output.
C. Regardless of the type manifested or cause, result is impaired pumping of the heart.
D. Decreased stroke volume stimulates sympathetic nervous system, resulting in increased vascular resistance with eventual left ventricular failure.

Assessment

✦ A. Effort dyspnea and fatigue due to elevated left ventricular diastolic pressure and low cardiac output.
B. Physical signs include pitting edema, sinus tachycardia, basal rales, low blood pressure, and possible enlarged liver.
C. Chest x-ray reveals cardiomegaly.

Treatment and Implementation

✦ A. Treatment begins with finding any specific cause (most often there is none) and treating it.
1. Therapy for heart failure and low cardiac output is implemented.
2. Combined afterload and preload reduction with ACE inhibitors, hydralazine, plus nitrates are the mainstay of treatment.
3. Digitalis, diuretics are also used in the treatment protocol.
✦ B. Nursing focus is aimed at improving cardiac output.
1. Bedrest and increased oxygenation.
   a. Gradually increase activity alternating with rest.
   b. Identify activities that cause shortness of breath and teach patient how to plan.
2. Monitor medications—compliance is vital to improved clinical status.

Surgical Procedures

Definition: Surgical procedures on the cardiac vessels, valves, or myocardium.

Characteristics

A. Common types of heart surgery.
✦ 1. Percutaneous transluminal coronary angioplasty (PTCA)—less invasive than bypass surgery and preferred as initial procedure.
   a. A catheter with a deflated balloon is threaded into artery at site of blockage.
   b. Balloon is inflated and opens artery by breaking up and compressing plaque against artery wall.
   c. Stent often placed to maintain patency.
2. Coronary bypass surgery—healthy sections of a leg or chest blood vessel are grafted distal to blocked area of coronary artery.
3. Commissurotomy of stenosed valve.
   a. Closed commissurotomy—finger inserted to dilate valvular opening.
   b. Open commissurotomy—dissection of scarred area by means of a scalpel.
4. Valve replacement—artificial, or prosthetic, valves; heterografts (porcine or bovine).
5. Transplantation—therapeutic option for severe heart disease.
   a. Immunosuppressant drugs decrease body's rejection of foreign protein (another's human heart).
   b. Patients must balance risk of rejection with risk of infection.
B. Major pre–cardiac surgery goals are to reduce anxiety, fear, and complications.

Assessment

A. Check that RN has obtained a health history and completed a physical assessment, which includes the patient's functional level, coping, and support systems.
B. Evaluate knowledge of operative procedure to prepare for preoperative teaching.
C. Assess vital signs, heart and lung sounds, other vital parameters for baseline data.

Implementation

✦ A. Observe for fluid and electrolyte imbalance.
1. Obtain lab specimens for hypokalemia and hyperkalemia.
2. Measure CVP for hypovolemia and volume overload.
3. Measure blood gases for acidosis and alkalosis.
4. Monitor hematocrit and hemoglobin lab values.
5. Weigh daily.
✦ B. Observe respiratory function.
1. Patient receives mechanical ventilation for varying length of time postoperatively.
   a. Endotracheal intubation with cuffed trach tube.
   b. Suction airway PRN.
   c. Auscultate for bilateral breath sounds.

d. Monitor pulmonary volumes; pulse oximetry.

2. Auscultate for abnormal lung sounds.

✦ C. Observe for circulatory complications.
1. Decreased blood pressure.
2. Tachycardia, thready pulse.
3. Weak peripheral pulses.
4. Decreased urine output.
5. Skin—cool, clammy, cyanotic.
6. Restlessness.
7. Elevated cardiac and central venous pressures.
8. Electrolyte imbalance.

D. Observe for signs of cardiac tamponade (mediastinal/chest tubes output over 100 mL/hr).

E. Place in semi-Fowler's position to facilitate cardiac and respiratory function.

F. Administer pain medication such as morphine sulfate IV.

✦ G. Monitor IV fluid and blood requirements by use of intracardiac pressures, blood pressure, urine output, hemoglobin, and hematocrit.
1. Keep CVP at 5–12 cm water pressure or 0–6 mmHg) or as directed by physician.
2. Monitor that urine is above 30 mL/hr.
3. Hematocrit maintained at 30–35.

✦ H. Maintain kidney function.
1. Keep urine output more than 30 mL/hr with IV fluids or plasma expanders.
2. Maintain blood pressure above 90 mmHg systolic.
3. Diuresis is common.
4. Report cloudy or pink urine.

✦ I. Maintain patent chest tubes.
1. Used to remove fluid and air from mediastinum/pleural space.
2. Maintain 20 cm H_2O suction.

✦ J. Maintain body temperature—patients are usually hypothermic following cardiac surgery.
1. Raise body temperature gradually.
a. Blankets used cautiously following hypothermic surgical procedure.
b. Monitor core temperature with PA catheter.
2. Patients at risk for developing fever caused by infection or postpericardiotomy syndrome.
a. Bedrest and anti-inflammatory agents primary treatment.
b. Keeping temperature below 100°F prevents increased metabolic rate, which increases cardiac workload.

K. Assess level of consciousness, pupil response, motor response.
1. Neurologic complications may result from extracorporeal perfusion or aorta clamping.
2. Orient patient frequently.

L. Administer anticoagulant therapy for valve replacements.

M. Monitor laboratory values for anticoagulation.
1. Partial thromboplastin time for heparin administration based on weight and sliding scale protocol.
2. Prothrombin time/INR for coumadin therapy.

N. Monitor for complications associated with valve replacement.
1. Conduction defects (may require temporary pacing).
2. Cardiac tamponade.
3. Supraventricular tachyarrhythmias (may use pacemaker overdrive).
4. Malfunction of prosthetic valve (murmur).

Pacemaker Insertion

Definition: A temporary or permanent device to initiate and maintain heart rate when patient's pacemaker is nonfunctioning.

Conditions Requiring Pacemakers
A. Conduction defect following open heart surgery.
B. Heart block (usually third degree).
C. Tachyarrhythmias.
D. Bradyarrhythmias.

Types of Pacemakers
✦ A. Permanent—electrodes inserted through central vein into apex of right ventricle.
1. Pulse generator implanted into subcutaneous tissue below clavicle.
2. Demand—most common type; functions only if patient's own pacemaker fails to discharge.
a. The pacemaker is set at a fixed rate and will discharge only if patient's own rate falls below it.
b. Used mainly in Adams–Stokes or bradyarrhythmias or following cardiac surgery.

✦ B. Temporary—external generator used for temporary conditions such as MI, drug toxicity, severe bradycardias.
1. Either chamber can be paced alone or both sequentially.
2. All methods use a pulse generator with replaceable batteries and an electrode or impulse conductor.

✦ Pacemaker Placement
A. Epicardial.
1. Electrodes are implanted on outside of left ventricle, and they barely penetrate myocardium.
2. Battery pack is placed subcutaneously in a skin pocket.
B. Endocardial implantation—pacing electrode inserted through neck vein and placed near apex of right ventricle.

1. Permanent—battery is implanted beneath skin.
2. Temporary—battery is located outside of skin.

Implementation

A. Preplacement.
1. Assess vital signs for baseline data.
2. Evaluate heart sounds to determine arrhythmias for baseline data.
3. Assess lung sounds.
B. Postplacement.
1. Observe for battery failure (pacemaker not firing as set).
   a. Faints easily.
   b. Hiccoughs.
   c. Rhythm change.
   d. Gradual decrease in pulse rate.
2. Observe for hematoma at site of insertion.
3. Observe for arrhythmias via cardiac monitoring.
4. Monitor vital signs.
✦ 5. Observe or counsel patient for pacemaker malfunction.
   a. Decreased urine output, edema, or weight gain.
   b. Dizziness or fatigue.
   c. Decreased blood pressure, slowed pulse rate.
   d. Chest pain.
   e. Shortness of breath.
6. Check for complications.
   a. Hemorrhage and shock.
   b. Infection.
C. Perform patient teaching.
1. Purpose and function of pacemaker.
2. Medication—dose and side effects.
3. How to monitor pulse rate.
4. Signs and symptoms of infection.
5. Wear MedicAlert bracelet and carry pacemaker ID card.

Inflammatory Diseases of the Heart

Definition: Conditions in which various microorganisms cause infection and inflammation of the structures of the heart. Damage to the valves of the heart is among the most serious consequences of inflammatory heart disease.

✦ Characteristics

A. Acute—fulminating disease caused by gram positive or gram negative or yeasts.
B. Subacute—slowly progressive disease of rheumatic or congenital lesions or prosthetic valve disease.
C. Types.
1. Infective endocarditis—an infection of the lining of the heart.
2. Pericarditis—inflammation of the pericardium.
3. Myocarditis—inflammation of the muscle of the heart walls.
4. Rheumatic fever—a systemic disease of connective tissue, which may involve the endocardium, myocardium, and pericardium.
5. Rheumatic heart disease—a chronic cardiac condition, which usually follows one or more episodes of rheumatic fever with valvular damage.

Assessment

✦ A. Signs of infection.
1. Fever and night sweats.
2. Chills.
3. Diaphoresis.
4. Lassitude.
5. Anorexia.
B. Tachycardia, regurgitant heart murmur.
C. Chest pain.
D. Dyspnea.
E. Check lab tests—increased WBC, ESR, blood culture.

Implementation

A. Administer specific antibiotic therapy for several weeks, as ordered.
B. Provide bedrest, decrease cardiac workload.
C. Administer salicylates.
D. Provide adequate nutrition, encourage fluids.

✦ Complications

A. Mitral stenosis—progressive thickening of the valve cusps, which results in narrowing of the lumen of the mitral valve.
B. Mitral insufficiency—distortion of the valve that allows backward flow of blood from ventricle to atrium.
C. Aortic stenosis—narrowing of the aortic valve opening due to fibrosis and calcification.
D. Aortic insufficiency—occurrence of blood flow back into the ventricle from aorta.
E. Tricuspid stenosis—progressive narrowing of tricuspid valve lumen.
F. Tricuspid insufficiency—occurrence of blood flow back into atrium from ventricle.

VASCULAR DISORDERS

Hypertension

✦ *Definition:* Sustained elevation of arterial pressure with either systolic pressure > 140 mmHg or diastolic pressure > 90 mmHg. (50 million people have this disease in the United States.)

Types

✦ A. Primary or essential—no known etiology (accounts for 90 percent).

✦ B. Secondary hypertension—directly related to another condition, such as:
   1. Renal disease.
   2. Endocrine disorders.
      a. Pheochromocytoma (adrenal tumor).
      b. Adrenal cortex lesions—hyperaldosteronism, Cushing's syndrome.
   3. Toxemia of pregnancy.
   4. Increased intracranial pressure.
   5. Congenital heart disease.
   6. Increased workload of the heart.
      a. Congestive heart failure.
      b. Myocardial infarction.

Assessment

A. Asymptomatic in early stage.

B. Risk factors: obesity; family history; age (> 60 years); race (two times more frequent in blacks); diabetes; smoking; gender.

✦ C. Common symptoms.
   1. Headache, dizziness, tinnitus.
   2. Fatigue, insomnia.
   3. Epistaxis, blurred vision, spots before eyes.

D. Identify if target organ involvement is present.
   1. Eyes—narrowing of arteries, papilledema (malignant hypertension), visual disturbances.
   2. Brain—mental and neurologic abnormalities, encephalopathy, CVA.
   3. Cardiovascular system—left ventricular hypertrophy and failure, angina, aggravation and acceleration of atherosclerotic process in coronary arteries and peripheral vessels.
   4. Kidneys—renal failure.

Implementation

A. Treat causes of secondary hypertension.

✦ B. Lifestyle changes.
   1. Diet—weight loss, decrease fat intake to < 30 percent of calories.
   2. Decrease sodium intake (1–3 g); adequate potassium/magnesium intake.
   3. Engage in regular aerobic exercise.
   4. Limit alcohol intake.
   5. Stop smoking.
   6. Do relaxation processes or meditation (reduce stress).

✦ C. Drug therapy.
   1. Diuretics—act on kidneys to increase urine output.
      a. Thiazides (Diuril, Esidrix, Enduron).
      b. Potassium sparing (Aldactone).
      c. Loop (potent) diuretics (Lasix, Edecrin, Bomex).

   2. Beta blockers (Inderal, Aldomet, Catapres, Ismelin), decrease contractility and myocardial workload.
   3. Vasodilators (Apresoline, Vasodilan).
   4. Angiotensin-converting enzyme (ACE) inhibitors (Captopril) allow blood vessels to dilate and help to prevent organ damage.
   5. Calcium channel blockers (Nifedipine) relax smooth muscles and block calcium flow into cells.
   6. Central alpha agonists (Clonidine) causes vasodilation.

✦ D. Emphasize to patient the importance of following medical treatment regimen.
   1. Weight control.
   2. Low-sodium diet.
   3. Change in lifestyle.
   4. Periodic medical checkups.
   5. Importance of compliance with program.
   6. Not to discontinue medication abruptly.
   7. Check with physician before taking any over-the-counter drugs.

Thromboangiitis Obliterans (Buerger's Disease)

✦ *Definition:* Chronic inflammation of arteries and veins, and secondarily, inflammation of nerves.

Assessment

✦ A. Pain, temperature, and color changes (cyanosis); alterations in skin of lower extremities at rest and especially after exercise.

B. Intermittent calf claudication—severe calf cramping following exercise; relieved upon resting.

C. Decreased pulse rates.

D. Complications of neuropathy, swelling, ulceration, gangrene.

Treatment and Implementation

A. Cessation of smoking.

B. Bilateral sympathectomy.

C. Low-dose aspirin.

D. Monitor use of vasodilator drugs (Trental) to increase blood supply to lower extremities.

E. Instruct patient to prevent injury to feet and maintain cleanliness to prevent complications.

Raynaud's Disease

Definition: A vasospastic condition of small, cutaneous digital arteries that occurs with exposure to cold or to strong emotion and affects fingers, toes, ears, nose, and cheeks.

Assessment

✦ A. Raynaud's disease—abnormality of the sympathetic nervous system where intermittent arteriolar vasoconstriction is evidenced by pain or coldness; bilateral or symmetric numbness.

✦ B. Raynaud's phenomenon—related to underlying collagen or connective tissue disease (lupus), there is intermittent pallor, cyanosis, rubor, and changes in skin temperature from cold or strong emotion; may be unilateral, but usually symmetric.

Implementation

✦ A. Encourage patient to stop smoking—increases vasoconstriction.

B. Vasodilator drugs—calcium channel blocker—nifedipine (Procardia). Causes coronary vasodilation by increasing myocardial oxygenation.

C. Encourage patient to avoid precipitating factors such as cold temperature and emotional stress.

D. Wear warm clothing in cold weather: boots, gloves, etc.

Deep Vein Thrombophlebitis

Definition: Formation of a clot in a vein—occurs most often in left leg (due to right common iliac artery compressing left common iliac vein).

Precipitating Causes

A. Stagnation of blood flow that occurs from inactivity, bedrest, or dehydration.

B. Change in clotting of blood.

C. Change in lining of blood vessel (trauma).

D. Incidence most common following abdominal or circulatory surgery, or fractures of leg or pelvis.

✦ Assessment

A. In superficial vein.
1. Vein hard to the touch, distended.
2. Skin reddened, hot, tender.

B. In deep vein.
1. Affected area swollen, tender.
2. Increased temperature, pulse, and white blood count.

C. Palpate peripheral pulses—presence of Homan's sign (now, not recommended as it may mobilize clot and it is not reliable).

Treatment and Implementation

✦ A. Take preventive measures.
1. Exercise.
2. Nonconstrictive clothing.
3. Footboard walking.
4. No "gatching" of bed.
5. No pillow under knees.
6. No calf massage.
7. Adequate hydration.

✦ B. Treatment.
1. Maintain strict bedrest 7–10 days.

2. Ensure proper fitting of elastic stockings.
3. Elevate affected limb slightly (20 degrees).
4. Administer anticoagulant drug therapy as ordered.
    a. Check lab values before giving drug.
    b. Coumadin prescribed for 3 months—dose adjusted to keep INR between 2.0 and 3.0.
    c. Observe for signs of bleeding—urine, stool, ecchymosis.
5. Apply heat to affected area if ordered.
6. Assist patient to do leg exercises in bed.
7. Monitor for pulmonary embolism.
    a. Cough; rapid, shallow respirations.
    b. Chest pain—worse with every breath.
    c. Tachycardia.

Varicose Veins

Definition: A condition in which the veins are dilated because of incompetent valves.

Precipitating Causes

A. Pregnancy.
B. Standing for long periods of time.
C. Poor venous return, history of DVT.
D. Heredity.
E. Obesity.
F. Prolonged and heavy lifting.

Assessment

A. Dull aching and heaviness in legs.
B. Swelling of ankles.
C. Browning of skin from blood, which has escaped from overloaded veins.
D. Ulceration.

Implementation

✦ A. Prevention—smoking, heavy lifting, overweight, etc.

B. Elevation of legs; wearing of nonconstrictive clothing and elastic stockings.

C. Surgery—vein ligation, stripping.

✦ Nursing Care for Vascular Problems

A. Limit disease and prevent complications.
B. Maintain adequate blood supply to affected areas.
1. Warmth.
2. Cleanliness.
3. Infection control.
4. Avoidance of heat and cold extremes.

C. Encourage patient to stop smoking.
D. Have patient wear nonconstrictive clothing and use body positions that protect affected areas from pressure.

E. Avoid emotional stress.
F. Teach patient to recognize an increase or extension of symptoms.

1. Increase of pain in extremities.
2. Changes in skin color.
3. Ulceration.
4. Change of temperature in extremities.

G. Assist patient to recognize limitations caused by disease.

Aortic Aneurysms

Definition: A localized abnormal dilatation of the vascular wall occurring most often in the ascending aorta and secondly in the aortic arch.

Characteristics

A. Causes.
   1. Trauma.
   2. Weakening of arterial wall due to atherosclerosis.
B. Hypertension and cigarette smoking are major risk factors.
C. Highest incidence in older men (25 percent also have peripheral vascular disease).
D. High mortality if not surgically treated.
E. Major cause of death is spontaneous rupture.

Assessment

✦ A. Evaluate symptoms to determine area involved.
   1. Thoracic aneurysm.
      a. Pain—sudden in onset with tearing or ripping sensation in thorax or anterior chest.
      b. Pain extends to neck, shoulders, lower back, or abdomen.
      c. Syncope.
      d. Pallor, perspiration.
      e. Dyspnea, increased pulse, cyanosis.
      f. Weakness, transient paralysis.
      g. Loss of pulses in affected extremities.
   2. Abdominal aneurysm.
      a. Pulsating mass in abdomen may be palpated.
      b. Systolic bruit over aorta.
      c. Tenderness on deep palpation.
      d. Large aneurysm may react as if it were renal calculi or lumbar disc disease.
      e. Lumbar pain radiating to flank and groin indicates impending rupture.
B. Assess vital signs to obtain baseline data.
C. Evaluate peripheral pulses.
D. Assess intensity of pain.
✦ E. Evaluate for dissecting aneurysms—simulates coronary occlusion.
   1. Originate in ascending aorta.
   2. Usually associated with severe hypertension.
   3. Pain described as tearing, referred pain.
F. Most accurate means for imaging are CT scan and MRI.

Implementation

✦ A. Maintain blood pressure at below 140 systolic if aneurysm is dissecting.
B. Administer propranolol to decrease force of contraction, as ordered.
C. Administer oxygen to prevent respiratory embarrassment.
D. Monitor fluid balance. Administer whole blood when needed, as ordered.
E. Prepare patient for immediate surgery if aneurysm is dissecting or for thoracic aneurysm. Abdominal aneurysm repair is not an emergency unless it is dissecting.
✦ F. Provide postoperative nursing management.
   1. Follow same procedures as for open heart surgery if patient has thoracic aneurysm; monitor vital signs and hemodynamic variables (CVP, PAP, PCWP).
   2. Observe circulatory status distal to graft site.
   3. Observe all peripheral pulses and temperature of extremities.
   4. Monitor renal function with accurate intake and output (cross-clamp of aorta during surgery).
   5. Observe for emboli to brain or lung.
   6. Monitor neurological signs.
   7. Monitor for complications.
      a. Hypertensive preoperatively, but can easily become hypotensive due to excessive bleeding.
      b. Acute renal failure—monitor I&O.
      c. Hemorrhage from graft site.
      d. Cerebral vascular accident.
      e. Paraplegia.
      f. Infection.

COMMON CARDIOVASCULAR DRUGS

Cardiac Glycosides (Digitalis, Digoxin, Lanoxin, Digitoxin)

✦ A. Therapeutic effects.
   1. Increases force of cardiac contraction.
   2. Slows heart rate.
   3. Slows conduction through AV node.
   4. Increases automaticity that may cause arrhythmias.
B. Used in heart failure.
   1. Increases contractility, which reduces oxygen need.
   2. Increases cardiac efficiency.
   3. Reduces heart size.
✦ C. Dosage individualized to patient and clinical situation; loading dose, then maintenance dose (usually 0.25 mg QD).
D. Precautions.
   1. Used with caution for patients with impaired renal or hepatic function.

2. Used with caution for patients with hypokalemia, which predisposes them to digitalis toxicity.

E. Side effects.
1. All types of cardiac arrhythmias.
   a. Bradycardia.
   b. Conduction disturbances.
2. Gastrointestinal effects.
   a. Anorexia.
   b. Nausea and vomiting.
   c. Diarrhea and/or constipation.
   d. Abdominal pain.
3. Central nervous system effects.
   a. Fatigue.
   b. Depression.
   c. Lethargy.
   d. Headache.
   e. Confusion, agitation.
4. Ophthalmic effects.
   a. Disturbed color perception.
   b. Halos circling dark objects.
5. Hypersensitivity.
   a. Pruritus.
   b. Urticaria.

✦ F. Nursing implementation.
1. Take apical pulse for one full minute; notify physician if above 120 or below 60.
   a. If below 60, hold dose and notify physician.
   b. If above 120, check for toxicity or arrhythmias.
2. Administer digitalis after meals to avoid gastric distress.
3. Monitor for toxicity in the elderly as they are more sensitive to digitalis.
4. Assist in designing instructional plan for patient.
   a. Drug action.
   b. Dosage.
   c. Keeping records.
   d. Method and timing for taking pulse.
5. Store in tightly covered, light-resistant containers.

✦ **Calcium Channel Blocking Agents (ion antagonists) (Cardizem, Verapamil, Procardia)**

A. Therapeutic effects.
1. Inhibits the influx of calcium ions across cell membrane.
2. Decreases heart rate as conduction is slowed through SA and AV nodes.
3. Increases myocardial oxygenation by causing coronary vasodilation.
4. Decreases peripheral vascular resistance by causing vasodilation of peripheral arteries.

B. Used for angina, usually when beta blocker and nitrate therapy are not effective, and as an antihypertensive.

C. Drugs.
1. Cardizem (diltiazem hydrochloride)—hypotension, nausea, edema, headache.
2. Procardia (nifedipine)—vertigo, nausea, peripheral edema, headache, and flushing, dyspnea.
   a. Do not discontinue suddenly.
   b. Give on empty stomach.
3. Calan, Isoptin (verapamil hydrochloride)—hypotension, peripheral edema, vertigo.
   a. Do not discontinue suddenly.
   b. Give on empty stomach.
   c. If patient depressed, notify head nurse.

✦ **Coronary Vasodilators—Nitrates**

A. Therapeutic effects.
1. Reduces vascular tone in arteries and veins.
2. Decreases peripheral arterial vascular resistance (afterload—calcium channel blockers and Apresoline).
3. Decreases venous blood return to heart (preload—vasodilators, diuretics and digitalis drugs).
4. Reduces myocardial oxygen consumption.

B. First line therapy for acute angina; heart failure related ischemic heart disease.

C. Side effects.
1. Flushed face.
2. Headache, common side effect.
3. Nausea and vomiting.
4. Vertigo and faintness.
5. Postural hypotension.

D. Drugs.
1. Short acting.
   a. IV—Tridil, Nitro-Bid, Nitrostat.
   b. Sublingual—nitroglycerin.
   c. Topical—Nitrol.
   d. Oral—Nitro-Bid.
2. Long acting.
   a. Sublingual—Cardilate, Isordil.
   b. Oral—Peritrate, Sorbitrate.
   c. Topical disk—Nitrodisc, Nitro-Dur, Transderm-Nitro.
3. Extended release—buccal tablets and capsules.

E. Nursing Implementation.
1. Development of tolerance is a problem.
2. Advise patient to take drug while sitting or lying down to prevent hypotension.
3. Drug should be replaced before 6-month expiration.
4. Instruct patient to notify physician if severe headache, weakness, blurry vision, irregular heart beat, or dry mouth is experienced.

✦ **Antihypertensive Drugs**

A. Therapeutic use—reduce blood pressure to normal or near normal without side effects—drugs come from several different categories of cardiac medications.

B. Drugs.

1. Thiazides (Diuril)—potentiates second drug when used in combination with other antihypertensive drugs.

2. Hydralazine (Apresoline).
   a. Effect—adrenergic blocker.
   b. Side effects—headache, tachycardia, and postural hypotension.

3. Methyldopa (Aldomet).
   a. Effect—decreases blood pressure.
   b. Side effects—postural hypotension.

4. Ganglionic blocking agents—pentolinium tartrate (Ansolysen), mecamylamine (Inversine).
   a. Effect: blocks parasympathetic and sympathetic ganglia.
   b. Side effect: postural hypotension.

5. Postganglionic blocking agents—guanethidine (Ismelin).
   a. Effect: blocks norepinephrine.
   b. Side effect: postural hypotension.

6. Diazoxide (Hyperstat).
   a. Effects: decreases peripheral vascular resistance in all circulatory beds; affects arterial smooth muscles.
   b. Use: hypertensive crisis only.
   c. Administration: IV, rapidly.
   d. Side effects: hypotension (rarely severe), GI disturbances, angina, atrial and ventricular arrhythmias, palpitations, headache, hyperglycemia, fluid retention due to reabsorption of sodium, propranolol potentiates action.

7. Sodium nitroprusside (Nipride).
   a. Effect: acts on vascular smooth muscle causing peripheral vasodilation. Effect occurs in 2 minutes but is transitory.
   b. Administration: IV infusion.
   c. Side effects: restlessness, agitation, muscle twitching, vomiting, or skin rash.

✦ ACE Inhibitors (Captopril [Capoten], Lotensin, Vasotec, Zestril, Univasc)

A. Action.

1. Effective for heart failure—improves cardiac function.

2. Works by suppressing the renin-angiotensin-aldosterone system.

B. Serious adverse effects have been reported—must be used with discrimination under close medical supervision.

1. Hypotension—especially with first dose.

2. Dry, irritating cough is often present.

3. Swelling of lips, tongue, and glottis may occur.

4. Warnings—proteinuria and agranulocytosis, renal insufficiency.

C. Instruct patient to follow certain protocol when taking an ACE drug.

1. Take medication at same time every day.

2. Move from lying to sitting to standing position slowly.

3. Avoid salt substitutes, which could lead to hyperkalemia (they are high in potassium).

4. Notify physician if cough, fatigue, or nausea develop.

✦ Diuretics

A. Therapeutic use—most diuretics block sodium and chloride reabsorption in ascending loop of Henle and distal tubule of the kidney and decrease ionic exchange of sodium in distal tubule, thereby excreting water.

B. Drugs.

✦ 1. Thiazides and thiazide-like drugs.
   a. Common drugs—chlorothiazide (Diuril), hydrochlorothiazide (Hydrodiuril), chlorthalidone (Hygroton).
   b. Administration—oral and parenteral.
   c. Advantages—potent by mouth; effective antihypertensives.
   d. Disadvantages or side effects—electrolyte imbalance; loss of potassium, hypotension.

✦ 2. Potassium-sparing agents.
   a. Common drugs—spironolactone (Aldactone), triamterene (Dyrenium).
   b. Administration—oral only.
   c. Advantages—conserve potassium.
   d. Disadvantages—usually not effective when used alone (best used with thiazides), and electrolyte imbalance.

✦ 3. Potent loop diuretics—moderate to severe volume overload.
   a. Common preparations—furosemide (Lasix), Bumex, Edecrin, Demadex.
   b. Administration—oral and parenteral.
   c. Advantages—rapid, potent action useful in cases of severe pulmonary edema and refractory edema.
   d. Disadvantages—allergic reactions, severe electrolyte imbalance (potassium and chloride loss), and hypovolemia.

C. Implications for nursing care.

1. Time administration to avoid nocturia and sleep interruption; give oral doses with food to decrease GI side effects.

2. Monitor intake and output.

3. Weigh daily.

4. Observe for postural hypotension.

5. Reduce potassium depletion by providing foods high in potassium (bananas, oranges).

6. Monitor for signs of fluid and electrolyte imbalance—dehydration.

✦ **Beta-Adrenergic Blockers (Propanolol, Lopressor, Inderal)**

A. Action.
1. Block cardiac response to sympathetic stimulation.
2. Pure beta or beta-1–specific action.
3. Carvedilal (alpha and beta blocker for heart failure).

B. Therapeutic effects.
1. Prevent chronic angina; used in unstable angina.
2. Slow heart rate, slow AV conduction, lower blood pressure.
3. Prolong life in postinfarction patients.
4. Prevent sudden death.
5. Improve left ventricular function.

C. Major side effects.
1. Bronchospasm (COPD).
2. Bradyarrhythmias.

Antihyperlipidemic Agents

A. Lipid-lowering compounds for patients with dangerously elevated cholesterol and low-density lipoprotein (LDL).

B. Bile acid sequestrants (Questran).
1. Binds with bile acids in the intestine and excreted in feces resulting in removal of LDL and cholesterol.
2. May interfere with absorption of certain drugs (thiazides, digoxin, beta-adrengic blockers) and fat soluble vitamins.

C. HMG-CoA reductase inhibitors (Mevacor, Pravachol, and Zocor) derived from fungi; Lescol is entirely synthetic; blocks systhesis of cholesterol.

D. Fibric acid derivatives (Atromid, Tricor, Lopid) inhibit liver synthesis of triglycerides and very low-density lipoprotein.

E. Nicotinic acid (niacin) (Nicobid, Niacor) decreases LDL levels and inhibits VLDL production in the liver.

F. Drugs are indicated in addition to diet for patients who have not responded well to nonpharmacologic measures.

✦ **Thrombolytic Agents**

A. Action is to activate formation of plasmin which digests fibrin and dissolves formed blood clots.

B. Stimulate conversion of plasminogen to plasmin (fibrinolysin).

C. Prescribed for acute pulmonary emboli, deep vein thrombosis, arterial thrombosis, and coronary thrombosis.

✦ D. Agents.
1. Streptokinase (Streptase); urokinase.
2. Tissue plasminogen activator (Activase).
3. APSAC, Eminase.
4. Reteplase (Retavase).

E. Major side effects.
1. Bleeding (increased fibrinolytic activity).
2. Ventricular dysrhythmias with coronary thrombosis.
3. Fever up to 100°F.
4. Allergic reactions; rash.

F. Contraindications for use.
1. Recent major surgery, GI bleed.
2. History of CVA.
3. Hepatic or renal disease.
4. Pregnancy.

✦ G. Nursing implementation.
1. Obtain TT, APTT, PT, fibrinogen level, and platelet count.
2. Infuse 250,000 IU over 30 minutes for loading dose.
3. Monitor infusion of 100,000 IU/hr (use controller or pump).
   a. 24 hours for pulmonary embolism.
   b. 24–72 hours for deep vein or arterial thrombosis.
4. Monitor closely for signs of bleeding and blood pressure.

Anticoagulant Drugs (Heparin Sodium, Coumadin, enoxaparin [Lovenox])

✦ A. Heparin sodium, given IV or sub q (inactivated orally).
1. Therapeutic effects.
   a. Blocks conversion of prothrombin to thrombin and fibrinogen to fibrin.
   b. Prolongs clotting time.
2. Uses.
   a. Prophylaxis.
   b. Treatment of thrombi and emboli.
3. Dosage individualized according to patient's partial thromboplastin time.
4. Contraindications.
   a. Bleeding tendency.
   b. Severe liver or kidney disease.
   c. Following brain surgery.
✦ 5. Antagonist.
   a. Protamine sulfate, 1 mg for each 100 U of heparin in last dose, if necessary.
   b. Effective within minutes.
6. Nursing care.
   a. Administer dosage ordered by physician according to patient's partial thromboplastin time (PTT at 50–80 seconds; normal is 39–53 seconds).
   ✦ b. Observe for any signs of bleeding in stools or urine or in emesis; report immediately.
   ✦ c. Utilize subcutaneous injection for administration.
      (1) Use lower abdominal skin area.
      (2) Administer drug at 90-degree angle; do not pull back on plunger.

(3) Do not massage area following injection.

◆ d. Observe for signs of toxicity.
   (1) Bruises or skin discoloration.
   (2) Frequent nosebleeds.
   (3) Hematuria.
   e. Instruct patient about precautions to take and observations to make when discharged.

◆ B. Coumadin, Dicumarol, miradon given orally.
   1. Therapeutic effects.
      a. Decreases prothrombin activity.
      b. Prevents utilization of vitamin K by the liver.
   2. Uses.
      a. Decreases clotting activity.
      b. Takes 24–72 hours for action to develop and continues for 24–72 hours after last dose.
      c. Prothrombin time (PT) kept at 18–30 seconds (normal is 12–14 seconds).
      d. INR kept between 2 and 3.
   3. Antagonist.
      a. Vitamin K—AquaMephyton IM or IV.
      b. Returns to hemostasis within 6 hours.
      c. Blocks action of Coumadin for 1 week.
   4. Nursing care.
      a. Check prothrombin time or INR before giving.
      b. Give at same time each day.
      c. Teach patient to avoid foods high in vitamin K (cabbage, cauliflower, spinach, and leafy vegetables), alcohol, ASA, NSAIDs, and Tylenol.
      d. Encourage patient to wear Med-Alert bracelet.

◆ **Antiarrhythmic Drugs (Quinidine, Pronestyl, Lidocaine, Amiodarone)**

A. Therapeutic effects.
   1. Increases recovery time of atrial and ventricular muscle.
   2. Decreases myocardial excitability.
   3. Increases conduction in cardiac muscle, Purkinje's fibers, and AV junction (exception: lidocaine).
   4. Decreases contractility (exception: lidocaine).
   5. Decreases automaticity.
B. Quinidine.
   1. Uses—atrial fibrillation, atrial flutter, supraventricular and ventricular tachycardia, premature systoles.
   2. Side effects.
      a. Hypersensitivity, thrombocytopenia.
      b. Cinchonism—nausea, vomiting, diarrhea, vertigo, visual disturbances, tinnitus.

   c. Sudden death from ventricular fibrillation.
   d. Congestive heart failure due to negative inotropism.
   e. Conduction disturbances.
C. Procainamide hydrochloride (Pronestyl).
   1. Uses—premature ventricular systoles.
   2. Side effects.
      a. Anorexia, nausea, vomiting, diarrhea.
      b. Systemic lupus erythematosus and agranulocytosis.
      c. Cardiac AV block.
D. Xylocaine (Lidocaine).
   1. Uses—ventricular tachyarrhythmias.
   2. Side effects.
      a. CNS disturbances—drowsiness, paresthesias, slurred speech, blurred vision, seizures, coma.
      b. Cautious use in patients with liver disease or low cardiac output (metabolism of drug slowed).
E. Amiodarone.
   1. Used for life-threatening arrhythmias unresponsive to other agents.
   2. Side effects: visual disturbances, bradycardia, hypotension, liver function abnormality.
   3. Potentiates digitalis toxicity.

◆ **Sympathomimetic Agents**

A. Therapeutic effects.
   1. Epinephrine HCL (Adrenalin): beta and alpha stimulation—increases heart rate and contractility.
   2. Isoproterenol HCL (Isuprel): beta stimulation.
      a. Increases heart rate, contractility, and oxygen consumption.
      b. Decreases peripheral vascular resistance.
      c. Bronchodilator.
   3. Dopamine (Depostat)—precursor of Norepinephrine.
      a. Raises blood pressure.
      b. Increases myocardial contractility.
      c. Increases cardiac output and perfusion.
      d. Dilates renal vessels.
   4. Dobutrex (dobutamine hydrochloride).
      a. Cardiac stimulation, but no real increase in heart rate.
      b. Increases cardiac output.
B. Uses.
   1. Epinephrine (Adrenalin) most commonly used for cardiac arrest.
   2. Isoproterenol (Isuprel).
      a. Cardiogenic shock with high peripheral vascular resistance.
      b. AV block—increases pacemaker automaticity and improves AV conduction.

3. Dopamine (Intropin)—precursor of Norepinephrine.
   a. Cardiogenic shock.
   b. Chronic cardiac failure with congestive heart failure.
4. Dobutrex (dobutamine hydrochloride).
   a. Organic heart disease.
   b. Cardiac surgical procedures.

C. Side effects.
   1. Epinephrine (Adrenalin).
      a. Chest pain, arrhythmias, tachycardia, hypertension.
      b. Hyperglycemia.
   2. Isoproterenol (Isuprel).
      a. Tachyarrhythmias, especially ventricular tachycardia.
      b. Hypotension when hypovolemia is not corrected.
      c. Headache, skin flushing, angina, dizziness, weakness.
   3. Dobutrex (dobutamine hydrochloride).
      a. Arrhythmias, palpitations, increased heart rate.

      b. Angina, chest pain, shortness of breath.
      c. Headache.

Peripheral Vasoconstrictors (Norepinephrine [Levophed], Aramine)

A. Effects.
   1. Alpha-adrenegic stimulation—peripheral vasoconstriction.
   2. Beta stimulation mild.
B. Uses.
   1. Elevates blood pressure.
   2. Used for hypotension, cardiac arrest.
C. Side effects.
   1. Anxiety (mimics reaction to stress), headache.
   2. Hypertension.
   3. Arrhythmias.
D. Nursing implementation.
   1. Carefully monitor blood pressure and vital signs.
   2. Check for IV infiltration—could cause tissue necrosis (central vein use preferred).
   3. Patient teaching.
      a. Recognition of side effects.
      b. Diet—high fiber to reduce constipation.

RESPIRATORY SYSTEM

The respiratory system is a group of related organs that together perform pulmonary ventilation. The act of breathing involves an osmotic and chemical process by which the body takes in oxygen from the atmosphere and gives off end products, mainly carbon dioxide, formed by oxidation in the alveolar tissues.

ANATOMY AND PHYSIOLOGY

Ventilation Tract

Nose
A. Structure.
  1. Septum divides nose into two cavities.
  2. Ciliated mucous membrane lines the cavities.
  3. Four pairs of sinuses drain into nose.
B. Function.
  1. Serves as passage for air.
    a. Filters.
    b. Warms.
    c. Moistens.
  2. Serves as organ of smell.
  3. Aids in phonation.

Pharynx
A. Structure.
  1. Tubelike structure.
  2. Composed of muscle.
  3. Ciliated mucous membrane lines the cavity.
  4. Divides into three areas.
    a. Nasopharynx—contains adenoids.
    b. Oropharynx—contains tonsils.
    c. Laryngopharynx.
B. Function.
  1. Serves as passage for air and food.
  2. Aids in phonation.

Larynx
A. Structure.
  1. Composed largely of cartilage held together by muscles.
  2. Major cartilages.
    a. Thyroid (forms Adam's apple).
    b. Epiglottis.
    c. Cricoid.
  3. Ciliated mucous membrane lines the structure.
  4. Contains vocal cords.
B. Function.
  1. Passage for air.
  2. Produces sound.

Trachea
A. Structure.
  1. Cylindrical structure.
  2. Walls consist of smooth muscle and C-shaped rings of cartilage.
  3. Divides at lower end into two primary bronchi.
B. Function—passage for air.

Pulmonic Organs

Lungs
A. Structure.
  1. Medial surface is roughly concave to allow room for mediastinal structures.
  2. Bronchi enter through slits (hili) in each lung.
  3. Left lung is partially divided by fissures into two lobes (upper and lower).
  4. Right lung is partially divided by fissures into three lobes (upper, middle, and lower).
  5. Visceral pleura covers outer surfaces.
  6. Interior consists of bronchial tree.
B. Function.
  1. Distribute air to alveoli.
  2. Exchange gas between air and blood.

Bronchi
A. Structure.
  1. Right mainstem bronchus (RMSB)—slightly larger and more vertical than left bronchus; most frequent route for aspirated materials.
  2. Left mainstem bronchus (LMSB)—branches off the trachea at a 45-degree angle.
  3. Walls contain incomplete cartilaginous rings at site where they enter lungs.
  4. Ciliated mucous membrane lines the structures.
  5. Primary bronchi divide into smaller branches (secondary bronchi) just past site of lung entry.
  6. Secondary bronchi continue to branch, forming small bronchioles.
  7. Bronchioles subdivide into smaller and smaller tubes and terminate into alveolar ducts and their several alveolar sacs.
B. Function—distribute air to lung's interior.

Alveoli
A. Structure—makes up the walls of alveolar sacs composed of single layer of tissue.
B. Function—gas exchange takes place between air and blood (oxygen and carbon dioxide).
  1. Contains substance known as surfactant.
  2. Keeps alveoli expanded—without surfactant, alveoli would collapse.

Thorax

A. Structure.
  1. The thorax (chest) is divided into three divisions, separated by partitions of pleura.
     a. Pleural divisions—each division occupied by a lung.
     b. Mediastinum—occupied by esophagus, trachea, large blood vessels, and heart.
  2. Pleura.
     a. Parietal layer lines entire thoracic cavity.
        (1) Adheres to internal surface of ribs, superior surface of diaphragm.
        (2) Partitions off mediastinum.
     b. Visceral layer covers outer surface of each lung.
     c. The two layers, separated only by a potential space (pleural space), contain just enough pleural fluid for lubrication.
B. Function—pleura allows for changes in chest size required for inspiration and expiration.

Principles of Pulmonary Ventilation

Respiratory Cycle Mechanics

A. Inspiration—active process.
  1. Diaphragm descends, external intercostal muscles contract.
  2. Chest expands, allowing air volume into the lungs as alveolar pressure decreases.
B. Expiration—passive process.
  1. Diaphragm ascends, external intercostal muscles relax.
  2. Chest becomes smaller, air moves out of lungs.
C. Atmospheric pressure—intrapulmonic pressure.
  1. Air moves into and out of the lungs because of the differences in air pressure inside and outside of the lung. (Atmospheric pressure—760 mm Hg.)
  2. During inspiration, air moves into the lungs. Intrapulmonic pressure (pressure within the lungs) is lower than atmospheric pressure.
  3. During expiration, intrapulmonic pressure is higher than atmospheric pressure.

Exchange Air Volume

A. Total lung capacity (TLC)—total volume of air that is present in the lungs after maximum inspiration.
B. Vital capacity (VC)—volume of air that can be expelled following a maximum inspiration.
C. Tidal volume (TV)—volume of air exhaled after a normal inspiration.
D. Expiratory reserve volume (ERV)—largest additional volume of air that can be forcibly expired after tidal air expiration.
E. Inspiratory reserve volume (IRV)—amount of air that can be forcibly inspired over and above a normal inspiration.
F. Residual volume (RV)—amount of air remaining in lung following maximal expiration.

Exchange of Gases

A. In lungs.
  1. Air and blood exchange gases through membrane of capillaries around alveoli.
  2. Oxygen enters blood from the alveolar air.
  3. Carbon dioxide enters alveolar air from the blood.
B. In tissues.
  1. Takes place between arterial blood flowing through tissue capillaries and cells.
  2. Oxygen diffuses out of the arterial blood into the cells.
  3. Carbon dioxide diffuses out of the cells into the blood.

Transportation of Gases in Blood

A. Oxygen combines with hemoglobin, the means of transportation, in blood to form oxyhemoglobin.
B. Half of the carbon dioxide is carried in the plasma as bicarbonate ions.
C. About one third of blood carbon dioxide combines with the hemoglobin to form carbaminohemoglobin.

Regulation of Respiration

A. Chemoreceptors—cells sensitive to changes in carbon dioxide concentrations in arterial blood.
  1. Above normal range (35–45 mm Hg) concentrations of carbon dioxide stimulate respirations.
  2. Below normal concentrations of carbon dioxide slow respirations.
  3. A decrease in arterial blood pH stimulates respirations.
B. Arterial blood pressure.
  1. A sudden rise in arterial blood pressure results in reflexive slowing of respirations.
  2. A sudden drop in arterial blood pressure results in reflexive increase in rate and depth of respirations.

Surfactant

A. Surface-active material that lines the alveoli and changes the surface tension, depending on the area over which it is spread.
B. Surfactant in the lungs allows the smaller alveoli to have lower surface tension than the larger alveoli.
  1. Results in equal pressures within both and prevents collapse.
  2. Production of surfactant depends on adequate blood supply.

C. Conditions that decrease surfactant.
1. Hypoxia.
2. Oxygen toxicity.
3. Aspiration.
4. Atelectasis.
5. Pulmonary edema.
6. Pulmonary embolus.
7. Mucolytic agents.
8. Hyaline membrane disease.

Compliance

A. Relationship between pressure and volume: elastic resistance, a measure of elasticity of lungs and thorax. This is determined by dividing the tidal volume by peak airway pressure (V_t PAP). Total compliance equals chest wall compliance plus lung compliance.
B. Conditions that decrease chest wall compliance.
1. Obesity—excess fatty tissue over chest wall and abdomen.
2. Kyphoscoliosis—marked resistance to expansion of the chest wall.
3. Scleroderma—expansion of the chest wall limited when the involved skin over the chest wall becomes stiff.
4. Chest wall injury—as in crushing chest wall injuries.
5. Diaphragmatic paralysis—as a result of surgical damage to the phrenic nerve, or disease process involving the diaphragm itself.
C. Conditions that decrease lung compliance.
1. Atelectasis—collapse of the alveoli as a result of obstruction or hypoventilation.
2. Pneumonia—inflammatory process involving the lung tissue.
3. Pulmonary edema—accumulation of fluid in the alveoli.
4. Pleural effusion—accumulation of pleural fluid in the pleural space compressing lung on the affected side.
5. Pulmonary fibrosis—scar tissue replacing necrosed lung tissue as a result of infection.
6. Pneumothorax—air present in the pleural cavity; lung is collapsed as volume of air increases.

DIAGNOSTIC PROCEDURES

✦ A. Pulmonary function tests.
1. Measurement of blood gases.
   a. An effective way to evaluate lung function and lung adequacy.
   b. Measure oxygen tension (arterial) (PaO_2) and carbon dioxide tension (arterial) ($PaCO_2$).

2. Measurement of lung air.
   a. Analyzes physical phenomena involved with the movement of the air in and out of the chest.
      (1) Vital capacity—measurement of the maximum amount of air that can be expired following a maximal inspiration.
      (2) Maximum breathing capacity—measurement of airway resistance within the lungs.
      (3) Timed vital capacity—the pattern of vital capacity as related to time.
   b. Measures the effectiveness of the mechanical processes and blood gases.
B. Chest x-ray.
1. Necessary in the assessment of respiratory disorders.
2. The view may be taken back to front (posteroanterior), side (lateral), or at an angle (oblique).
3. No specific preparation is necessary.
✦ C. Bronchoscopy.
1. A direct visual examination of the trachea, two major bronchi, and multiple smaller bronchi.
2. Flexible, fiberoptic scope (bronchoscope) is passed into the trachea, under local anesthesia.
3. A biopsy of tissue, specimen or sample of secretions can be obtained.
4. Preparation of patient.
   a. NPO 8–12 hours before procedure.
   b. Remove dentures.
   c. Provide mouth care.
   d. Explain process to patient so that he or she can relax and cooperate during procedure.
   e. Place patient supine with neck hyperextended.
5. Postprocedural care.
   a. NPO for several hours, until gag reflex returns.
   b. Encourage patient to expectorate.
   c. Advise patient to smoke and talk as little as possible; procedure may cause throat irritation, hoarseness.
✦ D. Sputum examination.
1. A microscopic examination of the cells of the sputum.
2. Sputum should be raised from deep within the bronchi such as sputum first expectorated in the morning.
3. If culture is to be grown, specimens need to be collected in a sterile container.
4. May require a 24-hour specimen.
5. Patient's mouth should be first washed out to remove food particles.

6. Note color, consistency, odor, and quantity of sputum.

✦ E. Gastric analysis.
1. Laboratory examination of stomach contents may include bronchial secretion the patient previously swallowed.
2. A gastric tube is inserted and stomach contents are aspirated.
3. Patient is NPO 8–12 hours prior to the procedure.

✦ F. Thoracentesis.
1. Removal of fluid from chest cavity.
2. Under local anesthesia an aspiration needle is inserted into the pleura.
3. Purpose is both diagnostic and therapeutic.
4. Nursing care.
  a. Assist patient to proper position.
  b. During procedure, observe patient for change of skin color and for changes in pulse and/or respiratory rate.
  c. After procedure, observe patient for change in respiratory rate and for coughing, expectoration of blood, or blood-tinged sputum.

G. Lung scintigraphy: measures concentration of gamma rays from lung after intake of isotope.

H. Perfusion studies: outline pulmonary vascular structures after intake of radioactive isotopes IV.

I. Biopsy of respiratory tissue.
1. May be done by needle, via bronchoscope, or an open lung procedure biopsy.
2. Nursing care: observe for hemothorax and/or pneumothorax.

✦ J. Tuberculin skin test.
1. Mantoux intradermal test (more reliable).
  a. 0.1 mL tuberculin injected intradermal; intermediate PPD.
  b. Test read 48–72 hours postintradermal wheal production.
  c. Erythema not important.
  d. Area of induration more than 10 mm: indicates positive reaction (patient has had contact with the tubercle bacillus). For HIV or severely immunosuppressed, test is positive if induration is more than 5 mm.
  e. Reactions of 5–9 mm require retest.
2. Tine test.
  a. Not recommended for diagnosis.
  b. Test read on third day.
  c. Mantoux test required if induration more than 2 mm.

✦ K. Arterial blood studies.
1. Arterial blood gases.
  a. Indicate respiratory function by measuring:
    (1) Oxygen (PO_2).
    (2) Carbon dioxide (PCO_2).
    (3) pH.
    (4) Oxygen saturation
    (5) Bicarbonate (HCO_3).
  b. Determine state of acid–base balance.
  c. Reveal the adequacy of the lungs to provide oxygen and to remove carbon dioxide.
  d. Assess degree to which kidneys can maintain a normal pH.
2. Normal arterial values.
  a. Oxygen saturation: 93–98 percent.
  b. PaO_2: 95 mmHg.
  c. Arterial pH: 7.35–7.45 (7.4).
  d. PCO_2: 35–45 mmHg (40).
  e. HCO_3 content: 24–30 mEq (25).
  f. Base excess: –3 to +3 (0).

Respiratory System Assessment

✦ A. Check for airway patency.
1. Clear out secretions.
2. Insert oral airway if necessary.
3. Position patient on side if there is no cervical spine injury.

✦ B. Listen to lung sounds.
1. Absence of breath sounds: indicates lungs not expanding, due to either obstruction or deflation.
2. Rales (crackling sounds): indicate vibrations of fluid in lungs.
3. Rhonchi (coarse sounds): indicate partial obstruction of airway.
4. Decreased breath sounds: indicate poorly ventilated lungs.
5. Detection of bronchial sounds that are deviated from normal position: indicates mediastinal shift due to collapse of lung.

✦ C. Determine level of consciousness; decreased sensorium can indicate hypoxia.

D. Observe sputum or tracheal secretions; bloody sputum can indicate contusions of lung or injury to trachea and other anatomical structures.

E. Evaluate vital signs for temperature, respiratory rate, pulse, and changes in skin color.

F. Evaluate for tightness or fullness in chest.

G. Determine degree of pain patient is experiencing.

H. Assess for respiratory complications.

I. Assess for other system complications. (*See* p. 257.)
1. Evaluate for polycythemia—increase in RBCs as a compensatory response to hypoxemia.
2. Observe for clubbing of fingers. Pathogenesis is not well understood.
3. Evaluate for cor pulmonale—enlargement of the right ventricle as a result of pulmonary arterial hypertension following respiratory pathology.
4. Evaluate for chest pain.
5. Assess for atelectasis.
6. Check for abdominal distention.
7. Assess for hypertension.

RESPIRATORY COMPLICATIONS

Abnormal Breathing Patterns
- Dyspnea—labored or difficult breathing.
- Hyperpnea—abnormal deep breathing.
- Hypopnea—reduced depth of breathing.
- Orthopnea—difficulty breathing in other than upright position.
- Tachypnea—rapid breathing.
- Stridor—noisy respirations as air is forced through a partially obstructed airway.

Cough
- Normally a protective mechanism utilized to keep the tracheobronchial tree free of secretions.
- Common symptom of respiratory disease.

Bronchospasm
- Bronchi narrow and secretions may be retained.
- Condition may lead to infection.
- Hemoptysis—expectoration of blood or blood-tinged sputum.
- ✦ Cyanosis—late sign of hypoxia, due to large amounts of reduced hemoglobin in the blood (PaO_2 of about 50 mm Hg)

Hypoxia (anoxia)—a deficiency of oxygen in body tissues

Hypercapnia
- Occurs when carbon dioxide is retained.
- High levels of oxygen depress and/or paralyze the medullary respiratory center.
- Peripheral chemoreceptors (sensitive to oxygen) become the stimuli for breathing.

Respiratory alkalosis or acidosis.

CHRONIC OBSTRUCTIVE PULMONARY DISEASES (COPD)

Definition: A broad category applied to respiratory disorders that obstruct normal ventilation pathways.

Chronic Asthma

Definition: An obstructive airway disease characterized by recurrent paroxysms of dyspnea with wheezing due to an inherited allergic tendency. More than 14.6 million people in the United States have asthma.

Assessment
A. Assess type of asthma.
   1. Mild intermittent.
   2. Mild persistent.
   3. Moderate persistent.
   4. Severe persistent.
B. Dyspnea, orthopnea.
C. Sense of tightness in the chest; feeling of impending suffocation.
D. A slight dry cough; wheezing.
E. Anxious expression.
F. Perspires freely.

Treatment and Implementation
A. Provide supportive respiratory care.
B. Identify and avoid known triggers for asthma.
C. Avoid aspirin and NSAIDS.
D. Teach peak flow monitoring.
✦ E. Administer drugs.
   1. Beta agonists: epinephrine, albuterol, terbutaline, isoetharine (Bronkosol).
   2. Methylxanthine, aminophylline, and derivatives.
   3. Corticosteroids.
   4. Anticholinergics (atropine).
   5. Mast cell inhibitors (cromolyn sodium).
   6. SRS-A leukotrienes cause airway inflammation; new leukotriene antagonists reduce symptoms dramatically (Accolate, Zyflo, Singulair).
   7. Observe for toxic effects of drugs.
F. Humidify inspired air; provide oxygen therapy only after a long attack and occurrence of cyanosis.
✦ G. Metered dose inhaler (MDI) therapy has advantages over nebulized medications for asthma patients.
H. Manage environment so that it is as free as possible from contributive factors to respiratory infection.
I. Provide rest.
J. Encourage fluids—3000 mL daily.
✦ K. Teaching principles.
   1. Stop smoking—this is the major irritant to the lungs and the major cause of death from cancer.
   2. Avoid irritants or allergens and pollutants when possible.
   3. Avoid high altitudes (where there is less oxygen).
   4. Teach pursed-lip breathing (helps to open airway) and stretching exercises.
   5. Monitor edema in legs and ankles, which may signify right-sided heart failure.

Chronic Bronchitis

✦ *Definition:* The hypersecretion of mucus by the bronchial glands; a chronic or a recurrent respiratory infection often following a long history of bronchial asthma or an acute respiratory infection.

Assessment
✦ A. Cigarette smoking is major cause. Cough is usually the earliest symptom; most marked on arising in the morning and just prior to going to bed.
B. Expectoration of thick, white, stringy mucus.
C. As the disease progresses, the sputum may become purulent, copious, and occasionally streaked with blood.
D. Possible sensation of heaviness in the chest.

E. Characteristic appearance is drawn, anxious, pale, and markedly dyspneic.

F. Speech characterized by short, jerky sentences.

G. Upright position often leaning slightly forward.

H. Distention of veins in neck during expiration.

✦ **Treatment and Implementation**

A. Provide prompt and effective treatment of predisposing factors; good treatment directly related to the control of cigarette smoking and air pollution.

B. Increase pulmonary ventilation by reducing bronchospasms with bronchodilators.

C. Administer expectorants, intermittent antibiotic therapy when infection occurs.

D. Monitor oxygen therapy using COPD precautions.

E. Postural drainage—chest physiotherapy.

F. Force fluids to 3000 mL to dilute secretions.

G. Teach self-care principles (pursed-lip breathing, avoid irritants, yearly flu vaccine, etc.).

Emphysema

✦ *Definition:* The permanent overdistention of the alveoli with resulting destruction of the alveolar walls. (Emphysema is a Greek word meaning "overinflated.")

✦ **Assessment**

A. Cough—may be present many years before dyspnea.

B. Dyspnea—chief complaint.

C. Increased sputum production.

D. Weight loss.

E. Hypoxia, hypercapnia.

F. Barrel chest.

G. Prolonged expiratory phase.

H. Wheezes, forced expiratory rhonchi.

I. Complications.
   1. Pulmonary hypertension.
   2. Right-sided heart failure.
   3. Spontaneous pneumothorax.
   4. Acute respiratory failure.
   5. Peptic ulcer disease, GERD.

Implementation

A. Monitor for signs of impending hypoxia.

B. Monitor for alterations in lung sounds.

C. Teach pursed-lip breathing exercises.

✦ D. Administer low concentration oxygen. Usually 2 L/min.

E. Monitor for signs of carbon dioxide narcosis.

✦ F. Monitor medications.
   1. Inhaled bronchodilators to dilate airways and improve gas exchange (beta-agonists such as Proventil, Ventolin, and Alupent).
   2. Systemic corticosteroids—controversial, used when bronchodilators are unsuccessful or in an acute attack.

✦ G. Provide hydration.
   1. Necessary to liquefy secretions present, or to prevent formation of thick, tenacious secretions.
   2. Hydration methods.
      a. Oral intake of fluids.
      b. IV administration of fluids.
      c. Humidification to tracheobronchial tree.
      d. Metered dose inhaler therapy.

H. Implications of humidification and aerosol therapy.
   1. Relief of bronchospasm and mucosal edema.
   2. Mobilization of secretions.

✦ I. Provide chest physiotherapy.
   1. Postural drainage used to promote gravitational drainage.
   2. Percussion and vibration is adjunct to postural drainage.
   3. Deep breathing and coughing.

Specialized Nursing Care

✦ **Chronic Pulmonary Disease**

A. When progress is slow, be patient, give attention to detail, and maintain interest and hope.

B. Give instruction for general health care.
   1. Principles of optimum nutrition for patient and family.
   2. A change in lifestyle and a realistic plan for adequate rest, recreation, and suitable work.
   3. The value of treatment program.
   4. Instructions concerning medications, breathing exercises, and avoidance of infection.

C. Observe and record symptoms.
   1. Amount of coughing, amount and character of sputum, degree of dyspnea and/or wheezing.
   2. Color, weight, and appetite of patient.
   3. Attitudes and sense of well-being.
   4. Complications and progression of illness.

D. Help adjust activities for the patient within framework of his or her tolerance.

✦ E. Positions for chest physiotherapy.
   ❖ **PROCEDURE** ❖
   1. To affect RUL and LUL, place patient upright.
   2. To affect RML, position patient on left side with head slanted down, right shoulder one-quarter turn onto pillow. Cup anteriorly over left nipple.
   3. To affect lingula LL, position patient on right side with head slanted down, left shoulder one-quarter turn onto pillow. Cup anteriorly over right nipple.
   4. To affect RLL and LLL, place patient in Trendelenburg's position, alternating sides, or prone.

✦ **Hypoxia**

A. Early symptoms.
  1. Restlessness.
  2. Headache.
  3. Visual disturbances.
  4. Slight confusion.
  5. Hyperventilation.
  6. Tachycardia.
  7. Mild hypertension.
  8. Dyspnea.
  9. Decreased pulse oximetry.
B. Advanced symptoms.
  1. Hypotension.
  2. Bradycardia.
  3. Metabolic acidosis (production of lactic acid).
  4. Cyanosis.
C. Chronic hypoxia.
  1. Polycythemia.
  2. Clubbing of fingers and toes.
  3. Thrombosis.

✦ **Administration of Oxygen   ❖ PROCEDURE ❖**

A. Conditions requiring oxygen therapy.
  1. Atmosphere hypoxia: oxygen therapy will correct depressed level of oxygen.
  2. Hypoventilation hypoxia: 100 percent oxygen will yield five times more oxygen into the alveoli than normal air.
B. Conditions where oxygen therapy is not corrective.
  1. Hypoxia caused by anemia, carbon monoxide poisoning, or abnormal hemoglobin transport.
  2. Inadequate tissue use of oxygen (cyanide poisoning).
  3. Chronic obstructive lung disease requires that oxygen be used with caution since oxygen could suppress respiratory drive and result in respiratory arrest.
C. Properties of oxygen.
  1. Colorless, odorless, and tasteless gas.
  2. Supports combustion.
✦ D. Oxygen delivery devices.
  1. Simple face mask.
    a. Requires fairly high oxygen flow to prevent rebreathing of carbon dioxide.
    b. FIO_2 is 35–60 percent and oxygen flow is 8–12L.
  2. Mask with reservoir bag.
    a. Partial rebreather—higher FIO_2 delivered because of reservoir—40–60 percent at 6–10 L.
    b. Nonrebreather—FIO_2 60–100 percent, with flow of 6–15 L.
    c. At flow less than 6 percent risk of rebreathing carbon dioxide increases.
  3. Venturi mask.
    a. Produces oxygen concentration of 24–50 percent at 2–4 to 6–8 L.

    b. Delivers fixed or predicted FIO_2.
    c. Used for COPD patients when accurate FIO_2 is necessary.
  4. Nasal prongs and cannula—produces oxygen concentration of 24–44 percent.
    a. Flow is 1–2 to 5–6 L.
    b. Fit small prongs into each nostril.
    c. Remove and clean every 8 hours.
    d. Easily tolerated by patients.
  5. Face tent.
    a. Produces oxygen concentration of 28–100 percent at oxygen flow 8–10 L.
    b. Well tolerated by patients.
    c. Convenient for providing humidified air.
  6. Intratracheal oxygen device used for long-term therapy.
✦ E. Side effects of oxygen therapy.
  1. Atelectasis.
    a. Nitrogen is washed out of the lungs when a high FIO_2 is delivered to patient.
    b. In alveoli free of nitrogen, oxygen diffuses out of the alveoli into the blood faster than ventilation brings oxygen into the alveoli.
    c. This results in a collapse (atelectasis) of the affected alveoli.
  2. Pulmonary oxygen toxicity.
    a. High FIO_2 delivered over a long period of time (48 hours) results in destruction of the pulmonary capillaries and lung tissue.
    b. The clinical picture resembles that of pulmonary edema.
  3. Retrolental fibroplasia.
    a. Blindness resulting from high FIO_2 delivered to premature infants.
    b. This condition is seen in prolonged FIO_2 of 100 percent when high levels of oxygen not needed.
  4. Carbon dioxide narcosis.
    a. Carbon dioxide narcosis can develop if hypoxic drive is removed by administering FIO_2 to return the arterial PO_2 to normal range.
    b. Symptoms of carbon dioxide narcosis.
      (1) Decreased mentation..
      (2) Flushed, pink skin.
      (3) Flaccid (sometimes twitching) extremities.
      (4) Shallow breathing.
      (5) Respiratory arrest.

Implementation

A. Check equipment.
  1. Eliminate kinks in tubing.
  2. Maintain proper positioning.

3. Check water supply in humidification bottle.

4. Adjust to proper liter flow.

B. Maintain safety measures.

1. No smoking or fire of any kind.

2. No materials that produce static electricity.

3. No electrical equipment; however, some hospital equipment may be safely used.

C. Monitoring a patient with oxygen.

❖ **PROCEDURE** ❖

✦ 1. Check order for type of therapy, use of catheter or cannula, and desired liter flow.

2. Place patient in semi- or high-Fowler's position to ensure adequate lung expansion.

3. Turn and reposition patient frequently to prevent pressure ulcers.

4. Encourage deep breathing and coughing exercises unless directed otherwise.

5. Ensure adequate hydration, especially if secretions are thick and tenacious.

6. Assess patient's progress by frequently checking vital signs, color, and level of consciousness.

7. Remain with patients who are frightened or anxious until they feel secure.

8. Use oxygen very conservatively on anyone with chronic lung disease—high levels of oxygen will knock out carbon dioxide center and lead to respiratory arrest.

   a. Ventilatory drive is hypoxemic.

   b. Start oxygen at 2 L/min.

✦ D. Using an oxygen analyzer.

❖ **PROCEDURE** ❖

1. Calibrate analyzer with room atmosphere prior to each reading.

2. Open tubing to the air, and compress two full times to fill analyzer.

3. Depress button. Analyzer should read 20 percent for room air. Adjust dial as necessary to obtain this reading.

4. Place tubing close to patient's nose.

5. Compress bulb three to six times, depress button, and read findings.

6. Based on reading, adjust oxygen flow.

7. Check analyzer with 100 percent oxygen at least one time per day.

✦ E. Using pulse oximetry.

1. Allows for continual monitoring of arterial blood gas (ABGs)—percent of hemoglobin oxygen saturation (SaO_2).

2. Sensor is applied to skin (noninvasive) and photodetector registers light passing through vascular bed.

3. Oxygen saturation level can be read on digital monitor.

4. Rotate site of clip-on probe every 4 hours and disposable probes every 24 hours.

ACUTE PULMONARY DISEASES

Common Cold (Coryza)

Definition: An infectious viral disease of the upper respiratory tract. It has a duration of 4–14 days and is endemic throughout the world.

Assessment

A. Sneezing.

B. Chills and slight fever.

C. Headache.

D. Watery eyes.

E. Dry, scratchy, sore throat.

F. Copious nasal discharge.

Treatment and Implementation

A. Encourage bedrest or extra sleep.

B. Advise avoidance of contact with others.

C. Force fluids.

D. ASA (aspirin) to relieve discomforts.

E. Instruct patient in proper use of tissues and preventive measures for spread of infection.

Pneumonia

Definition: Acute inflammation of the lungs due to infection caused by virus, bacteria, or fungus. Inflammation leads to replacement of air in the alveolar sacs by fluid or tissue and lung consolidation.

✦ **Characteristics**

A. Community acquired pneumonia.

1. Typical pneumonia.

   a. Bacterial pneumonia caused by *Streptococcus pneumoniae*.

   b. Communicable—most often young males are affected.

   c. *Haemophilus influenzae* is next most common organism.

✦ 2. Atypical pneumonia.

   a. Known etiology—fungus, virus, mycoplasma, rickettsial, chlamydia.

   b. More gradual onset.

B. Hospital acquired pneumonia (HAP)—leading cause of mortality from nosocomial infections. (*See* Infection Control chapter.)

1. Occurs 48 hours after hospitalization.

2. Common organisms are *Pseudomonas, Enterbacter, Staphylococcus aureus.*

C. Aspiration pneumonia—aspiration of material into mouth, then trachea and lungs.

D. Opportunistic pneumonia—patients with altered immune response very susceptible to respiratory infections.

Assessment

A. Complaint of tightness or fullness in chest.

B. Cough, dyspnea, or shortness of breath.

C. Increased vital signs, particularly temperature and respiratory rate.

D. Restlessness, fever, chills, diaphoresis.

Treatment and Implementation

✦ A. Administer antibiotics—given for 10–14 days (usually penicillin G IV, Bactrin, Vancomycin, Cephalosporin).

✦ B. Administer oxygen therapy according to O_2 saturation and ABGs.

C. Monitor IVs or force fluids to 3000 mL.

D. Keep patient ambulatory, if possible, or change position frequently if on bedrest. Elevate head of bed 30°.

E. Monitor vital signs.

F. Obtain throat, sputum, or blood cultures as ordered.

G. Monitor urinary output.

H. Check frequency of bowel movement.

I. Isolate patient if required.

J. Encourage expectoration.

Acute Respiratory Distress Syndrome (ARDS)

Definition: Sudden progressive form of acute respiratory failure from damaged alveolar-capillary membranes which have increased permeability.

Characteristics

A. Mortality rate is 50 percent.

B. Conditions that predispose to ARDS: aspiration, pneumonia, chest trauma, embolism and oxygen toxicity.

Assessment

A. Dyspnea, cough; shallow, increased respirations.

B. Cyanosis, hypoxemia.

C. Use of accessory muscles for breathing.

D. Decreased breath sounds, restlessness.

Treatment and Implementation

A. Oxygen therapy—may involve intubation and ventilation.

B. Prone positioning to increase PaO_2.

C. Monitor ABGs.

D. Maintain fluid balance.

Legionnaires' Disease

✦ *Definition:* An acute respiratory infection caused by gram-negative bacteria. The name was derived from an outbreak of the disease in Philadelphia in 1976 when members of the American Legion were attending a convention.

Assessment

A. The lungs are the organs most targeted by the bacteria.

   1. Primary entry into the body is through the lungs from air conditioners and cooling towers.

   2. The organisms are in infected water.

B. Early symptoms.

   1. Malaise.

   2. Mild headache.

   3. Dry cough.

C. Later symptoms.

   1. Fever and chills—unremitting until therapy.

   2. Other symptoms may be pleuritic pain, confusion, and impaired renal function.

Implementation

A. Diagnosis made from specific serum antibodies or by culture.

B. Monitor antibiotic therapy—erythromycin is drug of choice.

C. Nursing care is the same as for pneumonia.

Atelectasis

✦ A. Collapse of pulmonary alveoli, caused by mucous plug or inadequate ventilation.

B. May be diffuse and involve a segment, a lobe, or entire lung.

✦ Assessment

A. Asymmetrical chest movement.

B. Decreased or absent breath sounds over affected area.

C. Shortness of breath leading to cyanosis.

D. Painful respirations.

E. Increased vital signs: temperature (102°F), respiration, pulse.

F. Anxiety and restlessness.

Treatment and Implementation

✦ A. Preventive postoperatively.

   1. Turn every 30 minutes for patient at risk.

   2. Deep breathe and cough.

   3. Ambulate as soon as possible.

   4. Medicate to reduce pain.

B. Administer oxygen as ordered.

C. Monitor bronchodilators nebulized through IPPB.

Pleurisy

✦ *Definition:* Inflammation of the pleura that is usually a complication of pulmonary diseases.

Types

A. Acute fibrinous (dry pleurisy)—only small amounts of exudate are formed during the inflammatory process.

B. Pleurisy with effusion—large amounts of fluid are secreted and collect in the space between the pleural layers.

Assessment

A. Very sharp pain during respiration.
B. Pain gradually subsides as fluid is formed in pleural space.
C. Dry cough.
D. Fatigue, malaise.
E. Possible shortness of breath.
F. Tachycardia.

✦ Treatment and Implementation

A. Thoracentesis performed to remove fluid if condition is severe—relieves pressure by draining excess fluid.
B. Encourage bedrest.
C. Ventilate room well but maintain warmth.
D. Encourage coughing.
E. Position patient on side of the effusion.
F. Apply heat to painful area.
G. Monitor oxygen, maintain high-Fowler's position.

Influenza

Definition: Infectious epidemic disease of short duration that is caused by a virus.

Assessment

A. Sudden onset with variable individual symptoms.
B. Chills, high fever.
C. Severe headache, muscular aches.
D. Anorexia, weakness, apathy.
E. Sneezing, dry cough.
F. Sore throat, nasal discharge.

Treatment and Implementation

✦ A. Administer ASA for muscle aches and headache (unless patient is a child—then give Tylenol to prevent Reyes syndrome), and codeine to control cough.
B. Cool vapor steam inhalation.
C. Encourage bedrest.
D. Ventilate room well.
E. Take TPR every 4 hours during temperature elevation.
F. Provide large amounts of fluid.

CHRONIC LUNG CONDITIONS

Pulmonary Tuberculosis (TB)

Definition: An infectious disease of the parenchyma of the lung, bronchi, bronchioles, alveoli, pleurae, and bronchopulmonary lymph nodes that is characterized by the formation of tubercles. It is caused by the organism *Mycobacterium tuberculosis* (Koch's bacillus).

It is acquired by inhalation of disseminated air droplets of excretions from the nose, mouth, throat, and lungs of infected individuals.

Characteristics

A. Pathophysiology.
  1. Inhaled airborne droplets containing the bacteria infect the alveoli that become the focus of infection. Transmission requires close, frequent or prolonged exposure.
  2. After entrance of tubercle bacilli, the body attempts to wall off the organism by phagocytosis and lymphocytosis.
  3. Macrophages surround the bacilli and form tubercles.
  4. Tubercles go through the process of caseation—a necrotic process. (Cells become an amorphous cheeselike mass and may be encapsulated to form a nodule.)
  5. Caseous nodule erodes and sputum is released leaving an air-filled cavity.
  6. Initial lesion may disseminate by extension, via bloodstream or lymph system, and through bronchi.
✦ B. Diagnostic findings.
  1. Early AM sputum smear and culture acid-fast bacillus.
  2. Chest x-ray and bronchoscopy.
  3. Increased WBC and ESR.
  4. Mantoux skin test.

✦ Assessment

A. Insidious onset, early symptoms mild and non-specific.
B. Fatigue, malaise.
C. Anorexia, weight loss.
D. Elevated temperature, particularly in the late afternoon and evening.
E. Night sweats.
F. Initial nonproductive cough that later becomes productive of mucopurulent and blood-streaked sputum.
G. Hemoptysis (expectoration of blood from respiratory tract or lungs).
✦ H. Mantoux skin test: positive.
  1. PPD tuberculin injected intradermal.
  2. Test read in 48–72 hours. Induration of 10 mm or more means patient has had contact with the disease recently or in the past, or has recently been vaccinated with BCG.

✦ Treatment and Implementation

A. Maintain respiratory precautions.
  1. Patient not considered infectious 2–3 weeks after starting drug therapy.
  2. Teach patient how to prevent spread of disease.
B. Administer medications in single daily dose and on time—more effective.

C. Current drug regimen.
  1. First-line TB drugs: isoniazid (300 mg daily), INH, pyrazinamide is added for the initial 2 months, as well as rifampin (600 mg daily), RIF, followed by 4 months of INH and RIF.
  2. Ethambutol (15 mg/kg daily) and streptomycin (500 mg daily) added for 1–3 weeks.
  3. Six months of drug therapy is usually sufficient to kill tubercle bacilli.
  4. Second-line drugs used for resistant patients: capreomycin, kanamycin, para-aminosalicylic acid, etc.
D. Sputum smears obtained every 2–4 weeks until negative (usually 3–5 months).
E. Chemoprophylaxis—isoniazid and vitamin B_6 therapy for 6 months.
F. Compliance is major problem in eliminating TB—work with patient to adhere to drug regimen.
  1. Directly observed therapy (DOT) is observing every dose to be sure it is ingested.
  2. Continues for entire course of treatment.
G. Provide well-balanced diet—high protein, high carbohydrate, high vitamin B_6.

Cancer of the Lung

Definition: Pulmonary tumors are either primary or metastatic and interrupt the normal physiological functions of the lung.

Characteristics
A. Classification of lung cancer is designated by anatomic location or by histological pattern.
  1. Anatomic classification.
    a. Central lesions involve the tracheobronchial tube up to the distal bronchi.
    b. Peripheral lesions extend from the distal bronchi and include the bronchioles.
  2. Four histologic types.
    a. Squamous cell (epidermoid).
      (1) Most frequent lung lesions.
      (2) Affects more men than women.
      (3) Associated with cigarette smoking.
      (4) Lesion usually starts in bronchial area and extends.
      (5) Metastasis not usually a rapid process.
    b. Adenocarcinoma.
      (1) Usually develops in peripheral tissue (smaller bronchi).
      (2) Metastasizes by blood route.
      (3) May be associated with focal lung scars.
      (4) Affects more women than men.
    c. Small cell anaplastic or oat cell carcinoma.
      (1) Aggressive and spreads bilaterally.
      (2) Usually spreads to distant sites.
    d. Large cell (undifferentiated) carcinoma—usually spreads through the bloodstream; highly correlated with smoking.
B. Detection—pulmonary lesions are not usually detected by physical exam, and symptoms do not occur until process is extensive. Chest x-ray, CT scan, and MRI are very helpful in diagnosis.

Assessment
A. Pulmonary symptoms.
  1. Persistent cough (most common sign).
  2. Dyspnea.
  3. Bloody sputum.
  4. Long-term pulmonary infection.
  5. Atelectasis.
  6. Bronchiectasis.
  7. Chest pain.
  8. Chills, fever.
B. Systemic symptoms.
  1. Weakness.
  2. Weight loss.
  3. Anemia.
  4. Anorexia.
  5. Metabolic syndromes.
    a. Hypercalcemia.
    b. Inappropriate ADH.
    c. Cushing's syndrome.
    d. Gynecomastia.
  6. Neuromuscular changes.
    a. Peripheral neuropathy.
    b. Corticocerebellar degeneration.
  7. Connective tissue abnormalities.
    a. Clubbing.
    b. Arthralgias.
  8. Dermatologic abnormalities.
  9. Vascular changes.

TREATMENT

Diagnostic Evaluation
- Chest x-ray—a negative film does not rule out cancer
- Cytologic examination of sputum—to detect malignant cells
- Bronchoscopy—view of tracheobroncial tree; to stage cancer
- Percutaneious fine-needle aspiration—tissue for diagnosis
- Bone scan or bone marrow for metastasis; computed tomography may show primary tumor and metastasis
- Mediastinoscopy—examination of lymph nodes through a small incision over sternal notch

Management
- Surgery for localized tumors (Stage I and II)
- Radiation therapy
- Chemotherapy with multiple drugs (cisplatin and topoisomerase inhibitors)

◆ **Treatment and Implementation**
A. Comprehensive, supportive care of patient in the preoperative and postoperative state. (*See* section on care of the operative patient.)
B. Give appropriate information to patient to allay anxiety and clarify expectations.
C. Instruct patient in postoperative procedures to minimize complications.
D. Give psychological support.

CHEST INJURIES

Emergency Assessment of Respiratory Function

◆ A. Check for airway patency and ventilation.
B. Inspect thoracic cage for injury.
1. Inspect for contusions, abrasions, and deep open wounds.
2. Watch for movement of chest; asymmetrical movement indicates tension pneumothorax, hemothorax, fractured ribs, and/or flail chest.
C. Observe color; cyanosis indicates decreased oxygenation.
D. Observe type of breathing; stertorous breathing usually indicates obstructed respiration.
◆ E. Listen to lung sounds.
1. Absence of breath sounds indicates lungs not expanding, due to either obstruction or deflation.
2. *Crackles* or *rales* (crackling sounds) are produced by vibrations of fluid and indicate fluid in lungs.
3. *Rhonchi* (coarse rattlings) indicate partial obstruction of airway.
4. Decreased breath sounds indicate poorly ventilated lungs.
5. Bronchial sounds, deviated from normal position, indicate mediastinal shift due to collapse of lung.
F. Determine level of consciousness; decreased sensorium may indicate hypoxia.
G. Observe sputum or tracheal secretions; bloody sputum may indicate contusions of lung or injury to trachea and other anatomical structures.

Emergency Implementation

A. Take brief history from patient if feasible (or individual accompanying patient) to aid in total evaluation of his or her condition.
B. Assist with electrocardiogram to establish if there is associated cardiac damage.
◆ C. Maintain patent airway.
1. Place hand over nose and mouth to detect breathing; maintain adequate ventilation.

2. Clear out secretions; suction.
3. Insert either oral airway or endotracheal tube as necessary.
D. Position patient on side if no spinal injury.
◆ E. Seal off open chest wound immediately with pressure dressing to prevent air from entering thoracic cavity.
F. Maintain fluid and electrolyte balance.
1. When replacing blood and fluid loss, watch carefully for fluid overload as it can lead to pulmonary edema.
2. Record intake and output.
G. Maintain acid–base balance; assist with frequent blood gas determination as acid–base imbalances occur readily with compromised respirations or with mechanical ventilation.
H. Provide for relief of pain.
1. Use analgesics with caution as they depress respirations. (Demerol is rarely used now due to CNS neurotoxic effects.)
2. Morphine sulfate and other opioids can be used with careful monitoring
3. Nerve block used as necessary.

Open Wounds of the Chest

Pathophysiology
A. Air that enters the pleural cavity from the atmosphere causes collapse of lung.
B. Air entering and leaving the wound during inspiration and expiration can be detected.
C. Intrapleural negative pressure is lost, thereby embarrassing respirations. If not corrected promptly, this leads to hypoxia and death.

Implementation
A. Apply nonporous dressing to wound, taped on 3 sides to allow vent and prevent pneumothorax.
B. Place patient on assisted ventilation if necessary.
C. Prepare for insertion of chest tubes.
D. Place patient in high-Fowler's position (unless contraindicated) to help provide adequate ventilation.

Hemothorax or Pneumothorax

◆ *Definition:*   *Hemothorax* is an accumulation of blood within the pleural space. *Pneumothorax* is an accumulation of air within the pleural space. The blood or air accumulation builds up positive pressure in the pleural space and collapses the lung. *See* Figure 10-8.

Assessment
A. Sharp, sudden chest pain.
B. Decreased breath sounds.
C. Tracheal shift to unaffected side.
D. Dyspnea and respiratory embarrassment.
E. Hypotension, hypovolemic shock, tachycardia.

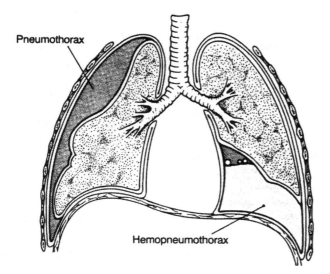

Fig.10-8

F. Elevated temperature, diaphoresis.
G. Asymmetrical expansion of the chest.

◆ **Treatment and Implementation**
A. A large bore needle may be inserted into the second intercostal space, midclavicular line, followed by aspiration of the fluid or air by means of a thoracentesis (emergency treatment).
B. Chest tubes may be inserted and connected to closed-chest drainage.
C. Observe vital signs continuously for shock and cardiac failure complications.
D. Assist patient to semi- or high-Fowler's position.
E. Reassure patient, who will be anxious.

Fractured Ribs

Definition: Fracture varies from simple to severe multiple breaks with flail chest and internal injuries; rib fracture is the most common chest injury.

Assessment
A. Pain and tenderness over fracture area especially on inspiration.
B. Bruises at injury site.
C. Respiratory distress resulting from bone splinters that have punctured lung, causing pneumothorax.
D. Shallow respirations, from splinting of chest, can cause a reduction in lung compliance as well as respiratory acidosis.

Treatment and Implementation
A. Decrease pain to promote chest expansion. Narcotics used with caution due to respiratory depression.
B. Encourage deep breathing and coughing to prevent respiratory complications such as atelectasis and pneumonia.

C. Observe for signs of hemorrhage and shock.
D. Intercostal nerve block is administered, if necessary, to decrease pain.

Flail Chest

◆ *Definition:* Unstable chest wall with respiratory impairment resulting from multiple rib fractures.

Assessment
A. Pain.
B. Dyspnea leading to cyanosis.
C. Detached position of flail chest moving in opposition to other areas of chest cage and lung.
   1. On inspiration, the affected chest area is depressed; on expiration, it is bulging outward.
   2. Opposing chest movement causes poor expansion of lungs and leads to carbon dioxide retention and respiratory acidosis.
D. Inability to cough effectively, which leads to accumulation of fluids and respiratory complications such as pneumonia and atelectasis.
E. Cardiac failure due to impaired filling of blood to the right side of the heart caused by the high venous pressure built up by paradoxical breathing.
F. Rapid, shallow, and noisy respirations.

◆ **Treatment and Implementation**
A. Progressive respiratory failure is treated with intubation and mechanical ventilation.
B. Positive end expiratory pressure (PEEP) used to improve oxygenation.
C. Suction as needed to prevent respiratory complications.
D. Pain medication as ordered.
E. Observe for signs of shock and hemorrhage. For patient on ventilator, use nasogastric tube to prevent abdominal distention and emesis, which can lead to aspiration.
F. Assist patient not on mechanical ventilator.
   1. Encourage turning, coughing, and hyperventilating every hour.
   2. Administer oxygen.
   3. Incentive spirometry.
   4. Suction as needed.

RESPIRATORY TRACT SURGICAL PROCEDURES

Submucous Resection (SMR)

Definition: Removal of part of deflected nasal septum.

Procedure
A. Lay back flap of mucous membrane.
B. Excise portion of septum.
C. Rationale.

1. Restore normal breathing space.
2. Permit more adequate sinus drainage.

Treatment and Implementation
A. Provide routine postoperative care.
B. Observe respiration.
C. Pack nasal cavity.
D. Apply mustache dressing.

Laryngectomy

◆ *Definition:*   Partial or total removal of larynx (epiglottis, thyroid cartilage, hyoid bone, cricoid cartilage, and part of trachea); may sometimes include removal of neck tissue.

Procedure
A. Bring out stump of trachea and suture to neck skin.
B. Close portion of pharynx.
   1. Procedure is permanent.
   2. Breathing through nose is eliminated.
C. If neck tissue and lymph nodes involved, radical neck resection performed.
D. Rationale: removal of benign or malignant tissue, tumors, or lymph nodes, if involved.

◆ Treatment and Implementation
A. Suction frequently with sterile technique until area has healed; then use clean technique.
B. Observe for hemorrhage from surgical site.
C. Instruct patient regarding means for communication.
   1. Patient will not be able to speak immediately after surgery.
   2. Inform patient of available speech rehabilitation after healing has occurred.
D. Feed through nasogastric tube.
E. Encourage normal eating patterns after healing has occurred.
F. Instruct patient how to care for opening.
G. Possibly refer patient to the Lost Cord Club.

Tracheostomy

Definition: Creation of an external opening into the trachea for insertion of a breathing tube.

Characteristics
A. Bypasses upper airway obstruction.
B. Facilitates removal of secretions.
C. Permits long-term mechanical ventilation.
D. Use as emergency measure for unconscious patients.

Procedure
A. Position patient so trachea is prominent.
B. Midline incision for tubal insertion.

Treatment and Implementation
◆ A. Care for and maintain cuffed tracheostomy tube.
   ❖ **PROCEDURE** ❖
   1. Deflating tracheal cuff is no longer a routine procedure.
   2. Hyperoxygenate patient before and after cuff is deflated with Ambu bag.
   3. Suction airway before deflating or inflating cuff.
      a. Always apply oral or nasal suction first, so that when cuff is deflated, secretions will not fall into lung from area above cuff.
      b. Catheter must be changed before tracheostomy suctioning.
   4. Humidification with tracheostomy mist mask if patient not on ventilator.
B. Observe for hemorrhage from tracheostomy site.
C. Change dressings (nonraveling type) and cleanse surrounding area with hydrogen peroxide at least every 4 hours.
◆ D. Care for and maintain tracheostomy tube.
   1. Removal of inner cannula for soaking in hydrogen peroxide solution to loosen mucus accumulation.
   2. Cleansing of inner and outer aspects of tube with brush.
   3. Sterile saline or water rinse; shake to dry.
   4. Suction of outer cannula before reinsertion.

THORACIC CAVITY SURGICAL PROCEDURES

Types of Procedures
A. Exploratory thoracotomy is an incision of the thoracic wall for locating bleeding, injuries, and/or tumors.
B. Thoracoplasty is the removal of ribs or portions of ribs to reduce the size of the thoracic space.
C. Pneumonectomy is the removal of entire lung.
D. Lobectomy is the removal of a lobe of the lung.
E. Segmented resection is the removal of one or more segments of the lung.
F. Wedge resection is the removal of a small, localized area of disease near the surface of the lung.

◆ Postoperative Implementation
A. Employ closed chest suction for all surgeries except pneumonectomy.
   1. In pneumonectomy, it is desirable that the fluid accumulate in empty thoracic space.
   2. Eventually the thoracic space fills with serous exudate, which consolidates, preventing extensive mediastinal shifts.

B. Maintain patent chest tube; drain by chest tube stripping (per facility protocol and/or physician's orders).

C. Maintain respiratory function—auscultate lungs.
   1. Encourage patient to turn, cough, and deep breathe.
   2. Suction if necessary.
   3. Oxygen therapy.
   4. Incentive spirometry.
   5. Mechanical ventilation if necessary.
   6. Observe for complications.

D. Ambulate patient to enhance adequate ventilation and prevent postoperative complications.

E. Provide range-of-motion exercises to all extremities for promotion of adequate circulation.

F. Monitor for signs of increased central venous pressure, which indicates impaired venous return to heart.

✦ G. Positioning of patient.
   1. Semi-Fowler's position to facilitate lung expansion when vital signs are stable.
   2. Specific positions that require readjustment every 1–2 hours.
      a. Pneumonectomy.
         (1) Position on operated side for back care only.
         (2) Position on back or unoperated side only. (Some physicians will allow positioning on either side after 24 hours.)
      b. Segmental resection or wedge resection.
         (1) Position on back or unoperated side.
         (2) Position enhances expansion of remaining pulmonary tissue.
      c. Lobectomy.
         (1) Turn to either side.
         (2) Expands lung tissue on both sides.

H. Encourage postoperative arm and shoulder exercises.
   1. Affected arm should be put through both active and passive range of motion every 4 hours.
   2. Exercises should start within 4 hours after surgery when patient has returned to room.
   3. Exercising prevents formation of adhesions.

Postoperative Complications

Respiratory Complications
✦ A. Causes.
   1. Inadequate ventilation.
   2. Airway obstructed by accumulation of secretion.
   3. Atelectasis (collapsed or airless lung) from underexpansion of lungs and anesthetic agents during surgery.
   4. Hypoventilation and carbon dioxide build-up from incisional splinting as a result of pain.

   5. Depression of CNS from overuse of medications.

B. Tension pneumothorax.
   1. Air leak through pleural incision lines.
   2. Mediastinal shift can occur.

C. Pulmonary embolism.

D. Bronchopulmonary fistula.
   1. Subcutaneous emphysema from escape of air into pleural space, which is then forced into subcutaneous tissue around incision.
   2. Inadequate closure of bronchus during resection.
   3. Alveolar or bronchiolar tears in surface of lung (particularly following pneumonectomy).

E. Atelectasis and/or pneumonia from airway obstruction or as result of anesthesia.

F. Possible respiratory arrest.

Circulatory Complications
A. Hypovolemia from loss of fluid or blood; can result in cardiac arrest.

B. Arrhythmias from underlying myocardial disease; can result in cardiac arrest.

C. Pulmonary edema from fluid overload of circulatory system.

TREATMENT FOR TRAUMATIC INJURY

Chest Tube Management

General Principles
A. Purpose is the removal of air and serosanguineous fluid from pleural space (following thoracic surgery) and to restore normal intrapleural pressure so lungs can re-expand.

B. Tubes are placed in pleural cavity and attached to water seal suction.

✦ C. Tubes are attached to water seal suction to maintain closed system.
   1. All connectors are taped.
   2. Bottle stoppers should fit tightly.
   3. Bottles kept below level of bed.
   4. Suction level maintained where ordered (be sure that bubbling is not excessive in the pressure-regulating bottle).
   5. Water level maintained in bottle.

✦ D. Mechanics of system.
   1. Used after some intrathoracic procedures.
   2. Chest tubes placed intrapleurally.
   3. Breathing mechanism operates on principle of negative pressure.
      a. Pressure in chest cavity is lower than pressure of atmosphere.
      b. An injury that breaks into chest cavity (such as stab wound) will cause atmospheric air to then rush into the cavity.

c. Vacuum must be applied to chest to reestablish negative pressure when chest has been open.

4. Closed water-seal drainage is method of reestablishing negative pressure.
   a. Water acts as a seal and keeps the air from being drawn back into pleural space.
   b. Open drainage system would allow air to be sucked back into chest cavity and cause collapse of lung.

5. Closed drainage is established by placing catheter into pleural space and allowing it to drain under water.
   a. The end of the drainage tube is always kept under water.
   b. Air will not be drawn up through catheter into pleural space when tube is under water.

6. Drainage can be accomplished with one, two, or three bottles.

7. Some physicians do not allow clamping or milking of chest tubes. Follow physician's orders.

Assessment

A. Before insertion perform baseline cardiopulmonary assessment.

B. Monitor vital signs, pulse oximetry.

C. Observe chest excursion.

D. Changes in level of consciousness.

E. Anxiety level.

F. Prepare patient for procedure.

Implementation ❖ PROCEDURE ❖

A. Assist physician in placement of tubes.
   1. Tubes placed in pleural cavity following thoracic surgery.
   2. Provides for removal of air and serosanguineous fluid from pleural space.

B. Attach to water-seal suction—maintains closed system.
   1. Tape all connectors.
   2. Ensure that all stoppers in bottles are tight fitting.

✦ C. Apply suction.
   1. Keep bottles below level of bed.
   2. Keep suction level where ordered (be sure that bubbling is not excessive in the pressure-regulating bottle).
   3. Maintain water level in bottle.

✦ D. Maintain patency—strip or milk chest tubes *only* with physician's orders.
   1. *Only if ordered*, milk chest tubes every 30–60 minutes if clots or debris present.
      a. Milk away from patient toward the drainage receptacle.
      b. Alternately compress and release drainage tubing between thumb and fore-

finger—this method prevents pressure changes.
      c. Continue going down tube in this method until reaching drainage receptacle.
   2. Milking may be ordered—stripping should be avoided unless specifically ordered.

✦ E. Maintain safety.
   1. Keep rubber-tipped hemostats at bedside so that tube can be clamped off near to chest insertion site. Clamping is controversial and no longer considered a routine clinical practice—check hospital policy.
   2. Clamp only to locate source of air leak when bubbling occurs in water-seal chamber; to prevent air from entering pleural space.
   3. Place on "waterseal" (stop suction) 24 hours prior to removal. Do *not* clamp before stopping suction as it may cause lung to collapse.

✦ F. Monitor intake and output.
   1. With Pleur-Evac suction equipment (Figure 10-9), visually measure chest drainage (holds up to 2800–3000 mL drainage). With two- or three-bottle suction, tape or bottle markings may approximate the amount of drainage (similar to Pleur-Evac).
   2. Change equipment only when the drainage chamber is full.

Chest Drainage Systems

Assessment

A. Assess patient's respiratory rate, rhythm, and breath sounds for signs of respiratory distress.

B. Check that all connections on tubing are airtight and suction control is connected.

C. Examine system to see if it is set up and functioning properly. (*See* Figures 10-9, 10-10, 10-11.)

D. Identify any malfunctions in system, i.e., air leaks, negative pressure, or obstructions.

Implementation

A. Maintain water-seal suction system.

B. Cessation of fluctuations indicates reexpansion of lung.

C. Chest tubes are used for lung reexpansion, bubbling will occur in the water-seal bottle.

✦ Three-Bottle Suction System

A. Maintain three-bottle/chambers suction system.

B. Most pleural drainage systems have 3 basic components.
   1. Collection chamber (bottle #1). Fluid and air from chest cavity drains into chamber. Air in this chamber is vented to the second chamber.
   2. Water-seal chamber (bottle #2). Acts as one-way valve so air drains from the chest cavity,

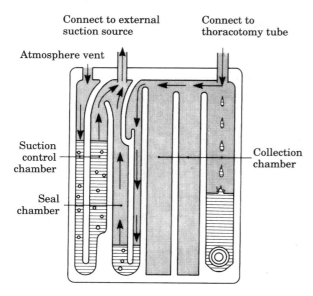

Fig. 10-9. Disposable water-seal suction equipment (Pleur-Evac).

THREE-BOTTLE SUCTION

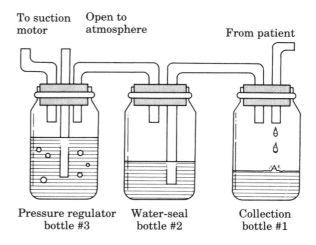

Fig. 10-10. Comparison of one-, two-, and three-bottle suction.

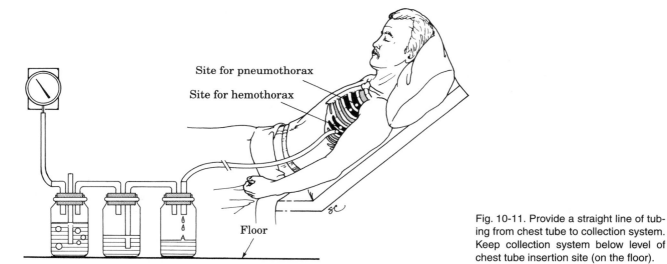

Fig. 10-11. Provide a straight line of tubing from chest tube to collection system. Keep collection system below level of chest tube insertion site (on the floor).

but can't return to the patient. Air bubbles out into water. Water level fluctuates as intrapleural pressure changes.

   3. Suction-control chamber (bottle #3). Amount of suction applied regulated by amount of water in chamber or depth of tubing in water, not by the amount of suction applied.

C. When control bottle fluid becomes too low, outside air is sucked into the system. Depth of control tube under water determines suction level of system.

D. Whenever suction is off, drainage system must be open, vented to the atmosphere.

   1. Intrapleural air can escape from the system.

   2. Vent prevents pressure buildup, which interferes with drainage from patient.

✦ CHECKPOINTS FOR CHEST TUBE AIR LEAKS

Continuous bubbling in water-seal chamber indicates an air leak.

- Insertion site: pinch tube at chest insertion site—bubbling stops in water-seal chamber if there is an air leak at insertion site.
- Tubing: pinch rubber connecting tube—bubbling stops if there is a leak at chest tube connector site.
- Water-seal drainage system: pinch rubber connecting tubing—bubbling continues if there is a leak in water-seal connection.
- Water-seal chamber: there should not be excessive continuous bubbling present; when patient exhales or coughs and air is forced out of pleural space, or when lung has reexpanded, bubbling occurs.

Mechanical Ventilation

Assessment

A. Assess respiratory status for need to use mechanical ventilation.

B. Identify type of mechanical ventilation needed.
1. Negative pressure ventilator.
    a. Helpful in problems of a neuromuscular nature, spinal cord injuries.
    b. Not effective in the treatment of increased airway resistance.
    ✦ c. Types—full body, chest, and chest–abdomen.
2. Positive pressure ventilator.
    a. Uses positive pressure (pressure greater than atmospheric) to inflate lungs—primary use in acutely ill patients.
    b. Types.
        (1) Pressure cycle.
            (a) Pressure ranges from 10–30 cm of water pressure.
            (b) Air is actively forced into lungs.
            (c) Expiration is passive.
        (2) Volume cycle.
            (a) Uses physiological limits.
            (b) Predetermined total volume is delivered irrespective of airway pressure.
            (c) Positive end expiratory pressure (PEEP) utilized to maintain positive pressure between expiration and beginning of inspiration.

C. Assess for complications of positive pressure therapy.
1. Respiratory alkalosis.
2. Gastric distention and paralytic ileus.
3. Gastrointestinal bleeding.
4. Diffuse atelectasis.
5. Infection.
6. Circulatory collapse.
7. Pneumothorax.
8. Suddent ventricular fibrillation.

Implementation

A. Monitor ventilator for complications.
B. Suction patient or check for kinks in tubing when pressure alarm sounds.
C. Monitor blood gas values frequently.
D. Maintain fluid therapy.
1. IV route.
2. Oral route if patient able to swallow.
E. Monitor intake and output.

Suctioning

A. Nasotracheal suctioning.
1. Equipment needed.
    a. Sterile suction catheter, usually No. 14 or No. 16 French.
    b. Sterile saline.
    c. Suction machine.
    d. Sterile gloves.
✦ 2. Procedure. ❖ **PROCEDURE** ❖
    a. Preoxygenate 1–2 minutes before beginning procedure.
    b. Lubricate catheter with normal saline.
    c. Insert catheter 6–8 inches into the nose.
    d. Do not apply suction while introducing catheter.
    e. When advanced as far as possible, begin suctioning by withdrawing catheter slowly, rotating it with pressure applied. (Usually a whistle-tip catheter or Y-connector tube is used to apply pressure.)

B. Tracheostomy suctioning.
1. Equipment needed.
    a. Same equipment as for nasotracheal.
    b. Sterile syringe (5 mL) and sterile saline for instillation into tracheostomy tube.
✦ 2. Procedure. ❖ **PROCEDURE** ❖
    a. Be sure that suction catheter is not more than half the diameter of the tracheostomy tube.
    b. Preoxygenate before beginning procedure.
    c. Lubricate with sterile saline.
    d. Insert catheter through tracheostomy tube for 8–12 inches with suction turned off.
    ✦ e. Suction for no more than 10 seconds.
    f. Rotate catheter while withdrawing it.
    g. Do not repeat procedure for at least 3 minutes, unless necessary to withdraw more secretions to permit adequate ventilation.
    h. Growing body of research advises against instilling saline into airway—increases chance of infection.

C. Closed suction system.
1. Suction catheter attached directly to ventilator tubing presents advantages over open system.
2. More effective—no need to disconnect patient from ventilator; thus, oxygenation is better.
3. Safer—catheter is enclosed in plastic sheath (a closed system) so risk of infection is decreased for both patient and nurse.

RESPIRATORY MEDICATIONS

✦ Sympathomimetic (Adrenergic) Bronchodilators

Definition: Relax smooth muscle and increase respirations by effect on beta-adrenegic receptor in bronchus.

A. Epinephrine (Adrenaline).
  1. Beta and alpha stimulant; relaxes bronchial smooth muscle.
  2. Routes: sub q, IV, MDI (metered dose inhalant).
  3. Used to treat severe bronchial attacks and for anaphylaxis.
  4. May cause arrhythmias, increased BP, urinary retention, increased blood sugar, headache.
B. Ephedrine sulfate.
  1. Relaxes smooth muscle of the tracheobronchial tree.
  2. Route: PO.
  3. Used for mild bronchospasm.
  4. Similar side effects as epinephrine.
C. Isoproterenol (Isuprel).
  1. Pure beta agonist; relaxes smooth muscle of tracheobronchial tree; relieves bronchospasms.
  2. Routes: IV, MDI.
  3. May cause marked tachycardia, arrhythmias, angina, palpitations.
D. Albuterol (Proventil, Ventolin).
  1. Very selective beta-2 agonist with rapid onset of action.
  2. Routes: PO, MDI (2–3 puffs every 4–6 hours).
  3. Minimal cardiovascular side effects.
E. Isoetharine (Bronkosol, Bronkometer).
  1. More beta-2 specific than Isuprel; relaxes smooth muscle of the tracheobronchial tree; less potent.
  2. Route: nebulized solution or MDI.
  3. Side effects similar to Isuprel, but appear less frequently; may cause tachycardia.
  4. Tolerance to bronchodilating effect may develop with too frequent use of medication.
F. Metaproterenol (Alupent).
  1. Relieves bronchospasm; has rapid onset.
  2. Routes: PO, MDI (2–3 puffs every 4–6 hours).
  3. Side effects same as isoetharine.
G. Terbutaline (Bricanyl, Brethine).
  1. Beta-adrenergic receptor agonist; bronchodilator; relieves bronchospasms associated with COPD, asthma; slow onset with PO meds.
  2. Routes: sub q, PO, Brethaire by MDI (2–3 puffs every 4–6 hours).
  3. May cause nervousness, palpitations; nausea if taken on an empty stomach.

✦ Anticholinergic Bronchodilators

Definition: Prevents bronchospasm caused by acetylcholine.
A. Ipratropium bromide (Atrovent).
  1. Greater bronchodilating effect than conventional beta-agonists. Primarily local and site specific; more potent than sympathomimetics in COPD, severe acute asthma.
  2. Route: MDI (2–3 puffs every 4–6 hours).
  3. Minimal side effects; dry mouth, cough.
B. Atropine.
  1. Prevents bronchospasm associated with asthma, bronchitis, and COPD.
  2. Routes: nebulizer 3–4 times/day.
  3. Monitor for tachycardia and hypertension.

✦ Methylxanthine Bronchodilators

Definition: Relaxes smooth muscle of tracheobronchial tree—less effective than inhaled beta-agonists; used later in treatment as additional bronchodilator.
A. Aminophylline.
  1. Relaxes smooth muscle of the tracheobronchial tree; bronchodilator.
  2. Routes: PO, IV, rectal suppository.
  3. Therapeutic serum level 8–20 µg/mL.
  4. May cause tachycardia, hypotension, arrhythmias, GI distress, tremors, anxiety, headache.
  5. Toxic levels cause arrhythmias, seizures.
B. Theophylline (Theo-Dur, Slo-bid, Uni-Dur).
  1. Long-acting bronchodilator—relaxes smooth muscle of the bronchi and pulmonary vessels.
  2. Routes: PO, rectally.
  3. Therapeutic serum level 10–20 µg/mL.
  4. Side effects similar to aminophylline.
C. Oxtriphylline (Choledyl).
  1. Similar to other bronchodilators.
  2. Route: PO.
  3. Less GI irritation than aminophylline.

✦ Leukotriene Inhibitors/Receptor Antagonists

Definition: Inhibit formation of leukotrienes, which cause airway inflammation, edema, bronchoconstriction, and mucus secretion.
A. Zafirlukast (Accolate), zileuton (Zyflo), and montelukast sodium (Singulair).
  1. Basic action is anti-inflammatory.
  2. Taken orally (not through MDI) so compliance is improved—used for long-term control, not acute asthma attack.
B. Side effects: headache, nausea, diarrhea, dizziness, fever, and myalgia.

✦ Antimediators (Mast Cell Stabilizers)/ Anti-inflammatory Agents

Definition: Mast cell stabilizers inhibit release of histamine; glucocorticoids reduce inflammation and act as a bronchodilator.

A. Cromolyn sodium (Intal, Nalcrom).
1. Used for younger patients with asthma.
2. Route:MDI, nebulizer, nasal spray.
3. Prevents bronchospasm when used before exercise or exposure to cold air.
B. Glucocorticoids (Beclovent, Vanceril, Beconase).
1. Used in conjunction with bronchodilators for treatment of bronchospasms—has anti-inflammatory effects, decreases mucous secretions. Aerosol use prevents systemic side effects of steroids.
2. Routes:
   a. Prednisone PO.
   b. Methylprednisolone PO, IV, hydrocortisone IV.
   c. Beclomethasone diproprionate (Beclovent, Vanceril) MDI.
   d. Triamcinolone (Azmacort) MDI.
3. Instruct patient to rinse mouth after MDI use to prevent oral candidiasis.
4. Side effects include increased appetite, sore throat, cough, thrush. Cushing-like appearance.

✦ Mucokinetic Agents

Definition: Reduces the viscosity of respiratory secretions by breaking down mucoproteins.
A. Acetylcysteine (Mucomyst).
1. Used to loosen secretions; reduces viscosity.
2. Routes: inhaled or instilled.
3. Instruct patient to rinse mouth after use.
B. Guaiafenesin.
1. Commonly used expectorant.
2. Route: PO.

✦ Antiprotozoal Drugs

Definition: Interferes with biosynthesis of deoxyribonucleic acid, ribonucleic acid, phospholipids, and proteins in susceptible organisms.
A. Pentamidine (NebuPent, Pentam 300) for prevention.
1. Prevention of *Pneumocystis carinii* pneumonia.
2. Routes: nebulizer (300 mg every 4 weeks).
3. If patient experiences fatigue, dizziness, or anxiety during inhalation, stop treatment and allow patient to rest.
4. Well tolerated, expensive; least effective form of prophylaxis.
B. Pentamidine for treatment.
1. Treatment of *Pneumocystis carinii*.
2. Route: IV or IM (4 mg/kg daily for 14 days).
3. Closely monitor for hypotension—place patient in supine position for IV administration.
4. May cause hyperglycemia, pancreatitis; nephrotoxic.
5. Screen for active TB before treating.

GASTROINTESTINAL SYSTEM

The alimentary tract's primary function is to provide the body with a continual supply of nutrients, fluids, and electrolytes for tissue nourishment. This system has three components: a tract for ingestion and movement of food and fluids; secretion of digestive juices for breaking down the nutrients; and absorption mechanisms for the utilization of foods, water, and electrolytes for continuous growth and repair of body tissues.

ANATOMY AND PHYSIOLOGY

Alimentary Tract

A. Mouth.
   1. Cheeks.
   2. Hard and soft palates.
   3. Muscles.
   4. Maxillary bones (jaw).
   5. Tongue—aids in chewing, swallowing, and speaking; contains taste buds.
   6. Salivary glands.
     a. Constant secretions form saliva.
     b. Three pairs of glands located in the mucous membrane of the oral cavity.
       (1) Parotid—below the ear.
       (2) Submaxillary—floor of mouth.
       (3) Sublingual—floor of mouth.
   7. Teeth—assist in mastication and in mixing saliva with food.
   8. Digestive process starts in the mouth.
B. Pharynx.
   1. Tubal structure that extends from the base of the skull to the esophagus.
   2. Serves as a passageway for air from nasal cavity to larynx and for food from mouth to esophagus.
   3. Parts.
     a. Nasopharynx.
     b. Oropharynx.
     c. Laryngopharynx.
C. Esophagus.
   1. Muscular canal.
   2. Extends from pharynx to stomach.
D. Stomach.
   1. Distensible pouch located between the esophagus and the duodenum.
   2. Divisions.
     a. Fundus, which forms upper portion, is located immediately below the cardiac sphincter.
     b. Body, which forms the largest and central portion.
     c. Pylorus forms the lower portion.
   3. Sphincters.
     a. Cardiac sphincter is muscle around the lower end of the esophagus where it opens into the stomach.
     b. Pyloric sphincter is muscle around the lower end of the stomach where it opens into the duodenum.
   4. Curvatures.
     a. Lesser curvature.
     b. Greater curvature.
   5. Layers.
     a. Serous coat is the outer layer, which forms the visceral peritoneum; the peritoneum folds and forms the omentum, which hangs over the intestines like an apron.
     b. Muscular layer formed of three directional (circular, longitudinal, and oblique) muscle fibers.
     c. Submucous layer contains blood vessels and lymphatics.
     d. Mucous layer contains microscopic glands, which assist in digestion.
   6. Glands.
     a. Mucous gland secretes mucus.
     b. Gastric gland secretes gastric juice containing hydrochloric acid and digestive enzymes.
   7. Function.
     a. Mechanical digestion.
       (1) Most digestion occurs near pyloric area where peristalsis is more forceful.
       (2) Peristalsis is stimulated by the vagus nerve.
     b. Chemical digestion—excretes gastric juice containing hydrochloric acid and enzymes.
E. Small intestine.
   1. Convoluted tube approximately 23 feet in length.
   2. General functions.
     a. Digestion and absorption.
     b. Receives bile and pancreatic juices.
   3. Segments.
     a. Duodenum begins at the pylorus and connects with the jejunum where it ends; it is approximately 10 inches long.
     b. Jejunum is the middle portion, which is approximately 8 feet long and lies coiled around the umbilical region.

c. Ileum is the terminal section that joins the colon at the ileocecal valve; it is approximately 12 feet long.

4. Folds.
    a. Extend around the intestinal lumen; most numerous in the duodenum but disappear in the lower ileum.
    b. Contain numerous villi through which products of digestion are absorbed. Each villus has an arteriole, venule, and lymph vessel.
    c. Folds provide a large surface area, which assists digestion, secretion, and absorption.

F. Large intestine.
    1. Extends from the ileocecal valve to the anus; it is 5–6 feet long and is wider than the small intestine.
    2. Segments.
        a. Cecum connects with the ileum at the ileocecal valve; appendix attaches to the distal end.
        b. Ascending colon continues up the right side of the abdomen to lower borders of the liver where it turns.
        c. Transverse colon continues from the ascending colon across the abdomen (front of stomach) to lower border of the spleen.
        d. Descending colon continues from the transverse colon down the left side of the abdomen to the brim of the pelvis.
        e. Sigmoid colon is the S-shaped portion, which extends to the rectum.
        f. Rectum is 6–8 inches long and ends at anus, the end of the digestive tract.
    3. General functions.
        a. Reabsorption of fluids, electrolytes, glucose, and urea.
        b. Mechanical digestion.
        c. Peristalsis and defecation.
        d. Elimination of wastes.

Accessory Organs

✦ A. Liver.
    1. Located in the right upper abdomen and protected by lower ribs.
    2. Largest organ in the body weighing about 3 pounds.
    3. General functions.
        a. Metabolism of carbohydrates, fats, and proteins.
        b. Detoxification of harmful substances in the blood.
        c. Breakdown of old blood cells.
        d. Constant secretion of bile, which drains from the liver through the hepatic duct into the common duct to the small intestine; bile is stored in the gallbladder.
        e. Stores glycogen and vitamins A, D, E, B, B$_{12}$, and K, and copper and iron.
        f. Produces and stores heparin and fibrinogen.

✦ B. Gallbladder.
    1. Small sac of smooth muscle located in a depression at the edge of the visceral surface of the liver.
    2. Functions as a reservoir for bile.
        a. Bile from the hepatic duct enters the gallbladder through the cystic duct for storage.
        b. Stored bile leaves the gallbladder through the cystic duct to flow through the common duct into the small intestine.
        c. The sphincter of Oddi guards the common entrance.
        d. Bile activates the pancreas to release its digestive enzymes and an alkaline fluid.

✦ C. Pancreas.
    1. Soft, pinkish-white organ that is 6 inches long and 1 inch wide; it adheres to the middle portion of the duodenum.
    2. Composed of exocrine and endocrine tissue.
        a. Exocrine cells secrete juices containing digestive enzymes.
        b. Endocrine cells secrete glucagon and insulin.
    3. Pancreatic juices contain enzymes for digesting proteins, carbohydrates, and fats.
        a. Trypsinogen to trypsin to act on proteins producing peptones, peptides, and amino acids.
        b. Pancreatic amylase acts on carbohydrates, producing disaccharides.
        c. Pancreatic lipase acts on fats, producing glycerol and fatty acids.

DIAGNOSTIC PROCEDURES

✦ Upper Gastrointestinal Roentgenography

A. Purpose.
    1. For visualizing GI tract.
        a. Structure and function of the esophagus.
        b. Size and shape of the right atrium.
        c. Size and shape of the stomach.
        d. Motility of the stomach.
        e. Ulcerations, tumor formations, and anatomic abnormalities of the stomach and small intestines.
        f. Emptying time of the stomach.
    2. For documenting in permanent records.

B. Procedure.
   1. Ingestion of barium or other contrast medium.
   2. Pass x-rays through the body so that GI tract will stand out in silhouette on film.
C. Preparation of the patient.
   1. NPO after midnight prior to the day of the test.
   2. Withhold medications.
   3. Explain procedure to the patient.

✦ **Barium Enema**
A. Purpose.
   1. For visualizing the lower intestinal tract.
   2. For revealing abnormalities of structure and motility of the cecum and appendix.
B. Procedure.
   1. Barium enema given.
   2. X-ray film taken.
C. Preparation of the patient.
   1. Evacuate the intestinal tract by enema, laxatives, or suppositories until returning solution is clear.
   2. NPO after midnight (some methods allow clear liquids for breakfast).
   3. Explain procedure to patient.

✦ **Endoscopy**
A. Purpose.
   1. For visualizing inside of body cavity to detect lesions.
   2. For taking biopsy.
   3. Secure washings for cytologic examination.
✦ B. Preparation of the patient.
   1. NPO after midnight.
   2. Ensure that a consent for the procedure is signed.
   3. Premedicate the patient.
   4. Give patient support during exam.
   5. Assist the physician.
   6. Topical anesthetic may be used to facilitate passage of the scope into the esophagus during exam. The anesthetic depresses the gag reflex.
C. Nursing care following an esophagogastroduodenoscopy (EGD).
   1. Withhold fluids or food by mouth until swallowing reflex returns.
   2. Observe carefully for swelling, hemorrhage, or dysfunction of the area.
   3. Prevent aspiration if vomiting occurs.

✦ **Gastric Analysis***
A. Purpose.
   1. For analyzing stomach contents for acid-fast bacilli, for volume, and for free acid.
   2. For detecting gastric bleeding.

B. Procedure.
   1. Insertion of nasogastric tube to aspirate stomach contents.
   2. Specimens obtained at varying times, usually at 10- and 20-minute intervals.
C. Preparation of the patient.
   1. NPO 6–8 hours prior to exam; administer gastric stimulant followed by dye.
   2. Collect specimens as ordered; label and send to lab. (Urine is analyzed to check amount of free acid in the stomach.)
   3. Remove nasogastric tube and provide oral hygiene.

Stool Analysis*

A. Purpose.
   1. For examining amount, consistency, color, shape, blood, fecal urobilinogen, fat, nitrogen, parasites, food residue, and other substances.
   2. For culturing bacteria and viruses.
✦ B. Procedure.
   1. Collect fresh, warm stool specimen for parasite analysis.
   2. Collect specimen in small amount for occult blood analysis (guaiac).
   3. Obtain a 24-hour collection for chemical analysis.
   4. Collect specimen in sterile container for C&S.
✦ C. Stool characteristics.
   1. Color.
      a. Foods (spinach, cocoa) produce dark red.
      b. Medicines (senna) produce yellow.
      c. Iron produces black.
      d. Upper GI bleeding produces tarry black.
      e. Fresh, lower tract bleeding produces bright red.
   2. Stool abnormalities.
      a. Steatorrhea may be indicated by bulky, greasy, foamy, and foul-odored stools.
      b. Biliary obstruction may be indicated by light gray or clay-colored stools.
      c. Ulcerative colitis may be indicated by loose stools with copious amounts of mucus and/or pus.
      d. Constipation or obstruction may be indicated by small, hard-massed stools.

Biopsy and Cytology
A. Specimens for microscopic examination are secured by endoscopy examination, cell scrapings, and needle aspiration.
B. Specimens are examined, and the laboratory then determines their origin, structure, functions, and the presence of malignant cells.

*See Chapter 7, Laboratory Tests.

Radionuclide Uptake

A. Radionuclides are used in diagnosis by measuring the localization of the substance, such as radioiodine in the thyroid, and the excretion of the material.

B. Various substances are studied, such as vitamin B_{12}, iron and fat, and major organs can be scanned.

C. Substances are tagged with radioactive isotopes to assess the degree of absorption.

Blood Examinations

A. Hematologic studies and electrolyte determinations reveal information about the general status of the patient.

B. Results of these examinations in conjunction with other assessment procedures and clinical symptoms help to localize the disorder.

✦ Gastrointestinal System Assessment

A. Evaluate patient's history regarding reported signs and symptoms.

B. Assess overall condition of patient including vital signs and level of consciousness.

C. Evaluate condition of mouth, teeth, gums, and tongue.
   1. Foul odor to breath may indicate diseased teeth, gums, or poor assimilation along gastrointestinal tract.
   2. Coated tongue may indicate chemical imbalance in system.
   3. Check voice for hoarseness.

D. Check for presence of gag reflex.

E. Assess general contour of abdomen with patient lying flat. Look for concave or protuberant abdomen.

F. Assess for bowel sounds: decreased, increased, or hypoactive.

G. Check bowel habits and/or alterations in bowel elimination.

H. Palpate abdominal muscles for tenderness or rigidity; evaluate all quadrants of abdomen.

I. Assess bowel motility.
   1. Hypermotility may be result of irritation of autonomic nervous system or inflammatory process.
   2. Hypomotility may be result of blockage, intestinal muscle weakness, or chemical agents.

J. Check for amount of flatulence patient reports, which indicates malfunction of system or dietary indiscretion.

K. Assess stool specimen.
   1. Check for presence of blood.
   2. Check for presence of mucus.
   3. Evaluate consistency, color, and odor of stool.

L. Assess urine for amount, color, and odor, and fluid intake per day.

M. Evaluate dietary program, i.e., type of foods, amount, etc.

N. Evaluate laboratory tests.

O. Note presence or absence of hemorrhoids.

P. Assess degree of sphincter control through patient reports of ability to control and regulate bowel movements.

Q. Assess for presence of pain along gastrointestinal tract and in accessory organs.
   1. Assess nonverbal signs, such as flinching, grimacing, etc.
   2. Evaluate onset, location, intensity, duration, and aggravating factors.

R. Palpate for rebound tenderness of spleen.

S. Check skin color for yellow tinge, pallor, or heavy flushing.

✦ T. Check for signs of dehydration.
   1. Dry mucous membranes.
   2. Poor skin turgor.
   3. Decreased urine output.
   4. Increased pulse.

U. Assess for signs of shock following trauma to abdomen.

V. Assess patient's knowledge of diagnostic tests or surgical interventions.

GASTROINTESTINAL DISORDERS

Anorexia

Definition: Loss or lack of appetite for food.

Causes

A. Anxiety, depression.

B. Improper fit of dentures.

C. Illness, physical discomfort.

D. Constipation.

E. Intestinal obstruction.

Implementation

A. Become familiar with patient's eating habits, i.e., likes and dislikes in food, cultural and religious beliefs regarding food.

B. When possible, permit patient to choose own food.

C. Show interest, but don't force patient to eat.

D. Provide a pleasant and inviting environment.

E. Serve small portions of attractively prepared food.

Nausea and Vomiting

Definitions: *Nausea* is the distressing feeling that is felt when nerves ending in stomach and other body parts are irritated; may lead to vomiting. *Vomiting* is ejection of stomach contents through mouth.

Characteristics

A. Vomiting centers in the body.
   1. Chemoreceptor emetic trigger zone.
   2. Center in the medulla.
B. Stimulation of vomiting center.
   1. Impulses from GI tract.
   2. Impulses from cerebral center.
   3. Chemicals in bloodstream.
   4. Increased intracranial pressure.
C. Causes
   1. Stress, fear, and depression.
   2. Pain.
   3. Acute febrile illness.
   4. Medications, food poisoning.
   5. Anesthesia.
   6. Diseases of the stomach.
   7. Intestinal obstruction.
   8. Pregnancy.
   9. Head injury.

✦ Implementation

A. Administer relief-giving drugs (antiemetics, phenothiazines).
B. Monitor fluid and electrolyte replacement.
C. Protect the patient from unpleasant sights, sounds, and smells.
D. Attempt to keep the stomach empty.
E. Promptly remove used equipment; change soiled linens and dressings.
F. Ventilate room and use unscented air fresheners.
G. Observe and record the character and quantity of emesis.

Constipation and Diarrhea

Definitions: Diarrhea is the rapid movement through intestines of loose, watery stools resulting from increased peristalsis. Constipation is the delay in the evacuation of feces, with passage of hard and dry fecal material.

Causes

A. Diarrhea—fecal impaction, ulcerative colitis, intestinal infections, drugs, or neurosis.
B. Constipation—lack of regularity, psychogenic causes, drugs, inadequate fluid intake, mechanical obstruction, lack of dietary bulk, or lack of exercise.

Implementation

✦ A. Administer laxatives for constipation.
   1. Bulk-forming/fiber (Metamucil, bran, pyllium seed) stimulates peristalsis.
   2. Milk of Magnesia alters stool consistency to stimulate peristalsis.
   3. Lubricants such as mineral oil to soften stool.

   4. Dulcolax to stimulate colon (or Cascara).
   5. Stool softener (Colace).
✦ B. Administer antidiarrheals for diarrhea.
   1. Mild diarrhea: oral fluids to replace lost fluids.
   2. Moderate diarrhea: drugs to decrease motility (Lomotil and Imodium).
   3. Severe diarrhea caused by infectious agent: antimicrobials and fluid replacement.
C. Administer anticholinergics (Atropine).
   1. Reduces bowel spasticity.
   2. Used to treat irritable bowel and diarrhea caused by peptic ulcer disease.
D. Provide fluids and electrolytes as needed to correct imbalance—IV therapy may be needed to replace fluids and electrolytes.
E. Diet high in nutrients and calories—vitamin supplements (A, D, E, & K).
F. Observe stools for color, odor, shape, consistency, amount, and presence of mucus, blood, or pus.
G. Provide perirectal skin care and prevent skin excoriation.

Oral Infections

Definitions: *Stomatitis* is an inflammation of the mouth. *Glossitis* is an inflammation of the tongue. *Gingivitis* is an inflammation of the gums.

Causes

A. Mechanical trauma.
B. Foods, drinks, allergies, or medications.
C. Poor oral hygiene.
D. Pathogens.
   1. Herpes simplex.
   2. Vincent's angina (trench mouth).

Assessment

A. Anorexia.
B. Excessive salivation.
C. Foul breath (halitosis).
D. Condition of gums, teeth, and tongue.

Treatment and Implementation

A. Remove causative factor.
B. Provide frequent, soothing oral hygiene.
C. Apply topical medications and administer systemic antibiotics.
D. Provide soft, bland diet.
E. Administer analgesic (may be topical application) 30 minutes before meals.
F. Avoid alcohol-based mouthwashes.

Esophageal Disorders

Definition: Local or systemic infection or chemical irritation from reflux of gastric juices into the lower esophagus.

Assessment

A. Heartburn.
B. Intolerance of spices.
C. Alcohol and caffeine intolerance.
D. Dysphagia.

Treatment and Implementation

A. Give oral antacids.
B. Provide bland diet.
C. Elevate head of bed; do not recline after meals.

Gastroesophageal Reflux Disease (GERD)

Definition: Backward flow (reflux) of gastric contents into the esophagus; suffered by 15 to 20% of adults.

Assessment

A. Assess for heartburn after meals.
B. Check for regurgitation of material into the mouth.
C. Assess for difficulty or pain in swallowing—pain may be severe.

Implementation

A. Monitor antacids (Maalox) for mild or moderate conditions.
B. Explain use of histamine H_2 receptor blockers (cimetidine, ranitidine) to reduce acid production.
C. Monitor use of proton-pump inhibitors (PPIs) such as Prilosec or Prevacid to reduce gastric sec-tretions and relieve symptoms.
D. Suggest dietary changes such as reduction in fat, coffee, spicy foods and cessation in smoking (which increases acidity).

Esophageal Varices

✦ *Definition:*   Tortuous dilation of veins in the lower esophagus caused by portal hypertension and often associated with cirrhosis of liver.

Assessment

A. Bleeding.
B. Hypotension.
C. Neck vein distention.
D. Observe for strain of coughing or vomiting, which could rupture esophagus.

Treatment and Implementation

A. Upper endoscopy evaluates and treats condition.
   1. Gastric lavage with normal saline to visualize varices.
   2. Varices may be banded or sclerosed.
      a. Varices are ligated with small rubber bands which occlude blood flow.
      b. Sclerosing agent injected into varices to induce inflammation and thrombosis.

✦ B. Placement of Sengstaken–Blakemore tube to exert pressure against ruptured vessels at 25 to 30 mm Hg.
   1. Maintain pressure in balloon tamponade.
   2. Do not deflate balloon (done only with physician's orders).
   ✦ 3. Keep scissors at bedside for safety—if tube causes obstruction, cutting will deflate balloon.
   4. Iced saline irrigations to vasoconstrict the small collateral vessels.
✦ C. Administer vitamin K replacement.
D. Observe vital signs watching for hemorrhage and shock.
E. Provide frequent oral hygiene.
F. Prevent nasal breakdown by keeping nostrils lu-bricated and clean.
G. Monitor fluid and nutritional balance.
H. Observe for complications of active bleeding.
   1. Hypovolemia.
   2. Hepatic encephalopathy from increased ammonia.

Esophageal (Hiatal) Hernia

✦ *Definition:*   Protrusion of a portion of the stomach through the diaphragm and into the thorax.

Causes

A. Congenital weakness of the diaphragm.
B. Trauma.
C. Relaxation of the muscles.
D. Intra-abdominal pressure (obesity, ascites, pregnancy).

✦ **Assessment**

A. Heartburn, substernal discomfort, and pain.
B. Dysphagia.
C. Vomiting.
D. Regurgitation (especially after large meals or in-gestion of spicy foods); reflux.

✦ **Implementation**

A. Provide small frequent meals (avoid highly sea-soned foods).
B. Maintain patient in upright position during and after meals.
C. Administer antacids after meals and at bedtime.
D. Elevate head of bed to avoid regurgitation while eating and for 30 minutes after.
E. Avoid anticholinergic drugs, which delay empty-ing of stomach.
F. Advise patient against constrictive clothing around the waist.
G. Advise patient against sharp and forward bends.
H. Surgery is indicated when there is risk of compli-cations or severe reflux.

Dyspepsia (Indigestion)

Definition: Imperfect digestion symptomatic of other GI diseases or disorders; characterized by heartburn and other abdominal discomforts.

Causes

A. Rapid ingestion.
B. Disease.
C. Altered gastric secretions.
D. Emotional problems.

Assessment

A. Heartburn.
B. Flatulence, feeling of fullness.
C. Nausea.
D. Eructations.

Implementation

A. Provide bland diet.
B. Administer antispasmodics, tranquilizers, and antacids.
C. Advise patient to modify current eating habits.

Acute Gastritis

Definition: Inflammation of the stomach by a local irritant.

Causes

A. Ingestion of corrosive or erosive substances (alcohol, aspirin, or contaminated food).
B. Acute systemic infections.
C. Radiotherapy or chemotherapy.
D. Infection.

Assessment

A. Epigastric burning and pain.
B. Nausea and vomiting.
C. Malaise.
D. Hemorrhage.
E. Anorexia.
F. Headache.

Treatment and Implementation

A. Attempt to eliminate the cause; treat symptomatically.
B. Administer antacids and phenothiazines.
C. Correct fluid and electrolyte balance; NPO for acute phase, then graduate to bland diet with fluid replacement.

Peptic Ulcer Disease (PUD)

✦ *Definition:* Ulceration in the mucosal wall of the stomach, pylorus, or duodenum. (*See* Table 10-2.)

Characteristics

A. No longer thought to be caused by excess stomach acid.
✦ B. Bacterial invasion of the mucosa caused by *Helicobacter pylori* bacterium.
  1. Found in more than 70 percent of gastric ulcer patients.
  2. Found in 95 percent of duodenal ulcers.
✦ C. Risk factors.
  1. Emotional and physical stress.
  2. Irregular, hurriedly ingested meals.
  3. Seasonal factor (spring and fall).
  4. Excessive smoking.

✦ **Table 10-2. COMPARISON OF DUODENAL AND GASTRIC ULCER**

	Chronic Duodenal Ulcer	Chronic Gastric Ulcer
Age	Usually 30 to 55	Usually 55 and over
Sex	Male:Female—2–3:1	Male:Female—1:1
Blood group	Most frequently type O	Blood group A
Social class	Executives, competitive leaders	Lower socioeconomic class
Incidence	80%	20%
General nourishment	Well nourished	Malnourished
Acid production in stomach	Hypersecretion	Normal to hyposecretion
Location	Within 3 cm of pylorus	Lesser curvature
Pain	2–3 hours after meals and at night	On an empty stomach or shortly after the meal
	Usually absent before breakfast—worsens as day progresses	Rarely is there pain at night
	Ingestion of food, antacids, or vomiting relieves pain	Relieved by antacids or vomiting
Vomiting	Uncommon	Common
Hemorrhage	Melena more common than hematemesis	Hematemesis more common than melena
Malignancy possibility	None	Usually < 10%

5. Drugs, e.g., salicylates, phenylbutazone, and steroids.
6. Hereditary factors.

Assessment
A. Boring, aching, gnawing, or burning epigastric pain.
B. Pain usually occurring 30 minutes to 3 hours after eating.
C. Weight loss from reduced intake or weight gain from excessive intake in effort to relieve pain.
D. Vomiting, which may result from pain or from pyloric obstruction due to ulcerations and to scarring that accompanies healing.
E. Occult blood in stool from bleeding.

✦ Implementation
A. Promote healing process by preventing complications.
B. Provide symptomatic relief and rest.
C. Eliminate irritating factors, e.g., alcohol, smoking, stress, and salicylates.
✦ D. Administer drugs.
  1. Antimicrobial therapy, antibiotics (Amoxil, tetracycline)—current therapy. One course of therapy treats ulcers caused by *Helicobacter pylori* infection.
  2. Histamine H_2 receptor antagonists (Pepcid, Tagamet, Zantac).
  3. Antacids, bismuth preparations—reduces gastric acidity.
  4. Anticholinergics—used for patients with severe pain in the morning.
  5. Sucralfate (Carafate) used when H_2 antagonists can't be given—adheres to ulcer surface.
  6. Proton pump inhibitor—blocks release of HCL—very effective, with 90 percent healing in 4 months.
E. Observe emesis and/or stool closely (iron preparations may also result in dark stools).
F. Provide diet that eliminates gas-producing, spicy foods—three meals per day; eliminate black pepper.
G. Observe and report significant physical and emotional responses to therapy.
H. Observe for indications of complications (i.e., hemorrhage, perforation).
I. Gastric surgery may be required if medical treatment is ineffective.

MALIGNANT CONDITIONS AND SURGICAL PROCEDURES

Malignant Tumors of the Mouth

Definition: Cancer of the mouth that usually affects the lips, tongue, or the mouth floor.

Predisposing Factors
A. Poor oral hygiene.
B. Chronic irritation.
C. Chemical and thermal trauma, i.e., tobacco, alcohol, and hot-spiced foods.

Assessment
A. Lesions that are painful, hard, and ulcerate.
B. Chronic irritation.
C. Metastasis by local extension.

Treatment
A. Surgical removal of tumor.
B. Radiation therapy.

Cancer of the Esophagus

Definition: Malignant tumors of the esophagus; carcinomas, constituting 4 percent of all malignant tumors along the GI tract, are the most common form of tumor.

Assessment
A. Risk factors.
  1. Smoking and alcohol.
  2. Men over age 50.
B. Dysphagia (most common).
C. Substernal pressure.
D. Benign lesions.

Treatment and Implementation
A. Surgical excision; radiation therapy.
B. Manage nutritional needs—gastrostomy feedings.
C. Monitor ability to handle secretions.
D. Watch for complications (rupture, hemorrhage).

Radical Neck Dissection

Definition: Removal of cancerous lymph nodes in the neck.

Assessment
✦ A. Patent airway.
  1. Observe for airway obstruction (wheezing, stridor, retraction).
  2. Observe for respiratory distress; stertorous, labored breathing; increased respirations; and cyanosis.
✦ B. Edema that could constrict trachea.
✦ C. Watch for difficulty in swallowing if allowed oral fluids. Difficulty may indicate nerve damage. If radical procedure, patient will probably be fed through either nasogastric tube, gastrostomy, or IV therapy.
✦ D. Hemorrhage, which could lead to respiratory embarrassment.
E. Vital signs for indications of bleeding and infection.

F. Infection—increase in temperature, foul odor to dressings.

G. Carotid rupture or chylous fistula—milky drainage.

H. Catheter drainage and suture lines.

I. Wound healing.

J. Lower facial paralysis indicating facial nerve injury.

K. Mental state for depression, damage to self-image, feelings of loss, etc.

Implementation

✦ A. Maintain adequate respiratory function.
   1. Place in high-Fowler's position.
   2. Monitor for respiratory distress.

B. Suction to prevent aspiration and pneumonia.

C. Administer oxygen as needed.

D. Encourage intake of fluids, which is necessary to thin secretions.

E. Provide care for laryngectomy (frequently performed with radical neck dissection).
   1. Use mist mask.
   2. Clean tube as you would tracheostomy tube.

F. Change dressings frequently to prevent infection.
   1. Drains are frequently placed in surgical site; Hemovac is the drain most commonly used.
   2. Observe for unusual drainage (amount, type, as well as odor).

G. Give oral hygiene every 2–4 hours.

✦ H. Develop means to communicate as patient will not be able to talk postoperatively if laryngectomy was also performed.
   1. Provide method of writing for the first few days.
   2. Explain to patient that hoarseness is usual for the first few weeks.
   3. Provide bell or readily accessible means of communication for patient who will be anxious following surgery.

I. Provide privacy for patient.

J. Develop nurse–patient relationship, for patient may be depressed, may suffer feelings of loss, and may need to verbalize concerns about self-image.

✦ K. Teach or follow through with rehabilitation exercises for head and shoulder.
   1. Rotate neck, tilt head to both sides, and drop chin to chest.
   2. Swing arm on operated side in arc to extend range of motion.

L. Provide general postoperative care.

Laryngectomy

Definition: Removal of larynx due to malignant tumors.

Characteristics

✦ A. Total laryngectomy and radical neck dissection—procedure of choice for cancer under following circumstances:

   1. If tumor does not extend more than 5 mm up base of tongue or below upper edge of cricoarytenoid muscle.
   2. If there is no evidence of distant metastasis.

B. Epiglottis, thyroid cartilage, hyoid bone, cricoid cartilage, and part of trachea are removed.

C. Stump of trachea is brought out to neck and sutured to skin. The pharyngeal portion is closed, and breathing through nose is eliminated.

D. Accompanied by radical neck dissection if neck tissue and lymph nodes are involved.

Assessment

A. Drainage from wound suction for amount, color, and odor.

B. Carotid artery hemorrhage.

C. Lungs for atelectasis and pneumonia.

Implementation

✦ A. Suction frequently with sterile technique until area has healed; then use clean technique.

✦ B. Place pressure on neck wound for hemorrhage around site.

C. Instruct patient regarding means for communication, as he or she will not be able to speak immediately postoperatively.

D. Speech rehabilitation is utilized after surgical area has healed.

Gastric Cancer

Definition: Malignant tumor of the stomach, a common cancer of the digestive tract; responsible for 20,000 deaths annually in the United States.

Assessment

✦ A. *Early stage of carcinoma produces no symptoms.*

✦ B. Weight loss and anorexia.

C. Vague feeling of fullness and sensation of pressure.

D. Anemia as a result of blood loss.

E. Occult blood in stools.

F. Vomiting if pylorus becomes obstructed.

G. Late stage produces symptoms that include ascites, palpable mass, metastatic pain.

Treatment

A. Surgical resection (mortality 5–12 percent).

B. Radiation therapy.

C. Chemotherapy.

Gastric Surgical Procedures

✦ A. Vagotomy—interruption of vagal innervation to reduce stimulation of hydrochloric acid production.

✦ B. Gastrectomy or partial gastrectomy (Billroth I and II)—removal of stomach portion that produces hydrochloric acid; anastomosis between remaining portion of stomach and small bowel (gastroenterostomy).

C. Gastrostomy, jejunostomy—creation of opening into the stomach or jejunum for general purpose of maintaining nutritional status of patient when conditions make use of normal food route not feasible.

Postoperative Implementation

✦ A. Provide routine care.
1. Observe and record vital signs.
2. Observe for signs of shock.
3. Check dressing for abnormal drainage or bleeding.
4. Provide bedrest.
5. Record intake and output.
6. Turn patient and encourage cough and deep breathing exercises every 2 hours.

B. Manage accessory equipment.
1. Foley and IV tubes.
2. Nasogastric tube in place (patient is NPO).
    a. Ensure patency.
        (1) Irrigate with normal saline.
        (2) Maintain proper suction pressure.
        (3) Maintain correct position.
    b. Observe and record color, consistency, amount, and unusual odor of gastric contents.

C. After anesthesia recovery, raise bed to semi-Fowler's position.

D. Following removal of NG tube, provide diet of warm liquids; provide soft diet.

E. Control pain but avoid irritating medications such as salicylates.

F. Change incisional dressings as needed.

G. Prevent constipation.

H. Ambulate first postoperative day unless specified otherwise.

I. Discourage smoking.

J. Protect patient from stressful situations.

Postoperative Complications

A. Hemorrhage.
1. Indications.
    a. Emesis with coffee-grounds color.
    b. Tarry black stools (melena).
    c. Hematemesis (vomiting of bright-red blood).
2. Treatment—possible surgical procedure.

✦ B. Perforation—erosion through stomach muscle into peritoneum.
1. Indications.
    a. Acute onset of severe, persistent pain that may be referred to shoulder or between the scapulae.
    b. Tender, boardlike rigidity of the abdomen.
    c. Thready, rapid pulse.
2. Treatment—surgical procedure.

✦ C. Pyloric obstruction (scarring, edema, or inflammation at the pylorus from healing of chronic ulcerations).
1. Indications.
    a. Nausea and projectile vomiting.
    b. Pain.
    c. Weight loss.
    d. Constipation.
2. Treatment—gastric decompression or surgical repair to relieve the stenosis (narrowing).

✦ D. "Dumping syndrome" (rapid emptying of large amounts of food into small bowel following gastrectomy).
1. Indications.
    a. Weakness, faintness.
    b. Diaphoresis.
    c. Palpitations.
2. Nursing care.
    a. Serve frequent meals of small proportions.
    b. Encourage drinking liquids between meals instead of with meals.
    c. Provide nutrients that are low in carbohydrates, high in proteins, and moderate in fats.
    d. Encourage 30-minute rest period lying down after meals.
    e. Discourage use of table salt and sugars.
    ✦ f. Vitamin B_{12} deficiency—loss of intrinsic factor due to surgery; requires B_{12} replacement throughout life.

Principles of Nursing Care for Gastrointestinal Surgery

Preoperative Care

A. Psychological care.
1. Allay fears regarding postoperative concerns.
2. Familiarize the patient with hospital procedures.
    a. Show method for getting in and out of bed.
    b. Teach leg exercises.
    c. Teach deep breathing and coughing exercises.
    d. Explain pain medication schedule.
    e. Discuss recovery room routines.
3. Encourage questions and feedback to determine what patient actually understands.
4. Include family in preoperative explanations.

✦ B. Physical care.
1. Report any change in vital signs.
2. Check and record each item on preoperative check list.
3. Give enema to cleanse the lower colon.
4. Remove all prostheses.
5. Encourage patient to void.

6. Administer preoperative medication (it will dry secretions and promote sense of well-being).
7. Put siderails up.
8. Remove valuables and place in safekeeping.

Postoperative Care

✦ A. Check airway for obstruction.
B. Evaluate the need for pain medication.
C. Check for presence and patency of tubes.
D. Monitor IV.
   1. Check flow rate and contents of bottle.
   2. Check insertion site for pain and signs of inflammation.
E. Examine dressing for color and amount of drainage; record in nurse's notes.
F. Check vital signs frequently.
✦ G. Observe for signs of hypovolemic shock.
   1. Drop in blood pressure.
   2. Increase in pulse or respirations.
   3. Change in color.
   4. Dyspnea.
H. Observe for first passage of flatus on all GI surgical patients. Bowel sounds or flatus indicate the return of peristalsis.
I. Record the time and amount of first voiding.
J. Turn patient every 2 hours.
   1. Encourage coughing and deep breathing.
   2. Support abdominal incision with pillow, hands, or blanket during patient coughing to reduce strain on incision and increase patient comfort.
K. Assist in ambulation as ordered.
L. Encourage taking of food as ordered and tolerated.
M. Evaluate need for medication every 3–4 hours for the first 24 hours; give freely.
N. Do not give morphine to patients with biliary or pancreatic disorders because it results in spasms of the smooth muscle.

✦ **Management of Nasogastric Intubation**
   ❖ **PROCEDURE** ❖

A. Purpose of intubation.
   1. Prevent postoperative vomiting after GI surgery.
   2. Provide feedings.
   3. Relieve abdominal distention as a result of bowel obstruction or paralytic ileus.
   4. Provide rest for the GI tract.
B. Tubal types.
   ✦ 1. Stomach tubes—flexible tubes introduced by way of nose to decompress stomach after surgery or for feedings.
      a. Salem sump—remove fluid accumulation.
      b. Levin tube—gastroduodenal catheter.
   2. Intestinal tubes—tubes placed in intestinal tract by way of nose to relieve gas pressure.

a. Miller–Abbott—double-channel intestinal tube.
b. Cantor tube—used for intestinal decompression.
✦ C. Nursing care.
   1. Provide frequent oral and nasal care.
   2. Maintain patency of tubes with irrigation of normal saline as ordered.
   3. Check for placement of tubes before irrigation.
   4. Observe color and amount of drainage.
   5. Record intake and output.
   6. Be alert to fact that vomiting or abdominal distention is an indication of obstruction.

LOWER GI DISORDERS

Diverticulosis and Diverticulitis

Definitions: Diverticula (blind pouches) formed in the intestinal mucosa and walls of the sigmoid. *Diverticulosis* is the presence of multiple diverticula. *Diverticulitis* is the inflammation of the diverticula. Confirmed by upper–lower GI series and sigmoidoscopy.

Assessment
A. Cramplike pain, usually left-sided.
B. Flatulence.
C. Nausea, vomiting, and fever.
D. Bowel irregularity.
E. Irritability, spasticity of intestine.

Implementation
A. Monitor diet.
   1. Provide high-fiber diet (with bran) that is high in protein, calories, vitamins, and iron for diverticulosis to increase stool bulk and reduce spasms.
   2. Low-fiber diet used in inflammatory phase of diverticulitis.
   3. Vitamin and iron supplements.
✦ B. Administer medications: antispasmodics, antibiotics, anticholinergics (Pro-Banthine), and bulk formers (Metamucil).
C. Administer pain medication (Talwin) rather than morphine or Demerol which increase colonic pressure.
D. Establish normal bowel habits for patient who has deviated from normal patterns.
E. Prepare for surgery as necessary.

Ulcerative Colitis

Definition: Chronic ulcerous and inflammatory disease of the colon and rectum, which commonly begins in the rectum and sigmoid colon and spreads upward; characterized by periods of exacerbation and remission.

Cause

A. Specific cause is unknown.
B. Autoimmune factors, allergic reactions, and emotional instability are potential causative factors.
C. Bacterial infections may be causal factor.

Assessment

A. Anemia and malnutrition.
B. Frequent stools that contain mucus, blood, and pus.
C. Anorexia, weight loss.
D. Cramplike pain.
E. Abdominal tenderness.

Treatment and Implementation

A. Relieve anxiety, i.e., provide quiet environment, remove stress factor; allow patient to ventilate feelings; monitor use of antianxiety medication.
✦ B. Monitor medications.
   1. Antibiotics for secondary bowel inflammation.
   2. Steroid therapy for inflammation, toxicity, and emotional symptoms.
   3. Anticholinergic drugs to relieve cramps and control diarrhea.
   4. New oral aminosalicylates have proven very effective.
   5. No cathartics in acute stage, as they may lead to perforation.
✦ C. Provide high-protein, high-calorie diet with high fiber.
   1. Avoid certain spices (pepper), gas-forming foods, and milk products.
   2. All foods should be cooked to reduce cramping and diarrhea.
   3. Vitamins (A and E), mineral (iron, zinc, calcium, and magnesium) supplements.
D. Replace fluid and electrolyte loss due to diarrhea; potassium chloride may need to be supplemented.
E. Administer IV therapy or TPN during acute phase.
F. Bedrest during acute phase.
G. Surgical treatment is indicated if medical management fails.

Complications

A. Dehydration.
B. Anemia and malnutrition (iron and vitamin K deficiency).
C. Magnesium and calcium imbalance.
D. Perforation, peritonitis, and hemorrhage.
E. Abscesses and strictures.
F. Hemorrhoids and anal fissures.
G. Tendency to bleed.

Inflammatory Bowel Disease

✦ *Definition:*   Also called regional enteritis or Crohn's disease. An inflammatory disease of the small intestine that is chronic and relapsing. The etiology is unknown, but may be related to altered immunologic reactivity.

Characteristics

A. May occur at all ages; usually observed in 20s or 30s.
B. High incidence in families and Jewish populations; low in African Americans.

Assessment

A. Continuous or episodic diarrhea and cramplike pain after meals.
B. Weight loss and malnutrition.
C. Chronic diarrhea that may contain pus, mucus, and blood.
D. Secondary anemia.
E. Check for complications:perforation, generalized peritonitis.

Treatment and Implementation

✦ A. Monitor appropriate diet.
   1. High calorie, high protein.
   2. Low residue, bland.
   3. Supplements of iron and vitamins (including vitamin B_{12}).
   4. Elimination of all milk and milk products.
✦ B. Administer medications.
   1. Antibiotics (Flagyl) to control infection.
   2. Anti-inflammatory drugs (corticosteroids) to reduce swollen membranes.
   3. Antidiarrheal agents to control diarrhea.
   4. Oral aminosalicylates (Asacol).
   5. Immunosuppressives to prevent relapses.
C. May require TPN to maintain nutritional status or surgical intervention.

Intestinal Obstruction

Definition: Impairment of the forward flow of intestinal contents by partial or complete blockage.

✦ **Causes**

A. Mechanical type of obstruction.
   1. Adhesions (fibrous bands of abdominal scar tissue that may become looped over a portion of the bowel).
   2. Incarcerated or strangulated hernias.
   3. Volvulus (twisting of the bowel).
   4. Intussusception (telescoping of bowel upon itself).
   5. Tumors.
   6. Hematoma.
   7. Fecal impaction.
B. Neurogenic type.
   1. Paralytic type.

2. Ileus (ineffective peristalsis due to toxic or traumatic disturbance of innervation to the bowel).

C. Vascular type.
1. Loss of blood supply to the bowel with resulting necrosis.
2. Mesenteric thrombosis.
3. Abdominal angina.

D. Pathophysiology.
1. Fluids and air collect proximal to obstruction.
2. Pressure increases in bowel.
3. Circulating blood volume is reduced—shock develops.

Assessment
◆ A. Small bowel obstruction. Mortality is 10 percent.
1. Cramplike pain in mid-abdomen—may be intermittent.
2. Nausea and vomiting.
3. Reverse peristalsis with possible fecal vomiting.
4. Abdominal distention.
5. Absence of stools.
6. Dehydration; signs of fluid and electrolyte imbalance.

◆ B. Large bowel obstruction.
1. Progression of symptoms slower than with small bowel obstruction.
2. Constipation.
3. Abdominal distention.
4. Cramplike pain in lower abdomen.

◆ C. Observe for paralytic ileus.
1. Dull–diffuse pain.
2. Bowel sounds absent or diminished.
3. Vomiting after eating.
4. Gaseous distention.

D. Presence and progression of distention and absence of flatus and stool.

E. Check lab tests: elevated hematocrit, BUN, and blood glucose; low potassium.

Treatment and Implementation
◆ A. A long, intestinal tube with weighted or balloon tip for intestinal decompression—may be inserted to remove gas and fluid.

B. Monitor parenteral fluids and electrolytes (dextrose and water; Na, K, and Cl).

C. Administer antibiotics to prevent secondary infection (peritonitis).

D. Note and record in chart.
1. Extent and nature of pain.
2. Characteristics, amount, and frequency of stools, emesis, and flatus.
3. Amount of intake and output; urinary output at 30 mL/hour or more.
4. Vital signs.

E. Possible surgery if medical therapy ineffective.

Colon Surgery
◆ A. Ileostomy.
1. Procedure—creation of opening into ileum brought through abdominal wall for purpose of eliminating bowel contents. Large intestine may or may not be removed.
2. Conditions that may lead to ileostomy.
   a. Ulcerative colitis.
   b. Crohn's disease.
◆ 3. Postoperative care.
   a. Observe and record vital signs.
   b. Need not irrigate for evacuation as stool is always in liquid state.
   c. Watch for excoriation of skin around stoma; condition may occur with ileostomy because of enzymatic action.
   d. Increase fluid intake because reabsorption in large bowel is absent.
   e. Provide low-residue, high-calorie diet; avoid foods that increase peristalsis or produce flatus.

◆ B. Colostomy.
1. Procedure—creation of abdominal stoma for bowel evacuation following removal of portion of lower (large) intestine.
2. Conditions indicating colostomy.
   a. Cancer—usually requires permanent colostomy.
   b. Traumatic injury—may require permanent or temporary colostomy.
   c. Diverticulitis or obstruction—usually requires temporary colostomy.
◆ 3. Preoperative care.
   a. Explain to patient the use of apparatus to be utilized in care of the colostomy.
   b. Reassure patient that nurse will give assistance in learning to care for the colostomy.
   c. Accept the patient's feelings about consequence of procedure; observe for depression, anxiety, and frustration.
   d. Provide high-calorie, low-residue diet for several days.
   e. Administer intestinal antibiotics (Kantrex, erythromycin) and neomycin (PO) to decrease bacterial content of colon and to soften and decrease bulk of contents of colon.
   f. Cleanse bowel by administering laxatives and enemas.
   g. Provide adequate fluids and electrolytes.
◆ 4. Postoperative care.
   a. Depends on which part of colon is involved; contents are liquid to formed.
   b. Patient has no voluntary control of bowel evacuation.

✦ Table 10-3. SURGICAL CORRECTIONS FOR THE COLON

Colostomy

A. Causes.
  1. Cancer of colon—permanent colostomy.
  2. Traumatic or congenital disruption of intestinal tract (permanent or temporary).
  3. Diverticulitis (double barrel)—can be reversed after inflammatory process is healed.
B. Procedure—portion of colon brought through abdominal wall.
C. Preoperative care.
  1. Provide high-calorie, low-residue diet for several days.
  2. Administer intestinal antibiotics, Kantrex, erythromycin, and neomycin (PO) to decrease bacterial content of colon and to soften and decrease bulk of contents of colon.
  3. Cleanse bowel by administering laxatives and enemas.
  4. Provide adequate fluids and electrolytes.
D. Postoperative care.
  1. Depends on which part of colon involved; contents are liquid to formed.
  2. Patient has no voluntary control of bowel evacuation.
  3. Ascending colostomy is hard to train for evacuation.
  4. Evacuate bowel every 24–48 hours.
     a. May irrigate with 200–500 mL at first—not commonly done today.
     b. Empty when ⅓–½ full.
  5. Control with diet and/or irrigation.
  6. Maintain skin care around stoma; use skin barrier.
  7. Assure proper fit and placement of appliance—⅛ inch from stoma.
  8. Normal fluid intake.
  9. Instruct patient in colostomy self-care.
  10. Suppositories may be given via colostomy.

Ileostomy

A. Causes.
  1. Ulcerative colitis.
  2. Crohn's disease (regional ileitis).
  3. Distal obstruction.
B. Procedure.
  1. Total colectomy and ileostomy (anything less gives only temporary relief).
  2. Portion of ileum brought through abdominal wall.
C. Preoperative care.
  1. Provide intensified fluid, blood, and protein replacement.
  2. Administer chemotherapy and antibiotics.
  3. If on steroids, maintain therapy after surgery and then gradually decrease.
  4. Provide low-residue diet in small, frequent feedings.
  5. Administer neomycin enemas.
D. Postoperative care.
  1. Contents always liquid (from small intestine).
  2. More chance of excoriation of skin around stoma.
  3. Provide increased fluids because of excessive fluid loss through stoma.
  4. Provide a low-residue, high-calorie diet until patient is accustomed to new arrangement for bowel evacuation; give B_{12}.
  5. Do not give suppositories via ileostomy.

Continent Ileostomy

A. Internal reservoir created by short segment of small intestines.
B. Nipple valve is formed from terminal ileum.
C. As reservoir fills, fecal pressure closes valve.
D. Patient catheterizes stoma 2–4 times a day.
E. Appliance may be needed if leaking occurs.

---

  c. Ascending colostomy is hard to train for evacuation.
  d. Evacuate bowel every 24–48 hours; irrigate with 200–500 mL at first.
  e. Control with diet and/or irrigation.
  f. Maintain skin care around stoma.
  g. Ensure proper fit and placement of appliance.
  h. Increase fluid intake.
  i. Support and guide patient in learning to care for body function, which henceforth will be accomplished differently.

See Table 10-3.

Appendicitis

Definition: Inflammation of appendix as a result of bacterial infection. May be classified as simple gangrenous or perforated.

Assessment
✦ A. Rebound tenderness (major symptom).
✦ B. Generalized and severe upper abdominal pain that localizes in right, lower quadrant.
  C. Anorexia, nausea, and vomiting.
  D. Slightly elevated temperature.
  E. Check diagnostic tests: elevated WBC, urinalysis, abdominal x-rays and ultrasound.

Surgical Procedure—Appendectomy

A. Preoperative care.
   1. Raise bed to semi-Fowler's position to relieve strain on abdomen.
   2. Give nothing by mouth—IV fluids may be given to maintain vascular volume.
   3. Insert nasogastric tube; rectal tube for flatus.
B. Postoperative care.
   1. Routine for abdominal surgery.
   2. NPO until bowel sounds are present.
C. Complications.
   1. Rupture.
   2. Peritonitis.
      a. Indications.
         (1) Severe abdominal pain localized in right lower quadrant.
         (2) Elevated temperature.
         (3) Elevated white cell count.
      b. Treatment.
         (1) Massive antibiotics.
         (2) GI decompression.
         (3) Bedrest.
         (4) High-Fowler's position to localize infection.
         (5) Nothing by mouth.

Hernia

Definition: Protrusion of part of an organ through the structures normally containing it.

✦ Types

A. *Inguinal*—occurring in the groin as result of increased abdominal pressure.
B. *Femoral*—occurring in the femoral canal.
C. *Umbilical*—occurring at the umbilicus.
D. *Incisional*—occurring at incisional site as a result of improper healing.

✦ Classifications

A. *Reducible*—can be replaced in normal cavity.
B. *Irreducible*—cannot be replaced in the normal cavity.
C. *Incarcerated*—resulting edema of the affected structures.
D. *Strangulated*—gangrenous condition results due to trapped blood supply.

Treatment and Implementation

A. Surgical repair—hernioplasty; herniorrhaphy.
B. Advise patient not to cough following surgical repair.
C. Take measures to prevent urinary retention.
D. Encourage patient to ambulate soon after surgery to prevent postoperative complications.

Hemorrhoids

Definition: Dilated varicose veins of the anal canal that cause discomfort and bleeding.

Types

✦ A. *Internal*—occurs above the internal sphincter, covered by mucous membrane.
   B. *External*—occurs outside the external sphincter, covered by anal skin.
   C. *Thrombosed*—infected, clotted, and painful.

Causes

A. Straining to evacuate when constipated.
B. Irritation and diarrhea.
C. Increased venous pressure from congestive heart failure.
D. Increased abdominal pressure as occurs in pregnancy.
E. Habitual toilet sitting (reading of magazines in the bathroom).

Assessment

A. Anal itching.
B. Painful bowel evacuation.
C. Bleeding with bowel evacuation.

Treatment and Implementation

✦ A. Treat constipation with diet, stool softeners, and laxatives.
   B. Maintain diet low in roughage and high in fiber.
   C. Relieve pain with heat, astringents, topical and systemic analgesics, and sitz baths.
   D. Treatments.
      1. Internal hemorrhoids ligated with rubber bands—tissue necroses and drops off.
      2. Cryosurgical hemorrhoidectomy.
      3. Infrared photocoagulation and laser therapy.
   E. Postoperative care of hemorrhoidectomy.
      1. Make routine observations including vital signs.
      2. Maintain meticulous perineal and rectal cleanliness.
      3. Apply topical anesthetics; give sitz baths for comfort.
      4. Maintain prone or on-side positions to prevent pressure and provide comfort.
      5. Administer medications before first postoperative bowel movement.
      6. Increase liquids and bulk with administration of stool softeners to decrease discomfort of first bowel movement.
      7. Give ordered enema with caution.
         a. Administer medications to relieve pain before giving enema.
         b. Use well-lubricated tip.
         c. Introduce tip with gentleness.

DIAGNOSTIC PROCEDURES FOR LIVER, GALLBLADDER, AND PANCREAS DISORDERS

Radiologic Techniques

✦ A. Cholecystogram.
   1. Purpose—visualize gallbladder by means of radiopaque dye given intravenously few minutes prior to exam or by means of Telepaque given orally the evening prior to exam.
   2. Preprocedural nursing care (using Telepaque).
      a. Give patient low-fat meal evening prior to exam.
      b. Give Telepaque according to body weight at 3–5-minute intervals with 240 mL of water (minimum).
      c. Give nothing by mouth after midnight.
✦ B. Cholangiography.
   1. Purpose—visualize bile ducts by means of contrast radiopaque dye injected directly into biliary tree.
   2. Preprocedural nursing care.
      a. Restrict fluids to concentrate dye.
      b. Clean intestinal tract.
   C. Liver scan—visualize liver tissue by means of administered radioiodine (^{131}I) or similar substances and scintiscan to reveal its concentration in the liver.

✦ Liver Biopsy

   A. Purpose—facilitate diagnosis by sampling liver tissues with needle aspiration to determine tissue changes.
✦ B. Preprocedural nursing care.
   1. Obtain baseline vital signs.
   2. Check test results of blood typing and prothrombin time; administer vitamin K as ordered.
   3. Maintain NPO regimen.
   4. Assemble equipment, have patient empty bladder, position patient, and assist the physician.
   C. Postprocedural nursing care.
   ✦ 1. Position patient on right side over biopsy site to prevent hemorrhage.
   2. Observe for complications (hemorrhage, shock).
   3. Measure and record vital signs.

✦ Laboratory Tests*

   A. Serum bilirubin level—abnormal amounts indicate biliary and liver disease leading to jaundice.
   B. Carbohydrate metabolism—glucose tolerance levels should return to normal within 1–2 hours.
   C. Blood ammonia—level rises in liver failure because liver converts ammonia to urea.
   D. Enzyme production—elevation of enzymes reflects organ damage (SGPT, SGOT, LDH).

See Chapter 7, Laboratory Tests.

   E. Prothrombin time—clotting ability reduced in liver cell damage.

DISORDERS OF THE LIVER, GALLBLADDER, AND PANCREAS

Jaundice

Definition: Symptom of liver disorder characterized by yellow pigmentation of the skin due to accumulation of bilirubin pigment in the blood. The degree of jaundice is best detected in the sclera of the eyes.

Characteristics

✦ A. Rapid rate of red blood cell destruction (hemolytic jaundice).
   B. Hepatocellular jaundice results from viral liver cell necrosis or cirrhosis of the liver, diseased liver cells.
   C. Obstruction due to inflammation, tumors, or cholestatic agents.

Assessment

✦ A. Laboratory findings include increased serum bilirubin and increased urobilinogen level, as well as increased SGOT and alkaline phosphatase.
   B. Yellow pigmentation of skin.
   C. Pruritus.

Implementation

   A. Relieve pruritus with starch baths, lotions, antihistamines, and mild sedatives.
   B. Provide emotional support.
   C. Prepare family for patient's altered skin and eye color.
   D. Remove mirrors from patient's line of sight.
   E. Encourage bedrest.

Viral Hepatitis

✦ *Definition:* Inflammation of the liver caused by a virus. With vaccinations, types A and B can be prevented.

Characteristics

✦ A. Type A hepatitis (HAV) (formerly infectious hepatitis).
   1. Transmitted by excreta, infected blood transfusion, contaminated syringes and needles, contaminated food products, and possibly by way of respiratory tract.
   2. Incubation is 20–50 days.
   3. Incidence—higher in fall and winter months.
   4. Infectious 3 weeks prior to and 1 week after becoming jaundiced.
✦ B. Type B hepatitis (HBV) (formerly serum hepatitis, SH virus).
   1. High-risk people are homosexuals, IV drug abusers, and medical workers.

2. Similar to but more severe than type A hepatitis.
3. Transmitted by oral, parenteral, or sexual route by means of infusion or ingestion from the blood or secretions of an infected person; and by contaminated equipment, such as needles, syringes, and dental instruments.
4. Incubation: 45–150 days.
5. Infected people can become carriers.
6. Active immunization—Heptavax B vaccine (three doses).

✦ C. Type C hepatitis (HCV) (formerly non-A, non-B).
1. Symptoms similar to other types.
2. Transmitted by contaminated blood.
   a. Incidence noted following gamma globulin injection.
   b. Incubation period 14–180 days.
3. May not show clinical jaundice.

D. Hepatitis D (delta agent).
1. Transmission same as hepatitis B.
2. Infections occur as coinfection with HBV or superinfection in HBV carrier.
3. Incubation: 15–60 days.

E. Hepatitis E.
1. Rare in the United States, but epidemic in India.
2. Transmitted through oral–fecal contaminated foods or water.

Assessment

A. Perform general assessment; keep in mind that patient is not immediately sick after being infected; onset depends on incubation period and degree of infection.

✦ B. Assess preicteric phase.
1. Signs are generally systemic.
   a. Lethargy and malaise.
   b. Anorexia, nausea, and vomiting.
   c. Headache.
   d. Abdominal tenderness and pain.
   e. Diarrhea or constipation.
   f. Low-grade temperature.
2. Above symptoms may precede jaundice or it may never appear.

✦ C. In anicteric hepatitis, patient has symptoms of disease and altered lab tests, but no jaundice.

✦ D. Assess icteric phase.
1. Dark urine and clay-colored stools generally occur a few days prior to jaundice.
2. Jaundice is first observable in the eyes.
3. Pruritus—usually transient and mild.
4. Enlarged liver with tenderness.
5. Nausea may continue with dyspepsia and flatulence.

✦ E. Assess posticteric phase.
1. Jaundice disappears.

2. The absence of clay-colored stools is an indication of resolution.
3. Fatigue and malaise continue.
4. Enlarged liver continues for several weeks.

Implementation

✦ A. Type A.
1. Wash your hands carefully, always wear gloves, and take precautions during stool and needle procedures.
2. Use disposable equipment or sterilized reusable equipment.
3. Isolate to prevent transmission of disease.
4. Provide diet.
   a. High-calorie, well-balanced diet; modified servings according to patient response.
   b. Protein decreased if signs of coma.
   c. Ten percent glucose IV if not taking oral foods.
   d. Vitamin K supplements if prothrombin time is abnormally long.
   e. Promote adequate fluid intake.
✦ 5. Instruct patient and family.
   a. Stress the importance of follow-up care.
   b. Stress the restricted use of alcohol.
   c. Stress that patient never offer to be a blood donor.
   d. Encourage gamma globulin for close contacts.
   e. Advise correction if any unsanitary condition exists in the home.
6. Bedrest during acute phase with bathroom privileges; reasonable activity level during subsequent phases.

✦ B. Type B.
1. Maintain bedrest until symptoms have decreased.
   a. Activities restricted while liver is enlarged.
   b. Activities discouraged until serum bilirubin is normal.
2. Provide well-balanced diet supplemented with vitamins.
3. Administer antacids for gastric acidity and soporifics for rest and relaxation.
4. Instruct patient and family in pathology of the disease and rationale for treatment.
5. Counsel patient to abstain from sexual activity during communicable period.

C. Type C, D, and E nursing care includes above interventions.

Cirrhosis

Definition: Progressive disease of the liver characterized by diffuse damage (degeneration) to the cells which cannot be recovered or reversed.

Types

+ A. Alcoholic or Laënnec's portal cirrhosis.
  B. Posthepatic cirrhosis (e.g., precipitated by viral hepatitis B or C or unknown cause).
  C. Biliary cirrhosis.

Assessment

A. History of gastrointestinal distress, fatigue, low resistance to infection, gradual failing health.
B. Emaciation and ascites due to malnutrition.
C. Edema of lower extremities.
D. Skin manifestations—spider angiomas, vitamin deficiencies.

+ **Implementation**

A. Provide diet adequate in proteins and carbohydrates, low in salt, and high in multivitamins (especially B).
B. Avoid administering sedatives and opiates and restrict use of alcohol.
C. Prevent infection by providing adequate rest during acute phase and environmental control.
D. Provide good skin care and control pruritus resulting from elevated BUN.
E. Measure and record and compare vital signs to previous measurement.
F. Evaluate level of consciousness and be alert to personality changes and signs of increasing stupor.

Hepatic Encephalopathy

Definition: Hepatic coma results from brain cell alterations due to buildup of ammonia levels.

+ **Assessment**

A. Impaired memory, attention, concentration, and rate of mental response.
B. Confusion, inappropriate behavior, and depressed level of consciousness.
C. Untidy appearance.
D. Flapping tremor upon dorsiflexion of the hand.
E. Disorientation leading to eventual coma.

Implementation

+ A. Observe, measure, and record neurologic status daily (ability to perform simple tasks such as writing one's signature diminishes as the blood ammonia level increases).
  B. Weigh patient daily because liver function decreases and ascites and edema increase.
  C. Measure and record intake and output.
  D. Administer sedatives (depressants) and analgesics sparingly because failing liver unable to detoxify them.
+ E. Temporarily decrease protein from the diet because the ammonia formed from the breakdown of proteins cannot be converted into urea for excretion.

1. Restrict protein to 60g/day.
2. Sodium intake may be restricted to less than 2g/day.
3. Supplement diet with bile salts.
4. Folic acid and iron to treat anemia; vitamin K to reduce risk of bleeding.

+ F. Monitor use of drugs.
  1. Antibiotics such as neomycin will destroy intestinal bacteria and reduce amount of ammonia produced.
  + 2. Lactulose acidifies colon contents and reduces blood ammonia (2 or 3 stools a day indicate lactulose is working).
  G. Avoid drugs (depressants, sedatives, narcotic analgesics) that are detoxified by the liver.

Cholecystitis with Cholelithiasis

+ *Definition: Cholecystitis*—Inflammation of the gallbladder caused by *cholelithiasis* (presence of gallstones). Estimated 25 million in the United States have gallstones; four times more common in women.

Assessment

A. Pain in upper right quadrant of abdomen that is moderate to severe with passage of stones.
B. Nausea and vomiting.
C. Intolerance to fat.
D. Fever.
E. Jaundice will occur if common bile duct obstructed with stones.
F. Edema from inflammation.
G. Laboratory values.
  1. Serum amylase and serum bilirubin elevated.
  2. White blood cell count elevated.
  3. Elevated alkaline phosphatase.

+ **Treatment and Implementation**

A. Administer drugs for control of pain (Demerol—morphine sulfate may increase pain by causing spasm of sphincter of Oddi).
+ B. Insert nasogastric tube for *low suction*—reduces distention.
  C. Give nothing by mouth (low-fat diet may be possible).
  D. Measure and record intake and output.
  E. Stones removed with *shock wave lithotripsy*—lithotriptor sends waves through a water bag, upon which patient is lying, to break up stones.
  F. Cholesterol stones removed through dissolution therapy with oral medication—chenodeoxycholic acid.
+ G. Postoperative nursing care for *cholecystectomy* (removal of gallbladder).
  1. Maintain T-tube, which provides for bile drainage from liver, allowing some of the bile to enter into the common duct. T-tube inserted into duct and connected to drainage bottle. ❖ **PROCEDURE** ❖

a. Ensure patency and avoid stress on the tube; carefully position after dressings are changed.
b. Use measures to control infection.
c. Note character and amount of drainage.
d. Clamp and release regimen as initial step in preparation for T-tube removal.
2. Prevent infection (patients are often obese and may have delayed healing).
3. Observe for indications of biliary obstruction, such as clay-colored stool, jaundiced sclera and/or skin.
4. Advise patient to remain on low-fat diet for at least 2–3 months. Also avoid alcohol and gas-forming foods.
H. *Laparoscopic cholecystectomy*—removal of gall-bladder through small puncture hole in abdomen.
1. Laser dissects gallbladder.
2. Patient discharged day of surgery—recovery 2–3 days.

Acute Pancreatitis

✦ *Definition:* Inflammation of the pancreas. Cause is unknown, although alcoholic indulgence or biliary tract disease are thought to be predisposing factors.

Assessment
A. Constant abdominal pain radiating to the back and flank, aggravated by fatty meal, alcohol, or lying in the recumbent position.
B. Nausea and vomiting, abdominal distention.
C. Low-grade temperature.
D. Possible jaundice (observe stool for fat or clay color).
E. Elevated glucose levels, serum lipase (rises within 2 to 12 hours), and amylase; bilirubin and alkaline phosphatase (due to compression of common duct).
F. Abnormal low serum levels of calcium, sodium, and magnesium due to dehydration and binding of calcium.
G. Elevated WBC (20,000–50,000).

✦ Treatment and Implementation
A. Give nothing by mouth to eliminate main stimulus to enzyme release.
B. Insert nasogastric tube to remove gastric secretions and air if nausea and vomiting or ileus is present. Keep on low suction.
C. Assess pain level (using a standard pain scale).
✦ D. Administer medications.
1. Synthetic analgesic for pain—avoid opiates—may cause spasms.
2. Anticholinergics (Pro-Banthine) to suppress vagal stimulation.
3. Sodium bicarbonate to reverse metabolic acidosis.

4. Histamine H$_2$ antagonists may be given to neutralize HCL secretion.
E. Monitor glucose levels with blood tests—may give regular insulin to treat hyperglycemia.
✦ F. Measure and record intake and output—maintain fluids and electrolytes.
1. Hypocalcemia—treated with calcium gluconate IV.
2. Hypokalemia—treated with potassium.
3. Hypomagnesemia treated with magnesium—can be life-threatening.
G. Aggressive respiratory care to prevent acute respiratory syndrome (ARDS).
H. Provide skin care.
I. Maintain quiet, nonstressful environment; bedrest; Fowler's position.
J. Observe and record vital signs every 15–30 minutes.
K. Weigh and record patient's weight.

Chronic Pancreatitis

Definition: Gland is fibrosed and ducts are obstructed following repeated attacks of acute pancreatitis. Alcohol abuse is the most common cause.

Assessment
A. Pain—persistent epigastric and left upper quadrant pain.
B. Anorexia, nausea, vomiting, and constipation.
C. Disturbance of protein and fat digestion; malnutrition, weight loss, abdominal distention, foul, fatty stools caused by decrease in pancreatic enzyme secretion.
D. Laboratory values: elevated serum amylase and lipase, increased glucose; decreased calcium and potassium.

Treatment and Implementation
✦ A. Monitor drugs.
1. Antacids (Maalox) to neutralize acid secretions.
2. Histamine antagonists (Tagamet and Zantac) to decrease HCl production so pancreatic enzymes are not activated.
3. Proton pump inhibitors (Prilosec) given to neutralize gastric acid.
4. Anticholinergics (atropine, Pro-Banthine) to decrease vagal stimulation.
5. Pancreatic enzyme replacements (Viokase, pancrelipase) with meals to aid digestion.
6. Narcotic analgesics are used for pain.
✦ B. Provide low-protein, low-fat, high-carbohydrate, bland diet.
C. Report any diabetic symptoms; insulin may be given; monitor blood glucose levels.
D. Monitor for potential complications—ascites, pleural effusion, GI hemorrhage, biliary tract obstruction.

GENITOURINARY SYSTEM

This system—the kidneys and their drainage channels—is essential for the maintenance of life. The organs of the GU system are responsible for excreting the end products of metabolism as well as regulating water and electrolyte concentrations of body fluids.

ANATOMY AND PHYSIOLOGY

Kidneys

A. Paired glandular organs located to the right and left of the midline, lateral to lower thoracic vertebrae, that have the ability to adapt to the body's changing needs for elimination of various substances.
B. Major functions.
   1. Excrete most of the end products of body metabolism.
   2. Maintain body acid–base and plasma electrolyte equilibrium.
   3. Produce enzymes that act on plasma substance, which is capable of raising blood pressure.
C. Composition.
   1. Nephrons—microscopic filtering units.
   2. Glomerulus—capillary clusters within nephron capsule; filtering unit of the nephron.
   3. Tubule—collecting channel in nephron that converts the fluid to urine as it goes to the pelvis of the kidneys.
   4. Pelvis—collecting funnel; leads into ureter.
D. Urine.
   1. Composed of excess water and other soluble waste materials that are not reabsorbed into the tubules.
   2. Characteristics of normal urine.
      a. Can be diluted or concentrated.
      b. Clear.
      c. Yellow-amber in color.
      d. Slightly acid.
      e. Specific gravity 1.010–1.025.
      f. Negative for bacteria, albumin, sugar, blood, ketones, or bilirubin.

Ureter

A. Paired tubes lined with mucosa connecting the kidneys with the bladder.
B. Conducts urine by rhythmic contractions.

Bladder

A. Round, hollow, membranous sac with muscular walls, located in the pelvis.
B. Extraperitoneal; however, peritoneum adheres to dome of bladder.
C. May hold 1000 mL in volume if outflow obstructed.

Urethra

A. Single tube that allows passage of urine from bladder to outside of body.
B. Female urethra approximately 3–5 cm in length.
C. Male urethra approximately 20 cm in length.

DIAGNOSTIC PROCEDURES

✦ A. Chemistry tests.
   1. Blood urea nitrogen (BUN) analysis will indicate the ability of the kidney to excrete waste products.
   2. Renal concentration tests.
      a. Evaluate ability of kidney to concentrate urine.
      b. Measured by specific gravity (normal range is 1.003–1.035 with normal usually at 1.010–1.025).
      c. If specific gravity stabilizes at 1.010, indicates kidney has lost ability to concentrate or dilute.
   3. Urine osmolarity—evaluates prescence of renal disease.
   4. Urinary sodium—24 hour test that determines amount of sodium excretion indicating fluid volume deficit, active renal failure and acid-base imbalance.
B. Urine analysis.
   1. Tests total function of renal system.
   2. Specific gravity—degree of concentration in urine.
   3. Urine pH: normal is 6–7 pH; lower than 6 is acidic, higher than 7 alkaline.
✦ C. Intravenous pyelogram (IVP)—injection of contrast dye for visualization on x-ray film of absence, presence, location, size, and configuration of each kidney, the filling of the renal pelvis, and outlines of the ureters.
D. Renal biopsy—needle inserted through renal tissue to extract tissue cells that are examined for evidence of malfunction; test can indicate the presence of disease, confirm a diagnosis, indicate prognosis, or give evidence of response to treatment.
E. Cystoscopy—direct visualization by cystoscope for purposes of inspection, biopsy, treatment, or removal of stones.
F. Retrograde pyelogram—insertion of cystoscope and placement of ureteral catheters followed by

injection of contrast dye into the catheters for visualization on x-ray film of ureters and kidneys.

G. Renal imaging.

　1. General term that includes flat plate of abdomen showing outline of kidneys, IVP, voiding cystourethrogram, retrograde pyelogram.

　2. Renal ultrasound—may be used to guide percutaneous needle biopsies of kidney.

Genitourinary System Assessment

✦ A. Check urinalysis findings to determine presence of infection, bleeding, signs of renal failure, or existing conditions.

　1. *Retention*—inability to expel urine from the bladder due to obstruction or loss of innervation.

　2. *Incontinence*—loss of voluntary control in discharge of urine.

　3. *Residual urine*—urine remaining in bladder after voiding.

　4. *Anuria*—suppression or failure of kidney to produce sufficient urine.

　5. *Oliguria*—amount and frequency of urination are diminished.

　6. *Hematuria*—blood in the urine, usually caused by infection or trauma.

✦ B. Assess pain for location, intensity, and precipitating factors.

　1. Ureteral pain is related to obstruction and is usually an acute manifestation.

　　a. Site of obstruction may be found by tracing the location of radiation of pain.

　　b. Pain may be severe and usually radiates down ureter into scrotum or vulva and to the inner thigh.

　2. Bladder pain is due to infection and overdistention of the bladder in urinary retention.

　3. Testicular pain is caused by inflammation or trauma, and is acute and severe.

　4. Pain in the lower back and leg may be caused by prostate cancer with metastasis to pelvic bones.

　5. Pain caused by renal disease.

　　a. Dull ache in flank, radiating to lower abdomen and upper thigh.

　　b. Pain may be absent if there is no sudden distention of kidney capsules.

C. Assess bladder for distention.

D. Examine the urinary catheter for abnormal findings.

E. Evaluate intake and output values.

F. Measure vital signs to determine presence of complications.

G. Assess patency of shunts.

H. Assess all body systems for potential alterations as a result of kidney problems.

　1. Peripheral edema.

　2. Hypertension.

　3. Eye disorders.

　4. Anemia.

　5. Lethargic or irritable condition.

　6. Congestive heart failure.

I. Observe for signs and symptoms of fluid and electrolyte imbalances.

J. Evaluate urinary test results for signs of renal abnormalities.

K. Assess patient's feelings about body image.

Male Examination

✦ A. Testicular self-exam (TSE).

　1. Instruct patient to perform monthly following warm bath. (Between ages 15 and 25, third highest cause of cancer deaths.)

　2. Rotate each testicle between thumb and forefinger, feeling for a firm surface.

　3. If painless lump is felt (*not* the epididymis), notify physician immediately.

✦ B. Prostate evaluation.

　1. Rectal exam annually beginning at age 40.

　2. Blood chemistry for cancer.

　　a. Prostatic acid phosphate (PAP)—elevated.

　　b. Prostate-specific antigen (PSA)— elevated; most sensitive tumor marker.

　　c. May be false positive readings.

　3. Ultrasound with biopsy if indicated.

Female Gynecological Examination

A. Pelvic examination.

　1. Inspection of external genitalia for signs of inflammation, bleeding, discharge, and epithelial cell changes.

　2. Visualization of vagina and cervix.

　3. Bimanual examination.

　4. Rectal examination.

✦ B. Papanicolaou smear.

　1. Diagnosis for cervical cancer.

　2. Vaginal secretions and secretions from posterior fornix are smeared on a glass slide.

　✦ 3. Pathological classifications.

　　a. Class I: no abnormal or atypical cells present.

　　b. Class II: abnormal or atypical cells present but no malignancy found; repeat Pap smear and follow-up if necessary.

　　c. Class III: cytology, suggests malignancy; additional procedures: biopsy, D and C.

　　d. Class IV: cytology, strongly suggests malignancy; additional procedures: biopsy, D and C.

　　e. Class V: cytology conclusive of malignancy.

✦ C. Breast self-examination (BSE).

　1. Perform 5 to 7 days after menses counting first day of menses as day one (less fluid is retained).

2. Instruct female patient to place pillow under the shoulder and, using three fingers, compress breast tissue in a circular motion.
   a. Examine entire breast including nipple area.
   b. Move pillow to other shoulder and repeat examination.
3. Remind patient to immediately report any lump, irregularity, edema, skin changes, discharge, or nipple changes.

✦ D. Mammography.
   1. X-ray of soft tissue to detect nonpalpable mass.
   2. Baseline (one time) age 35–39; yearly after age 40.

System Implementation

A. Maintain accurate measurement of intake and output.
B. Force or restrict fluids as ordered.
C. Observe and record characteristics of urine and times of voiding.
D. Record specific urinary complaints, e.g., urgency, burning, pain, frequency, bladder spasms, and inability to void (retention).
E. Strain all urine and take specimen to lab (if ordered) if renal lithiasis (stones) are suspected.
F. Maintain comfort of patient; position and provide analgesics and external heat for renal colic.

✦ **Specialized Catheter Care** ❖ **PROCEDURE** ❖
A. Maintain patency of catheters.
B. Types of urinary tract catheters.
   1. Foley catheter—designed with inflatable balloon that, upon inflation, anchors catheter within bladder.
   2. Three-way Foley catheter—provides for drainage of urine, balloon for anchoring, and a third channel to allow for irrigation of the bladder.
   3. Straight catheter—a simple rubber catheter that is inserted into bladder for drainage and then removed.
   4. Ureteral catheters—very small-gauge catheters inserted directly into ureters during cystoscopy for drainage of urine from the pelvis of the kidney or for injection of dye for diagnostic purposes; if left inserted, they are usually anchored with a Foley.

DISORDERS OF THE KIDNEY

Urinary Tract Infections

✦ *Definition:* A term that refers to a wide variety of conditions affecting the urinary tract in which the common denominator is the presence of microorganisms. A major health problem, especially among women; frequency rate is 20 percent among women.

Characteristics

A. Urine is sterile until it reaches the distal urethra.
B. Any bacteria can be introduced into the urinary tract resulting in infection, which may spread to any other part of the tract. *Escherichia coli* is most frequent organism.
C. The most important factor influencing ascending infection is obstruction of free urine flow.
   1. Free flow, large urine output, and pH are antibacterial defenses.
   2. If defenses break down, the result may be an invasion of the tract by bacteria.
D. Microscopic examination is completed for an accurate identification of the organism (especially important in chronic infections).
E. Most common health care problem in US—more common in women.

✦ **Assessment**

A. Examine urine laboratory tests.
   1. Urine cultures to find presence and number of bacteria.
   2. Urine colony count (over 100,000 mL indicates UTI).
B. Observe urine for color, consistency, and specific gravity.
C. Check blood or urine test to rule out STDs (which will produce similar symptoms).
D. Location, type, and precipitating factors leading to pain.

Treatment and Implementation

✦ A. Encourage fluids to 3000 mL.
✦ B. Administer urinary antimicrobials as ordered.
   1. Standard treatment—therapy for lower tract infection.
      a. Single-dose therapy effective in 80 percent.
      b. Trimethoprim (Primsol), sulfamethoxazole (Gantanol), or the quinolones (Cipro or Noroxin) may be used.
   2. Short-course therapy—3 or 4 days—more commonly prescribed.
   3. Longer course—10–14 days—for upper tract infections.
      a. Antibacterial may be prescribed with single-dose therapy.
      b. Urinary antiseptics may be used with antimicrobials.
   4. Action of antimicrobials—inhibits cell wall mucopeptide synthesis; interferes with enzyme needed for bacterial metabolism.
   ✦ 5. Adverse effects—hypersensitivity, nausea, vomiting, diarrhea, rash.

C. Fostomycin antibiotics (Monurol).
   1. Inhibits bacterial cell wall synthesis.
   2. Single dose treatment.
D. Administer antiseptics—interfere with vital processes of the bacteria.
   1. Medications: nitrofurantoin (Furadantin); methenamine salts (Hipres, Urised).
   2. Adverse effects—anorexia, nausea, vomiting.
E. Antispasmodics and analgesics may be used to relieve pain, frequency, urgency, and burning.
F. Encourage patient to void every 2–3 hours and to empty bladder—reduces urinary stasis and risk of reinfection.
G. Avoid beverages that irritate bladder.

Acute Renal Failure

Definition: Sudden loss of kidney function caused by failure of renal circulation or tubular or glomerular damage.

Causes

A. Dehydration.
B. Shock.
C. Traumatic injury.
D. Toxic agents, e.g., sulfonamides, arsenic.
E. Infection.

Assessment

✦ A. Decreased urine output (volume of less than 400 to 500 mL/24 hr), period of oliguria may be followed by periods of diuresis and then recovery.
B. Specific gravity may be fixed at 1.010–1.016 if renal failure occurs.
C. Hypertension may develop.
✦ D. Monitor serum levels of potassium, sodium, pH, PCO_2, and HCO_3—indication of complications.
E. Monitor urinalysis for proteinuria, hematuria, casts.
F. Nausea, vomiting, diarrhea, dehydration, and convulsions leading to coma.
G. Assess for signs of infection—may not have fever or increased WBC.

Treatment and Implementation

A. Treat cause of failure immediately.
B. Monitor body fluid volume and electrolytes.
C. Monitor urinary output (hourly basis may be indicated).
D. Weigh patient daily.
✦ E. Follow diet restrictions: moderate protein restriction (1g/Kg/day), restrict foods high in nitrogen, potassium, phosphate, sulfate, and sodium, with vitamin supplements.
F. Observe for complications of fluid overload, electrolyte disturbances, and CHF.

G. Maintain bedrest to decrease exertion and metabolic state; provide good skin care.

Chronic Renal Failure

Definition: Progressive impairment of kidney function that, without intervention, ends fatally in uremia.

Characteristics

A. Kidney dysfunction occurs in three stages.
   1. Diminished renal reserve—40 to 75% loss of function. No apparent symptoms.
   2. Renal insufficiency—increase in BUN and creatinine (10:1 ratio); 75 ot 90% loss of function.
   3. End-stage renal failure or uremia; less than 10% function.
B. In last stage renal failure normal regulatory function, secretory and hormonal functions are severely impaired.

Assessment

A. Weakness, fatigue, and headaches.
B. Anorexia, nausea, and vomiting, and hiccups.
C. Hypertension with renal and heart failure.
D. Anemia, azotemia (nitrogen retention in the blood).
E. Central nervous system signs (i.e., irritability, convulsions).
F. Low and fixed specific gravity of urine.

✦ Treatment and Implementation

A. Monitor intake and output.
B. Weigh patient daily.
C. Provide diet low in salt and low amounts of protein; prepare as attractively as possible.
D. Monitor blood pressure closely.
E. Provide emotional support because chronicity of disease may precipitate depression.
✦ F. Drugs are used to check for renal failure before patient is placed on dialysis.
   1. In most cases mannitol is tried.
      a. Has osmotic effect; increases urinary flow.
      b. 12.5 g of 25 percent solution given in 3 minutes; if flow rate can be increased to 40 mL/hr, patient is in reversible renal failure.
      c. Keep urine flow at 100 mL/hr with mannitol.
   2. Lasix (furosemide) and Edecrin (ethacrynic acid) may be used if mannitol is not effective.
   3. Antihypertensives, Epogen, iron supplements.
   4. Antacids treat hyperphosphatemia and hypocalcemia.
G. Electrolyte replacement: sodium, acidosis replacement of bicarbonate stores; potassium and phosphorus restricted.

Uremic Syndrome (Uremia)

✦ *Definition:*   The accumulation of nitrogenous waste products in blood due to inability of kidneys to filter out waste products.

Characteristics

A. May occur after acute or chronic renal failure.
B. Increased urea, creatinine, uric acid.
✦ C. Extensive electrolyte imbalances (increased K^+, increased Na^+, decreased Cl^-, decreased Ca^{++}, increased phosphorus).
D. Acidosis—bicarbonate cannot be maintained at adequate level.
E. Urine concentration ability lost.
F. Anemia caused by decreased rate of production of RBCs.

Assessment

✦ A. Signs of oliguria for 1–2 weeks (produces < 400 mL/day).
✦ B. Changes in urine characteristics.
   1. Urine contains protein, red blood cells, casts.
   2. Specific gravity of 1.010.
   3. Rise in urine solutes (e.g., urea, uric acid, potassium, magnesium).
C. Metabolic acidosis.
D. Hypotension or hypertension.
E. Gastrointestinal problems: stomatitis, nausea, vomiting, and diarrhea or constipation.
F. Respiratory complications.
G. Evaluate coma—with alterations of blood chemistry and acid load.

Implementation

A. Monitor restoration of blood volume.
B. Monitor fluid and electrolyte balance.
✦ C. Provide dietary regulation.
   1. Limit protein (.8g/kg) unless on peritoneal dialysis.
   2. Reduce nitrogen, potassium, phosphate, and sulfate.
   3. Limit sodium intake.
   4. Provide glucose to prevent ketosis.
   5. Control potassium balance to prevent hyperkalemia.
   6. Carbohydrate intake 100 g daily.

✦ Hemodialysis

A. Procedure permits passage through a semipermeable membrane of substances (urea, creatinine, and uric acid), which diffuse through the pores of the membrane in the machine.
   1. The blood, which contains the waste products, flows from the patient into the dialysis machine where it comes into contact with the dialysate.
   2. The waste products are removed through contact of the blood as it flows into the machine and comes in contact with the dialysate.
B. In essence, the dialysis machine becomes the patient's "kidney."

✦ Peritoneal Dialysis

A. Usually temporary, can be used for patient in acute, reversible renal failure.
   1. Treatment of choice for those unable or unwilling to undergo hemodialysis.
   2. Used for patients with diabetes or chronic heart disease who cannot use heparin or are not responsive to other treatments.
B. A method of separating substances by interposing a semipermeable membrane.
   1. The peritoneum is used as the dialyzing membrane and substitutes for kidney function during failure.
   2. Removes end products of protein metabolism (creatinine and urea).
C. Procedure allows for infusion of dialysate through a peritoneal catheter for "dwell time" in order that waste products in the blood may diffuse into the solution.
   1. The dialysate is in direct contact with blood supply of mesentery.
   2. After "dwell time," fluid is drained by gravity into receptacles, and sample is sent to laboratory for testing.
   3. The volume returned by gravity should equal or be in excess of the volume of the infusion.

✦ Continuous Ambulatory Peritoneal Dialysis (CAPD)

A. A variation of peritoneal dialysis developed to allow patient to be dialyzed while ambulatory.
B. Procedure for CAPD.
   1. Peritoneal catheter is inserted.
   2. 500–2000 mL of dialysate infused through catheter by gravity (10–20 minutes).
   3. The catheter is clamped, bag folded and placed in waistband of clothes.
   4. Every 4–6 hours, patient drains fluid from peritoneal cavity.
      a. Unclamp catheter.
      b. Place pouch to allow drainage by gravity —below level of abdomen.
      c. Drain for approximately 20 minutes.
      d. Reclamp catheter and remove bag with drainage.
      e. Examine drainage—a change in color may indicate infection (glucose in dialysate predisposes patient to infection).
   5. Aseptically attach a new bag of dialysate and repeat procedure.
   6. Repeat procedure 4–5 times daily.

7. Instruct patient to change tubing every 24 hours using strict aseptic technique.
C. Check for complications—peritonitis, dehydration, infection, hemorrhage.

Other Types of Peritoneal Dialysis
A. Continuous Cycling Peritoneal Dialysis (CCPD).
B. Intermittent Peritoneal Dialysis (IPD).
C. Nightly Peritoneal Dialysis (NPD).

Pyelonephritis

✦ *Definition:*   An acute or chronic infection and inflammation of one or both kidneys that usually begins in the renal pelvis.

Assessment
A. Attacks of chills and fever with malaise, headache.
B. Tenderness and dull, aching pain in the back.
C. Frequency and burning with urination.
D. Renal function—ability to concentrate urine and/or renal insufficiency (inability to excrete electrolytes).
E. Ultrasound or CT scan used to locate any obstruction.

Treatment and Implementation
A. Record characteristics, frequency, and amount of voiding.
B. Provide diet high in calories and vitamin supplements and low in protein if oliguria is present.
C. Give sufficient liquids to maintain urine volume of 1500 mL/24 hr.
D. Monitor drug therapy.
 1. Antibiotics—usually given for 2 weeks.
 2. Usual drugs: trimethoprin, ciproploxcin, gentamicin or a third generation cephalosporin.
E. Observe for edema and signs of renal failure.
F. Teach principles of optimum personal hygiene to prevent further infections.
G. Bedrest until asymptomatic.
H. Instruct patient to empty bladder regularly.

Acute Glomerulonephritis

✦ *Definition:*   Inflammatory disease of both kidneys that interferes with glomerular filtration; most commonly caused by repeated streptococcal infections in childhood.

✦ Assessment
A. Initially, symptoms may be mild—headache, malaise, and weakness; pharyngitis.
B. Oliguria and puffiness around the eyes; edema of legs or generalized.
C. Hematuria; proteinuria—2–8 g daily.
D. Moderate to marked hypertension.
E. Tenderness at costovertebral angle is common.
F. Diagnostic urinalysis indicates erythrocyte casts; hypoalbuminemia due to increased loss via urine; high specific gravity.

✦ Treatment and Implementation
A. Administer antibiotics (penicillin), antihypertensives, and loop diuretics.
B. Corticosteroids and immunosuppressives if disease progresses rapidly.
✦ C. Provide diet low in protein (40 g), if oliguria is severe.
 1. Protein should be the complete type (eggs, meat, fish, poultry, milk).
 2. High carbohydrates to spare protein and provide energy.
 3. Potassium and sodium usually restricted.
✦ D. Restrict fluids based on previous day's output; record intake and output.
E. Do not permit increase of activity until blood pressure and BUN are normal for 1–2 weeks.
F. Monitor vital signs continuously.
G. Weigh patient daily.
H. Observe for signs of overhydration, hypertension, renal failure, congestive failure and pulmonary edema.

SURGICAL INTERVENTIONS

Nephrectomy

Definition: Surgical removal of a kidney.

Indications
A. Severe injury producing irreparable damage to cells.
B. Chronic disease.
C. Permanent loss of kidney function.
D. Renal donor.

Implementation
A. Monitor, measure and record intake and output frequently.
B. Encourage patient to take fluids after bowel sounds return.
C. Observe for signs of hemorrhage and shock.
D. Provide care for incision and Penrose drain.
E. Administer medications.
 1. Antibiotics.
 2. Low-dose heparin to reduce risk of thrombophlebitis.
F. Turn, cough and hyperventilate; use incentive spirometer.
G. Encourage postoperative exercises and early ambulation.
H. Control environment against infection from visitors and personnel.

Nephrostomy

Definition: Creation of surgical opening into kidney and placement of a catheter in the renal pelvis for urinary drainage.

Implementation

A.   Record characteristics of drainage and urine.
B.   Check for bleeding at surgical site as this is major complication.
C.   Unless ordered, do not clamp catheter.
D.   Unless ordered, do not irrigate (never irrigate with force; use only 5–10 mL of sterile solution; be especially careful not to contaminate).
E.   In bilateral nephrostomy, maintain separate outputs.
F.   Maintain patency of tubes when positioning patient and when changing dressings.

Urolithotomy

◆ *Definition:*   Removal of stones (calculi) formed in the urinary system (urolithiasis).

◆ **Types**

A.   *Ureterolithotomy*—removal of calculi from ureter, which may be accomplished with use of cystoscope and stone crusher.
B.   *Pyelolithotomy*—removal of stone from kidney pelvis.

Implementation

A.   Force fluids.
B.   Strain all urine.
C.   Measure and record intake and output.
D.   Observe and record characteristics of urine and time of voiding.
E.   Prevent infection.
F.   Observe for perforation of bladder, abdominal rigidity, anuria, chills, fever, and urine retention.

BLADDER DISORDERS AND SURGERY

Cystitis

Definition: Inflammation of the bladder from infection or from obstruction of the urethra.

Assessment

A.   Frequency and urgency of urination.
B.   Burning sensation in urethra during urination.
C.   Suprapubic discomfort.
D.   Dark and odorous urine.
E.   Urinalysis reveals presence of bacteria and blood cells.

◆ **Treatment and Implementation**

A.   Attempt to remove cause of the condition (infection, obstruction).
B.   Administer antibiotic therapy: sulfamethoxazole is drug of choice (Bactrim, Septra).
C.   Collect uncontaminated urine specimen (catheterized or midstream).
D.   Maintain adequate fluid intake; force fluids if ordered—avoid urinary tract irritants (coffee, tea, citrus).
E.   Decrease patient's activity during the acute stage.
F.   Teach principles of optimum personal hygiene to prevent recurrent infection.

Suprapubic Cystostomy

◆ *Definition:*   Creation of surgical opening and placement of catheter into bladder for urinary drainage—diverts urine flow from urethra.

Implementation

A.   Change dressings frequently, and give skin care (avoid reinforcing and creating bulky, wet, odorous dressings that cause excoriation to the skin).
B.   Maintain patency of catheter when applying dressing or positioning patient.
C.   Provide clamp and release regimen until patient can void voluntarily.

Cystectomy

◆ *Definition:*   Removal of bladder (due to presence of tumors) with diversion of ureters into "bladder" constructed from loop of ileum, which is brought through abdominal wall as an ileostomy opening.

Implementation

A.   Provide routine postoperative care.
B.   Maintain nasogastric tube.
C.   Care for stoma with ileostomy procedure.
D.   Measure and record intake and output.
E.   Observe for development of fistula or dehiscence.
F.   Refer patient to enterostomy therapist and a visiting nurse association.

Prostatitis

◆ *Definition:*   Inflammation of the prostate gland caused by an infectious agent (bacteria, mycoplasma) or structure, hyperplasia.

Assessment

A.   Assess for peritoneal discomfort, burning, urgency, or frequency.
B.   Assess for generalized pain or pain associated with ejaculation or voiding.
C.   If acute, patient may have sudden onset of fever, chills, and pain.

Implementation

✦ A. Monitor broad spectrum antimicrobials (sensitive to causative agent)—may be tetracycline, doxycycline (10–14 days).

B. Maintain patient on bedrest until symptoms are alleviated.

C. Promote comfort with analgesics, antispasmodics, sedatives, sitz baths, rectal irrigations.

Benign Prostatic Hypertrophy (BPH)

✦ *Definition:* Enlargement of prostate gland from normal tissue usually in males over 50.

Assessment

A. Causes narrowing of urethra, which may result in obstruction.

✦ B. Clinical manifestations.
   1. Recurring infection and urinary stasis.
   2. Nocturia, frequency, dysuria, urgency, dribbling, retention, and hematuria.
   3. Hesitancy in starting urination.

Implementation

A. Treatment.
   1. Drug—finasteride (Proscar) reduces hypertrophy through inhibition of enzyme which blocks uptake of androgens; has severe side effects (impotence).
   2. Herbs (saw palmetto) and nutrients: magnesium, calcium, and zinc reduce hypertrophy.
   3. Monitor drug therapy if indicated.

B. Encourage fluids—2000–3000 mL/day.

C. Suggest diet high in minerals: calcium, magnesium, zinc, manganese.

D. Avoid drugs that could cause urinary retention (anticholinergics).

E. Provide postoperative care for removal of the hypertrophied fibroadenomatous portion of the prostate. (*See* Prostatectomy.)

Cancer of the Prostate

Characteristics

A. Type: androgen-dependent adenocarcinoma.

B. Clinical manifestations.
   1. Early symptoms similar to BPH.
   2. Urinary obstruction late in disease.
   3. Pain radiating from lumbosacral area down legs strongly indicative of cancer.

C. Many cancers so slow-growing the client will die of other diseases before the cancer spreads significantly.

✦ D. Prostate specific antigen (PSA) test shows concentration is proportional to total prostatic mass.
   1. Does not necessarily indicate malignancy.

✦ TREATMENT

✦ **Medical regimen.**
   1. Estrogen therapy or luteinizing hormone antagonist (Lupron) or antiandrogen agents may be given to slow rate of growth and extension of tumor.
   2. Orchiectomy decreases androgen production.
   3. Radiation to local lesion to reduce tumor: external beam radiation or implant.
   4. Do no procedure—monitor annually.

Surgical options.
✦ 1. Transurethral resection (TUR) most common intervention—removal of prostatic tissue by instrumentation through urethra.
   2. Suprapubic prostatectomy—removal of prostate by abdominal incision with bladder incision.
   3. Retropubic prostatectomy—low abdominal incision without opening bladder.
   4. Perineal prostatectomy (may be radical resection)—perineal incision between scrotum and anus for gland removal.
   5. Transurethral incision (TUIP)—instrument passed through urethra, one or two incisions made in prostate to reduce pressure and construction. Effective for treatment of BPH.
   6. Homium laser (Coherent Co.) may replace TUR for prostate surgery—advantages are less bleeding, fewer complications, and shorter hospital stay.

---

   2. Used routinely to monitor client's response to cancer therapy.

Prostatectomy

Definition: Removal of prostate gland.

Indications

A. Enlargement of prostate (benign prostatic hypertrophy), which interferes with free urinary bladder flow.
   ✦ 1. Symptoms of enlargement.
      a. Recurring infection.
      b. Urine stasis.
      c. Nocturia.
      d. Frequency.
      e. Dysuria.
      f. Straining to void.
   ✦ 2. Detected by PSA blood test and physical examination.

B. Malignancy of prostate gland.

Treatment and Implementation

✦ A. Medical regimen.
   1. Estrogen therapy may be given to slow rate of growth and extension of tumor.
   2. Radiation to local lesion to reduce tumor: external beam radiation or implant.
   3. Orchiectomy decreases androgen production.

✦ B. Surgical options.
1. Transurethral resection (TUR) most common intervention—removal of prostatic tissue by instrumentation through urethra.
2. Suprapubic prostatectomy—removal of prostate by abdominal incision with bladder incision.
3. Retropubic prostatectomy—abdominal incision without opening bladder.
4. Perineal prostatectomy—perineal incision.
5. Transurethral incision—1 or 2 incisions made in prostate to reduce pressure and constriction—effective treatment for BPH.
6. Homium laser may replace surgery for there is less bleeding, fewer complications, and shorter hospital stay.

Postoperative Implementation
✦ A. Maintain adequate bladder drainage via catheter.
1. Suprapubic catheter used following suprapubic prostatectomy.
2. Continuous bladder irrigation (or triple lumen catheter) is used following transurethral resection. ❖ **PROCEDURE** ❖
a. One lumen is used for inflating balloon (usually 30 mL), one for outflow of urine, and one for irrigating solution instillation.
b. Run solution in rapidly if bright red drainage or clots are present; when drainage clears, decrease to about 40 drops/minute.
c. If clots cannot be rinsed out with irrigating solution, irrigate with syringe as ordered (usually 50 mL).

✦ B. Provide fluids to prevent dehydration (2–3 L every 24 hours).
C. Provide high-protein, high-vitamin diet.
D. Observe for signs of hemorrhage and shock.
✦ E. Instruct patient in perineal exercises to regain urinary control.
1. Tense perineal muscles by pressing buttocks together; hold for as long as possible.
2. Repeat this process ten times every hour.
F. Ambulate early (after urine has returned to nearly normal color).
G. Observe for complications.
1. Epididymitis (most frequent).
2. Gram-negative sepsis.
H. Administer urinary antiseptics or antibiotics as ordered to prevent infection.
I. Provide wound care for suprapubic and retropubic prostatectomies (similar to that for abdominal surgery).
J. Provide sitz bath and heat lamp treatments to promote healing.

BLOOD AND LYMPHATIC SYSTEMS

The circulatory system, a continuous circuit, is the mechanical conveyor of the body constituent called blood. Blood, composed of cells and plasma, circulates through the body and is the means by which oxygen and nutritive materials are transported to the tissues and carbon dioxide and metabolic end products are removed for excretion.

System Assessment

A. Onset of symptoms, whether insidious or abrupt.
B. Petechiae, ecchymosis.
C. Bleeding time.
D. Fatigue and general weakness.
E. Chills or fever.
F. Dyspnea.
G. Ulceration of oral mucosa and pharynx.
H. Pruritus.
I. Skin color—pallor, yellow-cast, or reddish-purple hue.
J. Visual disturbances.
K. Hepatomegaly or splenomegaly.
L. Dietary deficiencies—ask questions about daily intake of foods.
M. Neurological symptoms.
   1. Numbness and tingling in the extremities.
   2. Personality changes.
N. Cardiovascular signs and symptoms.
   1. Hypotension or hypertension.
   2. Character of pulse.
   3. Capillary engorgement.
   4. Venous thrombosis.
O. Gastric distress and weight loss.

DISEASES OF THE BLOOD AND BLOOD-FORMING ORGANS

Megaloblastic (Pernicious) Anemia

Definition: A group of anemias caused by defective DNA synthesis and abnormal maturation.

Characteristics

✦ A. Primary cause is the absence of intrinsic factor.
✦ B. Causes related to:
   1. Deficiency of vitamin B_{12} or folic acid.
   2. Surgical resection of small intestine.
   3. Atrophy of gastric mucosa.
   4. Dietary deficiency—malabsorption disease.

   5. Bacterial or parasitic infections.
   6. Chemotherapy drugs.
C. Genetic predisposition (especially in northern Europe).
D. Diagnostic tests.
   1. RBC count, megaloblastic maturation.
   2. Bone marrow aspiration.
   3. Upper GI series.
   4. Schilling test (maintain NPO for 12 hours; collect 24-hour urine) for pernicious anemia.
   5. Gastric analysis—insertion of nasogastric tube, collection of aspirant, injection of histamine.

Assessment

A. Weakness, unsteady gait.
B. Dyspnea.
C. Palpitation, tachycardia.
D. Anorexia, dyspepsia.
E. Diarrhea.
F. Neurological distubance—numbness and tingling of extremities.
   1. Symptoms do not occur with folic acid deficiency.
   2. Distinction between deficiency in B_{12} must be made with deficiency in folic acid.
G. Pallor, slight jaundice.
H. Glossitis.
I. Mild hepatomegaly (enlarged liver).
J. Splenomegaly (enlarged spleen).

Treatment and Implementation

A. Provide safety measures if neurological deficit is present—assist with ambulation.
B. Avoid pressure on lower extremities due to circulation deficit (footcradle, etc.).
C. Avoid extremes of heat and cold.
✦ D. Administer B_{12} deep IM, as ordered (usually once a month) and folic acid (1 mg/day PO).
✦ E. Instruct in administration of B_{12}. This is a lifelong therapy.
F. Provide support and explain behavior changes to patient and family.

Aplastic Anemia

✦ *Definition:*   Deficiency of marrow stem cells resulting from bone marrow suppression.

Characteristics

A. Causes.
   1. Toxic action of drugs (Chloromycetin, sulfonamides, Dilantin, alkylating agents, antimetabolites, anticonvulsants).
   2. Exposure to radiation, chemicals.
   3. Diseases that suppress bone marrow or stem cell activity (leukemia and metastatic cancer).
B. Pancytopenia frequently accompanies RBC deficiency.

Assessment

A. Increased fatigue.
B. Lethargy.
C. Dyspnea.
D. Infection.
E. Low platelet and leukocyte count.

Treatment and Implementation

✦ A. Medical treatment.
    1. Bone marrow transplant and WBC transfusion are becoming more prevalent.
    2. Splenectomy (especially in severe thrombocytopenia).
B. Administer androgens and/or corticosteroids—now not commonly used due to toxic effects.
C. Monitor transfusion of fresh platelets (RBC transfusion may be introduced also).
D. Administer antibiotics when infection occurs.
E. Place patient in private room.
F. Protect from infections.
G. Prevent fatigue—provide for adequate rest periods.
H. Observe for complications.
I. Provide physical comfort measures.
J. Provide emotional support for patient and family.
K. Educate public in use of toxic pesticides and chemicals.

Purpuras

Definition: The extravasation of blood into the tissues and mucous membranes.

Characteristics

A. Idiopathic thrombocytopenic purpura is characterized by platelet deficiency.
B. Vascular purpura is characterized by weak, damaged vessels, which rupture easily.

Assessment

A. Petechiae.
B. Postsurgical bleeding.
C. Increased bleeding time.
D. Abnormal platelet count.
E. Ecchymosis.

Treatment and Implementation

A. Identify underlying cause if possible.
B. Complete steps to control bleeding.
C. Monitor transfusion of platelets.
D. Monitor administration of corticosteroids.

Agranulocytosis

✦ *Definition:*   An acute, potentially fatal blood disorder characterized by profound neutropenia. This condition is most commonly caused by drug toxicity or hypersensitivity.

✦ Assessment

A. Chills and fever.
B. Sore throat and flulike symptoms.
C. Exhaustion and depletion of energy.
D. Ulceration of oral mucosa and throat.

Implementation

A. Discontinue suspected chemical agents or drugs.
B. Isolate to reduce exposure to infections.
C. Administer corticosteroids if ordered.

Polycythemia Vera

✦ *Definition:*   A chronic disease of unknown etiology characterized by overactivity of bone marrow with overproduction of red cells and hemoglobin.

Assessment

A. Reddish-purple hue to the skin and pruritus.
B. Increased blood volume.
C. Capillary engorgement.
D. Hemorrhage.
E. Venous thrombosis.
F. Arterial hypertension.
G. Hepatomegaly and splenomegaly.

✦ Treatment and Implementation

A. Radiophosphorus (32P) in dosages based on body weight; initially IV, then orally.
B. Alkylating agent—busulfan.
C. Phlebotomy to remove 500–2000 mL of blood per week until hematocrit reaches 50 percent; repeated when hematocrit rises.
D. Monitor for complications—CVA, thrombocytosis.
E. Instruct patient to monitor for symptoms of iron deficiency.

Thrombocytopenia

Definition: Condition that is a lower than normal number of circulating platelets.

Characteristics

✦ A. Normal platelet count is 150,000 to 400,000/mm³. A count lower than 100,000 leads to this condition; lower than 60,000 may result in tendency to bleed.
B. Condition results from decreased platelet production, destruction of platelets (most common), decreased platelet survival, or sequestration of blood in the spleen.
C. Common causes of platelet destruction.
    1. Idiopathic thrombocytopenic purpura—production of an antibody that works against platelet antigen.
    2. Heparin induced—may develop when patient receives heparin for more than 5 days. Use of

low-molecular weight heparin may prevent this complication.

3. Certain drugs (alcohol, aspirin, chemotherapeutic agents, gold salts, sulfonamides, thiazides, penicillin, etc.) induce this condition, which will usually resolve 1–2 weeks after drug withdrawal.

Assessment

✦ A. Skin signs: petechiae (occurring only in platelet disorders), ecchymoses, and purpura.
B. History of menorrhagia, epistaxis.
C. Low platelet count, bleeding time, and bone marrow examination.

Implementation

✦ A. Monitor corticosteroid therapy—decreases antibody production. Inform patient not to stop medication suddenly.
B. Administer care following a splenectomy—removal of the organ responsible for destruction of antibody-coated platelets.
C. Monitor use of immunosuppressive drugs.
D. Monitor platelet transfusion—may be done for certain patients, especially for thrombocytopenic bleeding.
✦ E. Constantly monitor for bleeding tendency—when platelet count less than 60,000, avoid:
    1. Infections.
    2. Rectal temperature.
F. Apply pressure to venipuncture sites for 5 minutes.
G. Educate patient how to recognize signs and measures to prevent injury.
    1. Avoid trauma and contact sports.
    2. Use soft toothbrush—avoid trauma to gums.
    3. Use electric shaver.
    4. Avoid drugs that thin blood (aspirin).

Note: For sickle cell anemia and thalassemia, *see* Pediatric chapter.

Rupture of the Spleen

Definition: Traumatic bursting following violent blow or trauma to the spleen.

Assessment

A. Weakness due to blood loss.
B. Abdominal pain and muscle spasm particularly in the left upper quadrant.
C. Abdominal bleeding.
D. Rebound tenderness.
E. Referred pain to left shoulder.
F. Palpable tenderness.
G. Leukocytosis well over 12,000.
H. Progressive shock with rapid, thready pulse; drop in blood pressure; and pallor.

Treatment

A. Prepare patient for splenectomy.
B. Prevent infection.
C. Monitor vital signs closely.

NEOPLASTIC BLOOD AND LYMPHATIC DISORDERS

Leukemia

✦ *Definition:*   A disorder of blood-forming tissue characterized by proliferation of one type of white blood cell (granulocyte, lymphocyte, or monocyte), occurring in all races and developing at any age.

Characteristics

A. Increased proliferation process alters cell's ability to mature and/or function properly.
✦ B. Forms of leukemia.
    1. Acute myeloid leukemia (AML).
        a. Platelet deficiency, anemia present.
        b. Occurs usually at adolescence or after age 55.
    2. Chronic myeloid leukemia (CML).
        a. Increase in granulocytes and platelet cells.
        b. Disease of young adults (age 30–50)—may be genetic.
    3. Chronic lymphocytic leukemia (CLL).
        a. Decreased production of hematopoietic cells.
        b. Insidious onset, most common after age 50.
    4. Acute lymphocytic leukemia (ALL).
        a. Lymphoblast cells increase and other blood cells are reduced.
        b. Appears before age 15; highest incidence in 3–4 year olds.

Assessment

A. Diagnostic tests: bone marrow aspiration and differential blood count.
B. Poor appetite; generalized discomfort.
C. Ulceration of the mouth and pharynx.
D. High fever.
E. Diarrhea.
✦ F. Severe infection, e.g., pneumonia and septicemia.
G. Anemia with fatigue, lethargy, weakness, hypoxia, and pallor.
H. Bleeding gums, ecchymosis, and petechiae.
I. Splenomegaly, hepatomegaly, and lymphadenopathy.
J. Headache, disorientation, and convulsions.

Treatment and Implementation

◆ A. Specific drugs and combinations are given according to the specific type of leukemia and whether it is chronic or acute.

    1. AML or Acute—antimetabolites—interfere with cellular metabolic process (cytarabine, mitoxantrone, daunomycin, and/or idarubicin).

    2. CML or chronic—alkylating agents—damage DNA production of cells (chlorambucil, hydroxyurea, busulfan, etc.).

    3. CLL—chlorambucil, Cytoxan and glucocorticoids.

    4. ALL—induction therapy, then mercaptopurine (6-MP), methotrexate and vincristine. Prednisone is also given.

    5. Antibiotic agents—interfere with synthesis of RNA (adriamycin, caunarubicik, etc.).

    6. Enzymes—L-asparaginase.

    7. Hormones—estrogen, DES, progestins, androgens, etc.

    8. Combination drugs.

B. Blood transfusions as required.

C. Fluid and electrolyte balance.

D. High-calorie, high-vitamin diet.

E. Prevent infections, ulcerations.

F. Provide emotional support and client education.

Hodgkin's Disease

◆ *Definition:* A chronic, progressive, neoplastic, invariably fatal disease of unknown etiology, involving the lymphoid tissues of the body. It is most common between the ages of 20 and 40.

Signs and Symptoms

◆ A. Painless enlargement of the lymph nodes.

B. Severe pruritus.

C. Irregular fever.

D. Splenomegaly and hepatomegaly.

E. Jaundice.

F. Edema and cyanosis of the face and neck.

G. Pulmonary symptoms including dyspnea, cough, chest pain, cyanosis, and pleural effusion.

H. Progressive anemia with resultant fatigue, malaise, and anorexia.

I. Bone pain and vertebral compression.

J. Nerve pain and paraplegia.

K. Laryngeal paralysis.

L. Increased susceptibility to infection.

◆ M. Progresses in stages.

    1. Stage I: disease is restricted to single anatomic site, or is localized in a group of lymph nodes; asymptomatic.

    2. Stage II: two or three adjacent lymph nodes in the area on the same side of the diaphragm are affected.

    3. Stage IIE: symptoms appear; localized extra-lymphatic site on same side of diaphragm.

    4. Stage III: disease is widely disseminated on both sides of diaphragm into the lymph areas and organs.

    5. Stage IV: involvement of bone, bone marrow, pleura, liver, skin, gastrointestinal tract, central nervous system, and gradually the entire body.

N. B symptoms: fever over 38°C (100.4°F), night sweats, more than 10% weight loss.

Treatment and Implementation

◆ A. Radiation is used for stages I, II and IIE, and III in an effort to eradicate the disease.

B. Wide-field megavoltage radiation with doses of 3500–4000 roentgens over a 4–6-week period.

C. Recent results show improvement with a 2 to 4 month course of chemotherapy followed by radiation.

◆ D. Combination chemotherapy for stages III and IV and all B symptoms: doxorubicin, bleomycin, vinblastin and dacarbazine (ABVD). Prednisone (80 mg/day) may also be given.

E. Nursing care is supportive.

    1. Provide supportive relief from effects of radiation and chemotherapy.

        a. Side effects include nausea and vomiting.

        b. Controlled by premedication of sedatives and antiemetic agents.

    2. Assist patient to maintain as normal a life as possible during course and treatment of disease.

    3. Prevent infection as body's resistance is lowered.

    4. Continually observe for complications: pressure from enlargement of lymph glands on vital organs.

Non-Hodgkin's Lymphoma (NHL)

◆ *Definition:* A malignant disorder involving malignant B cells that originates from lymphoid tissues, but is not characterized as Hodgkin's disease.

Assessment

◆ A. Enlarged lymph nodes.

B. Gastrointestinal involvement: abdominal cramping, diarrhea, bowel obstruction.

C. Ureteral obstruction may cause hydronephrosis.

D. Diagnosis made by biopsy of suspicious nodes, then CT scan, bone marrow, and blood work determine stage.

E. Prognosis depends on cell type and ranges from excellent to poor.

    1. Good survival rate with low-grade localized lymphomas.

    2. Aggressive rate—one-third survival rate.

Treatment

A. Based on classification of disease—same as for Hodgkin's disease.

◆ B. Highly responsive to radiation with a high remission rate.

C. Single-agent or combination chemotherapy may be used for aggressive form.

1. ABVD combination: doxarubicin, bleomycin, vinblastine and dacarbazine.

2. Studies show this combination combined with prednisone given for 3 months is latest efficacious protocol.

D. Nursing implementation same as for Hodgkin's disease.

ENDOCRINE SYSTEM

The endocrine system is one of the integrative body systems that regulates body functions. It is made up of a series of glands that function individually or conjointly to integrate and control innumerable metabolic activities of the body. These glands automatically regulate various body processes by releasing chemical signals called hormones.

ANATOMY AND PHYSIOLOGY

Endocrine Glands

A. Secrete hormones directly into the bloodstream.
B. Located in various parts of the body.
C. Each gland has a specific function; actions of glands are also interrelated, influencing one another.
   1. Tropic hormones.
      a. Secreted by anterior lobe of pituitary gland.
      b. Influence several other glands' secretion of hormones.
   2. Target glands—those glands affected by tropic hormones.
      a. Thyroid—affects the rate at which all tissues metabolize.
      b. Adrenal cortex—essential to life. Secretes adrenocortical hormone.
      c. Gonads.
D. Also called *ductless glands* since they secrete directly into the bloodstream.

Hormones

A. Secreted in minute amounts but exert powerful influence on the body.
   1. Growth and development.
   2. Metabolism.
   3. Reproduction.
   4. Development of personality.
B. Influence is integrative and regulating; they control rate, but do not initiate cellular pro-cesses.
C. Effect of hormone on the body may occur in area far removed from secreting gland.

✦ Endocrine System Assessment

A. Assess for growth imbalance.
   1. Excessive growth.
      a. Pituitary or hypothalamic disorders.
      b. Excess adrenal, ovarian, or testicular hormone.
   2. Retarded growth.
      a. Endocrine and metabolic disorders; difficult to distinguish from dwarfism.
      b. Hypothyroidism.
B. Evaluate for obesity.
   1. Sudden onset suggests hypothalamic lesion (rare).
   2. Cushing's syndrome (with characteristic buffalo hump).
C. Assess abnormal skin pigmentation.
   1. Hyperpigmentation may coexist with depigmentation in Addison's disease.
   2. Thyrotoxicosis may be associated with spotty brown pigmentation.
   3. Pruritus is a common symptom in diabetes.
D. Check for hirsutism.
   1. Normal variations in body occur on nonendocrine basis.
   2. First sign of neoplastic disease.
   3. Indicates changes in adrenal status.
E. Evaluate appetite changes.
   1. Polyphagia is a common sign of uncontrolled diabetes.
   2. Indicates thyrotoxicosis.
   3. Nausea and weight loss may indicate addisonian crisis or diabetic acidosis.
F. Check for polyuria and polydipsia.
   1. Symptoms usually of nonendocrine etiology.
   2. If sudden onset, suggest diabetes mellitus or insipidus.
   3. May be present with hyperparathyroidism or hyperaldosteronism.
G. Assess mental changes.
   1. Though often subtle, may be indicative of underlying endocrine disorder.
      a. Nervousness and excitability may indicate hyperthyroidism.
      b. Mental confusion may indicate hypopituitarism, Addison's disease, or myxedema.
   2. Mental deterioration is observed in untreated hypoparathyroidism and hypothyroidism.
H. Assess metabolic status.
   1. Energy level.
   2. Fatigue.
   3. Heat or cold tolerance changes.
   4. Weight changes.
   5. Sleep pattern.
I. Assess for coma state.
   1. Drowsiness.
   2. Hyperpnea.
   3. Tachycardia.
   4. Subnormal temperature.
   5. Fruity odor to breath.
   6. Acetone in urine.
   7. Stupor leading to coma.

DIAGNOSTIC PROCEDURES

For endocrine blood tests, *see* Chapter 7, Laboratory Tests.

DISORDERS OF THE PITUITARY GLAND

Acromegaly

Definition: Overproduction of growth-stimulating hormone by the anterior lobe, occurring in adulthood after closure of the epiphyses of the long bones.

Assessment

✦ A. Excessive growth of short, flat bones.
   1. Large hands and feet.
   2. Thickening and protrusion of the jaw and orbital ridges.
   3. Coarse facial features.
   4. Pain in joints.
B. Increased diaphoresis.
C. Oily, rough skin.
D. Increased hair growth over the body.
E. Menstrual disturbances; impotence.
F. Symptoms associated with local compression of brain by tumor.
   1. Headache.
   2. Visual disturbances; blindness.
G. Related hormonal imbalances may develop.
   1. Diabetes mellitus.
   2. Cushing's syndrome.
H. Increased growth-stimulating hormone level as indicated by laboratory tests.

Treatment and Implementation

A. Provide emotional support.
   1. Encourage expression of patient's feelings.
   2. Avoid situations that may be embarrassing to the patient.
   3. Encourage family to give support to and to communicate with the patient.
B. Give frequent skin care.
C. Provide proper positioning and support for painful joints.
D. Test urine for glucose and acetone.
E. Be aware of possible needed treatment.
   1. Irradiation of the tumor.
   2. Hypophysectomy.
   3. Lifelong replacement of hormones as a result of above treatments.

Hypophysectomy

Definition: Excision of the pituitary gland. If tumors are small, an adenectomy may be performed.

Surgical Procedures

A. Craniotomy—for large, invasive tumors.
B. Microsurgery.
C. Cryohypophysectomy.

Implementation

A. General preoperative care.
   1. Emotional support.
   2. Explanation of procedure to be performed.
✦ B. General postoperative care.
   1. Administer care.
      a. Give corticosteroids on time.
      b. Encourage fluid intake of 2500+ mL/day unless otherwise instructed.
      c. Monitor vital signs.
   2. Check for signs of related hormonal disturbances and deficiencies.
      a. Adrenal insufficiency.
      b. Hypothyroidism and acute thyroid crisis.
      c. Diabetes insipidus.
      d. Severe hypoglycemia.
   3. Provide education to patient.
      a. Importance of continual medical supervision.
    ✦ b. Safe self-administration of replacement hormones.
         (1) Cortisone.
         (2) Thyroid.
         (3) Sex hormones.
         (4) Vasopressin tannate.
      c. Avoidance of over-the-counter drugs.
      d. Measures to prevent infections; prompt reporting to physician if infections appear.
      e. Recognition of stress and avoidance of stress-producing situations.
      f. Importance of Medic-Alert band and carrying emergency medications.
      g. Avoidance of forceful blowing of nose and of coughing.
   4. Need for emotional support and involvement of family in ongoing care.

Gigantism (Hyperfunction of Pituitary)

✦ *Definition:* Overproduction of growth-stimulating hormone by the anterior lobe, occurring in childhood prior to closure of the epiphyses of the long bones.

Assessment

A. Symmetrical overgrowth of the long bones.
B. Increased height in early adulthood of 8–9 feet.
C. Deterioration of mental and physical processes, which may occur in early adulthood.
D. Premature body-aging processes.

Treatment

A. Irradiation of pituitary.
B. Hypophysectomy.

Dwarfism

✦ *Definition:*   Underproduction of growth-stimulating hormone by the anterior lobe.

Characteristics
A. Symmetrical but severe retardation of physical growth.
B. Premature body-aging processes.

Treatment and Implementation
✦ A. Human growth-stimulating hormone injections (HGH).
B. Given if the imbalance is diagnosed and treated in early stage.

Diabetes Insipidus (DI)

✦ *Definition:*   Antidiuretic hormone (ADH) deficiency resulting from damage (head injury, brain surgery, infection of CNS) or tumors occurring in the posterior lobe of the pituitary gland.

✦ Assessment
A. Severe polyuria (as much as 20 L/day).
B. Severe polydipsia.
C. Dehydration.
D. Weight loss, muscle weakness, fatigue.
E. Laboratory values—low urinary specific gravity (1.001–1.005); inability to concentrate urine, serum sodium and vasopressin.

Treatment and Implementation
✦ A. Administer vasopressin tannate (Diabinese, Pitressin Tannate) IM or nasal spray.
B. Administer thiazide and related diuretics (Clofibrate) for mild cases.
C. Be aware that hypophysectomy may be required if tumor is present.
D. Provide adequate fluids; avoid fluids with diuretic-type actions.
E. Monitor diet: low sodium, low protein with diuretics.
F. Measure intake and output and weight.
G. Advise patient of importance of wearing Medic-Alert band.

DISORDERS OF THE ADRENAL GLAND

Addison's Disease

✦ *Definition:*   Hypofunction of adrenal cortex of adrenal gland, results in deficiency of steroid hormones (glucocorticoids, mineralocorticoids, and androgens).

Assessment
A. Slow and insidious onset: eventually fatal if untreated.
B. Lassitude, lethargy, fatigue, and generalized weakness.
C. Gastrointestinal disturbances, e.g., nausea, diarrhea, and anorexia.
D. Hypotension.
E. Increased pigmentation of the skin.
F. Emotional disturbances.
G. Weight loss.
H. Elevated serum potassium, decreased serum sodium, elevated BUN levels, and low blood glucose.

Treatment and Implementation
✦ A. Be aware that lifelong replacement therapy with synthetic corticosteroid drugs will be required.
B. Monitor vital signs QID—more often if patient is unstable.
✦ C. Weigh patient daily; keep accurate intake and output records—restoration of fluid and electrolyte balance is priority treatment.
D. Observe for side effects of replacement hormones.
  ✦ 1. Cortisone and hydrocortisone side effects.
    a. Sodium and water retention.
    b. Potassium depletion or hyperkalemia (may disappear with cortisol therapy).
    c. Drug-induced Cushing's syndrome.
    d. Gastric irritation (give medication with meal or antacid).
    e. Mood swings (depression).
    f. Local abscess at injection site when given IM (inject deeply into gluteal muscle).
    g. Addison's crisis, which might be produced by sudden withdrawal of medication.
  2. Fludrocortisone acetate side effects—the same as for cortisone and hydrocortisone, particularly sodium retention and potassium depletion.
  3. Deoxycorticosterone acetate side effects—sodium retention and potassium depletion.
E. Protect patient from exposure to infection.
F. Provide high-carbohydrate, high-protein diet in frequent small feedings.
G. Provide emotional support—assist patient to cope with stress.

Addisonian Crisis

Definition: Condition caused by adrenal insufficiency that may be precipitated by infection, trauma, stress, surgery, or diaphoresis with excessive salt loss.

Assessment
✦ A. Severe headache; abdominal, leg, and lower back pain.
B. Extreme, generalized muscular weakness.
C. Severe hypotension and signs of shock (rapid, weak pulse, pallor, weakness, rapid respirations).
D. Irritability and confusion.

E. Death from shock, vascular collapse, or hyper-kalemia.

Treatment and Implementation

✦ A. Monitor IV fluid replacement to restore fluid and electrolyte balance.

✦ B. Adrenocorticosteroid replacement—do not vary dosage or time from that ordered.

C. Monitor vital signs and intake and output continually and closely until crisis passes.

D. Take measures to protect patient from infection.

E. Do not allow patient to do anything for self and encourage remaining as quiet as possible; perform no unnecessary nursing procedures.

Cushing's Syndrome (Adrenocortical Hyperfunction)

Definition: Disease produced by hyperfunction of the adrenal cortices of the adrenal glands, resulting in hypersecretion of the glucocorticoid steroid hormones.

Assessment

✦ A. Abnormal adipose tissue distribution.
1. Moonlike fullness of face.
2. Buffalo hump (fatty swellings on body).
3. Obese trunk with thin extremities.

B. Reddish-purple striae of skin stretched with fat tissue.

C. Fragile skin; easily bruised.

D. Osteoporosis; susceptible to fractures.

E. Hyperglycemia; may eventually develop diabetes mellitus.

F. Mood swings from euphoria to depression.

G. High susceptibility to infections; diminished immune response to infections once they occur.

H. Lassitude and muscular weakness.

I. Masculine characteristics in females.

J. Electrolyte imbalance.
1. Metabolic alkalosis.
2. Potassium depletion.
3. Sodium and water retention.

K. Laboratory values.
1. Elevated blood glucose and glycosuria.
2. Elevated white blood count with depressed hyperkalemia.
3. Elevated plasma cortisone levels.
4. Elevated 17-hydroxycorticosteroids in urine.

Treatment and Implementation

✦ A. Take measures to protect from infections.

B. Protect patient from accidents or falls.

C. Give meticulous skin care, avoiding harsh soaps.

D. Provide low-calorie, high-protein, high-potassium diet.

E. Provide emotional support.
1. Encourage ventilation of patient's feelings.

2. Avoid reacting to patient's appearance.
3. Anticipate the needs of the patient.
4. Explain to patient that changes in body appearance and emotional lability should improve with treatment.

F. Measure intake and output; test for urinary glucose; weigh daily.

✦ G. Provide specialized care if *adrenalectomy* is necessary.
1. General preoperative care.
2. Postoperative care. (Bilateral surgery requires lifetime replacement of steroids; unilateral requires temporary steroid replacement for 6–12 months.)
   a. Frequent monitoring of vital signs and intake and output.
   b. Careful administration of parenteral fluids and medications as ordered.
   c. Strict adherence to sterile techniques when changing dressings.
   d. Observation for shock, hypoglycemia.

H. Be aware that chemotherapy may be administered for inoperable, cancerous tumors.

DISORDERS OF THE THYROID GLAND

Hypothyroidism (Myxedema)

Definition: Adult form of decreased synthesis of thyroid hormone resulting in a hypothyroid state.

Assessment

A. Occurs primarily in older age group, five times more frequent in women than in men.

✦ B. Slowed rate of body metabolism.
1. Lethargy, apathy, and fatigue.
2. Intolerance to cold, hypothermia, numbness and tingling of fingers.
3. Hypersensitivity to sedatives and barbiturates.
4. Weight gain.
5. Cool, dry, rough skin.
6. Coarse, dry hair.

C. Personality changes.
1. Forgetfulness and loss of memory.
2. Complacency.
3. Slowed speech.

D. Anorexia, constipation, and fecal impactions.

E. Interstitial edema.
1. Nonpitting edema in the lower extremity.
2. Generalized puffiness.

F. Decreased diaphoresis.

G. Menstrual disturbances (menorrhagia, infertility).

H. Cardiac complications.
1. Coronary heart disease.
2. Angina pectoris.

3. Myocardial infarction and congestive heart failure.
I. Anemia.
J. Below normal test results.
   1. PBI.
   2. ^{131}I.
   3. T_3 and T_4.
K. Elevated serum cholesterol level.

Treatment and Implementation

A. Administer thyroid replacement (initial small dosage, increased gradually).
✦ B. Individualize maintenance dosage.
   1. Desiccated thyroid.
   2. Sodium levothyroxine (Synthroid Sodium).
   3. Triiodothyronine (Cytomel).
   4. Natural thyroid from animal sources.
C. Observe for symptoms of overdosage in thyroid preparations.
   1. Myocardial infarction, angina, and cardiac failure, particularly in patients with cardiac problems.
   2. Restlessness and insomnia.
   3. Headache and confusion.
D. Provide time for patient to complete activities.
E. Provide warm environment with extra blankets and other modes of warming.
F. Give meticulous skin care.
G. Orient patient as to date, time, and place.
H. Take measures to prevent constipation.
I. Administer sedatives or narcotics as ordered by physician. (Usually one-half to one-third normal dosage is ordered.)
J. Myxedema coma is a serious condition resulting from persistent low thyroid production.
   1. Monitor for compromised respiratory function, hypotension, bradycardia.
   2. Administer thyroid IV and monitor effects.
K. Monitor arterial blood gases, pulse oximetry.

Hyperthyroidism (Thyrotoxicosis)—Graves' Disease

✦ *Definition:* A result of increased synthesis of thyroid hormone often accompanied by exophthalmic goiter.

Assessment

A. Occurs four times more frequently in women than in men; usually occurs between 20 and 40 years of age.
✦ B. Increased rate of body metabolism.
   1. Weight loss despite ravenous appetite and ingestion of large quantities of food.
   2. Intolerance to heat.
   3. Nervousness, jitters, and fine tremor of hands.
   4. Smooth, soft skin and hair.
   5. Diarrhea.
C. Personality changes.
   1. Irritability and agitation.
   2. Exaggerated emotional reactions.
   3. Mood swings from euphoria to depression.
D. Enlargement of the thyroid gland (goiter).
✦ E. Exophthalmos.
   1. Fluid collects around eye sockets, causing eyeballs to protrude.
   2. Condition not always in evidence.
   3. Usually does not improve with treatment.
F. Cardiac complications common: tachycardia, palpitations, atrial fibrillations, angina, CHF.
G. Above normal test results.
   1. PBI.
   2. ^{131}I.
   3. T_3 and T_4.
H. Relatively low serum cholesterol.

Treatment and Implementation

✦ A. Administer drugs if ordered by physician.
   1. Antithyroid drugs.
      a. Most common are propylthiouracil and methimazole (Tapazole).
      b. Possible side effect of agranulocytosis.
   2. Iodine preparations.
      a. Saturated solution of potassium iodide (SSKI).
      b. Lugol's solution—give in milk or juice through a straw to protect teeth.
      c. PIMA (potassium iodide).
      d. Alternative to iodides—lithium blocks hormone release.
   3. Radioiodine therapy.
      a. Useful for patients who are poor surgical risks and a safer treatment.
      b. Uptake of ^{131}I by thyroid gland results in destruction of thyroid cells.
      c. Myxedema may occur as complication.
   4. Propranolol and calcium antagonists; used preoperatively and to reverse toxic effects.
✦ B. Provide for adequate rest.
   1. Bedrest.
   2. Calming diversionary activities.
C. Provide cool, quiet, stable environment.
✦ D. Maintain diet high in calories, protein and vitamins; no stimulants; six small meals/day and snacks.
E. Weigh daily.
F. Provide emotional support to patient.
   1. Be aware that exaggerated emotional responses are a manifestation of hormone imbalance.
   2. Be sensitive to patient's needs.
   3. Avoid stress-producing situations.
G. Adhere to regular schedule of activities.

✦ H. Provide specialized care if *thyroidectomy* (subtotal or total removal of thyroid gland) is required—prevent thyrotoxicosis.
  1. Ensure that patient is in required preoperative state.
     a. Return of thyroid function tests to normal.
     b. Adequate nutritional status.
     c. Marked decrease in signs of thyrotoxicosis.
     d. Absence of cardiac problems.
  2. Provide postoperative care.
     a. Have tracheostomy tray, suction equipment, and oxygen equipment at bedside.
     b. Monitor vital signs carefully.
     c. Observe closely for signs of complications.
        (1) Bleeding—check vital signs, pressure on larynx, or hematoma around wound.
        (2) Respiratory distress.
        (3) Laryngeal nerve injury—respiratory obstruction, stridor, dysphagia, high-pitched voice.
        (4) Tetany and hypocalcemia.
        (5) Thyroid "storm."
     d. Raise bed to semi-Fowler's position; avoid strain to suture line.
     e. Encourage head and neck range-of-motion exercises when ordered.

Hashimoto's Thyroiditis

✦ *Definition:* An autoimmune disorder in which antibodies develop that destroy thyroid tissue.

Characteristics
A. Functional tissue is replaced with fibrous tissue and TH level decreases.
B. Decrease in TH levels prompt the gland to enlarge in order to compensate, causing a goiter.

Treatment and Implementation
Same as for Graves' disease.

Thyroid Storm (Thyroid Crisis)

Definition: Acute, potentially fatal hyperthyroid condition that may occur as a result of surgery, inadequate preparation for surgery, severe infection, or stress.

✦ **Assessment**
A. High fever (may rise to 106°F), diaphoresis, and dehydration.
B. Tachycardia, arrhythmias, pulmonary edema.
C. Gastrointestinal symptoms: pain, nausea, vomiting, jaundice, weight loss.
D. Irritability and restlessness leading to delirium and coma.

Treatment and Implementation
✦ A. Administer drugs and take special measures as ordered.
  1. Large doses IV of propranolol to control thyroid storm.
  2. Do not palpate thyroid gland.
  3. Antithyroid drugs and iodine preparations (SSKI PO).
  4. Adrenergic- and catecholamine-blocking agents.
  5. Glucocorticoids.
B. Decrease temperature, acetaminophen, external cold packs, cooling blanket.
C. Monitor vital signs, intake and output; observe for Na and K imbalance.
D. Take safety measures if agitated or comatose.
E. Provide calm, quiet environment.
F. Protect from infection, especially pneumonia.
G. Monitor ECG for arrhythmias.

DISORDERS OF THE PARATHYROID GLANDS

Hypoparathyroidism

Definition: Condition caused by acute or chronic deficient hormone production by the parathyroid gland.

Assessment
✦ A. Acute hypocalcemia.
  1. Numbness, tingling, and cramping of extremities.
  2. Acute, potentially fatal tetany.
     a. Painful muscular spasms.
     b. Seizures.
     c. Irritability.
     d. Positive Chvostek's sign.
     e. Positive Trousseau's sign.
     f. Laryngospasm.
     g. Cardiac arrhythmias.
✦ B. Chronic hypocalcemia.
  1. Poor development of tooth enamel.
  2. Mental retardation.
  3. Muscular weakness with numbness and tingling of extremities.
  4. Tetany.
  5. Loss of hair and coarse, dry skin.
  6. Personality changes.
  7. Cataracts.
  8. Cardiac arrhythmias.
  9. Renal stones.
C. Laboratory values.
  1. Low serum calcium levels.
  2. Increased serum phosphorus level.
  3. Low urinary calcium and phosphorus output.
  4. Increased bone density on x-ray examination.

Treatment and Implementation

A. General care.
   1. Same as for seizures and epilepsy.
   2. Maintain environment free of bright lights and noise.
 ✦ 3. Frequently check for increasing hoarseness.
   4. Observe for irregularities in urine.
   5. Force fluids as ordered.
B. Acute care.
 ✦ 1. Prepare for administration of slow drip IV calcium gluconate solution.
   2. Administer anticonvulsants and sedatives (phenytoin and phenobarbital).
   3. Prepare for tracheostomy if laryngospasm has caused obstruction.
C. Chronic care.
   1. Administer oral calcium salts (Os-Cal) and active form of vitamin D preparations.
   2. Provide high-calcium, low-phosphorus diet. (Warning—many high calcium foods are also high in phosphorus.)

Hyperparathyroidism

Definition: Abnormal, excessive hormone production by the parathyroid gland.

Assessment

A. Bone demineralization with deformities, pain, high susceptibility to fractures.
 ✦ B. Hypercalcemia.
   1. Calcium deposits in various body organs such as eyes, heart, lungs, and kidneys (stones).
   2. Gastric ulcers.
   3. Personality changes, depression, paranoia, and apathy.
   4. Nausea, vomiting, anorexia, and constipation.
   5. Polydipsia and polyuria.
   6. Hypertension, cardiac dysrhythmias.
 ✦ C. Primary hyperthyroidism—occurs when hyperplasia or adenoma is in one of the parathyroid glands.
 ✦ D. Secondary hyperparathyroidism (caused from malabsorption or renal failure) results in chronic hypocalcemia, which stimulates excessive hormone production.
   1. Cause is malabsorption—treatment is calcium supplements and vitamin D.
   2. Cause is renal failure—treatment is to lower phosphorous level, increasing calcium with oral supplements and vitamin D.

Treatment and Implementation

A. Be aware that subtotal surgical resection of parathyroid glands may be necessary.
 ✦ B. Administer additional oral calcium with vitamin D as ordered, for bone rebuilding processes may be required for several months.

C. Force fluids (include juices to make urine more acidic).
D. Take safety measures to prevent accidents and injury.
E. Provide a diet high in phosphorus.
F. Measure intake and output.
G. Observe urine closely for stones.
H. Observe for digitalis toxicity if patient is taking digitalis.

DISORDERS OF THE PANCREAS

Diabetes Mellitus (Types 1 and 2)

Definition: A group of disorders that have a variety of genetic causes, but have glucose intolerance as a common thread. Condition is caused by absence or lack of insulin or inability of cells to use insulin effectively.

Characteristics

✦ A. Classifications.
   1. Type 1—insulin-dependent diabetes mellitus (affects about 5% of all diabetics).
   2. Type 2—non–insulin-dependent diabetes mellitus (most common form—results when body produces insufficient insulin or there is insulin resistance with relative insulin deficiency).
   3. Gestational (GDM)—increased blood glucose levels during pregnancy.
   4. Other types: genetic defects of beta cell function, or insulin action, pancreatic disease, drug- or chemical-induced diabetes.
B. Distinguishing features of Type 1 and Type 2 diabetes. (*See* Table 10-4.)
C. Risk factors.
   1. Patient history—hereditary predisposition.
   2. Weight—presence of obesity.
   3. High stress levels.
D. Results of laboratory values.
 ✦ 1. Elevated fasting blood sugar > 126; postprandial blood sugar > 200; glucose tolerance test or tolbutamide (Orinase) tests.
   2. Fasting plasma glucose (FPG) < 100 mg/dL is normal and 100–125 mg/dL is prediabetes.
   3. Clinitest and Testape—not commonly used.
      a. Indicate presence of sugar in urine, i.e., 1+ to 4+.
      b. Acetest and Ketostix—may be positive for presence of acetone and ketones in urine.
   4. Glycosylated hemoglobin text (HgbA$_{IC}$).
      a. Monitors blood sugar and hemoglobin—determines how well diabetes is controlled.
      b. Reflects glycemic state over preceding 8–12 weeks.
   5. Elevated cholesterol and triglyceride levels.

Table 10-4. COMPARISON OF TYPE 1 AND TYPE 2 DIABETES

	Type 1	Type 2
Etiology	Unknown; autoimmune process involved	Heredity more relevant (100 percent of children contract NIDDM when both parents have it)
Cause	Absence of circulating insulin (in some cases, disease is mild and benign)	Insulin insufficient, not totally deficient; defective glucose-mediated insulin secretion
Onset	Usually abrupt—under age 35	Insidious, often over age 35
Weight	History of failure to gain despite voracious appetite	Linked to obesity and inactivity
Sex	Found in girls and boys equally	Most common in females
Cardinal signs	Polydipsia, polyphagia, polyuria	Polydipsia, polyphagia, polyuria
Other signs	Weakness, tiredness, urinary tract, infections, skin infections, blurred vision	Overweight, fatigue, frequent infections, blurred vision, impotence, absence of menstruation
Stability	Unstable; brittle—difficult to control	Stable with compliance; less difficult to control
Distinguishing feature	Honeymoon phase—symptoms decrease with a short remission	No honeymoon phase
Complications	Hyperglycemia, diabetic ketosis, and ketoacidosis	Neuropathy, retinopathy, uropathy
Treatment	Insulin and ADA diet, exercise	ADA diet alone; ADA and insulin, or ADA and oral hypoglycemic agents

6. Glycosylated hemoglobin test.
   a. Abnormally high in diabetes with chronic hyperglycemia.
   b. Values.
      (1) Normal 3.5–6.2 percent.
      (2) Good control < 7.5 percent.
      (3) Fair control 7.6–8.9 percent.
      (4) Poor control > 9.0 percent.

Assessment

A. Early symptoms.
   ✦ 1. Common to both Type 1 and Type 2.
      a. Polyuria.
      b. Polydipsia.
      c. Polyphagia.
      d. Blurred vision.
      e. Fatigue.
      f. Abnormal sensations (prickling, burning).
      g. Infections (vaginitis).
   ✦ 2. Type 1.
      a. Anorexia.
      b. Nausea, vomiting.
      c. Weight loss.
   3. Type 2.
      a. May be asymptomatic.
      b. Obese.
      c. Slow wound healing.
      d. Fatigue.
      e. Blurred vision.

Treatment

✦ A. Diet.
   1. The cornerstone of management, interdependent with medication and exercise.
   2. Attainment of normal weight may reduce symptoms.
   ✦ 3. Total calories are individualized.
      a. Stress high-complex carbohydrate foods—50–60 percent; focus is now on total carbohydrates—not source of carbohydrates.
      b. Water-soluble fiber (oat bran, pectin) important.
      c. Protein intake—10–20 percent of total calories from both animal and vegetable sources.
      d. Fat—20–30 percent of total calories; low saturated or mono-polyunsaturated fats; limit saturated fat to 10 percent or less of daily calories.
      e. Dietary ratio:5:2:1 carbohydrate to fat to protein.
   4. ADA exchange diet.
      a. Six exchange lists.
      b. Prescribed as to total calories and number of exchanges from each group.
   ✦ 5. Food Guide Pyramid including the basic food groups. (*See* Chapter 6.)
   ✦ 6. Carbohydrate counting is a new nutritional tool used to maintain blood glucose levels.

Table 10-5. INSULIN TYPES AND ACTION				
Types	**Source**	**Onset**	**Peak**	**Duration**
Rapid Acting				
Humalog® (Lispro)	Human	5–15 min	60–90 min	3–5 hrs
Novolog® (Aspart)				
Short Acting				
Novolin R	Human	0.5–1 hr	2–4 hrs	5–7 hrs
Humulin R	Human			
Intermediate Acting				
Humulin N (NPH)	Human	1–2 hrs	6–12 hrs	16–24 hrs
Novolin N (NPH)	Human	2 hrs	6–8 hrs	16–22 hrs
Mixture				
Humulin 70/30	Human (70% NPH, 30% Regular)	30 min	2–12 hrs	24 hrs
Novolin 70/30	Human (70% NPH, 30% Regular)			
Humulin 50/50	Human (50% NPH, 50% Regular)			
Humalog 75/25	(75% lispro protamine suspension 25% lispro)	15 min	1 hr	24 hrs
NovolinL	Human	3–4 hrs	4–12 hrs	16–20 hrs
Long Acting				
Humulin Ultralente	Human	6–8 hrs	12–16 hrs	20–30 hrs
Lantus (glargine)		4–6 hrs	no peak	24 hrs

NPH = neutral protamine Hagedorn. Note: The time of insulin may vary in different clients.

Human insulin is biologically engineered through the process of recombinant-DNA technology; it is modified human insulin.

Source: Smith, S., Duell, D., & Martin, B. (2008). *Clinical Nursing Skills*, 7th ed. Upper Saddle River, NJ: Prentice Hall Health.

a. Count grams of carbohydrates.
b. Measure servings or choices.
c. Use the glycemic index, which describes how much blood glucose level rises with a specific food when compared with an equivalent amount of glucose. (*See* Chapter 6.)

✦ B. Medications.
   1. Insulin types: *See* Table 10-5.
  ✦ 2. *Insulin pump*—a battery-operated device worn on a belt—delivers low-dose insulin at a continuous rate through a needle inserted in sub q tissue.
      a. Uses regular insulin, 50 percent continuous delivery and 50 percent divided into three premeal bolus doses.
      b. Amount calculated by two to four glucose monitoring tests/day.
      c. This method useful for conscientious, active person who is responsible.
   3. Insuline pens.
      a. Prefilled insulin cartridge loaded into penlike holder.

      b. Dial dose.
   4. Jet injectors.
      a. Delivers insulin through skin.
      b. No needles.
  ✦ 5. Oral hypoglycemic drugs—improve sensitivity to insulin.
      a. First generation sulfonylureas.
         (1) Thought to stimulate beta cells to increase insulin release.
         (2) Tolbutamide (Orinase), short acting.
         (3) Chlorpropamide (Diabinese), long acting.
         (4) Acetohexamide (Dymelor), intermediate acting.
         (5) Tolazamide (Tolinase), intermediate acting.
      b. Second-generation sulfonylureas.
         (1) Glyburide (Micronase), intermediate acting.
         (2) Glipizide (Glucotrol), short acting.
      c. Nonsulfonylureas.
         (1) Metformin (Glucophage).
         (2) Acarbose (Precose).

(3) Tryglitazone (Rezulin).

(4) Repaglinide (Pranslin).

(5) Advandia and actos.

C. Exercise.

1. Decreases body's need for insulin.

2. Regular, ongoing activities important.

3. Administer 10 g CHO before exercise.

Common Problems in Regulation

✦ A. *Somogyi phenomenon* or rebound effect: insulin causes hypoglycemia at night, which rebounds to hyperglycemia in early morning.

1. Symptoms: night sweats, restlessness, early morning nausea, headaches, and confusion.

2. Treated by gradually lowering insulin dosage while monitoring blood glucose.

✦ B. *Dawn phenomenon:* blood glucose is normal until 3 AM and then begins to rise in early morning. Treated by altering time and dose of insulin by 1 or 2 units.

Implementation

A. Administer meticulous skin care, particularly of lower extremities.

B. Take measures to protect patient from infection, injury, stress.

C. Observe for signs of insulin reaction and ketoacidosis.

D. Take second voided specimen for accurate sugar and acetone urine test.

E. Measure intake and output.

F. Provide emotional support.

1. Encourage patient to verbalize feelings.

   a. Necessity for changes in lifestyle, diet, and activities.

   b. Possible change in self-image and self-esteem.

   c. Fear of future and complications.

2. Encourage involvement of family.

✦ G. Educate patient—the key to effective self-management.

1. Determine patient's current status.

   a. Level of knowledge.

   b. Cultural, socioeconomic, and family influences.

   c. Daily dietary and activity patterns.

   d. Emotional and physical status and effect on current ability to learn.

✦ 2. Inform patient about insulin and insulin injections. (*See* Table 10-5.)

   a. Keep insulin at room temperature; refrigerate extra supply of insulin.

   b. Rotate insulin bottle gently prior to drawing up insulin.

   c. Use sterile injection techniques.

   d. Abdominal injection sites preferred for rapid and consistent absorption.

✦ (1) Rotating injection sites recommended for patients using pork or beef insulin. Rotation *within* sites recommended for those using human or purified pork insulin.

(2) Injection site should be 1 inch from previous injection site.

(3) Wait 30 seconds after slowly injecting insulin to prevent leakage.

(4) Aspiration before and massaging after injection no longer recommended.

   e. Watch for signs of hypo- and hypergycemia.

✦ 3. Self-monitoring of blood glucose level (SMBG) is important teaching.

✦ a. Balancing blood glucose levels results in fewer complications.

   b. Protocol is to take blood glucose levels two to four times/day.

   (1) Glucose monitors are small and easy to use—Lancets and lasers are used to obtain blood sample.

   (2) Continuous noninvasive glucose monitoring system soon will be available.

   c. Pattern control is the goal.

   d. Teach patient to use a diary or log to record results.

4. Oral medications.

   a. Take medications regularly.

   b. Watch for hypoglycemic reactions occurring with sulfonylureas.

   c. Be aware that alcohol ingestion in conjunction with sulfonylureas produces Antabuse effects.

5. Advise patient to take all possible measures to prevent infection and injury.

   a. Report infection or injury promptly to physician.

   b. Maintain meticulous skin care.

   c. Maintain proper foot care.

   d. Be aware that insulin requirements may need to be increased when suffering from infections.

   e. Be prepared for impairment of healing process.

   f. Avoid tight-fitting garments and shoes.

   g. Avoid "bathroom surgery" for corns and calluses.

✦ 6. Stress the importance of diet.

   a. No variation in meal times.

   b. Importance of patient's individual dietary goals.

   c. Incorporation of diet into life style, cultural and socioeconomic food patterns, and daily activities.

   d. Need for increase of intake when vigorously exercising.

7. Stress the importance of exercise.
   a. Regularity and amount of exercise important.
   b. Sporadic, vigorous activities should be avoided.
   c. With careful planning, participation in most activities and sports is possible.
   d. Give 10 g of CHO before exercise and every hour during exercise.
   e. Increased or decreased food intake might be required according to anticipated level of activity.
8. Advise patient to wear Medic-Alert band or carry other identification regarding diabetic status.
9. Advise patient to carry a form of concentrated sugar at all times.

Complications

✦ A. *See* Table 10-6.
B. Ketoacidosis (DKA)—*See* following information.
C. Infections.
D. Vascular disease.
  ✦ 1. Microangiopathy—affects basement membrane of almost all small blood vessels throughout body.
    a. Retinopathy—impairment of retinal circulation causing vision loss.
    b. Nephropathy—renal disease, the result of chronic diabetes.
    c. Tight control of blood sugar—using smaller and more frequent doses of insulin will reduce complications by 50–60 percent.
  2. Large vessel.
    a. Coronary heart disease.
    b. Atherosclerosis, arteriosclerosis.
E. Neuropathy—general deterioration that affects peripheral and ANS.
F. Cataracts.

Insulin Reaction (Hypoglycemia)

✦ *Definition:* Condition that is the result of excess secretion of insulin by the beta cells of the pancreas gland, not enough food, or exercise activity, leading to an abnormally low blood glucose—below 50 mg.

Assessment

A. Personality changes.
  1. Tenseness.
  2. Nervousness.
  3. Irritability.
  4. Anxiousness.
  5. Depression.
B. Excessive diaphoresis.
C. Excessive hunger.

D. Muscle weakness and tachycardia.
E. May be associated with "dumping syndrome" following gastrectomy.
F. May occur prior to development of diabetes mellitus.
G. Laboratory values—low blood sugar during hypoglycemic episodes.

Treatment and Implementation

✦ A. Administer oral carbohydrate if patient is alert—glucagon sub q or IV if not alert; carbohydrates by mouth when patient awakens.
B. Provide patient teaching for diet, medications, prevention of condition.

Insulin Resistance

Definition: Most common cause is obesity—requires daily insulin of 200 units.

Assessment

A. Monitor blood glucose level.
B. Hyperglycemia.

Treatment and Implementation

A. Administer purer insulin.
B. Monitor prednisone.
C. Patient must monitor for hypoglycemia during treatment.

Ketoacidosis

✦ *Definition:* One of the most serious results of poorly managed diabetes. The two major metabolic problems that are the source of this condition are hyperglycemia and ketoacidemia, both due to insulin lack associated with hyperglucagonemia.

Assessment

A. Onset of condition.
  1. Acute or over several days.
  2. Result of stress, infection, surgery, or lack of effective insulin.
  3. Overeating may contribute to but does not cause onset.
  4. Life-threatening situation.
B. Symptoms.
  1. Hyperglycemia, glycosuria, ketosis, ketonuria.
  2. Low CO_2 combining power.
  3. Polyuria, polydipsia, and dehydration.
  4. Nausea, vomiting, and anorexia.
  5. Flushed, warm skin.
  6. Blurred vision.
  7. Acetone odor (sweet) on breath.
  8. Kussmaul respirations (rapid, deep).
  9. Cardiac failure and coma.

Table 10-6. COMPLICATIONS ASSOCIATED WITH DIABETES

Clinical Manifestations	Diabetic Hypoglycemia	Hyperglycemic Hyperosmolar Ketoacidosis (DKA)	Nonketotic Coma (HHNK)
	Type 1	**Type 1**	**Type 2**
Cause	Too much insulin or too little food	Absence or inadequate insulin	Uncontrolled diabetes or oral hypoglycemic drugs
Onset	Rapid (within minutes)	Slow (about 8 hours)	Slow (hours to days)
Appearance	Exhibits symptoms of fainting	Appears ill	Appears ill
Respirations	Normal	Hyperpnea (Kussmaul's breathing) from metabolic acidosis	No hyperpnea—unless lactic acidosis is present
Breath odor	Normal	Sweetish due to acetone	Normal
Pulse	Tachycardia	Tachycardia	Tachycardia
Blood pressure	Not specified	Lowered blood pressure	Decreased blood pressure
Hunger	Hunger pangs in epigastrium	Loss of appetite	Hunger
Thirst	None	Increased	Increased, dehydration
Vomiting	Nausea; vomiting rare	Common	Common
Eyes	Staring, double vision	Appear sunken	Visual loss
Headache	Common	Occasionally	Occasionally
Skin	Pallor, perspiration, chilling sensation	Hot, dry skin	Hot, dry skin
Muscle action	Twitching common, unsteady gait	Twitching absent	Twitching absent
Pain in abdomen	None	Common	Common
Mental status	Confusion, erratic, change in mood, unable to concentrate	Malaise, drowsy, confusion, coma	Confused, dull, coma
Lab findings			
Sugar in urine	None after residual is discarded	Present	Present
Blood sugar	Below 50–70 mg/dL	High, 350–900 mg/dL	Very high, 800 mg/dL up to 2400 mg/dL
Ketones	Absent	High	Absent
Ketones in blood plasma	Absent	4+ present	Absent

C. Ketoacidotic coma is usually preceded by a few days of polyuria and polydipsia.
   1. Associated symptoms: fatigue, nausea and vomiting, mental stupor.
   2. Physical assessment indicates dehydration, rapid breathing, and fruity order of acetone to breath.

Treatment and Implementation

✦ A. Maintain fluid and electrolyte balance.
   1. Normal saline IV until blood sugar reaches 250–300 mg; then a dextrose solution (5 percent glucose) is started.
   2. Potassium added to IV after renal function is evaluated and hydration is adequate.

B. Provide insulin management.
   1. Give one-half dose IV and one-half dose sub q.
   2. Give with small amounts of albumin as insulin adheres to IV tubing.
   3. Hourly dosage depends on S&A and blood glucose levels.

C. Maintain patent airway and adequate circulation to brain.

D. Monitor vital signs every 1–2 hours; arterial blood gases hourly until pH is 7.2+.

E. Obtain hourly glucose and acetone urine tests.

F. Test blood glucose level q 1–2 hours. Keep sugar and acetone at 1+.

G. Maintain personal hygiene.

H. Protect from injury if comatose; keep patient warm.

INTEGUMENTARY SYSTEM

The integumentary system comprises the enveloping membrane or skin of the body. It consists of the outer epidermis and inner layer of dermis. The hair, nails, and various glands are outgrowths of the skin. The skin performs many vital body functions that include protection against negative elements in the environment and reception of temperature, touch, and pressure.

ANATOMY AND PHYSIOLOGY

Skin

A. Skin comprises about 15 percent of the body weight and forms a barrier between the internal organs and the external environment.
B. The epidermis, dermis, and subcutaneous tissue comprise the skin's three layers.
C. Skin is the largest sensory organ of the body. It contains nerves and specialized sensory organs sensitive to pain, touch, pressure, heat, and cold.
D. Chief pigment is melanin, produced by basal cells.
E. Skin harbors bacterial flora.
   1. Bacteria normally present in varying amounts.
   2. Organisms are shed with normal exfoliation of skin; bathing and rubbing may also remove bacteria.
   3. Normal pH of skin (4.2–5.6) retards growth of bacteria.
   4. Damaged areas of skin are potential points of entry for infection.
F. Functions of skin.
   1. Protection.
   2. Temperature regulation.
   3. Sensation.
   4. Storage.

Hair

A. Keratinous structures growing out of tubular invaginations of the epidermis called hair follicles.
B. Hair goes through cyclic changes of growth, atrophy, and rest.
C. Melanocytes present in the bulb of each hair account for color.
D. All parts of the body except the palms, soles of the feet, distal phalanges of fingers and toes, and the penis are covered with some form of hair.

Sweat Glands

A. Aggregate of cells that produce a liquid (perspiration) salty to the taste and with a pH ranging from 4.5–7.5.
B. Contains duct that opens out at the surface of the skin.
C. Chief components of sweat are water, sodium, potassium, chloride, glucose, urea, and lactate.

Integumentary System Assessment

✦ A. Assess color.
   1. Assess color of skin, including deviations from the normal range within individual's race.
      a. Use a nonglare daylight or 60-watt bulb.
      b. Note especially the bony prominences.
      c. Observe for pallor (white), flushing (red), jaundice (yellow), ashen (gray), or cyanosis (blue) coloration.
      d. Check mucous membranes to be accurate.
   2. Observe for increased or decreased areas of pigmentation.
   3. Observe for various skin discolorations: ecchymosis, petechiae, purpura, or erythema.
B. Evaluate skin temperature.
   1. Palpate skin (especially areas of concern) for temperature.
   2. Note changes in different extremities.
✦ C. Assess turgor.
   1. Observe skin for its ease of movement and speed of return to original position.
   2. Observe for excessive dryness, moisture, wrinkling, flaking, and general texture.
   3. Observe for a lasting impression or dent after pressing against and removing finger from skin—indicates edema or fluid in the tissue.
D. Assess skin sensation.
   1. Ability to detect heat, cold, gentle touch, and pressure.
   2. Note complaints of itching, tingling, cramps, or numbness.
E. Assess signs of poor nutrition.
   1. Rough, dry, scaly skin.
   2. Pigmentation or irritation.
   3. Bruises or petechiae.
F. Observe cleanliness.
   1. Observe general state of hygiene. Note amount of oil, moisture, and dirt on the skin surface.
   2. Note presence of strong body odors.
   3. Investigate hair and scalp for presence of body lice.
G. Assess integrity (intactness of skin).
   1. Note intactness of skin. Observe for areas of broken skin (lesions) or ulcers.

2. Assess any lesion for its location, size, shape, color(s), consistency, discomfort, odor, and sensation associated with it.

H. Assess skin conditions.

✦ **Skin Lesions**

A. Primary lesions.
1. *Bulla*—large vesicle; elevation filled with serous fluid.
2. *Erythema*—form of macula showing redness over skin.
3. *Lichenification*—thickening of affected tissue.
4. *Macule*—flat, discolored patch of various colors and shapes on skin.
5. *Papule*—raised, solid elevation of skin, usually smaller than 1 cm.
6. *Pustule*—small elevation of skin filled with purulent fluid.
7. *Telangiectasis*—dilation of capillary, producing visible, red, irregular line.
8. *Vesicle*—elevation of skin filled with clear, serous fluid; "blister."
9. *Wheal*—irregularly shaped elevation that is caused by edema.

B. Secondary lesions.
1. *Crust*—dried serum from open lesion mixed with surface dirt and dead cells; "scab."
2. *Scale*—flake of dry epidermis.

General Implementation

A. Determine type of lesion or area of altered tissue.
1. Primary lesion is initial, or first, lesion.
2. Secondary lesion is a result of a change or complication that involves a primary lesion.

B. Provide psychological support.
1. Encourage patient to express feelings.
   a. May be embarrassed about appearance.
   b. May be fearful of scarring.
   c. May be depressed about long duration and chronicity of disorder.
2. Accept patient as he or she is; nonverbal communication is therapeutic (touch).

C. Take measures to prevent damage to healthy skin.
1. Prevent scratching—keep skin clean.
   a. Keep fingernails smooth and short.
   b. Encourage patient to wear cotton gloves as reminder not to scratch.
   c. Restrain if ordered.
2. Use hot and cold applications with caution.
3. Promote high fluid intake to maintain hydration and prevent skin breakdown.

D. Take measures to prevent secondary infections.
1. Use medical aseptic technique.
2. Maintain isolation if lesions are infectious.
3. Careful handwashing.

E. Take measures to reverse inflammatory process.
1. Relieve symptoms.
   a. Control room temperature and humidity.
   b. Decrease local irritation.
2. Give medication and treatment as needed.

ALLERGIC REACTIONS

Contact Dermatitis

Definition: Skin reaction caused by contact with a substance to which the skin is sensitive. Reaction is characterized by inflammation as evidenced by itching, redness, and skin lesions.

Causes

A. Contact with chemicals.
1. Clothing (especially woolens).
2. Cosmetics.
3. Household products (especially detergents).
4. Industrial substances (paints, dyes, cements).

B. Contact with toxic irritants: poison oak, poison ivy, or poison sumac.

Assessment

A. Papules.
B. Vesicles.
C. Severe itching (pruritus).

Preventive Measures

A. Avoid irritant or remove irritating clothing.
B. Do not use detergent.
C. Wear rubber gloves for household chores.
D. Make request of industry to provide protective clothing; or allow change of job site for highly sensitive individuals.

Treatment and Implementation

A. Cleanse skin of plant oils.
B. Apply lotion.
C. Administer steroids for severe reactions.
D. Apply cold wet dressings of Burow's solution to relieve itching.

Eczema (Atopic Dermatitis)

✦ *Definition:* Superficial inflammatory process involving primarily the epidermis.

Assessment

A. Local eruptions.
1. Erythema, papules, vesicles may be present.
2. Area may be edematous, weeping, eroded, and/or crusted.

B. Swelling of regional lymph nodes.
C. May occur at any age, but particularly common in infancy, especially those with hereditary allergic tendencies.

D. Runs a chronic course with remission and exacerbation.
   1. Patient usually becomes irritable.
   2. Skin may be thickened, scaled, and fissured.

Treatment and Implementation

A. Seek the cause, which may be foods, emotional problems, or familial tendencies.
B. There is no cure—goal is to reduce pruritus and inflammation, and to hydrate and lubricate skin.
✦ C. Do not allow the patient to be vaccinated for smallpox; isolate from individuals recently vaccinated.
✦ D. Control skin eruptions.
   1. Encourage patient to withhold scratching.
   2. Apply wet dressings soaked in aluminum acetate or give therapeutic baths (no soaps during acute stages).
   3. Apply corticosteroids 1% to 2½% as anti-inflammatory agent.
   4. Recent topical treatment of zinc spray shows excellent results.

BACTERIAL INFECTIONS

Acne Vulgaris

Definition: A disorder of the skin with eruption of papules or pustules primarily due to increased production of sebum from the sebaceous glands. Affects adolescents and young adults.

Characteristics

A. Noninflammatory type composed of whiteheads and blackheads in the follicular duct.
B. Inflammatory acne pustules with possible scarring.
C. Affected by hormone levels (androgen), which lead to blocking of secretions with subsequent blackheads.

Medical Implications

A. Oral contraceptives are FDA approved.
B. Desquamation preparations, which allow free flow of sebum.
✦ C. Accutane—specifically for severe acne.
   1. Active ingredient is risotretinoin, a retinoid and relative of vitamin A.
   2. Absolutely contraindicated during pregnancy—causes birth defects.
   3. Blood tests recommended every few weeks to monitor for liver damage or high fat levels in the blood.
   4. There may be an association between drug and mental health problems such as suicide.
D. Retin-A (tretinoin)—a topical cream to reduce scarring from acne.

E. Mechanical removal by an extractor.
F. Complete cleansing with regular or Neutrogena soap and clean towels.
G. Mild facial erythema via sunlight or lamp.
H. Topical antibiotics.
I. Systemic tetracycline for some cases.
J. Dermabrasion for selected cases, to reduce scarring.

Implementation

A. Teach good skin and scalp hygiene.
B. Have patient avoid squeezing, rubbing, picking.
C. Have patient avoid greasy cleansing creams and cosmetics.
D. Support a high-protein, low-fat diet.
   1. Fatty foods, white sugar, nuts, and chocolate may be avoided, but research has not verified food impact.
   2. Diet not as important a therapy as in the past.
   3. Eliminate seaweed products, which aggravate condition.
E. Encourage patient to get adequate rest and sunshine.
F. Provide emotional support for body image and relationship problems.

Cellulitis

Definition: Infection of the dermis or subcutaneous tissue caused by either streptococcal or staphylococcal organisms—may follow surgical wound, impetigo, trauma, or otitis media.

Assessment

A. Swelling, erythema.
B. Leukocytosis.
C. Pain and itching.

Implementation

A. Monitor systemic antibiotics—effective for the condition.
B. Elevate the extremity to reduce dependent edema.
C. Apply heat to extremity to promote blood circulation.
D. Encourage rest to decrease muscular contractions to limit extension of organism into circulatory system.

Impetigo

Definition: Bacterial disease caused by *Streptococcus* or *Staphylococcus* or combined infection.

Assessment

A. Local vesicles.
B. Pustules evolving from vesicles that become crusted.

Treatment and Implementation

A. Prevent the spread of disease.

B. Dry the lesions by exposure to air (use compresses of Burow's solution to remove the crusts so as to allow better exposure to air).

C. Apply local antibiotic ointments.
1. Bacitracin or mupirocin.
2. If no responses to topical antibiotic cream, systemic drug (erythromycin) is used.

D. Caution family to use only hexachlorophene soap, to use other hygienic care materials, and to use separate towels to prevent the spread of the disease.

Furuncle (Boil)

Definition: Bacterial inflammation of skin caused by *Staphylococcus* infection of a hair follicle.

Assessment

A. Onset is sudden; the skin becomes red, tender, and hot around the hair follicle.

B. The center forms pus, and the core may be extruded spontaneously or by excision and manipulation.

Treatment and Implementation

A. Isolate towels, soap, and clothing; necessary to maintain scrupulous cleanliness.

B. Administer systemic antibiotics if a series of furuncles occur and if ordered.

C. Check for presence of diabetes mellitus. Should be ruled out only after tests prove negative.

Lyme Disease

Definition: A multisystem inflammatory disorder caused by an infection acquired through ticks that live in wooded areas and survive by attaching themselves to animal and human hosts.

Assessment

A. Disease is caused by the spirochete, *Borrelia burgdorferi*.

B. Disease has many and varied symptoms and is difficult to diagnose because it masquerades as other illnesses.

✦ C. Following a tick bite, the first symptoms occur several days to a month later.
1. Assess for a small red pimple, macule, or papule that spreads into a ringed-shaped rash in 4–20 days. Rash may be large or small, or not occur at all (making diagnosis difficult).
2. Assess for flulike symptoms: headache, stiff neck, muscle aches, and fatigue.

D. Assess for the second stage occurring several weeks following the bite: central nervous system abnormalities (about 15 percent); heart disease symptoms (8 percent), or joint pain (arthritis).

E. Assess for third stage symptoms: arthritis progresses and large joints are usually involved (50 percent).
1. Lingering Lyme arthritis may be caused by lingering infection or immune response.
2. A test called the polymerase chain reaction (PCR) identifies persistent Lyme arthritis that may persist even after aggressive antibiotic therapy.

Implementation

A. Blood test may detect the disease but is usually negative during the early phases.
1. Once diagnosis is confirmed, administer antibiotics—dosage depends on severity of symptoms.
2. Penicillin-type drugs given as soon as possible—shortens course of disease.

B. Prevention is the best treatment.
1. Avoid areas that contain ticks—those that are wooded, grassy, especially in the summer months.
2. Wear tight-fitting clothing and spray body with tick repellent.
3. Examine entire body for ticks upon return home; if tick is located, remove with tweezers and wash skin with antiseptic; preserve tick for examination.

VIRAL INFECTIONS

Herpes Simplex

Definition: Viral condition (cold sore) caused by herpesvirus that may occur on lips, face, or genitalia.

Assessment

✦ A. Herpes I.
1. Local burning, tingling, itching followed by tiny vesicles.
2. Local erythema.
3. Most commonly occurs on lips.

✦ B. Herpes II.
1. Most often cause of genital infection.
2. Transmitted primarily through sexual contact.

Implementation

A. Keep lesion dry and clean.

B. Advise patient to avoid sexual or direct contacts.

C. Encourage patient to request physician to periodically reexamine lesion.

D. Herpes, type II—use Acyclovir cream or PO (200 mg PO ×5 for 5 days).

Herpes Zoster (Shingles)

Definition: Acute infectious process caused by viral invasion of central nervous system.

Assessment

A. Pain and discomfort with fever.

B. Cutaneous lesions (usually located along major nerve root) appear in 3–4 days.

Implementation

A. Apply drying lotions.

B. Administer medications.
1. Analgesics for pain.
2. Antiviral agents (Acyclovir).
3. Anti-inflammatory drugs (NSAIDs).

BURNS

Definition: Destruction of skin layers by thermal, chemical, or electrical agents.

Classification of Burns

✦ A. Degree of burn—determined by depth of tissue destruction. Categories are similar to, but not the same as, prior categories of first, second and third degree burns.
1. Superficial partial thickness (first degree)
   a. Involves epidermis.
   b. Area is red or pink.
   c. Moderate pain.
   d. Spontaneous healing.
2. Deep partial thickness (second degree).
   a. Involves epidermis and dermis to the basal cells.
   b. Blistering.
   c. Severe pain.
   d. Regeneration in 1 month.
   e. Scarring may occur.
3. Full thickness (third-degree).
   a. Involves epidermis, dermis, and subcutaneous tissue and may extend to the muscle in severe burns.
   b. White, gray, or black in appearance.
   c. Absence of pain.
   d. Edema of surrounding tissues.
   e. Eschar formation.
   f. Grafting needed due to total destruction of dermal elements.
✦ B. Extent of burn.
1. Rule of Nines (Figure 10-12). Good for rapid estimation of extent of body surface area (BSA) involved.
2. Lund/Browder method—more accurate for calculating fluid replacement.
3. Palm method—patient with scattered burns may have percentage calculated with this method.
✦ C. Classification according to the percentage of body area destroyed.

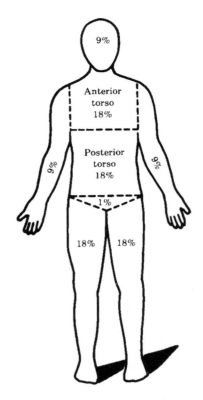

Fig.10-12 Rule of Nines

1. Major burns—35 percent or more of the body has sustained second-degree burn and 10 percent has sustained third-degree burn; further complicated by respiratory involvement, smoke inhalation, fractures, and other tissue injury.
2. Moderate burns— < 10 percent of the body has sustained third-degree burn and 15–25 percent has sustained second-degree burn.
3. Minor burns— < 15 percent of the body has sustained second-degree burn and < 2 percent has sustained third-degree burn.
4. Estimation of percentage of total body surface involved with "Rule of Nines."
✦ D. Fluid replacement formulas.
1. Brooke Army formula—colloids, electrolytes and glucose for first 24 hours.
2. Parkland/Baxter—lactated Ringer's only for first 24 hours. Day 2, colloids added.
3. Consensus formula—lactated Ringer's solution first 24 hours.
4. Evans formula—colloids, electrolytes, and glucose for first 24 hours.
✦ E. Classification according to cause.
1. Thermal burns: flame burns, scalding with hot liquids, or radiation.
2. Chemical burns: strong acids or strong alkali solutions.
3. Electrical burns.
   a. Most serious type of burn.

b. Body fluids may conduct an electrical charge through body (look for entrance and exit area).

c. Cardiac arrhythmias may occur.

d. Toxins are created postburn that injure kidneys.

e. Voltage and ampere information important in history taking.

Problems Associated with Burns

A. Fluid and electrolyte imbalance.
1. Edema appears around the wound as a result of damage to capillaries.
2. There is a loss of fluid at the burn area.

B. Pulmonary changes from inhalation injury.
1. Pulmonary edema.
2. Obstruction of the air passages from edema of the face, neck, trachea, and larynx.
3. Restriction of lung mobility from eschar on chest wall.

C. Renal changes.
1. In burns of 15–20 percent of the body surface, there is a decreased urinary output, which must be avoided or reversed.
2. Urinary tract infections are frequent.

D. Gastrointestinal changes.
1. Acute gastric dilation.
2. Paralytic ileus.
3. Curling's ulcer that produces "coffee ground" aspirant.

E. Factors that determine seriousness of burn.
1. Age.
   a. Below 18 months.
   b. Above 65 years.
2. General health.
3. Site of burn.
4. Associated injuries (fractures).
5. Causative agents.

Treatment and Implementation

✦ A. Maintain patent airway—monitor for tracheal or laryngeal edema.

✦ B. Maintain aseptic area—prevent infection.
1. Use meticulosis handwashing technique or antiseptic gel before and after care.
2. Cap, gown, mask, and clean or sterile gloves are precaution protocol.

✦ C. Provide fluid replacement therapy.
1. Resuscitative phase.
   a. First 24–48 hours postburn, fluid shifts from plasma to interstitial space.
   b. Potassium levels rise in plasma.
   c. Blood hemoconcentration and metabolic acidosis occur.
   d. Fluid loss is mostly plasma.
   e. Nursing responsibilities.
      (1) Monitor vital signs frequently.
      (2) Monitor urinary output (50–100 mL/hr; minimum output is 30 mL/hr)—notify RN or physician if urinary output less than 30 mL/hr.
      (3) Give one half of total fluids in first 8 hours or as ordered.
2. Acute or intermediate phase.
   a. Capillary permeability stabilizes and fluid begins to shift from interstitial spaces to plasma.
   b. Hypokalemia, hypernatremia, hemodilution, and pulmonary edema are potential dangers.
   c. Nursing responsibilities.
      (1) Monitor CVP.
      (2) Observe lab values.
      (3) Maintain adequate urine output.

D. Assess pain level frequently and relieve pain with morphine sulfate as ordered. Give small doses frequently. Give IV.

E. Assess peripheral circulation.

F. Provide adequate heat to maintain patient's temperature.

G. Promote good body alignment: begin range of motion early—prevent contractures.

✦ H. Administer antacids, H_2 receptor antagonists, and sucralfate (Carafate) to prevent stress ulcer.

✦ I. Provide adequate nutrition.
1. Give twice normal amount of calories.
2. Give three to four times normal requirement of protein.
3. Give nutritional supplements (Ensure) and vitamin/mineral supplements.

J. Maintain wound dressings.
1. Initial excision: mainly for electrical burns.
2. Occlusive dressings.
   a. Painful and costly.
   b. Decreases water loss.
   c. Limits range-of-motion exercises.
   d. Helps to maintain functional position.
   e. Advent of topical antibiotics has led to decreased use.
3. Exposure method.
   a. Allows for drainage of burn exudate.
   b. Eschar forms protective covering.
   c. Use of topical therapy.
   d. Skin easily inspected.
   e. Range-of-motion exercises easier to perform.

✦ K. Apply topical preparations to wound area.
1. Mafenide (Sulfamylon 5 to 10%).
   a. Exerts bacteriostatic action against many organisms.
   b. Penetrates tissue wall.
   c. Dressings not needed when used.
   d. Breakdown of drug provides heavy acid load. Inhibition of carbonic anhydrase

compounds situation. Monitor ABGs for acidosis. Individual compensates by hyperventilating.
  e. Alternate use with Silvadene.
2. Silvadene (1%)
  a. Broad antimicrobial activity.
  b. Effective against yeast.
  c. Inhibits bacteria resistant to other antimicrobials.
    (1) Not usually used prophylactically.
    (2) Given for specific organism.
    (3) Not helpful first 48 hours due to vessel thrombosis.
  d. Can be washed off with water.
  e. Assess for leukopenia after 2–3 days—may resolve automatically.
3. Silver nitrate (0.5%)—used for many years but decreasing in use.
L. Administer systemic antibiotics when there is wound sepsis or positive cultures.
M. Debridement and eschar removal daily.
N. Provide long-term care.
  1. Maintain good positioning to prevent contractures.
  2. Provide adequate rest.
  3. Prevent infection.
  4. Maintain adequate protein and caloric intake to promote healing.
  5. Monitor hydration status.
  6. Protect skin grafts.
O. Monitor for complications.
  1. Congestive heart failure and/or pulmonary edema.
  2. Sepsis.
  3. Acute respiratory failure.
✦ P. Types of skin grafts.
  1. Homograft or allograft—from cadaver or other person.
  2. Xenograft—from an animal (usually pigs).
  3. Autograft—from self.
  4. Biosynthetic covering—mimics skin.
  5. Cultured epithelial autograft (CEA) from patient's cells, which are grown in the laboratory.
  6. Integra—artificial skin.
Q. Provide psychological support (as important as physical care).
  1. Deal with the patient's fear of disfigurement and immobility from scarring.
  2. Provide constant support, as plastic repair is lengthy and painful.
  3. Involve the family in long-term planning and day-to-day care.

Isolation Protocol   ❖ Procedure ❖

✦ A. Protocol for entering isolation room.
  1. Wash hands.
  2. Put on gown and tie.
  3. Put on and tie mask.
  4. Put on goggles or face shield.
  5. Don gloves.
✦ B. Protocol for leaving isolation room.
  1. Untie gown at waist.
  2. Take off gloves.
  3. Untie gown at neck.
  4. Pull gown off and place in laundry hamper.
  5. Take off goggles.
  6. Take off mask.
  7. Leave room and wash hands.

COLLAGEN DISEASES

Lupus Erythematosus

✦ *Definition:* Collagen disease of the connective tissue that leads to a skin rash. The disease may involve any organ of the body.

Characteristics
A. One-half million in the United States have disease, mostly women.
B. Etiology unknown.
C. Onset may be insidious or acute.

Assessment
✦ A. Discoid eruption—a chronic, localized scaling erythematous skin eruption over nose, cheeks, and forehead, producing characteristic "butterfly" appearance.
B. Fever, malaise, and weight loss.
C. Exacerbation and remission of symptoms.
D. Sensitivity to sunlight (photophobia).
✦ E. Systemic (disseminated) lupus erythematosus may involve multiple organs and lead to death.
  1. Pericarditis common manifestation (30 percent); myocarditis also present (25 percent).
  2. Lung and pleural involvement common (40–50 percent).
  3. Vascular system often involved with inflammation producing lesions on fingertips, elbows, toes, etc.
  4. Lymphadenopathy occurs in half the patients.
  5. Neuropsychiatric symptoms are often present and require intervention.

Treatment and Implementation
✦ A. Protect patient from sunlight and avoid antibiotic ointments that may spread the lesions.
B. Administer steroid treatment to prevent progression of the disease.
C. Advise patient that strict personal hygiene is an absolute requirement.
D. Be aware that there is no development of immunity and recurrence is common.

MALIGNANT TUMORS OF THE SKIN

Basal Cell Epithelioma

✦ *Definition:*   Tumor arising from the basal layer of the epidermis. Lesion is a small, smooth papule with telangiectasis and atrophic center.

Assessment
A.   Starts as a small, smooth papule and grows slowly.
B.   Central area may become depressed and ulcerated, forming a classic rodent ulcer.
C.   Locally invasive and seldom metastasizes.

Treatment and Implementation
A.   Surgical excision is preferred.
B.   Radiation therapy is administered for lesions of the eyelid and nose.
C.   Watch for potential malignancy in other locations.

Squamous Cell Carcinoma

✦ *Definition:*   Tumor of the epidermis that frequently arises out of keratosis and is considered an invasive cancer. The lesion begins as erythematous macules or plaques with indistinct margins; surface often becomes crusted.

Assessment
A.   Lesions enlarge more rapidly than in basal cell epithelioma and may metastasize.
B.   A nodular tumor usually appears on the lower lip, tongue, head, or neck.

Treatment
A.   Excision is preferred.
B.   Irradiation.

Melanoma

Definition: Malignant pigmented tumor (the most malignant of all cutaneous lesions) that arises out of melanocytes and is often fatal. May arise from so-called blue-black mole and becomes an invasive cancer.

Treatment
A.   Surgical excision preferred.
B.   Cancer-destroying drugs (chemotherapy) may be used.

MUSCULOSKELETAL SYSTEM

Skeleton provides body with support and protection. The skeleton is used in locomotion but requires muscles to supply source of power and added support. Musculoskeletal system assists in unifying actions of whole body and helps it adjust to environmental changes.

ANATOMY AND PHYSIOLOGY

Skeletal System

A. System of separate bones (206) bound together by ligaments.
B. System responsible for supporting, moving, and giving shape to the body.
   1. Supports surrounding tissues and provides body with framework.
   2. Protects vital organs and soft tissues.
   3. Provides leverage and source of attachment for skeletal muscles.
   4. Forms erythrocytes, granular leukocytes, and thrombocytes in red marrow of bone.
   5. Stores calcium and other minerals.

Classification

A. According to body region.
   1. Axial skeleton—includes head and trunk, which form central axis to which appendicular skeleton is attached.
      a. Composed of 80 bones.
      b. Includes skull, spine, ribs, sternum, and hyoid bone.
   2. Appendicular skeleton—includes shoulder girdle, arm bones, pelvic girdle, and leg bones.
      a. Composed of 126 bones.
      b. Shoulder (pectoral girdle from which arms hang).
         (1) Consists of two clavicles (collarbones).
         (2) Consists of two scapulae (shoulder blades), which are attached to clavicle.
      c. Arm bones.
         (1) Humerus (upper arm bone) is connected at elbow to ulna and radius (lower arm bones).
         (2) Carpals make up wrist.
         (3) Metacarpals form hand palm.
         (4) Phalanges form finger bones.
      d. Pelvic girdle (hip).
         (1) Pelvis formed from pelvic girdle, plus bones of sacrum and coccyx.
         (2) Encircles and protects genitourinary organs.
         (3) Sockets in girdle fit femur leg bone.
      e. Leg bones.
         (1) Constructed similarly to arm bones but heavier and stronger.
         (2) Femur (thigh bone) extends from pelvis to knee.
         (3) Tibia and fibula extend from knee to ankle.
         (4) Knee is separate bone (patella).
         (5) Ankle bones (tarsals); foot bones (metatarsals); toe bones (phalanges).
B. According to shape.
   1. Long bones—made up of a shaft (diaphysis) and two flared ends (epiphyses); include radius and femur.
   2. Short bones include carpals and tarsals.
   3. Flat bones include ribs and skull.
   4. Irregular bones include vertebrae.

Development

A. The bonelike tissue of very young is mostly cartilage.
B. Cartilage is replaced by bone tissue through process of ossification.
   1. Calcium collects in cartilage and becomes hardened.
   2. Some cartilage cells break loose so that channels develop in bone shaft.
   3. Blood vessels enter channels carrying small cells of connective tissue; some tissue cells (osteoblasts) form true bone.
      a. Osteoblasts enter hardened cartilage, forming layers of hard bone.
      b. Other cells work to tear down old bone structure (osteoclasts) so osteoblasts can rebuild with new bone.
C. Bone-growth process occurs by mechanism of cartilage formation followed by replacement of cartilage with hard material.
   1. Cartilage grows over hardened bone.
   2. Cartilage hardens with addition of calcium.
   3. Process continues until full growth of body is reached.
D. Amount of calcium deposited and reabsorbed into blood is regulated by the parathyroid and thyroid glands.

Structure

A. Bone is formed of dense connective tissue.
   1. Tissue consists of bone cells (osteocytes).
   2. Cells embedded in matrix made up of calcified intercellular substance.

3. Bone consists of 50 percent water and 50 percent solid matter.
4. Calcium phosphate is the basic bone chemical that gives hardness and strength.

B. Bone is comprised of concentric cylindrical layers.
   1. Periosteum (the exterior covering, outer layer)—thin, tough membrane of fibrous tissue.
      a. Supports tendons connecting muscle to bone.
      b. Serves as protective sheath.
      c. Serves to extend blood supply to bone.
   2. Compact bone layer—dense hard layer of bone tissue.
      a. Fibrous composition to give resiliency to bone.
      b. Compact tissue tunneled by central canal or hollow cavity.
         (1) Marrow (soft tissue, medulla) contained in compact bone hollow.
         (2) Contains fine branching canals (haversian system) through which small blood vessels and lymphatics run.
         (3) Porous bone layer—spongy (cancellous) tissue that contains spongelike hollows.

Joints

A. A joint, also called an articulation, is a union or junction of two or more bones.
B. Function of joint is skeletal flexibility and motion.
C. Classification—according to structural variations that allow for different kinds of movement.
   1. Diarthroses—joint is freely movable.
      a. This type of joint is a cavity enclosed by a capsule lined with synovial membrane that secretes a lubricant.
      b. Capsule is reinforced by ligaments.
      c. Articular cartilage covers ends of bones.
   ✦ d. Types of joint movement make for structural variations.
         (1) Hinge type allows single directional movement (elbows and knees).
         (2) Ball-and-socket type allows bending (hip).
         (3) Saddle type allows multidirectional shifting (joint at base of thumb).
         (4) Pivot type allows rotary movement (articulation between radius and ulna).
         (5) Gliding type allows limited sliding of bones against each other (wrist, ankle, intervertebral joints).
   2. Synarthroses—joint is immovable.
      a. Tissue grows between articulating surfaces.
      b. Includes suture lines of skull.
   3. Amphiarthroses—joint with minimal movement.

Muscular System

A. System of fibers (more than 600) attached to bones and marked by striation.
B. System allows body movement under control of voluntary nervous system.
   1. Provides for body movement, locomotion.
   2. Provides support for the body.
   3. Performs body functions such as partial production of heat.

Classification

A. According to location—posterior tibial allows inversion of foot.
B. According to direction of fibers—muscle of tongue allows for change in shape for eating.
C. According to action—flexor muscle of toe allows toe to bend on itself, extensor muscle of toe allows extension of toe.
D. According to size and shape—trapezius of neck and shoulder allows for elevation and rotation of shoulder.
E. According to number of origin heads—biceps of arm allow for flexing and turning arm upward.
F. According to points of attachment—sternocleido-mastoid allows for flexion and rotation of head.

Cell Structure

A. Fibers of voluntary muscles grouped together in sheath of connective tissue.
B. Each bundled group of muscle fibers surrounded by connective tissue sheath.
C. Sheath tissue may be continuous with fibrous tissue that extends from the muscle as a tendon.

Properties

A. Excitability—capacity of muscle to respond to stimulus without intervention of motor nerves.
B. Contractility—ability of muscle to shorten, tighten, and contract.
C. Tonicity—ability of muscle to maintain steady contraction, which determines its firmness.
D. Extensibility—ability of muscle to stretch in response to applied force.
E. Elasticity—ability of strained muscle to regain original size and shape when applied force is removed.

Contraction

A. For muscle contraction and other fine movements to occur, muscle tissue must be stimulated.
   1. Each fiber receives own neural impulse from somatic motor neuron.
   2. Signal of impulse along nerve muscle fiber changes chemical to mechanical energy.
   3. Each fiber has stored supply of fuel for contraction energy source.

a. Stimulus releases calcium to cause fiber filament movement.

b. Nerve stimulates breakdown of ATP.

B. Area where motor neuron ends in muscle fiber is called myoneural junction.

Movement

A. Skeletal muscles produce body movement by pulling on bones.

B. Bones serve as levers, and joints serve as fulcrums of these levers.

1. Each muscle has a point of origin and a point of insertion that are usually attached to bone.

2. The point of origin is the more fixed point of attachment.

3. The point of insertion is the more movable end.

C. Muscles that move a body part usually do not extend over that part.

D. Skeletal muscles usually perform with group action; some contract while others relax.

1. Prime movers are muscles responsible for the primary movement of contraction.

2. Antagonists are muscles that exert an action opposing that of prime mover.

3. Synergists are muscles that enhance action of prime mover.

E. Accessory parts.

1. Ligaments—cordlike connective tissue that holds bones together.

2. Tendons—attach muscles to bones.

MUSCULOSKELETAL DISORDERS

Fractures

Definition: A break in the continuity of bone.

Characteristics

A. Causes.

1. Direct application of force at site.

2. Distant application of force but transmitted to fracture site.

3. Sudden muscle contraction.

4. Spontaneous break as result of disease (bone decalcification).

B. Source of weakened bones resulting in fractures.

1. Fatigue—muscles cannot absorb force.

2. Bone neoplasms—malignant cells replace normal tissue.

3. Metabolic disorders—poor mineral absorption or hormonal changes.

4. Prolonged bedrest or disuse.

✦ C. Classification.

1. According to severity.

a. *Simple* (closed)—a break is present but no external wound in skin.

b. *Compound* (open)—a break is present and there is external wound in skin over or leading to fracture site.

c. *Comminuted*—bone has splintered into fragments.

d. *Greenstick*—one side of the bone broken but the opposite side is bent.

e. *Compression*—fractured bone compressed by other bones.

2. According to direction and location.

a. *Oblique*—break runs in slanting direction.

b. *Spiral*—break coils around bone.

c. *Extracapsular*—break occurs outside the joint.

d. *Intracapsular*—break occurs inside the joint.

Assessment

✦ A. Cardinal signs of a fracture.

1. Pain or tenderness over involved area.

2. Loss of function or movement.

3. Deformity.

B. Other signs.

1. Crepitation—sound of grating bone fragments.

2. Ecchymosis or erythema.

3. Edema.

4. Muscle spasm.

C. Possible shock.

Treatment and Implementation

A. Objectives.

1. Regain correct alignment through reduction.

2. Maintain alignment.

3. Regain function of affected part.

B. Emergency implementation.

1. Keep limb or part stable until immobilized.

2. Take measures to prevent shock.

3. Cover open wound with dry and clean or sterile dressing.

✦ C. Fractures treated by reduction; broken ends pulled into alignment and continuity of bone established so healing can occur.

1. Methods of reduction.

a. Closed—fractured bone brought into alignment by manual manipulation; no incision made.

b. Open—surgical incision made and bone aligned under direct visualization; also performed to cleanse open fracture or to stabilize alignment with inserted fixators.

2. Forms of alignment.

a. Closed—application of cast, splint, and/or traction.

b. Open—fixation with metallic pins, wires, screws, plates, nails, or rods.

✦ Principles of Cast Care ❖ PROCEDURE ❖

A. After application of cast, allow 24–48 hours for drying; for synthetic cast, allow 30 minutes—60 minutes for weight-bearing.
   1. Cast will change from dull to shiny substance when dry.
   2. Heat can be applied to assist in drying process.
B. Do not handle cast during drying process as indentations from fingermarks can cause skin breakdown under cast.
C. Keep extremity elevated to prevent edema and promote venous return.
D. Provide for smooth edges surrounding cast.
   1. Prevents crumbling and breaking down of edges.
   2. Stockinet can be pulled over edge and fastened down with adhesive tape to outside of cast.
E. Observe casted extremity for signs of circulatory impairment. Cast may have to be cut if edematous condition continues.
F. Observe for signs of complications: pain, swelling, discoloration, tingling or numbness, diminished or absent pulse, cool to touch, etc.
   1. *Circulation*—report if:
      a. Digits are swollen, pale, blue or cold.
      b. Delayed capillary refill (> 2 seconds).
   2. *Motion*—report if:
      a. Pain on passive movement.
      b. Strength is unequal in both extremities.
   3. *Sensation*—report if:
      a. Pain increases with passive motion of digits or when extremity is elevated.
      b. Patient complains of numbness or pins and needle sensation.
G. If there is an open, draining area on affected extremity, a window (cut-out portion of cast) can be utilized for observation and/or irrigation of wound.
H. Keep cast dry; it can break down when water comes in contact with plaster.
   1. Plastic bags or plastic coated bed Chux can be utilized during the bath or when using bedpan, to protect cast material.
   2. Synthetic cast can be cleaned—does not easily break down.
I. Utilize isometric exercises to prevent muscle atrophy and to strengthen the muscle.
J. Position patient with pillows to prevent strain on unaffected areas.
K. Turn every 2 hours to prevent complications. Encourage to lie on abdomen 4 hours a day.

Crutch Walking ❖ PROCEDURE ❖

A. Purpose—provide support during ambulating when lower extremities unable to support body weight.
B. Safety factors.
   1. Measure 1½ to 2 inches from axillary fold to floor (4 inches in front and 6 inches to side of toes).
   2. Handpiece adjusted to allow 30-degree elbow flexion.
   3. Rubber suction tips on crutches.
   4. Wear well-fitting shoes with nonslip soles.
C. Techniques for teaching crutch walking.
   1. Four-point gait: move right crutch, left foot, left crutch, right foot.
   2. Three-point gait: move crutches and affected leg forward, move unaffected leg forward.
   3. Upstairs: crutches and unaffected leg on same level; put weight on crutch handles and lift unaffected leg to first step; put weight on unaffected leg and lift other leg and crutches to step.
   4. Downstairs: uninjured leg and crutches on same step; put crutches on first step; put weight on crutch handles and transfer unaffected leg to first step.

Using a Cane ❖ PROCEDURE ❖

A. Purpose.
   1. Provide greater stability and speed when walking.
   2. Relieve pressure on weight-bearing joints.
   3. Provide force to push or pull body forward.
B. Safety factors.
   1. Handle at level of greater trochanter.
   2. Elbow flexed at 25- to 30-degree angle.
   3. Lightweight material.
   4. Rubber suction tip.
C. Techniques for walking with cane.
   1. Hold cane close to body.
   2. Hold in hand on stronger or unaffected side.
   3. Place cane 12 inches in front of foot and to the side.
   4. Move stronger leg forward to cane.

The Immobilized Patient

✦ A. Prevent respiratory complications.
   1. Have patient cough and deep breathe every 2 hours.
   2. Turn every 2 hours if not contraindicated.
   3. Provide suction if needed.
✦ B. Prevent thrombus and emboli formation.
   1. Apply antiembolic stockings; CPM.
   2. Initiate isometric and isotonic exercises.

3. Start anticoagulation therapy, if indicated.
4. Turn every 2 hours.
5. Observe for signs and symptoms of pulmonary and/or fat emboli.
◆ C. Prevent contractures.
1. Start range-of-motion exercises to affected joints QID, all joints BID.
2. Provide footboard and/or footcradle.
3. Position and turn every 2 hours.
◆ D. Prevent skin breakdown.
1. Massage with lotion once a day to prevent drying.
2. Use alcohol for back care to toughen skin.
3. Massage elbows, coccyx, heels BID.
4. Turn every 2 hours.
5. Alternate pressure mattress, sheepskin.
6. Use Stryker boots or heel protectors.
7. Use elbow guards.
◆ E. Prevent urinary retention and calculi.
1. Encourage fluids.
2. Monitor intake and output.
3. Administer urinary antiseptic (Mandelamine, etc.) if ordered.
4. Offer bedpan every 4 hours.
◆ F. Prevent constipation.
1. Encourage fluids.
2. Provide high-fiber diet.
3. Administer laxative or enema.
4. Offer bedpan at same time each day—encourage to establish good bowel habits.
G. Provide psychological support.

Acute Compartment Syndrome

Definition: An injury that causes swelling due to bleeding and edema which, in turn, causes increased pressure within the "compartment" that compromises circulation to the involved tissues.

Assessment

A. Monitor extremity for:
1. Pain—is it out of proportion to the injury? Does it increase on active and passive motion?
2. Pallor.
3. Paresthesia or numbness.
4. Cold extremity compared to the other extremity.
5. Pulselessness in affected extremity.
B. Measure compartment pressure using an intra-compartmental monitor (normal is less than 10 mmHg; 20 mmHg or more may cause ischemia).
C. Pain is unrelieved by pain medication.
D. Check if pain is increased with elevation of the extremity or when pressure is applied.
E. Assess for late signs: diminished or absent pulses, coolness, pallor or opening wound to the outside.

Implementation

A. Following an injury, remain vigilant to the possibility of compartment syndrome.
B. Position limb at level of patient's heart (elevation higher may increase ischemia).
C. Initiate IV line and administer pain medication.
D. Do not apply cold or heat without orders—may further compromise circulation.
E. Prepare for surgery—fasciotomy to release pressure and skin grafting to decrease risk of sepsis.

Traction

A. Traction is force applied in two directions.
B. Purpose is to reduce and/or immobilize a fracture, to provide proper bone alignment and regain normal length, or to reduce muscle spasm.
C. *See* Table 10-7 for types of traction.

◆ **Skeletal Traction**

A. Mechanical—applied to bone, using pins (Steinmann), wires (Kirschner), tongs (Crutchfield), Gardner Wells, Halo external fixation.
B. Most often used in spine immobilization and to stabilize cervical vertebrae.
C. Nursing care.
◆ 1. Observe pin or tong insertion site for drainage, odors, erythema, edema (usually indication of inflammatory process or infection).
2. Watch for skin breakdown if bandage is used to apply traction.
3. Cover end of pins or wires with rubber stoppers or cork to prevent puncture of nursing personnel or patient.
4. Cleanse area surrounding insertion site of pin or tongs with hydrogen peroxide or Betadine. Some physicians order antibiotic ointments to be applied to area.

◆ **Balanced Suspension Traction**

A. Thomas splint with Pearson attachment is used in conjunction with skin or skeletal traction (used particularly with skeletal traction for fractured femur).
B. Balanced suspension traction is produced by a counterforce other than the patient.
C. Nursing care. ❖ **PROCEDURE** ❖
1. Maintain proper alignment and check traction mechanism.
2. Protect skin from excoriation, particularly around the top of Thomas splint. Pad with cotton wadding or ABDs.
3. Prevent pressure points around the top of Thomas splint by keeping patient pulled up in bed.
4. Maintain at least 20-degree angle from thigh to the bed.
5. Provide footplate to prevent foot drop.

Type	Position	Purpose
Table 10-7. TYPES OF TRACTION		
Skin Traction		
Cervical	Flat in bed or head of bed elevated 15–20 degrees	Relieve muscle spasms and compression in upper extremities and neck
Buck's	Head of bed elevated 10–20 degrees for ADLs, knee flexed	Preop for fractured hip, relieve muscle spasms before hip surgery
Bryant's	Flat with 45–90-degree hip flexion and buttocks raised 1 inch from mattress, legs extended	Stabilize fractured femur; correct congenital hip in young children weighing less than 30 lbs.
Russell's	Foot of bed slightly elevated—30 degrees	Stabilize fractured femur prior to surgery, some knee injuries
Pelvic girdle	Head of bed elevated, knee gatch elevated to same level (William's position, 45 degrees)	Relieve low back, hip, or leg pain; reduce muscle spasm, herniated disc
Cervical Tongs		
Blackburn, Gardner–Wells, Crutchfield, Vinke Tongs	Spine immobilized, bedrest, supine position	Provide for hyperextension; traction allows vertebrae to slip back into position
Halo Traction	Flat, low-Fowler's in bed, ambulate, or sit up	Stabilize fractured or dislocated cervical vertebrae
Balanced Suspension		
Steinmann pin, Kirschner wires, used with Thomas splint and Pearson attachment	Low-Fowler's, either side or back	To align bone and approximate fractures of femur, tibia, fibula
External Fixation Devices		
Hoffman	Any position is possible with device	Manages complex fractures with soft tissue damage
Synthes	Allows mobility and active exercise	Offers stability for comminuted fractures

6. Keep heels clear of Pearson attachment to prevent skin breakdown and pressure ulcers.
7. Position patient frequently from side to side (as ordered).
8. Unless contraindicated, head of bed can be elevated for comfort and facilitating adequate respiratory functions.
9. Place overbed table on unaffected side.

Halo Traction

A. Immobilization device for spinal injury.
B. Used after cervical or upper thoracic vertebral injury.
C. Halo ring is attached to a vest by vertical bars and ring is attached to the skull.
D. Nursing care. ❖ **PROCEDURE** ❖
   1. Complete a neurologic assessment.
      a. Cranial, peripheral nerves at base of skull—this area is prone to injury.
      b. Check motion and sensation.
   2. Check alignment—neck should not be flexed or extended.
   3. Safety issues.
      a. Keep Allen wrench taped to front of vest in case of emergency (need for CPR).
      b. Patient is top heavy with limited view— remove obstacles when walking.
      c. Have emergency tracheostomy tray and bag-valve-mask available on unit.
      d. Never use bars of halo brace to move patient.
   4. Inspect pin site for drainage, crusting or inflammation.
   5. Provide skin care under vest.

Skin Traction

A. Traction applied by use of elastic bandages, moleskin strips, or adhesive.
B. Used most often in alignment or lengthening (for congenital hip displacement, etc.).
C. Most common types.
   1. Russell traction.
   ✦ 2. Buck's extension (most common).
      ❖ **PROCEDURE** ❖
      a. Pull is exerted in one plane.
      b. Used for temporary immobilization.
      c. Apply moleskin or adhesive material to leg. Follow with application of Ace wrap.
      d. Attach a foot block with a spreader and rope, which goes into a pulley.
      e. Attach weight to pulley and hang freely over edge of bed. (Not more than 8–10 pounds of weight can be applied.)

f. Observe and readjust bandages for tightness and smoothness (can cause constriction, which leads to edema or even nerve damage).

g. Do not apply Buck's over or under a calf compression device. Foot pumps are allowed to prevent DVT.

✦ 3. Cervical traction (used for whiplashes and cervical spasm). ❖ **PROCEDURE** ❖

a. Use head harness (or halter).

(1) Pad chin.

(2) Protect ears from friction rub.

b. Elevate head of bed and attach weights to pulley system over head of bed.

c. Observe for skin breakdown.

(1) Powder areas encased in the halter.

(2) Place back of head on padding.

✦ 4. Pelvic traction (used for low back pain). ❖ **PROCEDURE** ❖

a. Apply girdle snugly over patient's pelvis and iliac crest; attach to weights.

b. Observe for pressure points over iliac crest.

c. Keep patient in good alignment.

d. May raise foot of bed slightly (12 inches) to prevent patient from slipping down in bed.

Traction Apparatus and Nursing Care

A. Care of traction apparatus. ❖ **PROCEDURE** ❖

✦ 1. Weights should hang freely and not touch the floor.

2. Pulleys should not be obstructed.

3. Ropes in the pulley should move freely.

4. Knot should be secured in rope to prevent slipping.

✦ 5. Proper body alignment (up in bed, in direct line with traction) and proper countertraction should be maintained.

6. Weights should not be removed or lifted without specific order. (Exceptions are pelvic and cervical traction that patients can remove at intervals.)

7. Sharp edges from traction apparatus should be covered with hollowed out rubber balls to prevent injury to nursing personnel if they bump into equipment.

✦ B. Care of patient in traction. ❖ **PROCEDURE** ❖

1. Maintain correct alignment.

✦ 2. Maintain counterbalance or correct pull.

a. Pull is exerted against traction in opposite direction (balanced suspension).

b. Pull is exerted against a fixed point.

c. Bed is elevated under area involved to provide the countertraction.

3. Provide firm mattress or bedboards.

4. Observe for complications.

5. Provide range-of-motion exercises for unaffected extremities.

✦ 6. Observe for circulatory impairment.

a. Blanching of nailbeds (color should return quickly when nailbeds are depressed).

b. Extremity should be pink and warm.

c. Check for edema in affected extremity.

d. Patient should be able to wiggle finger or toes.

e. Patient should not have tingling or loss of sensation in affected extremity.

✦ 7. Prevent foot drop.

a. Provide footplate.

b. Encourage dorsiflexion exercises.

8. Provide overhead trapeze to allow patient to assist in activities (turning, moving up in bed, using bedpan, etc.).

9. Prevent postoperative complications.

External Fixation Devices

A. Devices used for stabilizing bone or joint.

B. Device has metal frame and percutaneous pins.

C. Provides traction without ropes or weights so patient has mobility.

Implementation

A. Check pin site for signs of infection.

B. Provide pin site care.

C. Check neurovascular status (circulation, motion & sensation) every 4 hours; patient may have extensive soft tissue and vessel damage.

D. Instruct patient to keep extremity elevated if edema is present.

Hip (Proximal) Fracture

Definition: Bone discontinuity of proximal end of femur, intracapsular or extracapsular, which occurs most frequently in elderly women.

Characteristics

A. Intracapsular—within the joint, capsule, head or neck of femur.

1. Treated by internal fixation.

2. May require total hip replacement.

B. Extracapsular—trochanteric fracture outside the joint.

1. Fracture of greater trochanter—treated by balanced suspension traction.

2. Intertrochanteric fracture—treated initially by balanced suspension traction.

Preoperative Implementation

A. Provide care similar to patients in skin traction.

B. Give special care if patient's increased age is a factor.

C. Observe for elimination regularity.

D. Encourage proper exercises.

E. Maintain proper positioning.

F. Assist patient with eating; nourishing diet essential for healing process.

Operative Procedure

A. Surgical fixation with nails, plates, or screws.

B. Possible prosthesis.

Postoperative Implementation

✦ A. Turn patient from unaffected side to back as routine; a physician's order is required to turn from side to side.

✦ B. Turn patient with hip prosthesis by always placing pillows between legs to avoid adduction.

✦ C. Elevate head (may be limited to 30 to 40 degrees) to avoid acute hip flexion.

D. Introduce quadricep and gluteal setting muscle exercises; encourage use of overhead trapeze for assistance in moving.

E. Take measures to protect patient when moving from bed to chair (patient not to bear weight on affected leg).

F. Provide routine postoperative measures to ensure patient's comfort.

G. Take measures as necessary to prevent complications.

Hip Arthroplasty (Total Hip Replacement)

Definition: Amputation of femoral head with implantation of a steel ball and stem and placement of polyethylene or metal cupin for the acetabulum; its purpose is the alleviation of pain and the restoration of movement for those with osteoarthritis or rheumatoid arthritis.

Postoperative Implementation

✦ A. Keep operative leg in abduction to prevent flexion by use of pillows or abductor splints.

1. Positioning is important (every 2 hours).

2. Turn patient about 45 degrees with aid of trapeze and pillows. Do not elevate bed more than 30–45 degrees.

3. Do not turn to affected side unless specific orders.

4. Maintain anti-rotation boot (if indicated) while patient is supine; remove when patient is turned.

✦ B. Keep Hemovac in place until drainage has substantially decreased (24–96 hours).

1. Drainage should be 30 mL in 8 hours after 48 hours.

2. Check dressing to ensure patency of Hemovac.

3. Observe drainage for signs of hemorrhage or infection.

✦ C. Prevent edema and thrombus formation from venous stasis.

1. Incidence of deep vein thrombosis is 45–70 percent.

2. Use antiembolic stockings or continuous passive motion (CPM).

3. Readjust antiembolic stockings at least every 4–8 hours.

4. Change position frequently by raising and lowering head of bed. When ordered, tilt bed to change positions.

✦ D. Ambulate patient carefully at bedside—first or second postoperative day.

1. Do not allow patient to bear weight on affected hip.

2. Up with walker second postoperative day.

3. Avoid positions with 60–90-degree flexion, such as sitting straight up in a chair.

4. Start physical therapy 3–4 days.

E. Monitor antibiotics used to prevent infection.

Arthroscopy (Knee Surgery)

Definition: Incision of joint for removal of cartilage.

Implementation

A. Encourage and assist with bed exercises.

✦ B. Begin quad-setting, straight-leg raising exercises (should be done for 5 minutes every 30 minutes).

1. Quad-setting exercises—tightening or contracting the muscles of anterior thigh (knee cap is drawn up toward thigh).

2. Straight-leg raising—lifting leg straight off the bed, keeping knee extended and foot in neutral position.

C. Encourage and assist with dorsiflexion and plantar flexion of feet and ankles.

D. Apply ice bags to knee to reduce edema as necessary.

E. Help patient out of bed first postoperative day (use three-point crutch-walking gait without weight bearing).

F. Give routine postoperative care as necessary.

Total Knee Replacement

Definition: Implantation of a metallic upper portion, which substitutes for the femoral condyle, and a lower, high-polymer plastic portion, which substitutes for the tibial joint surfaces.

Implementation

A. Control pain—patient may have epidural or PCA for first 24 hours, then oral analgesics.

B. Monitor dressing and drainage if closed (wound drainage system is used).

1. Record and measure intake and output accurately.
2. Observe for hemorrhage and infection.

C. Promote mobility.
   ✦ 1. CPM may be ordered postop—moderate flexion and extension.
   2. Provide quad-setting and straight-leg raising exercises every hour; encourage general bed exercises; passive range-of-motion.

D. Patient usually has a cast or splint—provide care.

E. Do not dangle leg; may result in dislocation.

F. Instruct patient how to walk with crutch—will be out of bed in 2–3 days.

G. Provide general postoperative care. Monitor for pulmonary embolism (anticoagulant therapy may be ordered).

Amputation

Definition: Surgical removal of part or all of an extremity; connecting bones may be separated at joint (disarticulation).

Types

A. Closed, or flapped—skin closed over bone end of stump.

B. Open, or guillotine—skin not closed over stump end in order that drainage can occur.

Preoperative Implementation

A. Support patient emotionally and listen to patient's expressed concerns regarding limb loss.

✦ B. Help patient strengthen muscles of upper extremity (if lower extremity affected) as preparation for crutch walking.
   1. Extend and flex arms while holding weights.
   2. Do push-ups if condition permits.

✦ C. Inform patient of possible occurrence of phantom pain following surgery. The sensation may last from a few hours to a longer period of time.

Postoperative Implementation

✦ A. Delayed fitting of prosthesis. ❖ **PROCEDURE** ❖
   1. Observe stump for excessive bleeding (keep tourniquet ready in event of hemorrhage).
      a. Reinforce or change dressing only if ordered.
      b. Observe drainage, especially if Penrose drain inserted.
   ✦ 2. Elevate extremity.
      a. Elevation of foot of bed for first 24 hours ONLY is preferred to prevent hemorrhage and reduce edema.
      b. Avoid dependent positioning of stump to prevent edema and discomfort.
      c. Keep tourniquet at bedside to control hemorrhage if it occurs.

3. Turn patient to prone position first postoperative day for brief period and gradually increase time.
4. Exercise all extremities.
5. Assist with transfer of patient to wheelchair.
6. Assist with and encourage crutch walking several days postoperatively.
7. Apply Ace bandage properly (avoid tightness while maintaining tension); helps to condition stump.
8. Observe for signs of depression; listen to patient's expression of feelings.
9. Encourage physical and psychological progress.

✦ B. Immediate fitting of prosthesis.
   1. Immediate fitting causes less pain and hastens healing.
   2. Immediately following surgery, sterile dressing is applied to stump followed by rigid plastic dressing.
   3. Prosthetic device is attached.
   4. If cast falls off, wrap stump immediately with Ace bandage and call physician; normally, cast will be changed and reapplied 10–14 days postoperatively.
   5. Observe for drainage and mark site with pen.
   6. Elevate extremity stump for only 24 hours.
   7. Assist patient in dangling and walking first day postoperatively (first use parallel bars, then crutches).
   8. Be aware that exercises are usually not required because of early ambulation.

Laminectomy, Discectomy

Definition: Removal of posterior arch of vertebrae, or the nucleus of the disc; performed on the cervical or lumbar area of vertebra for removal of spinal cord tumors or herniated disc.

Postoperative Implementation

A. Observe neurovascular signs—blanching, color, warmth of lower or upper extremities.
   1. Observe for sensation and motion in lower extremities.
   2. Check patient's ability to move toes and feet.

✦ B. Monitor dressing for clear or bloody drainage.
   1. Use Dextrostix to test leakage. If positive for glucose, a strong indication it is CSF.
   2. Leaking CSF increases risk of infection to wound and meninges.

C. Place pillow between patient's legs and turn patient from side to side as a unit (log roll) every 2 hours.

D. Head of bed is usually kept flat for lumbar laminectomy but elevated for cervical laminectomy.

E. Roll patient onto bedpan (as used with fractures), supporting back with pillow.

F. Assess bowel sounds—patient will be NPO until flatus and bowel sounds present.

✦ G. Give assistance in preparation for ambulation—1 to 2 days. ❖ **PROCEDURE** ❖
   1. Turn patient on side.
   2. Reach under shoulder that is resting on bed.
   3. Help raise patient as he or she uses arms to push up from bed.
   4. Help patient swing over edge of bed.

H. Instruct patient in proper movement and position.
   1. Turn as a unit.
   2. Sit with back straight.
   3. When necessary to reach floor with hands, squat and maintain straight back.

I. Give routine postoperative care.

J. Encourage fluid intake and diet rich in nutrients; increase intake of fruits, vegetables, and fiber to prevent constipation.

Spinal Fusion

Definition: Removal of bone from iliac crest for fusing with spinal vertebrae.

Postoperative Implementation

✦ A. Keep patient supine for first 8 hours to reduce possibility of compression ordered by physician (most physicians order patient to be off back first 48 hours).

B. Monitor both surgical sites.

C. Brace is applied when patient is ambulated; beginning of ambulation varies from 3–4 days to 8 weeks, depending on extent of fusion.

✦ D. Patient is not to lift, bend, stoop, or sit for prolonged periods for at least 3 months.
   1. Grafts are stable by 1 year.
   2. Some limitation to flexion of spine, depending on extent of fusion.

E. Provide routine care as for postlaminectomy.

Harrington Rod Fusion

Assessment

A. Circulatory impairment.

B. Pain.

C. Signs of fluid and electrolyte imbalance.

D. Clinical manifestations of immobility.

Implementation

✦ A. Keep patient flat in bed (no leg dangling or head elevation).

B. Provide cast care for full body cast.

✦ C. Log roll every hour, 30 degrees to either side, for at least 4 days.

D. Assist in pain control.

1. Severe pain first few days.
2. Pain for several weeks.
3. Pain medication routinely every 3–4 hours for 5 days.
4. Positioning.
5. Relaxation exercises.

E. Provide necessary care for complications of immobility.

F. Monitor signs of fluid and electrolyte imbalance, and record intake and output.

G. Provide diet high in protein, iron, and thiamine, and low in calcium.

Osteoarthritis

Definition: Degeneration of articular cartilage in the joints resulting from prolonged wear and tear on joint surfaces.

Predisposing Factors

A. Aging.

B. Faulty body posture, joint trauma.

C. Familial tendency.

D. Being female (females more frequently affected than males).

E. Obesity.

Assessment

A. Onset usually insidious and gradual.

B. Stiffness of joints.

C. Aching of joints (more noticeable after exercise).

D. Limited joint movement.

E. Nodular bony enlargements on the distal joints of fingers (Heberden's nodes).

F. Occurs usually in hip, knee, vertebra, and finger joints.

Treatment and Implementation

A. Arrange for weight reduction if indicated.

B. Provide rest periods; avoid excessive exercise of joints.

C. Apply warm moist packs; give tub baths and paraffin dips.

D. Assist with exercise program to improve posture.

E. Provide range-of-motion exercises.

✦ F. Administer medications as ordered.
   1. Anti-inflammatory drugs, e.g., phenylbutazone, acetylsalicylic acid.
   2. Analgesics, e.g., acetylsalicylic acid.
   3. Corticosteroid intra-articular injections.
   4. NSAIDs—COX-2 inhibitors (Vioxx and Celebrex).

G. Be aware of possible need for surgical procedure (synovectomy, arthrodesis, or arthroplasty).

H. Instruct patient in use of proper body mechanics.

I. Advise patient to avoid emotional stress to lessen strain on muscles and joints.

J.   Encourage patient to engage in prescribed exercises, to take prescribed medications, and to avoid being overweight.

Rheumatoid Arthritis

✦ *Definition:*   Chronic systemic disease affecting any or all of the body systems and characterized by recurrent inflammation involving the linings of the joints.

Characteristics
A.   Joint capsule progressively changes and ankylosis occurs.
B.   Actual cause is unknown; suspected causes may be an autoimmune disorder or hereditary factors.
C.   Usual onset is 30–50 years of age but may occur at any age.

Assessment
A.   Easily fatigued.
B.   Loss of weight.
C.   Joint pain and stiffness, especially in the morning.
D.   Painful and stiff joints that become swollen, reddened, and tender.
E.   Subcutaneous nodules over bony prominences.
F.   Anemia.
G.   Periods of remission and exacerbation.

Treatment and Implementation
✦ A.   Encourage adequate rest periods; extent of rest depends on current status of disease.
   1.   During day as necessary.
   2.   Use of firm mattress and no pillows; improper positioning of joints can result in contracture.
   3.   Use of splints for supporting joints.
   4.   Relief from emotional stress.
✦ B.   Administer medications as ordered.
   1.   Anti-inflammatory analgesics (*see* Osteoarthritis medications): salicylates, NSAIDs.
   2.   Corticosteroids, e.g., prednisone; adjunct therapy.
   3.   Intra-articular corticosteroid injections into joint.
   4.   Gold salts—effective after 3 to 4 months.
   5.   Alternative to gold salts—pencillamine (Cuprimine) has anti-inflammatory action.
   6.   Antimetabolics (methotrexate, Cytoxan) for patients who don't respond to NSAIDs.
   7.   Low-dose antibiotics, e.g., tetracycline, is effective with some patients.
C.   Apply moist heat, i.e., baths, packs, paraffin dips.
D.   Encourage exercise of joints within limits of tolerance.
E.   Be aware of possible need for surgery (*see* Osteoarthritis).
F.   Discuss aspects of the disease with the patient in a realistic and optimistic manner.
G.   Assist patient in maintaining independence.
H.   Advise patient to call on physician for any problems; caution against promises for quick cures, whatever the source.

Osteoporosis

✦ *Definition:*   Decrease in the amount of bone capable of maintaining structural integrity of the skeleton. Loss of bone mass is associated with aging.

Characteristics
A.   Factors that contribute to condition.
   1.   Bone remodeling results in increased bone mass until age 35; thereafter, bone mass decreases; fragility and risk of fractures increased.
✦   2.   Nutritional factors contribute to development.
    a.   Lack of vitamin D.
    b.   Deficient calcium (minimum 800 mg; for women with decreased bone mass, 1200 mg).
    c.   Low estrogen levels after menopause.
   3.   Excessive intake of drugs (corticosteroids).
   4.   Coexisting medical conditions (malabsorption, lactose intolerance, alcohol abuse, renal failure).
   5.   Immobility causes bone to be reabsorbed faster than it is formed.
B.   Diagnostic tests.
   1.   Routine x-ray when there is 25–45 percent demineralization.
   2.   Single-photon absorptiometry identifies degree of bone mass in wrist.
   3.   Dual-photon absorptiometry identifies bone loss at hip or spine.
   4.   Laboratory studies exclude other diagnoses.
   5.   Quantitative computed tomography of the spine is the most sensitive test to detect osteoporosis.
   6.   Dual-energy x-ray absorptiometry (DEXA) of lumbar spine or hip measures bone density.

Assessment
A.   Backache with pain radiating around trunk.
B.   Skeletal deformities.
C.   Pathologic fractures.
D.   Lab findings.
   1.   Serum calcium, phosphorus, and alkaline phosphatase are usually normal.
   2.   Parathyroid hormone may be elevated.

Treatment and Implementation
A.   Provide pain control: application of heat and cold, medications.
✦ B.   Prevent fractures.
   1.   Instruct in safety factors—watch steps, avoid use of scatter rugs.

2. Keep siderails up to prevent falls.
3. Move gently when turning and positioning.
4. Assist with ambulation if unsteady on feet.
✦ C. Medications which may be ordered.
1. Estrogen—decreases rate of bone resorption—and progesterone at menopause; treatment currently controversial as studies suggest a significant increase in cancer risk.

2. Calcium and vitamin D—support bone metabolism.
D. Instruct in regular exercise program.
1. Range-of-motion and weight-bearing exercises.
2. Ambulation several times per day.
E. Instruct in good use of body mechanics.
F. Provide diet high in protein, calcium, vitamin D.

MEDICAL-SURGICAL NURSING REVIEW QUESTIONS

1. A patient's hemoglobin is 10 gm/dL and the hematocrit is 30 percent. Based on these lab results, the highest priority nursing goal would be to

   1. Promote skin integrity.
   2. Conserve the patient's energy.
   3. Prevent constipation.
   4. Encourage mobility.

2. The nurse has an order to remove a patient's nasogastric tube. The correct nursing action related to this procedure would be to

   1. Put on sterile gloves after untaping the tube from the patient's face.
   2. Instill 30 mL of normal saline before removing the tube.
   3. Pull the tube out slowly and gently.
   4. Pull the tube out quickly while keeping it pinched.

3. In completing a full assessment on a patient, it is important to identify breathing patterns. The breathing pattern depicted in the drawing is

   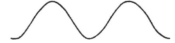

   1. Bradypnea.
   2. Tachypnea.
   3. Biot's.
   4. Kussmaul's.

4. The nurse knows there is a need for further teaching when the patient taking Coumadin says

   1. "I cannot eat foods high in vitamin K, such as leafy vegetables."
   2. "I can take aspirin for my 'aches and pains'."
   3. "I need to have a prothrombin time before I return to the doctor."
   4. "I need to report any bleeding to the doctor."

5. The nurse is teaching a type 1 diabetic patient to self-test her blood glucose. The nurse tells her that if she obtains a result that is over 250 mg/dL, she should

   1. Test her urine for ketones.
   2. Reduce the amount of food that she eats.

   3. Increase her dose of regular insulin by 5 units.
   4. Do nothing unless the results remain elevated for 2 days.

6. A patient with a history of pernicious anemia has been admitted to a long-term care facility. There are no orders written. The LVN would ask the charge nurse to question the physician about obtaining medical orders for

   1. Folic acid.
   2. Iron.
   3. Vitamin B_6.
   4. Vitamin B_{12}.

7. The nurse will know that the patient on a sodium-restricted diet needs more teaching after hearing which of the following statements?

   1. "I must check food labels for preservatives."
   2. "I must check labels on any over-the-counter drugs I use."
   3. "I can drink all the milk I want."
   4. "I can eat all the fresh fruits and vegetables I want."

8. A patient is experiencing tachycardia. The nurse's understanding of the physiological basis for this symptom is explained by which of the following statements?

   1. The demand for oxygen is decreased because of pleural involvement.
   2. The inflammatory process causes the body to demand more oxygen to meet its needs.
   3. The heart has to pump faster to meet the demand for oxygen when there is lowered arterial oxygen tension.
   4. Respirations are labored.

9. Which nursing diagnosis should receive highest priority in a patient who is receiving the chemotherapeutic agent cisplatin (Platinol)?

   1. Risk of infection.
   2. Activity intolerance.
   3. Altered oral mucous membranes.
   4. Altered nutrition: less than body requirements.

10. A patient in hepatic coma has orders for phenobarbital. The nurse knows that this drug is preferred to a depressant drug because it is

1. Excreted by the kidney.
2. Not as strong as a depressant drug.
3. Relaxing for an agitated patient.
4. Safe when the blood ammonia level is up.

11. A female patient with a tentative diagnosis of urinary tract infection has been admitted to the unit. The nurse knows that the most important factor influencing ascending infection is

    1. Not enough fluid intake.
    2. Obstruction of free urine flow.
    3. A change in pH.
    4. Presence of microorganisms.

12. When administering a tepid bath to reduce a patient's temperature, the patient begins to shiver. The intervention would be to

    1. Continue with the bath, as this helps dissipate the heat.
    2. Stop the bath briefly and place a warm blanket on the patient to stop shivering.
    3. Stop the bath, as the body is attempting to produce heat.
    4. Warm the solution, continue the bath, and change the location of cloth placement.

13. A patient is about to be discharged on the drug bishydroxycoumarin (Dicumarol). Of the principles below, which one is the most important to teach the patient before discharge?

    1. He should be sure to take the medication before meals.
    2. He should shave with an electric razor.
    3. If he misses a dose, he should double the dose at the next scheduled time.
    4. It is the responsibility of the RN to do the teaching for this medication.

14. The patient with myasthenia gravis is being treated with an anticholinergic drug, neostigmine (Prostigmin). In administering this drug, the most important nursing measure is to

    1. Give the medication exactly on time.
    2. Give the medication with plenty of water.
    3. Monitor the patient's intake and output.
    4. Monitor the patient's vital signs before and after the medication.

15. A patient is admitted with a diagnosis of atelectasis. Assessing for immediate postoperative complications, the nurse knows that a complication likely to occur following unresolved atelectasis is

    1. Hemorrhage.

2. Infection.
3. Pneumonia.
4. Pulmonary embolism.

16. A cyanotic patient with an unknown diagnosis is admitted to the emergency room. In relation to oxygen, the first nursing action would be to

    1. Wait until the patient's lab work is done.
    2. Not administer oxygen unless ordered by the physician.
    3. Administer oxygen at 2 L flow per minute.
    4. Administer oxygen at 10 L flow per minute and check the patient's nailbeds.

17. A patient is started on ASA therapy. She tells the nurse that she is having a great deal of gastrointestinal distress. The therapeutic response would be to

    1. Inform the charge nurse so the physician can change to another drug.
    2. Explain that this happens frequently and there is nothing to be concerned about.
    3. Ask the patient when she takes the drug during the day.
    4. Tell the patient to take an antacid with the drug.

18. A patient with a diagnosis of gout will be taking colchicine and allopurinol BID to prevent recurrence. The most common early sign of colchicine toxicity that the nurse will observe for is

    1. Blurred vision.
    2. Anorexia.
    3. Diarrhea.
    4. Fever.

19. An employee at the local factory comes to the nurse's office with a large furuncle (boil) on his left upper arm. He has come to the office with this same complaint over the past 6 months. In addition to specific care for the boil itself, the nursing intervention should include

    1. Advising the patient to bathe more regularly.
    2. Doing nothing else, as furuncles are not related to any other disease process.
    3. Calling in all employees and checking them for furuncles.
    4. Encouraging the patient to see his family physician as recurrent boils may be a sign of underlying disease.

20. The nurse is inserting a Foley catheter into a male patient. How far should the catheter be inserted before inflating the balloon?

1. 3–4 inches.
2. 5–6 inches.
3. 7–9 inches.
4. 10–12 inches.

21. The importance of providing instructions to women on self-examination of the breast is best reflected in which of the following statements?

    1. The majority of breast abnormalities are first discovered by women.
    2. Once a lesion has been discovered, the informed patient may monitor the progress of the abnormality herself.
    3. Breast cancer occurs much more often in women than men and is a major cause of death in women.
    4. The high mortality rate of breast cancer can be most effectively reduced by early detection and adequate surgical treatment.

22. The priority assessment for a patient with acute infective (bacterial) endocarditis is

    1. Presence of a heart murmur.
    2. Emboli.
    3. Fever.
    4. Congestive heart failure.

23. A 53-year-old female patient has returned to the unit following a laparoscopic cholecystectomy. She complains of right shoulder pain. The nurse would explain to the patient that this pain is

    1. Common following this type of operation.
    2. Expected after general anesthesia.
    3. Unusual and will be reported to the surgeon.
    4. Indicative of a need to use the incentive spirometer.

24. The nurse would chart that a patient is experiencing Cheyne–Stokes respiration when he has

    1. Periods of hyperpnea alternating with periods of apnea.
    2. Periods of tachypnea alternating with periods of apnea.
    3. An increase in both rate and depth of respirations.
    4. Deep, regular, sighing respirations.

25. Basilar crackles are present in a patient's lungs on auscultation. The nurse knows that these are discrete, noncontinuous sounds that are

    1. Caused by the sudden opening of alveoli.
    2. Usually more prominent during expiration.
    3. Produced by air flow across passages narrowed by secretions.
    4. Found primarily in the pleura.

26. In developing a nursing care plan for a patient with Buerger's disease, it is important to include

    1. Buerger–Allen exercises.
    2. Exercises to increase collateral circulation.
    3. Thigh-high TEDs at all times.
    4. Side effects of drug therapy.

27. The nurse is collecting data on a patient with joint pain. The nurse knows that a patient who is in the early stages of rheumatoid arthritis is most likely to complain of pain, swelling, and limitation of motion in the

    1. Hips.
    2. Knees.
    3. Hands.
    4. Spine.

28. The nurse would expect to find an improvement in which of the blood values as a result of dialysis treatment?

    1. High serum creatinine levels.
    2. Low hemoglobin.
    3. Hypocalcemia.
    4. Hypokalemia.

29. A 50-year-old patient has a tracheostomy and requires tracheal suctioning. The first intervention in completing this procedure would be to

    1. Change the tracheostomy dressing.
    2. Provide humidity with a trach mask.
    3. Apply oral or nasal suction.
    4. Deflate the tracheal cuff.

30. The exercise that would be most beneficial for a patient with COPD is

    1. Controlled coughing.
    2. Whistling while exhaling.
    3. Deep breathing.
    4. Incentive spirometry.

31. The nurse is teaching a type 1 diabetic patient about her diet, which is based on the exchange system. The nurse will know the patient has learned correctly when she says that she can have as much as she wants of

    1. Lettuce.
    2. Tomato.
    3. Grapefruit juice.
    4. Skim milk.

32. A patient with a bile duct obstruction is jaundiced. The priority intervention to control the itching associated with jaundice is to

1. Be sure the patient's nails are clean and short.
2. Maintain the room temperature at 72°–75° F.
3. Provide tepid water for bathing.
4. Use alcohol for back rubs.

33. When using nasotracheal suction to clear a patient's airway of excessive secretions, a principle of the suctioning procedure is to

1. Lubricate the catheter with sterile petrolatum.
2. Insert the catheter with a finger on the vent.
3. Place a finger over the vent intermittently while withdrawing the catheter.
4. Limit suctioning to 30 seconds or less.

34. A patient with an admitting diagnosis of head injury has a Glasgow Coma Score of 3 - 5 - 4. The nurse's understanding of this test is that the patient

1. Can follow simple commands.
2. Will make no attempt to vocalize.
3. Is unconscious.
4. Is able to open his eyes when spoken to.

35. The nursing diagnosis that would have the highest priority in the care of a patient who has become comatose following a cerebral hemorrhage is

1. Impaired physical mobility.
2. Altered nutrition: less than body requirements.
3. Ineffective airway clearance.
4. Constipation.

36. Part of a plan of care for a patient with increased intracranial pressure is to maintain an adequate airway and to promote gas exchange. To accomplish these goals, an effective nursing action is to

1. Encourage the patient to cough vigorously.
2. Avoid hypercapnia in the patient.
3. Suction the patient nasotracheally at frequent intervals.
4. Pack gauze in the nares when there is drainage from the nose.

37. The patient has orders for Nitropaste Ointment, 1 inch every 6 hours. He complains of a headache after each application. The nursing intervention is to

1. Check the blood pressure for hypertension.
2. Decrease the dose to ¾ inch.
3. Give an analgesic such as acetaminophen (Tylenol) as ordered PRN.
4. Apply the paste only every 8 hours.

38. Based on nursing knowledge, the nurse is aware that an epidural hematoma is characterized by

1. A long period of unconsciousness followed by complete lucidity.
2. A short period of unconsciousness followed by a lucid period, followed by rapid deterioration.
3. Slowly developing signs of increasing intracranial pressure.
4. No complaints of headaches.

39. A patient has a retention catheter in place. The priority intervention to prevent bladder infection is to

1. Keep the collection bag dependent of the tubing.
2. Keep the collection bag higher than the abdomen.
3. Flush the catheter frequently.
4. Monitor closely antibiotics as ordered.

40. A patient is admitted following an automobile accident in which he sustained a contusion. The nurse knows that the significance of a contusion is that

1. It is reversible.
2. Amnesia will occur.
3. Loss of consciousness may be transient.
4. Laceration of the brain may occur.

41. A male patient complaining of persistent lower back pain for several months has been admitted for a workup prior to a laminectomy. After a myelogram, which uses a water-soluble dye, the nurse will position him in a

1. Side-lying position.
2. Supine position with the head of the bed elevated.
3. Dorsal recumbent position with the head flat.
4. Prone position.

42. The most appropriate nursing intervention for a patient requiring a finger probe pulse oximeter is to

1. Apply the sensor probe over a finger and cover lightly with gauze to prevent skin breakdown.
2. Set alarms on the oximeter to at least 100 percent.
3. Identify if the patient has had a recent diagnostic test using intravenous dye.
4. Remove the sensor between oxygen saturation readings.

43. A female patient is admitted with a diagnosis of seizure disorder. A priority in protecting the patient against injury during a seizure is to

1. Restrain her arms so that she won't hit herself.
2. Use a padded tongue blade so that she won't injure her tongue.
3. Keep her on her back so that she can breathe.
4. Position her on her side to facilitate drainage.

44. When a patient is in liver failure, which of the following behavioral changes is the most important assessment to report?

    1. Shortness of breath.
    2. Lethargy.
    3. Fatigue.
    4. Nausea.

45. A 55-year-old patient with severe epigastric pain due to acute pancreatitis has been admitted to the hospital. The patient's activity at this time should be

    1. Ambulation as desired.
    2. Bedrest in supine position.
    3. Up ad lib and right side-lying position in bed.
    4. Bedrest in Fowler's position.

46. A 25-year-old female patient with a lower urinary tract infection is admitted to the hospital. Her history indicates she has suffered from repeated infections. The initial data collection will most likely reveal

    1. Frequency and dysuria.
    2. Fever and chills.
    3. Malodorous, cloudy urine.
    4. Leukocytosis and back pain.

47. The most common cause of bladder infection in the patient with a retention catheter is contamination

    1. Due to insertion technique.
    2. At the time of catheter removal.
    3. Of the urethral/catheter interface.
    4. Of the internal lumen of the catheter.

48. The nurse will know a patient with lupus erythematosus understands principles of self-care when she can discuss

    1. Drying agents.
    2. Moisturizing agents.
    3. Antifungal creams.
    4. Solar protection.

49. A patient in acute renal failure receives an IV infusion of 10 percent dextrose in water with 20 units of regular insulin. The nurse understands that the rationale for this therapy is to

    1. Correct the hyperglycemia that occurs with acute renal failure.
    2. Facilitate the intracellular movement of potassium.
    3. Provide calories to prevent tissue catabolism and azotemia.
    4. Force potassium into the cells to prevent arrhythmias.

50. The priority assessment for signs of circulatory impairment in a patient with a fractured femur is to determine if the patient can

    1. Cough and deep breathe.
    2. Turn himself in bed.
    3. Perform biceps exercises.
    4. Wiggle his toes.

51. A 38-year-old female patient is admitted to the emergency room after breaking her right wrist in a fall. Before administering the NSAID ketrololac tromethamine (Toradol) for pain, the nurse would assess for

    1. Any eye problems such as glaucoma.
    2. Presence of peptic ulcer disease.
    3. Currently taking birth control pills.
    4. An allergy to Tylenol.

52. When a patient is being instructed in crutch walking using the swing-through gait, the most appropriate directions are

    1. "Look down at your feet before moving the crutches to ensure you won't fall as you move them."
    2. "Place one crutch forward with the opposite foot and then place the second crutch forward followed by the second foot."
    3. "Move both crutches forward then lift and swing your body past the crutches."
    4. "Use the crutch bar to balance yourself to prevent falls."

53. A cast placed on a patient's leg has dried. If the drying process were completed, the nurse would observe the cast to be

    1. Dull and gray in appearance.
    2. Shiny and white in appearance.
    3. Cool to the touch and gray in appearance.
    4. Warm to the touch and white in appearance.

54. A patient in the early stages of progressive renal failure is admitted to the hospital. The initial assessment will probably reveal

    1. Oliguria, nausea, elevated urine specific gravity.
    2. Anuria, weight gain, hypertension.
    3. Polyuria, low urine specific gravity, polydipsia.
    4. Hematuria, proteinuria, oliguria.

55. The nurse will assess for the most significant complication in patients undergoing chronic peritoneal dialysis, which is

    1. Pulmonary embolism.
    2. Hypotension.

3. Dyspnea.

4. Peritonitis.

56. The most important teaching the nurse should do for a patient to have well managed intermittent hemodialysis is

1. Diet and fluid compliance between sessions will help control the development of complications.
2. To manage his blood pressure between hemodialysis treatments.
3. His energy level should be monitored following each session.
4. Excess fluid will not be removed during hemodialysis.

57. A 12-year-old patient has just been returned to the unit following a tonsillectomy. A priority nursing intervention during the postoperative period is to

1. Administer oral analgesics every 4 hours.
2. Place the patient in a semi-Fowler's position.
3. Apply warm compresses to the surgical site.
4. Provide cool water or apple juice to drink.

58. A patient with a history of cholecystitis is now being admitted to the hospital for possible surgical intervention. The orders include NPO, IV therapy, and bedrest. In addition to assessing for nausea, vomiting, and anorexia, the nurse should observe for pain

1. In the right lower quadrant.
2. After ingesting food.
3. Radiating to the left shoulder.
4. In the right upper quadrant.

59. A patient scheduled for colostomy surgery will have a preoperative diet ordered that will include

1. Broiled chicken, baked potato, and wheat bread.
2. Ground hamburger, rice, and salad.
3. Broiled fish, rice, squash, and tea.
4. Steak, mashed potatoes, raw carrots, and celery.

60. A patient with chronic renal failure is on continuous ambulatory peritoneal dialysis (CAPD). Which nursing diagnosis would have the highest priority?

1. Powerlessness.
2. Risk for infection.
3. Imbalanced nutrition: less than body requirements.
4. Deficient fluid volume.

61. A patient has been receiving digoxin (Lanoxin) 0.125 mg daily for a week. When the nurse visits him at home, the patient tells the nurse about several problems that have been developing over the last few days. The nurse, in assessing for digoxin toxicity, will ask the patient about

1. Constipation.
2. Urinary frequency.
3. Loss of appetite.
4. Ankle edema.

62. A patient is scheduled for a kidney transplant. A medication she will probably take on a long-term basis that will require specific patient teaching to ensure compliance is

1. Corticosteroids.
2. Antibiotics.
3. Anticoagulants.
4. Gamma globulin.

63. Which of the following statements is true of skeletal traction?

1. Neurovascular complications are less apt to occur than with skin traction.
2. The patient has less mobility than he does with skin traction.
3. Fractures can be reduced because more weight can be used than with skin traction.
4. It is preferred for children because fracture fragment alignment is so important.

64. Russell's traction is easily recognized because it incorporates a

1. Sling under the knee.
2. Cervical halter.
3. Pelvic girdle.
4. Pearson attachment.

65. When evaluating all forms of traction, the nurse will check that the direction of pull is controlled by the

1. Patient's position.
2. Rope/pulley system.
3. Amount of weight.
4. Point of friction.

66. Following surgery, the patient's surgeon orders a Foley catheter to be inserted. The first intervention is to

1. Clean the perineum from front to back.
2. Check the catheter for patency.
3. Explain to the patient that she will feel slight, temporary discomfort.
4. Arrange the sterile items on the sterile field.

67. A patient has had a cystectomy and ureteroileostomy (ileal conduit). The nurse is assigned

this patient in the postoperative period. Which of the following observations indicates an unexpected outcome and requires priority care?

1. Edema of the stoma.
2. Mucus in the drainage appliance.
3. Redness of the stoma.
4. Feces in the drainage appliance.

68. A patient requires that a bronchoscopy procedure be done. Due to his physical condition, he will be awake during the procedure. As part of the pretest teaching, the nurse will instruct him that before the scope insertion, his neck will be positioned so that it is

1. In a flexed position.
2. In an extended position.
3. In a neutral position.
4. Hyperextended.

69. The major rationale for the use of acetylsalicylic acid (aspirin) in the treatment of rheumatoid arthritis is to

1. Reduce fever.
2. Reduce inflammation of the joints.
3. Assist the patient in range-of-motion activities without pain.
4. Prevent extension of the disease process.

70. A patient with chronic lymphocytic leukemia is started on chemotherapy. Monitoring the administration of these drugs, the nurse would suggest dietary guidance to

1. Have a liquid diet before the treatments.
2. Consume fluids and foods high in bulk and fiber several hours before the treatment.
3. Encourage the patient to eat a high-starch meal just before the treatment.
4. Encourage large, rather than small, frequent meals.

71. Lactulose is ordered for a 68-year-old patient hospitalized with hepatic failure. The nurse knows that the primary action of this drug is to

1. Prevent constipation.
2. Decrease the blood ammonia level.
3. Increase intestinal peristalsis.
4. Prevent portal hypertension.

72. A patient is receiving Dexamethasone (Decadron). The nurse, in assessing for the outcome of this intervention, will observe for

1. Enhanced immune response.
2. Decreased inflammation in cerebral edema.

3. Reversed signs and symptoms of septic shock.
4. Delayed complications of hepatic coma.

73. In developing a nursing care plan for a patient with multiple sclerosis, the nurse would *not* include

1. Preventative measures for falls.
2. Interventions to promote bowel elimination.
3. Instructions on doing only moderate activities.
4. Techniques to promote safe swallowing.

74. Which one of the following conditions could lead to an inaccurate pulse oximetry reading if the sensor is attached to the patient's ear?

1. Artificial nails.
2. Vasodilation.
3. Hypothermia.
4. Movement of the head.

75. Patient education is an important component of the total nursing care plan. The primary purpose of patient education is to

1. Collect client data.
2. Determine readiness to learn.
3. Assess degree of compliance.
4. Increase patient's knowledge that will affect health status.

76. Thrombolytic therapy would be appropriate for which of the following conditions?

1. Continual blood pressure above 200/120.
2. History of diabetic retinopathy.
3. History of significant kidney disease.
4. Myocardial infarction.

77. While on a camping trip, a friend sustains a snake bite from a poisonous snake. The most effective initial intervention would be to

1. Place a restrictive band above the snake bite.
2. Elevate the bite area above the level of the heart.
3. Position the patient in a supine position.
4. Immobilize the limb.

78. Which one of the following rules for charting narrative notes does not fit into acceptable charting procedures?

1. Each entry should be signed with the nurse's name and professional status.
2. Objective facts are more relevant than nursing interpretation.
3. Behaviors rather than feelings should be charted.
4. Use of the word *client* or *patient* is important to designate particular entries.

79. There is a physician's order to irrigate a patient's bladder. The priority nursing measure to ensure patency is to

    1. Use a solution of sterile water for the irrigation.
    2. Apply a small amount of pressure to push the mucus out of the catheter tip if the tube is not patent.
    3. Carefully insert about 100 mL of aqueous Zephiran into the bladder, allow it to remain for 1 hour, and then siphon it out.
    4. Irrigate with 20 mL of normal saline to establish patency.

80. When assessing an ECG, the nurse knows that the P-R interval represents the time it takes for the

    1. Impulse to begin atrial contraction.
    2. Impulse to traverse the atria to the AV node.
    3. SA node to discharge the impulse to begin atrial depolarization.
    4. Impulse to travel to the ventricles.

81. When a patient has suffered severe burns all over his body, the most effective method of monitoring the cardiovascular system is

    1. Cuff blood pressure.
    2. Arterial pressure.
    3. Central venous pressure.
    4. Pulmonary artery pressure.

82. A female patient has orders for an oral cholecystogram. Prior to the test, the nursing intervention would be to

    1. Provide a high-fat diet for dinner, then NPO.
    2. Explain that diarrhea may result from the dye tablets.
    3. Administer the dye tablets following a regular diet for dinner.
    4. Administer enemas until clear.

83. The practical nurse knows there is a need for further teaching when the hemodialysis patient with an arteriovenous fistula in the left arm says

    1. "I can carry heavy packages in my right arm."
    2. "You cannot take my blood pressure in my left arm."
    3. "I can wear several bracelets to cover the scar on my left arm."
    4. "You can start the IV in my right arm."

84. Knowing that a patient has the diagnosis of heart failure (HF), what symptoms would the nurse assess during data collection?

    1. Crackles, bradycardia, arrhythmias.

    2. Cyanosis, crackles, gallop rhythm.
    3. Anxiety, bronchospasm, pedal edema.
    4. Diaphoresis, orthopnea, sensorium changes.

85. Moving a patient from the bed to a chair, the first intervention is

    1. Dangling with feet on the floor at his bedside.
    2. Putting nonslip shoes or slippers on patient's feet.
    3. Rocking the patient and pivot.
    4. Positioning patient so that he is comfortable.

86. When a patient has peptic ulcer disease, the nurse would expect a priority intervention to be

    1. Assisting in inserting a Miller–Abbott tube.
    2. Assisting in inserting an arterial pressure line.
    3. Inserting a nasogastric tube.
    4. Inserting an IV.

87. A type 1 diabetic patient tells the nurse she doesn't like what is on her dinner tray and refuses to eat it. The best intervention is to

    1. Call the physician for a different diet order.
    2. Obtain a regular diet tray from the kitchen and remove all sugar and desserts.
    3. Order a sandwich and soup from the kitchen and make a referral to the dietician.
    4. Ask the kitchen staff to send another diabetic meal tray for the patient.

88. A physician has written orders to test nasogastric drainage every hour for a patient on mechanical ventilation. The nurse recognizes the importance of this action because

    1. The NG tube may become dislodged.
    2. The pH should be maintained below 5.
    3. Stress ulcers are frequently associated with mechanical ventilation.
    4. It will determine if the antacids are working.

89. A patient in hepatic coma has orders for lactulose to reduce blood ammonia. The nurse would evaluate the medication and understand that it is working when

    1. Watery diarrhea occurs.
    2. The patient has two to three stools/day.
    3. The patient is constipated.
    4. Dehydration occurs and can be observed in the patient's skin condition.

90. The nurse is to assess the capillary refill time of a patient who has a leg cast. When the nurse compresses one of the patient's toenails and releases

the compression, the nurse would expect the color to return to the nail within

1. 1 second.
2. 3 seconds.
3. 10 seconds.
4. 15 seconds.

91. A patient has a 1000 mL bag of D5/0.45 NS hung at 10 AM/1000hrs. His 24 hour IV orders are for 3 bags of 1000 mL. What time should the second bag be hung? _____ PM.

92. While caring for a patient who had a left leg above-the-knee amputation several days earlier, the patient cheerfully begins talking about getting back to the "old tennis courts" for a "set or two." His emotional acceptance of this condition can be interpreted as

1. Denying his altered body image.
2. Adjusting well to his altered mobility.
3. Accepting his loss.
4. Beginning to deal with his limitations.

93. The nurse is assigned to work with a patient diagnosed as having pernicious anemia. In evaluating the diet for the patient, the nurse would know the patient understands dietary parameters when he chooses

1. Meat, milk, cheese.
2. Whole grains, cereals.
3. Fruits, green leafy vegetables.
4. Organ meats, yellow vegetables.

94. After application of a leg cast following a fracture, the patient is unable to feel pressure on his toes and complains of tingling. These signs indicate

1. Pressure on a nerve.
2. Phantom pain syndrome.
3. Overmedication with an analgesic.
4. Improper alignment of the fracture.

95. When evaluating the patient's understanding of a low-potassium diet, the nurse will know he understands if he says that he will avoid

1. Pasta.
2. Raw apples.
3. Dry cereal.
4. French bread.

96. Urecholine (bethanechol chloride) is ordered PRN for a patient following a transurethral resection (TUR). Which of the following conditions would need to be present for the nurse to administer this drug?

1. Complaints of bladder spasms.

2. Complaints of severe pain.
3. Inability to void.
4. Frequent episodes of painful urination.

97. The milliliters of drug that should be used to give 0.5 g if the label on the bottle reads 5 g in 10 mL is _____ mL.

98. After removing the fecal impaction, the patient complains of feeling lightheaded and the pulse rate is 44. The priority intervention is to

1. Monitor vital signs.
2. Place in shock position.
3. Call the physician.
4. Begin CPR.

99. A patient is to receive 65 mg of gentamicin (Garamycin). Available is a solution containing 80 mg/2 mL. How much of this solution should the nurse draw up?

1. 0.6 mL.
2. 1.2 mL.
3. 1.6 mL.
4. 2.5 mL.

100. The laboratory result that should be monitored regularly in a patient who is receiving gentamicin (Garamycin) is

1. Serum creatinine.
2. Serum calcium.
3. Platelets.
4. White blood cell (WBC) count.

101. Which nursing action is the most critical when caring for a patient who is receiving continuous nasogastric tube feedings?

1. Warming the feeding to room temperature.
2. Maintain accurate records of intake and output.
3. Flushing the tube with water every 4 hours.
4. Keeping the patient in a semi-Fowler's position.

102. A patient with thrombophlebitis should be positioned so that his legs are

1. Dependent.
2. Flat on the bed.
3. Elevated about 30 degrees.
4. Elevated about 60 degrees.

103. A patient has reported to the ambulatory surgical center for a hernia repair. While in the preoperative area, the patient tells the nurse he is very nervous about the surgery. The best response by the nurse is

1. "What did the physician tell you she is planning to do?"
2. "Do you usually get nervous about new experiences?"
3. "Your physician is very competent and will help you get better."
4. "Tell me how you are feeling right now."

104. A hypothyroid patient has orders for all of the following medications. The nurse would evaluate the patient most closely following administration of which medication?

   1. Morphine sulfate.
   2. Ibuprofen (Motrin).
   3. Levothyroxine (Synthroid).
   4. Digoxin (Lanoxin).

105. A patient has been receiving chemotherapy for the treatment of breast cancer. She is now to start receiving daily injections of filgrastim (Neupogen). The nurse would assess for a therapeutic response to this drug by monitoring which laboratory test result?

   1. Blood urea nitrogen (BUN).
   2. Potassium.
   3. Platelets.
   4. WBC.

106. A patient with COPD has developed secondary polycythemia. Which nursing diagnosis would be included in the care plan because of the polycythemia?

   1. Fluid volume deficit related to blood loss.
   2. Impaired tissue perfusion related to thrombosis.
   3. Activity intolerance related to dyspnea.
   4. Risk for infection related to suppressed immune response.

107. The nurse is teaching a patient with a new colostomy how to apply an appliance to a colostomy. How much skin should remain exposed between the stoma and the ring of the appliance?

   1. ⅛ inch.
   2. ½ inch.
   3. ¾ inch.
   4. 1 inch.

108. Which of the following blood chemistry results would the nurse expect to find elevated in a patient with right-sided heart failure?

   1. Ammonia.
   2. Albumin.
   3. LDH.
   4. CK.

109. You are taking the blood pressure of a patient with hypertension. Place the steps in correct order for performing the skill.

   1. Place the bell of the stethoscope on the medial antecubital fossa.
   2. Place the diaphragm of the stethoscope on the medial antecubital fossa.
   3. Inflate the cuff.
   4. Listen for the first Korotkoff sound.
   5. Deflate the cuff until you hear the first sound.

110. A patient with pulmonary edema is admitted to the unit. Which of the following physician's orders should the nurse question?

   1. Administer furosemide (Lasix) 20 mg IV immediately.
   2. Administer oxygen at 3 L/min via nasal prongs.
   3. Keep the head of the patient's bed in low-Fowler's position.
   4. Weigh the patient every day.

111. In preparation for discharge of a patient with arterial insufficiency and Raynaud's disease, patient teaching instructions should include

   1. Walking several times each day as part of an exercise routine.
   2. Keeping the heat up so that the environment is warm.
   3. Wearing TED hose during the day.
   4. Using hydrotherapy for increasing oxygenation.

112. Assessing the urine of a patient with suspected cholecystitis, the nurse expects that the color will most likely be

   1. Pale yellow.
   2. Greenish-brown.
   3. Red.
   4. Yellow-orange.

113. The treatment prescribed for the burned area of skin before skin grafting can take place will include

   1. Silver nitrate soaks for 24 hours.
   2. Burn irrigations with Sulfamylon.
   3. Warm soaks with sterile water.
   4. Germicidal soap scrubs to the affected area.

114. When a patient asks the nurse why the physician says he "thinks" the patient has tuberculosis, the nurse explains to him that diagnosis of tuberculosis can take several weeks to confirm. Which of the following statements supports this answer?

1. A positive reaction to a tuberculosis skin test indicates that the patient has active tuberculosis, even if one negative sputum is obtained.
2. A positive sputum culture takes at least 3 weeks, due to the slow reproduction of the bacillus.
3. Because small lesions are hard to detect on chest x-rays, x-rays usually need to be repeated during several consecutive weeks.
4. A patient with a positive smear will have to have a positive culture to confirm the diagnosis.

115. The nurse is counseling a patient with the diagnosis of glaucoma. She explains that if left untreated, this condition leads to

1. Blindness.
2. Myopia.
3. Retrolental fibroplasia.
4. Uveitis.

116. A patient is admitted with a diagnosis of esophageal varices. When collecting data, the nurse will expect to find which of the following conditions that contributed to the diagnosis?

1. Decreased prothrombin formation.
2. Decreased albumin formation by the liver.
3. Portal hypertension.
4. Increased central venous pressure.

117. A nursing assessment for initial signs of hypoglycemia will include

1. Pallor, blurred vision, weakness, behavioral changes.
2. Frequent urination, flushed face, pleural friction rub.
3. Abdominal pain, diminished deep tendon reflexes, double vision.
4. Weakness, lassitude, irregular pulse, dilated pupils.

118. One of the major goals of therapy for a patient with peptic ulcer disease is to

1. Talk about the recent stressful situations, which may have contributed to the ulcer formation.
2. Understand the pathogenesis of the ulcer.
3. Accept that stress will negatively affect the condition.
4. Discover what foods caused pain.

119. The physician has ordered a 24-hour urine specimen. After explaining the procedure to the patient, the nurse collects the first specimen. This specimen is then

1. Discarded, then the collection begins.

2. Saved as part of the 24-hour collection.
3. Tested then discarded.
4. Placed in a separate container and later added to the collection.

120. When a head injury patient has fluid draining from the left ear, the nurse will immediately position the patient with the head of his bed

1. Elevated and his head turned to the left.
2. Flat and his head turned to the right.
3. Flat and his head turned to the left.
4. Elevated and his head turned to the right.

121. As the nurse is completing evening care for a patient, he observes that the patient is upset, quiet, and withdrawn. The nurse knows that the patient is scheduled for diagnostic tests the following day. An important question to ask the patient is

1. "Would you like to go to the dayroom to watch TV?"
2. "Are you prepared for the test tomorrow?"
3. "Have you talked with anyone about the test tomorrow?"
4. "Have you asked your physician to give you a sleeping pill tonight?"

122. Assessing a patient's shunt for patency by using a stethoscope and the nurse's hand, the nurse would expect to feel and hear

1. A loud bruit and feel the area cool to touch.
2. The sound of rushing blood and feel the area warm to touch.
3. No sound, but feel the area warm to touch.
4. A regular heartbeat and feel the area cool to touch.

123. What should be the priority goal when a patient assessment indicates the presence of a reddened, tender, painful area on the patient's calf?

1. Maintain a patent airway.
2. Prevent infection.
3. Foster fluid and electrolyte balance.
4. Promote venous return.

124. The patient has arrived in the recovery room following a lobectomy. As the nurse assigned to care for the patient during the immediate postoperative period, the first intervention will be to

1. Take the patient's temperature, blood pressure, respirations, and pulse for baseline data.
2. Check that the IV is running on time and that the correct solution is infusing.

3. Administer oxygen through an appropriate supply device.
4. Connect the Pleur-evac to suction.

125. Following an amputation, the advantage to the patient for an immediate prosthesis fitting is

1. Ability to ambulate sooner.
2. Less chance of phantom limb sensation.
3. Dressing changes are not necessary.
4. Better fit of the prosthesis.

126. Evaluating the effectiveness of preoperative teaching before colostomy surgery, the nurse expects that the patient will be able to

1. Describe how the procedure will be done.
2. Exhibit acceptance of the surgery.
3. Explain the function of the colostomy.
4. Apply the colostomy bag correctly.

127. A nursing care plan for a patient with a suprapubic cystostomy would include

1. Placing a urinal bag around the tube insertion to collect the urine.
2. Clamping the tube and allowing the patient to void through the urinary meatus before removing the tube.
3. Catheter irrigations every 4 hours to prevent formation of urinary stones.
4. Limiting fluid intake to 1500 mL/day.

128. Following a treadmill test and cardiac cath-eterization, the patient is found to have coronary artery disease, which is inoperable. He is referred to the cardiac rehabilitation unit. During his first visit to the unit he says that he doesn't understand why he needs to be there because there is nothing that can be done to make him better. The best nursing response is

1. "Cardiac rehabilitation is not a cure but can help restore you to many of your former activities."
2. "Here we teach you to gradually change your lifestyle to accommodate your heart disease."
3. "You are probably right but we can gradually increase your activities so that you can live a more active life."
4. "Do you feel that you will have to make some changes in your life now?"

129. A patient admitted for possible bleeding in the cerebrum has vital signs taken every hour to monitor the neurological status. Which of the following neurological checks will give the nurse the best information about the extent of bleeding?

1. Pupillary checks.
2. Spinal tap.
3. Deep tendon reflexes.
4. Evaluation of extrapyramidal motor system.

130. Patient teaching following cataract surgery should include

1. The eye patch will be removed in 3–4 days, and the eye may be used without difficulty.
2. They must use only one eye at a time to prevent double vision.
3. They will be able to judge distances without difficulty.
4. Contact lenses will be fitted before discharge from the hospital.

131. Preoperative teaching for a patient scheduled for a laryngectomy should include the fact that

1. The patient will continue to be able to breathe and smell through the nose.
2. The patient will be fed through a permanent gastrostomy tube.
3. The patient will be able to speak again, but it will not be the same as before surgery.
4. Oral fluids will be eliminated for the first week following surgery.

132. The main complication following a nephrostomy that the nurse must assess for is

1. Bleeding from the nephrostomy site.
2. Cardiopulmonary involvement following the procedure.
3. Difficulty in restoring fluid and electrolyte balance.
4. Contamination of the site.

133. Hemorrhage is a major complication following oral surgery or radical neck dissection. If this condition occurs, the most immediate nursing intervention would be to

1. Notify the surgeon immediately.
2. Treat the patient for shock.
3. Put pressure over the common carotid and jugular vessels in the neck.
4. Immediately put the patient in high-Fowler's position.

134. Following laminectomy surgery, the patient returns from the recovery room to the surgical unit. The nurse would assess for the most common complication following anesthesia

1. Atelectasis.
2. Pneumonia.

3. Paralytic ileus.

4. Edema.

135. A patient just received a diagnosis of carcinoma. While making morning rounds the day before surgery, the nurse observes the patient crying. An appropriate response would be to

1. Ignore the crying, as the nurse realizes the patient may not want to talk.
2. Acknowledge the patient by saying, "Good morning," as the nurse passes the door and observe if she seems to wish to talk.
3. Go in the room and ask her why she is crying.
4. Go in the room, sit down, and stay quietly with her.

136. When auscultating the apical pulse of a patient who has atrial fibrillation, the nurse would expect to hear a rhythm that is characterized by

1. The presence of occasional coupled beats.
2. Long pauses in an otherwise regular rhythm.
3. A continuous and totally unpredictable irregularity.
4. Slow but strong and regular beats.

137. To achieve the desired outcome of fracture healing, which nursing goal should receive the highest priority?

1. Maintain immobilization and alignment.
2. Provide optimal nutrition and hydration.
3. Promote independence in activities of daily living.
4. Provide relief from pain and discomfort.

138. A 34-year-old patient is admitted with a diagnosis of hypoparathyroidism. One of the parameters the nurse will assess the patient for is hypocalcemia. If present, the nurse would expect to observe

1. Negative Chvostek's sign.
2. Hyperventilation.
3. Generalized edema.
4. Spasms of hands and feet.

139. The nurse, collecting data for a nursing history from a newly admitted patient, learns that he has a Denver shunt. This suggests that he has a history of

1. Hydrocephalus.
2. Renal failure.
3. Peripheral occlusive disease.
4. Cirrhosis.

140. For a patient with the diagnosis of acute pancreatitis, the nurse would include which critical component as part of the care plan?

1. Testing for Homan's sign.
2. Measuring the abdominal girth.
3. Performing a glucometer test.
4. Straining the urine.

141. The nurse collects the following information when taking a nursing history from a postmenopausal patient. The data reveals a risk factor for the development of osteoporosis when the patient

1. Has diabetes mellitus, type 2.
2. Has been on prednisone (Deltasone) for 3 months.
3. Swims laps in a pool, three times per week.
4. States she was never pregnant.

142. For a patient in a long leg cast, which nursing intervention should receive the highest priority?

1. Handle the cast with the palms of the hands.
2. Keep the cast uncovered until it is dry.
3. Elevate the limb so the toes are higher than the hip.
4. Petal the cast edges with adhesive tape.

143. The nurse has been teaching a patient to use crutches. Which statement made by the patient indicates a need for more teaching?

1. "I will not look down to watch my feet while I'm walking."
2. "I will place my weight on the hand grips."
3. "I will put my weak leg down first when going down stairs."
4. "I will raise the placement of the hand grips on the crutches as I get stronger."

144. A 40-year-old patient is to be discharged and she wishes to walk outside. The nurse explains that the reason patients are discharged in a wheelchair is for

1. Comfort.
2. Convenience.
3. Safety.
4. Rehabilitation.

145. To perform the skill, "turning to the side-lying position," the nurse would lower the head of the bed, elevate the bed to working height, move the patient to the nurse's side of the bed, and flex the patient's knees. The next intervention would be to

1. Roll the patient on his side.
2. Reposition the patient.
3. Place one hand on the patient's hip and the other on his shoulder.
4. Reposition the patient's arms so they are not under his body.

146. While the IV fluids are infusing via infusion pump, the nurse monitors the system every hour and suspects a significant amount of air has entered the tubing. The first action is to

1. Immediately shut off the IV and notify the charge nurse.
2. Increase the drops per minute to flush the air out.
3. Place the patient on his left side.
4. Place the patient in an upright position.

147. The charge nurse instructs the LVN to admit a new patient from the ER because all of the RNs are busy. The most appropriate response is

1. "I will be happy to help out; I know everyone is busy."
2. "I will put the patient in bed and orient him to the environment only."
3. "I'm sorry, I can't help you because my license doesn't allow me to admit patients."
4. "I will admit the patient but I will need to document that I'm working outside my license parameters in case there is a problem."

148. In teaching a newly diagnosed diabetic patient about insulin self-injection, the nurse teaches that the injection site currently believed to be the best, because it provides the most rapid insulin absorption, is the

1. Arms.
2. Abdomen.
3. Thighs.
4. Buttocks.

149. A patient who is in respiratory failure requires endotracheal intubation and a ventilator. Nursing care while on the ventilator should include

1. Suctioning the endotracheal tube every 2 hours.
2. Encouraging the patient to talk about his anxiety.
3. Keeping the endotracheal tube securely taped to the face.
4. Offering small sips of water as needed for oral comfort.

150. The nurse is preparing a patient for a myelogram using metrizamide (Amipaque), a water-soluble contrast material. The nurse will know the patient understands the postmyelogram care regimen when she says

1. "I will need to keep my head elevated for at least 8 hours."
2. "I will need to lie flat for 12 to 24 hours."
3. "I will not be allowed to drink much liquid for 12 hours."
4. "I expect to have some itching and a stiff neck for a few days."

MEDICAL-SURGICAL NURSING
Answers with Rationale

1. (2) These test results indicate anemia. Impaired oxygen-carrying capacity of red blood cells causes cellular hypoxia and results in fatigue. Conserving energy limits oxygen expenditure and minimizes fatigue. Increased mobility (4) increases the demand for oxygen and contributes to fatigue. Although hypoxic tissues are more vulnerable to breakdown, protecting the integumentary system (1) is not as high a priority as is the promotion of overall oxygenation. Constipation (3) is not a problem in anemia.

NP:P; CN:PH; CA:M; CL:A

2. (4) Removing the tube quickly while keeping it pinched lessens the risk of gastric secretions falling into the trachea during removal. Instilling 20–30 mL of air, rather than normal saline, into the tube will also help prevent aspiration of gastric secretions. Unsterile gloves are worn for this procedure.

NP:I; CN:PH; CA:M; CL:A

3. (1) Bradypnea—slow, regular respirations; rate is below 10/minute. Tachypnea is increased rate, above 24/minute. Biot's are abrupt interruptions between a faster, deeper rate. Kussmaul's respirations are deep, gasping breaths.

NP:P; CN:PH; CA:M; CL:A

4. (2) Aspirin can potentiate the anticoagulant effect. Analgesics without salicylates such as acetaminophen (Tylenol) should be used instead.

NP:E; CN:PH; CA:M; CL:A

5. (1) An elevated blood sugar may be accompanied by ketoacidosis; therefore, it is important to test for urinary ketones when the blood glucose is over 250 mg/dL. Reducing intake (2) may provoke hypoglycemia in a type 1 diabetic. Any change in insulin dosage (3) needs to be medically prescribed. The patient should not wait 2 days before taking action (4) when the blood sugar is high.

NP:I; CN:PH; CA:M; CL:A

6. (4) In pernicious anemia, a person cannot absorb vitamin B_{12} because of a deficiency of the intrinsic factor. The person must regularly receive vitamin B_{12} parenterally to prevent neurologic deficits. The other listed nutrients are not effective in the treatment of pernicious anemia.

NP:I; CN:PH; CA:M; CL:A

7. (3) Milk has a high sodium content and would be restricted on a sodium-restriction diet. It is necessary to check all labels for sodium content, such as preservatives. Fresh fruits and vegetables have minimal sodium content.

NP:E; CN:PH; CA:M; CL:A

8. (3) The arterial oxygen supply is lowered and the demand for oxygen is increased, which results in the heart's having to beat faster to meet body needs for oxygen.

NP:P; CN:PH; CA:M; CL:C

9. (1) Cisplatin may depress the bone marrow, thereby interfering with the production of WBCs. The resultant leukopenia can be life threatening; therefore, risk of infection is the highest priority. The other nursing diagnoses, although appropriate for this patient, would be of lower priority.

NP:P; CN:PH; CA:M; CL:A

10. (1) Depressant drugs are detoxified by the liver, which is already compromised. Phenobarbital is excreted by the kidney, so it is a safer medication.

NP:P; CN:PH; CA:M; CL:C

Coding for Questions/Answers Abbreviations: **Nursing Process: NP,** Data Collection: D, Planning: P, Implementation: I, Evaluation: E, **Client Needs: CN,** Safe, Effective Care Environment: S, Health Promotion and Maintenance: H, Psychosocial Integrity: PS, Physiological Integrity: PH, **Clinical Area: CA,** Medical Nursing: M, Surgical Nursing: S, Maternal/Newborn Nursing: MA, Pediatric Nursing: P, Psychiatric Nursing: PS, **Cognitive Level: CL,** Knowledge: K, Comprehension: C, Application: A, Analysis: AN

11. (2) Free flow of urine together with large urine output and normal pH are antibacterial defenses. If free flow is obstructed, the infection will most likely ascend up the tract.

NP:P; CN:PH; CA:M; CL:C

12. (3) Stop or modify the bath to prevent shivering. Shivering is a method of producing body heat. Continuing with the bath would be detrimental for the patient. Stopping the bath briefly is also not advised.

NP:I; CN:PH; CA:M; CL:A

13. (2) Dicumarol is an anticoagulant drug and one of the dangers involved is bleeding. Using a safety razor can lead to bleeding through cuts. The drug should be given at the same time daily but not related to meals. Due to danger of bleeding, missed doses should not be made up. The LVN is prepared to do this patient teaching.

NP:P; CN:PH; CA:M; CL:A

14. (1) The drug should be given exactly on time. If the drug is given late, the patient could have a myasthenic crisis and be unable to swallow the drug. If the drug is given early, the patient may have a cholinergic crisis.

NP:I; CN:PH; CA:M; CL:A

15. (3) Pneumonia is a major complication of unresolved atelectasis and must be treated along with vigorous treatment for atelectasis. Hemorrhage (1) and infection (2) are not related to this condition. Pulmonary embolism (4) could result from deep vein thrombosis.

NP:D; CN:PH; CA:M; CL:C

16. (3) Administer oxygen at 2 L/min and no more, for if the patient is emphysemic and receives too high a level of oxygen, he will develop CO_2 narcosis and the respiratory system will cease to function.

NP:I; CN:PH; CA:M; CL:A

17. (3) It is important to find out whether the drug is taken on a full or empty stomach. Gastric irritation is a common side effect of ASA therapy. It can be decreased by taking the drug with meals. An antacid can be given with the drug at bedtime; however, the nurse cannot arbitrarily tell the patient to do so as it takes a physician's order.

NP:D; CN:PH; CA:M; CL:A

18. (3) Diarrhea is by far the most common early sign of colchicine toxicity. When given in the acute phase of gout, the dose of colchicine is usually 0.6 mg PO q hr (not to exceed 10 tablets) until pain is relieved or gastrointestinal symptoms ensue.

NP:D; CN:PH; CA:M; CL:C

19. (4) Sometimes recurrent boils are symptoms of an underlying disease process such as glycosuria. Bathing (1) will not influence the course of the boils, and (3) they are not communicable.

NP:I; CN:PH; CA:M; CL:AN

20. (3) The male urethra is 6–8 inches long. Accepted procedure is to insert the catheter until urine begins to flow, then advance the catheter 1–2 inches more before attempting to inflate the balloon.

NP:P; CN:PH; CA:M; CL:K

21. (4) Health professionals have the responsibility to provide clear guidelines focused on the prevention and early treatment of breast cancer. Self-examinations following menstruation coupled with annual screening examination by the physician is very effective in detecting early breast cancer.

NP:D; CN:PH; CA:M; CL:C

22. (2) While all of the symptoms may be present, the major complication with this condition is that of emboli. If emboli arise in the right heart chambers, they will terminate in the lungs; left chamber emboli may travel anywhere in the arterial tree. The nurse should constantly monitor for this complication.

NP:D; CN:PH; CA:M; CL:AN

23. (1) Carbon dioxide is insufflated into the abdomen during a laparoscopic cholecystectomy. It may irritate the diaphragm and cause referred shoulder pain. This patient's complaint is a common response to this type of operation, so telling the patient will be reassuring and will help to decrease the anxiety accompanying the pain.

NP:I; CN:PH; CA:M; CL:C

24. (1) Periods of hyperpnea alternating with apnea is a breathing pattern that is easily missed if the patient's respirations are not observed for a few minutes. It may indicate disorders of cerebral circulation, increased cerebral pressure, and/or injury to the brain tissue.

NP:D; CH:PH; CA:M; CL:K

25. (1) Basilar crackles are usually heard during inspiration and are caused by sudden opening of alveoli.

NP:D; CH:PH; CA:M; CL:C

26. (1) Buerger-Allen exercises improve peripheral arterial circulation which is specific for treatment of Buerger's disease. Drug therapy is the treatment of choice for Raynaud's disease; therefore, instructing about the side effects of these agents is not important.

NP:P; CN:PH; CA:M; CL:K

27. (3) Rheumatoid arthritis typically begins with inflammatory changes in the small joints of the hands, wrists, and feet.

NP:D; CN:PH; CA:M; CL:C

28. (1) High creatinine levels will be decreased. Anemia is a result of decreased production of erythropoietin by the kidney and is not affected by hemodialysis (2). Hyperkalemia and high base (bicarbonate) levels are present in renal failure patients (3) and (4).

NP:I; CN:PH; CA:M; CL:A

29. (3) Before deflating the tracheal cuff, the nurse will apply oral or nasal suction to the airway to prevent secretions from falling into the lungs. Dressing change (1) and humidity (2) do not relate to suctioning.

NP:I; CN:PH; CA:M; CL:A

30. (2) Whistling while exhaling prevents the bronchi from collapsing, thereby permitting more effective exhalation of trapped carbon dioxide. The other exercises do not foster exhalation of carbon dioxide.

NP:P; CN:PH; CA:M; CL:C

31. (1) Lettuce contains primarily water and fiber, and is considered a "free food" in the American Dietetic Association exchange lists. The other listed foods contain significant amounts of carbohydrates and/or protein and must be computed into the diet plan.

NP:E; CN:PH; CA:M; CL:AN

32. (3) Itching is made worse by vasodilation. Tepid water prevents excessive vasodilation. Warm environmental temperatures (2) promote vasodilation. Alcohol (4) not only produces vasodilation, but is drying to the skin, which further compounds the problem of itching. Keeping the nails clean and short (1) will help prevent skin irritation and infection if the patient scratches, but will not prevent the itching from occurring.

NP:P; CN:PH; CA:M; CL:A

33. (3) To prevent trauma to the mucous membranes lining the airway, suction should be applied only while withdrawing the catheter. The catheter should be lubricated with a water-soluble substance to prevent lipoidal pneumonia. Suctioning attempts should be limited to 10 seconds to prevent hypoxia.

NP:I; CN:PH; CA:M; CL:A

34. (4) A Glasgow Coma Score of 3 - 5 - 4 means that the patient is able to open his eyes when spoken to and can localize pain, attempting to remove noxious stimuli when motor function is tested. He is not able to follow commands (1). He is able to vocalize, but is confused. Verbal response is usually tested by asking the patient to state who he is, where he is, or the date.

NP:E; CN:PH; CA:M; CL:AN

35. (3) An unconscious person is unable to independently maintain a clear airway; therefore, the highest priority should be given to planning and providing nursing interventions that promote effective airway clearance. The other nursing diagnoses are of lower priority.

NP:P; CN:PH; CA:M; CL:AN

36. (2) Hypercapnia leads to vasodilation, thus increasing cerebral blood flow and increasing intracranial pressure. The patient should not be encouraged to cough vigorously (1), as this will also raise the intracranial pressure. An intact autoregulation mechanism provides for sharp fluctuation in intracranial pressure, as might occur during coughing or sneezing in the patient without increased intracranial pressure; however, patients with increased intracranial pressure have compromised autoregulation.

NP:I; CN:PH; CA:M; CL:A

37. (3) Headaches are a frequent side effect of nitroglycerin medications, so giving a mild analgesic would be indicated. The nurse would not change the dose or frequency without a physician's order.

NP:I; CN:PH; CA:M; CL:A

38. (2) Epidural hematomas classically present with a brief period of unconsciousness, followed by a lucid interval of varying duration, and finally followed by rapid deterioration of the level of consciousness, accompanied by complaints of a severe headache.

NP:P; CN:PH; CA:M; CL:C

39. (1) Infection due to catheter presence is most commonly associated with migration to the bladder along the internal lumen after contamination. The

collection bag should be below the abdomen (2). Frequent flushing will not necessarily prevent infection if contamination is present (3). If infection occurs antibiotics will be prescribed (4).

NP:I; CN:PH; CA:S; CL:A

40. (4) Laceration, a more severe consequence of closed head injury, occurs as the brain tissue moves across the uneven base of the skull in a contusion. Contusion causes cerebral dysfunction, which results in bruising of the brain. A concussion causes transient loss of consciousness and retrograde amnesia, and is generally reversible.

NP:D; CN:PH; CA:M; CL:K

41. (2) Patients must have the head of the bed elevated to prevent the contrast medium from irritating cervical nerve roots and cranial structures. Patients may sit up in a chair following the procedure if they are comfortable.

NP:I; CN:PH; CA:M; CL:A

42. (3) Patients may experience inaccurate readings if dye has been used for a diagnostic test. Dyes use colors that tint the blood, which causes inaccurate readings.

NP:I; CN:PH; CA:M; CL:A

43. (4) The major goal in protecting the seizure patient from injury is to always maintain an adequate airway. Placing the patients in a side-lying position assists in preventing aspiration. Current treatment of seizures no longer advocates the use of a padded tongue blade during a seizure (2) because of possible injury to teeth. Restraints (1) may also cause injury.

NP:P; CN:PH; CA:M; CL:C

44. (2) Lethargy may indicate impending encephalopathy and dictate the need for patient safety measures. Fatigue (3) is expected due to anemia, shortness of breath (1) due to ascites, and nausea (4) due to GI vascular congestion, but these are not as grave as lethargy.

NP:D; CN:PH; CA:M; CL:AN

45. (4) The pain of pancreatitis is made worse by walking and supine positioning. The patient is more comfortable sitting up and leaning forward.

NP:I; CN:PH; CA:M; CL:C

46. (1) Frequency and dysuria are the most specific symptoms of lower urinary tract infection while answers (2) and (3) are more indicative of upper urinary tract infection. Cloudy urine may indicate microscopic hematuria, while odor may be related to diet.

NP:D; CN:PH; CA:M; CL:C

47. (4) Infection due to catheter presence is most commonly associated with migration to the bladder along the internal lumen of the catheter after contamination. Keeping the collection bag dependent of the tubing is important to prevent reflux and contamination. The other distractors are potential, but not as common, causes of infection.

NP:E; CN:PH; CA:M; CL:C

48. (4) It is most important that the patient with lupus protects herself from sun exposure with large brimmed hats, long sleeves, and sunscreen cream. Keeping the skin moist and clean are also important, but lesions are best prevented by sun protection.

NP:E; CN:PH; CA:M; CL:C

49. (2) Dextrose with insulin helps move potassium into cells and is immediate management therapy for hyperkalemia due to acute renal failure. An exchange resin may also be employed. This type of infusion is often administered before cardiac surgery to stabilize irritable cells and prevent arrhythmias; in this case, KCl is also added to the infusion.

NP:P; CN:PH; CA:M; CL:C

50. (4) The only activity that will indicate a complication that is directly related to impairment in circulation due to a fractured femur is the inability to wiggle his toes.

NP:D; CN:PH; CA:S; CL:A

51. (2) Toradol can cause GI toxicity, ulceration, or hemorrhage, especially in patients with a history of ulcers or bleeding. Salicylate levels can be increased in the serum and bleeding times can be prolonged with use of the drug. The other conditions are not affected by the medication. An allergy to Tylenol is not related.

NP:D; CN:PH; CA:S; CL:A

52. (3) This is the procedure for using the swing-through gait. Patients are instructed to look straight ahead when walking with crutches. Looking down (1) can lead to falls and uneven gait. Putting pressure from the arm on the crutch bar can cause nerve damage.

NP:I; CN:PH; CA:S; CL:C

53. (2) The cast will be shiny and cool to the touch when dry. It will have a dull appearance (1) when wet.

NP:D; CN:PH; CA:S; CL:K

54. (3) Early in progressive (chronic) renal failure, the tubules lose ability to concentrate urine so there is increased urinary output with urine of low specific gravity and concomitant increase in fluid intake. This stage goes unnoticed by most patients.

NP:D; CN:PH; CA:M; CL:K

55. (4) Peritonitis is a grave complication with peritoneal dialysis. Hemodialysis may be necessary until infection clears. Excess fluid and protein effluent into the peritoneum also complicate care. Use of aseptic technique is essential.

NP:E; CN:PH; CA:M; CL:A

56. (1) It is essential that the end-stage renal patient adhere to all aspects of the medical regimen. Only excess solutes and fluid are removed with dialysis. Blood pressure management needs to be consistent, not just between treatments, aspects of care concerning concomitant anemia, and phosphate/calcium/vitamin D imbalance, as well as protein restriction and fluid restriction, must be carried out at all times. The dialysis patient continues to be uremic and has multisystem problems that continue despite dialysis.

NP:P; CN:PH; CA:M; CL:AN

57. (4) Apple juice or water is given as soon as the patient is awake and not hemorrhaging. Avoidance of citrus juices will prevent irritation of the operative site. The patient should be placed on his abdomen or side to facilitate drainage and prevent aspiration. Ice bags are applied to the neck to prevent edema and bleeding.

NP:I; CN:PH; CA:S; CL:A

58. (4) Pain occurs 2–4 hours after eating fatty foods and is located either in the epigastric region or in the upper right quadrant of the abdomen.

NP:D; CN:PH; CA:M; CL:C

59. (3) The patient's diet should be low residue and high calorie. Foods high in carbohydrates are usually low residue; chicken without skin is acceptable. Any salad, fresh vegetables, or grains would be considered high residue.

NP:P; CN:PH; CA:S; CL:C

60. (3) There is a high risk of infection in patients receiving CAPD because microorganisms can enter the body by migrating around, or through, the peritoneal dialysis catheter. They may also enter through contaminated dialysate solutions. The other diagnoses are not life threatening for a patient on CAPD.

NP:P; CN:PH; CA:M; CL:A

61. (3) Anorexia is a common and early manifestation of digoxin toxicity. The other complaints are not related to digoxin.

NP:E; CN:PH; CA:M; CL:A

62. (1) Prednisone, a corticosteroid, is the usual drug of choice. The other medication classifications are not used in the routine care of transplant patients.

NP:P; CN:PH; CA:S; CL:C

63. (3) Because more weight can be applied with skeletal traction, it can be used to reduce fractures and maintain alignment. It is not used commonly in the elderly because of prolonged immobilization. It is not preferred for children because some displacement of fracture fragments is desirable to prevent growth disturbance. Frequently, patients have more mobility than they do with skin traction, because balanced suspension is often incorporated with skeletal traction.

NP:P; CN:PH; CA:S; CL:K

64. (1) Russell's traction is a type of skin traction that incorporates a sling under the knee that is connected by a rope to an overhead bar pulley. It is frequently used to treat femoral shaft fractures in the adolescent.

NP:D; CN:PH; CA:S; CL:K

65. (2) The rope/pulley and weight system is arranged so that fracture fragments are in the desired approximate position for healing. The patient's position should always rest in line with the traction pull. The line of pull must never be interfered with by changing the position of a pulley and extension bar.

NP:D; CN:PH; CA:S; CL:C

66. (3) It is necessary to give the patient an adequate explanation for any procedure. This will result in less anxiety and more cooperation from the patient.

NP:I; CN:PH; CA:S; CL:C

67. (4) The ileal conduit procedure incorporates implantation of the ureters into a portion of the ileum that has been resected from its anatomical position and now functions as a reservoir or conduit for

urine. The proximal and distal ileal borders can be resumed. Feces should not be draining from the conduit. Edema (1) and a red color of the stoma are expected outcomes in the immediate postoperative period, as is mucus from the stoma (2).

NP:E; CN:PH; CA:S; CL:AN

68. (4) Hyperextension brings the pharynx into alignment with the trachea and allows the scope to be inserted without trauma.

NP:I; CN:PH; CA:M; CL:A

69. (2) Aspirin acts as an anti-inflammatory drug and thus reduces the inflammation of the joint. In doing so, it also relieves pain. Aspirin does not prevent extension of the disease (4). While aspirin reduces fever (1), this is not the major reason for its use in the treatment of rheumatoid arthritis.

NP:P; CN:PH; CA:M; CL:K

70. (2) Food and fluids would be consumed several hours before treatments. Because of possible problems with constipation, the foods need to be high in bulk and fiber. Small and frequent rather than large meals (4) are encouraged to counter nausea and anorexia.

NP:I; CN:PH; CA:M; CL:A

71. (2) Lactulose decreases blood ammonia levels in patients with hepatic coma. It is thought to decrease the colon pH through bacterial degradation.

NP:E; CN:PH; CA:M; CL:C

72. (2) Decadron decreases inflammation by stabilizing leukocyte lysosomal membranes. It also suppresses the immune response and is contraindicated in patients with infection, cirrhosis, and debilitating disease.

NP:P; CN:PH; CA:M; CL:AN

73. (4) Patients with multiple sclerosis do not usually have difficulty swallowing; therefore, techniques to promote safe swallowing would not be included on a care plan. The three other responses are important aspects in patient care and should be included in the care plan.

NP:P; CN:PH; CA:M; CL:C

74. (3) Hypothermia or fever may lead to an inaccurate reading. Artificial nails may distort a reading if a finger probe is used. Vasoconstriction can cause an inaccurate reading of oxygen saturation. Arterial saturations have a close correlation with the reading from the pulse oximeter as long as the arterial saturation is above 70 percent.

NP:D; CN:PH; CA:M; CL:A

75. (4) The primary purposes of patient education include increasing knowledge, increasing self-esteem, improving patient's ability to make decisions, and facilitating behavioral changes.

NP:P; CN:PH; CA:M; CL:K

76. (4) For patients with an MI, thrombolytic therapy minimizes the infarct size through lysis of the clot in the occluded coronary artery. The patent artery then promotes perfusion of the heart muscle. The other three responses are all contraindications for the use of thrombolytic agents.

NP:P; CN:PH; CA:M; CL:A

77. (2) Elevation of the limb and transport to the nearest hospital for antivenom is the best intervention. A restrictive band 2–4 inches above the snake bite has now been found not to be the intervention.

NP:I; CN:PH; CA:M; CL:A

78. (4) The word *patient* or *client* should not be used, as the chart belongs to the patient; thus, adding it to the chart is redundant.

NP:E; CN:PH; CA:M; CL:K

79. (4) Normal saline is the fluid of choice for irrigation. It is never advisable to force fluids into a tubing to check for patency (2). Sterile water (1) and aqueous Zephiran (3) will affect the pH of the bladder as well as cause irritation.

NP:I; CN:PH; CA:M; CL:A

80. (4) The P-R interval is measured on the ECG strip from the beginning of the P wave to the beginning of the QRS complex. It is the time it takes for the impulse to travel to the ventricle.

NP:D; CN:PH; CA:M; CL:C

81. (4) Pulmonary artery pressure is the most effective method of monitoring the cardiovascular system for this patient. Patients with a large percentage of burned body surface often do not have an area where a cuff can be applied. Cuff blood pressures (1) are also affected more by peripheral vascular changes. Pulse monitoring is not accurate enough to detect subtle changes in the system. Central venous pressures (3) are less than optimal because changes in left heart pressure (sign of pulmonary edema) are often not reflected in the right heart pressures.

NP:P; CN:PH; CA:M; CL:A

82. (2) Diarrhea is a very common response to the dye tablets. A dinner of tea and toast is usually given to the patient. Each dye tablet is given at 5-minute in-

tervals, usually with one glass of water following each tablet. The number of tablets prescribed will vary, because it is based on the weight of the patient.

NP:I; CN:PH; CA:M; CL:C

83. (3) The patient should be taught not to do any activities or wear anything that could interfere with the free flow of blood through the arteriovenous fistula.

NP:E; CN:PH; CA:M; CL:A

84. (2) Cyanosis is a result of impaired oxygen–carbon dioxide exchange at the alveolar level. Advent of the gallop (S3, S4) rhythm indicates that the patient is in HF. Cerebral/mental changes (4) often occur but they are due to hypoxia rather than edema. Changes in the lungs (1, 3) occur because of increased fluid that expands in the interstitial spaces and decreased oxygen transport, not because of airway changes.

NP:D; CN:PH; CA:M; CL:A

85. (1) Before moving the patient, dangling at the bedside is important. This procedure stabilizes the patient and allows the nurse time to assess whether he develops vertigo from a drop in blood pressure.

NP:I; CN:PH; CA:M; CL:C

86. (3) An NG tube insertion is the most appropriate intervention because it will determine the presence of active gastrointestinal bleeding. A Miller–Abbott tube (1) is a weighted, mercury-filled ballooned tube used to resolve bowel obstructions. There is no evidence of shock or fluid overload in the patient; therefore, an arterial line (2) is not appropriate at this time, and an IV (4) is optional.

NP:I; CN:PH; CA:M; CL:A

87. (4) The patient must have the correct carbohydrates, fats, and proteins determined by the specific diet plan so a new tray should come from the kitchen. Substituting food may not provide the correct balance.

NP:I; CN:PH; CA:M; CL:A

88. (3) Mechanical ventilation may cause stress ulcers, so checking the pH to maintain it above 5 will yield information about whether or not the patient requires antacids. Below 5, the pH would be too acidic and this condition could cause a stress ulcer.

NP:P; CN:PH; CA:M; CL:AN

89. (2) Two to three stools/day indicates that the lactulose is working to acidify the colon contents and reduce blood ammonia. If watery diarrhea occurs (1), there is a drug overdose.

NP:E; CN:PH; CA:M; CL:AN

90. (2) Normal capillary refill time is 3 seconds or less. Prolonged refill time is indicative of circulatory impairment.

NP:D; CN:PH; CA:S; CL:C

91. The second bag should be hung at 6 PM/1800 hours. Each bag will cover 8 hours of a 24-hour order.

NP:P; CN:PH; CA:M; CL:A

92. (1) Denial is the first stage in the grief process. The patient does not yet fully comprehend the loss that has occurred. He is protecting himself from painful feelings.

NP:E; CN:PS; CA:S; CL:A

93. (1) Vitamin B_{12} comes from animal products. Patients with pernicious anemia have a B_{12} deficiency. Patients either need frequent B_{12} injections or they must drastically increase the foods that provide B_{12} in sufficient quantity.

NP:E; CN:H; CA:M; CL:A

94. (1) Because the patient cannot feel sensory stimuli, a blockage of the nerves between the central nervous system and the peripheral system is suspected.

NP:D; CN:PH; CA:S; CL:C

95. (2) Raw apples are high in potassium, while white enriched and French bread (4), dry cereal (3), and pasta (1) are foods low in potassium.

NP:E; CN:PH; CA:M; CL:C

96. (3) Urecholine stimulates the parasympathetic nervous system. It increases the tone and motility of the smooth muscles of the urinary tract. It is used frequently following a TUR when the patient has a lack of muscle tone and is unable to void. Bladder spasms can be relieved with belladonna or opium suppositories.

NP:E; CN:PH; CA:S; CL:AN

97. The answer is 1.0 mL. Dose on hand is in 10 mL, so to calculate the amount to give, divide the dose desired by the dose on hand and multiply by 10 mL. Example: 0.5 g ÷ 5 g = 0.1, then × 10 = 1 mL.

NP:P; CN:PH; CA:M; CL:C

98. (2) The patient requires treatment for shock. Vital signs are monitored (1) after placing the patient in the shock position; then the physician is called for orders (3).

NP:I; CN:PH; CA:M; CL:A

99. (3) This computation can be done using the formula of D (dose desired) ÷ H (dose on hand) × V (volume). Therefore, $65 \div 80 \times 2 = 1.625$ mL.

NP:I; CN:PH; CA:M; CL:C

100. (3) Gentamicin, a potent aminoglycoside antibiotic, has the potential for causing nephrotoxicity. Renal function studies such as the serum creatinine and BUN should be monitored regularly to detect impaired renal function.

NP:E; CN:PH; CA:M; CL:AN

101. (4) Protecting the airway from aspiration is a high priority when caring for a patient receiving nasogastric tube feedings. Keeping the patient in an upright position helps prevent aspiration of gastric contents. The other actions are correct but are less critical.

NP:P; CN:PH; CA:M; CL:A

102. (3) Elevating the legs about 30 degrees promotes venous return and reduces leg edema. Elevation beyond 45 degrees reduces arterial flow and causes sharp flexion at the hip, thereby reducing venous return. Leaving the legs flat on the bed or dependent promotes edema formation and venous stasis. Patients with arterial, rather than venous, insufficiency benefit from a dependent position.

NP:P; CN:PH; CA:M; CL:A

103. (4) This response encourages the expression of feelings, which may help reduce the patient's anxiety. Answer (1) does not focus on the patient's feelings and is not a useful initial response. Answer (2) is a closed question, which discourages expression of feelings. Answer (3) is inappropriate because it negates the patient's feelings, is a stereotypical response, and expresses the nurse's opinion, which is irrelevant to the situation.

NP:I; CN:PS; CA:S; CL:A

104. (1) Hypothyroidism reduces the metabolic rate and prolongs the sedative effects of medications. Narcotics are especially dangerous and should be given in smaller doses. The patient must be closely monitored for signs of oversedation and respiratory depression.

NP:E; CN:PH; CA:M; CL:A

105. (4) Filgrastim stimulates the production of WBCs. It is given to patients experiencing bone marrow depression with leukopenia secondary to cancer chemotherapy.

NP:E; CN:PH; CA:M; CL:A

106. (2) Chronic hypoxia associated with COPD may stimulate excessive RBC production (polycythemia). This results in increased blood viscosity and the risk of thrombosis. The other nursing diagnoses are not applicable in this situation.

NP:P; CN:PH; CA:M; CL:C

107. (1) A colostomy appliance should be cut to fit the stoma so that there is no pressure placed on the stoma by the appliance and there is a minimum amount of skin exposed to fecal drainage. Leaving ⅛ inch of skin exposed conforms to these criteria.

NP:I; CN:PH; CA:S; CL:K

108. (3) The liver becomes engorged with blood in right-sided heart failure. Liver function studies, such as the LDH, an enzyme production test for the liver, will be abnormally elevated in 40 percent of the patients. Serum bilirubin is also frequently increased. Ammonia (1) and albumin (2), also liver tests, will not be elevated.

NP:E; CN:PH; CA:M; CL:C

109. The steps are 3, 1, 5, 4. The bell is used rather than the diaphragm to hear the Korotkoff sounds. The American Heart Association recommends that noting Korotkoff's sounds are the best index of blood pressure.

NP:I; CN:PH; CA:M; CL:A

110. (3) Oxygen would be ordered; however, the patient should be in an orthopneic or high-Fowler's position to facilitate respiratory effort. Diuretics are administered to decrease circulatory overload.

NP:E; CN:PH; CA:M; CL:AN

111. (2) The patient's instructions should include keeping the environment warm to prevent vasoconstriction. Wearing gloves, warm clothes, and socks will also be useful in preventing vasoconstriction, but TED hose (3) would not be therapeutic. Walking will most likely increase pain.

NP:E; CN:H; CA:M; CL:C

112. (4) The presence of bile in the urine would lead to a yellow-orange or brown colored urine.

NP:D; CN:PH; CA:M; CL:K

113. (4) In addition to the germicidal soap scrubs, systemic antibiotics are administered to prevent infection of the wound. Silver nitrate is not a common treatment today.

NP:P; CN:PH; CA:M; CL:C

114. (2)   Answer (2) is correct because the culture takes 3 weeks to grow. Usually, even very small lesions can be seen on x-rays due to the natural contrast of the air in the lungs; therefore, chest x-rays do not need to be repeated frequently (3). Patients may have positive smears but negative cultures if they have been on medication (4). A positive skin test indicates the person has been infected with tuberculosis but may not necessarily have active disease (1).

NP:I; CN:PH; CA:M; CL:C

115. (1)   The increase in intraocular pressure causes atrophy of the retinal ganglion cells and the optic nerve, and leads eventually to blindness.

NP:I; CN:H; CA:M; CL:K

116. (3)   As the liver cells become fatty and degenerate, they are no longer able to accommodate the large amount of blood necessary for homeostasis. The pressure in the liver increases and causes increased pressure in the venous system. As the portal pressure increases, fluid exudes into the abdominal cavity. This is called *ascites*.

NP:D; CN:PH; CA:M; CL:C

117. (1)   Weakness, fainting, blurred vision, pallor, and perspiration are all common symptoms when there is too much insulin or too little food—hypoglycemia. The signs and symptoms in answers (2) and (3) are indicative of hyperglycemia.

NP:D; CN:PH; CA:M; CL:C

118. (3)   A nursing goal is to promote physical rest and reduce stress. Discussing stressful situations may cause the patient to become anxious and delay ulcer healing. Discussing the pathogenesis of ulcer disease (1, 2) will not help the patient to relax. Identification of substances that cause pain (4) will assist in planning for teaching. Dietary teaching should include incorporating the patient's food preferences into such a regimen.

NP:E; CN:H; CA:M; CL:A

119. (1)   The first specimen is discarded because it is considered "old urine" or urine that was in the bladder before the test began. After the first discarded specimen, urine is collected for 24 hours.

NP:I; CN:PH; CA:M; CL:C

120. (1)   It is important to decrease intracranial pressure (head of bed elevated) and to allow for drainage (head turned to left). All of the other responses are incorrect because the position would not facilitate cerebral drainage or ear drainage.

NP:I; CN:PH; CA:M; CL:A

121. (3)   An important assessment question is to find out how the patient feels about the tests to be performed. Learning if he has talked with anyone about his concerns or fears will help the nurse assess the patient's resources for emotional support and whether the patient needs to talk about his fears or feelings.

NP:I; CN:PS; CA:M; CL:C

122. (2)   If the shunt is patent, it will feel warm to the touch and the nurse will hear the sound of rushing blood and a loud bruit. The nurse can also feel the thrill by palpating over the fistula site.

NP:D; CN:PH; CA:S; CL:C

123. (4)   These symptoms may indicate the presence of thrombophlebitis; therefore, promoting venous return is the priority nursing goal. The other goals are not relevant to this assessment finding.

NP:P; CN:PH; CA:M; CL:A

124. (4)   Closed chest drainage is used for lobectomies to reestablish negative pressure in the chest. Because the breathing mechanism operates on the principle of negative pressure, this is an essential action. The other interventions would follow this one.

NP:I; CN:PH; CA:S; CL:AN

125. (1)   When the prosthesis is in place immediately following surgery, the patient can stand up several hours postoperatively and walk the next day. The operative site is closed to outside contamination and benefits from improved circulation due to ambulation.

NP:P; CN:PH; CA:S; CL:C

126. (3)   Successful teaching can be validated when the patient is able to repeat the information. A description of the surgery is irrelevant and application of the bag will be done later. Acceptance of the surgery (2) is an emotional issue.

NP:E; CN:PH; CA:M; CL:C

127. (2)   Allowing the patient to void naturally will be done prior to removal of the catheter to ensure adequate emptying of the bladder. Irrigations (3) are not recommended, as they increase the chances of the patient's developing a urinary tract infection. Any time a patient has an indwelling catheter in place, fluids should be encouraged (unless contraindicated) to prevent stone formation.

NP:P; CN:PH; CA:M; CL:C

128. (1)   Such a response does not give false hope to the patient but is positive and realistic. This answer

tells the patient what cardiac rehabilitation is and does not dwell on his negativity about it.

NP:I; CN:PH; CA:M; CL:A

129. (1) Pupillary checks reflect function of the third cranial nerve, which stretches as it becomes displaced by blood, tumor, etc.

NP:D; CN:PH; CA:M; CL:A

130. (2) The function of the lens is that of accommodation, the focusing of near objects on the retina by the lens; therefore, only the remaining lens will function in this capacity, depending on whether a cataract is present.

NP:P; CN:PH; CA:S; CL:C

131. (3) Most of the laryngectomy patients will use esophageal speech or a mechanical device for communication. They can usually begin to take oral fluids sometime after 48 hours. They are generally fed by an intravenous or nasogastric tube prior to oral feedings. Because the larynx is removed, it will be impossible to breathe through the nose.

NP:P; CN:PH; CA:S; CL:C

132. (3) While all the other conditions may be complications, bleeding from the site is the main concern. The procedure is done to achieve relief from infection caused by urinary stasis, which may have resulted in kidney congestion.

NP:D; CN:PH; CA:S; CL:A

133. (1) Putting pressure over the vessels in the neck may be lifesaving because a severe blood loss can occur rapidly, leading to shock and death. The surgeon would be notified as soon as possible.

NP:I; CN:PH; CA:S; CL:AN

134. (1) Even before pneumonia (2), atelectasis may occur as a result of the alveoli's not being expanded. This leads to an alteration in gas exchange. Paralytic ileus (3) could result from any surgery, especially if the patient ingests food before the bowel is functioning properly.

NP:E; CN:PH; CA:S; CL:A

135. (4) The most effective communication technique in this case would be silence; support the patient nonverbally, accept her, and open up the opportunity for an expression of feelings.

NP:I; CN:PS; CA:PS; CL:C

136. (3) In atrial fibrillation, multiple ectopic foci stimulate the atria to contract. The AV node is unable to transmit all of these impulses to the ventricles, resulting in a pattern of highly irregular ventricular contractions.

NP:D; CN:PH; CA:M; CL:C

137. (1) Maintaining the prescribed immobilization and body alignment will keep the fracture fragments in close anatomical proximity, thereby promoting functional fracture healing. This goal should receive the highest priority. The other goals, although applicable in the care of a patient with a fracture, do not have as high a priority in meeting this particular desired outcome.

NP:P; CN:PH; CA:S; CL:A

138. (4) Calcium produces a sedative effect on nerve cells and is essential for the transmission of nerve impulses. A deficit of calcium produces abnormal muscle contractions and is manifested by carpopedal spasms. Acute muscular spasms (tetany) may be potentially fatal. Chvostek's sign (1) would be positive if hypocalcemia is present. Edema (3) or hyperventilation (2) would not be noted with this diagnosis.

NP:D; CN:PH; CA:M; CL:A

139. (4) The Denver shunt is a type of peritoneovascular shunt used in the treatment of patients who have cirrhosis with ascites. The shunt diverts ascitic fluid from the abdomen into the jugular vein or the vena cava.

NP:D; CN:PH; CA:M; CL:C

140. (3) Hyperglycemia is a common finding in acute pancreatitis because the islet cells may not be able to produce adequate amounts of insulin. An important component of the treatment is to administer regular insulin to treat the hyperglycemia.

NP:P; CN:PH; CA:M; CL:AN

141. (2) Glucocorticoids, such as prednisone, promote protein catabolism and are a known risk factor for the development of osteoporosis. Swimming (3) would be an exercise to reduce risk of osteoporosis.

NP:D; CN:PH; CA:M; CL:A

142. (3) Although all of the interventions are appropriate in the care of a patient with a casted limb, it is most critical to maintain limb elevation. This nursing action prevents edema, which could compress blood vessels and nerves.

NP:I; CN:PH; CA:S; CL:A

143. (4) The hand grips should be placed so that the elbows are flexed at 20–30 degrees when standing

with the crutches. This placement should not be changed as long as the patient continues to need crutches. The other statements indicate effective learning.

NP:E; CN:H; CA:S; CL:C

144. (3) Transportation by wheelchair can prevent falls and injury; therefore, safety is the important issue.

NP:I; CN:PH; CA:M; CL:K

145. (3) Before rolling the patient on his side, the nurse's hands must be in the correct position to turn. Answer (4) would be the final intervention.

NP:I; CN:PH; CA:M; CL:C

146. (3) The first action is to move the patient to his left side and lower the head of the bed. In this position, air will rise to the right atrium. The charge nurse should then be notified.

NP:I; CN:PH; CA:M; CL:A

147. (2) Licensed vocational/practical nurses can only assist in the admission of patients. They can orient the patient to the environment, take vital signs, and weigh patients. They do not make *initial* assessments or develop initial care plans. They can update patient assessments and do standard care plans.

NP:I; CN:S; CA:M; CL:A

148. (2) Studies have shown that insulin is most rapidly and consistently absorbed from the subcutaneous tissue of the abdomen. The current thinking, therefore, is that insulin injections should be rotated among sites on the abdomen alone (with the exception of 1 inch around the umbilicus), rather than among the other available anatomic sites, i.e., arms (1), thighs (3), and buttocks (4).

NP:P; CN:H; CA:M; CL:C

149. (3) The endotracheal tube must be kept in place because it is the conduit between the ventilator and the patient's lungs. Also, accidental extubation can produce laryngospasm. Suctioning is done only as needed, rather than on a fixed schedule (1). An intubated patient cannot speak (2) or swallow (4) safely.

NP:P; CN:PH; CA:M; CL:A

150. (1) The head must be kept elevated because this drug could provoke a seizure if it reaches the brain in a bolus form. After myelography that uses an oil-based contrast medium (Pantopaque), patients are kept flat. Forcing fluids helps prevent postmyelogram headache by replacing lost spinal fluid. Itching suggests an allergic reaction, while a stiff neck suggests meningeal irritation; neither is an expected response to a myelogram.

NP:E; CN:PH; CA:M; CL:C

Emergency Nursing

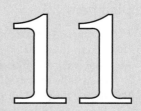

EMERGENCY AND FIRST AID NURSING*

Disasters

Definition: A catastrophe, which may be either natural or man-made in origin.

A.   General guidelines: keep calm, take time to think, then take appropriate action.

✦ B.   Every hospital on every floor now has a Disaster Plan posted with specific instructions for staff actions.

C.   First steps to take in a disaster—gather the following items:
1.   Water.
2.   Canned or sealed packaged foods that do not require refrigeration or cooking.
3.   Medicines needed by family members.
4.   First aid kit.
5.   Blankets or sleeping bags.
6.   Flashlights.
7.   Battery-powered radio.
8.   Covered containers for toilet and/or garbage.

D.   Precautions after a disaster.
1.   Use caution in entering a building or working indoors.
2.   Check for gas leaks.
3.   Stay away from fallen or damaged electrical wires.

Water, Food, and Sanitation Principles

✦ A.   Care and use of water.
1.   Allocate 1 quart of water per day per person.
2.   Strain rusty water through a paper towel or several thicknesses of clean cloth.
3.   Methods of purifying water.
a.   Boil 3–5 minutes.
b.   Add four purifying tablets per gallon of water.
c.   Add 8 drops chlorine to 1 gallon of water and let stand for 30 minutes.
d.   Add 10 drops bleach to 1 gallon of water and let stand for 30 minutes.
e.   Use 12 drops tincture of iodine per 1 gallon of water.

B.   Care and use of food.
1.   One-half normal intake is adequate except for growing children and pregnant women.
2.   Store in covered containers.

C.   Sanitation.
1.   Emergency toilet facility can be made by using a watertight container with snug-fitting cover.
2.   After each use, pour or sprinkle household disinfectant to decrease odor and germs.

*See Disaster Nursing Chapter.

D.   Garbage—dispose of garbage by wrapping in newspaper and placing in airtight container.
E.   Insect control.
1.   Maintain cleanliness.
2.   Spray with insect repellent if available.

First Aid Care

Definition: Immediate care given to a person who has been injured or suddenly taken ill, when medical assistance is not available.

✦ A.   First aid training can mean the difference between life and death, temporary and permanent disability, and rapid recovery and long hospitalization.

B.   General directions for giving first aid.
1.   Decisions and actions vary according to:
a.   Circumstances.
b.   Number of persons involved.
c.   Immediate environment.
d.   Availability of medical assistance.
e.   Availability of equipment and supplies.
2.   Improvise—make do with what is available.

✦ 3.   Set priorities.
a.   Sorting of casualties.
(1)   Sorting is done by most responsible person.
(2)   Rapid initial evaluation of the victims' general condition to determine most seriously injured person.
b.   Priorities of treatment.
(1)   First priority is victim needing immediate attention in order to survive.
(2)   Second priority is victim needing immediate surgery.
(3)   Third priority is victim who requires surgery but can tolerate a delay.

✦ 4.   Cardinal rules.
a.   Establish airway.
b.   Stop bleeding.
c.   Treat for shock.
d.   Preserve function of injured area.
e.   Give comfort.
f.   Preserve cosmetic appearance.

5.   When calling for assistance, give following information.
a.   Identify problem.
b.   Relate what is currently being done.
c.   Give your name and name of victim.
d.   Give location of accident.
e.   Relate number of persons involved.
f.   Give phone number you are calling from.

6.   Once first aid is begun, remain with victim until qualified persons arrive or victim is able to care for self.

7.   Do not make a diagnosis.

◆ C.   Dressings—applied over wounds.
   1.   Function.
      a.   Assist in controlling bleeding.
      b.   Absorb blood and wound secretions.
      c.   Prevent additional contamination.
      d.   Ease pain.
   2.   Sterilizing dressings.
      a.   Place in moderate oven (350°) for 3 hours.
      b.   Press clean cloth with iron.
◆ D.   Bandage—used to hold dressing or splint in place.
   1.   Material used.
      a.   Usually gauze, cloth, or elastic.
      b.   Emergency—handkerchief, belt, tie.
   2.   General principles for applying bandages.
      a.   Snug but not so tight as to interfere with circulation.
      b.   Leave fingertips and toes exposed when splint or bandage applied.
      c.   Check for swelling, color changes, and coldness in extremities.

SHOCK STATES

Definition: An abnormal physiological state in which there is insufficient circulating blood volume for the size of the vascular bed, thereby resulting in circulatory failure and tissue anoxia.

Classifications of Shock States

A.   Low blood flow states.
   1.   Hypovolemic shock.
      a.   Absolute hypovolemia—lowered intravascular volume.
         (1)   Blood loss—from trauma, surgery, etc., is most common cause.
         (2)   Plasma loss from burns; fluid loss from diarrhea, vomiting, etc.
      b.   Relative hypovolemia—shift of fluid volume out of vascular space into extravascular space.
         (1)   Etiology: pooling of fluids.
         (2)   Internal bleeding or massive vasodilation.
   2.   Cardiogenic shock.
      a.   Myocardial dysfunction that results in compromised cardiac output.
      b.   Causes.
         (1)   Systolic dysfunction: inability to pump blood forward.
         (2)   Diastolic dysfunction: ventricles unable to adequately fill (cardiac tamponade).
         (3)   Arrhythmias.
         (4)   Structural abnormalities (valvular stenosis or regurgitation).

B.   Maldistribution of blood flow.
   1.   Distributive shock is caused by massive vasodilation and pooling of blood.
   2.   Types of distributive shock include septic, neurogenic, and anaphylactic shock.
   3.   Results in decreased cardiac output.

General Shock Assessment

Early Shock

A.   Assess early stages, regardless of cause.
   1.   Decreased tissue perfusion.
   2.   Cellular hypoxia.
   3.   Increased sympathetic nervous system activity.
◆ B.   Oliguria—usually the first sign of shock.
   1.   Kidneys receive 25 percent of cardiac output, so if urine volume drops acutely, assume cardiac output has dropped.
   2.   If volume falls below 30 mL/hr, notify physician immediately.
◆ C.   Hypotension.
   1.   Due to compensatory peripheral vasoconstriction (not evident initially, but it does appear in late shock).
   2.   Narrowing pulse pressure—due to systolic pressure falling and diastolic pressure being maintained (early symptom of hypovolemic shock).
   3.   Traditional criteria—systolic blood pressure below 70 mm Hg.
◆ D.   Tachycardia—caused by heart's responding to increased sympathetic activity.
◆ E.   Tachypnea—use pulse oximeter for accurate assessment.
   1.   Medulla is stimulated by buildup of lactic acid through anaerobic metabolism.
   2.   As blood pH is lowered, the respiratory rate increases in an effort to blow off excess carbon dioxide and return body to acid–base balance.
F.   Cool, dry, or moist skin.
   1.   Caused by peripheral vasoconstriction.
   2.   Blood is supplied to vital organs rather than to skin.
G.   Sensorium changes—due to brain cell hypoxia.
   1.   Restlessness.
   2.   Apprehension and anxiety.
   3.   Lethargy.
   4.   Confusion.
   5.   Semiconsciousness to coma.
H.   Excess thirst is present caused by loss of fluids or blood volume, as well as peripheral vasoconstriction, which decreases salivary secretions.
I.   Fatigue and muscle weakness—result of shift from aerobic to anaerobic metabolism leading to lactic acid buildup.

Severe Shock

✦ A. Blood pressure—below 70 mm Hg and narrowing of pulse pressure (body loses ability to compensate and blood pressure drops rapidly).

B. Shallow, irregular respirations.

C. Tachycardia.

D. Level of unconsciousness; progresses to coma as blood supply to brain cells decreases.

E. Dilated, fixed pupils due to decreased oxygen to brain.

F. Anuria as blood supply to kidneys decreases sharply.

G. Cyanotic skin, mucous membranes, and nailbeds—indicates poor prognosis.

INDIVIDUAL SHOCK STATES

Hypovolemic Shock

✦ **Characteristics**

A. Initial—15% volume loss: no signs/symptoms; body begins to respond to imbalance of O_2 supply and demand.

B. Compensatory or 2nd stage—volume loss increases from 15% to 30%: body activates mechanisms to maintain homeostasis. Clinical symptoms manifest.

C. Progressive or 3rd stage—30% to 40% blood loss: as the compensatory mechanisms fail, requires immediate interventions. Decreased perfusion and altered cellular permeability.

D. Refractory—more than 40% volume loss: profound hypotension and hypoxemia; life-threatening.

Treatment and Implementation

✦ A. Prepare fluids to treat shock state.

1. First-line treatment is crystalloids: hypertonic, hypotonic, or isotonic fluids.

2. Prepare patient for IV fluid, colloids-plasma expanders, blood replacement, and drugs (vasodilator).

B. Start IV fluid with D_5W. When adequate kidney function is assessed, physician may change to Ringer's lactate (this is more isotonic).

✦ C. Place patient in supine position with legs elevated, head on pillow.

1. Trendelenburg's position compromises ventilation and baroreceptor mechanisms.

2. If respirations are compromised, raise bed 30–45 degrees.

D. Provide oxygen via nasal catheter, mask, or cannula—concentration moderate; monitor SaO_2 with pulse oximeter.

✦ E. Record vital signs every 15 minutes. Changes may take place slowly except in massive hemorrhage changes can progress rapidly.

✦ 1. Blood pressure.

a. Decreased BP is usually late sign of shock.

b. Orthostatic hypotension develops before systemic hypotension.

c. Systolic BP below 80 mm Hg indicates inadequate coronary artery blood flow.

d. Progressive drop in BP with a thready, increasing pulse indicates fluid loss.

e. Decreased BP with strong, irregular pulse indicates heart failure.

✦ 2. Respirations.

a. Become rapid and shallow early in shock (compensation for tissue anoxia).

b. Slow breathing (below 4/min) appears late in shock after compensatory failure.

c. Emergency respiratory equipment (ventilator, trach tubes, etc.) should be available.

✦ 3. Temperature.

a. Below normal with hemorrhagic shock.

b. Gradually increasing temperature indicates sepsis.

✦ 4. Central venous pressure.

a. CVP line should be inserted in subclavian vein.

b. If below 5 cm H_2O indicates shock condition.

c. If CVP decreases early, it is usually a sign of shock.

F. Insert Foley catheter for hourly urine volumes.

1. Record intake and output.

✦ 2. Notify physician if total urine output is below 30 mL/hr.

G. Monitor skin changes.

1. Change in skin temperature and color reflect changes in tissue oxygenation and perfusion.

a. Cold, clammy skin indicates peripheral vascular constriction.

b. Flushing and sweating reflects overheating, which indicates increased metabolic rate and the need for oxygen.

✦ c. Pallor and cyanosis indicate tissue hypoxia.

2. Observe for restlessness—indicates hypoxia.

H. Place enough light covering over patient to prevent chilling, but not enough to cause vasodilation.

I. Treat the cause of the shock (stop bleeding, prepare for surgery, etc.).

Cardiogenic Shock

Characteristics

✦ A. Causes.

1. Massive myocardial infarction with 40–60 percent muscle damage.

2. Inadequate blood supply, compensatory mechanism, or changes in microcirculation leads to clinical manifestations.

B. Pathophysiology.
  1. Decreased contractility.
  2. Decreased arterial blood pressure, causing sympathetic nervous system stimulation, which produces vasoconstriction and opens AV shunts.
  3. Oxygen transport impairment causes increased anaerobic metabolism.
     a. Result is increased lactate.
     b. Increased lactate causes metabolic acidosis.
  4. Decreased cerebral perfusion.
  5. Decreased renal perfusion, resulting in renal failure.
  6. Myocardial ischemia leads to further pump failure.

✦ **Assessment**
  A. Cold and clammy skin—vasoconstriction.
  B. Tachycardia—(weak and feeble) sympathetic stimulation; arrhythmias leading to cardiac arrest.
  C. Blood pressure, if less than 80 mm Hg systolic.
  D. Restlessness—cerebral anoxia due to decreased cardiac output.
  E. Increased left ventricular pressure.
  F. Measure urinary output. May be < 30 mL/hr due to poor renal perfusion.
✦ G. Assess for heart failure symptoms.
  1. Pallor or cyanosis.
  2. Hypoxia.
  3. Orthopnea.
  4. Dyspnea.
  5. Pitting edema.
  6. Distended neck veins.
  7. Pulmonary congestion.
  H. Acidemia—decreased pH of the blood.
  I. Differentiate from hypovolemic shock.
  1. Pulmonary capillary wedge pressure and CVP are increased in cardiogenic shock.
  2. Pulmonary capillary wedge pressure and CVP are normal or low in hypovolemic shock.

Treatment and Implementation
✦ A. Monitor drugs for improvement of left ventricular function.
  1. Inotropic drugs: dobutamine, dopamine (precursor of norepinephrine)—causes vasoconstriction peripherally but increases renal perfusion, BP, and raises cardiac index.
  2. Norepinephrine (epinephrine) if dopamine is ineffective (monitor for tachycardia, arrhythmias).
✦ B. Monitor use of Nipride or Amrinone.
  1. Drug lowers peripheral vascular resistance—dilates arteries and veins.
  2. Decreases cardiac workload and increases cardiac output.
✦ C. Maintain arterial blood pressure—vasopressors.

  1. Intra-arterial blood pressure monitoring necessary to obtain accurate reading.
  2. Cuff pressures may be low (false reading) due to vasoconstriction and poor Korotkoff sounds.
  3. Evaluate distal pulses.
✦ D. Assist RN in monitoring Swan–Ganz catheter to assess heart failure.
  1. Balance and calibrate transducer.
  2. Connect catheter to a transducer and pressure monitor.
  3. Obtain measurements.
    ✦ a. Catheter positioned in pulmonary artery through percutaneous puncture.
       (1) PAP measures: systolic (15–25 mm Hg), diastolic (3–12 mm Hg), and mean pressure (10–20 mm Hg—mean of 15 mm Hg).
       (2) High PA pressures indicate (L) ventricular failure.
    ✦ b. Pulmonary capillary wedge pressure (PCWP) is measured by inflating the distal balloon. PCWP pressures range from 14–18 mm Hg. High PCWP pressures indicate (L) ventricular failure.
       c. Cardiac output is measured by attaching the catheter to the computer monitor and injecting a bolus of IV fluid with a controlled temperature into the bloodstream.
  ✦ 4. Implement nursing interventions for Swan–Ganz catheter.
    a. Apply sterile dressing over site.
    b. Monitor patient's vital signs and status.
    c. Evaluate distal pulses in cannulated extremity (usually radial pulse).
    d. Monitor PA pressures continuously and record with vital signs. (Transducer should be at the level of the right atrium.)
    e. Obtain PCWP pressures as ordered.
    f. Monitor for complications.
       (1) Arrhythmias (especially PACs, PVCs).
       (2) Pulmonary infarction caused by wedging.
       (3) Pulmonary emboli.
       (4) Infection.
       (5) Pneumothorax.
       (6) Abnormal wave forms.
✦ E. Maintain ventilation and oxygenation.
  1. Patent airway.
  2. Oxygen administration.
  3. Artificial ventilation, if necessary.
  4. Arterial blood gases, to determine effect of therapy.
  F. Establish fluid and electrolyte acid–base balance.
  1. Replace fluid if hypovolemic.

2. Correct acidosis—for example, $NaHCO_3$.

3. Maintain urinary output— > 30 mL/hr.

G. Control pain and restlessness—IV analgesia most effective.

H. Treat arrhythmias—result of tissue hypoxia, acidosis, electrolyte imbalance, underlying disease, and drug therapy.

I. Decrease cardiac workload.

1. Physical and emotional rest.

2. Psychological support.

3. Comfortable position—flat with pillow, or semi-Fowler's position if patient has difficulty breathing.

Septic Shock

Assessment

◆ A. Stage 1: sepsis (*warm shock*)—may appear to be mild infection.

1. Mental confusion may be first sign.

2. Flushed, pink face warm to the touch; dry skin.

3. Normal blood pressure; pulse and respirations slightly increased.

4. Temperature—may be normal or slightly elevated (hyperfusion increases heat loss, which may prevent high temperature).

5. May not appear to be shock.

6. Check results of complete blood count—blood culture to determine organism.

◆ B. Stage 2 (*cool shock*).

1. Low cardiac output with vasoconstriction: tachycardia; blood pressure drops; PO_2 is dropping.

2. Does not appear pink and warm—cool and pale skin.

3. Hyperventilation; tachypnea.

4. Urine output—may drop to 30 mL/hr.

5. Thirst.

◆ Treatment and Implementation

A. Administer broad spectrum antibiotics as ordered—begin STAT (do not wait for regular medication times).

1. Continue to check IV site frequently—if evidence of infection, get a new site.

2. Check BUN level regularly.

◆ B. Take vital signs hourly. Stages can progress rapidly.

C. Observe continually for change in pattern: blood pressure down, pulse and respirations up. Notify charge nurse immediately.

◆ D. Check PO_2 and pH—patient may go into metabolic acidosis. Notify charge nurse if pH falls below 7.35.

E. Administer oxygen as ordered—concentration should be moderate; pulse oximeter reading useful for SaO_2.

F. Give frequent skin care to prevent breakdown.

◆ G. Check I&O frequently; pay attention to amount of urine from catheter.

1. If urine output falls below 33 mL/hr, notify charge nurse immediately.

2. Prevent fluid overload by calculating previous hourly urine output plus 30 mL/hr.

H. Administer aspirin or cooling blanket if necessary to control fever.

I. Monitor drugs that may be ordered.

1. Inotropic drugs (dopamine)—if tissue perfusion is inadequate.

2. Norepinephrine (Levophed)—potent vasoconstrictor if dopamine does not raise mean arterial blood pressure.

3. Naloxone (Narcan)—may be ordered to treat gram-negative septic shock—attacks bacterial endotoxin, which causes cellular destruction.

J. Provide appropriate psychological support.

1. Patient is frightened, so remain in the room.

2. Explain all procedures and attempt to alleviate anxiety.

K. Observe for complications or reversal in improvement of shock state.

1. Respiratory: dyspnea, cyanosis, intercostal retractions (shock lung).

2. Cardiac: heart failure—may require digitalis.

3. Renal: oliguria—may require mannitol.

Neurogenic (Spinal) Shock

Definition: Massive vasodilation and pooling of blood due to failure of peripheral vessels (imbalance of parasympathetic/sympathetic vascular tone) (also see Spinal Cord Injury).

Characteristics

A. Interference with sympathetic nervous system (head injury).

B. Injury to the spinal cord or as a result of spinal anesthesia.

C. Severe pain, drugs, or hypoglycemia causing vasomotor center depression.

Assessment

A. Assess for hypoglycemia, bradycardia or hypothermia.

B. Assess vital signs; hypotension.

C. Loss of reflex activity in spinal cord below injury level (areflexia).

D. Paralytic ileus.

Implementation

A. Monitor airway, breathing, circulation (ABC) measures (hypotension, bradycardia).

B. Fluid resuscitation to increase blood pressure.

C. Monitor vasoconstrictors to increase blood pressure.

D. Monitor atropine-like drugs to block vagal effects causing bradycardia.

E. If hypothermia present, requires warming measures.

Anaphylactic Shock

Characteristics

✦ A. Caused by hypersensitivity to allergen (allergic reaction to medication, bee sting, etc.).

B. Antigen–antibody reaction.

C. Increased cell membrane permeability—histamine is released, causing marked vasodilatation.

D. Bronchiolar constriction and hypoxia.

E. Pooling of blood, causing decreased venous return.

F. Decreased cardiac output and hypoxia.

Assessment

✦ A. Dyspnea, respiratory difficulty, cyanosis, wheezing.

✦ B. Vertigo, decreased blood pressure, increased pulse.

C. Local edema.

D. Urticaria (occasional).

E. Flushed face.

F. Apprehension or anxious feelings.

Treatment and Implementation

✦ A. Maintain patent airway.

B. Identify causative agent.

✦ C. Position patient for optimal cerebral perfusion (flat or 30-degree elevation if dyspneic).

✦ D. Administer epinephrine, sub q.
1. Dilates bronchioles and constricts arterioles.
2. Side effects: tachycardia, CNS stimulation.
3. Rapid acting.

E. Administer oxygen.

F. Administer antihistamine (Benadryl).
1. Relieves itching, wheals, congestion of nasal mucosa.
2. Side effect: dries mucous membranes.

✦ G. Maintain IV of NS or lactated Ringer's to support perfusion—as much as 2000 mL in 1 hour.

H. Administer corticosteroids.
1. Reduce formation of cellular proteins and decrease edema.
2. Side effects: same as any steroids.

I. Administer aminophylline—bronchodilator; controls bronchospasms.

Snake Bite

Assessment

A. Assess extent of envenomation: rattlesnakes, copperheads, cottonmouths (pit vipers) are responsible for 98 percent of venomous bites.

B. Signs.
1. Blood oozing from wound.
2. One or two distinct puncture wounds.
3. Edema and discoloration.
4. Numbness around bite within 5–15 minutes.
5. Painful and enlarged lymph nodes.

C. Reactions to poisonous snakes occur within 30–60 minutes.

D. Advanced signs indicating shock.
1. Nausea, vomiting.
2. Ecchymosis, blebs, blisters.
3. Bleeding.
4. Weakness, vertigo, clammy skin.
5. Diaphoresis, chills.
6. Visual disturbance; seizure.

Treatment and Implementation

✦ A. Seek emergency treatment: within 30–60 minutes of medical help.
1. Immobilize area with support or sling.
2. Do not apply tourniquet.
3. Do not allow patient to physically exert self as this hastens spread of venom.
4. Do not incise area or apply suction.

✦ B. In-hospital treatment.
1. Monitor vital signs.
2. Test for sensitivity to horse serum.
3. Judge severity of envenomation before giving antivenin; dose based on severity.
   a. Minimal pit viper bite: 1–5 ampules of antivenin (Crotalidae) IM.
   b. Moderate bite: 5–9 ampules IV drip.
   c. Severe bite: 9 ampules IV drip immediately and up to 20 ampules over next 4–24 hours, until edema ceases and symptoms improve.
4. Administer tetanus toxoid.
5. Administer analgesics for pain.
   a. ASA for mild pain.
   b. Codeine or Demerol for severe pain.
6. Administer antibiotics.
   a. Initial dose: ampicillin, erythromycin, or tetracycline 500 mg.
   b. Maintain 250 mg q 4 h for 24 hours.
7. Type and cross match blood.
8. Monitor blood coagulation studies.

Bee Sting

✦ Assessment

A. Tightness in chest, difficulty swallowing or breathing.

B. Generalized swelling and itching.

C. Erythema and hives.

D. Feeling of heat throughout body.

E. Weakness, vertigo.

F. Nausea, vomiting, abdominal cramps.

Treatment and Implementation ❖ Procedure ❖

A. Remove stinger with tweezers or by scraping motion with fingernail. Do not squeeze venom sac.

✦ B. When patient goes into full-blown anaphylactic shock, immediately administer epinephrine 1:1000 solution sub q as ordered.
1. Adult: 0.25–0.3 mL at sting site and same amount in unaffected arm.
2. Child: 0.01 mL/kg (maximum 0.25 mL at each site).

C. Repeat injections as ordered one to three times at 20-minute intervals until blood pressure and pulse rise toward normal.
1. Adult: 0.3–0.4 mL.
2. Child: < 20 kg, 0.10–0.15 mL; > 20 kg, 0.15–0.3 mL.

D. Cleanse sting area and apply ice to relieve pain and edema.

✦ E. Administer pressor agents as ordered if blood pressure does not stabilize following two to three sub q injections of epinephrine.
1. Aramine or Levophed are drugs of choice.
2. Administer IV drip at 30–40/min.

✦ F. Monitor IV solution of D_5W with 250 mg aminophylline and 30–40 mg Solu-Cortef to support circulation and prevent shock.

G. Observe for signs of laryngospasm or bronchospasm. Be prepared to assist with a tracheostomy.

H. Keep patient warm and positioned supine with head and feet slightly elevated.

I. Administer a rapid-acting antihistamine: Benadryl 50 mg IM as ordered.

COMMON EMERGENCIES

Wounds

Definition: Break in the continuity of the tissue of the body, either internal or external.

A. Classification.
1. Open—break in the skin or mucous membrane.
2. Closed—injury to underlying tissues without a break in the skin or mucous membrane.

B. Types of open wounds.
1. Incised.
2. Contused.
3. Lacerated.
4. Punctured.

C. The RYB wound classification classifies open wounds that are healing—not usually an emergency.
1. Red wounds (R) are in the inflammatory, proliferative, or maturation phase of healing.
2. Yellow wounds (Y) are infected or contain fibrinous slough and aren't ready to heal.

3. Black wounds (B) contain necrotic tissue and aren't ready to heal.
4. Treatment options are based on wound color.

✦ D. First aid for open wounds.
1. Stop bleeding immediately.
2. Protect wound from contamination and infection.
3. Provide shock care.
4. Obtain medical attention.

✦ E. Techniques to stop severe bleeding.
1. Direct pressure.
2. Elevation.
3. Pressure on supplying artery.
4. Tourniquet.

F. Characteristics of closed wounds.
1. No break in skin.
2. Blood loss may be from outer openings of body cavities.
3. Usually caused by an external force.
4. Victim demonstrates signs of internal bleeding.

✦ G. First aid for closed wounds.
1. Check for fractures and other internal injuries.
2. Treat for shock.
3. Do not give fluids by mouth if internal injuries are suspected.
4. Apply ice to small areas of closed wounds.

✦ H. Measures to prevent contamination or infection of wounds.
1. Do not remove cloth pad initially placed on wound.
2. Do not cleanse deep wounds that require medical attention.
3. Use sterile dressing or cleanest dressing available.
4. Do not remove deeply embedded objects.

Choking

Definition: Temporary or permanent asphyxia due to obstruction of the airway.

✦ A. Signs and symptoms.
1. Violent choking.
2. Alarming attempts at inhalation.
3. Cyanosis of face, neck, and hands.
4. Cessation of breathing.
5. Inability to speak.
6. Unconsciousness.

✦ B. First aid measures.
1. Remove object if possible.
2. Allow victim to assume position of comfort.
3. Encourage coughing.
4. Use Heimlich maneuver (*see* p. 373).
5. Artificial respirations if breathing ceases.
6. Obtain medical assistance.

Poisoning

Definition: Introduction into the body or onto the skin surface of any solid, liquid, or gas that tends to impair health or to cause death.

◆ A. First aid treatment.
   1. Call doctor or poison control center. Give the following information.
      a. Age of victim.
      b. Name and amount of poison taken.
      c. Whether or not victim vomited.
   2. If victim is conscious, give antidote, if known.
   3. Induce vomiting (syrup of ipecac) if material ingested is not strong acid or petroleum product. With these substances, use activated charcoal.
   4. If inhaled gases, remove victim to fresh air.
   5. If contact poison, wash exposed areas.
   B. Follow-up treatment as prescribed.

Frostbite and Cold Exposure

◆ A. Signs and symptoms.
   1. White or grayish-yellow skin.
   2. Pain.
   3. Blisters.
   4. Area cold and numb.
   5. Mental confusion.
◆ B. First aid treatment.
   1. Cover area.
   2. Rewarm area quickly.
   3. Do not rub.
   4. Elevate affected area.

Heat Exhaustion

Definition: Response to heat characterized by fatigue and weakness; occurs when intake of water cannot compensate for loss of fluids through sweating.

◆ A. Signs and symptoms.
   1. Pale, clammy skin.
   2. Profuse perspiration.
   3. Headache.
   4. Nausea.
   5. Dizziness.
   6. Fainting.
◆ B. First aid treatment.
   1. Offer victim sips of salt water—one-half glass every 15 minutes for 1 hour.
   2. Have victim lie down and elevate feet.
   3. Place in cool environment.
   4. Apply cool, wet cloths.

Heatstroke

Definition: Response to heat characterized by extremely high body temperature due to disturbance in sweating mechanism.

◆ A. Signs and symptoms.
   1. High body temperature—104° or higher.
   2. Hot, red, dry skin.
   3. Rapid, strong pulse.
   B. First aid treatment—cool body quickly.

Burns*

Definition: Injury of the skin, subcutaneous tissue, muscle, and/or bones caused by heat, chemical agent, or radiation.

◆ A. Classification of burns.
   1. First-degree—red skin, mild swelling and pain, rapid healing.
   2. Second-degree—red or mottled skin, blisters, considerable swelling, wet appearance due to loss of plasma, and severe pain.
   3. Third-degree—deep tissue destruction, white or charred appearance, complete loss of all layers of skin. Skin graft needed for healing.
◆ B. First aid treatment for first-degree burn.
      ❖ **PROCEDURE** ❖
   1. Apply cold water or submerge in cold water.
   2. Prevent contamination.
   3. Avoid greasy substances.
   4. Apply aloe vera gel if available.
   C. First aid treatment for second-degree burn.
   1. Immerse burn, if fairly small area, in cold water for 1–2 hours.
   2. Apply clean cloths.
   3. Blot area dry.
   4. Do not break blisters.
   5. Do not apply antiseptic preparations or home remedies.
   6. Elevate affected extremities.
   7. Seek medical attention.
◆ D. First aid treatment for third-degree burns.
   1. Do not attempt to remove clothing from burned area.
   2. Cover burn with sterile dressing.
   3. Elevate involved extremities.
   4. Do not immerse burn in water or apply ice water to it.
   5. If medical help is not quickly available, and victim is conscious and not vomiting, give victim, at 15-minute intervals, a solution of ½ teaspoon of salt and ½ teaspoon of soda in a quart of water.

Fracture

Definition: A break or crack in a bone.
   A. Types of fractures.
   1. Open—bone ends protrude through skin.

*See Burns, Hospital Treatment in Chapter 10.

2. Closed—bone cracked or broken but does not protrude through skin.

◆ B. Signs and symptoms.
   1. Victim heard or felt bone snap.
   2. Abnormal or false motion in body area.
   3. Differences in shape and length of corresponding bones.
   4. Obvious deformities.
   5. Swelling.
   6. Discoloration.
   7. Pain or tenderness to touch.

◆ C. First aid measures.
   1. Prevent motion of injured parts and adjacent joints.
   2. Elevate involved extremities.
   3. Apply splints.

D. Splinting—device used to immobilize extremity or trunk when a fracture is suspected.

   ❖ PROCEDURE ❖
   1. Purpose.
      a. Immobilize part.
      b. Decrease pain.
      c. Reduce chance of shock.
      d. Protect against further injury during transportation.
   2. Principles.
      a. Ensure splint is long enough to extend past joint on either side of suspected fracture.
      b. Place pad between splint and skin.
      c. Immobilize joints above and below location of suspected fracture.
      d. Apply splint to extremity; do circulation checks to fingers/toes.

See Fractures in Chapter 10.

Sprain

Definition: Injury to a joint ligament or a muscle tendon in region of a joint.

◆ A. Signs and symptoms.
   1. Swelling.
   2. Tenderness.
   3. Pain on motion.
   4. Discoloration.

◆ B. First aid measures.
   1. Do not allow walking if ankle or knee sprained.
   2. Elevate limb for 24 hours.
   3. Apply ice first 24 hours.
   4. If swelling and pain persist, seek medical attention.

C. Common athletic injuries (even those that require clinical attention) use the formula RICE.
   1. Rest—immobilize injured part.
   2. Ice—apply ice to dull pain and reduce blood flow.

3. Compression—apply pressure with towel or elastic bandage.
4. Elevation—for first day or two keep injured area elevated.

Strain

Definition: Injury to a muscle as a result of overstretching.

◆ A. Signs and symptoms.
   1. Pain on motion.
   2. Discoloration.

B. First aid measures.
   1. Bedrest.
   2. Heat.
   3. Bed board (with back sprain).

Dislocation

Definition: Injury to capsule and ligaments of a joint that results in displacement of a bone end at a joint.

◆ A. Signs and symptoms.
   1. Swelling.
   2. Obvious deformity.
   3. Pain upon motion.
   4. Tenderness to touch.
   5. Discoloration.

B. First aid measures.
   1. Splint and immobilize affected joint in position as found.
   2. Do not reduce dislocation or correct deformity near a joint.
   3. Apply sling if appropriate.
   4. Elevate affected part if possible.

EMERGENCY TREATMENTS

Cardiopulmonary Resuscitation (CPR)

◆ **Suspect Unconsciousness**

A. Check responsiveness.
   1. Shake shoulders.
   2. Shout "Are you OK?"
B. Call for help.
C. Establish airway.
   1. Position victim on flat, firm surface.
   2. Rescuer: next to victim at approximately the same level.
   3. Use head tilt, chin lift, or jaw thrust.
      a. Apply head-tilt, jaw-thrust, or chin-lift method (if neck injury even remotely possible).
      b. Infant or toddler: tilt head back without hyperextension; use normal, horizontal alignment, flat surface.

Respiratory Management

A. Airway obstruction.
   ✦ 1. Food or other foreign body aspirant (if known cause of unconsciousness). ❖ **PROCEDURE** ❖
      a. Tilt head—hyperextend neck and chin forward.
      b. One attempt to ventilate will not be successful if obstructed.
      c. If not successful, reposition head and reattempt to ventilate.
      d. If not successful, presence of foreign body is assumed.
      e. Turn patient to one side and finger-probe for obstruction only if patient is *not* breathing.
   2. If this method proves unsuccessful, institute Heimlich maneuver.

B. Evaluate respiratory function.
   1. Maintain open airway.
   2. Observe for respiratory activity.
      a. Put ear down near mouth.
      b. Look for chest movement.
      c. Feel for air flow with cheek.
      d. Listen for exhalation.

✦ C. Administer ventilations. ❖ **PROCEDURE** ❖
   1. Maintain open airway.
   2. Use barrier device if available—form tight seal.
   3. Adult management.
      a. Replace victim's dentures (if any).
      b. Pinch off nostrils.
      c. Fit mouth-to-mouth tight seal.
   4. Infant or toddler management.
      a. Encircle nose and mouth.
      b. Maintain tight seal.
      c. Take fresh breath; do not allow complete deflation of lungs (stairstep volume).
      d. Maintain position.
      e. Assess volume: adult—800 mL minimum; infant—cheek full puffs.
   5. Administer slow breaths (2 seconds each breath).
      a. Give breaths slowly to allow time for chest to expand.
      b. Observe that each ventilation causes chest to rise and fall, hear and feel exhalation.
      c. Continue breaths at rate of 5 seconds (12 breaths/minute).
      d. Between breaths, release seal for exhalation.
      e. Check carotid pulse for 5–10 seconds.

✦ Abdominal Thrust (Heimlich) Maneuver

A. Place patient in sitting or standing position. Stand behind and place arms around waist of patient.

B. Make a fist and place it halfway between xiphoid and umbilicus.
C. Place other hand on top of fist and perform a quick upward thrust.
D. Repeat this maneuver three more times before returning to first method of removing a foreign body.
E. Repeat entire procedure until open airway is obtained or advanced life support service is available.

Circulatory Management ❖ **PROCEDURE** ❖

✦ A. Take major pulse.
   1. Adult—carotid preferably (check for 5–10 seconds) and femoral as alternate.
   2. Palpate one side, with two fingers, for 5 seconds.
✦ B. If no pulse present, immediately attach *automated external defibrillator* (AED), if available.
✦ C. If no AED available, begin CPR.
   1. For adults.
      a. Place heel of hand on midline, lower half of sternum, 2 fingerwidths above xiphoid.
      b. Place other hand on top.
      c. Interlace fingers or extend off rib cage.
      d. Administer 15 compressions at a rate of 100/min; compress chest at depth of 1½ to 2 inches.
      e. Count compressions using first 15 letters of alphabet "a, b, c," etc. through "o" or "off." (Protocol changed from "one and two" to "a, b, c," etc. in 2003.)
      f. Release pressure between compressions for cardiac refilling, but do not take hands off chest between compressions.
   2. For children.
      a. Place hand on midline sternum, midway between xiphoid process and cricothyroid notch.
      b. Use heel of one hand only.
      c. Rate 80/min, depth 1 to 1½ inches.
   3. For infants.
      a. Place fingers on midline sternum, midway between xiphoid process and cricothyroid notch.
      b. Use two fingers only.
      c. Rate 100/min, depth ½ to 1 inch.
      d. Count compressions: one, two, three, four.
✦ D. CPR protocol.
   1. Shake and shout.
   2. Open airway.
   3. Look, listen, and feel for breathing.
   4. Call code.
   5. Ventilate patient with two slow breaths.
   6. Check carotid pulse for 5–10 seconds.

7. Initiate CPR at 15 cardiac compressions to 2 ventilations at rate of 100 compressions per minute.

8. Check for carotid pulse after 1 minute. If absent, continue CPR.

✦ Interpolation (Compressions: Ventilations)

A. Lone rescuer: pause for 2 ventilations after every 15 chest compressions.

B. Two rescuers: continue 15:2 but note that when airway is protected, may change to 1 ventilation after every 5 chest compressions.

C. Changing roles. ❖ **PROCEDURE** ❖

1. Rescuer A, compressor sets pace and maintains rhythm using alphabet, "a," "b," "c," etc. (Using the alphabet is a faster rate of compression, 100/minute).

2. Compressor observes need for and institutes change.

3. Rescuer B checks carotid pulse after 1 minute, then every few minutes.

4. Rescuer giving breaths gets into position to give compressions.

5. Rescuer giving compressions moves to victim's head after fifth compression, counts pulse for 5 seconds.

6. If no pulse, rescuer checking pulse states, "No pulse, start CPR," gives a breath, and CPR is begun again.

✦ CPR Evaluation

A. In process. ❖ **PROCEDURE** ❖

1. Check major pulse after 1 minute of CPR; should be equal to 6 sets of 15:2 by one rescuer.

2. Check major pulse every 4–5 minutes thereafter.

3. Check pupils every 4–5 minutes; optional if third trained person present (not always a conclusive indicator).

4. Observe for abdominal distention (all age groups).
   a. If evident, reposition airway and reduce force of ventilation.
   b. Maintain a volume sufficient to elevate ribs.

5. Ventilator must check carotid pulse frequently between breaths to evaluate perfusion.

6. Ventilator must observe each breath for effectiveness.

7. If respiratory arrest only, check major pulse after each minute (12 breaths) to ensure continuation of cardiac function.

B. After termination.

1. Diagnosis made (no pulse, no respirations) and intervention instituted within 1 minute after unconsciousness.

2. Assistance summoned and entry into Emergency Medical System done promptly and efficiently.

3. Proper CPR performed until acceptable termination.

5. No delay in CPR longer than 5 seconds for extraordinary circumstances (intubation, transportation down stairs).

6. Victim outcome.
   a. Condition.
   b. Potential for cardiac rehabilitation.
   c. Secondary complications (fractured ribs, ruptured spleen, lacerated liver, etc.).

✦ Termination of CPR

A. Successful resuscitation.

1. Spontaneous return of adequate life support.

2. Assisted life support.

B. Transfer to emergency vehicle (other trained rescuers assume care).

C. Pronounced dead by physician.

D. Exhaustion of rescuer(s).

✦ Automated External Defibrillator (AED)

A. Place AED near victim's left ear.

B. Turn on AED power switch if not automatically part of opening AED and lift monitor screen up.

C. Open defibrillatory pads and connect to cables and to victim's chest (after removing clothing on torso).

D. Stop CPR (if second rescuer performing).

E. Press "analyze" control.

1. If ventricular fibrillation present, message will indicate.

2. Loudly state "ALL CLEAR."

3. Deliver shock, press "analyze" control, and repeat shock second and third times if indicated.

F. Continue CPR for 1 minute.

G. Recheck pulse—if absent, repeat sets of three stacked shocks.

EMERGENCY NURSING QUESTIONS

1. An earthquake has just occurred and the hospital has sustained a great deal of damage. The first action is to

   1. Call for help for the patients who are the most critical.
   2. Find the disaster instructions posted on every unit in the hospital and follow instructions.
   3. Return to the central staff room for instructions.
   4. Wait until you receive instructions.

2. If medical care is not available and someone is injured, the first nursing intervention should be to

   1. Determine the priority action.
   2. Call 911.
   3. Don't get involved because of legal ramifications.
   4. Improvise—make do according to the circumstances.

3. A 6-year-old child is brought into the emergency department with a jellyfish sting on his leg. He is screaming with pain. The first emergency intervention is to

   1. Bathe the lesion in vinegar and apply shaving cream.
   2. Bathe the area with fresh water.
   3. Administer an antihistamine as ordered.
   4. Administer a tetanus shot, as ordered.

4. A female patient comes to the emergency room. The nurse's immediate assessment reveals that the patient is bleeding profusely from a deep laceration on her left lower forearm. The *first* action is to

   1. Apply a tourniquet just below the elbow.
   2. Apply pressure directly over the wound.
   3. Call for the physician to check the wound.
   4. Place the patient in shock position.

5. The first maneuver for the nurse to use when checking for airway obstruction is to

   1. Tilt the head and lift the chin.
   2. Attempt to ventilate.
   3. Turn the patient to the side.
   4. Do a jaw thrust.

6. The nurse can best establish whether a patient is unconscious by observing the patient's response to

   1. Verbal stimuli.
   2. Light in the eyes.
   3. Pinching the earlobe.
   4. Opening the airway.

7. Administering care to a patient in hypovolemic shock, the sign that the nurse would expect to observe is

   1. Hypertension.
   2. Cyanosis.
   3. Oliguria.
   4. Tachypnea.

8. When a patient experiences a severe anaphylactic reaction to a medication, the nurse's initial action is to

   1. Start an IV (standard orders)
   2. Assess vital signs.
   3. Place the patient in a supine position.
   4. Prepare equipment for intubation.

9. A patient has burns on the front and back of both his legs and arms. The approximate percentage of his body that has been involved is

   1. 27 percent.
   2. 36 percent.
   3. 45 percent.
   4. 54 percent.

10. While assessing a patient who is being treated with a heating pad or hot compress, the first sign of possible thermal injury is

    1. Tingling sensation in the extremities.
    2. Redness in the area.
    3. Edema.
    4. Pain.

11. Proper depth of compressions for an infant (under 12 months) who is receiving CPR would be

    1. ½ to 1 inch.
    2. ¼ to ¾ inch.
    3. 1 to 1½ inches.
    4. 1½ to 2 inches.

12. A systolic blood pressure of 60 mm Hg or less would indicate shock in which of the following patient age groups?

    1. 5 years old or younger.
    2. 5 to 12 years old.

3. 12 to 16 years old.
4. 16 to 20 years old.

13. The nurse assessing a patient for shock observes that the earliest symptom of shock is

    1. Hypertension.
    2. Increased urine output.
    3. Narrowing pulse pressure.
    4. Warm, moist skin.

14. A 20-year-old female patient is admitted in a comatose state to the emergency room. Her vital signs are BP 140/80, P 110, R 30 and labored. A Medic-Alert bracelet indicates that she is a diabetic. If the nurse were assessing her for ketoacidosis, one significant symptom would be

    1. Oliguria.
    2. Acetone odor to breath.
    3. Kussmaul breathing.
    4. Sensorium change.

15. When caring for an unconscious patient, the nurse's *primary* concern must always be

    1. Airway protection and adequate respiratory status.
    2. Decreasing intracranial pressure.
    3. Fluid balance and cardiac stability.
    4. Maintaining range of motion and muscle tone.

EMERGENCY NURSING

Answers with Rationale

1. (2) The first action is to follow instructions posted in the Disaster Planning poster. If everyone follows these guidelines, there will be less confusion and patients will receive the care they require. The other options would all follow the first action.

   NP:I; CN:S; CA:M; CL:AN

2. (1) Setting the priority is the first action; for if a person is bleeding, then stopping the bleeding is a critical action that could save a life. Calling for help or calling 911 (2) would come after assessing the priorities. It is a professional responsibility to get involved (3) if circumstances are critical. Improvising (4) would also come after setting priorities.

   NP:I; CN:S; CA:M; CL:A

3. (1) A standard jellyfish kit contains vinegar and shaving cream. The vinegar is to bathe the lesion to reduce pain, and the cream is applied so that cysts will adhere to the cream and be scraped off. Seawater, not fresh water (2), is used to bathe the lesion because fresh water will cause the cysts to fire. Later, the child may be given an antihistamine (3) if the sting was severe; he would require a tetanus shot (4) only if he were not up to date with tetanus.

   NP:I; CN:S; CA:M; CL:A

4. (2) The first action is to apply direct pressure to the wound. If the bleeding continues, additional actions must be taken. They include placing the patient in shock position (4) and perhaps applying a tourniquet (1).

   NP:I: CN:S; CA:M; CL:A

5. (1) If airway obstruction is suspected, the first action is to tilt the head by pressing backward and lifting the chin. Then, the nurse would attempt to ventilate (2). To open the airway, a jaw thrust (4) is done.

   NP:I; CN:S; CA:M; CL:A

6. (1) A patient's response (or lack thereof) to verbal stimuli is the best indicator of unconsciousness. An unconscious patient's pupils may continue to react to light. Pinching the lobe of the ear (3) offers little in the way of pain stimuli. Opening the airway (4) is not an appropriate stimulus.

   NP:D; CN:PH; CA:M; CL:C

7. (3) In shock, there is decreased blood volume through the kidneys. This is evidenced by a decrease in the amount of urine excreted. The body has numerous compensatory mechanisms that assist in keeping the blood pressure normal for a short time.

   NP:D; CN:PH; CA:M; CL:A

8. (3) The shock position is necessary to maintain vital signs. The other interventions would be implemented in order (2), then (1) start an IV and prepare for intubation.

   NP:I; CN:S; CA:M; CL:A

9. (4) The patient's burns cover approximately 54 percent of his body surface. Each arm is 9 percent (18 percent) and each leg is 18 percent (36 percent).

   NP:D; CN:PH; CA:M; CL:C

10. (2) Redness, or erythema, is the first sign of possible injury. This is an important observation to prevent a burn injury.

    NP:D; CN:S; CA:M; CL:A

11. (1) The proper depth of compression for infant CPR is ½ to 1 inch. This is done midsternum, using only two fingers or the thumbs, if the chest is encircled by the rescuer's hands. (3) Compression depth for a child is 1 to 1½ inches; for an adult (4) is 1½ to 2 inches.

    NP:P; CN:S; CA:M; CL:K

Coding for Questions/Answers Abbreviations: **Nursing Process: NP,** Data Collection: D, Planning: P, Implementation: I, Evaluation: E, **Client Needs: CN,** Safe, Effective Care Environment: S, Health Promotion and Maintenance: H, Psychosocial Integrity: PS, Physiological Integrity: PH, **Clinical Area: CA,** Medical Nursing: M, Surgical Nursing: S, Maternal/Newborn Nursing: MA, Pediatric Nursing: P, Psychiatric Nursing: PS, **Cognitive Level: CL,** Knowledge: K, Comprehension: C, Application: A, Analysis: AN

12. (2) A systolic blood pressure of 60 mm Hg or less found in children 5 to 12 years old would indicate shock.

NP:P; CN:S; CA:M; CL:C

13. (3) Narrowing pulse pressure and hypotension are two early signs of shock. Decreased, not increased, urine output is present as well as cool, moist skin caused by vasoconstriction.

NP:D; CN:S; CA:M; CL:A

14. (2) As acetone is liberated through the breakdown of fat, it is volatile and is blown off by the lungs, creating the characteristic fruity odor of the breath. Polyuria (not oliguria), polydipsia, and polyphagia are early symptoms. Kussmaul breathing is a sign of early shock as the body attempts to return to acid–base balance. Sensorium change would occur later.

NP:D; CN:PH; CA:M; CL:A

15. (1) As neuro status deteriorates, the airway *must* be assured to avoid compromising oxygenation or aspiration. Hypoxia will exacerbate brain injury. The other answers are appropriate goals *after* airway patency is assured.

NP:I; CN:PH; CA:M; CL:AN

Oncology Nursing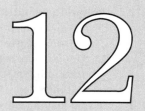

ONCOLOGY CONCEPTS

Cancer Incidence and Trends

A. Cancer—a definition.
1. Term represents a group of more than 100 neoplastic diseases that involve all body organs.
2. One or more cells lose their normal growth-controlling mechanism and continue to grow uncontrolled.

✦ B. Second leading cause of death in the United States after heart disease.
1. Ranks fourth for males and first for females as cause of death; second after accidents as cause of death for children.
2. Greatest increase seen in lung cancer—consistent with smoking patterns.

✦ C. Incidence rate.
1. 1.2 million in the United States are diagnosed with cancer every year.
2. Number of cancer deaths increased by 11 percent during past 40 years. It is predicted that incidence of cancer in the USA could double by 2050 due to growth and aging of population.
3. Leading causes of cancer death are: lung, prostate, and colorectal for males; lung, breast, and colorectal for females.

Identified Causes and Risk Factors

A. Multiplicity theory: multiple factors lead to the development of cancer; 60–90 percent thought to be related to environmental factors.
B. Carcinogens: agents known to increase susceptibility to cancer.
1. Chemical carcinogens: asbestos, benzene, vinyl chloride, by-products of tobacco, arsenic, cadmium, nickel, radiation, etc.
2. Iatrogenic chemical agents: DES, chemotherapy, hormone treatment, immunosuppressive agents, radioisotopes.
3. Radiation carcinogens: x-rays, sunlight (ultraviolet light), nuclear radiation.
4. Viral factors: herpes simplex, Epstein–Barr, hepatitis B, and retroviruses.
5. Genetic factors: hereditary or familial tendencies.
6. Demographic and geographic factors.
7. Dietary factors: obesity, high-fat diet, diets low in fiber, diets high in smoked or salted foods, preservatives and food additives, alcohol.
8. Psychological factors: stress.
9. Age.

Preventive Measures

✦ A. Optimal dietary patterns and lifestyle changes.
1. Avoid obesity (at 40 percent overweight, there is a 55 percent increased risk of cancer in females and 33 percent in males).
2. Decrease fat intake of both saturated and unsaturated fats—maximum 30 percent of total calories.
3. Increase total fiber in diet—decreases risk of colon cancer—and increase cruciferous vegetables (cabbage, broccoli, carrots, brussels sprouts).
4. Increase vitamin A—reduced incidence of larynx, esophagus, and lung cancers.
5. Increase vitamin C—aids tumor encapsulation and promotes longer survival time.
6. Increase vitamin E—inhibits growth of brain tumors, melanomas, and leukemias.
7. Decrease alcohol consumption.
8. Avoid salt-cured, smoked, or nitrate-cured foods.

✦ B. Minimize exposure to carcinogens.
1. Avoid smoking—thought to be a cause of 75 percent of lung cancers in the United States.
2. Avoid oral tobacco—increases incidence of oral cancers.
3. Avoid exposure to asbestos fibers and constant environmental dust.
4. Avoid exposure to chemicals.
5. Avoid radiation exposure and excessive exposure to sunlight.

C. Obtain adequate rest and exercise to decrease stress.
1. Chronic stress associated with decreased immune system functioning.
2. Strong immune system responsible for destruction of malignant cells as they develop.

Early Detection Methods

A. Risk assessment (*see* Risk Factors).
B. Health history and physical assessment.
C. Screening methods.
1. Tests such as a mammography, Pap test, sigmoidoscopy, prostate exam, PSA blood test, fecal occult test for blood (50 years and older).
✦ 2. Self-care practices: breast self-examination (BSE) done every month; testicular self-examination (TSE) done every month in the shower; skin inspection.
D. Teaching patient the seven early warning signs of cancer (use mnemonic **CAUTION**).
1. Change in bowel or bladder habits.
2. Any sore that does not heal.
3. Unusual discharge or bleeding.
4. Thickening or lump in breast or elsewhere.
5. Indigestion or difficulty swallowing.
6. Obvious change in wart or mole.
7. Nagging cough or hoarseness.

Identifying Neoplasms

Characteristics

A. Benign neoplasms: usually encapsulated, remain localized, and are slow growing.

B. Malignant neoplasms: not encapsulated, will metastasize and grow, and exert negative effects on host.

C. Categories of malignant neoplasms.
   1. Carcinomas—grown from epithelial cells; usually solid tumors (skin, stomach, colon, breast, rectal).
   2. Sarcomas—arise from muscle, bone, fat, or connective tissue—may be solid.
   3. Lymphomas—arise from lymphoid tissue (infection-fighting organs).
   4. Leukemias and myelomas—grow from blood-forming organs.

D. Mechanisms of metastasis.
   1. Metastasis occurs via lymphatics—spreads along lymph channels to mass in lymph nodes (e.g., breast to axillary nodes) or spread diffusely.
   2. The bloodstream may carry cells from one site to another (e.g., liver to bone, etc.).
   3. Direct spread of cancer cells (seeding) where there are no boundaries to stop the growth (e.g., ovary and stomach).
   4. Transplantation is the transfer of cells from one site to another.

Diagnosis

A. Diagnostic studies will depend on suspected primary site.

B. Laboratory and radiologic tests often identify a problem first.
   1. Radiographic procedures (e.g., tomography, CT, contrast studies).
   2. Ultrasonography.
   3. Radioisotopic scanning studies (e.g., brain scan, gallium imaging).
   4. Magnetic resonance imaging (MRI).
   5. Biologic response markers (useful for diagnosing primary tumors).
   6. Other laboratory tests (enzyme tests, such as acid phosphatase).

C. Biopsy: definitive diagnosis of cancer.
   1. Excisional biopsy—removes all suspicious tissue.
   2. Incisional biopsy—removes a sample of tissue from a mass.
   3. Needle aspiration—aspiration of small amount of core tissue from a suspicious area.
   4. Exfoliative cytology—cells in tissue or secretions are evaluated by PAP method.

Grading

A. Grading refers to classifying tumor cells—done by biopsy, cytology or surgical excision.

Table 12-1. MALIGNANT AND BENIGN TUMOR COMPARISON

	Malignant	Benign
Cell Type	Abnormal from those of tissues	Close to those of original tissues
Growth	Variable and rapid; infiltrates surrounding tissues in all directions	Slow and noninfiltrating, expansive
Encapsulated	Infrequent, rare	Frequent
Metastasis	Through blood, lymph, or new tumor sites	Absent—remains localized
Effect	Terminal without treatment	Can become malignant or obstruct vital organs
Recurrence	Frequent	Rare
Vascularity	Moderate-to-marked	Slight

B. Tissue specimens are evaluated as frozen or permanent sections by a pathologist.

C. Tumor grading is only one factor in developing a treatment plan—refers to degree of abnormality of cancer cells compared to normal cells.

D. Cancer's grade and stage reveal the extent to which disease has progressed (stage) and its microscopic features (grade).

E. Results from biopsy and other diagnostic procedures (blood tests, x-ray studies, endoscopic procedures) will determine extent of disease staging and grade.

Staging: How Cancer Is Classified

A. Staging describes the extent or metastasis of a malignant tumor; also quantifies severity of disease.

✦ B. A useful system of staging for carcinomas is the TNM system.
   1. T: Primary tumor.
   2. N: Regional nodes.
   3. M: Metastasis.

C. Primary tumor (T).
   1. T_0: no evidence of primary tumor.
   2. Tis: carcinoma in situ.
   3. T_1, T_2, T_3, T_4: progressive increase in tumor size and involvement.
   4. Tx: tumor cannot be assessed.

Table 12-2. GUIDELINES FOR GRADING TUMORS

The American Joint Commission on Cancer has recommended the following guidelines for grading tumors.

Grade	Differentiation	Dysplasia
GX	Cannot be assessed	
G1 Low	Well-differentiated	Mild dysplasia, cells differ slightly from normal cells
G2 Intermediate	Moderately well-differentiated	Moderate dysplasia, more abnormal
G3 High	Poorly differentiated	Severe dysplasia
G4 High	Undifferentiated	Anaplasia, cell of origin unable to be determined

NB: Some cancers also have special grading systems; for example, the Gleason system to describe the degree of differentiation of prostate cancer cells. The Gleason system uses scores ranging from Grade 2 to Grade 10. Lower Gleason scores describe well-differentiated, less aggressive tumors. Higher scores describe poorly-differentiated, more aggressive tumors.

CLINICAL STAGING OF TUMORS

Stage 0:	Cancer in situ
Stage I:	Tumor limited to tissue of origin; localized tumor growth
Stage II:	Local spread limited
Stage III:	Extensive local and regional spread
Stage IV:	Metastasis

D. Involvement of regional nodes (N).
   1. N_0: regional lymph nodes not abnormal.
   2. N_1, N_2, N_3, N_4: increasing degree of abnormal regional lymph nodes.
   3. Nx: regional lymph nodes cannot be assessed clinically.
E. Metastatic development (M).
   1. M_0: no evidence of distant metastasis.
   2. M_1, M_2, M_3, M_4: increasing degree of distant metastasis.
   3. Mx: not assessed.

TREATMENT METHODS

A. Broad goals.
   1. Goal of therapy is to cure the patient—eradicate the tumor.
   2. When cure is not possible, controlling or arresting tumor growth becomes the goal—to prolong survival.
   3. Palliation or alleviation of symptoms is a third goal.
B. The gold standard for cancer treatment remains surgery, radiation therapy, chemotherapy, and combined approaches.

Surgery

A. Useful as primary treatment for localized cancer (breast, colon, melanoma of skin, etc.).
   1. Highest rate of cure for localized disease.

   2. Disadvantage—deforming or debilitating to patient.
✦ B. Types of treatment.
   1. Local excision: simple surgery with small margin of normal tissue surrounding tumor.
   2. En bloc dissection or wide excision: removal of tumor, nodes, tissues, and any contiguous structures.
   3. Surgery on cancer in situ.
      a. Electrosurgery—application of electrical current to destroy cancerous cells.
      b. Cryosurgery—deep freezing with liquid nitrogen.
      c. Chemosurgery—application of chemotherapeutic agents layer by layer with surgical excision.
      d. CO_2 laser—use of laser for local excision.
   4. Other forms of surgery.
      a. Palliative surgery—promotes comfort and quality of life without cure.
      b. Prophylactic—removal of tissue or organs that may develop cancer.

Implementation
A. Preoperative care.
   1. Promote health status prior to surgery.
      a. Malnourished patient is at risk for infection, delayed wound healing, and dehiscence.
      b. Mental status may impact results of surgery.
   2. Provide emotional support prior to surgery.
      a. Encourage talking about fears and anxieties.
      b. Provide accurate information—clarify level of knowledge.
      c. Assess family needs and provide information and support.
✦ B. Postoperative care.
   1. Provide traditional postop care (*see* Chapter 10).

2. Provide for physical comfort.
   a. Enteral feeding.
   b. Pain relief.
   c. Positioning and activity.
   d. Wound care and healing.
3. Provide emotional support.
   a. Allow for grief process—encourage expression of fears.
   b. Discuss change in body image—support increase in self-esteem.
   c. Provide accurate information.
4. Support rehabilitation process.
   a. Encourage family involvement.
   b. Refer patients and families to appropriate resources.
   c. Complete discharge planning.

Radiation Therapy

Definition: Use of high energy moving through space or medium to interrupt cellular growth.

◆ A. Indications.
   1. Used to treat solid tumors—ionizing radiation transfers energy to molecules present in cancer cell.
   2. Different tissues have different radiosensitivities—rapidly dividing tissues (testes, ovaries, lymphoid tissues, and bone marrow) are more sensitive.
◆ B. Types of ionizing radiation.
   1. Electromagnetic—radiation in wave form.
      a. X-rays—linear accelerators deposit maximum dose 5 cm or more below the skin.
      b. Electrons—delivered by machines.
      c. Gamma rays—delivered by machines that contain radioactive sources (Cobalt-60, Cesium-137) or radioactive substances (seeds, threads, or liquids).
   2. Particulate—radiation in the form of heavy particles.
      a. Beta particles—high speed electrons (Phosphorus-32; Strontium-90).
      b. Protons, neutrons, and alpha particles accelerate subatomic particles through body tissue.
      c. A new option in radiation is intensity-modulated radiation therapy (IMRt).
         (1) Delivers a high dose of radiation to the tumor, but spares vital, healthy tissue around it.
         (2) Heralded as greatest breakthrough in cancer management in 25 years.

◆ **External Radiation**
   A. Teletherapy—external source of radiation. (Machine is a distance from patient—most common type of treatment).

   B. Types.
      1. Natural radioactive source—gamma rays delivered via machine to lesion.
      2. Machine is the linear accelerator—high-voltage electric current delivers electrons to patient.
   C. Side effects: fatigue—major systemic effect; headache; nausea and vomiting; skin irritation or injury, scaling, erythema, dryness.

Implementation
A. Offer psychological support.
   1. Tell patient what to expect from treatment.
   2. Explain radiotherapy room.
   3. Tell patient of possible side effects and ways to minimize them.
◆ B. Promote diet: high protein, high carbohydrate, fat free, and low residue.
   1. Foods to avoid: tough, fibrous meat; poultry; shrimp; all cheeses (except soft); coarse bread; raw vegetables; irritating spices.
   2. Foods allowed: soft-cooked eggs, ground meat, pureed vegetables, milk, cooked cereal.
   3. Increase fluids.
   4. Diet supplement to increase calorie and fluid intake.
   5. Remind patient not to eat several hours before treatment.
   C. Administer medications.
   1. Compazine—nausea.
   2. Lomotil—diarrhea.
◆ D. Provide skin care—radiodermatitis occurs 3–6 weeks after start of treatment.
   1. Avoid creams, lotions, perfume to irradiated areas unless ordered by physician; aloe vera cream or gel may be recommended for radiation burn.
   2. Wash with lukewarm water, pat dry (some physicians allow mild soap).
   3. Avoid exposure to sunlight or artificial heat such as heating pad.
   4. Cornstarch may be used for itchy skin; aloe vera gel for radiation burns.
◆ E. Observe for "wet" reaction.
   1. Weeping of skin due to loss of upper layer.
   2. Promote rest after therapy.
   3. Cleanse area with warm water and pat dry BID.
   4. Apply antibiotic lotion or steroid cream if ordered.
   5. Expose site to air.

Internal Radiation
A. Implantation of radioactive substance within a tumor or close to it.
◆ B. Types.
   1. Unsealed sources: isotopes (^{131}I and ^{32}p).
      a. Liquid and administered orally.

      b.   Half-life generally short but varies with isotope.

      c.   Precautions important during high-risk period (usually first 4 days).

  2. Sealed sources: radium needles, radon seeds, and ^{137}Cs.

      a.   Radioactive substance encased in metal capsule placed in body cavity.

      b.   Delivers radiation directly to tumor.

      c.   Even though implant is sealed, special precautions are instituted.

◆ C. Side effects.

  1. Occur when normal cells are damaged.

  2. Acute side effects occur during or shortly after radiation therapy; chronic effects occur months or years following therapy.

  3. Common side effects from radiation therapy: alopecia (hair loss), mouth dryness, mucositis, esophagitis, nausea and vomiting, diarrhea, cystitis, erythema, and dry and wet desquamation.

  4. Factors influencing degree of side effects.

      a.   Body site irradiated.

      b.   Radiation dose—higher dose given, the more potential side effects.

      c.   Extent of body area treated (larger area, more potential for side effects).

      d.   Method of radiation therapy.

Implementation

◆ A. Maintain bedrest when radiation source in place.

  1. Restrict movement to prevent dislodging radiation source.

  2. Do not turn or position patient except on back (when cesium needle in tongue or cervix).

  B. Administer range-of-motion exercise QID.

  C. Take vital signs every 4 hours (report temperature over 100°F).

◆ D. Observe for untoward effects: dehydration or paralytic ileus (if cervical implant).

  E. Observe and report skin eruption, discharge, abnormal bleeding.

  F. Provide clear liquid diet (low residue is sometimes ordered) and force fluids.

◆ G. Insert Teflon Foley catheter as ordered (radiation decomposes rubber) to avoid necessity of bedpan.

  H. Avoid direct contact around implant site; avoid washing areas, etc.

◆ I. Observe frequently for dislodging of radiation source (especially linen and dressings).

  ◆ 1. When radiation source falls out, do not touch with hands. Pick up source with foot-long applicator.

  2. Put source in lead container and call head nurse–physician.

  3. If unable to locate source, call head nurse–physician immediately and bar visitors from room.

◆ J. After source is removed:

  1. Administer Betadine douche as ordered if cervical implant.

  2. Give Fleet enema.

  3. Patient may be out of bed.

  4. Avoid direct sunlight to radiation areas.

  5. Administer cream to relieve dryness or itching.

  K. Instruct that patient may resume sexual intercourse within 7–10 days.

  L. Notify head nurse if nausea, vomiting, diarrhea, frequent urination or bowel movements, or temperature above 100°F is present.

Radiation Safety Measures

◆ A. General guidelines for radiation safety measures.

  1. Wear radiation badges to monitor total amount of radiation exposure. Cumulative dose (measured in millirems) not to exceed 1250 every 3 months.

  2. Observe for displacement or dislodgment of radiation source every 4–6 hours.

  3. Check that sealed lead container is kept in patient's room in case of accidental dislodgment.

  4. Collect body waste until it can be determined radiation source is not dislodged.

  5. Radiation source removed at prearranged time—after removal, patient is no longer radioactive.

  6. Do not allow persons under age 18 or pregnant women to visit or care for patients with radioactive implant.

  7. Never touch a dislodged sealed source—use long-handled tongs or contact radiation safety personnel.

  8. Mark patient's room and chart with radiation safety precautions.

◆ B. Follow special principles of time, distance, and shielding.

  ◆ 1. Minimize time.

      a.   Radiation exposure proportional to amount of time spent with patient.

      b.   Care planned to be delivered in shortest amount of time to meet goals—be efficient with time.

      c.   Review procedures before beginning them.

  ◆ 2. Maximize distance.

      a.   Intensity of radiation related to distance from patient.

      b.   Duration of safe exposure increases as distance is increased; work as far away from source as possible.

  ◆ 3. Utilize shielding.

      a.   Use lead shields or other equipment to reduce transmission of radiation.

b.   Store radioactive material in lead-shielded container when not in use.

✦ C.   Follow radiation precautions for isotope implant.
1.   All body secretions considered contaminated—use special techniques for disposal.
2.   If patient vomits within first 4 hours—everything vomitus touches is considered contaminated.
3.   Use disposable gown, dishes, etc.
4.   Limit contact with hospital personnel and visitors.

Chemotherapy

Characteristics

A.   The medical management of cancer includes the use of chemotherapy. First used in the early 1950s, there are now more than 80 effective drugs available.
1.   Chemotherapy is method of choice when there is suspected or confirmed spread of malignant cells.
2.   Method used when the risk of recurrence systemically is high.
3.   May be used as palliative measure to relieve pain or increase comfort.
B.   Mechanism of action—chemotherapeutic agents eradicate cells, both normal and malignant, that are in the process of cell reproduction.

Drug Classification

A.   Drugs classified by group into those that act on a certain phase of cell reproduction (cell cycle specific) or those that do not (cell cycle nonspecific).
✦ B.   Cell cycle–specific agents: antimetabolites and mitotic inhibitors or plant alkaloids.
1.   Act on the cell during a particular phase of reproduction.
2.   Most effective in tumors where a large number of cells are dividing.
3.   Divided doses produce greater cytotoxic effects (not all cells will be in the same phase at the same time).
4.   Antimetabolites—methotrexate, 6-mercaptopurine, 5-fluorouracil, Azacytidine, cytarabine, Hydrea.
5.   Plant alkaloids—vincristine, vindesine, vinblastine, teniposide.
✦ C.   Cell cycle nonspecific drugs: alkylating agents, antitumor antibiotics, and nitrosoureas.
1.   Act on cells during any phase of reproduction—some drugs will attack cells in the resting phase (not actively dividing).
2.   Agents are dose dependent—the more drug given, the more cells destroyed.
3.   These drugs are more toxic to normal tissue because they are less selective.

4.   Alkylating agents—Cytoxan, Myleran, melphalan (L-pam), thiotepa, Platinol.
5.   Antitumor antibiotics—Adriamycin, dactinomycin.
6.   Nitrosoureas—streptozocin, methyl CCNU, BCNU, DCNU.
D.   Other miscellaneous agents (such as procarbazine) are used in the chemotherapy group, but their exact mechanism of action is unknown.
E.   Hormones (estrogens, androgens, progestins) are used in therapy to affect the hormonal environment—Decadron, DES, tamoxifen, prednisone.
1.   Affect the growth of hormone-dependent tumors.
2.   Antihormones (tamoxifen) block tumor growth by depriving the tumor of the necessary hormones.
F.   Combination chemotherapy.
1.   Drugs used in combination for synergistic activity.
✦ 2.   Many protocols include three or four drugs. (Example: the protocol for Hodgkin's lymphoma is based on four drugs: doxarubicin, bleomycin, vinblastine and dacarbazine (ABVD).)
3.   Latest studies at Stanford University suggest that 4 or 5 chemotherapy drugs combined with prednisone given for 3 (instead of 6) months are an efficacious protocol for Hodgkin's lymphoma.

Chemotherapeutic Administration

✦ A.   Chemotherapeutic agents are administered through a variety of routes.
1.   Oral route—used frequently. Safety precautions must be observed.
2.   Intramuscular and sub q used infrequently as drugs are not vesicants.
3.   Intravenous is the most common route.
a.   Provides for better absorption.
b.   Potential complications: infection, phlebitis.
4.   Central venous catheter infusion—used for continuous or intermittent infusions.
5.   Venous access devices (VADs)—used for prolonged infusions.
6.   Intra-arterial route—delivers agents directly to tumor in high concentrations while decreasing drug's systemic toxic effect.
7.   Intraperitoneal—used for ovarian and colon cancer. High concentration of agents delivered to peritoneal cavity via a catheter, then drained.
B.   Factors for deciding dosage and timing of drugs.
1.   Dosage calculated on body surface area and kilograms of body weight.
2.   Time lapse between doses to allow recovery of normal cells.

3. Side effects of each drug and when they are likely to occur.
4. Liver and kidney function, as most antineoplastics are metabolized in one of these organs.

C. Oncology is one area that is benefitting from the field of pharmacogenomics—targeted medicine based on genetic makeup.
   1. Breast cancer—Herceptin targets a protein and stops growth in a certain type of cancer.
   2. Many fewer side effects than chemotherapy.

Chemotherapy Safety Guidelines

✦ A. Antineoplastic drugs are potentially hazardous to personnel and may have teratogenic and/or carcinogenic effects.

✦ B. Safety guidelines have been issued by the Occupational Safety and Health Administration (OSHA).
   1. Obtain special training for drug administration.
   2. Wear surgical latex gloves with a thickness of at least 0.007 and a disposable, closed, long-sleeved gown.
   3. Use Luer-Lok syringes.
   4. Label all prepared drugs appropriately.
   5. Double bag chemotherapy drugs once prepared, before transport.
   6. Have equipment ready to clean up any accidental spill.
   7. Dispose of all materials in marked containers labeled hazardous waste.
   8. Dispose of all needles and syringes intact.
   9. Be sure to follow your facility's policies and procedures when preparing to administer chemotherapy.
   10. Double-check the chemotherapy orders with another oncology nurse
   11. Read material safety data sheets (MSDS) prior to administration.
   12. Use personal protective equipment (PPE).
   13. Wash your hands both before you put on and after you take off gloves.
   14. After infusion is complete, promptly dispose of any equipment that contained the drug in a puncture-proof container that's clearly marked.
   15. Chemotherapy agents may be excreted in body fluids, these may be contaminated for 48 hours after the last drug dose. Wear PPE when handling such excreta, and wash your hands after removing your gloves.
   16. Check your facility's policies about handling linen that's been contaminated with chemotherapy.
   17. If a chemotherapy drug comes into contact with your skin or a patient's skin, thoroughly wash the affected area with soap and water, but don't abrade the skin with a scrub brush.
   18. If the drug gets in your eye(s), flush with copious amounts of water for at least 15 minutes while holding back your eyelids. Then get evaluated by employee health or the ED.

C. When infusing vesicant drugs, monitor IV carefully and, at first sign of extravasation, remove IV and implement Rx protocol.

Side Effects of Chemotherapy and Nursing Management

A. Side effects occur primarily due to the mechanism of action of potent drugs on normal cells.

✦ B. Skin and mucosa, protective linings of the body, are damaged; mucositis (cells of the mucosa are affected)—may extend from oral cavity and stomatitis through GI tract.

✦ C. Alopecia, or hair loss, caused by damage to rapidly dividing cells of the hair follicles.
   1. Hair loss begins 2–3 weeks after chemotherapy and continues through the cycles of chemotherapy; regrowth occurs following the course of therapy.
   2. Nursing interventions include applying scalp hypothermia (ice cap) and scalp tourniquet to reduce the amount of drug reaching the hair follicle—may prevent hair loss.

✦ D. Nausea, vomiting, and anorexia are common.
   1. Support changes in food preferences, additional or less seasoning, small and more frequent meals.
   2. Antiemetic drugs (Reglan) may counteract these symptoms.
   3. Offer high calorie and protein supplements.
   4. Diarrhea is related to toxicity of the drugs on the mucosal lining; diet bland and low residue.
   ✦ 5. Constipation may be related to drugs (vinblastine and vincristine) because nerve endings in GI tract are affected. Patient should add more fiber and liquid to diet.

✦ E. White blood cell and platelet suppression.
   1. White blood cell suppression—leukopenia (less than 5,000/mm^3 when normal white blood cell count is 5,000–10,000/mm^3).
   2. Platelet suppression to below normal (< 150,000/mm^3 when normal is 150,000 to 300,000/mm^3).
      a. A number < 50,000/mm^3 makes the patient susceptible to bleeding gums and nose, easy bruising, heavier menstrual flow, etc.
      b. Tell patient precautions: soft toothbrush, avoidance of douches and enemas, care with trimming nails.

F. Red blood cell suppression—anemia (may not be severe).

CANCER NURSING

✦ A. Key stress periods for patient with cancer are: time of diagnosis, period of hospitalization, and release from the hospital.
  1. Shock and fear are the major reactions.
  2. Severe depression is experienced by some patients.
  3. Emotional pain of the diagnosis initially outweighs physical component of the cancer.
B. Adjustment to cancer depends on past life experiences.
C. Phases of psychological adaptation to terminal illness include: denial, anger, bargaining, depression, and acceptance.
D. The patient will experience a range of feelings and defense mechanisms.
  ✦ 1. Denial may occur initially with the diagnosis; this is a protective mechanism necessary until the diagnosis can be confronted.
    a. Allow patient to be in denial until he or she is ready to face reality.
    b. Provide opportunities for the patient to confront her illness—be open to questions and clarification.
  2. Fear and anxiety may manifest in physical symptoms: insomnia, nausea, vomiting, diarrhea, headaches, etc.
  3. Anger and resentment, especially in the initial phases of the disease, may be a healthy way of expressing feelings.
  4. Depression may be considered normal for a period of time following surgery.
    a. Observe for the signs of depression.
    b. Because suicide is always a risk with depression, interventions should be aimed at safety for the patient.

Psychosocial Aspects of Caring for the Cancer Patient

✦ A. Talk with the patient so that he or she will not feel they have to cope alone—provide emotional support to help allay fears and anxieties.
✦ B. Always be honest with the patient—provides the foundation for a nurse–patient relationship.
  1. Accurate information can be followed by an open discussion of disease, prognosis, the patient's feelings, etc.
  2. Knowing the truth enables patient to begin to accept situation.
✦ C. Assist patient to cope with pain.
  1. The nature of cancer pain falls into two categories: chronic and intractable pain.
  2. Assess the severity of pain using a 5 or 10 point scale (0 being pain free and 5 or 10 being worst possible pain).
  3. Stay with patient, especially when the pain is severe.
  4. Respect patient's response to pain and believe what patient tells you.
D. Provide general comfort measures.
  1. Position for proper alignment.
  2. Use touch and massage for painful areas.
  3. Exercise extremities gently to maintain range of motion.
  4. Maintain patency of tubes and keep free of infection using meticulous handwashing and aseptic technique.
  5. Preserve the patient's energy by prioritizing activities.
  6. Assist the patient to obtain adequate rest at night and during the day to reduce fatigue.
✦ E. Support family of patient as they move through the grieving process.

Table 12-3. 3 STEP ANALGESIC LADDER

The 3 step analgesic ladder proposed by the World Health Organization (WHO) is often followed in managing pain.

Step	Pain Intensity on a 0–10 Point Pain Scale	Drugs of Choice	Pain Management
1	Pain is mild and is described by patient at 1–3	Nonopioids for mild pain (e.g., aspirin, acetaminophen, NSAIDs)	Provide appropriate and concurrent treatment for cause of pain; use adjuvant drugs* as needed
2	Pain is moderate and is described by patient at 4–6	Opioids for mild-to-moderate pain (e.g., codeine, oxycodone)	Pain persists or increases Add Step 2 opioid; continue Step 1 drugs and add adjuvant drugs as needed
3	Pain is moderate-to-severe and is described by patient at 7–10	Opioids for moderate-to-severe pain (e.g., morphine, hydromorphone, methadone)	Pain persists or increases Replace Step 2 opioid with Step 3 opioids; continue Step 1 drugs and add adjuvant drugs as needed

* Examples of adjuvant drugs: tricyclic antidepressants, antiseizure drugs, anxiolytics, antihistamines, benzodiazepines, caffeine, dextroamphetamine, corticosteroids.

✦ F.　Introduce the hospice concept—provides care for the terminally ill patient and family.

Medication Management

A.　Drug therapy is cornerstone of cancer pain management—begins with least potent and progresses to opioids as pain intensifies.

   1.　May go from ASA and NSAIDs to codeine and hydrocodone to intraspinal morphine.

   2.　Evaluate patient continually for opioid side effects (constipation, nausea, vomiting, sedation, and urinary retention) that would interfere with goal of therapy.

B.　DO NOT undermedicate for cancer pain.

   1.　Undertreatment with analgesics has been identified as a major problem (70–80 percent) for cancer patients—and nursing has a crucial responsibility to correct this problem.

   2.　Two forms of undertreatment: physicians underprescribe and nurses routinely administer less than half the amount patients could receive.

ONCOLOGY NURSING QUESTIONS

1. A patient has just received a report from her physician that describes a tumor that was recently biopsied. If the result she receives is listed as "To, No, Mo," the patient will know that she has

   1. No evidence of a primary tumor, lymph node involvement, and metastasis.
   2. No primary tumor, but evidence of a degree of distant metastasis.
   3. A primary tumor and regional nodes involved.
   4. Carcinoma in situ.

2. The nurse is assessing a patient with a radiation implant and observes that the implant has been dislodged. The nurse cannot immediately locate the implant. The first nursing action is to

   1. Search for the implant in the bed covers and place it in a lead container.
   2. Call the charge nurse and bar all visitors from the room.
   3. Pick up the source with a foot-long applicator.
   4. Notify the radiation safety team.

3. A patient experiencing severe, intractable pain from cancer complains that the pain medication is not handling the pain at all. The nurse has given the patient all of the medicine she can receive. The next nursing action is to

   1. Emotionally support the patient and tell her she will receive the next dose of medication as soon as possible.
   2. Contact the charge nurse immediately and intervene on the patient's behalf to have the pain dose increased or changed.
   3. Suggest the patient try breathing or other alternative techniques to cope with the pain.
   4. Explore the nature of the pain and help the patient perceive it in a different way.

4. Cancer is the second major cause of death in the United States. What is the first step toward effective cancer control?

   1. Increasing government control of potential carcinogens.
   2. Changing habits and customs that predispose the individual to cancer.
   3. Conducting more mass screening programs.
   4. Educating public and professional people about cancer.

5. When a patient has terminal cancer, morphine sulfate is an agent used for patient controlled analgesia (PCA). The nurse caring for the patient knows that the usual concentration available in a vial injector is _____ mg/mL or _____ mg/mL.

6. A female patient was admitted to the hospital for biopsy of the left breast and a possible mastectomy. The patient has just returned from surgery after having a mastectomy with reconstruction on the left side. The nurse will position the patient in

   1. Low-Fowler's, turned to the affected side.
   2. Semi-Fowler's, affected arm elevated.
   3. Semi-Fowler's, turned to unaffected side.
   4. Prone position.

7. When the nurse is counseling a patient about preventive measures for cancer, one of the most important behaviors to emphasize is to

   1. Decrease fat intake.
   2. Avoid exposure to the sun.
   3. Avoid smoking.
   4. Obtain adequate rest and avoid stress.

8. A patient has just completed a course in radiation therapy and is experiencing radiodermatitis. The most effective method of treating the skin is to

   1. Wash the area with soap and warm water.
   2. Apply a cream or lotion to the area.
   3. Leave the skin alone until it is clear.
   4. Avoid all creams or lotions to the area.

9. The nurse is teaching a class on cancer prevention and treatment. Of the following symptoms, which one is an early warning sign of cancer?

   1. Heartburn.
   2. Fever, chills, and cough.
   3. Change in bowel or bladder habits.
   4. Persistent headache.

10. A 45-year-old patient has just been admitted to the hospital for an abdominal hysterectomy following a diagnosis of uterine cancer. Results of lab tests indicate that the patient's white blood cell count is 9800/mm^3. The most appropriate intervention is to

    1. Call the operating room and cancel the surgery.
    2. Notify the surgeon immediately.

3. Take no action as this is a normal value.
4. Call the lab and have the test repeated.

11. A patient has possible malignancy of the colon, and surgery is scheduled. The rationale for administering neomycin preoperatively is to

    1. Prevent infection postoperatively.
    2. Eliminate the need for preoperative enemas.
    3. Decrease and retard the growth of normal bacteria in the intestines.
    4. Treat cancer of the colon.

12. Of the following screening methods for prevention of cancer, the most important one for the female patient to be aware of is

    1. Magnetic resonance imaging (MRI).
    2. Breast self-examination.
    3. Risk assessment.
    4. Sigmoidoscopy.

13. A female patient has a cesium needle implanted in her cervix. She asks the nurse if she may get out of bed to go to the bathroom. The appropriate response is to tell her

    1. She may not get out of bed while the needle is implanted.
    2. She may get out of bed with the nurse's help.
    3. The nurse will have to get a physician's order for her to get out of bed.
    4. She must stay in bed, but she can move around to be more comfortable while the needle is implanted.

14. A patient with cancer that has metastasized to the liver is started on chemotherapy. His physician has specified divided doses of the antimetabolite. The patient asks why he should take the drug in divided doses. The appropriate response is

    1. "There really is no reason; your doctor just wrote the orders that way."
    2. "This schedule will reduce the side effects of the drug."
    3. "Divided doses produce greater cytotoxic effects on the diseased cells."
    4. "Because these drugs prevent cell division, they are more effective in divided doses."

15. A patient is suffering from severe side effects from chemotherapy. She is experiencing nausea, vomiting, and anorexia. In addition to antiemetic medications, the nurse might suggest

    1. Eliminating salt and spices in the diet.
    2. Drinking fluids only between, not with, meals.

3. Low-protein meals.
4. High-calorie and high-protein supplements.

16. For a patient who has received a diagnosis of skin cancer, the type that has the poorest prognosis because it metastasizes so rapidly and extensively via the lymph system is

    1. Basal cell epithelioma.
    2. Squamous cell epithelioma.
    3. Malignant melanoma.
    4. Sebaceous cyst.

17. Alkylating drugs are used as chemotherapeutic agents in cancer therapy. The nurse understands that these drugs stop cancer growth by

    1. Damaging DNA in the cell nucleus.
    2. Interrupting the production of necessary cellular metabolites.
    3. Creating a hormonal imbalance.
    4. Destroying messenger RNA.

18. Antineoplastic drugs are dangerous because they affect normal as well as cancer tissue. Normal cells that divide and proliferate rapidly are more at risk. Which of the following areas of the body would be least at risk?

    1. Bone marrow.
    2. Nervous tissue.
    3. Hair follicles.
    4. Lining of the GI tract.

19. While the nurse is orienting a patient scheduled for surgery, the patient states she is afraid of what will happen the next day. The most appropriate response is to

    1. Assure her that the surgery is very safe and problems are rare.
    2. Encourage her to talk about her fears as much as she wishes.
    3. Explain that her physician is one of the best and she has nothing to worry about.
    4. Explain that worrying will only prolong her hospitalization.

20. A patient has had a partial colectomy because of a diagnosis of cancer. Surgery began at 7:30 AM. She returned to the unit at 1:30 PM. During a 6:00 PM assessment, the nurse observed all of the following. A priority concern that would require the earliest intervention is a

    1. Dressing that is moderately saturated with serosanguineous drainage.
    2. Warm and reddened area on the patient's left calf.
    3. Distended bladder that is firm to palpation.
    4. Decrease in breath sounds on the right side.

ONCOLOGY NURSING

Answers with Rationale

1. (1) The staging of the cancer according to cancer classification means that there is no evidence of a primary tumor (To), regional lymph nodes are not abnormal (No), and there is no evidence of distant metastasis (Mo).

   NP:E; CN:PH; CA:M; CL:C

2. (2) The first nursing action is to bar all visitors from the room and notify the charge nurse who will notify the physician. It is important not to contaminate yourself by searching for the implant. The physician will notify the radiation team and make decisions about reimplanting the radiation source in the client.

   NP:I; CN:S; CA:M; CL:AN

3. (2) It is the nurse's responsibility to intervene with the charge nurse and physician and report that the pain medication is not providing adequate pain relief. Undertreatment with analgesics has been identified as a major problem for cancer patients, and studies have shown that physicians frequently underprescribe. The other responses will help support the patient, but they will not be effective enough to relieve severe pain.

   NP:I; CN:PH; CA:M; CL:A

4. (4) The most important step in controlling cancer is educating the public about cancer and its warning signs. Education will have an effect on early diagnosis and treatment.

   NP:P; CN:H; CA:M; CL:C

5. Morphine sulfate in doses of 1 mg/mL or 5 mg/mL can be used for PCA.

   NP:P; CN:PH; CA:M; CL:C

6. (2) The most therapeutic position is semi-Fowler's with the affected arm elevated to prevent edema and promote drainage. The patient should be turned only to the back and unaffected side.

   NP:I; CN:S; CA:S; CL:A

7. (3) Avoiding smoking is a primary cancer preventive behavior. Smoking is believed to be the cause of 75 percent of lung cancers in the United States. All of the other behaviors are also important preventive measures, but tobacco is a known carcinogen.

   NP:I; CN:H; CA:M; CL:C

8. (4) Irradiated areas are very sensitive; all creams and lotions, which would serve to irritate the skin, should be avoided. The area should be washed with lukewarm water; a mild soap may be used, but most physicians prefer clear water.

   NP:P; CN:PH; CA:M; CL:C

9. (3) A change in bowel or bladder habits is one of the seven early warning signs of cancer. Indigestion or difficulty swallowing is a sign, as is a nagging cough or hoarseness.

   NP:D; CN:PH; CA:M; CL:K

10. (3) The normal WBC count is 5000–10,000/mm^3. If the results were abnormally high or low, the surgeon would have to be notified and the surgery may be canceled. Tests with abnormal results are not routinely repeated unless the results are grossly abnormal.

    NP:I; CN:PH; CA:S; CL:AN

11. (3) Neomycin suppresses normal bacterial flora, thereby "sterilizing" the bowel preoperatively to decrease the possibility of postoperative infection. It cannot prevent infection (1). Neomycin does not influence the need for preoperative enemas (2) or treat cancer of the colon (4).

    NP:P; CN:PH; CA:S; CL:A

Coding for Questions/Answers Abbreviations: **Nursing Process: NP,** Data Collection: D, Planning: P, Implementation: I, Evaluation: E, **Client Needs: CN,** Safe, Effective Care Environment: S, Health Promotion and Maintenance: H, Psychosocial Integrity: PS, Physiological Integrity: PH, **Clinical Area: CA,** Medical Nursing: M, Surgical Nursing: S, Maternal/Newborn Nursing: MA, Pediatric Nursing: P, Psychiatric Nursing: PS, **Cognitive Level: CL,** Knowledge: K, Comprehension: C, Application: A, Analysis: AN

12. (2) Breast self-examination (BSE) is the most important method to instruct the patient about, because it is a primary prevention method. It is performed every month (whereas a mammogram is done every year after age 50), and many breast lumps are first found by the woman when she is examining her breasts. An MRI (1) would be done for diagnosis. Risk assessment (3) and sigmoidoscopy (4) are also important preventive measures, but in priority fall below a BSE.

    NP:D; CN:H; CA:M; CL:K

13. (1) While the sealed source is implanted, the patient must remain on bedrest, and movement is restricted to prevent dislodging the radiation source. The patient must remain on her back and should not turn or move in bed.

    NP:I; CN:S; CA:M; CL:A

14. (3) Because not all cells will be in the same phase at the same time, divided doses will produce greater cytotoxic effects. This schedule will not reduce the side effects of the drug. Even though the drugs may prevent cell division, divided doses will not affect this characteristic.

    NP:I; CN:PH; CA:M; CL:A

15. (4) The most effective deterrent to the nausea and vomiting is to offer the patient high-calorie and high-protein supplements. If diarrhea is a problem, eliminating spices (1) would be helpful. Food preferences of the patient may also encourage eating (additional seasoning; small, more frequent meals; etc.). Not including fluids with meals (2) may be helpful, but it is not known to help nausea and vomiting.

    NP:I; CN:PH; CA:M; CL:A

16. (3) Malignant melanoma has the poorest prognosis. Basal cell epithelioma (1) and squamous cell epithelioma (2) are both superficial, easily excised, slow-growing tumors. A sebaceous cyst (4) is a benign (nonmalignant) growth.

    NP:D; CN:PH; CA:M; CL:K

17. (1) Alkylating agents affect production of DNA which, in turn, disrupts cell growth and division. Answers (3) and (4) are not applicable, since these drugs do not create an imbalance in hormones or destroy RNA. Antimetabolites, such as Methotrexate, act on the cell during a particular phase of production.

    NP:P; CN:PH; CA:M; CL:C

18. (2) Nervous tissue is least at risk. Answers (1), (3), and (4) are the cells that are most vulnerable because they have rapid cell division and proliferation similar to cancer cells. The nervous tissue cells do not have rapid cell division.

    NP:D; CN:PH; CA:M; CL:C

19. (2) Allowing the patient to express her fears results in a decrease in anxiety and a more realistic and knowledgeable reaction to the situation. Studies have shown that the less anxiety the patient has about the surgery, the more positive the postoperative results. Answers (1) and (3) are false reassurance and nontherapeutic.

    NP:I; CN:PS; CA:PS; CL:A

20. (3) Inability to void after surgery is a common problem resulting from anesthesia or pain medication and requires an early intervention. It is important to be aware of the patient's output for several reasons: to ensure adequate intake, to detect renal problems, and to assess for blood pressure problems. Solution to this problem is catheterization, based on a physician's order. The dressing (1) should be closely observed but is not presently a problem. The area on the calf (2) may be developing throbophlebitis and should be reported to the physician immediately. The breath sounds (4) can be improved by turning, coughing, and deep breathing.

    NP:D; CN:PH; CA:S; CL:AN.

Geriatric Nursing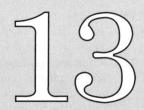

GENERAL CONCEPTS

General Principles

Terminology
A. Geriatrics—concerned with the diseases and care of patients with diseases of old age.
B. Gerontology—study of normal aging process.
C. Aging—natural continuous process.
   1. Begins at birth.
   2. Is common to all living organisms.
D. Old age.
   1. Young old—61 to 70 years.
   2. Middle old—70 to 80 years.
   3. Very old—80 to 90 years.
E. Elderly elderly—75 years or over.

Profiles
A. In 2030, the U.S. popuation will include 35 million persons over age 65, 21% of the total population.
   1. In 2010, "baby boomers" will reach senior status.
   2. The number of persons over 65 is projected to grow to 40 million by 2010, an increase of 20%.
   3. Yearly income of 15 to 25 percent is at or below the poverty level.
   4. Two to 10 percent are alcohol abusers.
B. Cost of health care for the aged.
   1. Only 5 to 6 percent are institutionalized; nursing home population has increased to 1.8 million.
   2. Twenty-five percent of all prescription drugs are dispensed to persons over 65.
   3. Diseases may be multiple and chronic (over 40 percent have more than one illness concurrently).
   4. Disability results more readily when an aging person becomes ill.
   5. Response to treatment is diminished.
   6. Resistance is lower due to the aging process—person is more susceptible to disease.
   7. The aged have less resistance to stressors: mental, environmental, and physical.
   8. Poor health care is prevalent.
      a. Less than one-third have annual checkups.
      b. Many see health care as a service to be used only during life crisis.
      c. Many see more than one doctor, so care is fragmented.
C. Increased life expectancy up from 77 years in 2000.
   1. Advanced health care.
   2. Decreased infant/child mortality.
   3. Improved nutrition and sanitation.
   4. Increased infectious disease control.
✦ D. Causes of death.
   1. Heart disease is major cause.
   2. Cancer is second.
   3. Stroke/CVA is third.
   4. In 2001, leading causes of death decreased: stroke down by almost 5%, heart disease 4%, cancer 2% and accidents 2%.
E. Major fears of the aged.
   1. Physical and economic dependency.
   2. Chronic illness.
      a. Arthritis.
      b. Hypertension.
      c. Hearing deficit.
      d. Heart disease.
   3. Loneliness.
   4. Boredom resulting from not being needed.

Aging Process

Theories of Aging
A. Individualized process.
   1. Each person ages at a different rate.
   2. Each person ages in a different manner.
   3. No single factor has been found to cause or prevent aging.
B. Biological theories.
   1. Genetic programming and/or mutations.
   2. "Wear and tear"—overexertion and stress cause body cells to wear out.
   3. Cellular changes caused by free radical oxidation.
   4. Cross-link—chemical bondage of elements.
   5. Exposure to radiation, pathogens, nutritional deficiencies.
   6. Errors in the RNA and DNA leading to cell mutation.
C. Psychosocial theories.
   1. Activity.
      a. Aging will increase in direct proportion to decrease in activity.
      b. Optimum pattern is to continue in lifestyle of middle age.
   2. Adaptation to stress—genetic makeup and personal learning to deal with stress.
   3. Personality continuity—basic personality or behavior patterns are unchanged by aging.
   4. Disengagement—society and individual withdraw from each other.
   5. Environment—toxins and pollutants.

Physiological Changes
A. Cells.
   1. Fewer in number.
   2. Larger in size.
   3. Decreased total body fluid due to decreased intracellular fluid.
✦ B. Nervous system.
   1. Decreased speed of nerve conduction.

FACTORS THAT INFLUENCE AGING

- Heredity.
- Nutrition.
- Health status.
- Life experiences.
- Environment.
- Stress.

---

2. Delay in response and reaction time, especially with stress.
3. Diminution of sensory faculties.
   a. Decreased vision.
   b. Loss of hearing.
   c. Diminished sense of smell and taste.
   d. Greater sensitivity to temperature changes, with low tolerance to cold.
C. The ear.
   1. Age related changes resulting in hearing loss may be related to insults from noise, vascular disease, nutrition, ototoxic drugs and pollution exposure.
   ◆ 2. Presbycusis.
      a. Progressive hearing loss in inner ear.
      b. High-frequency tones are lost first.
      c. Sounds are distorted; difficulty understanding words when other noises in background.
      d. Fifty percent of those over age 65.
   3. Tympanic membrane atrophic, sclerotic.
   4. Cerumen accumulates; may impact due to increased amount of keratin.
D. The eye.
   ◆ 1. Presbyopia—loss of accommodation from loss of elasticity of lens.
   2. Pupil sphincter sclerosis with loss of light responsiveness.
   3. Cornea more spherical.
   4. Lens more opaque.
   5. Increased light perception threshold.
      a. Adapt to darkness more slowly.
      b. Difficult to see in dim light.
   6. Decreased visual field; less peripheral vision.
   7. Decreased color discrimination on blue/ green end of scale.
   8. Tearing is decreased—"dry" eyes.
E. Changes in vital signs.
   1. Increased systolic and diastolic blood pressure.
   2. Heart and respiratory rate may be unchanged.
   3. Prone to hypothermia.
F. Cardiovascular system.
   1. Heart valves thicken and become rigid; mild fibrosis and calcification.

2. Cardiac output decreases 1 percent per year after age 20 due to decreased heart rate and stroke volume.
3. Vessels lose elasticity.
   a. Less effective peripheral oxygenation.
   b. Position change from lying to sitting or sitting to standing can cause blood pressure to drop up to 65 mm Hg.
4. Blood pressure increases due to increased peripheral vessel resistance.
   a. Systolic may normally be 170.
   b. Diastolic may normally be 95.
   c. Hypertension, over 120/80, common in elderly.
G. Respiratory system.
   1. Respiratory muscles lose strength and become rigid.
   2. Ciliary activity decreases.
   3. Lungs lose elasticity.
      a. Residual capacity increases.
      b. Larger on inspiration.
      c. Maximum breathing capacity decreases; depth of respirations decreases.
   4. Alveoli increase in size, reduce in number.
   5. Arterial blood oxygen pO_2 decreases to 75 mm Hg.
   6. Arterial blood carbon dioxide pCO_2 unchanged.
   7. Coughing ability is reduced.
   8. Decline in immune response.
   9. System less responsive to hypoxia and hypercardia.
   10. Ability to maintain acid-base balance decreases.
H. Gastrointestinal system.
   1. Tooth loss.
      a. Periodontal disease major cause of loss after 30 years of age.
      b. Other causes include poor dental health, poor nutrition.
      c. Gingival retraction.
   2. Taste sensation decreases.
      a. Chronic irritation of mucous membranes.
      b. Atrophy of up to 80 percent of taste buds.
      c. Lose sensitivity of those on tip of tongue first: sweet and salt.
      d. Lose sensitivity of those on sides later: salt, sour, bitter.
   3. Esophagus dilates, motility decreases, lower sphincter pressure decreases.
   4. Stomach.
      a. Hunger and thirst sensations decrease.
      b. Secretion of gastric acid decreases.
      c. Emptying time decreases.
   5. Peristalsis weakens and constipation is common.

6. Absorption function is impaired.
    a. Body absorbs less nutrients due to reduced intestinal blood flow and atrophy of cells on absorbing surfaces.
    b. Decrease in gastric enzymes affects absorption.
7. Liver.
    a. Smaller with decreased storage space.
    b. Decreased blood flow.
    c. Ezymes decrease.
    d. Ability to regenerate decreases.
8. Pancreas.
    a. Ducts become distended.
    b. Lipase production decreases.

I. Genitourinary system.
1. Kidneys.
    a. Smaller due to nephron atrophy.
    b. Renal blood flow decreases 50 percent.
    c. Glomerular filtration rate decreases 50 percent.
    ✦ d. Tubular function diminishes.
        (1) Less able to concentrate urine; lower specific gravity.
        (2) Proteinuria 1+ is common.
        (3) Blood urea nitrogen (BUN) increases to 21 mg%.
    e. Renal threshold for glucose increases.
    f. Potential for dehydration increases.
    g. Excretion of toxins and drugs decreases.
    h. Nocturia, frequency and urgency increases.
✦ 2. Bladder.
    a. Muscle weakens; decreased sphincter control.
    b. Capacity decreases to 200 mL or less, causing frequency.
    c. Emptying is more difficult, causing increased retention.
3. Prostate enlarges to some degree in 75 percent of men over 65; difficulty initiating urine stream.
4. Vulva atrophies.
5. Vagina.
    a. Mucous membrane becomes dryer.
    b. Elastic tissue decreases so surface is smooth.
    c. Secretions become reduced, more alkaline.
    d. Flora changes.
6. Sexuality.
    a. Older people are sexual beings also.
    b. There is no particular age at which a person's sexual functioning ceases.
    c. Frequency of genital sexual behavior (intercourse) may tend to decline gradually in later years, but capacity for expression and enjoyment continues far into old age.

J. Endocrine system.
1. Production of most hormones is reduced.
2. Parathyroid function and secretion are unchanged.
3. Pituitary.
    a. Growth hormone present but in lower blood levels.
    b. Reduced ACTH, TSH, FSH, LH production.
✦ 4. Reduced thyroid activity.
    a. Decreased basal metabolic rate.
    b. Reduced ^{131}I uptake.
5. Reduced aldosterone production.
6. Reduced gonadal secretion of progesterone, estrogen, testosterone.

K. Integumentary system.
1. Skin is less effective as a barrier.
    a. Decreased ability to retain water.
    b. Decreased temperature regulation.
    c. Decreased sensory receptors.
2. Wrinkles due to loss of subcutaneous fat.
3. Scalp hair thins and grays.
4. Hair in nose and ears thickens.
5. Skin composition changes.
    a. Skin pigmentation increases due to clustering of melanocytes.
    b. Elasticity lessens due to decreased hydration and vascularity.
6. Fingernails become hard and brittle.
7. Toenails become overgrown and horny.
8. Sweat glands decrease in number and function.

✦ L. Musculoskeletal system.
1. Bone loses density, brittleness increases.
2. Kyphosis with backward tilt of head occurs.
3. Intervertebral discs narrow, height diminishes by 1–4 inches (2.5–10 cm).
4. Hips, knees, wrists flex.
5. Discs thin so height decreases.
6. Joints enlarge and stiffen.
7. Tendons shrink and sclerose with decrease in tendon jerks.
8. Muscle fibers atrophy.
    a. Person moves more slowly.
    b. Muscle cramps and/or tremors occur.

Psychological Changes

A. Factors that influence these changes.
1. Physiological changes primarily, especially those of the sense organs.
2. General health.
3. Educational level.
4. Heredity.
5. Environment.
B. Drastic personality change is rare.
1. More often honest expression of how one feels.
2. "Rigidity" may be due to other factors such as diseases.
C. Memory.
1. Old memories unchanged.

2. Short-term or recent memory may be poor.
D. Cognitive skills.
    1. Unchanged with information, mathematics, and verbal expressions.
    2. Reduced performance on spatial perceptions and psychomotor skills.

Psychosocial Changes/Adjustments

A. Retirement.
    1. Worth often judged by productivity.
    2. Identity connected to job role.
B. Sense or awareness of mortality.
C. Alteration in living style, i.e., nursing home, moving in with children.
D. Economic deprivation.
    1. Increased cost of living on a fixed income (Social Security).
    2. Increased need for costly medical care.
E. Chronic disease and disability.
F. Social isolation, loneliness.
G. Sensory deprivation (blindness and deafness).
H. Nutritional deprivation.
I. Series of losses, i.e., relationships, friends, family.
J. Loss of physical strength and agility.
    1. Body image altered.
    2. Self-concept altered.
K. Organic brain changes.

Evaluation of the Elderly Patient

Assessment

A. Purpose.
    1. Determine patient's self-care capacities/limitations.
    2. Provide basis for individualized nursing care plan.
    3. Aid in avoiding stereotyping and labeling patient.
    4. Give patient time to answer.
B. Baseline assessment.
    ✦ 1. Temperature.
        a. May be as low as 95°F.
        b. Sublingual most accurate.
    ✦ 2. Pulse.
        a. Rate, rhythm, volume.
        b. Apical (for one minute so premature beats are not missed), radial, pedal, other sites as indicated by disorder.
    3. Respirations.
        a. Rate, rhythm, depth.
        b. Irregularity common.
    ✦ 4. Arterial blood pressure.
        a. Lying, sitting, standing, and in both arms.
        b. Postural hypotension common.
    5. Weight—gradual loss in late years.
    6. Orientation level.
    7. Memory.

8. Sleep pattern.
    a. Sleep disturbance.
    b. Depression–inability to sleep.
9. Psychosocial adjustment.
C. Nervous system.
    1. Facial symmetry.
    2. Level of alertness—presence of organic brain changes.
        a. Not all elderly persons become senile.
        b. Most people have memory impairment.
        c. The change is gradual.
    3. Eyes: movement, clarity, presence of cataracts.
    4. Pupils: equality, dilation, construction, dryness.
    5. Visual acuity—decreases with age.
        a. Do not test facing window.
        b. Use handheld chart.
        c. Check condition of glasses.
    6. Sensory deprivation.
    7. Hearing acuity.
        a. Hearing aid.
        b. Tinnitus.
        c. Cerumen in outer ear—do not clean.
    8. Presence of pain.
D. Cardiovascular system.
    1. Peripheral circulation, color, warmth.
    2. Auscultate apical pulse.
    3. Check for jugular vein distention.
    4. Dizziness.
    5. Fainting.
    6. Edema.
E. Respiratory system.
    1. Chest excursion.
    2. Auscultate chest/lung/breath sounds.
    3. Describe cough, if present; describe sputum.
    4. Rib cage deformity.
F. Gastrointestinal system.
    1. Nutritional status.
    2. Dietary and fluid intake.
    3. Anorexia, indigestion, nausea, vomiting.
    4. Chewing, swallowing.
    5. Condition of teeth, gums, buccal cavity.
    6. Auscultate bowel sounds.
    7. Palpate for distention, dilated colon.
    8. Constipation, diarrhea.
G. Genitourinary system.
    1. Urine: appearance, color, odor.
    2. Bladder distention, incontinence.
    3. Frequency, urgency, hesitancy.
    4. Fluid intake, output.
    5. Dysuria.
    6. Sexuality.
        a. Lack of opportunities for expression.
        b. Social stigma toward activity.
H. Integumentary system.
    1. Skin.
        a. Temperature, degree of moisture.

      b.   Intactness, open lesions, tears.

      c.   Turgor.

      d.   Pigmentation alterations.

  2. Bruises, scars.

  3. Condition of nails.

  4. Condition of hair.

  5. Infestations.

I. Musculoskeletal system.

  1. Contractures.

      a.   Muscle atrophy.

      b.   Tendon shortening.

      c.   Lack of adequate joint motion.

  2. Mobility level.

      a.   Ambulate with or without assistance or devices.

      b.   Limitations to movement.

      c.   Muscle strength.

      d.   Gait.

  3. Range of motion of joints.

  4. Paralysis.

  5. Kyphosis.

J. Psychosocial.

  1. Exhibits increasing dependency.

  2. Concerns focus increasingly on self.

  3. Displays narrower interests.

  4. Needs tangible evidence of affection.

K. Life story.

L. Immunization history.

✦ Implementation

A. Provide adequate lighting.

  1. Natural lighting best.

  2. Avoid glare.

  3. Night-light at all times in bathrooms, halls.

B. Encourage sensory stimulation.

  1. Large-print books.

  2. Changes in environment.

  3. Colors patient can see.

C. Maintain reality orientation.

  1. Calendars.

  2. Clocks.

  3. One-to-one visits.

✦ D. Provide circulatory care.

  1. Avoid tight/restrictive clothing.

  2. Change position, especially from horizontal to vertical.

  3. Provide warmth by applying blankets and clothing.

  4. Encourage activity to increase circulatory stimulation.

  5. Provide support and use safety measures during transfer.

  6. Use gentle friction during bath.

E. Provide respiratory care.

  1. Clean nares if nasal passages are clogged.

  2. Protect from draughts.

  3. Promote respiratory activity with exercises.

      a.   Deep breathing.

      b.   Forced expiration.

      c.   Coughing.

      d.   Inflatable toys.

  4. Oxygen therapy caution: check for carbon dioxide narcosis.

      a.   Confusion.

      b.   Profuse perspiration.

      c.   Visual disturbance.

      d.   Muscle twitching.

      e.   Hypotension.

      f.   Cerebral dysfunction.

F. Provide gastrointestinal care.

  1. Stimulate appetite.

      a.   Small, frequent feedings of high quality.

      b.   Attractive meals.

      c.   Wine, if allowed.

      d.   Female, 1600 calories; male, 2200.

      e.   Hot foods hot; cold foods cold.

      f.   Preferred foods if possible; ethnic choices.

  2. Lessen/prevent indigestion.

      a.   Fowler's position for meals.

      b.   Antacids contraindicated.

      c.   Smaller meals without gas formers.

      d.   Adequate fluids.

  3. Prevent constipation.

      a.   Ensure adequate bulk, and fiber; fluid in diet.

      b.   Encourage activity.

      c.   Ensure regular and adequate time for bowel movement.

      d.   Provide privacy and normal positioning.

      e.   Administer laxative or suppository if above not effective.

✦ G. Provide genitourinary care.

  1. Adequate fluid intake: 2000 to 3000 mL daily.

  2. Incontinence prevention.

      a.   Offer opportunity to void every 2 hours.

      b.   Keep night-light in bathroom to prevent falls.

      c.   Schedule diuretics for maximum effect during daylight hours.

      d.   Limit fluids near and at bedtime.

  3. Sexuality.

      a.   Provide counseling if desired.

      b.   Provide opportunity for desired sexual expression.

      c.   Encourage touching and companionship (important for older people).

✦ H. Provide integumentary care.

  1. Bathing.

      a.   Have patient take complete bath only twice a week due to dryness of skin.

      b.   Use superfatted soap or lotions to aid in moisturizing.

  2. Clip facial hairs for female patients if desired.

3. Handle gently to prevent skin tears, bruising, and pressure ulcers.
4. Cut toenails unless contraindicated.
   a. Mycosis of nails.
   b. Medical/surgical disorder.

I. Provide musculoskeletal care.
1. Ambulate within limitations.
2. Alter position every 2 hours; align correctly.
3. Prevent osteoporosis of long bones by providing exercises against resistance.
4. Provide active and passive exercises.
   a. Rest periods necessary.
   b. Paced throughout the day.
5. Provide range-of-motion exercises to all joints three times a day.
6. Educate family that allowing the patient to be sedentary is not helpful.
7. Encourage walking, which is best single exercise for the elderly.

J. Provide psychosocial care.
1. Encourage psychological activity to aid sense of normality.
2. Encourage life review.
3. Assist in selecting and attending activities.
4. Foster touching, which is a very useful tool in establishing trust.
5. Provide dignity and the feeling of worth.
6. Foster the wellness approach to life.

✦ K. Maintain safety precautions.
1. Siderails when in bed.
   a. Often awaken disoriented for various reasons.
   b. Fall easily due to weakened muscles.
   c. Orthostatic hypotension.
2. Bed in low position when not giving direct patient care.
3. Handrails in bathrooms and halls.
4. Uncluttered rooms and floors.
5. Adequate, nonglare lighting.
6. Restraints when necessary.

COMMON CONDITIONS IN THE AGED

Depression

✦ *Definition:*   State of mind wherein person loses interest in life and finds no pleasure in activities; feels hopeless and sad.

Etiology
A. Reaction to life event.
B. Reaction to environment.

Characteristics
✦ A. Seven to eleven percent of community-based elderly are depressed—1 to 2 percent suffer from major depression.

B. Most commonly ignored disorder in elderly.
C. Course usually 2 weeks to 6 months, varies day to day.

Assessment
A. Mental status examination.
1. Often can answer correctly.
2. Can spell "world" backward.
3. May not try to answer.
B. Major symptoms.
1. Difficulty remembering and concentrating.
2. Poor task performance.
3. Alterations in appetite and weight, sleep patterns.
4. Feels worthless, self-reproach.
5. Loss of motivation, lethargic.

Implementation
✦ A. Safety precautions for suicide risk (75 to 85 year olds, suicide rate is 53:100,000).
✦ B. Antidepressants.
1. Check cautions regarding drug use in the elderly.
2. Few manufacturers have included geriatric dose in literature; start with half dose.
C. *See* specific interventions for depression in Chapter 16.

Dementia

Definition: Acquired impairment of memory and other intellectual abilities secondary to structural brain damage; this damage may be microscopic.

Characteristics
✦ A. Diagnostic criteria—must meet one criterion numbered 1 through 5.
1. Sufficiently severe loss of intellectual abilities to interfere with social or occupational functioning.
2. Memory impairment, usually short-term memory.
3. Impairment of abstract thinking or impaired judgment or disturbance of higher cortical function or personality change.
4. Cloudy state of consciousness.
5. Presence of a specific organic etiology or presumed presence.
B. Onset slow, insidious, unrelated to specific situation.
C. Gradual degeneration.
D. Mental status examination.
1. Early in the disease will attempt to find the right answer.
2. Later will not understand question.
3. The more severe the dementia, the more errors.
✦ E. Symptoms.
1. Paranoid accusations.

2. Personality changes, withdrawn.
3. Confusion noted by others but not by the patient.
4. Unaware of memory loss.
   a. Begins with recent-memory loss.
   b. Later problem with coding and retrieving information.
5. Oblivious to failures.

Dementia, Alzheimer's Type (DAT)

Definition: Degeneration of all layers of the cortex and atrophy of the cerebrum.

Characteristics

A. Etiology is unknown.
B. Most common dementia in the elderly (50 to 70 percent); one in 10 persons over age 65.
C. Incidence in United States is 1.2 million over age 65; by 2050 over 14 million will develop this disease.
D. Diagnosis by exclusion.
   1. No other diagnosis applicable.
   2. Specific data from brain autopsy.
      a. Neurofibrillary tangles.
      b. Neuritic plaques.
      c. Amyloid clusters.

Assessment

A. Possible predisposing factors.
   1. Genetic.
   2. Familial history of Down syndrome.
   3. Enzyme deficiency.
   4. Immune system deficiency.
   5. Slow growing virus.
   6. Aluminum toxicity.
   7. Head trauma.
   8. Acetylcholine (a neurotransmitter) deficiency.
✦ B. Symptoms.
   1. Physical health appears good.
   2. Onset slow; progressive decline.
   3. Restless, irritable.
   4. Aphasia, can produce words but not sentences.
   5. Intellectual impairment.
   6. Disoriented to person, place, and time.
   7. Motor ability declines.
   8. Incontinent.
   9. Doesn't recognize staff or family.

Implementation

✦ A. Institute safety precautions.
B. Verbal communication
   1. Use short words, simple sentences, verbs and nouns.
   2. Call patient by name and identify yourself.
   3. Speak slowly, clearly; wait for response.
   4. Ask only one question, give one direction at a time.

✦ THREE CLINICAL STAGES OF DAT

- Early stage: patient is forgetful, confused, irritable and family begins to notice changes.
- Middle stage: increased memory loss, recall of recent events diminishes, ADLs become difficult to accomplish. Aggressiveness and social inappropriateness present. Wandering increases.
- Late stage: severely disoriented, delusional and paranoid. Patient may not speak, forgets family members and becomes increasingly helpless.

---

   5. Repeat, do not rephrase.
C. Nonverbal communication.
   1. Use gestures, move slowly.
   2. Stand directly in front of patient, maintain eye contact.
   3. Move or walk with patient.
   4. Listen actively; show interest.
   5. Chart all phrases and nonverbal techniques used and use those that "work."
D. Maintain the patient's physical activity within limits of safety.
   1. Walk outside if grounds are fenced, alarmed, or if accompanied.
   2. Exercises with simple commands.
   3. Active games.
   4. Balance activities, dance.
   5. Activities of daily living.
E. Mental stimulation.
   1. Simple hobbies.
   2. One-to-one contact.
   3. Reality orientation.
   4. Play word, number games.
F. Encourage self-care, give cues. Pantomime brushing teeth instead of brushing patient's teeth.
G. Put families in touch with support groups such as Alzheimer's Disease and Related Disorders Association, Inc. (ADRDA) chapters.

Associated Degenerative Diseases

✦ A. Multi-infarct dementia.
   1. Second most common dementia in the elderly.
   2. Focal neurological signs and symptoms.
   3. History of significant cerebrovascular disease.
✦ B. Korsakoff's syndrome.
   1. Varied symptoms associated with chronic alcoholism.
   2. Often associated with Wernicke's encephalopathy.
C. Dementia with Lewy Bodies (DLB).
   1. This form of dementia is named for the development of lewy bodies in the cerebral cortex.
      a. The appearance of parkinsonism symptoms caused by effects on the extrapyramidal tract of the CNS.

b. Symptoms include intermittent confusion, lapses of consciousness and psychiatric problems.

2. Patients may have this form of dementia alone (less common) or concurrent with DAT (20 to 30%).

D. Creutzfeldt-Jakob Disease.
   1. Suspected cause is an infection of a prion spread after transplant (cornea) or injection of human growth hormone.
   2. A new variant of this disease known as mad cow disease (bovine spongiform encephalopathy or BSE) was identified in 1996 and may be linked to eating contaminated beef.

E. Vascular dementia.
   1. Type of dementia involving intermittent emboli or infarcts that destroy brain tissue.
   2. This form accounts for about 19% of dementias.
   3. Characteristics include abrupt onset with numerous remissions and exacerbations; patient may also have a history of diseases affecting other organs.

F. Huntington's chorea—genetically transmitted disorder.
   1. Characterized by onset of symptoms after the age of 30.
   2. Progressive mental and physical deterioration is inevitable.

G. Paresis—central nervous system degeneration caused by invasion of brain cells from *Treponema pallidum* (syphilis).
   1. Infection may have occurred much earlier but remained untreated by penicillin.
   2. Symptoms reflect general brain disorder deterioration.

Implementation

A. Meet both physical and psychological needs.
B. Help patient maintain contact with reality.
   1. Give feedback.
   2. Avoid chatter.
   3. Personalize interaction.
   4. Supply stimulation to motivate patient.
   5. Keep patient from becoming bored and distracted.
C. Assist patient in accepting the diagnosis.
   1. Be supportive.
   2. Maintain good communication.
   3. During denial phase, listen and accept; do not argue.
   4. Assist development of awareness.
   5. Help patient develop the ability to cope with his or her altered identity.
D. Focus of interactions with patient.
   1. Conduct short, frequent contacts with patient.
   2. Use concrete ideas in communicating with the patient.

PSYCHOLOGICAL REACTIONS TO BRAIN SYNDROME DISORDERS

- Changes in self-concept.
- Anger and frustration as reactions to forced changes in various life roles.
- Denial used as a defense.
- Depression.
- Limitations accepted.
- "Sick" role assumed.
  a. Becomes dependent.
  b. Lacks motivation.

---

3. Maintain a reality orientation by allowing the patient to talk about his or her past and to confabulate.
4. Acknowledge the patient as an individual.

E. Provide a safe, stable, consistent environment.
F. Assess the patient's disabilities, and help to develop a nursing plan to deal with them.
G. Become a member of the rehabilitation team.

Urinary Incontinence

Definition: Involuntary release of urine of such severity as to have social and/or hygienic consequences.

Characteristics

A. Ten million adults are incontinent—over half the residents of nursing homes and one-third of elderly living at home are affected.
B. Prevalence rises with age.
C. This condition is not a normal consequence of aging; it is a symptom signaling the presence of other problems.
✦ D. Types.
   1. *Stress incontinence*—result of sudden increase in intra-abdominal pressure, which pushes urine out of the bladder.
   2. *Urge incontinence*—leakage of urine before one reaches the toilet, usually caused by uncontrolled contraction of the bladder.
   3. *Overflow incontinence*—constant dribble of urine results when bladder is not completely emptied during voiding.
   4. *Functional incontinence*—nonorganic; impaired mobility, depression, and dementia can prevent patient from reaching bathroom.

Assessment

A. Pattern of problem—*see* types of incontinence.
   1. Decreased bladder tone/volume.
   2. Muscle tone—urgency and frequency.
B. Presence of other problems, disease states, or change in physical health.
   1. Congestive heart failure.
   2. Urinary tract infection.

3. Pneumonia.
4. Stool impaction.
C. Effects of medication(s).
D. Environmental problems.
1. Access to toilet.
2. Restraints.
3. Privacy.
4. Response of staff/family.
E. Skin condition.
F. Emotional coping in relation to the problem.

Treatment and Implementation

◆ A. Monitor drug therapy.
1. Anticholinergic (Pro-Banthine).
2. Antispasmodic (Ditropan) to inhibit bladder contractions.
B. Postop care following surgery to strengthen pelvic muscles, repair a damaged urethra, remove an obstruction.
C. Provide appropriate skin care.
D. Establish toileting schedule.
1. Easy access.
2. Appropriate clothing, patient's own, if possible.
◆ E. Assist patient to learn Kegel exercises.
1. Will help to control stress and urge incontinence.
2. Steps are to contract pubococcygeus muscle, hold contraction for 10 seconds, relax for 10 seconds. Work up to 25 repetitions three times a day.
F. Provide protection plan for accidents.
1. Accidents are embarrassing and often limit excursions and social activities.
2. Prevent problems and avoid disrupting patient's life.
G. Devise ways to build patient's self-esteem.
1. Positive reinforcement.
2. Plan activities that patient can enjoy.

PROBLEM AREAS FOR ELDERLY PATIENTS

Impaired Mobility–Disability

Definition: The elderly can suffer impaired mobility and disability due to decreased physical function and/or accidents.

Characteristics

A. Nearly 23 percent of older people living in the community have some degree of disability.
1. Those 85 and older constitute a disproportionate share of those who are dependent in physical functioning.
2. Those 85 and older constitute 27 percent of those who have impaired mobility.

◆ B. Impaired mobility can lead to many subsequent problems: depression, negative self-image, dependent behavior, loss of independence, etc.
C. Effects of disability.
1. Impact upon the individual's body image.
a. Physical appearance.
b. Bodily sensations.
2. Behavior during reaction period.
a. Appears confused and disorganized.
b. Denies disability exists.
c. Overreacts to situations and physical condition.
d. Assumes false positive attitude.
e. Becomes self-centered.
f. Becomes depressed.
g. Mourns loss of function or body part.
3. Adaptation and adjustment.
a. Revises body image by modifying former picture of self.
b. Reorganizes values.
c. Accepts degree of dependency.
d. Accepts limitations imposed by disability.
e. Begins to develop realistic goals.

Assessment

A. Specific source of disability or impaired mobility.
B. Presence of accompanying disease state: arthritis, stroke, dementia, diabetes, CHF, COPD.
C. Strength and function of limbs and joints.
D. Stability of gait.
E. Presence of pain.
F. Condition of skin.
G. Drug effects—sedation, incontinence, orthostatic hypotension.
H. Motivation for rehabilitation.
I. Nutritional status.
J. History of falls.

Implementation

A. Develop nursing care plan to meet patient's needs.
B. Focus on disability or impaired mobility.
C. Establish supportive relationship.
◆ D. Teach activities of daily living.
1. Activities that must be accomplished each day for the individual to care for own needs and be as independent as possible.
2. Ascertain best assistive aid for patient.
3. Demonstrate and encourage individual to practice.
4. Increase activities as individual progresses and is able to assume activity.
5. Give positive reinforcement for all effort expended.
◆ E. Prevent deformities and complications.
1. Turn and position in good alignment.
a. Prevent contractures.

b. Stimulate circulation.

c. Prevent thrombophlebitis.

d. Prevent pressure ulcers.

2. Prevent edema of extremities.

3. Promote lung expansion.

Sensory Impairment

A. Elderly experience loss of function in the senses.

1. Ability to taste declines after age 40; taste buds are fewer in number, and there is less saliva flow.

2. Ability to smell declines.

3. Hearing fades, especially in high-frequency ranges.

4. Regulation of body temperature is less efficient.

✦ B. Major diseases or degeneration of organs occurs.

1. Vision loss—*See* eye conditions in Medical–Surgical Nursing Implications.

a. Glaucoma—increased pressure causes damage to optic nerve, leading to blindness.

b. Cataracts—clouding of the lens leading to blurred vision.

c. Retinal detachment.

d. Macular degeneration—macula cells fail to function, which causes loss of central vision.

✦ 2. Hearing loss—*See* ear surgery in Medical–Surgical Nursing Implications.

a. Otosclerosis requiring a stapedectomy.

b. Hearing loss due to accumulation of earwax—requires periodic irrigation of auditory canal.

Nutrition

A. Physiological requirements change (decrease) with age.

1. Nutrition intake must meet two major demands.

a. Normal structural repair.

b. Energy production for functional needs.

2. Met by protein and amino acids and adequate calorie intake.

B. Many elderly do not feel thirsty; thus, they do not drink adequate water—dehydration is common.

✦ C. Many elderly are deficient in nutrients, especially protein, B vitamins, vitamins A and C, iron, and calcium.

1. Change in diet often responsible.

a. Senses of taste and smell decrease, thus less conscious of hunger.

b. Teeth in poor condition or dentures don't work properly.

c. Physical disabilities or lack of mobility, unable to buy groceries.

d. Loss of interest in eating.

e. Limited income affects buying nutritious food.

2. System cannot assimilate nutrients as well as when younger.

a. Reduced hydrochloric acid, reduced stomach activity.

b. Decreased salivary flow.

D. Health status affects nutritional state.

1. Chronic diseases: heart disease, cancer, diabetes, gastrointestinal problems, etc.

2. Drugs: antacids, antidepressants, anticonvulsants, cathartics, diuretics, antimicrobials, etc.

E. Decreased physical activity and metabolic changes reduce caloric needs.

F. Financial resources, emotional and physical state affect nutritional status.

Assessment

A. Hydration status, body weight, edema.

B. Anemia.

C. Appetite.

D. Ability to feed self—physical and mental.

1. Dentition.

2. Mastication.

3. Swallowing.

4. Desire to eat.

E. Fatigue, energy reserve.

F. Constipation.

G. Compliance to special diets.

H. Effects of drugs on nutrition.

1. Gastrointestinal irritation.

2. Food–drug interactions.

3. Some drug side effects are nausea and vomiting.

I. Skin and mucous membrane condition.

Implementation

A. Offer/give oral fluids in small amounts every hour.

B. Plan diet to be high in nutrients.

1. Give foods with high fiber content.

2. Balance of vitamins and minerals.

3. Use lemon, vinegar, herbs on foods (rather than salt) to stimulate appetite.

C. Devise tools and plates that assist self-feeding.

D. Serve meals with others present to reduce isolation.

✦ Elder Abuse and Neglect

Characteristics

A. Over 1 million older adults are estimated to be abused or neglected. Abuse occurs in about 2% of the population.

◆ B. Forms of elder abuse.
1. Physical:intentionally inflicted injury or pain.
2. Emotional: verbal harassment, intimidation, denigration, or isolation.
3. Neglect:deteriorating health, dehydration, malnutrition, failure to provide food or services or care necessary to maintain health and safety; pressure ulcers, dirt, body odor, over- or undermedication.
4. Financial: improper or unauthorized use of funds or property or power of attorney.

C. Suspect abuse if patient has unexplained injuries or conflicting stories from patient and caregiver.
◆ 1. Abuse associated with substance abuse, depression, caregiver strain.
2. Typical victim is older woman, widowed, Caucasian, low income and dependent on abuser for some aspect of care.

D. Abuse is seldom reported to authorities, even though pattern is often repeated.

E. All states have enacted elder abuse laws designed to protect older or vulnerable adults from abuse.

◆ F. Majority of states require nurses and other health care providers to report cases of suspected elder abuse.
1. Standard for reporting is "reasonable" belief.
2. Most states provide immunity from civil and criminal liability.
3. Support suspicions with documentation and witnesses.

◆ **Assessment**
A. Ask patient and caregiver to explain injury.
1. If patient appears to be a victim, separate from caregiver and question.
2. Follow up by documenting and report according to facility policy.

B. Assess physical injuries for abuse.
1. Multiple injuries or fractures.
2. Bruises or burns.
3. Sprains or dislocations (frequent falls).

C. Assess for neglect.
1. Deteriorating health, failure to thrive.
2. Dehydration or malnutrition.
3. Pressure ulcers.
4. Over- or undermedication.

D. Question patient about emotional or financial abuse.

Implementation
◆ A. Report all cases of suspected elder abuse even if there is no direct evidence—just a "reasonable" belief abuse is present.

B. Promote family problem-solving actions to resolve situation.

Medications

◆ A. Twenty-five percent of all prescriptive drugs are used by the elderly, and this does not include over-the-counter drugs.

B. Eighty percent of people age 65 and over have at least one chronic medical problem that requires medications (one-third have three or more chronic problems).

C. The typical elderly American takes between four and seven prescription drugs each day in addition to over-the-counter drugs.

D. Elderly (13 percent of the population) suffer 50 percent of all drug side effects (estimated 17 per 100,000 population).
◆ 1. Increased risk for drug toxicity.
a. Renal excretion altered—kidneys cannot process drugs as well.
b. Liver enzymes altered.
c. Diminished blood circulation to liver.
d. Receiving multiple drugs that compete for binding and interact.
e. CNS more sensitive to drugs.
(1) Drugs interfere with neurotransmitters (chemicals) that regulate brain function.
(2) Side effects result in confusion in elderly.
f. Altered body mass and ratio of fat to muscle.
g. Elderly receive greater peak and longer duration of action from analgesics than younger adults.
2. Iatrogenic illness can be caused by drug therapy.
3. Most commonly abused drugs.
a. Tranquilizers most frequently abused.
b. Sleeping pills.
c. Medications to control pain.
d. Laxatives.

E. Major problems with prescriptive drugs in the elderly.
◆ 1. Drug interactions—people who use multiple physicians and pharmacies run risk of taking drugs that interact to cause adverse reactions.
2. Medication errors—the more medications a person takes, the greater the risk of medication error (people over age 75 take an average of 17 prescriptions annually).
3. Opioids—produce greater analgesic effect in elderly.
◆ a. Opioid therapy should be initiated with 25–50% lower dose than that given to adults.
◆ b. Monitor for respiratory depression and reduced arterial O_2 saturation in elderly.

c. Monitor for other side effects: sedation, hypotension, urinary retention, constipation, etc.

✦ 4. Noncompliance—not taking right dose at right time or discontinuing drug without consultation; common due to lack of understanding about reason to take drug and general knowledge base of drug action.

5. Unpredictable drug action—physiological changes in the elderly associated with age and disease may alter effects of the drugs.

6. Drug side effects not recognized—elderly not aware or do not understand potential dangerous side effects of drugs.

7. Inadequate monitoring—elderly often alone or not monitored consistently so drug problems are not identified.

8. Cost of drugs—multiple medications are costly for many elderly, so they stop taking drugs.

F. Elderly often receive less analgesic medications, which may lead to inadequate pain relief.

Administration of Medications

A. Oral route.
  1. Check for mouth dryness.
     a. Drug may stick and dissolve in mouth.
     b. Drug may irritate mucous membrane.
  2. Place patient in sitting position.
  3. Crush tablets if they are very large.
  4. Do not open capsules.
  5. Do not crush enteric-coated tablets.
  6. Check with pharmacy for liquid preparations if patient has difficulty swallowing tablets.

B. Suppository.
  1. Position for comfort.
  2. May take longer to dissolve due to decreased body core temperature.
  3. Do not insert suppository immediately after removing from refrigerator.

C. Parenteral.
  1. Site may ooze medication or bleed due to decreased tissue elasticity.
  2. Do not use immobile limb.
  3. Danger of overhydration with IV.

D. Self-administration.
  1. Check compliance with amounts and times.
  2. Color code to facilitate proper administration.

Assessment

A. Changes in mental status.
B. Vital signs.
  1. Orthostatic blood pressure.
  2. Apical pulse.
C. Urine production, retention.
D. Hydration and appetite.
E. Visual disturbances.
F. Swallowing ability.
G. Evaluate effects of drug.
  1. Laboratory studies.
  2. Signs and symptoms for toxic/interaction effects of drugs.
H. Bowel function.
I. Effects of nutrition and foods on drug response.

Implementation

✦ A. No alcohol or alcohol-based elixirs when receiving benzodiazepines or antihistamines.
B. Method of administering drugs.
  1. Deep breathing and relaxation to reduce use of analgesic drugs.
  2. Position patient sitting with head slightly flexed to reduce chance of aspiration.
✦ C. Administering tablets.
  1. Do not crush time-released or enteric-coated tablets.
  2. Crush large tablets if not contraindicated.
  3. Give with textured foods (nectar, applesauce) if not contraindicated.
D. Stroke victim—give drug on functional side of mouth.

Drug–Food Interactions for Elderly

A. Certain foods, vitamins/minerals, and natural remedies can interfere with therapeutic effects of drugs.
  1. Reduce absorption of drug.
  2. Interfere with cellular action.
✦ B. Medication regimen affected by nutrition may put patient at risk.
  1. Important to assess patient's diet.
  2. Monitor potential vitamin–drug interactions.
  3. Monitor for nutrient depletion (vitamin B) caused by certain drugs.
C. Review patient's prescriptive and over-the-counter drugs.
  1. Review in relation to normal dietary intake.
  2. Consider vitamin/mineral intake and supplements in terms of decreasing effect of medications.
  3. Check lab values for problems.
✦ D. Review herbs patient is taking because interaction with medications may be dangerous. (See Drug-Herb table in Pharmacology chapter.)
E. Document findings so health care team is informed of diet–drug plan.
✦ F. Food sources of vitamins and minerals.
  1. Folic acid sources: liver, kidney, fresh vegetables.
  2. Niacin sources: yeast, meat, fish, milk, eggs, green vegetables, and cereal grains.
  3. Pantothenic acid sources: meat, vegetables, cereal grains, legumes, eggs, milk, fish, and fruit.

4. Pyridoxine hydrochloride (vitamin B_6) sources: cereal grains, legumes, vegetables, liver, meat, and eggs.
5. Cyanocobalamin (vitamin B_{12}) sources: animal foods, liver, kidney, fish, shellfish, meat, and dairy foods.
6. Ascorbic acid (vitamin C) sources: fresh fruits and vegetables.
7. Vitamin A sources: eggs, milk, cream, butter, organ meats, fish.
8. Vitamin D source: activated in body by sunlight.
9. Vitamin E sources: vegetable oils, whole grains, animal fats, eggs, and green vegetables.
10. Vitamin K sources: green leafy vegetables, spinach, broccoli, cabbage, and liver.

LAB VALUES—ELDERLY PATIENTS

✦ Urinalysis

A. Protein.
   1. Normal 0–5 mg/100 mL—rises slightly.
   2. May reflect changes in kidney or subclinical urinary tract infection.
B. Glucose.
   1. Normal 0–15 mg/100 mL—declines slightly.
   2. May reflect changes in kidney.
C. Specific gravity.
   1. 1.010—changes to 1.024 by age 80 (which means elderly have more concentrated urine).
   2. Thirty to 50 percent decline in number of nephrons affects ability to concentrate urine.

✦ Hematology

A. Hemoglobin.
   1. Men 13–18 g/100 mL—drops to 10–17 g/100 mL.
   2. Women 12–16 g/100 mL—no change.
B. Hematocrit.
   1. Men 45 to 52 percent—no change.
   2. Women 37 to 48 percent—no change.
C. Leukocytes.
   1. 4300–10,800/mm^3—drops to 3100–9000/mm^3.
   2. As bone marrow diminishes, hematopoiesis declines.
D. Lymphocytes.
   1. 500–2400/mm—T lymphocytes fall.
   2. 50–200/mm^3—B lymphocytes fall.
E. Platelets, prothrombin time (PT), and partial thromboplastin time (PTT)—no change.

✦ Blood Chemistry Tests That Change with Age

A. Blood urea nitrogen (BUN).
   1. Men 10–25 mg/100 mL—increases, may be as high as 69 mg/100 mL.
   2. Women 8–20 mg/100 mL—increases.
   3. Renal function decreased due to decline in cardiac output, renal blood flow, and glomerular filtration rate.
B. Creatinine.
   1. 0.6–1.5 mg/100 mL—increases as high as 1.9 mg/100 mL in men and women.
   2. Endogenous creatinine production as lean body mass shrinks.
   3. Drugs excreted by urinary system may cause toxicity if creatinine level too high.
C. Creatinine clearance.
   1. 104–132 mL/min.
   2. Referenced interval—men's formula for age: 140 – age × kg body weight ÷ 72 × serum creatinine.
   ✦ 3. Reduced levels may result in toxicity when drugs are excreted by the kidneys.
D. Glucose tolerance.
   1. 1 hour: 160–170 mg/100 mL.
      2 hours: 115–125 mg/100 mL.
      3 hours: 70–110 mg/100 mL.
   2. With age, results rise more quickly in first 2 hours, then drop to baseline more slowly.
   3. Alcohol, MAO inhibitors, and beta blockers can all cause a rapid fall in glucose.
E. Fasting serum glucose.
   1. 70–115 mg/dL increases with age.
   2. Elderly more prone to glucose intolerance and diabetes.
F. Thyroxine (T_4) 4.5–13.5 µg/100 mL, and triiodothyronine (T_3) 90–220 mg/100 mL; both decrease by 25 percent.

TEACHING GOOD HEALTH CONCEPTS TO THE ELDERLY

A. Regular exercise—elderly must continue to exercise regularly to maintain health (can increase function by 50 percent through exercise).
B. Nutritious diet—intake of adequate nutrients and calories to maintain body.
   1. Malnutrition in elderly contributes to high incidence of chronic disease.
   2. Obesity contributes to increased health risks (heart disease, hypertension).
   3. Diet adequate to maintain normal body weight, low fat, and include all four food groups for minimal nutrients, vitamins, and minerals.
C. No smoking—smokers die earlier than nonsmokers and have a higher incidence of heart disease, heart attack, cancer, and chronic lung disease.
D. Moderate alcohol intake—high alcohol intake is a health risk that leads to liver disease, nervous system damage, gastrointestinal problems.

E. Prevention of health problems—yearly physical examinations are important for the elderly to diagnose early disease process.
1. Check warning signs of cancer, heart disease (hypertension).
2. Pap smear and mammogram for women as precaution against cancer.

F. Managing stress—stress is associated with increased incidence of heart disease, hypertension, cancer, and other diseases.

G. Maintain contact with friends for support—studies show that isolated elders have more health problems and die earlier than people who have close attachments.

GERIATRIC NURSING QUESTIONS

1. An elderly patient has been admitted to the orthopedic unit with an intracapsular fracture of the right hip sustained after a fall on the ice. Buck's extension is applied, and arrangements are being made for hip prosthesis surgery in the morning. The purpose for the application of Buck's extension at this time is to

   1. Reduce the fracture.
   2. Relieve muscle spasms.
   3. Keep the knee extended.
   4. Stabilize the fractured hip.

2. An elderly patient with infectious hepatitis (hepatitis A) and his family are being instructed by the nurse in prevention techniques. The single most important action to prevent this disease is

   1. Not to eat out in public places.
   2. Good personal hygiene.
   3. Thorough handwashing.
   4. Active immunization.

3. The signs of pacemaker malfunction that the nurse would include in discharge teaching for a patient with a new pacemaker are

   1. Increased urine output, headache.
   2. Regular, slow pulse.
   3. Weakness, fatigue.
   4. Disorientation, confusion.

4. An elderly patient with heart disease has orders for daily diuretics. Serum potassium levels should be evaluated for a patient on diuretics. If the potassium level were low, the nurse would expect to find

   1. Dyspnea.
   2. Skeletal muscle weakness.
   3. Hypertension.
   4. Headache.

5. A 70-year-old patient with organic brain syndrome, dementia type, is frequently incontinent, even when he is fully dressed. An initial plan to deal with this behavior is to

   1. Remind the patient to tell the nurse when he has to urinate.
   2. Put the patient in diapers.
   3. Take the patient to the bathroom on a 2-hour schedule.

   4. Tell the patient that he must remember to go to the bathroom before he wets his pants.

6. After a Foley catheter was inserted for 2 days, it was removed by the nurse. The nurse will evaluate for the response considered to be normal at this time, which would be

   1. Dribbling after the first several voidings.
   2. Urgency and frequency for several days.
   3. Frequent voidings in small amounts.
   4. Retention of urine for 10- to 12-hour periods.

7. An elderly female patient with newly diagnosed osteoporosis requires counseling prior to discharge. The most important components of the discharge plan are

   1. Instruction in safety factors to prevent injury.
   2. Monitoring medications.
   3. Instruction in regular exercise and diet.
   4. Appropriate use of body mechanics.

8. A 63-year-old male patient with a history of alcohol abuse has been admitted with a diagnosis of acute pancreatitis. After completing data collection, the priority nursing diagnosis would be

   1. Deficient fluid volume due to fluid losses into body spaces.
   2. Impaired oxygenation due to rapid respirations.
   3. Risk for infection due to decreased immune response.
   4. Imbalanced nutrition, less than requirements, due to decreased intake.

9. A 78-year-old patient who suffered a cerebrovascular accident (CVA) is in a long-term facility. She has developed a pressure ulcer. The nurse is applying a wet-to-damp dressing. The rationale for using this type of dressing is to

   1. Prevent the dressing from leaking on the bedclothes.
   2. Prevent damage to granulating tissue when removing the dressing.
   3. Enable the dressing to almost dry on the ulcer to promote healing.
   4. Assist in debriding the wound.

10. A 60-year-old female patient has received the diagnosis of hypertension. Her blood pressure is

160/100. Which of the following symptoms would the nurse expect to find during data collection?

1. Dizziness and flushed face.
2. Drowsiness and confusion.
3. Faintness when getting out of bed.
4. Ataxia and tachycardia.

11. A patient in a long-term care facility has the diagnosis of Alzheimer's disease. His care plan should include the goal of assisting him to participate in activities that provide him a chance to

1. Interact with other patients.
2. Compete with others.
3. Succeed at something.
4. Get a sense of continuity.

12. A 72-year-old patient diagnosed with Ménière's disease has been admitted to the medical–surgical unit. He asks the nurse if he can get up and go to the bathroom any time he needs to. The most appropriate response is

1. "Yes, whenever you wish, you may go."
2. "No, you are on strict bedrest."
3. "Please ring for assistance when you wish to get out of bed."
4. "We will have to check with the physician."

13. Oxygen is ordered for a 70-year-old patient hospitalized for heart failure. Which of the following methods of administration will deliver the highest concentration of oxygen?

1. Venturi mask.
2. Nasal prongs.
3. Oxygen catheter.
4. Mask with reservoir bag.

14. After the patient has recovered from coronary bypass surgery, her physician has advised a low-cholesterol diet. The nurse will know that the patient understands this diet when she includes foods such as

1. Meats, especially organ meats, and dairy products.
2. Eggs, cheese, fruits, and vegetables.
3. Vegetables, fruits, lean meats, and vegetable oils.
4. Raw or cooked vegetables, fruits, and red meat.

15. An elderly patient is in a long-term care facility. She had a left-sided CVA 4 weeks ago and has been bedridden since that time. A sign or symptom indicating a possible complication of immobility is

1. A reddened area over the sacrum.
2. Stiffness in the left leg.

3. Difficulty moving her left arm.
4. Difficulty hearing low voices.

16. A patient, age 70, is admitted with the diagnosis of organic brain syndrome, dementia type. Assessing his condition, the nurse would expect that his prognosis would be

1. Good, because the condition tends to be reversible.
2. Unpredictable because the condition may reverse.
3. Poor because symptoms are reduced intellectual capacity, emotional stability, memory, and judgment.
4. Poor because the condition will rapidly progress.

17. An 87-year-old patient is admitted to the hospital complaining of weakness and shortness of breath. Her diagnosis is heart failure. As the nurse is assessing the patient's condition, which of the following signs will indicate that she is in left-sided heart failure?

1. Fatigue, dyspnea, and wheezing.
2. Hepatomegaly and oliguria.
3. Increased pulmonary artery pressure.
4. Peripheral edema such as sacral edema.

18. The visiting home health nurse is assigned to a patient who just had cataract surgery. A care plan would include instructions to

1. Maintain bedrest for at least 2 days with bathroom privileges only.
2. Keep the head up and straight and not to look down.
3. Deep breathe and cough four times a day.
4. Lie only on the affected side when in bed.

19. Instructing a 60-year-old patient with long-term diabetes on preventing chronic complications of retinopathy or nephropathy, an important principle to teach is to

1. Visit the physician frequently for checkups.
2. Obtain frequent lab values of BUN and creatinine.
3. Complete frequent blood glucose testing.
4. Maintain stable blood glucose levels.

20. The nurse is assessing a 75-year-old patient who is taking digitalis. Assessing for digitalis toxicity, the nurse would identify

1. Anorexia, nausea, vomiting.
2. Diarrhea, headache, vertigo.
3. Nausea, vomiting, diarrhea.
4. Vomiting, diarrhea, vertigo.

GERIATRIC NURSING

Answers with Rationale

1. (2) The purpose of Buck's extension application following hip fracture is immobilization to relieve muscle spasm at the fracture site and thereby relieve pain. Any movement of fracture fragments will aggravate severe muscle spasm and pain. Skin traction such as this is not used to reduce a fracture (1) and it is not important to keep the knee extended (3). Bryant's or Russell's traction will stabilize a fractured femur, not the hip (4).

    NP:P; CN:PH; CA:S; CL:C

2. (3) Thorough handwashing is the most important action to prevent the transmission of hepatitis A. Good personal hygiene (2) is also important, but it does not replace handwashing. Contaminated food (1) is a mode of transmission. Passive immunization is prevention.

    NP:I; CN:S; CA:M; CL:K

3. (3) Weakness and fatigue are symptoms that indicate hypoxia to the tissues. The patient should be taught to recognize these as symptoms of pacemaker malfunction.

    NP:E; CN:PH; CA:M; CL:A

4. (2) Skeletal muscle weakness is a result of low potassium levels in the blood; potassium is required for normal muscle function. Hypotension may occur, as well as cardiac arrhythmias and tachycardia. Dyspnea (1) and headache (4) are specific indications of hypokalemia.

    NP:E; CN: PH; CA:M; CL:A

5. (3) Because the patient cannot remember to tell the nurse or remember himself to go to the bathroom, the best plan is to take him on a schedule. This is preferable to dressing him in diapers (2), even though this may eventually have to be done.

    NP:P; CN:PS; CA:PS; CL:AN

6. (1) Dribbling may be normal until the sphincter muscles regain their tone. If the catheter had been in place for several weeks, (3) might have been the most appropriate response. Urgency and frequency (2) are symptoms of a bladder infection.

    NP:E; CN:PH; CA:M; CL:C

7. (3) This is a new diagnosis, so regular exercise (especially weight-bearing) and a diet high in protein, calcium, and vitamin D, with avoidance of alcohol and coffee, are the most important components of the plan to prevent extension of the condition.

    NP:P; CN:H; CA:M; CL:C

8. (1) Because of the autodigestion of pancreatic and surrounding tissue, there is interstitial hemorrhage, local vascular drainage, increased vascular permeability, and vasodilation. Fluid loss will lead to fluid volume deficit. The patient will be placed on bedrest, a nasogastric tube inserted, and analgesics will be used liberally for extreme pain.

    NP:P; CN:PS; CA:PS; CL:AN

9. (2) Wet-to-damp dressings prevent damage to new tissue when the dressing is removed. A wet-to-dry dressing debrides the wound (4). This dressing is not to prevent leaking (1), and allowing the dressing to almost dry (3) will not support new tissue.

    NP:P; CN:PH; CA:M; CL:C

10. (1) Cardinal symptoms are dizziness and flushed face as well as headache, tinnitus, and epistaxis. Drowsiness and confusion (2) occur in hypertensive crisis, and faintness (3) would occur in hypotension.

    NP:D; CN:PH; CA:M; CL:C

11. (3) It is essential that the patient participate in activities that provide him with immediate success and increase his self-esteem. Interaction with oth-

---

Coding for Questions/Answers Abbreviations: **Nursing Process: NP,** Data Collection: D, Planning: P, Implementation: I, Evaluation: E, **Client Needs: CN,** Safe, Effective Care Environment: S, Health Promotion and Maintenance: H, Psychosocial Integrity: PS, Physiological Integrity: PH, **Clinical Area: CA,** Medical Nursing: M, Surgical Nursing: S, Maternal/Newborn Nursing: MA, Pediatric Nursing: P, Psychiatric Nursing: PS, **Cognitive Level: CL,** Knowledge: K, Comprehension: C, Application: A, Analysis: AN

ers (1) is important but is secondary to improving his self-esteem.

NP:P; CN:PS; CA: PS; CL:C

12. (3)   The patient may be on bedrest (although not strict) due to the extreme vertigo he may experience. Because of the dizziness, he should ring for assistance if he does wish to get up to go to the bathroom. This is a safety intervention to prevent the patient from falling.

NP:I; CN:S; CA:M; CL:A

13. (4)   A liter flow of 8 to 10 will provide an FIO_2 of 70 to 100 percent. The reservoir bag contains a high level of oxygen. As the patient inhales, oxygen is taken in from the bag. The Venturi mask (1) delivers a fixed FIO_2, usually 24 to 35 percent. A 38 to 44% FIO_2 is the maximum amount of oxygen delivered through prongs (2).

NP:D; CN:PH; CA:M; CL:K

14. (3)   These food choices will provide the lowest cholesterol content. Whole milk, dairy products, and fatty meats are all high in cholesterol.

NP:E; CN:PH; CA:M; CL:C

15. (1)   A reddened area over the sacrum may be the first sign of a pressure ulcer. If it is recognized at this stage and nursing actions are taken to avoid additional pressure (frequent turning, massaging the skin, etc.), the ulcer may be prevented. Answers (2) and (3) can be expected with left-sided CVA and (4) is usually an expected development with an elderly person.

NP:E; CN:PH; CA:M; CL:A

16. (3)   Dementia has a poor prognosis, is usually progressive and irreversible, and the symptoms are closely related to the patient's basic personality. All of the characteristics in (3) fit the picture of organic brain syndrome. The condition may or may not progress rapidly (4), but will generally deteriorate.

NP:D; CN:PS; CA:PS; CL:K

17. (1)   In left-sided heart failure, congestion occurs mainly in the lungs. It is caused by inadequate ejection of the blood into the systemic circulation. Dyspnea, sneezing, coughing, rales, and fatigue are common symptoms. The other answers refer to right-sided failure.

NP:D; CN:PH; CA:M; CL:C

18. (2)   Keeping the head straight and avoiding looking down will prevent increasing intraocular pressure. The nurse would practice breathing exercises with the patient but will not encourage coughing (3), as this could cause an increase in intraocular pressure in the operative eye.

NP:P; CN:PH; CA:S; CL:A

19. (4)   The most important principle to teach the patient is the necessity of maintaining stable blood glucose levels. Frequent testing is part of the picture (3), but unless the levels are stabilized, testing itself is not enough.

NP:I; CN:H; CA:M; CL:C

20. (1)   Anorexia is the initial symptom associated with digitalis toxicity. Nausea and vomiting are very common symptoms also.

NP:D; CN:PH; CA:M; CL:A

Maternal/Newborn and Gynecological Nursing

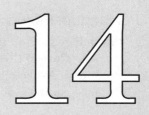

FEMALE REPRODUCTIVE SYSTEM

ANATOMY

External Genitalia
A. Collectively called the vulva.
B. Visible structures.
   1. Mons veneris (mons pubis).
   2. Labia majora.
   3. Labia minora.
   4. Clitoris.
   5. Vestibule.
   6. Urethral meatus.
   7. Skene's and Bartholin's glands.
   8. Hymen.
   9. Perineum.

Internal Organs
A. Located in pelvic cavity.
B. Reproductive structures.
   1. Uterus—a muscular organ with a central cavity.
      a. Functions.
         (1) Structure of fetal development.
         (2) Site of menstrual shedding.
      b. Sections.
         (1) Corpus (body)—lies below tubal insertion and composed of three layers.
            (a) Perimetrium—external layer.
            (b) Myometrium—middle layer.
            (c) Endometrium—internal layer.
         (2) Fundus—lies above tubal insertion.
   2. Cervix—canal located between internal and external os.
      a. Internal os opens into body of uterine cavity.
      b. External os opens into vagina.
   3. Fallopian tubes.
      a. Two slender muscular tubes extending laterally from the cornu of uterine cavity to ovaries.
      b. Passageways through which ova reach uterus.
   4. Ovaries.
      a. Flat, oval-shaped organs.
      b. One ovary located on each side of uterus.
      c. Functions.
         (1) Develop and expel ova.
         (2) Secrete estrogen and progesterone.

   5. Vagina.
      a. Canal extending from lower part of vulva to cervix.
      b. Functions.
         (1) Allows for passage of menstrual blood.
         (2) Allows for passage of fetus.
         (3) Provides site for copulation.

Support Structure (Pelvis)
A. Important in obstetrics.
   1. Passage through which baby passes at birth.
   2. Disproportions between fetus and size of pelvis make vaginal delivery difficult or impossible.
B. Bone formations.
   1. Two innominate bones.
   2. Sacrum.
   3. Coccyx.
C. Pelvic cavities.
   1. False pelvis—shallow extended portion above brim that supports abdominal viscera.
   2. True pelvis—portion that lies below pelvic brim; divided into three sections.
      a. Pelvic outlet.
      b. Mid-pelvis.
      c. Pelvic inlet.
◆ D. Pelvic types.
   1. Gynecoid—nearly round or blunt; typical of normal female.
   2. Android—wedge-shaped; typical of male.
   3. Anthropoid—oval-shaped.
   4. Platypelloid—oval-shaped, transversely.
E. Measurements of the pelvis.
   1. Diagonal conjugate—distance between sacral promontory and lower margin of symphysis pubis. Measurement > 12.5 cm adequate.
   2. True conjugate, or conjugate vera—distance from upper margin of symphysis to sacral promontory. Measurement > 11 cm adequate.
   3. Tuberischial diameter—transverse diameter of outlet. Measurement > 8 cm adequate.
   4. Size determination.
      a. X-ray pelvimetry is most accurate means of determining size of pelvis.
      b. X-ray pelvimetry is contraindicated to avoid undue exposure of mother and infant unless pelvic contraction is suspected.

PHYSIOLOGY

Menstruation and the Menstrual Cycle
A. Menstruation.
   1. Culmination of menstrual cycle.
   2. Discharge of blood, mucus, and epithelial cells from the uterus.

B. Menstrual cycle.
   1. Occurrence—usually between ages 12 and 45.
   2. Duration—about 28 days but varies from 21 to 35 days; ovulation occurs about 14 days before beginning of menstruation.
C. Menstrual cycle regulated primarily through phasic hormonal control of pituitary, ovaries, and uterus.
   ✦ 1. Proliferative phase.
      a. Follicle-stimulating hormone (FSH), secreted by anterior pituitary during the first half of the menstrual cycle, stimulates the development of the graafian follicle.
      b. As graafian follicle develops, it produces increasing amounts of follicular fluid containing a hormone called estrogen.
      c. Estrogen stimulates buildup or thickening of the endometrium.
      d. As estrogen increases in the bloodstream, it suppresses secretion of FSH and favors the secretion of the luteinizing hormone (LH).
      e. LH stimulates ovulation and initiates development of the corpus luteum.
   ✦ 2. Secretory phase.
      a. Follows ovulation, which is the release of mature ovum from the graafian follicle.
      b. Rapid changes take place in the ruptured follicle under the influence of LH.
      c. Cavity of the graafian follicle is replaced by the corpus luteum (mass of yellow-colored tissue).
      d. Main function of the corpus luteum is to secrete progesterone and some estrogen.
      e. Progesterone acts upon the endometrium to bring about secretory changes that thicken and maintain the endometrium during the early phase of pregnancy, should a fertilized ovum be implanted.
   ✦ 3. Menstrual phase.
      a. Corpus luteum degenerates in about 8 days unless the ovum is fertilized.
      b. There is a cessation of progesterone and estrogen produced by corpus luteum and blood levels drop.
      c. Endometrium degenerates and menstruation occurs.
      d. The drop in blood levels of estrogen and progesterone stimulate production of FSH and a new cycle begins.
      e. Basal body temperature dips then rises about a day after ovulation has occurred (0.5–1.0° F increase).
D. Discomforts associated with menstruation.
   1. Breast tenderness and feeling of fullness.
   2. Tendency toward fatigue.
   3. Temperament and mood changes—because of hormonal influence and decreased levels of estrogen and progesterone.
   4. Discomfort in pelvic area, lower back, and legs.
   5. Retained fluids and weight gain.
✦ E. Abnormalities of menstruation.
   1. Dysmenorrhea (painful menstruation).
      a. May be caused by psychological factors: tension, anxiety, preconditioning (menstruation is a "curse" or should be painful).
      b. Physical examination is usually done to rule out organic causes.
   2. Treatment.
      a. Oral contraceptives—produce anovulatory cycle.
      b. Mild analgesics such as aspirin.
      c. Urge patient to carry on normal activities to occupy her mind.
      d. Dysmenorrhea may subside after childbearing.
   3. Amenorrhea (absence of menstrual flow).
      a. Primary—over the age of 17 and menstruation has not begun.
         (1) Complete physical necessary to rule out abnormalities.
         (2) Treatment aimed at correction of underlying condition.
      b. Secondary—occurs after menarche—does not include pregnancy and lactation.
         (1) Causes include psychological upsets or endocrine conditions.
         (2) Evaluation and treatment by physician is necessary.
   4. Menorrhagia (excessive menstrual bleeding)—may be due to endocrine disturbance, tumors, or inflammatory conditions of the uterus.
   5. Metrorrhagia (bleeding between periods)—symptom of disease process, benign tumors, or cancer.
F. Counseling guidelines.
   1. Assist with providing education about the physiology of normal menstruation and correct misinformation.
   2. Assist with providing education about abnormal conditions associated with menstruation—absence of menstruation, bleeding between menstrual periods, etc.
   3. Assist with providing education related to normal hygiene during menstruation.
      a. Importance of cleanliness.
      b. Use of perineal pads and tampons.
      c. Continuance of normal activities.

DEVELOPMENT OF THE FETUS

Fertilization

Definition: A gamete is a matured sex cell (ovum or spermatozoon) that has undergone maturation and is ready for fertilization.

A. Fertilization takes place when two essential cells (sperm and ovum) unite; usually occurs in outer third of fallopian tube.

B. Each reproductive cell (one gamete) carries 23 chromosomes.

✦ C. Each sperm carries two types of sex chromosomes, X and Y; when united with female, X chromosome determines the sex of the child (XY—male; XX—female). *See* Table 14-1.

D. After fertilization, the fertilized egg descends to the uterus within 3 days.

Fetal Development (Table 14-2)

A. Embryo is the fertilized ovum during the first 2 months of development.

B. Fetus is product of conception from 2 months to time of birth.

C. Implantation occurs about the seventh day after fertilization.

D. During embryonic development, cells arrange themselves into three layers.

E. Fetal membranes and amniotic fluid.
  1. Fetal membranes (those which surround the fetus) are composed of two layers.
    ✦ a. Amnion (glistening inner membrane) forms early, about the second week of embryonic development; encloses the amniotic cavity.
    b. Chorion is the outer membrane.
  ✦ 2. Amniotic fluid forms within the amniotic cavity and surrounds the embryo. Usually consists of 500–1000 mL of fluid at the end of pregnancy.
    a. Amniotic fluid is slightly alkaline and contains fetal urine, lanugo from fetal skin, epithelial cells, and sebaceous materials.
    b. Function of the fluid is to provide an optimum temperature and environment for fetus and provide a cushion against injury; fetus also drinks the fluid, probably as much as 600 mL/day near term.
    c. Probably bidirectional maternal-fetal exchange.

✦ F. Placenta and fetal circulation.
  1. Placenta—organ that provides for the exchange of nutrients and waste products between mother and fetus and acts as an endocrine organ. The placenta provides oxygen and removes carbon dioxide from the

✦ Table 14-1. MULTIPLE PREGNANCIES	
Double Ovum	**Single Ovum**
Dizygotic or fraternal twins	Monozygotic or identical twins
Ova from same or different ovaries	Union of a single ovum and a single sperm
Same or different sex	Same sex
Brother or sister resemblance	Identical genetic pattern
Two placentas but may be fused	One placenta
Two chorions and two amnions	One chorion and one amnion

fetal system (because its respiratory system is not yet functioning) as well as maintaining fetal fluid/electrolyte and acid/base balance.

  a. Placenta develops by the third month.
    (1) Formed by union of chorionic villi and decidua basalis.
    (2) Fetal surface smooth and glistening.
    (3) Maternal surface red and fleshlike.
    (4) Exchange takes place between mother and fetus through diffusion.
    ✦ (5) Materials passed through placenta in addition to nutrients are drugs, antibodies to some diseases, and certain viruses. Large particles such as bacteria cannot pass through barrier.
    ✦ (6) Hormones produced by the placenta.
      (a) Chorionic gonadotropin can be detected in the urine about 15 days after implantation. This hormone stimulates the corpus luteum to maintain endometrium.
      (b) Estrogen and progesterone.
  b. Umbilical cord extends from fetus to center of fetal surface of placenta.
    (1) Main vessels in the umbilical cord are two arteries and one vein.
    (2) The umbilical cord is protected by mucoid connective tissue termed *Wharton's jelly*.
    (3) Average cord is 2 cm (0.8 in) diameter and 55 cm (22 in) length.
  ✦ 2. Circulation.
    a. Vein carries oxygenated blood.
    b. Arteries carry venous blood.
    c. There are three bypasses in fetal circulation.
      (1) Two bypasses exist because the lungs are not functioning.
        (a) Ductus arteriosus, between pulmonary artery and aorta.

Table 14-2. FETAL GROWTH	
Age	**Development**
End of 1 month or 4 weeks	→ Form of embryonic disc No clearly defined features Body systems rudimentary form Cardiovascular system functioning
End of 2 months or 8 weeks	→ Head greatly enlarged, about the size of rest of body Some fetal movement as a result of beginning neuromuscular development Facial features becoming distinct Body covered with thin skin
End of 3 months or 12 weeks	→ Teeth forming under gums Center ossification appearing in most bones Fingers and toes are differentiated and bear nails Kidneys able to secrete Eyes have lids, which are fused shut until six months Fetus swallows Sex distinguishable Fetal heart heard with ultrasonic equipment
End of 4 months or 16 weeks	→ Lanugo appears over body Meconium in intestines Face has human appearance Size about 6 inches long; weight about 3.5 oz
End of 5 months or 20 weeks	→ Skeleton begins to harden Buds of permanent teeth develop Vernix caseosa makes appearance Fetal movements stronger and felt by mother Fetal heart rate heard with fetoscope Size about 10 inches long; weight about 11 oz
End of 6 months or 24 weeks	→ Fat beginning to deposit beneath skin Body and head better proportioned Eyebrows and eyelashes appear Size about 12 inches long; weight about 1½ lbs
End of 7 months or 28 weeks	→ Skin reddish and covered with vernix Size about 14 inches long; weight about 2½ lbs May be viable if born at this time, though still immature
End of 8 months or 32 weeks	→ Nails are firm and extend to end of digits Lanugo begins to disappear Size about 16 inches long; weight about 4 lbs Increased chance for survival if born at this time
End of 9 months or 36 weeks	→ Increased fat deposits under skin Increased development Size about 18 inches long; weight about 5 lbs Chances for survival are good
End of 10 months or 40 weeks	→ Full term Little lanugo Smooth skin Size about 20 inches long; weight 7 to 7½ lbs Optimum time for survival

      (b) Foramen ovale, between right and left atrium.

  (2) Ductus venosus bypass exists because the fetal liver is not used for exchange of waste; connects umbilical artery to inferior vena cava; allows most fetal blood to bypass liver.

      d. Bypasses must close following birth to allow blood to flow through the lungs for respiration and through the liver for waste exchange.

G. A multiple pregnancy is one in which two or more embryos are contained in the amniotic sac. May be the result of fertilization of a single ovum or two separate ova.

✦ H.   Calculation of expected date of delivery or confinement (EDC).

✦ 1.   Nägele's rule—count back 3 months from first day of last menstrual period (LMP) and add 7 days.

Example: LMP July 18
EDC April 25

2.   Pregnancy usually does not terminate on the exact EDC. If using Nägele's rule, it may vary from 1 week before to 2 weeks after the expected date. If ultrasound used (BPD) between 17–24 weeks' gestation, the expected date is usually ± 5 to 7 days.

MATERNAL CHANGES DURING PREGNANCY

Physiological Changes

Reproductive Organs

✦ A.   Uterus increases in weight from 2 ounces to about 2 pounds at the end of gestation and increases in size five to six times.
1.   Changes in tissue.
   a.   Hypertrophy of muscle cells and development of new muscles.
   b.   Development of connective and elastic tissue, which increases contractility.
   c.   Increase in the size and number of blood vessels.
   d.   Hypertrophy of the lymphatic system.
   e.   Growth of the uterus is brought about by the influences of estrogen during the early months and the pressure of the fetus.
2.   Other changes.
   a.   Contractions occur throughout pregnancy, starting from very mild to increased strength.
   b.   As the uterus grows, it rises out of the pelvis, displacing intestines, and may be palpated above the symphysis pubis.
B.   Ligaments.
1.   Broad ligaments located in the pelvis.
2.   They become elongated and hypertrophied to help support and stabilize uterus during pregnancy.
C.   Cervix.
1.   Becomes shorter, more elastic, and larger in diameter.
2.   Marked thickening of mucous lining and increased blood supply.
3.   Edema and hyperplasia of the cervical glands and increased glandular secretions.
4.   Mucous plug expelled from cervix as cervix begins to dilate at onset of labor.

✦ D.   Vagina.
1.   Increased vascularity, deepening of color to dark red or purple (*Chadwick's sign*).
2.   Hypertrophy and thickening of muscle and mucosa.
3.   Loosening of connective tissue.
4.   Increased vaginal discharge.
5.   Secretions have high pH and are less acidic (4.0–6.0 pH).
E.   Perineum.
1.   Increased vascularity.
2.   Hypertrophy of muscles.
3.   Loosening of connective tissue.
F.   Ovaries and tubes.
1.   Usually one large corpus luteum present in one ovary. Produces hormones (estrogen and progesterone) until week 10–12.
2.   Ovulation does not take place.

Breasts

A.   Changes in tissue.
1.   Extensive growth of alveolar tissue, necessary for lactation.
2.   Montgomery's glands enlarge.
B.   Other changes.
1.   Increase in size and firmness; become nodular.
2.   Nipples become more prominent, and areolae deepen in color.
3.   Superficial veins grow more prominent.
4.   At the end of third month, colostrum appears.
5.   After delivery, anterior pituitary stimulates production and secretion of milk.

Abdomen

A.   Contour changes as the enlarging uterus extends into the abdominal cavity.
B.   *Striae gravidarum* usually appear on the abdomen as pregnancy progresses.

Skin

A.   Pigmentation increases in certain areas of the body.
1.   Breasts—primary areolae deepen in color.
✦ 2.   Abdomen—*linea nigra*, dark streak down the midline of the abdomen, especially prominent in brunettes.
✦ 3.   Face—*chloasma*, the "mask of pregnancy" pigmentation, distributed over the face; usually disappears after pregnancy.
4.   Face and upper trunk—occasionally spider nevi or palmar erythema develops with the increase in estrogen.
B.   Increased sebaceous and sweat gland activity.
C.   Pigmented areas on abdomen and breast usually do not completely disappear after delivery.

Circulatory System

✦ A. Considerable increase (about 50 percent) in volume of blood as a result of:
1. Increased metabolic demands of new tissue.
2. Expansion of vascular system, especially in the reproductive organs.
3. Increased steroid hormones, which cause retention of sodium and water.

B. Increase in plasma volume is greater than increase in red blood cells and hemoglobin, although dilution is not sufficient to cause anemia (low hemoglobin in pregnancy usually caused by iron-deficiency anemia).

C. Heart increases in size, and cardiac output is increased 25 to 50 percent.

D. Blood pressure *should not* rise during pregnancy.

E. Fibrinogen concentration increases until term.

✦ F. Folic acid and iron requirements are increased to meet demands of increased blood supply and growing fetus (need cannot be met by diet alone; supplement usually given).

G. Palpitations may be experienced during pregnancy due to sympathetic nervous disturbance and intra-abdominal pressure caused by enlarging uterus.

Respiratory System

A. Thoracic cage is pushed upward and the diaphragm is elevated as the uterus enlarges.

B. Thoracic cage widens to compensate so that vital capacity remains the same or is increased.

C. Oxygen consumption is increased 15 percent to support fetus and tissue.

D. Shortness of breath may be experienced in latter part of pregnancy due to pressure on diaphragm caused by enlarging uterus and decreased CO_2 levels.

Digestive System

A. Nausea, vomiting, and poor appetite are present in early pregnancy because of a decreased gastric motility.

B. Constipation is due to a decrease in gastrointestinal motility, reduced peristaltic activity, and the pressure of the uterus; it may be present in latter half of pregnancy.

C. Flatulence and heartburn may be present as a result of decreased gastric acidity and decreased motility of the gastrointestinal tract.

Urinary System

A. Kidneys.
1. Kidney and renal function is increased.
2. Renal blood flow and glomerular filtration is increased by 50%.

B. Bladder and ureters.
1. Blood supply to the bladder and pelvic organs is increased.
2. Pressure of uterus on bladder causes frequent urination during early pregnancy.
3. Relaxation of smooth muscles during pregnancy leads to dilatation of ureters and renal pelvis; may cause urine stasis.
4. A decrease in bladder tone is caused by hormonal influences; a decrease in bladder capacity occurs because of crowding. Such decrease may lead to complications during pregnancy and in the postpartum period (UTI, urinary retention).

Joints, Bones, Teeth, and Gums

A. Softening of pelvic cartilage occurs, probably due to the hormones relaxin, progesterone, and estrogen.

B. Postural changes occur as upper spine is thrown forward to compensate for increased abdominal size (Lordosis).

C. Demineralization of teeth does not occur as a result of normal pregnancy but may be related to poor dental hygiene.

D. Increased vascularity of gums due to hormonal changes with tendency to bleed easily.

Endocrine System

✦ A. Placenta produces the hormones human chorionic gonadotropin (HCG) and placental lactogen (HPL).
1. Production of estrogen and progesterone is taken over from the ovaries by the placenta/fetal unit after the second month.
2. Normal cycle of production of estrogen and progesterone by ovaries is suspended until after delivery.

B. Anterior lobe of pituitary gland enlarges slightly during pregnancy.

C. Adrenal cortex enlarges slightly.

D. Thyroid enlarges slightly and thyroid activity increases.

E. Aldosterone levels gradually increase beginning about the 15th week.

Metabolism

✦ A. Weight gain.
1. Progressive gain to ensure fetal growth and development and stores for successful lactation.
2. Pattern of weight gain important.
3. Recommendation determined by prepregnancy weight (normal: 11.5–16 kg or 25.3–35.2 lb).

B. Some of the weight gain is caused by retention of fluid and by deposits of fatty tissue.

C. Water metabolism.
 1. Tendency to retain fluid in body tissues, especially in the last trimester.
 2. Reversal of fluid retention usually takes place in the form of diuresis in the first 24 hours postpartum.
D. Basal metabolic rate increases.
E. Carbohydrate metabolism—increased need to spare protein.

Emotional Changes

✦ Altered Emotional Characteristics

A. Quick mood changes and a certain amount of emotional lability is common.
B. Emotional reactions may change during pregnancy; may range from early rejection of pregnancy to that of elation.
C. Pregnant women may become more passive and introverted in second trimester.
D. A woman may be puzzled by changes in her feelings and needs reassurance from the nurse that these are normal reactions about which one need not feel guilty.
E. Father of the baby needs to be informed that the woman's emotional lability, attitudes, and feelings toward sex are emotional reactions of pregnancy and will pass.
F. The woman may have fears and worries about the baby and herself and needs to be able to express her feelings to the nurse.

Taking on the Parental Role

A. Pregnant woman may fantasize or daydream to "experience" the role of mother before the actual birth occurs.
B. Takes on adaptive behaviors that are best suited to her own personality and situation.
✦ C. Experiences a "letting go" of her former role (e.g., as a career woman).
 1. May experience ambivalence about letting go of her old role to take on the new one.
 2. Desire to have a baby influences adjustment and acceptance of the maternal role.
D. Father may also experience ambivalence about taking on new role and sharing wife's attention with new baby.

Childbirth Preparation

Theories of Childbirth

A. Factors that influence pain in labor.
 1. Preconditioning by "old wives' tales," fantasies, and fears. Accurate information about the childbirth process can often alleviate effects of preconditioning.

 2. Pain produces stress, which in turn affects the body's functioning. Interpretations of and reactions to pain can be altered by a refocusing of attention and by conditioning.
 3. Feelings of isolation. Social expectations and tension may also increase feelings of pain.
✦ B. Childbirth education classes.
 ✦ 1. Read method (original natural childbirth movement). (This theory is not subscribed to today.)
 ✦ 2. Lamaze method (psychoprophylactic method).
 a. Basic thrust is education and training.
 b. Instruction in anatomy, the physiology of the reproductive system; an extensive study of labor and delivery; replacement of misinformation and superstition with facts.
 c. Training that consists of controlled breathing and neuromuscular exercises.
 d. Husband, family member, or a friend is included in the class and serves as coach.
 3. LeBoyer birth method (introduced in the 70s to reduce stress to infant with warm room environment with soft lighting, and a warm bath immediately after birth).
 4. Other: Water birth; Bradley method; scientific relaxation methods for childbirth.

Nutritional Guidelines for Pregnancy

A. Influences upon dietary habits and nutrition.
 1. Food—many emotional connotations originating in infancy.
 2. Eating habits influenced by:
 a. Emotional factors.
 b. Cultural factors.
 c. Religious beliefs.
 d. Nutritional information.
 e. Age—especially adolescent and aged.
 f. Physical health.
 g. Personal preferences.
B. Nutritional needs in pregnancy. *See* Appendix 14-4.
 1. Influenced by above factors.
 2. Must supply caloric, nutritional, and fluid needs of mother as well as promote optimum fetal growth.
 3. May be complicated by:
 a. Poor maternal nutrition before pregnancy.
 b. Medical complications prior to pregnancy (diabetes, anemia).
 c. Complications resulting from pregnancy (toxemia, anemia).
 d. Pica (cravings).
✦ C. Weight gain in pregnancy.
 1. Average weight gain recommended—25–35/40 lbs. (even for obese patients)—24 pounds.
 a. First trimester—3–4 pounds.

b. Second trimester—10 pounds.

c. Third trimester—10 pounds.

2. Weight gain accounted by:

a. Product of conception.

Fetus—average size	7.5 pounds
Placenta	1.5
Amniotic fluid	2
Uterus	2.5
Breasts	1
Extracellular fluid	3
Blood volume	3
	20.5 pounds

b. Rest of weight gain deposited as fat stores or fluid representing energy stored for lactation.

D. Alcohol consumption.

1. There is no "safe" level of alcohol consumption during pregnancy.

2. It is recommended that women abstain from any alcohol during first trimester.

3. Alcohol passes the placental barrier within minutes of consumption—the effects of alcohol on the fetus will vary according to the stage of fetal development.

✦ E. Revised daily food guide.

1. Iron and folacin (folic acid)—cannot be ingested in sufficient quantities by dietary means. Must be supplemented during pregnancy.

✦ 2. 300 additional calories needed to meet recommended allowances.

3. Protein intake includes both animal and vegetable protein.

a. Vegetable protein may be omitted in those whose income will allow by increasing animal servings to three 3-oz servings.

b. One serving at least should be red meats.

4. Whole grain items are better choices than enriched breads and cereals. They contain more magnesium, zinc, folacin, and vitamin B_6.

5. At least 2 tablespoons of fat or oils should be consumed daily for vitamin E and essential fatty acids.

F. Special diets.

1. Adolescents.

a. Have high proportion of low-birth-weight infants.

b. Dietary habits often poor.

c. Plan menu to include necessary items around foods they like.

d. Stress balanced diet—avoid empty calories.

✦ 2. Sodium.

a. Presently sodium restriction is not recommended.

b. Sodium is essential in maintaining increased body fluids needed for adequate placental flow, increased tissue requirements, and renal blood flow.

c. If moderate salt intake is necessitated, avoid highly salted foods such as canned soups, potato chips, soda pop.

3. Weight control.

a. Presently, weight loss in pregnancy is discouraged.

b. Even obese patient should gain 24 pounds to ensure adequate nutrition for fetal growth.

c. Strict dieting may lead to ketosis, which has proven harmful to fetal brain.

d. Stress careful dietary planning to include essential nutrients and avoid empty calories.

e. Weight reduction program should begin *after* lactation only.

SIGNS AND DISCOMFORTS OF PREGNANCY

✦ **Presumptive Signs (Subjective Changes)**

A. Cessation of menstruation (amenorrhea).

B. Breasts increase in size with feeling of fullness; nipples more pronounced, areola darker.

C. Nausea and vomiting ("morning sickness") appear in about 50 percent of pregnant women and usually disappears at the end of the third month.

D. Frequent urination (desire to void) usually occurs in the first 3–4 months. Pressure on the bladder from an enlarged uterus gives the sensation of a distended bladder.

E. Quickening (first perception of fetal movement) occurs between 16th and 18th week.

F. Fatigue with periods of drowsiness and lassitude during first 3 months.

✦ **Probable Signs (Objective Changes)**

A. Enlargement of the abdomen usually occurs after the third month when the fetus rises out of the pelvis into the abdominal cavity.

B. Increased pigmentation of skin, chloasma, linea nigra, and striae gravidarum.

C. Changes in internal organs.

1. Change in shape, size, and consistency of the uterus.

2. *Hegar's sign*—softening of the isthmus of the uterus, occurs about 6th week.

3. *Goodell's sign*—softening of the cervix, occurs beginning of the second month.

4. *Chadwick's sign*—vaginal changes, discoloration and thickening of vaginal mucosa.

D. *Braxton Hicks* contractions—slight, irregular contractions usually not felt by the woman until 7 months, but contractions begin in the early weeks of pregnancy and continue through gestation.

E. *Ballottement*—pressure on an organ giving a sudden push to the fetus and feeling it rebound in a few seconds to the original position; usually possible in the fourth to fifth month.

F. Outline of the fetus by abdominal palpation (a probable sign, because a tumor may simulate fetal parts).

G. Positive pregnancy test is based upon the secretion of chorionic gonadotropin in the urine of a pregnant woman; it is usually detectable 10 days after the first missed menstrual period.

H. Amenorrhea by week 4.

✦ Positive Signs

A. Apparent after 18th to 20th week.

B. Auscultation of fetal heart rates (120–160) with stethoscope or ultrasonic equipment. (*Note:* With ultrasonic equipment, fetal heart rate may be heard at 12 weeks.)

C. Active fetal movements are perceptible by the examiner.

D. Ultrasound examination showing fetal outline by 5 weeks' gestation.

Pseudocyesis (Pseudopregnancies)

A. The emotional control of physiological functioning that is psychological in origin; woman believes she is pregnant when she is not.

B. Clinical manifestations.
1. Amenorrhea, breast changes, and secretion of colostrum.
2. Enlargement of abdomen.
3. Reports of quickening.
4. Appears any age, but more common in older women.

C. Treatment.
1. Uncover underlying emotional problem.
2. Offer continued emotional support as this is important.

Physical Examination

✦ A. Initial examination.
1. Complete history is recorded (past pregnancies, medical history, family history).
2. Physical examination of pelvis, breasts, and abdomen.
3. Assess for risk factors: age, socioeconomic, ethnicity, prepregnancy history, multiple pregnancy, late prenatal care, pre- or coexisting medical problems, substance abuse.
4. Blood pressure, urinalysis, blood work including Rh factor, rubella titer, Pap smear, slide for gonorrhea and chlamydia, serology for syphilis (VDRL), HIV, hepatitis.
5. Diet and health instructions are given to patient.

✦ B. Subsequent examinations are usually done once a month until the last trimester, then more frequently.
1. Weight and blood pressure taken; urine tests for protein and sugar content made.
2. Palpation of abdomen.
3. Auscultation of fetal heart tones.
4. Observation for untoward signs and symptoms.
5. Screen and treatment of beta-hemolytic streptococci (GBS) culture—if positive, treat woman before delivery.
6. Continuing health care and instructions.

C. *See* Table 14-3 for pregnancy discomfort and relief measures.

COMPLICATIONS OF PREGNANCY

✦ Danger Signals

A. Bleeding from vagina.

B. Escape of amniotic fluid denoting premature rupture of membranes.

C. Abdominal pain.

D. Contractions increasing in strength, duration, and proximity before term.

E. Dizziness or blurring of vision.

F. Persistent headache.

G. Edema of face and fingers.

H. Persistent and severe vomiting.

I. Chills and elevated temperature.

J. Absence of or significant and consistent decrease in fetal movement.

K. Decrease or absence of fetal heart tones.

Abortion

Definition: Abortion is the expulsion of the fetus before it is viable; abortion may be spontaneous or induced.

✦ Categories of Abortion

A. Threatened—some loss of blood and pain without loss of products of conception.

B. Imminent—bleeding profuse, contractions severe, bearing-down sensation; without intervention, products of conception will be lost.

C. Inevitable—bleeding, contractions, ruptured membranes, and cervical dilatation.

D. Incomplete—portion of products of conception remain in uterine cavity.

E. Complete—all products of conception expelled.

F. Habitual—abortion in three or more succeeding pregnancies.

Table 14-3. MAJOR DISCOMFORTS OF PREGNANCY AND RELIEF MEASURES

Discomfort	Trimester Most Prominent	Relief Measures
Nausea and vomiting	1st	Instead of 3 large meals daily, have 5 or 6 small, frequent meals
		In between meals, have couple of crackers or a piece of toast without fluid
		Avoid foods high in carbohydrates, with a strong odor, or fried and greasy
		Plan rest period after meals
		If nausea occurs at regular intervals when stomach is empty, plan ahead by eating 20–30 minutes earlier
Urinary frequency	1st and 3rd	Wear perineal pads if there is a leakage
Heartburn	2nd and 3rd	Avoid fatty, fried, and highly spiced foods
		Have small frequent feedings
Abdominal distress	1st, 2nd, and 3rd	Eat slowly, chew food thoroughly, take smaller helpings of food
Flatulence	2nd and 3rd	Maintain daily bowel movement
		Avoid gas-forming foods
Constipation	2nd and 3rd	Drink sufficient fluids
		Eat fruit and foods high in roughage
		Exercise moderately
Hemorrhoids	3rd	Apply ointments, suppositories, warm compresses
		Avoid constipation
		Rest
Insomnia	3rd	Exercise moderately to promote relaxation and fatigue
		Change position while sleeping
Backaches	3rd	Rest
		Improve posture
		Use a good abdominal support and wear comfortable shoes
		Do exercises such as squatting, sitting, and pelvic rock
Varicosities, legs and vulva	3rd	Avoid long periods of standing or sitting with legs crossed
		Sit or lie with feet and hips elevated
		Move about while standing to improve circulation
		Wear support hose
Edema of legs and feet	3rd	Elevate feet while sitting or lying down
		Avoid standing or sitting in one position for long periods
Cramps in legs	3rd	Extend cramped leg and flex ankles, pushing foot upward with toes pointed toward knee
		Increase calcium intake
Pain in thighs or aching of perineum	3rd	Alternate periods of sitting and standing
		Rest
Shortness of breath	3rd	Sit up
		Lie on back with arms extended above bed
Supine hypotensive syndrome	3rd	Change position to left side to relieve pressure of uterus on inferior vena cava
Vaginal discharge	3rd	Practice proper cleansing and hygiene
		Avoid douche unless recommended by physician
		Observe for signs of vaginal infection common in pregnancy

G. Therapeutic—medically terminated for woman's physical or emotional health.

H. Criminal—termination of pregnancy outside medical or approved facilities.

Etiology

A. Abnormalities of fetus.

B. Abnormalities of reproductive tract.

C. Injuries—physical and emotional shock.

D. Endocrine disturbances.

E. Acute infectious diseases.

F. Maternal diseases.

G. Psychogenic problems.

Assessment

A. Vaginal bleeding.

B. Intermittent contractions and pain, which usually begin in the small of the back; abdominal cramping.

C. Passage of tissue.

D. Psychological state of patient.

Treatment

A. Notification of physician immediately.

B. Endocrine therapy (usually progesterone if deficiency).

C. Correction of abnormalities or disturbances of reproductive tract.

D. Avoidance of stress and exertion during early pregnancy.

E. Bedrest and sedation; avoid climbing stairs and coitus until at least 2 weeks after bleeding stops.

F. Oxytocic drug may be given to hasten process of abortion, if it is inevitable, and to promote contraction of uterus after abortion.

G. Medication for pain if necessary.

H. Blood available for transfusion.

I. Dilatation and curettage may be necessary in an incomplete abortion.

✦ J. Administration of RhoGAM in Rh-negative women.

K. Maintain sterile technique in all examinations and treatments.

Implementation

A. Offer emotional support and comfort; do not say, "Everything will be all right," if there is loss of the fetus.

B. Save all perineal pads and expelled tissue for examination.

C. Observe for and report signs of shock.

D. In criminal abortions, observe for serious complications such as septic shock, thrombophlebitis, and renal failure.

Habitual Abortion

Definition: Habitual abortion is the condition in which the patient has spontaneously aborted three or more consecutive times.

Etiology

A. Endocrine disturbances.

B. Blood incompatibilities.

C. Incompetent cervical os.

D. Chromosomal abnormalities.

E. Abnormalities of reproductive tract.

F. Fibromas of uterus.

G. Psychological.

Treatments

A. Hormone therapy (estrogen and progesterone) and thyroid therapy for endocrine disturbances.

B. Shirodkar procedure (internal os constricted by encircling suture, which is removed when labor begins) for incompetent cervical os.

C. Surgical correction of abnormalities, if possible, and removal of fibromas.

D. Psychotherapy for psychological cause.

Hydatidiform Mole

Definition: Benign neoplasm of the chorion in which chorionic villi degenerate; become filled with a clear, viscid fluid; and assume the appearance of grapelike clusters involving all or parts of the decidual lining of the uterus.

Incidence

A. Rare, occurs once in every 1000–1500 pregnancies except in Asia, where it is far less rare (1 in 250).

B. Usually there is no fetus found.

C. Incidence increases with advanced maternal age.

Etiology

A. May be pathological ova.

B. High incidence in Asia may be due to a protein deficiency in diet.

C. Significance of disease is loss of pregnancy and remote possibility of developing choriocarcinoma from the tissue.

✦ Assessment

A. Pregnancy appears normal at first.

B. Bleeding varies from spotting to profuse. Anemia may result from blood loss.

C. Rapid enlargement of the uterus.

D. Nausea and vomiting appear earlier; usually are more severe and last longer.

E. Severe preeclampsia may develop in the early part of the second trimester.

F. PIH may occur with the rapid expansion of the uterus.

G. Characteristic vesicles may be passed.

Diagnosis

A. Test for increased titer of chorionic gonadotropin. It is best to collect a 24-hour specimen for the total daily output.

B. Ultrasound, which will give positive diagnosis in the first trimester.

C. Amniography—x-ray following injection with contrast dye.

Treatment and Implementation

✦ A. Evacuation of uterus as soon as positive diagnosis is made (by dilatation and curettage or vacuum curettage suction).

B. Follow-up visits to physician for examination, because hydatidiform mole may lead to choriocarcinoma of uterus.

C. Observe for hemorrhage.

D. Provide emotional support for there may be fear of malignancy or patient may feel the loss of the baby.

E. Patient should avoid pregnancy for 1 year from negative test.

Extrauterine (Ectopic) Pregnancy

Definition: A pregnancy that develops outside the uterus. Usually cannot develop longer than 10–12 weeks.

Process of Pregnancy

✦ A. Although the fertilized ovum usually attaches to the uterine lining, it may become implanted at any point between the graafian follicle and the uterus.

B. Tubal pregnancy is the most common form (95 percent) but the ovum may attach to an ovary, the abdomen, or interligaments.

C. Implantation.
 1. Ovum attaches to tube and erodes into mucosa wall, as it would to the endometrial lining of the uterus.
 2. Tube increases in size and stretches.
 3. Pregnancy usually terminates during the first 3 months.
  a. Spontaneous tubal abortion.
  b. Tubal rupture.
  c. Death and disintegration of products of conception within the tube.

Etiology

A. Progress of ovum through tube is delayed for some reason.

B. Tubal deformities that are either congenital or due to disease such as gonorrhea.

C. Tumors pressing against the tube.

D. Adhesions from previous surgery.

E. Tubal spasms.

F. Migration of ovum to opposite tube.

Assessment

A. Woman may or may not know she is pregnant.

B. May have history of missed periods and "spotting."

C. May have slight abdominal pain.

D. Early signs of pregnancy may be present.

E. Uterus enlarges and decidua develops due to hormonal influence.

✦ F. Often first symptom is a sudden, excruciating, one-sided lower abdominal pain.
 1. Often first indication of ruptured tube.
 2. 50% experience referred right shoulder pain.

✦ G. May feel faint and have signs of shock as a result of hemorrhage into the peritoneal cavity.

H. May have little external bleeding.

I. Laboratory tests and ultrasound.

Treatment and Implementation

A. Immediate removal of the affected tube.

B. Blood transfusions may be necessary.

C. Observe for signs of shock and give treatment for shock as necessary.

D. Provide emotional support; patient may be frightened and feel the loss of the pregnancy.

Placenta Previa

✦ *Definition:*   A placenta develops so that it partially or completely covers the internal os when ovum implants low in the uterus toward the cervix. Occurs once in every 200 deliveries.

Types

A. Complete—os entirely covered.

B. Partial—only part of os covered.

C. Marginal—margin overlaps os.

Etiology

A. Occurs more often in multiparas.

B. Occurs more often with increased age of woman.

Assessment

✦ A. Painless, bright red vaginal bleeding after the seventh month without precipitating cause.

B. Bleeding may be intermittent.

C. As internal os begins to dilate, the part of placenta that overlies the os separates and leaves gaping vessels so that bleeding occurs.

D. Uterus usually remains soft and flaccid.

Diagnosis

A. History of painless bleeding begins late in pregnancy.

B. Localization of placenta by ultrasound.

C. Sterile vaginal or pelvic examinations are usually not done as part of diagnosis until adequate preparation has been made. Ultrasound assists in diagnosis.

✦ Treatment and Implementation

A. Immediate hospitalization.

B. Placed on bedrest in quiet, restful room.

C. Blood is typed and cross-matched for possible transfusion.

✦ D. Treatment depends upon type of placenta previa, condition of woman, and viability of baby.
 1. Mechanical pressure applied to placental site by bringing down baby's head and occluding blood vessels; usually accomplished by the rupture of membranes.
 2. Delivery by cesarean section.

E. If baby is small and bleeding stops, delivery is usually postponed.

F. Count perineal pads.

G. Observe for hemorrhage.

H. Give emotional support, explain procedures, and help allay fears.

I. Carefully monitor fetal heart tones with external monitor.

J. Monitor carefully postpartum for bleeding.

Abruptio Placentae

✦ *Definition:*   A separation of the placenta from the normal implantation site in upper segment of uterus before birth of baby. Occurs once in 90 pregnancies and accounts for 15 percent of perinatal mortality.

✦ **Types**

A. Complete—placenta becomes completely detached from uterine wall.

B. Partial—portion of placenta becomes detached from uterine wall.

C. Central—placenta separates centrally and blood is trapped so bleeding is concealed.

D. Hemorrhage.
   1. External—blood escapes from the vagina.
   2. Concealed—blood is retained in uterine cavity.

Etiology

A. Trauma.

B. Chronic vascular renal disease.

C. High parity.

D. Cocaine use.

E. Hypertensive disease.

Assessment

✦ A. Dark vaginal bleeding accompanied by abdominal pain is chief external sign.

✦ B. Concealed signs.
   1. Intense, cramplike uterine pain.
   2. Uterine tenderness and rigidity.
   3. Lack of alternate contraction—relaxation of uterus.
   4. Fetal heart tones indicate bradycardia or are absent.

C. Early and late signs of shock: restlessness, narrowing pulse pressure, increased pulse rate, pallor, changes in levels of consciousness.

Treatment and Implementation

A. Depends upon severity and extent of labor.

✦ B. Treatment for blood loss and shock.
   1. Moderate bleeding—rupture membranes to hasten delivery and help control bleeding.
   2. Severe—immediate cesarean section.
   3. Blood drawn for coagulation studies because of risk of DIC.

C. Keep patient on bedrest.

D. Carefully monitor contractions (electronic monitor), fetal heart rate, and vital signs, CVP.

E. Maintain record of intake and output.

F. Nursing actions after delivery.

   1. Observe closely for hemorrhage and DIC.
   2. Carefully record intake and output; observe for anuria or oliguria. Anuria may develop as a result of decreased kidney perfusion.

Hyperemesis Gravidarum

✦ *Definition:*   Pernicious vomiting during pregnancy.

Assessment

A. Usually develops during the first 3 months of pregnancy.

B. Persistent nausea and vomiting.

C. May have abdominal pain and hiccups.

D. Considerable weight loss (5 percent of pregnancy weight).

E. May become severely dehydrated, caused by excessive vomiting.

F. May have depletion of essential electrolytes because of unreplaced loss of sodium chloride and potassium.

G. Metabolic acidosis may develop.

H. Blood urea nitrogen increases.

Etiology

A. Cause unclear, but may be caused by the addition of new substances to the body system such as a toxicity or maladjustment of the maternal metabolism.

B. Human chorionic gonadotropin (HCG) increases and is believed to play a role in this condition.

C. Increased incidence of Helicobacteri pylori (stomach ulcers).

Treatment and Implementation

A. Aimed at reducing the severity of symptoms.

B. Give frequent feedings in small amounts every 2 hours; dry foods preferred; provide low-fat meals; offer liquids between or after meals.

C. Avoid giving spicy or fried foods.

D. Give antiemetics as prescribed along with a tranquilizer or a sedative.

E. If vomiting is persistent:
   1. Patient is usually hospitalized.
   2. Dehydration and starvation are treated by administration of parenteral fluids, TPN, and vitamin supplements.
   3. Rest and sedatives are prescribed.

F. Use tact and understanding of the patient's problem.

G. Carefully record intake and output; maintain IVs.

H. Observe for acetone odor on breath.

I. Reduce stimuli and restrict visitors if necessary.

J. Monitor fetal heart rate.

Pregnancy-Induced Hypertension (PIH)

✦ *Definition:*   A group of conditions (formerly called toxemias) that usually appear after the 20th week;

occurs in 7–10 percent of all pregnancies. The major symptoms—hypertension, proteinuria, and edema—most frequently occur in young or elderly primigravidas, women with deficient diets, multiple pregnancies, polyhydramnios, and in long-standing diabetes.

Preeclampsia

Definition: An acute, hypertensive disease peculiar to pregnancy that may be mild or severe.

Assessment

A. Usually appears after the 6th month.
◆ B. Major symptoms are hypertension, proteinuria, and edema, which may appear separately or together. Two of the three symptoms are usually needed for diagnosis.
C. Mild.
   1. Blood pressure above 140/90 or systolic 30 mm Hg and diastolic 15 mm Hg above normal on two occasions, 6 hours apart.
   2. Edema.
   3. Proteinuria (0.3 g/L in 24 hours).
D. Severe.
   1. Blood pressure 160/110 or above, or systolic 50 mm Hg above normal.
   2. Massive edema with excessive weight gain.
   3. Proteinuria (5 g or more in 24 hours).
   4. Oliguria (400 mL or less in 24 hours).
   5. Visual disturbances.
   6. Headache.
   7. Vasospasms.
   8. Hemoconcentration.
   9. Epigastric pain (usually a late sign).
   10. CNS irritability (hyperreflexia).

Treatment and Implementation

◆ A. Mild.
   1. Patient usually remains at home.
   2. Extra rest is prescribed.
   3. Adequate fluid intake is maintained.
   4. Highly salted food is avoided.
   5. Weight is checked daily.
   6. Physician should be notified if further symptoms occur.
   7. Increased calcium supplement reduces vascular and uterine muscle tone.
   8. Begin low-dose use of aspirin in women with a history of severe preeclampsia.
◆ B. Severe.
   1. Antihypertensive, sedative drugs.
   2. High-protein diet; moderate salt—sodium intake is usually not restricted, but patient should avoid use of highly salted foods.
   3. Fluid and electrolyte replacement.
   4. Maintain bedrest.

◆ 5. Monitor magnesium sulfate IV (given to prevent seizures); administer sedatives if ordered.
   a. Observe for toxic dose: hypotonia, loss of deep tendon reflexes.
   b. Check serum levels of $MgSO_4$: 4–7 mEq/dL.
6. Observe for signs of central nervous system irritability and hyperactivity.
7. Take and record vital signs.
8. Measure and record intake and output.
9. Check weight at same time each day.
10. Test urine for proteinuria—24-hour urine for total protein and creatinine clearance.
11. Limit visitors.
12. Maintain seizure precautions.
13. Provide diversional activities.

Eclampsia

Definition: A more severe form of toxemia usually accompanied by convulsions and even coma.

Assessment

A. Severe edema with tremendous weight gain.
B. Scanty urine.
C. Urine may contain red blood cells, varied casts, and protein 3+ or greater with two random samples.
D. Blood pressure may rise to 160/110 or above on two occasions, 6 hours apart.
E. There may be visual disturbances, blurring, or even blindness, caused by edema of the retina.
F. Severe epigastric pain.
G. Convulsions (both tonic and clonic).
H. Labor may begin; fetus may be born prematurely or die.

Treatment and Implementation

A. Prevent and/or control convulsions.
   1. Quiet, dark room.
   2. Use seizure precautions.
   3. Have suction available.
   4. Use padded siderails.
B. Promote diuresis; measure and record intake and output.
C. Take and record vital signs.
D. Provide oxygen as necessary.
E. Maintain IV of magnesium sulfate (obtain blood levels every 4 hours); give fluid if ordered.
F. Monitor fetal heart rate.
G. Observe carefully for anuria and convulsions after delivery.
H. Have emergency medications at bedside, i.e., magnesium sulfate, calcium gluconate (antidote for magnesium sulfate toxicity).
I. *See* Appendix 14-3 for drugs normally used during toxemia.

HELLP Syndrome

Definition: Hemolysis, Elevated Liver enzymes, and Low Platelet count; a syndrome that is an unusual variation of PIH.

Etiology

A. This syndrome (identified first in 1982) occurs with no warning and no regular signs of eclampsia.
B. Epigastric pain may be first symptom—occurs before 36th week.
C. Check platelet count (low); liver enzymes (elevated); proteinuria (1+ to 4+).

Treatment and Implementation

A. Variation of PIH—check treatment under this topic.
B. Women with HELLP should give birth as soon as possible (induced labor or cesarean).
C. With PIH treatment, patient recovers in 4–5 days.

Polyhydramnios

✦ *Definition:* An excessive amount of amniotic fluid. Usual normal amount is 500–1000 mL. In polyhydramnios there is over 1500–2000 mL, which is excessive.

Etiology

A. Actual cause is unknown. Occurs frequently in:
  1. Fetal malformations.
  2. Diabetes.
  3. Erythroblastosis.
  4. Multiple pregnancies.
  5. Toxemias.
B. Diagnosis usually made through clinical observation of the greatly enlarged uterus.

Assessment

A. Related to pressure of the enlarged uterus or adjacent organs.
B. Edema of the lower extremities.
C. General abdominal discomfort.
D. Occasional shortness of breath.

Treatment

A. Amniocentesis offers only temporary relief.
B. Delivery.

Fetal Demise (Death)

Assessment

A. Cessation of fetal movement.
B. Absence of fetal heart tones.
C. Failure of uterine growth.
D. Low urinary estriol.
E. Negative pregnancy test that may remain positive for a few weeks due to elevated human chorionic gonadotropin.

F. X-ray (overlapping of skull bones).
G. Uterus feels smaller.

Treatment and Implementation

✦ A. Labor usually begins spontaneously a few weeks after death of fetus.
B. Labor may be induced if it does not occur spontaneously.
C. Watch patient closely for signs of disseminated intravascular disease from prolonged retention of the dead fetus.
D. Provide emotional support to parents.
E. Guide parents in planning future pregnancies.
F. Observe for hemorrhage.
G. Observe for psychological disturbances; refer for psychological counseling.

MEDICAL CONDITIONS AND PREGNANCY

High-Risk Pregnancy

✦ *Definition:* A pregnancy that refers to any condition that may interfere with the normal development or delivery of the fetus, or to any preexisting maternal disease that may increase the risk of pregnancy.

✦ Predisposing Factors

A. Under age 17, over age 35, or unmarried.
B. Parity (having borne five or more pregnancies).
C. Previous conditions.
  1. Previous infant death, premature birth, or congenital malformations.
  2. History of cardiac disease, diabetes, renal disease, or other maternal conditions.
  3. Difficulty in conceiving.
  4. Substance or alcohol addiction.
  5. Less than a year since last pregnancy.
  6. Rh incompatibility and sensitization.

Conditions Leading to High Risk

A. During pregnancy.
  1. Infection.
  2. Bleeding.
  3. Pregnancy-induced hypertension.
B. Intrapartum conditions.
  1. Premature labor.
  2. Abnormal fetal positions.
  3. Premature rupture membranes.

Cardiovascular Disease

Characteristics

A. Pregnancy expands plasma volume, increasing cardiac output and load on heart.

B. Most deaths are caused by cardiac failure, when blood volume is at a maximum in the last weeks of the second trimester.

C. Heart failure occurs infrequently in labor.

D. Over age 35, there is an increase in the incidence of heart failure and death.

Management During Pregnancy

A. With proper management, mortality is minimal.

B. Patient should avoid acute infections, especially respiratory infections.

C. Patient should rest frequently—8–10 hours' sleep.

✦ D. Strenuous activities such as rigorous exercise, stair climbing, heavy cleaning, and straining should be avoided.

✦ E. Patients in Class III and over may be hospitalized before labor for controlled rest and diet.

F. If patient decompensates or has distress symptoms with exertion, she should remain on bedrest or in a chair.

G. Salt intake may or may not be restricted. Diuretics may be prescribed if signs of heart failure occur. The use of highly salted foods is discouraged.

H. Iron, folic acid, and vitamin supplements are important; fluids and high fiber to promote soft stools.

I. Digitalis treatment when indicated.

J. Emotional stress should be avoided.

Management During Labor

✦ A. Observe for signs that cardiac function is deteriorating, such as pulse rate over 110 or respiratory rate over 24; heart murmurs.

B. Relieve pain and anxiety.

C. Vaginal delivery usually preferred.

D. Patient may decompensate in early postpartum phase.

Implementation

A. Educate about special needs and danger signals during pregnancy and postpartum.

B. Be alert for signs of decompensation during pregnancy, especially in the second trimester.

✦ C. During labor.
   1. Check vital signs every 15 minutes or more often as needed.
   2. Keep patient in bed and preferably lying on one side or in semirecumbent position.

   3. Administer oxygen as necessary.
   4. Provide calm atmosphere and emotional support to alleviate fears.
   5. Administer pain medications as ordered to reduce discomfort during labor.
   6. Be alert for signs of impending heart failure.
   7. Monitor fetal heart tones.

D. Careful observation during postpartum period.

E. Counsel during postpartum to have help at home and planned rest periods.

Diabetes

Definition: A chronic metabolic disease caused by a disturbance in normal insulin production.

Characteristics

✦ A. In 3–6 percent of pregnant women, tendency to develop gestational diabetes.
   1. Abnormalities disappear after pregnancy.
   2. Diet is cornerstone of intervention—insulin therapy is used when diet does not control condition.

✦ B. Maternal glucose crosses placenta, but insulin does not.

C. Pregnant women should be screened for glucose levels—normal is between 60 and 120 mg/dL.

✦ D. White's Classifications.
   1. Class A—abnormal glucose tolerance test, indicative of latent or gestational diabetes.
   2. Class B—diabetes beginning after age 20.
   3. Class C—diabetes at ages 10–19 years, or beginning in adolescence after age 10.
   4. Class D—diabetes of long duration, or onset in childhood before the age of 10.
   5. Class F—nephropathy, including capillary glomerulosclerosis.
   6. Class H—heart involvement.
   7. Class R—malignant retinopathy.
   8. Class T—pregnant after renal transplant.

E. Implications of diabetes in pregnancy.
   1. Diabetes is more difficult to control.
   2. There is a tendency to develop acidosis.
   3. Patient is prone to infection.
   4. Toxemia, hemorrhage, and polyhydramnios are more likely to develop.
   5. Latent diabetes may develop into full-blown diabetes.
   6. Insulin requirements are increased.
   7. Premature delivery is more frequent.
   8. Infant may be overgrown but have functions related to gestational age rather than size.

✦ 9. Infant is subject to hypoglycemia, hyperbilirubinemia, respiratory distress syndrome, and congenital anomalies (incidence is 5–10 percent).

DIABETES SUGGESTED DIET

- Daily calories. 2000–2500 kcal. (Severe calorie restriction may lead to ketosis.)
- Protein. 12–20 percent or 0.8 g/kg unless renal disease is present.
- Carbohydrate. 55–60 percent, primarily complex carbohydrates.
- Fat. < 20–30 percent total calories.
- Fiber. 300 g/day to control glycemia and constipation—also satisfies appetite.

---

10. Stillborn and neonatal mortality rates are high, but may be reduced by proper management and control of diabetes.

Implementation

A. Reinforce teaching the effects of diabetes on the mother and fetus during pregnancy and the reasons for frequent testing of blood glucose.

✦ B. Emphasize dietary control (usually provided with 3 meals and 3 snacks), good nutrition, and health practices.

✦ C. If hospitalized:
    1. Maintain insulin on regular schedule.
    2. Test blood for glucose level.
    3. Provide adequate diabetic diet as prescribed by physician.
    4. Frequent home monitoring of blood glucose.
    5. Monitor fetal heart rate.
    6. Check vital signs, especially blood pressure QID and PRN.
    7. Weigh daily at the same time each day.
    8. Keep accurate records of intake and output.
    9. Provide support and explanations to help allay fears and reduce anxiety.
    10. Watch for symptoms of hyperglycemia or hypoglycemia.

D. In labor.
    ✦ 1. Monitor fetal status continuously for signs of distress.
    2. Carefully regulate insulin and provide IV glucose as labor depletes glycogen.

E. Postpartum.
    ✦ 1. Close observation for insulin reaction—precipitous drop in insulin requirements usual—hypoglycemic shock may occur.
    2. Close observation for early signs of infection.
    3. Close observation for postpartum hemorrhage.

Anemia

Definition: Decrease in the numbers of erythrocytes and reduction in hemoglobin.

Characteristics

A. Hemoglobin < 12 g/dL in nonpregnant women and < 10 g/dL in pregnant women (lower values in pregnancy due to hemodilution).

B. 90 percent caused by iron deficiency (HGB level 10 g/dL, HCT 37 percent or below).

Implementation

A. Patient tires easily and looks pale; monitor for rest.

B. Hemoglobin values are usually checked routinely in antepartum care.

C. Usually treated by diet and an iron supplement; ferrous sulfate 0.3 gm TID or Imferon if condition is severe.

Urinary Tract Infection

Definition: Bacteria entering the urinary tract by way of the urethra causing infection.

Characteristics

✦ A. Usually occurs after the fourth month or in early postpartum—affects 10 percent of maternity patients.

B. Causes.
    1. Pressure on ureters and bladder.
    2. Hormonal effects on tone of ureters and bladder.
    3. Displacement of bladder.

C. Kidneys as well as ureters may be involved.

✦ Assessment

A. Frequent micturition.

B. Paroxysms—pain in kidney or flank pain.

C. Fever and chills.

D. Catheterized urine specimen contains bacteria and pus.

Treatment and Implementation

A. Maintain patient on bedrest.

B. High fluid intake.

C. Antibiotic treatments.

D. Monitor urinary antispasmodics and analgesics.

Infectious Diseases

Rubella

✦ A. In the first trimester, rubella may cause congenital anomalies.

✦ B. Vaccine is available and should be given to children from age 1 to puberty or to the mother in early postpartum, while she is still hospitalized. (Vaccine should not be given if pregnancy is suspected.)

✦ C. Titer should be checked before pregnancy or on first prenatal visit.

Acute Infectious Diseases

A. Diseases such as influenza, scarlet fever, toxoplasmosis, and cytomegalovirus may be transmitted to the fetus.

B. Diseases may cause abortions or malformations in early pregnancy, premature labor or infant death in later pregnancy.

C. Check for elevated temperature, sore throat, cough, skin rash.

Sexually Transmitted Diseases

Chlamydia

A. Caused by *Chlamydia trachomatis;* produces infections in both men and women (fallopian tubes, cervix, urethra) and can develop into PID.

✦ B. Most common sexually transmitted disease (STD) in the United States; 5 million people contract disease each year.
  1. High-risk women: young, nonwhites with multiple sex partners and women not using barrier contraceptives.
  2. Chlamydia is not a reportable disease in 50 percent of states.

C. Sensitive to antibiotics (azithromycin or doxycycline).

D. Spread through sexual contact. Incubation period 5–10 days or longer (28 days; gonorrhea is only 2–10 days).

E. Symptoms: discharge—vaginal or urethral burning, lower abdominal pain or testicular pain, bleeding or pain with coitus; 33 percent of women report no symptoms.

F. Treatment is antibiotics—doxycycline 100 mg 2×/day for 7 days; erythromycin (base) 500 mg 4×/day for 7 days as second choice (take with meals); penicillin does not cure chlamydia.

G. Education of men and women about transmission, symptoms, and prevention is important nursing teaching.

Syphilis

✦ A. A chronic, infectious disease caused by *Treponema pallidum.*
  1. May cause abortion or premature labor.
  2. Infection is passed to the fetus after the fourth month of pregnancy as congenital syphilis.

✦ B. VDRL test for syphilis on first prenatal visit.
  1. Incubation period is 10 to 90 days—primary stage (nonreactive VDRL); secondary stage (reactive VDRL).
  2. May repeat at a later date, as disease may be acquired after initial visit.

✦ C. Treatment—during pregnancy, 2.4 million units of procaine penicillin G with 2 percent aluminum monostearate, IM, normally in divided doses.

D. All cases of syphilis must be reported to health authorities for treatment of contacts.

Gonorrhea

✦ A. Common contagious bacterial disease caused by *Neisseria gonorrhoeae.*

B. Incidence has been steadily rising as a result of increase in premarital sex—transmission by sexual intercourse.

C. May be mildly symptomatic in women and may persist unsuspected; male may have painful urination, pelvic pain, fever, and mucopurulent discharge.

✦ D. May cause salpingitis after third month if left untreated; PID is complication.

E. Slide for gonorrhea usually done on first prenatal visit.

F. Important to treat sexual partner, as patient may become reinfected.

G. Infection may be transmitted to baby's eyes during delivery, causing blindness.

✦ H. Soon after birth all newborns have prophylactic treatment of 1 percent silver nitrate or an antibiotic preparation, usually erythromycin.

I. Treatment—same as for syphilis. Other antibiotics may be used for sensitivity to penicillin.

Herpes Simplex Virus

A. Caused by the *herpes simplex virus* (HSV).
  1. Type 1—involves external genitalia, vagina, cervix.
  2. Type 2—development and draining of painful vesicles.

✦ B. 45 million in the United States have been diagnosed.

C. Treatment—symptomatic—no specific cure identified. Safe use of acyclovir has not been established for pregnant women.

✦ D. Virus is lethal to fetus if inoculated during vaginal delivery. Usual mode of delivery is C-section.

Veneral (Genital) Warts (HPV)

✦ A. Almost 1 million Americans develop this sexually transmitted infection each year—major STD of 1990s. Caused by the *human papillomavirus* (HPV).

B. The virus affects cervix, urethra, penis, scrotum, and anus.

C. Warts appear 1 or 2 months after exposure, transmitted through intimate sexual contact.
  ✦ 1. Symptoms are large wartlike growths on genitals (no symptoms other than lesions) and cervical cell changes.
  2. HPV associated with up to 90 percent of cervical malignancies.

D. There is no cure for HPV—treatment is cryotherapy, liquid nitrogen, or electrocautery to remove lesions.

E. Key is prevention—similar to any other STD: limit sexual contacts and use condoms.

Human Immunodeficiency Virus (HIV)

A. A retrovirus that may develop into acquired immune deficiency syndrome (AIDS).

B. Contracted through exchange of body fluids, it has a long latency period before progressing to AIDS.

C. History of belonging to high-risk group (drug use, prostitution).

D. Pregnancy associated with slight reduction of helper T cells—may increase possibility of opportunistic infections.

✦ E. HIV transmitted to 30 percent of exposed infants—risk increases with low T cell count.

F. Symptoms of seropositivity (mononucleosis-like symptoms) or ARC (pre-AIDS condition); severely compromised immune system (indicates presence of AIDS).

G. History of risk behaviors; assess for signs of STDs and CMV.

H. Complete post-test counseling if patient tests HIV positive.

I. Counsel importance of continued medical care during pregnancy.

J. Maintain body fluid precautions for all contact with patient and teach patient precautions.

K. Assess signs and symptoms of illness and serum tests.

L. *See* Newborn with (HIV) AIDS, page 458.

Adolescent Pregnancy

✦ A. More than 1 million teenagers become pregnant every year and 85 percent are unintended.

✦ B. Risk to mother and fetus is increased.
1. Crisis of pregnancy compounds the crises of adolescence related to physical, emotional, social development.
2. Patient may be unwed, which may cause additional problems.
3. Physical development may not be complete.

C. Nursing care.
1. Encourage early antepartum care.
2. Provide health instruction on pregnancy, nutrition, hygiene, infant care, and childbirth preparation.
3. Observe frequently for complications.
4. Provide emotional support and counseling.

LABOR AND DELIVERY

Definition of Terms

A. Labor is the process by which the products of conception are expelled from the body.

B. Delivery refers to the actual birth.

C. Adaptive processes.
1. During latter months of pregnancy, the fetus adapts to the maternal uterus enabling it to occupy the smallest space possible.
2. The term attitude refers to the posture the fetus assumes in utero.
3. Fetal lie is the relationship of the long axis of the baby to the long axis of the mother.

Presentation

✦ A. A term used to describe that part of the fetus that enters the true pelvis first.

✦ B. Cephalic—presentation of any part of fetal head—occurs in 95 to 97 percent of births.
1. May be vertex, face, or brow.
2. Vertex most common and most favorable for delivery. Head is sharply flexed in the pelvis with chin near chest.

✦ C. Breech—presentation of buttocks or lower extremities.
1. Types.
   a. Complete or full—buttocks and feet present (baby in squatting position).
   b. Frank—buttocks only present, or legs are extended against anterior trunk with feet touching face.
   c. Incomplete—one or both feet or knees presenting, footling single or double, or knee presentation.
2. May rotate to cephalic during pregnancy but possibility lessens as gestation nears term.
3. May be rotated by physician but usually returns to breech position.

✦ D. Transverse lie: long axis of infant lies at right angles to longitudinal axis of mother (delivery by C-section).

Position

A. A term used to describe the relationship of the fetal presenting part to the maternal bony pelvis.

B. Position is determined by locating the presenting part in relationship to the pelvis.

C. Woman's pelvis is divided into four imaginary quadrants (right anterior, right posterior, left anterior, and left posterior).

✦ D. Most common positions (abbreviations usually used).
1. **LOA** (left occiput anterior)—occiput on left side of maternal pelvis and toward front, face down, favorable for delivery.
2. **LOP** (left occiput posterior)—occiput on left side of maternal pelvis and toward rear or face up.
   a. Usually causes back pain during labor.
   b. May slow the progress of labor.
   c. Usually rotates before delivery to anterior position.

d.   May be rotated in delivery room by physician.

3.   **ROA** (right occiput anterior)—occiput on right of maternal pelvis, toward front, face down, favorable for delivery.

4.   **ROP** (right occiput posterior)—occiput on right side of maternal pelvis, face up. Same problems as LOP.

E.   Means of assessing fetal position during labor.

✦ 1.   Leopold's maneuver—method of abdominal palpation to determine information about the fetus such as presentation, engagement, position, and rough estimate of fetal size.

2.   Vaginal examination.

3.   Rectal examination (rarely done at this time).

Engagement—Lightening

✦ A.   Largest diameter of presenting part has passed into the inlet of the maternal pelvis. Usually takes place 2 weeks before labor in primiparas, but often not until labor begins in multiparas.

B.   May be assessed by Leopold's maneuver or vaginal or rectal examination.

Station

A.   Degree to which presenting part has descended into pelvis is determined by the station (the relationship between the presenting part and the ischial spines).

B.   Assessed by vaginal or rectal examination.

✦ C.   Measured in numerical terms.

1.   At level of spines: 0 station.

2.   Above level of spines: –1, –2, –3 cm.

3.   Below level of spines: +1, +2, +3 cm.

D.   Other terms used to denote station.

1.   High—presenting part not engaged.

2.   Floating—presenting part freely movable in inlet of pelvis.

3.   Dipping—entering pelvis.

4.   Fixed—no longer movable in inlet but not engaged.

5.   Engaged—biparietal plane passed through pelvic inlet.

Premonitory Signs of Labor

Physical Signs of Impending Labor

A.   Premonitory signs—physiologic changes that take place the last several weeks of pregnancy, indicating that labor is near.

✦ B.   *Lightening*—descent of the uterus downward and forward, which takes place as the presenting part descends into the pelvis.

1.   Time in which it takes place varies from a few weeks to a few days before labor. In multigravida, it may occur during labor.

2.   Sensations.

a.   Relief of pressure on diaphragm, and breathing is easier.

b.   Increased pelvic pressure leading to leg cramps, frequent micturition, and pressure on rectum.

✦ C.   *Braxton Hicks* contractions.

✦ 1.   May become quite regular but do not effectively dilate cervix, thus often called false labor.

2.   True labor has regular, painful contractions that continue with walking.

3.   Usually are more pronounced at night.

4.   May play a part in ripening the cervix.

D.   Decrease in weight—there is usually a decrease in water retention due to hormonal influences.

E.   Cervical changes—cervix usually becomes softer, shorter, and somewhat dilated. May be dilated 1–2 cm by the time labor begins.

F.   Bloody show.

1.   Tenacious mucous vaginal discharge, usually pinkish or streaked with blood, which is expelled from the cervix as it shortens and begins to dilate.

2.   Labor usually begins within 24–48 hours.

G.   Rupture of membranes.

1.   May break any time before labor or during labor. Occasionally, they remain intact and are ruptured by the physician during labor (amniotomy).

2.   May gush or trickle.

3.   Patient usually advised to come to the hospital as labor may begin within 24 hours.

4.   If labor does not begin spontaneously, it is induced to avoid intrauterine infections.

Implementation

✦ A.   Test vaginal secretions for alkalinity with Nitrozine paper—normal vaginal pH is acidic—confirms rupture.

B.   Keep patient on bedrest if ordered.

C.   Watch for signs of infection.

D.   Watch for signs of labor.

E.   Watch for prolapse of cord.

F.   Monitor fetal heart rate regularly.

G.   Observe amniotic fluid for foul odor or signs of fetal distress (meconium staining); record time, amount, color, and odor, if present.

Assessment of Fetal Maturity and Placental Function

✦ Studies for Delivery Capability

A.   Estriol excretion.

1.   Estriol level increases as the fetus grows and decreases when growth ceases.

2.   Provides guide to placental functioning and fetal well-being.

3. Measured by 24-hour urine specimen or serum estriol levels.

✦ B. Amniocentesis.
1. Introduction of a needle through the abdominal and uterine wall and into the amniotic cavity to withdraw fluid for examination.
2. Preparation of patient.
   a. Have patient empty bladder.
   b. Take fetal heart rate.
   c. Make patient comfortable.
   d. Explain and give reassurance that the procedure will not harm the baby.
   e. Prepare abdomen with antiseptic solution.
   f. Have necessary equipment available.
✦ 3. Indications.
   a. Sex of baby.
   b. Certain congenital defects such as Down syndrome.
   c. State of fetus affected by Rh isoimmunization.
   d. Fetal maturity.
✦ C. Phosphatidylglycerol (PG).
1. Second most abundant phospholipid in surfactant.
2. Recently, lung maturity is determined by combination of L/S ratio and PG.
✦ D. Lecithin/sphingomyelin (L/S ratio).
1. Test for fetal maturity by examining the ratio of two components of surfactant— lecithin and sphingomyelin.
2. Lecithin major constituent of surfactant in the lungs.
   a. 13th week, sphingomyelin is higher than lecithin.
   b. Lecithin increases slowly until 35th week when it is two or more times sphingomyelin —infant lungs are now mature.
E. Sonography.
1. Used to measure biparietal diameter of the fetal skull after 16 weeks (should be measured weekly when growth retardation is suspected).
2. Can determine position of placenta.
✦ F. Ultrasound.
1. A diagnostic test of intermittent high frequency sound waves that reflect off tissues according to varying densities.
   a. Most common diagnostic procedure— 70 percent women in the United States.
   b. Evaluates both functional and structural characteristics.
2. Advantages—technique is noninvasive, non-damaging, and painless.
3. Purpose—to differentiate tissue mass and do serial studies. Determines fetal movements, breathing, heart valve capability.

4. Results—detects placental location (amniocentesis, placenta previa), gestational age, presence of twins, fetal growth.
5. Procedure—patient instructed to have a full bladder; test takes 20–30 minutes to complete. Near term, anticipate supine hypotension, nausea, and vertigo.
✦ G. Contraction stress test (oxytocin challenge test).
✦ 1. Test designed to measure the fetus reaction to uterine contractions.
2. Performed on high-risk patients (postmature diabetes).
3. If placental flow is normal, fetus remains oxygenated during uterine contractions.
4. Placental insufficiency produces characteristic late deceleration pattern during contraction. Fetal bradycardia is < 120 beats/min.
✦ 5. Procedure. ❖ **PROCEDURE** ❖
   a. Measured dosage of oxytocin by infusion pump; piggybacked into main IV line.
   ✦ b. Dosage is increased q 15–20 minutes until patient has three uterine contractions of at least 40 seconds in 10 minutes.
   c. Oxytocin is then discontinued.
   d. Patient is monitored with external fetal monitor. Baseline fetal heart rate is established prior to beginning the test.
   e. Apply external monitor and obtain baseline fetal heart rates.
   f. Observe for complications.
      (1) Fetal heart rate below 120.
      (2) Sustained uterine contractions.
      (3) Supine hypotensive syndrome.

Chorionic Villus Sampling (CVS)

✦ A. Diagnostic capability similar to amniocentesis; results reflect fetal chromosome, enzyme, and DHA.
✦ B. Advantage is that diagnostic information available before end of first trimester of pregnancy; disadvantage is increased risk of pregnancy loss.
C. A transcervical approach used to aspirate chorionic villi from the placenta through endocervix.
D. Syringe contents (villi) inspected microscopically and prepared for culture; results are available in 1–2 weeks.

Alpha-Fetoprotein (AFP)

✦ A. Principal screening procedure for detection of neural tube defect (spina bifida, hydrocephalus, done at 16–18 weeks; incidence is 1/1000–2000 births in the United States).
1. Low levels detect Down syndrome and maternal hypertensive states.

2. High levels detect open neural tube defects (risk of which can be reduced with mother supplementing diet with folic acid prior to and during first trimester); risk of premature delivery, toxemia, fetal distress, Rh isoimmunization.

B. Mother's blood is analyzed for amount of AFP that liver normally re-releases at a known and increasing amount as pregnancy proceeds.

C. Procedure allows families to choose whether to have a child with an identified birth defect.

Induction of Labor

Mammary Stimulation Test (MST)

✦ A. Also called Breast Self-Stimulation Test (BSST). Purpose—start contractions without the use of oxytocin.

B. Preferred method to oxytocin infusion because it is noninvasive.

C. Procedure—manual stimulation of mother's nipples triggers release of oxytocin to induce contractions.
1. Contractions similar to those with spontaneous labor.
2. Nerve impulses cause release of endogenous oxytocin.
3. Contractions begin within 15–30 minutes.
4. Assess FHR for prolonged decelerations.
5. Perform test in or near delivery room.

Oxytocin Infusion

A. Indications for use.
1. Patient overdue (2 weeks or more); placental functions reduced.
2. Severe preeclampsia.
3. Diabetes.
4. Premature rupture of membranes (should deliver within 24 hours).
5. Uncontrolled bleeding.
6. Rh sensitization (rising titer).
7. Excessive size of fetus.

✦ B. Prerequisites for successful induction.
1. Fetal maturity.
2. Cervix amenable to induction (at times, patient may be induced for several days consecutively with rest at night to ripen cervix, if it is desirable to deliver fetus because of complications).
3. Normal cephalopelvic proportions.
4. Fetal head engaged.

✦ C. Danger signals.
1. Prolonged uterine contractions (over 90 seconds with less than 30 seconds rest period between). Safety intervention is to turn off IV—check with RN.
2. Sustained uterine contractions.

3. Fetal heart tones above 160 or below 120; change in heart rhythm.
4. Hemorrhage and shock.
5. Elevated blood pressure.
6. Abruptio placentae.

Process of Labor and Delivery

Theories Pertaining to Cause of Labor

A. Absolute causes unknown.

B. Alterations in hormonal balance of estrogen increases contractility; progesterone decreases uterine contractility.

C. Degeneration of the placenta so that it no longer provides necessary elements to fetus.

D. Overdistention of uterus incites a stimulus that triggers release of oxytocin and initiates contractions.

E. High levels of prostaglandins near term may stimulate uterine contractions.

F. It may be a combination of several of these physiological occurrences that produce the type of contraction necessary for true labor.

Forces That Produce Labor

A. Muscular contractions originate primarily in muscles of uterus and secondarily in abdominal muscles.

B. Uterine muscles contract during first stages and bring about effacement and dilatation of the cervix.

C. Abdominal muscles come into play after complete cervical dilatation and help to expel the baby.

Duration of Labor

A. Varies according to individual.

✦ B. Average.
1. Primipara—up to 18 hours; some may be shorter, others longer.
2. Multipara—up to 8 hours; some may be shorter, others longer.

C. Length of labor depends on:
1. Effectiveness of contractions.
2. Amount of resistance baby must overcome to adapt to the pelvis.
3. Stretching ability of soft tissue.
4. Preparation and relaxation of mother (fear and anxiety can retard progress).

Uterine Contractions

A. Characteristics.
1. *Involuntary*—cannot be controlled by will of mother.
2. *Intermittent*—periods of relaxation between contractions. Intervals allow mother to rest and also allow adequate circulation of uterine blood vessels and oxygenation of fetus.

3. *Regular*—occur once true labor is established.
4. Discomfort in back (usually starts low and radiates around to abdomen).
5. Increase in discomfort from intensity, frequency, and duration of contractions as labor progresses.

B. Methods for monitoring contractions.
1. Place finger lightly on the fundus of the uterus (the most contractile portion), and relate what you feel in your fingers to seconds and minutes on a clock. Uterus becomes firm, then hardens, and then decreases in hardness.
✦ 2. Use electronic monitoring device (*see* fetal monitoring procedure, page 440).
   a. External (less accurate)—done with a pressure-sensitive button placed over the uterine fundus.
   b. Internal (catheter inserted into uterine cavity, which measures internal pressures); relays information to a graph.

✦ C. Contractions are monitored for frequency, duration, and intensity.
1. *Frequency*—measure by timing contractions from the beginning of one contraction to the beginning of next.
2. *Duration*—measure time at beginning of contraction to the completion of the contraction. Cannot be measured exactly by feeling with the hand.
3. *Intensity*—measure by internal fetal monitoring device; cannot be measured by feeling.
4. Contractions may be described as mild, moderate, or intense.

D. Purpose of contractions.
1. To propel presenting part forward.
2. To bring about effacement and dilatation of the cervix.

Effacement and Dilatation

✦ A. *Effacement*—process by which cervical canal is progressively shortened to a stage of complete obliteration. Progresses from a structure of 1–2 cm in length to almost complete obliteration.
✦ B. *Dilatation*—process by which external os enlarges from a few millimeters to approximately 10 cm.
C. All that remains of the cervix after effacement and dilatation is a paper-thin circular opening about 10 cm in diameter.
D. Effacement and dilatation may be measured by vaginal or rectal examination.

Changes in the Uterus

A. Uterus usually becomes differentiated in two distinct portions as labor progresses.
1. Upper portion is contractile and becomes thicker.

2. Lower portion is passive, becomes thinner and more expanded.

B. Boundary between the two segments is termed the *physiologic retraction ring*.

False Labor

✦ A. Signs.
1. Irregular contractions.
2. Contractions that may cause discomfort.
3. Discomfort is usually located in abdomen.
4. Labor usually does not intensify.
5. Discomfort may be relieved by walking.
6. Contractions do not bring about appreciable changes in cervix.

B. Sometimes difficult to differentiate false labor from true labor until woman is observed for several hours in the hospital.
C. Signs of true labor.
1. Contractions increase in frequency, intensity, and duration.
2. Progressive cervical effacement and dilatation.
3. Progressive descent of presenting part.
4. Presence of bloody show.
5. Contractions increase in intensity with walking.

Signs of Imminent Delivery

A. Increase in bloody show.
B. Nausea, vomiting, and shaking.
C. Pressure on rectum, and woman feels the urge to push (involuntary bearing down).
D. Deep grunting sound from woman.
E. Woman states she is ready to deliver.
F. Bulging of the perineum.

Four Stages of Labor

Stage One

A. Stage one begins with first true labor contraction and ends with complete cervical dilatation.
✦ B. *Phase one: latent (effacement) phase*.
1. Begins with onset of regular contraction pattern.
2. Dilatation 3 to 4 cm; membranes usually intact.
3. Contractions are mild and become well established.
4. Contractions are 5–15 minutes apart and last about 10–30 seconds. Averages 6.4 hours.
5. Cervix thins.
6. Usually some bloody show.
7. Station is anywhere from –2 cm to –1 cm in multipara; at 0 in primigravida.
8. Woman may be quite comfortable, talkative, alert, and cheerful.

9. Woman has lots of energy and feels she can cope with labor.
10. Auscultate fetal heart rate every 30 min to 1 hour.
11. Check vital signs every 4 hours or more frequently.

◆ C. *Phase two: active (dilatation) phase.*
   1. Dilatation 4–8 cm.
   2. Dilatation is more rapid.
   3. Contractions are 3–5 minutes apart, last 30–45 seconds.
   4. Increase in bloody show.
   5. Station varies from 0 to +1 cm.
   6. Woman becomes tired and less talkative and shows lack of energy.
   7. Woman may need coaching on breathing/relaxation techniques, or analgesia (anesthesia).

◆ D. *Phase three: transitional phase.*
   1. Dilatation slows as it reaches 8–10 cm.
   2. Contractions are intense and close (1½ to 2 minutes apart, lasting 60–90 seconds).
   3. Station +1 or +2 cm.
   4. Copious bloody show.
   5. Desire to bear down or defecate.
   6. Membranes may rupture spontaneously if they have not done so previously; physician may rupture them artificially.
   7. Woman's attention and feelings are inner-directed; she feels exhausted and no longer able to cope.
   8. Signs of restlessness, shaking, nausea, vomiting, trembling, burping, or crying may be present.

Stage Two

A. Stage two begins with complete dilatation (10 cm) and ends with birth of baby.
◆ B. Mechanism of labor and delivery.
   ◆ 1. Sequence of movements of presenting part through birth canal. Head usually enters transverse and must rotate LOA or ROA for birth.
   2. *Engagement*—head enters pelvis.
   3. *Descent*—movement that occurs simultaneously with passage of head through pelvis.
   4. *Flexion*—occurs as head descends and meets with resistance. In extreme flexion the smallest diameter of the head presents.
   5. *Internal rotation*—head usually enters with long diameter conforming to long diameter of inlet (usually transverse position) and must be rotated before it can emerge from outlet (head rotates so that smallest diameter presents to conform to pelvis).

6. *Extension*—follows internal rotation. The head, which is flexed as it passes through birth canal, must extend for birth.
7. *External rotation or restitution*—soon after birth, the head rotates to either mother's right or left side (fetal position before birth).
8. *Expulsion*—with delivery of shoulders, rest of body is expelled spontaneously.

C. Stage of expulsion.
   1. Expulsion brought about by contractions of uterine and abdominal muscles.
   2. Contractions are every 2–3 minutes, last 60–90 seconds.

Stage Three

◆ A. Stage three, or placental stage, begins with birth and ends with delivery of placenta.
B. Phase of placental separation.
   1. Usually takes place with next few contractions after birth.
   2. Usually begins at center but may begin at edges.
   3. Some bleeding usually accompanies separation of placenta.
C. Phase of expulsion.
   1. May be expulsed spontaneously by mother, but is usually expressed manually by the physician after separation is complete.
   ◆ 2. Mechanisms.
      a. *Schultze* (most common)—placenta is inverted on itself, and the shiny fetal surface appears; 80 percent separate in center.
      b. *Duncan*—descends sideways and the maternal surface appears.

Stage Four

A. Stage four begins with delivery of placenta and ends when postpartum condition of the mother is stabilized.
B. First hour after birth is critical.

NURSING CARE IN LABOR AND DELIVERY

Phase One: Latent Phase (Dilatation to 3–4 cm)

Admission

A. Details of care vary from hospital to hospital.
B. Check vital signs—temperature, pulse, respirations, and blood pressure.
C. Check fetal heart tones (FHT).
D. Determine intactness of membranes.
E. Give prep (perineal shave) and enema (if ordered by physician).

F. See that appropriate forms are completed.

G. Encourage woman to void; check urine for sugar and acetone.

H. Determine frequency, intensity (mild, moderate, severe), and duration of contractions.

I. Determine amount and character of bloody show.

J. Determine amount of cervical dilatation, effacement, station, presentation, and vaginal discharge.

K. Keep call bell within easy reach.

✦ After Admission

A. Maintain bedrest if membranes have ruptured. (In some hospitals, the patient may be allowed out of bed with ruptured membranes if the baby's head is well engaged and the patient is otherwise all right.)

B. Note frequency, duration, and strength of contraction every 30 minutes or PRN.

C. Auscultate FHT every 15 minutes or PRN.

D. Check blood pressure every 30 minutes or PRN.

E. Check vital signs once per shift or more often if needed.

F. Periodic vaginal examination as indicated.

G. Observe for ruptured membranes and take FHT immediately if membranes rupture.

H. Reinforce breathing techniques or teach breathing techniques if woman has had no classes.

I. Keep family informed of progress.

J. Encourage the presence of patient's husband or a significant other person.

K. Provide support based upon woman's knowledge of the labor process.

L. Reduce stimuli if woman wants to rest.

M. Start IV if ordered; usually NPO.

✦ Phase Two: Active Phase (Dilatation 3–4 to 8 cm)

A. Encourage breathing techniques.

B. Maintain IV fluids.

C. Encourage voiding.

D. Auscultate FHT every 15 minutes or PRN.

E. Monitor contractions.

F. Take blood pressure every 30 minutes or PRN.

G. Periodic vaginal examination to determine progress.

H. Observe amount and character of show.

I. Urge mother to stay off back to avoid supine hypotensive syndrome, and to lie on side.

J. Administer medications as ordered. Tranquilizing drugs may be given in early labor, but analgesics are not usually given until labor is well established.

K. Assist with anesthesia, if given, and monitor blood pressure and FHT.

L. Continue giving patient support and information.

✦ Phase Three: Transitional Phase (Dilatation 8 to 10 cm)

A. Continue with care listed above.

B. Explain progress to patient and encourage her to continue with breathing and relaxing techniques.

C. Discourage bearing-down efforts until dilatation is complete.

D. Encourage deep ventilation prior to and after each contraction.

E. Monitor contractions lightly with fingers as abdomen is sensitive.

F. Accept irritable behavior and aggression; continue supportive care.

G. Help patient to push when ready.

H. Observe for signs of imminent delivery, and transfer patient to delivery room when ready.

Fetal Assessment

Fetal Distress

A. Signs.
   - ✦ 1. FHT above 160 or below 120 beats/min.
   - ✦ 2. Meconium-stained fluid (during hypoxia, bowel peristalsis increases, and meconium is likely to be passed).
   - 3. Fetal hyperactivity.

✦ B. Immediate nursing interventions.
   1. Discontinue oxytocin if it is infusing.
   - ✦ 2. Turn patient to left side; if no improvement, turn to right side. This procedure relieves pressure on umbilical cord during contractions and pressure of uterus on the inferior vena cava.
   - ✦ 3. Administer oxygen at 6–7 L/min per orders.
   4. Report findings to charge nurse or physician immediately.

Vena Caval Syndrome (Supine Hypotensive Syndrome)

Assessment

✦ A. Assess for shocklike symptoms that occur when venous return to the heart is impaired by weight of gravid uterus causing partial occlusion of the vena cava (reduced cardiac output).
   1. Hypotension.
   2. Tachycardia.
   3. Sweating, dizziness, pallor.
   4. Nausea and vomiting.
   5. Air hunger.

B. Check for risk factors—multiple pregnancies, obesity, polyhydramnios.

C. Fetal distress; caused by reduced flow of blood to placenta from reduced cardiac output.

Implementation

✦ A. Assist mother to turn to left side (using a wedge pillow) to shift weight of fetus off inferior vena cava.

✦ B. Provide oxygen with tight mask at 6–7 L/min if recovery is not immediate after positioning.

✦ C. Monitor fetal heart rate to determine fetal status.

Signs of Complications of Labor

✦ A. Fetal distress.
   1. Fetal tachycardia—persistent fetal heart rate above 160 or an increase in the basal rate, 20–30 beats/min.
   2. Fetal bradycardia—below 120 beats/min.

B. Absent, minimal, or irregular FHT.

C. Foul-smelling or meconium-stained amniotic fluid.

D. Fetal hyperactivity.

E. Elevated temperature in woman.

F. Dehydration.

G. Hemorrhage.

H. Inadequate uterine relaxation between contractions—> 90 seconds and < 30 seconds between contractions.

I. Anxiety in woman.

J. Distended bladder.

Fetal Monitoring

Characteristics

✦ A. Two types of electronic fetal monitoring.
   1. External (EFM) and internal (IFM)
   2. Continuous data readout of fetal heart rate and uterine contraction pattern.

B. Ultrasound transducer picks up motion of the fetal heart valves—provides external recording.

C. Pressure-sensitive button placed over the uterine fundus—external monitoring of uterine contraction.

D. Heart rate sounds and uterine contractions are translated into electrical impulses reproduced on a printout strip on the fetal monitor.

✦ E. Types of external fetal monitors.
   1. Abdominal electrodes—elicit fetal and maternal heart rates.
   2. Phonotransducer—picks up fetal heart tones.
   3. Ultrasonic transducer—picks up fetal heart tones.
   4. Tocotransducer—monitors uterine activity.

Implementation ❖ PROCEDURE ❖

✦ A. Preparation.
   1. Explain procedure to patient.
   2. Plug tocotransducer into monitor inlet.
   3. Turn monitor on and press printout button.
   4. Move stylus to zero. The printout is divided into two parts. The uterine activity waveform is found on the right side.

✦ B. Placement of external uterine contraction monitor.
   1. Place external tocotransducer over uterine fundus. (Locate fundus using Leopold's maneuvers.)
   2. Position the tocotransducer in place with belt. (Powder belt first to avoid irritating skin.)
   3. When patient is free of contractions, tighten belt until stylus on monitor moves to the 50 mm Hg mark on the right side of the printout.
   4. Turn control knob until stylus moves back to the 10 mm Hg mark.
   5. Test tocotransducer by pressing down on transducer. If the baseline recorder moves, tocotransducer is functioning properly.
   6. Record frequency and duration of contractions as required by hospital policy.

C. Placement of external fetal monitor.
   1. Apply water-soluble gel to underside of transducer.
   2. Position transducer on uterus over area of fetal back.

✦ D. Monitoring uterine activity.
   1. *Normal fetal heart rate:* 120–160 beats/min; determine baseline.
   2. *Early deceleration:* 10–20 beat drop in rate usually within normal range of 120–160 beats/min.
   3. *Late deceleration:* decrease in fetal heart rate of 10–20 beats/min—usually indicates fetal distress.
   4. *Variable deceleration:* no uniformity in pattern—may indicate cord compression.
   5. *Loss of beat-to-beat variation:* baseline is smooth—may be serious sign of fetal anoxia.
   6. *Bradycardia:* any persistent drop of 20 beats below baseline or under 120 beats/min—may be indicative of fetal distress.
   7. *Tachycardia:* increase of 10 percent over baseline or over 160 beats/min—an ominous sign—requires intervention stat due to fetal hypoxia.

Nursing Responsibilities

Birthing Room Care

A. If separate delivery room used, transfer woman carefully from bed to delivery table; place in lithotomy position.

B. On birthing bed or delivery table, pad stirrups to avoid pressure to popliteal veins and pressure areas. Gently raise both legs simultaneously into stirrups to avoid ligament strain. Adjust stirrups and drape patient.

C. Provide patient with handles to pull on as she pushes.

✦ D. Cleanse vulva and perineum using sterile technique, commonly referred to as perineal "wash down."

✦ E. Auscultate FHT every 5 minutes or after each push—transient fetal bradycardia not unusual due to head compression.

✦ F. Check blood pressure and pulse every 15 minutes PRN.

G. Allow baby's father in room, and position him at the head of bed.

H. Encourage patient and keep her informed of advancement of baby.

I. Encourage patient to take a deep breath before beginning to push with each contraction and to sustain push as long as possible (long pushes are preferable to frequent short pushes).

✦ **Postpartum Care**

A. Palpate fundus every 15 minutes and PRN for first hour.

✦ B. Massage fundus gently if it is not firm.

✦ C. Check TPR and blood pressure upon admission; check blood pressure every 15 minutes and PRN for first hour.

D. Encourage voiding and measure amount.

E. Check lochia for color, consistency, and amount.

F. Inspect perineum and episiotomy for signs of bleeding, unusual redness, or swelling.

G. Weigh pads if unusual bleeding noted.

H. Allow mother and baby's father the privacy to talk.

I. Encourage mother to rest.

J. Provide medications for pain as ordered and needed.

K. Chart all pertinent data.

L. Maintain intake and output the first 24 hours or until patient is voiding a sufficient quantity.

OPERATIVE OBSTETRICS

Obstetrical Procedures

Episiotomy

✦ A. An incision made into the perineum during delivery to facilitate the birth process.

B. Types.

1. Midline—incision from the posterior margin of the vaginal opening directly back to the anal sphincter.
   a. Healing is less painful.
   b. Incision is easy to repair.
2. Mediolateral—incision made at 45-degree angle to either side of the vaginal opening.

a. Healing process is quite painful.
b. Incision is harder to repair.

C. Purpose.

1. To spare the muscles of perineal floor from undue stretching and tearing (lacerations).
2. To prevent the prolonged pressure of the baby's head on perineum.

D. Method.

1. Generally done during contraction when the baby's head pushes against perineum and stretches it.
2. Blunt scissors are used.
3. Mother is usually given an anesthetic (regional, local, or inhalation).

Assisted Delivery: Forceps or Vacuum

A. Baby is extracted from the birth canal by the physician with the use of a specially designed instrument; cervix must be fully dilated.

✦ B. Types.

1. Low forceps—presenting part at or below pelvic floor.
2. Mid forceps—presenting part below or at the level of the ischial spine.
3. Vacuum extraction: soft silicone cup applied to fetal head; used during prolonged second stage; preferred if borderline CPD.

C. Indications.

✦ 1. Fetal distress.
2. Poor progress of fetus through the birth canal.
3. Failure of the head to rotate.
4. Maternal disease (heart disease, acute pulmonary edema, infection), or exhaustion.
5. Woman unable to push (as with regional anesthesia, epidural–spinal combined, or epidural).

D. Complications.

1. Lacerations of the vagina or the cervix; there may be oozing or hemorrhage.
2. Rupture of the uterus.
3. Intracranial hemorrhage and brain damage to the fetus.
4. Facial paralysis of the fetus.

Cesarean Delivery

A. Incision into abdominal wall and uterus to enable the delivery of an infant.

✦ B. Types.

1. Classical—vertical incision through the abdominal wall and into the anterior wall of the uterus.
2. Low segment transverse—transverse incision made into lower uterine segment after abdomen has been opened.
   a. Incision made into part of uterus where there is less uterine activity and blood loss is minimal.

b. Less incidence of adhesions and intestinal obstruction.
3. Cesarean hysterectomy—abdomen and uterus are opened, baby and placenta are removed, and then the hysterectomy is performed. Conditions indicating hysterectomy:
   a. Presence of diseased tissue or fibroids.
   b. An abnormal Pap smear.
   c. Ruptured uterus.
   d. Uncontrolled hemorrhage, abruptio placentae, uterine atony, or other disorders.

C. Indications.
1. Fetal distress unrelieved by other measures.
2. Uterine dysfunction.
3. Certain cases of placenta previa and premature separation of placenta.
4. Prolapsed cord.
5. Diabetes or certain cases of toxemia.
6. Cephalopelvic disproportion.
7. Malpresentations such as transverse lie.

Nursing Management

Preoperative Care

A. Discuss and reassure to decrease anxiety.
B. Pre-op teaching and support to patient and family.
C. Prep IV, Foley catheter inserted, operative procedure permission signed.

Postoperative Care

◆ A. Take vital signs (blood pressure, pulse, and respiration) every 5 minutes until stable, then every 15 minutes for 2–3 hours.
B. Observe site of incision for bleeding every 15 minutes for 2–3 hours.
C. Palpate fundus for location and tone every 15 minutes for 2–3 hours.
D. Check lochia for amount and color every 15 minutes for 2–3 hours.
E. Reinforce abdominal dressing as necessary.
F. Observe drainage from Foley catheter (amount, color, pressure of blood, and other aspects).
G. Check level of consciousness.
H. Measure intake and output.
I. Assist patient to deep breathe, cough, and turn.
J. Change perineal pad as needed.
K. Reassure the patient that the delivery is over, and give her information regarding the condition of the baby. (If something is wrong with the baby, usually the physician will first discuss this with parents.)
L. Help ambulate patient (usually the first postpartum day).
M. Give stool softener as ordered and needed.
N. Encourage patient to talk about delivery and baby.
O. Reinforce physician's teaching about care at home.
1. Planned rest periods.
2. Avoidance of heavy lifting for 4–6 weeks.
3. Signs of infection.
4. Care of the breasts.
5. Avoidance of constipation.
6. Nutritive diet.
7. Arrangements for postpartum checkup in 4–6 weeks.

COMPLICATIONS OF LABOR AND DELIVERY

Dystocia

◆ *Definition:* Prolonged and difficult labor and delivery, i.e., it extends for 24 hours or more after the onset of regular contractions.

Classification

◆ A. Dystocia may be classified in several ways; although the divisions are artificial, they are useful in looking at the processes involved.
1. Dysfunctions of powers or forces with respect to the uterus and abdominal muscles.
2. Abnormalities of the passengers (the fetus and placenta).
3. Abnormalities of the passages (bony and soft tissue).
4. May be a combination of two or more dysfunctions and abnormalities.
B. Characteristics.
1. True labor begins but fails to progress.
2. Dystocia may occur during latent or active phase of labor.
3. It is important to look at the rate of progress as well as the overall length of labor, i.e., is the patient slowly progressing or is she arrested at one spot?

Dysfunctional Labor

◆ A. Prolonged latent phase—time required to dilate cervix to 4 cm is prolonged; primipara over 20 hours, multipara 14 hours.
1. Causes or contributing condition.
   a. Oversedation.
   b. "Unripe" cervix.
   c. False labor.
   d. Uterine dysfunction or abnormalities.
2. Treatment and nursing care.
   a. Encourage rest as woman is usually exhausted.
   b. Narcotic agent is given to stop labor and promote rest.

✦ Table 14-4. COMPLICATIONS AND SIGNS OF DISTRESS IN THE MOTHER: PROLONGED LABOR

Complication	Signs of Distress	Possible Nursing Care
Infection	Elevated temperature and pulse	Maintain sterile technique while doing vaginals Keep vaginals to a minimum Administer antibiotics as ordered
Exhaustion	Loss of emotional stability Lack of cooperation	Provide supportive therapy and comfort measures to promote relaxation and relieve tension Encourage rest Administer sedation as ordered
Dehydration	Dry tongue and skin Concentrated urine Acetonuria	Monitor IV fluids Place a wet cloth to the patient's mouth Make a frequent check of bladder elimination

---

✦ Table 14-5. COMPLICATIONS AND SIGNS OF DISTRESS IN THE FETUS: PROLONGED LABOR

Complication	Signs of Distress	Possible Nursing Care
Asphyxia	Irregular heart rate Heart rate above 160 or below 120 Passage of meconium if fetus is in the vertex position	Administer oxygen to the mother Constantly observe and monitor FHT Check for prolapse of the cord Prepare delivery room equipment for possible resuscitation of the baby at birth
Generalized infection	Irregular heart rate Heart rate above 160 or below 120	Administer antibiotics to the mother Keep vaginals to a minimum Follow same care (except cord check) as asphyxia

---

c. Vaginal examination is made to determine fetal position and station.

d. X-ray pelvimetry is made to determine the disorder.

e. Performance of amniotomy (artificial rupture of membranes) if conditions are favorable for vaginal delivery.

f. Oxytocin is given as a stimulant.

g. Labor usually progresses normally after rest and stimulation by oxytocin.

✦ B. Prolonged active phase—dilatation slower than 1.2 cm/hr for primigravida; dilatation slower than 1.5 cm/hr for multigravida.

1. Causes.

a. Cephalopelvic disproportion (CPD).

b. Malpositions.

c. Excessive sedation or anesthesia.

d. Unknown causes.

2. Treatment and nursing care.

a. Usually no active treatment is given if dilatation is regular unless labor will be prolonged over 24 hours; then give supportive therapy.

b. Cesarean section may be indicated in CPD or for labor over 24 hours.

C. Arrested phase—lack of progress.

1. Causes.

a. CPD.

b. Malposition of the fetus.

c. Excessive sedation and anesthesia.

d. Uterine abnormalities.

2. Medical treatment and nursing care.

a. Vaginal examination to determine position and station of fetus.

b. X-ray pelvimetry to determine CPD.

c. Provide rest for exhausted patient.

d. Cautious use of oxytocic stimulation if malposition, CPD, and other abnormalities are ruled out.

e. Cesarean section if appropriate.

D. Complications of prolonged labor (*see* Tables 14-4 and 14-5).

✦ Other Causes of Dysfunctional Labor

A. Tetanic uterine contractions—contraction lasting over 90 seconds. May lead to fetal asphyxia or uterine rupture.

B. Precipitate delivery—labor of 3 hours' or less duration. May lead to injury of mother and fetus due to trauma.

C. Rupture of the uterus—splitting of the uterine wall accompanied by extrusion of all or part of uterine contents into the abdominal cavity. Baby usually dies, and mortality rate in mothers is high due to blood loss.

1. Signs of rupture.

a. Acute abdominal pain and tenderness.
b. Presenting part no longer felt through cervix.
c. Feeling in patient that something has happened inside her.
d. Cessation of labor pains (no contractions).
e. Bleeding usually internal; may be some external bleeding.
f. Signs of shock (pale appearance, pulse weak and rapid, air hunger, and exhaustion).

2. Treatment.
   a. Laparotomy to remove fetus.
   b. Hysterectomy, although uterus may be sutured and left in.
   c. Blood transfusions.
   d. Antibiotics to prevent infection from traumatized tissues.

Implementation

A. Promote rest (darken room, reduce noise level).
B. Position patient for comfort.
C. Give patient a back rub.
D. Provide clean linen and gown; allow patient to bathe or shower if permissible.
E. Promote oral hygiene.
F. Give patient reassurance and support.
G. Explain procedures to the patient.
H. Let mother express feelings and emotions freely.
I. Watch for signs of exhaustion, dehydration, and acidosis.
J. Monitor vital signs.
K. Monitor FHT.
L. Monitor contractions for frequency, intensity and duration.
M. Watch for signs of excessive bleeding and fetal distress.
N. Administer medications as ordered.

Abnormalities of the Fetus and Placenta

✦ Abnormal Presentations and Positions

✦ A. Occiput posterior position.
   1. Usually prolongs labor because baby must rotate a longer distance (35 degrees or more) to reach symphysis pubis.
   2. Possible results.
      a. Persistent occiput posterior (head does not rotate).
      b. Deep transverse arrest (head arrested in transverse position).
   3. Treatment.
      a. Head usually rotates itself with contraction.
      b. Rotation may be done by physician manually or with forceps.

✦ B. Breech prolongs labor because soft tissue does not aid cervical dilatation as well as the fetal skull.
C. Face presentation is rare; results in increased prenatal mortality.
   1. Chin must rotate so it lies under symphysis pubis for delivery.
   2. If baby is delivered vaginally, the face is usually edematous and bruised, with marked molding.
   3. Cesarean section is indicated if face does not rotate.
D. Transverse lie.
   1. Long axis of fetus at right angles to long axis of mother.
   2. Spontaneous conversion may occur. Cesarean section is the usual method of delivery.

Excessive Size of Fetus

A. Disproportion between the size of the fetus and the size of the pelvis when fetus is 10 pounds or over.
B. Head is usually large and less moldable.
C. Size of shoulders may also complicate delivery.
D. Causes.
   1. Multiparity—birth weight may progress with each pregnancy.
   2. Maternal diabetes.
E. Size of fetus may be determined by sonography and x-ray.
F. Treatment.
   1. Vaginal delivery if disproportion is not too great. Usually, there are fetal injuries— brachial plexus, dislocated shoulder.
   2. Cesarean section indicated if proportion too great.
G. Fetal abnormalities.
   1. Hydrocephalus.
   2. Tumors.

Abnormalities of Passage

Cephalopelvic Disproportion

A. Disproportion may be in inlet, mid-pelvis, or outlet.
B. Pelvis is considered contracted if it is reduced enough in size to interfere with normal delivery.
C. Trial labor may be done in borderline cases.
D. Determined by x-ray of pelvis (pelvimetry).
E. Cesarean delivery is the usual method of treatment.

Other Complications of Labor

Premature Labor and Delivery

A. Occurs when pregnancy terminates after the period of viability but usually before the end of the 36th week.

B. Betamethasone or some other drug is administered to the mother to hasten fetal maturity by
stimulating development of lecithin when membranes are ruptured and premature labor cannot
be arrested.

Prolonged Pregnancy

A. Pregnancy of over 42 weeks' gestation.
B. Complications.
  1. Amniotic fluid decreases and vernix caseosa
     disappears; infant's skin appears dry and
     cracked.
  2. Infant may weigh less.
  3. Chronic hypoxia due to placental dysfunction.
  4. Infant may pass meconium due to hypoxia.
C. Determination of gestational age usually made to
   ascertain actual duration of pregnancy by means
   of estriol studies, sonography.
D. Contraction stress test (oxytocin challenge test) to
   determine fetus's ability to tolerate labor.
E. Labor stimulated with oxytocin.
F. Cesarean section if induction contraindicated.

Prolapsed Umbilical Cord

✦ A. Descent of prolapsed cord through cervical canal
   alongside the presenting part; may even protrude
   from the vagina.
B. Causes.
  1. Ruptured membranes before engagement.
  2. Abnormal presentations.
  3. Premature infant—presenting part does not
     fill the birth canal and allow for more space.
  4. Polyhydramnios.
C. Symptoms.
  1. Abnormal fetal heart pattern.
  2. Cord may be palpated or seen on vaginal
     examination.
D. Complications—cord is compressed between presenting part and pelvis resulting in fetal
   asphyxia.
✦ E. Immediate treatment and nursing care.
  1. Move presenting part so that it is elevated off
     umbilical cord.
     a. Place patient in knee–chest position or
        modified Sims' with hips elevated on
        pillows.
     b. If experienced (or call for another nurse),
        insert fingers (in sterile glove) into vagina
        to lift presenting part off umbilical cord.
  2. Maintain patient on absolute bedrest.
  3. Cover exposed cord with sterile dressing if
     available.
  4. Auscultate FHT every 2 minutes.
  5. Stay with patient and offer support.
  6. Cesarean section is prescribed if cervix is not
     dilated enough to allow the baby to pass.
     Haste is important.

Emergency Delivery

Definition: Rapid or sudden labor of less than 3
hours' duration, from onset of cervical changes to delivery of infant.

Assessment

A. Obtain rapid history by asking focused questions.
  1. "Do you want to push?"
  2. "Have your membranes ruptured?"
  3. "Are you bleeding?"
  4. "Have you had a baby born quickly before?"
B. Assess ability to understand your directions.
C. Evaluate resources (proximity of physician and/or
   other assistance).
D. Psychological state and need for support at this
   time.
✦ E. Signs and symptoms of impending delivery.
  1. Desire to push.
  2. Frequency of strong contractions.
  3. Heavy bloody show.
  4. Membranes ruptured.
  5. Bulging rectum.
  6. Presenting part visible.
  7. Severe anxiety.
F. Observe for above signs continually as labor may
   progress with unexpected rapidity.

Implementation

ASSISTING WITH DELIVERY

✦ A. Never leave mother unattended during this time
   and never hold baby back. Have another employee
   notify the physician and bring the emergency
   delivery pack to room.
B. Reassure mother that you will remain with her
   and provide care until the physician arrives.
C. Put on sterile gloves if they are available and if
   there is time.
✦ D. Break membranes immediately if they have not
   done so spontaneously.
E. Have mother pant rather than push to avoid rapid
   delivery of the head.
✦ F. With a clean or sterile towel (if available), support
   baby's head with one hand applying gentle pressure to the head to prevent sudden expulsion and
   undue stretching of the perineum or brain
   damage to the infant.
✦ G. If cord is draped around baby's neck, with free
   hand gently slip it over head.
H. If bulb syringe is available, gently suction baby's
   mouth; wipe blood and mucus from mouth and
   nose with towel, if available.
I. Shoulders are usually born spontaneously after
   external rotation. If shoulders do not deliver spontaneously, ask mother to bear down to deliver
   them.

J. Support the baby's body as it is delivered.

K. All manipulation should be gentle to avoid injury to mother and baby.

✦ CARE AFTER DELIVERY

A. After delivery, hold baby securely over hand and arm with head in a dependent position to allow fluid and mucus to drain.

B. If baby does not cry spontaneously, gently rub baby's back or the soles of baby's feet. Do not hit baby on the back.

C. Dry baby to prevent heat loss.

✦ D. Place the baby on the mother's abdomen to provide warmth. The weight on the uterus will help it to contract.

E. Palpate mother's abdomen to make sure uterus is contracting.

F. Watch for signs of placental separation.

G. Support placenta in your hand after it is expelled.

H. Clamp the cord after it stops pulsating if clamp or ties are available. Cord need not be cut; there will be no bleeding from the placental surface.

I. Wrap the baby in a blanket.

J. Put the baby to the mother's breast. This reassures the mother that the baby is all right and helps contract the uterus.

K. Check the uterus after delivery of the placenta. Make sure the uterus is contracting.

L. Keep an accurate record of the time of birth and other pertinent data.

M. If baby is delivered unassisted, in bed, before the nurse arrives (precipitate delivery), the nurse should immediately:
    1. Check the baby to make sure breathing is established.
    2. Check the mother for excessive bleeding.

N. Comfort mother.

OBSTETRIC ANESTHESIA AND ANALGESIA

General Characteristics

A. No optimum anesthesia exists.

✦ B. One of the major causes of maternal death; other three are hemorrhage, infection, and eclampsia.

C. History and physical should be obtained before administering anesthesia.

D. Should be NPO before use.

E. Should be administered by trained personnel.

F. Choice of the type of anesthesia in obstetrics is determined by the specific patient situation and condition.

General Inhalation Anesthetics

A. Advantages.
    1. May anesthetize patient rapidly.
    2. Depth and duration can be controlled.
    3. Effects are rapidly dissipated in both infant and mother.
    4. These anesthetics cause uterine relaxation when necessary for manipulation.
    5. Inhalation anesthetics are preferred in hypovolemic patient and in patient whose condition prohibits the use of regional anesthetics.

B. Disadvantages.
    1. Woman is not awake for delivery.
    2. Brings about respiratory depression of the infant.
    3. May cause emesis and aspiration in the patient.
    4. May be flammable.

C. Common types.
    1. Ether—seldom used.
    2. Halothane—used in selected cases only.
    3. Penthrane—analgesia and light anesthesia; it may be used as a self-administered analgesic.
    4. Sodium thiopental (Pentothal)—IV anesthesia used as an adjunct in induction of anesthesia.
    5. Trichloroethylene (Trilene) is often used in self-administration by mask during labor and delivery. Never leave patient alone when she is using self-administered anesthesia.

✦ Regional Analgesia and Anesthesia

A. Drugs given to block the nerves carrying sensation from the uterus to the pelvic region.

B. Some common agents used.
    1. Novocaine.
    2. Xylocaine.
    3. Pontocaine.
    4. Carbocaine.

C. Vasoconstrictor agents (e.g., epinephrine) are commonly used in conjunction with regional anesthetics.
    1. Slow absorption and prolong the effect of the anesthetic.
    2. Prevent secondary hypotension.
    3. Opioids often used with anesthetic agent to produce analgesia (i.e., morphine, fentanyl).

D. Two principal types of regional anesthesia are nerve root block and peripheral nerve block.

E. Nerve root block.
    1. General considerations.
        a. Usually relieves pain completely if administered properly.
        b. Provides vasodilation below the anesthetic level, which may be responsible for a decrease in blood pressure.
        c. Does not depress the respiratory center, and therefore does not harm the patient unless hypotension in the patient is severe enough to interfere with adequate uterine blood flow.

d. May cause postspinal headache.

e. Contraindicated in a hypovolemic patient or in the case of central nervous system disease.

f. Drug may impede labor if given too early (before 5–6 cm dilatation).

g. Special skill of anesthesiologist required to administer drug.

h. Infant may need forceps delivery because the mother usually cannot push effectively due to level of anesthesia.

2. Types.
   a. Epidural–spinal combined.
   b. Lumbar epidural.
   c. Spinal block.

◆ 3. Nursing care.
   a. Assist patient to a knee–chest position over a bolster or on her left side with head flexed and knees drawn up.
   b. Monitor blood pressure every 3–5 minutes until stabilized; then every 30 minutes or PRN.
   c. Auscultate FHT.
   d. If hypotension does occur:
      (1) Turn mother to one side, off the inferior vena cava.
      (2) Give oxygen by mask.
      (3) Notify physician.
   e. Watch for signs of dizziness, nausea, faintness, and palpitations.

F. Peripheral nerve block.
   1. General considerations.
      a. May be done by attending physician (does not require an anesthesiologist).
      b. Local injection of anesthetic to block peripheral nerve endings.
      c. Less effective in relieving pain than nerve root block.
      d. May cause transient bradycardia in fetus, possibly due to rapid absorption of the drug into fetal circulation.
      e. Usually there are no maternal side effects.
      f. Needle guide such as Iowa trumpet usually used.
   2. Types.
      a. Local infiltration anesthesia.
      b. Pudendal block.
   ◆ 3. Nursing management.
      a. Measure vital signs.
      b. Auscultate FHT.
      c. Assist patient to a dorsal recumbent position.
      d. Offer reassurance and support during procedure.
      e. Auscultate FHT every 5 minutes for 15–30 minutes and every 30 minutes thereafter.

POSTPARTUM PERIOD

Physiology of the Puerperium

Definition: Period of 4–6 weeks following delivery in which the reproductive organs return to the normal, nonpregnant state.

Uterus

A. Involution—rapid diminution in the size of the uterus as it returns to the nonpregnant state.

B. Lochia—discharge from the uterus, consisting of blood from vessels of the placental site and debris from the decidua.

C. Placental site—blood vessels of the placenta become thrombosed or compressed.

Cervix and Vagina

A. Cervix—remains soft and flabby the first few days, and the internal os closes.

B. Vagina—usually smooth walled after delivery. Rugae begin to appear when ovarian function returns and estrogen is produced.

Ovarian Function and Menstruation

A. Ovarian function depends upon the rapidity in which the pituitary function is restored.

B. Menstruation—usually returns in 4–6 weeks in a nonlactating mother.

Urinary Tract

A. May be edematous and contain areas of submucosal hemorrhage due to trauma.

B. May have urine retention due to loss of elasticity and tone and loss of sensation from trauma.

C. Diuresis—mechanism by which excess body fluid is excreted after delivery. Usually begins within the first 12 hours after delivery.

Breasts

A. Proliferation of glandular tissue during pregnancy due to hormonal stimulation.

B. Usually secrete colostrum the first 2–3 days postpartum; enhances immunity and nutrition of infant. Breast millk usually produced by 3rd day.

C. Pituitary stimulates secretion of prolactin after placental hormones inhibiting the pituitary are no longer present.

D. In 3–4 days, breasts become firm, distended, tender, and warm (engorged), indicating production of milk.

E. Milk usually produced in response to sucking of infant.

Blood

A. White blood cells increase 25,000 to 30,000 during labor and early postpartum period and then return to normal in a few days.

B. Decrease in hemoglobin, red blood cells, and hematocrit; usually return to normal in 1 week.

C. Elevated fibrinogen levels usually return to normal within 1 week.

Nursing Care of the Postpartum Patient

Assessment

✦ A. Vital signs every 8 hours and PRN—decreased blood pressure, increased pulse, or temperature over 100.4°F; use pain scale to evaluate comfort.

✦ B. Fundus for consistency and level. Massage fundus lightly with fingers if it is relaxed.

✦ C. Lochia for amount, color, consistency, and odor. Watch for hemorrhage.

D. Perineum for redness, discoloration, or swelling.

E. Episiotomy for healing; check for drainage.

F. Breasts for engorgement or redness; cracking or inverted nipples.

G. Emotional status of new mother for depression or withdrawal.

H. Problems with flatus or elimination and bladder or bowel retention.

I. Morther-infant feeding quality.

J. Assess for thrombophlebitis (Homan's sign).

K. Blood values: Hgb, Hct, WBC, Rh.

Other Nursing Considerations

A. May administer drug to inhibit lactation (if ordered and if it has not been given immediately postpartum). Rarely, if ever, used today.

B. Apply breast binder or bra after 24 hours for 7 days.

✦ C. Administer RhoGAM as ordered within 72 hours postpartum to Rh-negative mother who has delivered an Rh-positive fetus (direct Coombs' negative) and who is not sensitized.

D. Maintain intake and output until patient is voiding a sufficient quantity without difficulty; usually the first two voids are measured.

E. Teach mother perineal care and give perineal care until mother is able to do so.

F. Encourage ambulation as soon as ordered and as patient is able to tolerate it, giving assistance the first time.

G. Encourage verbalization of mother's feelings about labor, delivery, and baby.

H. Give warm sitz baths as ordered.

Emotional Aspects of Postpartum Care

The Maternal Role as Outlined by Rubin

✦ A. *Taking-in phase* (first 2–3 days).
1. Mother's primary needs are her own; she needs sleep and food.
2. Mother usually is quite talkative. She wants to discuss labor and delivery. She is assimilating and appropriating experience.
3. Nurse can listen and help the patient interpret events to make them more meaningful.
4. Important for nurse to interpret future mother-child relationship at this important time.

✦ B. *Taking-hold phase* (from the third postpartum day to about 2 weeks); the phase varies with each individual.
1. Emphasis is on present.
2. Mother is impatient and wants to get on with reorganization of her life.
3. Less passive and more in control of situation.
4. Begins to take hold of "mothering" task, which takes priority over all else.
5. May be unsure of herself. It is important for nurse to reassure mother and not make her feel awkward.
6. Success at this time is important for the future mother–child relationship.
7. Important time for nurse to share information without making mother feel inadequate.

✦ C. *Letting-go phase*—usually occurs after discharge from hospital.
1. Mother may feel a deep loss over the separation of the baby from part of her body; she may grieve over this loss.
2. Mother may be caught in dependent–independent role; she wants to feel safe and secure yet wants to make decisions. Teenage mother needs special consideration because of the conflicts taking place within her as part of adolescence.
3. Mother may feel resentful and guilty about the baby causing so much work.
4. May have difficulty adjusting to the mothering role.
5. May feel conflict between the roles of mother and wife.
6. May feel upset and depressed at times—postpartum blues (*see* Postpartum Depression, pg. 451).
7. May be concerned about her other children.
8. Important for nurse to encourage vocalization of these feelings and give positive reassurance.

Role of the Baby's Father

A. Encourage the father or significant other to hold and care for the baby.

B. Encourage parents to take turns caring for the baby at night so that the mother can rest once she is home.

C. Explain the feelings that are normal to the mother at this time, e.g., tension, fatigue, insecurity in the mothering role, and her need to be dependent and independent.

Breast-Feeding

Nursing Management

✦ A. Conditions of breast indicating breast-feeding should be postponed.
  1. Tenderness and hardness.
  2. Pain and redness.
  3. Cracking of nipples.
  B. Feeding procedure.
  ✦ 1. Put baby to breast as soon as mother's and baby's conditions are stable (on the delivery table in some hospitals, or within 6–12 hours in others).
  2. Have mother assume comfortable position sitting or lying down.
  3. Guide baby to breast.
  4. Gently press breast away from baby's nose; stimulate rooting reflex if necessary.
  ✦ 5. Usually the baby is nursed 2–3 minutes at each breast the first time, gradually building to 10 minutes or so on each side in later feedings.
  6. Release suction by inserting a finger into the baby's mouth (the breast will become sore if baby is pulled off it).
  7. Burp baby after feeding at each breast.
  8. Stay with mother each time she nurses until she feels secure or confident with the baby and feedings.
  9. Baby should not nurse more than every 2 hours.
  ✦ C. Teaching mother principles of breast-feeding.
  1. Explain to the mother that the baby's stool will be yellow and watery; that it is not uncommon for nursing infants to have three to four stools each day or even one for each feeding.
  2. Dry the breast after feeding and allow it to air occasionally, especially if it is sore.
  3. Use general hygiene and wash the breast once daily.
  4. Encourage the mother to eat a well-balanced diet (additional 500 calories) and drink 3000 mL of fluid daily.
  5. Explain to the mother that she may offer sterile water but not formula to the baby between feedings. (The baby will not be hungry if given formula then and will not nurse well later.)
  6. Formula may be given at feeding time, or the mother may express milk manually and put it in a bottle if she plans to be away during feeding time.
  7. Breasts may leak between feedings or during coitus. Place a washcloth or pad in brassiere.
  8. Uterine cramping may occur the first few days after delivery while nursing as oxytocin stimulation causes the uterus to contract.
  9. Medications or drugs should be avoided unless specified by the physician (drugs are passed to infant through breast milk).
  10. Some foods such as cabbage or onions may alter the taste of milk or cause gas in the infant.
  11. Birth control pills are usually avoided while nursing as they decrease milk production and are passed to the infant in the milk.

CLINICAL PROBLEMS IN THE PUERPERIUM

Postpartum Hemorrhage

Definition: A blood loss of 500 mL or more during or 24 hours after vaginal birth; 1000 mL in cesarean birth. The leading cause of maternal death in the world.

✦ **Causes**
  A. Lacerations of the cervix or of the high vaginal walls, with oozing from blood vessels.
  B. Retained placental tissue or incomplete separation of the placenta. This is the most frequent cause of late postpartum hemorrhage. (May occur from 12–21 days after delivery.)

Assessment
✦ A. Uterine atony is the *primary cause* of early postpartum hemorrhage.
  1. Boggy, relaxed uterus.
  2. Dark bleeding.
  3. Passage of clots.
✦ B. Lacerations of the reproductive tract is the *second cause* of early postpartum hemorrhage.
  1. Lacerations of cervix or vaginal walls.
  2. Oozing of bright red blood from blood vessels.
✦ C. Retained placental tissue is a *third cause* and most frequent cause of late postpartum hemorrhage (occurs 24 hours to 6 weeks after delivery).
  1. Boggy, relaxed uterus.
  2. Dark bleeding.
✦ D. Check for signs and symptoms of shock.
  1. Air hunger (difficulty in breathing).
  2. Restlessness.
  3. Weak, rapid pulse.
  4. Rapid respirations.
  5. Decrease in blood pressure.
  E. Compare admission and postpartum lab values (hemoglobin, hematocrit, clotting time, platelets).

Treatment and Implementation
  A. Recognize abnormal bleeding and determine source.
  B. Monitor intravenous solutions, blood, or volume expanders.

C. Administer oxytocin or other uterine stimulants (methergine, Egotrate, Hemabate, or Prostin as ordered) if uterus is boggy.

D. Assist with laceration repair.

E. Assist with removal of retained placental tissue.

F. Prevent infection.

G. Hysterectomy may be indicated if bleeding cannot be controlled.

H. Check for clotting defect.

✦ I. Monitor vital signs every 15 minutes or until stable.

✦ J. Palpate fundus every 15 minutes or PRN while bleeding continues; then every 2–4 hours.

✦ K. Gently massage fundus until firm. Be careful not to overmassage.

L. Weigh pads and linen.

M. Provide for warmth.

N. Measure intake and output.

Disseminated Intravascular Coagulation (DIC)

Definition: Uncontrolled bleeding that occurs as a result of abruptio placentae, missed abortion, fetal death, or amniotic fluid embolism.

Etiology

A. Thromboplastin from placental tissue enters bloodstream and fibrinogen and clotting factors are used up, which results in bleeding.

B. Signs of shock and uncontrolled bleeding.

Treatment and Implementation

A. Assist with monitoring heparin injections and administration of fresh-frozen plasma and/or platelets.

B. Administer oxygen at 2–3 L as ordered.

Postdelivery Infection

Definition: An infection in the uterus within 28 days as a consequence of abortion or labor and delivery.

Causes

A. Organisms that were introduced during labor and delivery.

B. Bacteria normally present in vaginal tract.

Predisposing Factors

A. Cesarean for this major risk.

B. Weakened resistance due to prolonged labor and dehydration.

C. Traumatic delivery.

D. Excessive vaginal examinations during labor.

E. Premature rupture of membranes.

F. Excessive blood loss.

G. Poor health status; anemia.

H. Intrauterine manipulation.

I. Retained placental fragments.

Assessment

A. Elevated temperature of 100.4°F or more.

B. Discomfort in the abdomen and tenderness.

C. Burning on urination.

D. Foul-smelling lochia or discharge; decreased amount.

E. Pelvic pain.

F. Chills.

G. Rapid pulse.

H. Malaise.

Endometritis

Definition: An inflammation of the lining of the uterus.

General Considerations

A. Most frequent site of infection.

B. Uterus may be boggy, relaxed, and tender.

C. If untreated, may spread through lymphatic system to whole body, causing septicemia.

Treatment and Implementation

A. Antibiotics.

B. May have pelvic examination.

C. Establish adequate drainage of uterus.

D. Monitor IV fluids if ordered.

E. Encourage fluid intake (3000–4000 mL) if not contraindicated.

F. Administer medications as ordered.

G. Provide high-calorie nutritive diet.

H. Place patient in Fowler's or semi-Fowler's position as ordered. Position of patient may impede extension of infection from moving upward in pelvis.

I. Provide emotional support to mother, who is usually in isolation and unable to see baby.

Deep Vein Thrombosis (Thrombophlebitis)

Definition: A vascular occlusion of a vessel of the pelvis or lower extremity.

Characteristics

A. Development of thrombi at placental site that become infected, causing inflammation of the deep pelvic veins.

B. Thrombophlebitis may be confined to blood vessels in uterine wall, or it may extend to ovarian, hypogastric, or femoral veins.

C. Femoral thrombophlebitis, commonly called "milk leg," may originate in a leg vein.

Assessment

✦ A. Discomfort in abdomen and pelvis.

✦ B. Tenderness localized on one side of the pelvis.

✦ C. Femoral symptoms usually do not appear until the second week or later.

   1. Edema and pain in affected leg.

   2. Chills and low-grade fever.

D. Assess for redness and pain in calf. (Homan's sign no longer considered reliable.)

Treatment and Implementation

✦ A. Administer antibiotics until temperature stable. Encourage fluids.

B. Give anticoagulants (heparin) as ordered.

C. Provide bedrest and diversion.

D. Apply warm compresses as ordered (for 15–20 minutes). Now considered controversial.

E. Bed cradle—keep bedclothes off leg.

F. Antiembolic stockings.

G. Elevate affected leg.

✦ H. Never massage leg, and teach patient not to do so.

I. Teach patient to watch for signs of excessive bleeding.

J. Allow patient to express fears and concerns.

K. Watch for signs of pulmonary embolism.

Urinary Tract Infection

Definition: Urinary tract infections are usually caused by coliform bacteria and may occur soon after delivery.

Assessment

✦ A. Monitor bladder frequently during recovery period to start preventive measures.

B. Suprapubic or perineal discomfort.

C. Frequent urination.

D. Burning sensation on urination.

E. Elevated temperature.

F. Urine contains pus, bacteria, and red blood cells on microscopic examination.

G. Pain in flank area.

Treatment and Implementation

✦ A. Observe patient closely postpartum for full bladder or residual urine.
   1. Palpate bladder for distention.
   2. Palpate fundus (full bladder displaces fundus upward and to the sides).

B. Institute measures to help patient void.

C. Insert catheter as ordered, using sterile technique.

✦ D. Encourage fluids to 3000 mL/day.

E. Administer drugs as ordered: antibacterials, antispasmodics (NegGram, Mandelamine, Furadantin).

F. Obtain urine specimens for microscopic examination.

G. Provide emotional support to patient, and allow her to express feelings about her illness and the baby.

Mastitis

Definition: An infection in breast tissue due to invading organisms, usually *Staphylococcus*.

Causes

A. Infected hands of mother or attendants.

B. Bacteria normally present in lactiferous glands.

C. Fissure in nipples.

D. Bruising of breast tissue.

E. Stasis of milk or overdistention may injure tissue, but does not cause infection in itself.

F. Infected baby.

✦ ### Assessment

A. Chills.

B. Fever 103°F (39.5°C) or above.

C. Elevated pulse rate.

D. Lobe may become hard to the touch, red, and painful.

E. May progress to abscess if untreated.

✦ ### Treatment and Implementation

A. Administer antibiotics as ordered (may be based on culture of breast milk).

B. Apply ice pack as ordered.

C. Bedrest for first few days.

D. Increase fluid intake (2000–3000 mL).

E. Make sure mother is wearing snug-fitting, supportive brassiere.

F. Teach mother to empty breast every 4 hours if nursing is to be discontinued.

G. Wash hands before touching patient's breast, and teach mother careful handwashing and care of the breast.

H. May require incision and drainage if abscess develops.

I. Some physicians recommend that breast-feeding be stopped; others favor discontinuance with artificial removal of milk for a few days.

Postpartum Depression (PPD)

Definition: Intense and prolonged feelings of sadness, crying, fear, irritability, severe anxiety, panic attacks or spontaneous crying.

Characteristics

A. Lasts longer than postpartum blues, which usually last several weeks.

B. Occurs in about 8%–26%; greatest risk round 4th week PP or just prior to initiation of menses, and upon weaning.

C. Not associated with depression during pregnancy.

D. Woman often cannot continue normal parenting tasks, which can increase guilt feelings.

E. Usually requires medical intervention and medication.

F. Symptoms of psychosis (paranoia, hallucinations) requires psychiatric interventions.

Assessment

A. Assess for risk factors: primiparity, ambivalence toward pregnancy, history of PPD or psychiatric illness, stressful life events, lack of supportive relationships, personal expectations and perceptions of self.

B. Observe for signs of depression.
   1. Note severity and duration.
   2. Ask appropriate questions, which show sensitivity to the negative feelings and thoughts that may occur.

C. May utilize PPD checklists or screening scales.

Implementation

A. Anticipatory guidance: realistic information regarding possible negative feelings and reactions that often occur, detrimental effect of the perfect mother or perfect newborn expectations.

B. Encourage family to seek early and/or continue interventions.
   1. Call if notice symptoms.
   2. Take medication (depending on symptoms—tranquilizers, mood elevators, phenothiazines).
   3. Provide emotional support (encourage verbalization, support positive self-image, participate in support groups).

C. Implement followup interventions to ensure safety (self or newborn).

D. Discuss possible strategies for mother and family to prevent PPD.
   1. Don't be ashamed of having emotional problems after the baby is born—about 15% have this problem. Be open and share knowledge about PPD with close friends and family.
   2. Adhere to good health habits: well-balanced diet/hydration, exercise regularly, 7–8 hours of sleep.
   3. Have realistic expectations—don't try to be a "supermom."

NEWBORN

Immediate Care of the Normal Newborn

Principles of Maintenance

✦ A. *Always handle newborn with gloves until after the first bath with antibacterial soap (CDC guidelines).* Standard Precautions essential to observe as newborn may have HIV-positive mother.

✦ B. Maintain body temperature.
   1. Place infant in radiant warmer, wrap in warm blankets, or give to mother to hold.
   2. Wipe off fluid, mucus, and excessive vernix.
   3. Avoid excessive exposure.
   4. Wrap infant in warm blankets.
   5. Transfer to the nursery as soon as possible, after parents have seen and held infant.

✦ C. Maintain respiration—assess if resuscitation is needed.
   1. Suction mucus as needed with bulb or suction catheter attached to mucus trap.
   2. Place infant on side, in modified Trendelenburg's position, to facilitate drainage of mucus.
   3. Provide oxygen as needed.

✦ D. Prevent infection.
   1. Eye care—apply broad-spectrum antibiotic ointment (erythromycin) to prevent eye infection in the infant (or apply 2 drops of 1 percent silver nitrate in conjunctival sacs). This is now rarely used. Mother may be infected with gonorrhea or chlamydia.
   2. Cord care—use sterile gauze to cover.

✦ E. Administer medications, as ordered, within first 4 hours after birth.
   1. Vitamin K—according to infant weight.
   2. Hepatitis B vaccine if ordered and only if consent is signed by parents—use still controversial.

General Observations

✦ A. Apgar scoring, 1 and 5 minutes (*see* Table 14-6); based on the scoring method developed by Virginia Apgar.

B. Congenital malformations.

C. Umbilical cord—two arteries and one vein.

D. Meconium staining—skin, nails.

E. Abnormal cry or no cry.

F. Injuries caused by birth trauma—dislocated shoulder, edema of scalp, lacerations.

G. Respiratory—nasal flaring, retractions, expiratory grunt.

H. Neurological status—reflexes, tremors, and twitching.

Implementation

A. Clamp the cord if so requested by the physician; should be clamped 1 inch from the base or left longer if the mother is Rh negative (in case of possible blood exchange).

B. Identify the baby with bands.

C. Show the baby to the parents and allow them to hold the infant with help (if not contraindicated).

D. Observe the mother's reactions to baby.

E. Monitor heel-stick blood glucose immediately after birth and PRN.

F. Transfer the baby to the admitting nursery with appropriate data.

Care in the Nursery

✦ A. Care at admission and during the first 12 hours.

Table 14-6. APGAR SCORING			
Sign	**0**	**1**	**2**
Heart tone	Absent	Slow (less than 100)	Over 100
Respiratory effort	Absent	Slow, irregular	Good, crying
Muscle tone	Flaccid	Some flexion of extremities	Active motion
Reflex irritability	No response	Cry	Vigorous cry
Color	Blue, pale	Body pink, extremities blue	Completely pink

Apgar scoring system is a method of evaluating a newborn's condition at 1 and 5 minutes after birth.

- Newborns who score 7–10 are considered free of immediate danger.
- Newborns who score 4–6 are moderately depressed.
- Newborns who score 0–3 are severely depressed.

Scores less than 7 at 5 minutes, repeat every 5 minutes for 20 minutes. Infant may be intubated unless 2 successive scores of 7 or more occur.

1. Check axillary temperature (normal is 36.5°–37°C or 98.6°F).
   a. Axillary is a safer method than rectal for a newborn.
   b. Some hospitals recommend the first temperature by rectal method to assess patency of rectum, but alternative methods can be used (rubber catheter, first bowel movement).
2. Weigh and measure—total length and head circumference.
3. Place in heated crib.
4. Check respiratory rates every hour for 4–5 hours and PRN.
5. Check for nasal flaring, retractions, expiratory grunt, breath sounds.
6. Check apical pulse every hour for 2–3 hours; watch for above 180 or below 100.
7. Keep bulb syringe available and suction as needed.
8. Bathe and dress baby when his or her temperature is stable.
9. Place in an open crib when baby's temperature is stable.
✦ 10. Administer first feeding as ordered; usually sterile water is given to evaluate feeding capability.
11. Assess baby for congenital defects.

B. Routine nursing care.
1. Assessment.
   ✦ a. Observe for jaundice—check general skin color, blanching, sclera of the eyes.
   ✦ b. Check for respiratory difficulty—mucus, flaring of nostrils, grunting, and other signs.
   c. Note tremors, twitching, muscle tone, and reflexes.
   d. Take baby's temperature each shift.
   e. Check baby's weight daily.
   f. Note amount voided and number of stools.
   g. Check for signs of infection on the skin and cord.
2. Apply alcohol to cord daily PRN.
3. Circumcision care.
   a. Observe for bleeding.
   b. Change petroleum gauze as necessary.
   c. Keep area clean to prevent infection.
✦ 4. If infant has feeding (protein source) in hospital, PKU test can be done while infant is in hospital. If not, arrange appointment for mother to have test done.
   a. PKU test important to determine if baby can metabolize the amino acid, phenylalanine.
   b. If PKU present, can result in mental retardation.
5. Provide for nutrition and hydration.
6. Teach mother how to hold and burp the baby.
7. Use proper handwashing between babies to prevent spreading infection.
8. Isolate babies with known or suspected infections.
9. Be sure that the mother understands the doctor's orders regarding care of the infant before she goes home and plans follow-up visits to the physician.

Physical Characteristics

Respiratory Status

A. Infant's respiratory system must function immediately after loss of placental function; adequate maturation at birth is necessary.
✦ B. Normal respiration is about 30–50; over 60 or below 30 may indicate a problem.
   1. Respiration may be slightly elevated during crying episodes or shortly afterwards.
   2. Tachypnea is earliest symptom of many neonatal problems (respiration above 60).

Circulatory Status

✦ A.   Ductus arteriosus, ductus venosus, and foramen ovale should close (may not be complete for 1 or 2 days).

B.   Peripheral circulation may be sluggish (there may be mottling, acrocyanosis).

C.   Heart rate may be variable—normal 120–160; it may be as high as 180 with crying or below 120 when resting.

D.   Anemia is common in early months because of the decrease in erythropoiesis and breakdown of red blood cells.
   1.   Baby may need an iron-supplemented formula.
   2.   RDA for iron is 6 mg/day from birth to 6 months.

✦ E.   Physiologic jaundice—normal level less than 1 mg/100 mL blood.
   1.   Jaundice visible in the skin, sclera.
   2.   Does not become visible until the second or third day after birth.
   3.   Caused by impairment in the removal of bilirubin—deficiency in the production of glucuronide transferase, which is needed to convert indirect insoluble bilirubin to direct water-soluble bilirubin and then excreted.
   4.   Jaundice begins to decrease by the sixth or seventh day.
   5.   Infant may require treatment, although usually does not if watched carefully. If needed, usual treatment is phototherapy.

F.   When clinical jaundice persists beyond 7 days (for term infants) or 14 days (for premature infants), usual treatment is phototherapy.

✦ G.   Transitory deficiency in the ability of the blood to clot.
   1.   Bacteria in the intestines are necessary for the production of vitamin K.
   2.   Bacteria are not present in the intestines during the first few days after birth.
   3.   Vitamin K IM usually given after birth to aid in blood coagulation.

Ability to Maintain Body Heat

A.   The baby suffers a large loss of heat because he is wet at birth and because of the coolness of the delivery room.
   1.   The infant should be placed immediately in a radiant warmer and dried off.
   2.   Place a knit cap on infant's head to maintain body heat.

B.   Temperature may be taken by rectum or axilla (usually taken by rectum the first time to check for patent anus).

Weight

✦ A.   Infants usually lose between 5 and 10 percent of their body weight the first few days because of low fluid intake and loss of excess fluid from tissue.

B.   They usually regain weight lost within 7–14 days.

Head

A.   Head or face may be asymmetrical due to birth trauma.

B.   Molding of head may be present (elongation of head as it passes through birth canal to accommodate pelvis); usually disappears in about a week.

✦ C.   Caput succedaneum—diffuse swelling of soft tissues of scalp caused by an arrest in circulation in those tissues present over the cervix as it dilates.

✦ D.   Cephalohematoma—extravasation of blood beneath periosteum of one of the cranial bones because of a ruptured blood vessel during the trauma of labor and delivery.

E.   Anterior and posterior fontanel.
   1.   Should be open.
   2.   Should neither bulge (may indicate intracranial pressure) nor be depressed (may indicate dehydration).

F.   Ears well formed and cartilage present.

Gastrointestinal System

A.   Salivary glands immature.

B.   May have Epstein's pearls (white raised areas on palate caused by an accumulation of epithelial cells).

C.   May have transient circumoral cyanosis.

D.   Infant stools.
   1.   Meconium plug—thick gray-white mucus passed before meconium.
   ✦ 2.   Meconium—sticky, black, tarry-looking stools, consisting of mucus, digestive secretions, vernix caseosa, and lanugo; usually passed during the first 24 hours after birth.
   ✦ 3.   Transitional stool passed second to fifth day; greenish-yellow color and loose (partly meconium and partly milk).
   4.   Number of stools varies. Breast-fed infants usually have more bowel movements—yellow, golden, pasty.
   5.   Bottle-fed stools: pale, yellow-light brown, formed, foul smelling.
   6.   Stools should be observed for color, frequency, and consistency.

E.   Regurgitation following feeding is common. It may be reduced by frequent burping during feedings.

Genitourinary System

A.   Check presence of voiding.

B.   Uric acid crystals (pink or reddish spots) may appear on diaper due to high uric acid secretion.

C. Genitalia.
 1. Female.
  a. May have heavy coating of vernix between labia.
  b. Usually has mucus discharge. Mucus may be blood tinged due to elevated hormonal levels in mother (pseudomenstruation).
 2. Male.
  a. Size of penis and scrotum vary.
  b. Testicles should be descended or in inguinal canal.
  c. Circumcision—surgical removal of the foreskin of penis by physician.
   (1) Usually performed by the second or third day.
   (2) Observe for bleeding from postoperative site.
   (3) Observe for postoperative voiding.

Skin

A. Should be pinkish color or consistent with ethnic background.
✦ B. Acrocyanosis (cyanosis of extremities) may be present for the first hour or two after birth. Persistent blueness may indicate complications such as heart disease.
✦ C. Lanugo and vernix caseosa may be present.
D. Petechiae may be present because of the trauma of birth.
✦ E. Milia—secretions of sebaceous materials in obstructed sebaceous glands (may be present and will disappear).
F. Hemangiomas may be present on nape of neck or upper eyelids.
G. Skin may appear dry or cracked.
✦ H. Mongolian spots—bluish pigmented areas present on the buttocks of babies of Asian, African-American, or Mediterranean heritage.

Effects of Maternal Hormones

✦ A. Maternal hormones may cause enlargement of breast in both male and female infants, and "witches' milk," a milklike substance, may be excreted from the breasts.
B. Vaginal bleeding in female infant.
C. Hypertrophy of vulva or prostate.

Neurological System

A. Muscle tone.
 1. Fist usually kept clenched.
 2. Baby should offer resistance when change in position is attempted.
 ✦ 3. Head should be supported when baby is lifted.
 4. Muscles should not be limp.
B. Cry.
 ✦ 1. Cry should be loud and vigorous.

 2. Baby should cry when hungry or uncomfortable.
C. Hunger.
 1. Usually becomes fretful and restless at 3–4-hour intervals.
 2. May suck fingers or anything placed near mouth.
D. Sleep.
 ✦ 1. Sleeps about 20 out of 24 hours.
 2. Often stirs and stretches while sleeping.
E. Senses.
 1. Eyes.
  a. Eyelids may be edematous or have purulent discharge from the chemical irritation of silver nitrate.
  b. Light perception is present.
  c. Eye movement is uncoordinated.
  d. Usual color of eyes is blue-gray.
  e. May have subconjunctival hemorrhages, which disappear in a week or two.
 2. Nose.
  a. Newborn breathes through nose.
  b. Sense of smell is present.
 3. Ears—hearing is present at birth.
 4. Taste is present at birth.
 5. Touch is present at birth. Responds to stimuli and discomfort.
F. Assess gestational age (using Ballard tool).
G. Immunity.
 ✦ 1. May receive from the mother some passive immunity to infectious diseases, such as measles, mumps, and diphtheria.
 2. Capacity to develop own antibodies is slow during first few months.
 3. Has little resistance to infection.
 4. Imunizations: hepatitis B vaccine is recommended **only** if mother is a carrier.

Feeding the Newborn

Schedules of Feeding

✦ A. First feeding. ❖ **PROCEDURE** ❖
 1. May be breast-fed on the delivery table.
 2. Colostrum is not irritating if aspirated and is absorbed by the respiratory system.
 3. First feeding in first hour of life. Latest to feed is usually within 2–3 hours after birth, when normal low blood sugar occurs.
 4. Usually a test feeding of 5–10 drops of sterile water is made to evaluate feeding capability. Glucose is no longer given (to prevent aspiration pneumonia).
 5. Give full-strength formula or breast milk as soon as newborn shows an interest.
B. Subsequent feeding.
 1. Routine schedule—3–4-hour feedings.

2. Self-demand—baby is fed according to his or her needs (when hungry), usually every 3–6 hours.

Calories and Fluid Needs

A. Fluid—140–160 mL/kg of body weight in 24 hours. More fluids should be given in hot weather or when the baby has an elevated temperature.

✦ B. Caloric needs—approximately 20 kcal/oz formula for term infant or 105–108 kcal/kg/day for newborn.

HIGH-RISK INFANTS

Preterm (Premature) Newborn

Definition: An infant born before a 37-week gestation period, weighing less than 2500 gm, and measuring less than 18½ inches (47 cm) long with a head circumference less than 13 inches (33 cm).

Assessment

A. Skin is thin and capillaries are easily seen.

B. Lanugo is prominent; hair on the head is fine and fuzzy.

C. Little subcutaneous fat.

D. Body temperature is unstable and may be below normal.

E. Head is large in comparison to the rest of the body.

F. Poor muscle tone—muscles appear limp; baby assumes froglike position when placed on abdomen.

G. Feeble cry.

H. Gagging and sucking reflexes may be weak.

I. Jaundice appears later than in the normal newborn, and it may be more severe and last longer (2 weeks).

J. Renal function immature.

✦ K. Moro reflex is developed; grasp is feeble; rooting is present.

✦ Potential Complications

A. Heightened capillary fragility and increased tendency toward hemorrhage.

B. Lack of immunity and lack of resistance to infection.

C. Poor ability to tolerate fats because of immaturity of digestive system.

D. Tendency toward periods of apnea because of immaturity of nervous system.

E. Tendency to develop respiratory distress, hypoglycemia, anemia, hypocalcemia.

F. High proportion of body surface to weight; leads to an increase in the loss of body fluids.

G. Immaturity of retina—leads to development of retrolental fibroplasia with increased levels of oxygen consumption.

H. Immaturity of liver—difficulty detoxifying medications.

I. Sucking varies, although it is usually present at 32 weeks; poor coughing ability, gagging, and swallowing.

Implementation

✦ A. Provide immediate care to infant.
  1. Give immediate attention in delivery room and transport to nursery to maintain heat.
     a. Maintain skin temperature at about 36°C or 97.6°F in isolette or heated crib.
     b. Gradually wean infant from heated environment and monitor temperature closely until stable.
     c. Warming infant too quickly may cause apneic spells.
  2. Administer humidity (distilled water) usually between 40 and 70 percent as ordered. *See* Table 14-7.

✦ B. Evaluate respiratory status.
  1. Check respiratory rate—every hour and PRN.
  2. Observe for the following signs of respiratory distress.
     a. Color of skin; circumoral pallor, cyanosis.
     b. Flaring of nares.
     c. Grunting retractions.
     d. Diminished breath sounds.
  3. Auscultate breath sounds with stethoscope.
  4. Analyze oxygen concentration 1–2 hours or as necessary to prevent retrolental fibroplasia and to ensure adequate oxygenation.
  5. Observe for periods of apnea and stimulate by gently rubbing chest or tapping foot.
  6. Percuss, vibrate, and suction as ordered to remove mucus.
  7. Reposition every 2 hours to promote aeration in lobes of lung and facilitate drainage.

C. Monitor blood gases and electrolytes frequently; IV regulated by infusion pump to prevent circulatory overload.

✦ D. Monitor feedings.
  1. Initiate feedings as ordered (usually begin with sterile water or breast milk); progress to breast milk or full-strength formula as tolerated.
  2. Use preemie nipple on bottle.
  3. Give gavage feeding if respirations are about 60 breaths/min.
     a. Use preemie nipple if bottle feeding.
     b. Infants often require alternate feedings of gavage and bottle feeding.

E. Maintain intake and output, including stool, and weigh daily.

F. Organize care to conserve energy with rest periods after each feeding.

Table 14-7. THE PREMATURE INFANT

Need	Nursing Implementation
Needs of Family	
Keep separation to a minimum	Allow parents to visit baby frequently; as soon as possible, allow parents to help care for infant.
Provide data on baby's progress	Answer questions openly, provide up-to-date information on baby's progress.
Express feelings and concerns	Allow parents to talk freely about infant, give support as needed and help parents to accept reality of situation.
Provide information	Explain specialized care to parents. Have them report to pediatrician any of following symptoms: diarrhea, vomiting, lack of appetite, or elevated temperature. Help mother to feel confident in care of infant before discharge.
Needs of Infant	
Warmth	Immediate attention in delivery room and transporting to nursery to maintain heat. Maintain temperature at about 36°C or 97.6°F in isolette or heated crib. Gradually wean infant from heated environment and watch temperature closely until stable.
Oxygen and humidity	Administer oxygen (should be warmed and humidified). Administer humidity (distilled water) usually between 40 and 70 percent as ordered. Check respiratory rate—q 1 h and PRN. Observe for signs of respiratory distress, color, flaring, grunting retractions, skin color, auscultate breath sounds with stethoscope. Analyze oxygen concentration q 2–4 h or as necessary to prevent retrolental fibroplasia and to ensure adequate oxygenation. Observe for periods of apnea and stimulate by gently rubbing chest or tapping foot; percuss, vibrate, and suction as ordered to remove mucus. Reposition q 2 h to promote aeration of all lobes of lung and facilitate drainage. Monitor blood gases and electrolytes frequently. (Oxygen administration is determined by blood gases.)
Nutrition and hydration	May require IV feedings through umbilical catheter until stabilized. IV regulated by infusion pump to prevent circulatory overload. Initiate feedings as ordered (usually begin with sterile water or glucose water). Progress to dilute formula or breast milk to full strength formula as tolerated. Usually gavage feeding if respirations are about 60 breaths/min. Use preemie nipple if bottle feeding. Infants often require alternate feedings of gavage and bottle feeding. Maintain intake and output including stool; weigh daily and organize care to conserve energy with rest periods after each feeding. Measure head circumference and length at least once a week.
Prevention from infection	Maintain aseptic technique. Strict isolation techniques with infected babies. Prevent skin breakdown—change position, careful cleansing and handling. Observe for signs of infection—vomiting, jaundice, lack of appetite, lethargy; cover IV sites.
Maintenance of circulatory functioning	Check heart rate by apical pulse for a full minute q 1–2 h. Frequently check for bleeding from umbilical catheter. Apply pressure to puncture site as necessary to prevent bleeding. Administer vitamin K as ordered after birth to prevent hemorrhage.
Mothering and physical stimulation	Gently stroke and talk to baby when giving care. Hang colorful mobiles or other nonharmful objects in crib. Hold baby during feeding as soon as condition permits. Encourage parents to hold, cuddle, feed, and diaper baby as soon as baby's condition permits.

G. Measure head circumference and length at least once a week.

H. Observe for signs of infection: vomiting, jaundice, lack of appetite, and lethargy.

I. Maintain aseptic technique and strict isolation techniques with infected babies.

J. Prevent skin breakdown: change position, careful cleansing and handling.

K. Check heart rate by apical pulse for a full minute every 1–2 hours.

L. Frequently check for bleeding from umbilical catheter.
  1. Apply pressure to puncture site as necessary to prevent bleeding.
  2. Administer vitamin K as ordered after birth to prevent hemorrhage.
  3. Frequently check monitors if monitored electronically.

M. Gently stroke and talk to baby when giving care.

N. Hang colorful mobiles or other nonharmful objects in crib.

O. Hold baby during feeding as soon as condition permits.

P. Provide for family's needs to be met.
  1. Allow parents to visit baby frequently; as soon as possible, involve parents in infant care to promote parent-to-infant attachment.
  2. Answer questions openly, provide up-to-date information on baby's progress.
  3. Allow parents to talk freely about infant, give support as needed, and help parents to accept reality of situation.
  4. Explain specialized care to parents. Have them report to pediatrician any of the following symptoms: diarrhea, vomiting, lack of appetite, or elevated temperature.
  5. Allow mother to feel confident in caring for infant before discharge. Explain to mother infant's special needs. *See* Table 14-7.
  6. Encourage parents to hold, cuddle, feed, and diaper baby as soon as baby's condition permits.

Small for Gestational Age

Definition: Refers to infants who are significantly undersize (below 10th percentile) for gestational age. Also called intrauterine growth retardation (IUGR).

Characteristics

A. Postmature infants.

B. Defective embryonic development.

C. Placental insufficiency.

D. Associated factors: diabetes, toxemia, maternal infection, maternal malnutrition, cigarette smoking, multiple gestation.

✦ E. Infant appearance.
  1. Little subcutaneous tissue.

  2. Loose, dry, scaling skin.
  3. Appears thin and wasted; old for size.
  4. May be meconium staining of skin, nails.
  5. Sparse hair on head.
  6. Active, alert, seems hungry.
  7. Cord dries more rapidly than normal infants.

Assessment

✦ A. *Hypoglycemia:* nervousness, pallor, apnea, temperature instability, high-pitched cry.

✦ B. *Cold stress:* lethargy, poor feeding pattern, cold to touch, respirations increased.

C. *Asphyxia:* may have been deprived while in utero or aspirated amniotic fluid. Infant may require resuscitation at birth.

D. *Polycythemia:* usually asymptomatic but may have tachycardia, tachypnea, respiratory distress.

Implementation

A. Provide care similar to preterm infant until the infant is stabilized.

B. Protect from cold stress: keep warm, usually in isolette.

C. Perform tests for glucose levels.

D. Weigh daily and maintain intake and output.

Newborn with (HIV) AIDS

A. Don gloves and gown to protect self from contamination—Standard Precautions.

B. Wait until newborn's temperature is stable in the nursery to provide care.

C. Wash infant carefully with antibacterial soap.

D. Administer cord care with alcohol, iodine solution or antibacterial ointment.

E. Wrap infant in clean blanket.

F. Dispose of gloves and gown in plastic bag.

✦ G. Principles of care for mother of HIV baby.
  1. Breast feeding is discouraged when mother tests positive for HIV.
  2. Circumcisions are not done on infants with HIV positive mothers until infant's status is determined.
  3. Immunizations with live vaccine (oral polio, MMR) should not be done until child's status confirmed. If child infected, live vaccine will not be given. Inactivated polio vaccine (IPV) will be administered.
  4. Excellent hygiene procedures should be carried out in the home.
  5. Inform the care giver exposed to infant's body fluids of the potential for infection transmission.
  6. Teach the importance of good handwashing techniques.
  7. Facilitate referral to community agencies and support groups as needed.

DISEASES AFFECTING THE NEWBORN

Respiratory Distress Syndrome

Definition: A group of clinical symptoms signifying that the infant is experiencing problems with the respiratory system.

Etiology
✦ A. Symptoms are the result of a decrease in the amount of surfactant in the infant's lungs as a result of one of the following conditions.
1. Prematurity—immaturity of lungs, decreased number of mature alveoli, and inability to produce surfactant.
2. Hypoxia and acidosis.
3. Hypothermia.
4. High concentration of oxygen.
B. Respiratory distress syndrome is the most common cause of death in infants.

Assessment
✦ A. Increased respirations—> 60/min.
B. Retractions—sternal and intercostal.
C. Cyanosis.
D. Expiratory grunting; increased number of apnea episodes.
E. Lack of activity.
F. Inability to take in sufficient oxygen leading to low oxygen and hypoxemia.
G. Respiratory acidosis due to retention of carbon dioxide as a result of inadequate pulmonary ventilation.
H. Metabolic acidosis due to increased production of lactic acid and decreased pH.
I. Result of x-ray examination.
1. Atelectasis—collapsed portions of lung.
2. Fibrinous membrane that lines alveolar ducts and terminal bronchioles; membrane is formed by transudation of fluid from pulmonary tissue.

✦ Implementation
A. Primarily supportive.
B. Maintain warmth—infant usually placed in isolette or open crib with overhead warmer. Skin temperature is maintained at minimum 97.7°F (36°C).
C. Provide for nutrition and hydration—usually give IV glucose fluids during acute periods, then gradually increase feedings as tolerated.
D. Administer oxygen for hypoxemia, warmed and humidified, in lowest concentration possible, via hood, nasal prongs, endotracheal tubes, or bag and mask.
1. Oxygen may be given at atmospheric or increased airway pressure.
2. Check and change nasal prongs frequently if used.
3. Analyze oxygen concentration.
E. Apply continuous positive pressure to lungs during spontaneous breathing.
F. Apply positive pressure to lungs during expiratory cycle when using the mechanical ventilator (used for severe cases).
G. If infant requires an endotracheal (ET) tube: loosely tape and check endotracheal tube frequently for correct placement and connection at adaptor site.
H. Procedure for suctioning infant with endotracheal tube. ❖ **PROCEDURE** ❖
✦ 1. Disconnect from respirator at site of adaptor.
2. Instill few minims to 0.5 mL of sterile normal saline into tube to loosen secretions.
3. Suction no longer than 5 seconds using sterile catheter.
4. Ventilate infant as needed during procedure.
5. Reconnect tube to respirator; be certain it is in place and adaptor is secure.
6. Auscultate chest for breath sounds.
I. Provide postural drainage and percussion and suction as ordered.
J. Surfactant replacement therapy is now available to decrease severity of RDS—given via endotracheal tube.
K. Keep parents informed of infant's progress.
L. Allow parents to visit child as much as possible and express their feelings about child's illness.
M. Gently stroke and talk with child while giving care.

Hyperbilirubinemia

Definition: An abnormal elevation of bilirubin in the newborn (above 12.9 mg/100 mL for formula-fed infants and 15 mg/100 mL for breast-fed or premature infants).

Etiology
A. Functional immaturity of the liver—usually appears after 24 hours and disappears after 10 days.
B. Bacterial infections.
✦ C. ABO and Rh incompatibilities—usually show up in the first 24 hours and may be severe.
D. Enclosed bleeding, such as hematoma, from trauma of delivery.
E. May lead to Kernicterus—a deposit of yellow pigment in basal ganglia of the brain—irreversible brain damage.

Assessment
A. Jaundice, progressing from head to extremities.
B. Pallor.

C. Infant is lethargic and feeds poorly.

D. Urine is concentrated, and stools are light in color.

E. If untreated, infant may progress to muscular rigidity or flaccidity, increased lethargy, high-pitched cry, respiratory distress, decreased Moro's reflex, and spasms.

Treatment and Implementation

A. Observe infant carefully for signs of increased jaundice.

B. Observe for and prevent acidosis/hypoxia and hypoglycemia, which decrease binding of bilirubin to albumin and contribute to jaundice.

✦ C. Maintain adequate hydration and offer fluids between feedings as ordered.
   1. Infant may be on forced fluids to aid in the excretion of bilirubin.
   2. Phototherapy can cause loose stools, so there is a danger of dehydration.

D. Maintain temperature at 97.6°F to avoid cold stress.

E. Take measures to avoid infection.

✦ F. Treatment with phototherapy—fluorescent light breaks down bilirubin into water-soluble products. ❖ PROCEDURE ❖
   1. Do not clothe infant.
   ✦ 2. Cover infant's eyes to prevent retinal damage.
   3. Change baby's position every 2 hours to ensure adequate exposure.
   4. Remove infant from light and remove eye patches during feedings.
   5. Carefully examine eyes for signs of irritation from eye patches.
   6. Keep an accurate record of hours spent under fluorescent lights.

G. Meet emotional needs of infant.

H. Reinforce physician's instruction to parents and allow parents to express concerns and feelings.

I. Exchange transfusion may be done; considered only when bilirubin reaches extremely high levels (20 mg/mL in full-term infant and 16 mg/mL in premature infant).
   1. No "safe" level of bilirubin to prevent kernicterus.
   2. Consider combination of bilirubin and neurological age.

Hemolytic Disease of the Newborn

Definition: Alteration, dissolution, or destruction of red blood cells.

Etiology

✦ A. Rh incompatibility—Rh antigens from the baby's blood enter the maternal bloodstream. The mother's blood does not contain Rh factor, so she produces anti-Rh antibodies. These antibodies are harmless to the mother but attach to the erythrocytes in the fetus and cause hemolysis. Exchange of fetal and maternal blood takes place primarily when the placenta separates at birth.
   1. Problem may begin in early pregnancy; it may be mild to severe and can cause the death of the fetus.
   2. Sensitization usually does not occur with the first pregnancy.
   ✦ 3. Diagnosis of Rh incompatibility.
      a. Begins in pregnancy, with discoveries of antibodies in an Rh negative mother's blood by means of *indirect Coombs' test*.
      b. Titration is used to determine the extent to which antibodies are present.
      c. Analysis of amniotic fluid (which is golden in color) for bilirubin determines the severity of the disease (the higher the bilirubin content, the more severe the disease).
      d. Testing of cord blood (*direct Coombs' test*) determines the presence of maternal antibodies attached to baby's cells.

B. ABO incompatibility—usually less severe.

Assessment

A. Anemia—caused by destruction of red blood cells.

B. Jaundice—develops rapidly after birth (before 24 hours).

C. Edema—usually seen in stillborn infants or those who die shortly after birth, most likely due to cardiac failure.

Treatment

✦ A. Immunization against hemolytic disease with Rho(D)-immune globulin (RhoGAM) to the mother as ordered (now given at 28 weeks and postpartum—may also be given at 24 weeks' gestation).

B. For mild forms, treat as for hyperbilirubinemia.

C. For severe, give exchange transfusion after birth or intrauterine. Use Rh negative blood.

Infants of Diabetic Mothers (IDM)

General Considerations

A. May be delivered early to prevent intrauterine death (after 36 weeks).

B. Often delivered by cesarean section.

C. Children with diabetic mothers have a higher incidence of congenital anomalies than the general population.

D. High incidence of hypoglycemia, respiratory distress, hypocalcemia, and hyperbilirubinemia.

Assessment

✦ A. Baby is usually excessively large in size and weight due to excess fat and glycogen in tissues.
1. High blood sugar levels in mother cross the placenta and enter the baby's bloodstream, elevating blood sugar levels.
2. High blood sugar stimulates infant's metabolic system to store glycogen and fat and increase the production of insulin.
3. High levels of insulin deplete glucose levels, which leads to hypoglycemia (occurs 1–3 hours after birth).
B. May have puffy appearance of face and cheeks.
C. Enlarged heart, liver, and spleen.
D. Lethargy.
E. Irregular respiration.

Implementation

✦ A. Observe for signs of hypoglycemia—twitching, difficulty in feeding, lethargy, apnea, seizures, cyanosis, and high-pitched cry.
✦ B. Observe for signs of respiratory distress—tachypnea, cyanosis, retractions, grunting, nasal flaring.
✦ C. Observe for hypocalcemia (may be caused by prematurity or stress); tremors.
D. Care is the same as for a premature infant.
E. Initiate feedings with sterile water, then formula or breast milk within 2–4 hours after birth, as ordered by physician.
F. Oral glucose may be given after glucose reading.

Hypoglycemia

✦ *Definition:* Abnormal low level of sugar in the blood (blood glucose value of 40 mg/dL).

Characteristics

A. Placental dysfunction.
B. Diabetes in mother.
C. Cold stress.
D. Renal disease, cardiac disease, preeclampsia, or chronic infection in the mother.
E. Small-for-gestational-age infants.
F. Post-term infant.
G. Asphyxia at birth.
H. Infection in infant or any condition that stresses the metabolic rate and increases the need for glucose.

Assessment

A. Cyanosis.
B. Increased respiratory rate.
✦ C. Twitching, nervousness, or tremors.
D. Lethargy and poor muscle tone.
E. Unstable temperature.
✦ F. Shrill or intermittent cry.
G. Feeding problems.

H. Apneic periods.
I. Blood sugar values: normal is 45–100/100 mL of blood; usually around 60–75/100 mL.
1. Term infant: 30–40 mg/100 mL blood.
2. Preterm: 20 mg/100 mL blood.
J. Monitor screening that is done with heel-stick test with laboratory studies as a follow-up.

Implementation

✦ A. Prevent low blood glucose through early feedings (immediate breast feeding, D_5W or $D_{10}W$).
✦ B. Administer glucose orally or IV, depending on baby's condition—IV started with 5–10 percent glucose, the highest safe concentration (as ordered).
✦ C. Perform close monitoring of blood sugar values every 1–2 hours.
D. Give care as for other high-risk infants.

Drug-Dependent Newborn

General Considerations

A. There is a direct relationship between the duration of the maternal addiction and dosage and the severity of symptoms in the infant.
✦ B. Heroin addicted mother: infant may appear normal at birth with a low birth weight.
1. Withdrawal within 72 hours—may not begin until 2 weeks after birth.
2. Infant appears less ill than when mother is taking methadone.
3. Heroin causes early maturity of the liver.
✦ C. Mother on methadone.
1. Withdrawal 1–2 days to 1 week or more; most evident 48–72 hours and may last 6 days to 8 weeks.
2. Infant may appear to be very ill.
3. May develop jaundice due to prematurity.
✦ D. Mother addicted to cocaine, a stimulant.
1. Infant evidences decreased interactive behavior, feeding problems, irregular sleep patterns, diarrhea.
2. Seven out of 1000 mothers will have infants with major deformities—especially of the kidneys.

Assessment

✦ A. Irritability and tremors.
B. Disruption of normal sleep patterns.
✦ C. Persistent high-pitched, shrill cry.
D. Sneezing, nasal stuffiness.
E. Respiratory distress.
F. Fever.
G. GI symptoms.
1. Diarrhea.
2. Vomiting.
3. Poor feeding.

H. Excess sweating.

I. Increased muscle tone.

J. Sucking of fist.

K. Convulsions (rare).

✦ **Implementation**

A. Monitor respiratory and cardiac rates every 30 minutes and PRN.

B. Take temperature every 4–8 hours and PRN.

C. Administer medications as ordered—paregoric (narcotic opiate), phenobarbital, Valium, or tincture of opium.

D. Reduce external stimuli and handle infant infrequently.

✦ E. Maintain warmth and swaddle infant in blanket. Hold firmly and close to body during feedings and when giving care.

F. Pad sides of crib to protect infant from injury.

G. Administer small, frequent feedings as ordered.

H. Suction if necessary.

I. Cleanse buttocks and anal area carefully.

J. Measure intake and output.

K. Keep mother informed of infant's progress.

L. Promote mother's interest in infant.

✦ Fetal Alcohol Syndrome (FAS)

Characteristics

A. Maternal alcohol abuse throughout pregnancy results in fetal alcohol syndrome.

1. Most serious cause of teratogenesis.

2. In affected infants, growth is retarded; they are microcephalic with severe mental retardation.

✦ B. Lesser amount of alcohol ingested throughout pregnancy results in less severe symptoms called fetal alcohol effect (FAE).

1. Prenatal and/or postnatal growth retardation.

2. Developmental delay.

3. May not be diagnosed until early childhood.

Assessment

✦ A. Respiratory distress and apnea.

B. Cyanosis.

C. Seizures.

D. Major brain dysfunction symptoms.

Implementation

✦ A. Position on side to facilitate drainage of secretions.

1. Keep resuscitation equipment at bedside.

2. Have suction available, especially following feeding.

B. Administer small feedings and burp well.

C. Avoid heat loss.

D. Reduce environmental stimuli.

GYNECOLOGY

Examination

A. Pelvic exam.

1. Inspection of external genitalia for signs of inflammation, bleeding, discharge, and epithelial cell changes.

2. Speculum may be inserted for visualization of vagina and cervix.

3. Bimanual examination is done—gloved fingers of one hand inserted into vagina while abdomen palpated with other hand.

4. Rectal exam.

B. Breast exam may also be done when woman comes in for pelvic.

C. Papanicolaou smear.

1. Diagnosis for cervical cancer.

2. Vaginal secretions and secretions from posterior fornix are swabbed and smeared on a glass slide.

Conditions of the Vulva

Vulvitis

A. An inflammation of the vulva that usually occurs in conjunction with other conditions such as vaginal infections and venereal disease.

✦ B. Signs and symptoms.

1. Burning pain during urination.

2. Itching.

3. Red and inflamed genitalia.

4. Discharge.

C. Treatment and nursing care.

1. Apply soothing compresses and give colloidal baths.

2. Administer medicated creams.

3. Administer sedatives (antihistamines).

Cancer of the Vulva

A. Signs and symptoms.

1. Long-standing pruritus (itching).

2. Foul-smelling discharge.

3. Bleeding.

4. Pain.

B. Treatment and nursing care.

1. Vulvectomy is the preferred treatment.

2. Immediate postoperative care.

a. Observe dressings for signs of hemorrhage.

b. Check vital signs until stable.

c. Assist patient to turn, cough, and deep breathe every 2 hours.

d. Give pain medications as ordered.

e. Observe drainage, and empty Hemovac as necessary.

f. Record intake and output.

g.   Maintain IV.

h.   Maintain catheter care to reduce incidence of infection.

i.   Position for comfort.

3.   Convalescent care.

a.   Encourage patient to verbalize feelings related to change in body image.

b.   Irrigate wound as ordered, using solution as prescribed (usual solution is sterile saline or hydrogen peroxide), which cleans area and improves circulation.

Conditions of the Vagina

✦ Vaginal Infections

A.   Vagina normally protected from infection by acidic environment.

B.   Leukorrhea (whitish vaginal discharge) normal in small amounts at ovulation and prior to menstruation.

C.   *Trichomonas vaginalis*—overgrowth of protozoan normally present in vaginal tract due to normal pH alteration.

D.   Moniliasis—fungal (yeast) infection caused by *Candida albicans*.

1.   Thrives in carbohydrate-rich environment; common in poorly controlled diabetes.

2.   Antibiotic or steroid therapy reduces protective organisms normally present.

E.   Treatment—medications and vaginal inserts as prescribed.

Conditions of Ovaries and Pelvic Cavity

Endometriosis

✦ A.   Abnormal growth of endometrial tissue outside the uterine cavity.

B.   This condition is a common cause of infertility.

C.   Etiological theories.

1.   Embryonic tissue that remains dormant until ovarian stimulation after menarche.

2.   Endometrial tissue transported from the uterine cavity through the fallopian tubes during menstruation.

3.   Endometrial tissue transported by lymphatic tissue during menstruation.

4.   Accidental transfer of endometrial tissue to pelvic cavity during surgery.

D.   Signs and symptoms.

1.   Lower abdominal and pelvic pain during menstruation due to distention of involved tissue and surrounding area by blood (symptoms are acute during menstruation).

2.   Dysmenorrhea—usually steady and severe.

3.   Abnormal uterine bleeding.

4.   Pain during intercourse.

5.   Back and rectal pain.

E.   Treatment and nursing care.

1.   Pregnancy may delay growth of lesions but symptoms usually recur after pregnancy.

2.   Hormone therapy with oral contraceptives usually eliminates menstrual pain and controls endometrial growth.

3.   Surgical intervention; total hysterectomy may be indicated.

4.   Provide emotional support.

✦ Pelvic Inflammatory Disease (PID)

A.   An inflammatory condition of the pelvic cavity that may involve ovaries, fallopian tubes, vascular system, or pelvic peritoneum.

B.   Etiology.

1.   *Staphylococcus* or *Streptococcus*.

2.   Venereal disease.

3.   Tubercle bacilli.

✦ C.   Signs and symptoms.

1.   Elevated temperature.

2.   Nausea and vomiting.

3.   Abdominal and low-back pain.

4.   Purulent, foul-smelling vaginal discharge.

5.   Leukocytosis.

✦ D.   Treatment and nursing care.

1.   Take measures to control the spread of infection.

2.   Place patient in semi-Fowler's position for dependent drainage.

3.   Take and record vital signs every 4 hours.

4.   Administer antibiotics, douches, and abdominal heat as ordered.

5.   Note nature and amount of vaginal discharge.

6.   Avoid use of tampons and urinary catheterization to prevent the spread of infection.

7.   Promote good nutrition and fluid intake.

8.   Explain rationale for treatment.

Cancer of the Ovary

A.   Malignancy may occur at all ages—risk increases after age 40.

✦ B.   The most deadly form of reproductive cancer; etiology not understood and lack of warning symptoms.

✦ C.   Early diagnosis important (survival rate is 87 percent).

1.   Usually detection is by chance, not screening.

2.   Tumor marker, CA-125, may be useful, but many false negatives occur.

✦ D.   Cancer is staged according to the involvement of tissue and may involve one or both ovaries. (*See* Oncology chapter for more complete explanation.)

1.   Stage I—limited to the ovaries.

2.   Stage II—pelvic extension.

3.   Stage III—metastasis outside pelvis or positive retroperitoneal lymph nodes.

4.   Stage IV—distant metastasis.

E. Laparotomy is used for diagnosis and treatment—surgery is primary treatment;

F. Chemotherapy may be used for Stage I; radioactive instillation for Stage II.
   1. Chemotherapeutic drugs include: cyclophosphamide, cisplatin, carboplatin, or paclitaxel.
   2. Cisplatin and paclitaxel most commonly used because of clinical benefits and manageable toxicity.
   3. Leukopenia, neurotoxicity, and fever may occur with treatment.
   4. Paclitaxel can cause cardiac effects.

G. Nursing care is the same as for any major abdominal surgery with the exception of psychosocial implications of cancer.

Implementation

✦ A. Provide immediate postoperative care.
   ❖ **PROCEDURE** ❖
   1. Observe dressings for signs of hemorrhage.
   2. Check vital signs until stable.
   3. Assist patient to turn, cough, and deep breathe every 2 hours.
   4. Give pain medications as ordered.
   5. Observe drainage and empty Hemovac as necessary.
   6. Record intake and output.
   7. Maintain IV.
   8. Maintain catheter care to reduce incidence of infection.
   9. Position for comfort.

B. Provide convalescent care.
   1. Encourage verbalization regarding change in body image.
   2. Irrigate wound as ordered, using solution as prescribed (usual solution is sterile saline) which cleans area and improves circulation.
   3. Prevent wound infection.

C. Instruct patient on discharge teaching.
   1. Signs of infection—foul-smelling discharge, elevated temperature, swelling.
   2. Nutritious diet and planned rest periods.
   3. Wound irrigation and dressing change.
   4. Importance of follow-up care by physician.

Conditions of the Uterus

Displacements

✦ A. Retroversion and retroflexion—backward displacement of the uterus.
   1. May cause difficulty in getting pregnant.
   2. Treatment consists of moving the uterus to the normal position by shortening its ligaments.

✦ B. Prolapse (usually occurs in multiparas).
   1. Weakening of uterine supports causes the uterus to slip down into the vaginal canal; the uterus may even appear outside the vaginal orifice.
   2. Prolapse often causes urinary incontinence or retention.
   3. Treatment.
      a. Pessary—instrument that keeps the uterus in place by exerting pressure on ligaments; usually used in patients of advanced age.
      b. Surgery to reposition uterus and shorten ligaments; or hysterectomy.

Tumors

✦ A. Benign fibroid tumors.
   1. Occur in 20–30 percent of all women between the ages of 25 and 40.
   2. Symptoms include menorrhagia, back pain, urinary difficulty, and constipation.
   3. Fibroid tumors may cause sterility.
   4. Treatment.
      a. Removal of tumors, if they are small.
      b. Hysterectomy is performed when there are large tumors.

✦ B. Malignant tumors of the reproductive system (second highest cause of death in the female).
   1. Cancer of the cervix—most common type of cancer in the reproductive system.
      a. Usually appears in females between the ages of 30 and 50.
      b. Signs and symptoms include bleeding between periods—may be noted especially after intercourse or douching; leukorrhea.
      c. May become invasive and include tissue outside the cervix, fundus of the uterus, and the lymph glands.
      d. Treatment depends on extent of the disease.
         (1) Hysterectomy.
         (2) Radiation.
         (3) Radical pelvic surgery in advanced cases.
   2. Cancer of the endometrium (fundus or corpus of uterus).
      a. Usually not diagnosed until symptoms appear; Pap smear inadequate for diagnosis.
      b. Progresses slowly; metastasis occurs late.
      c. Treatment.
         (1) Early—hysterectomy.
         (2) Late—radium and x-ray therapy.

Hysterectomy

✦ Types

A. Total—removal of the entire uterus but retention of fallopian tubes and ovaries.

B. Panhysterectomy—removal of the entire uterus, ovaries, and fallopian tubes.
C. Radical hysterectomy—wide removal of vaginal, cervical, uterosacral, and other tissue along with the uterus.
D. Cervical.
E. Abdominal.
F. Vaginal.

✦ **Postoperative Implementation**
A. Immediate care.
  1. Observe incisional site for bleeding and reinforce dressings as needed.
  2. Monitor vital signs frequently.
  3. Administer pain medications as ordered.
  4. Monitor IV fluids as ordered.
  5. Provide for hygienic care.
  6. Catheter care to prevent infection (observe amount and color of drainage).
  7. Assist patient to cough, turn, and deep breathe.
  8. Promote methods for decreasing pelvic congestion.
    a. Apply antiembolic stocking.
    b. Avoid high-Fowler's position.
  9. Measure intake and output.
  10. Apply range-of-motion exercises.
B. Common complications.
  1. Hemorrhage.
  2. Infection.
  3. Pneumonia.
  4. Paralytic ileus.
  5. Thrombophlebitis.
  6. Changes in body image.

Anterior and Posterior Colporrhaphy
A. Purpose.
  ✦ 1. Repair of cystocele—downward displacement of the bladder toward the vaginal entrance caused by tissue weakness, injuries in childbirth, and atrophy associated with aging.
  ✦ 2. Repair of rectocele—anterior sagging of rectum and posterior vaginal wall caused by injuries to the muscles and tissue of the pelvic floor during childbirth.
B. General postoperative care of the patient with cystocele and rectocele repair.
  1. Observe for foul-smelling discharge from vaginal area or operative site.
  2. Two methods of caring for perineal sutures.
    a. Sutures left alone until healing begins; thereafter, daily vaginal irrigations with sterile saline.
    b. Sterile saline douches twice daily beginning with the first postoperative day.
  3. Observe for urinary retention and catheterize as necessary.

4. Prepare patient for discharge with instruction in perineal hygiene (no douching or coitus until advised by physician), and in detection of signs of infection.

Pelvic Exenteration
A. A surgical procedure that is performed for widespread cancer that cannot be controlled by other means.
✦ B. Three types of pelvic exenteration.
  1. Anterior pelvic—the removal of the reproductive organs, pelvic lymph nodes, adnexa, pelvic peritoneum, bladder, and lower ureter. Ureters are implanted in the small intestines or the colon.
  2. Posterior pelvic—removal of the reproductive organs, vagina, adnexa, colon, and rectum. Pelvic lymph nodes may also be removed.
  3. Total pelvic—removal of the reproductive organs, pelvic floor, pelvic lymph nodes, perineum, bladder, rectum, and distal portion of sigmoid colon. A substitute bladder is made from a segment of the ileum. Patient will have a permanent colostomy.
C. Care of the patient undergoing pelvic exenteration.
  1. Exercise general postoperative procedures.
  2. Observe surgical site for drainage and reinforce dressings as necessary; patient may have drainage tubes connected to suction from incision area.
  3. Apply antiembolic stockings.
  4. Encourage patient to express feelings.

✦ **Patient Receiving Radiation Therapy**
A. Radiation therapy is treatment with radioactive substance given to break down cancerous tissue.
B. Therapy procedure.
  1. Radioactive cobalt, radium, or iridium inserted into endocervical canal by radiotherapist.
  2. Supplemented by external radiation.
C. Nursing care.
  1. Provide low-residue diet to prevent bowel movement and dislodging of radium.
  2. Inspect catheter to make sure it is draining (distended bladder will be in the path of radiation).
  3. Observe for unusual or profuse vaginal discharge.
  4. Instruct patient to lie on side or on back with head slightly elevated on pillow.
  5. Administer skin care to prevent tissue breakdown.
  6. While giving nursing care, encourage patient to talk and express anxieties.
  7. Measure intake and output.

8. Observe patient for side effects, e.g., nausea, vomiting, anorexia, and redness or blistering of skin in pelvic area.

9. Check vital signs and observe for elevated temperature.

Tumors of the Breast

Clinical Findings

A. Nontender lump in breast, usually in upper outer quadrant.

B. Dimpling of breast tissue surrounding nipple.

C. Asymmetry, with affected breast being higher.

D. Nipple bleeding or retraction.

Implementation

✦ A. Begin giving emotional support preoperatively and continue during postoperative period.
    1. Patient will have altered body image.
    2. Patient may be extremely depressed.

✦ B. Position in semi-Fowler's position with the affected arm elevated to prevent edema.

C. Turn, cough, and hyperventilate to prevent respiratory complications.

D. Turn only to back and unaffected side.

E. Hemovac placed frequently.
    1. Maintain suction.
    2. Record amount of drainage.
    3. Record drainage characteristics.

✦ F. Prevent complications of contractures and lymphedema by encouraging range-of-motion exercises early in postoperative period.

G. IV fluids should not be administered in affected arm.

✦ H. Monitor vital signs for prevention of complications such as infection and hemorrhage. Take blood pressure on unaffected arm only.

BREAST SURGERY

Breast Conserving Therapy
- Surgical procedures: lumpectomy, wide excision, partial mastectomy, segmental mastectomy, quadrantectomy.
- Removal of involved breast tissue and some surrounding tissue and axillary lymph nodes.

Total Mastectomy
- Removal of breast tissue only.
- Performed for carcinoma in situ, typically ductal.

Modified Radical Mastectomy
- Removal of breast tissue and axillary lymph nodes.
- Pectoralis major and minor muscles remain intact.

Radical Mastectomy
- Removal of breast tissue and pectoralis major and minor.
- Axillary lymph node dissection.

I. Pressure dressings should be reinforced. Observe for signs of restriction from dressing.
    1. Impaired sensation.
    2. Color changes of skin.

J. If skin grafts were applied, treat as for any other graft.

K. Encourage visit from Reach for Recovery Group.

THERAPEUTIC ABORTION

General Considerations

✦ A. Legality.
    1. Abortion is now legal in all states as the result of a Supreme Court decision in January 1973.
    2. It is regulated in the following manner.
        a. First trimester—decision between patient and physician.
        b. Second trimester—decision between patient and physician (state may regulate who performs the abortion and where it can be done).
        c. Third trimester—states may regulate and prohibit abortion except to preserve the health or life of the mother.

✦ B. Indications for abortion.
    1. Medical—psychiatric condition; chronic hypertension or disease in the mother (e.g., nephritis, severe diabetes, cancer, or acute infection such as rubella); possible genetic defects in the infant or severe erythroblastosis fetalis.
    2. Nonmedical—socioeconomic reasons, unmarried, financial burden, too young to care for infant, rape.

C. Preparation of the individual.
    1. Advise patient of available sources of abortion.
    2. Inform patient as to what to expect from the abortion procedure.
    3. Provide emotional support during decision-making period.
    4. Maintain an open, nonjudgmental atmosphere in which the individual may express concerns or guilt.
    5. Encourage and support the individual after the decision is made and after surgery.
    6. Give information about contraceptives.

D. Complications and effects.
    1. Abortion should be performed before the twelfth week, if possible, because complications and risks are lower during this time.
    2. Complications.
        a. Infection.

b.   Bleeding.

c.   Sterility.

d.   Uterine perforation.

Abortion Techniques

✦ A.   First trimester.

1.   Dilatation and curettage (D&C).

a.   Cervical canal is dilated with instruments of increasingly large diameter.

b.   Fetus and accessory structure is removed with forceps.

c.   Endometrium is scraped with curette to assure that all products of conception are removed.

d.   Process usually takes 15–20 minutes.

2.   Vacuum aspirator.

a.   Hose-linked curette is inserted into dilated cervix.

b.   Hose is attached to suction.

c.   The vacuum aspirator lessens the chance of uterine perforation, reduces blood loss, and reduces the time of the procedure.

✦ B.   Second trimester abortion.

1.   Intra-amniotic injection or amniocentesis abortion.

a.   Performed after the 14th–16th week of pregnancy.

b.   50–200 mL of amniotic fluid are removed from the amniotic cavity and replaced with hypertonic solution of 20–50 percent saline that is installed through gravity drip over a period of 45–60 minutes.

c.   Increased osmotic pressure of the amniotic fluid causes the death of the fetus.

d.   Uterine contractions usually begin in about 12 hours, and the products of conception are expelled in 24–30 hours.

e.   Oxytocic drugs may be given if contractions do not begin.

f.   Complications.

(1)   Infusion of hypertonic saline solution into uterus.

(2)   Infection.

(3)   Disseminated intravascular coagulation disease may develop during procedure.

(4)   Hemorrhage.

✦ 2.   Hysterotomy.

a.   Incision is made through abdominal wall into uterus.

b.   Procedure is usually performed between the 14th and 16th week in pregnancy.

c.   Products of conception are removed with forceps.

d.   Uterine cavity is curetted.

e.   Tubal ligation may be done at same time.

f.   Patient usually requires several days of hospitalization.

g.   Operation requires general or spinal anesthesia.

3.   Prostaglandins.

a.   These hormonelike acids cause abortion by stimulating the uterus to contract.

b.   They may be administered IV into the uterine cavity through the cervical canal, into the posterior fornix of the vagina, or after 12 weeks into the amniotic cavity. The IV method is least effective and has many possible side effects.

C.   Nursing care.

1.   Administer preoperative medications.

2.   Ensure that patient understands the procedure.

3.   Offer emotional support and let patient express feelings.

4.   Monitor IV.

5.   Check vital signs postoperatively.

6.   Check for excessive bleeding.

7.   Administer pain medications as ordered.

8.   Instruct patient to watch for signs of excessive bleeding (more than a normal menstrual period) and infection (elevated temperature, foul-smelling discharge, persistent abdominal pain).

9.   Administer oxytocic drug as ordered.

10.   Administer RhoGAM as ordered for an unsensitized Rh-negative patient.

11.   Offer fluids as tolerated after vital signs are stable and patient is alert and responsive.

12.   Counsel regarding birth control methods.

CONTRACEPTIVE METHODS

Natural Contraceptive Methods

A.   Periodic abstinence: 75 percent effective.

1.   Based on following principles.

a.   Ovulation usually occurs 14 days before period begins.

b.   An ovum may be fertilized 12–24 hours after release from ovary.

c.   Sperm survives only 24–48 hours in the uterine environment.

d.   If coitus is avoided during the fertile period, pregnancy should not occur.

2.   Cervical mucus (Billings): couple avoids intercourse during peak 72-hour period of cycle, when mucus becomes clear, stringy, stretchable, and slippery.

B.   Coitus interruptus: 60 percent effective.

1.   Requires withdrawal of penis before ejaculation.

2.   Pre-ejaculatory fluid may contain sperm.

C. Lactation—unreliable.
   1. Breast-feeding has contraceptive effect.
   2. Prolactin's inhibition of luteinizing hormone, which maintains menstruation.

✦ Mechanical Methods

A. Condom: 95–98 percent effective with proper application.
   1. Acts as mechanical barrier by collecting sperm and not allowing contact with vaginal area.
   2. Prevents spread of disease.
B. Diaphragm: 80 percent effective; with proper use, 94 percent.
   1. Functions by blocking external os and closing access to cervical canal by sperm. It is a mechanical barrier.
   2. Must be used in conjunction with vaginal cream or jelly to be effective.
   3. Toxic Shock Syndrome may occur—remove 6–8 hours after intercourse and do not use during menstruation.
C. Contraceptive sponge: 80–90 percent effective.
   1. Inserted deep into vagina, sponge releases spermicide—leave in place 6 hours after intercourse.
   2. Decreases risk of STDs.
   3. May be risk of developing Toxic Shock Syndrome.
D. Cervical cap: 90 percent effective.
   1. Rubber cap with spermicide placed over cervical opening.
   2. May decrease risk of STD.
✦ E. Intrauterine devices: 95 percent effective.
   1. Medicated with coppor or progesterone.
      a. More rapid transport of ovum through tube reaching endometrium before it is "ready" for implantation.
      b. IUD may cause substances to accumulate in uterus and interfere with implantation.
      c. IUD may stimulate production of cellular exudate, which interferes with the ability of sperm to migrate to fallopian tubes.
   2. Usually made of soft plastic or nickel-chromium alloy.
   3. Complications: perforation of uterus; infection; increased incidence of PID; spotting between periods; heavy menstrual flow or prolonged flow; and cramping during menstruation.

✦ Chemical Methods

A. Oral contraceptives (combined or single hormone): 99 percent effective.
   1. Contraceptive effect occurs by:
      a. Artificially raising the blood levels of estrogen and/or progesterone, thereby preventing the release of FSH and LH. Without FSH, the follicle does not mature and ovulation fails to take place.
      b. Endometrial changes.
      c. Alteration in cervical mucus, making it hostile to sperm.
      d. Altered tubal function.
   2. Types of birth control pills.
      a. Combined: contains both estrogen and progesterone.
      b. Sequential (mimics normal hormonal cycle): estrogen given alone for 15–16 days, followed by combination of estrogen and progestin for the next 5 days.
      c. Progestin only (99+% effective) (called mini-pill) contains less progestin and no estrogen, so it is slightly less effective.
   3. Other types of combined hormones.
      a. Injection—Lunelle given every month.
      b. Transdermal patch—given every week × 3.
      c. Vaginal ring delivers hormones; worn for 3 weeks.
   4. Minor side effects, which usually diminish within a few months: breast fullness and tenderness; edema, weight gain; nausea and vomiting; chloasma; and breakthrough bleeding.
   ✦ 5. More serious side effects: thrombophlebitis; pulmonary embolism; hypertension.
B. Chemical agent: Nonoxynol-9 or octoxynol-9.
   1. Agent acts by killing or paralyzing sperm; may kill STD agents.
   2. Agent acts as a vehicle for spermicide as well as a mechanical barrier through which sperm cannot swim.
   3. Available forms are foams, creams, jellies, or suppositories.
✦ C. Implants: more than 99 percent effective.
   1. Norplant—under skin releases progestin for up to 5 years.
   2. Depo-Provera—injection of a progestin every 12 weeks.
D. Emergency postcoital contraception.
   1. Within 72 hours of sex inhibits ovulation.
   2. Copper T-380A IUD is inserted within 5–7 days after sex—prevents implantation.

Operative Sterilization Procedures

✦ A. Vasectomy.
   1. Surgical procedure with local anesthesia on outpatient basis.
      a. Incision made over ductus deferens on each side of scrotum; sperm ducts isolated and severed.
      b. Ends ligated, lumen coagulated, clipped, or polyethylene tubing used with a stopcock for potential reversal.
   2. Patient instruction for care.

a. Apply ice with pain or swelling.

b. Use scrotal support for 1 week.

c. Inform patient that it takes 4–6 weeks and 3–36 ejaculations to clear sperm from ductus.

d. Sperm samples (two or three) should be checked for sperm count.

e. Patient rechecked at 6 and 12 months to ensure fertility has not been restored by recanalization.

3. Possible side effects of procedure.

a. Hematoma, sperm granulomas, and spontaneous reanastomosis.

b. For those who wish to reverse process, 30–85 percent are successful.

✦ B. Tubal ligation most common method (removal of uterus and ovaries is permanent method of sterilization).

1. Accomplished by abdominal or vaginal procedures; most common method is transection of fallopian tubes.

a. Tubes are isolated, then crushed, ligated, or plugged (newer reversible procedure).

b. The postpartal and mini-laparotomy procedures require hospitalization.

c. Laparoscopic sterilization requires an incision at the umbilicus; the tube is coagulated and may be transected.

2. Complications of procedure include bowel perforation, infection, hemorrhage, and adverse anesthesia effects.

a. Reversal of tubal ligations results in overall pregnancy rate of 15 percent.

b. Three-quarters of these pregnancies result in live births, and 10 percent are tubal pregnancies.

✦ Appendix 14-1. PRENATAL INSTRUCTIONS

Nutrition

A. It is important that adequate nutrition is maintained.

B. *See* Appendix 14-2 for specific guidelines.

Use of Drugs

A. All drugs can be expected to cross the placenta and affect the fetus.

B. Greatest danger occurs in first trimester, especially when organs are developing (organogenesis).

C. Many other effects of drugs on the fetus are unknown and may not be evident for years.

D. Pregnant women should refrain from taking drugs during pregnancy; even commonly used drugs such as aspirin should only be taken by physician's order.

E. Nicotine in cigarettes may retard the growth of fetus.

1. Causes vasoconstriction of woman's vessels resulting in decreased placental flow.

2. Increases carbon dioxide levels in blood and reduces oxygen-carrying capacity.

F. *See* Appendix 14-3 for an outline on drugs that adversely affect fetus.

Exercise, Relaxation, and Rest

A. Exercise in moderation is beneficial but should never be carried on past the point of fatigue.

B. May participate in sports if they are part of the woman's usual activity and there are no complications present.

C. Fatigue is common in early pregnancy.

D. Frequent rest periods, at 10–15-minute intervals, are helpful in avoiding needless fatigue.

E. Relaxation and stress reduction important to maintain emotional stability during pregnancy.

✦ Appendix 14-2. RECOMMENDED DAILY DIETARY ALLOWANCES FOR PREGNANCY AND LACTATION

	Pregnancy		Lactation		Function	Sources
	14 to 18	Adult	14 to 18	Adult		
Calories	2400	2300	2600	2500	Meet increased nutritional needs as well as body maintenance	All foods; important to emphasize food values of foods and avoid empty calories
Protein	60 gm	60 gm	65 gm	65 gm	Augment maternal tissues—breasts, uterus, blood Growth and development of placenta and fetal tissue Constant repair and maintenance of maternal tissue	All essential amino acids may be found in milk, meat, eggs, and cheeses Other sources, though not complete protein by themselves: tofu, whole grains, legumes, nuts, peanut butter
Iron	30+ mg	30+ mg	*	*	Essential constituent of hemoglobin Part of various enzymes Fetal development and storage, especially later part of pregnancy	Good sources: liver, kidney, heart, cooked dry beans, lean pork and beef, dried fruits such as apricots, peaches, prunes, and raisins Fair sources: spinach, mustard greens, eggs
Calcium	1200 mg	1200 mg	1200 mg	1200 mg	Skeletal tissue Bones; teeth Blood coagulation Neuromuscular irritability Myocardial function Fetal stores, especially last months	Good sources: milk, cheese, ice cream, yogurt Fair sources: broccoli, canned salmon with bones, dried beans, dark leafy vegetables
Magnesium	320 mg	320 mg	355 mg	355 mg	Cellular metabolism Structural growth	Whole grains, milk, nuts, dark green vegetables, legumes
Phosphorus	1200 mg	1200 mg	1200 mg	1200 mg	90% compounded with calcium Rest distributed throughout cells—involved in energy production, building and repairing tissue, buffering	Whole grain items: cereals, whole wheat bread, brown rice; milk
Sodium	0.5 gm	0.5 gm	0.5 gm	0.5 gm	Metabolic activities Fluid balance and acid–base balance Cell permeability Muscle irritability	Table salt, meat, eggs, carrots, celery, beets, spinach, salted nuts, carbonated beverages
Iodine	125 µg	125 µg	125 µg	125 µg	Necessary for health: mother and fetus; prevents goiter in mother; decreases chance of cretinism in infants	Iodized table salt, cod liver oil
Vitamin A	5000 IU	5000 IU	6000 IU	6000 IU	Tooth formation and skeletal growth Cell growth and development Integrity of epithelial tissue Vision—light/dark adaptation Fat metabolism	Good sources: butter, egg yolk, fortified margarine, whole milk, cream, kidney, and liver Fair source: dark green and yellow vegetables such as sweet potatoes, pumpkin, mustard greens, collards, kale, bok choy, carrots, cantaloupe, apricots

Appendix 14-2. *(Continued)*

	Pregnancy		Lactation		Function	Sources
	14 to 18	**Adult**	**14 to 18**	**Adult**		
Riboflavin	1.4 mg	1.4 mg	1.6 mg	1.6 mg	Enzyme systems Tissue functioning Tissue oxygenation and respiration Energy metabolism Excreted in breast milk	Good sources: kidney, liver, heart, milk Fair sources: cheese, ice cream, dark leafy vegetables, lean meat, poultry
Thiamine	1.4 mg	1.4 mg	1.4 mg	1.4 mg	Carbohydrate metabolism Normal appetite and digestion Health of nervous system	Good sources: enriched and whole-grain products—bread and cereals, dried peas, beans, liver, heart, kidney, nuts, potatoes, lean pork Fair sources: eggs, milk, poultry, fish, vegetables
Niacin	18 mg	18 mg	17 mg	17 mg	Cell metabolism	Good sources: fish, lean meat, poultry, liver, heart, peanuts, peanut butter Fair sources: enriched and whole-grain cereals and bread, milk, potatoes
Folic acid	600 g	600 g	500 g	500 g	Cell growth Important to prevent neural tube defect Enzyme activities in production of protein Deficiency results in megaloblastic anemia in 1 to 4% of pregnant women in the United States	Dark green and leafy vegetables Liver, peanuts, whole-grain cereals
Vitamin B_{12}	2.6 mg	2.6 mg	2.8 mg	2.8 mg	Deficiency may result in pernicious anemia	Found only in animal sources
Pyridoxine Vitamin B_6	1.9 mg	1.9 mg	2.0 mg	2.0 mg	Essential coenzyme with amino acids Deficiency may lead to hypochromic microcytic anemia	Animal and vegetable protein such as meat, fish, beans, nuts and seeds, milk and milk products
Vitamin D	500 IU	500 IU	500 IU	500 IU	Influences absorption, retention, and utilization of calcium and phosphorus Formation of bones, teeth, and other tissue	Good sources: fortified milk, butter, egg yolk, liver, fish oils
Vitamin C Ascorbic acid	80 mg	85 mg	115 mg	120 mg	Production of intracellular substances necessary for development and maintenance of normal connective tissue in bones, cartilage, and muscles Role in metabolic processes involving protein and tissues Increases absorption of iron	Good sources: citrus fruits and juice, broccoli, cantaloupe, collards, mustard and turnip greens, peppers Fair sources: asparagus, raw cabbage, other melons, spinach, prunes, tomatoes, canned or fresh chilies

* Iron needs during lactation are not different from those of a nonpregnant female (18 mg/day taken with vitamin C to increase assimilation), but continued supplementation following birth is important to replenish iron stores depleted by pregnancy.

✦ Appendix 14-3. COMMON DRUGS IN OBSTETRICS AND GYNECOLOGY

Name of Drug and Action	Uses and Side Effects	Nursing Implications
Oxytocin, Syntocinon, Pitocin Classification: oxytocic Produces rhythmic contractions of uterine musculature Dosage: varies with method and purpose of administration. IV: 10–40 USP units in 1000 mL 5% dextrose in saline solution infused at rate of 0.5–0.75 mL/min. Calibrated pump 2.5 USP units in 50 mL 5% D/W. Start at 1 μ/min and increase as necessary	Used to induce or augment labor, constrict uterus, and decrease hemorrhage after delivery and postabortion Stimulates contractile tissue in lactating breast to eject milk Side effects: water intoxication, allergic reactions, death due to uterine rupture, pelvic hematomas, bradycardia Excessive contractions more frequent than every 2½ minutes or lasting longer than 40–60 seconds	Observe for signs of sensitivity and overdose Monitor strength and duration of uterine contractions Check FHT every 15 minutes and PRN Take pulse and blood pressure every hour Contractions of 90 seconds with no resting period—stop infusion immediately and notify physician
Methergine Classification: oxytocic, ergot alkaloid Produces constrictive effects on smooth muscle of uterus (more prolonged constrictive effects as compared to rhythmic effects of oxytocin); has minimal vasoconstrictive effect Usual IM dose: 0.2 mg; may be repeated in 2–4 hrs; usual oral dose 0.2 mg 3–4×/day for 2 days	Used primarily after delivery to produce firm uterine contractions and decrease uterine bleeding May be used to prevent postabortal hemorrhage Side effects include nausea, vomiting, dizziness, increased blood pressure, dyspnea, and chest pain	Check blood pressure and pulse before administration of medication (do not give if BP is > 140/90), and check vital signs frequently after administration Injectable form deteriorates rapidly when exposed to lights and heat; do not use if discoloration occurs Do not administer with Percodan—hallucinations
Hemabate Classification: oxytocic, prostaglandin Stimulates uterine contractions Used as a method of controlling hemorrhage Usual IM dose: 0.25 mg repeated up to maximum 5 doses, may be repeated q 15–90 min	Control of refractory causes of postpartal hemorrhage caused by uterine atony; generally used after failed attempts at control of hemorrhage with oxytoxic agents Side effects include nausea, vomiting, diarrhea, headache, flushing, bradycardia, bronchospasm, wheezing, cough, chills, and fever	Monitor blood pressure, pulse, and respiratory status Administer in deep muscle mass, rotate sites Contraindicated in women with active cardiovascular, renal or liver disease, or asthma
Apresoline (hydralazine hydrochloride) Classification: antihypertensive Relaxes vascular smooth muscle, decreases peripheral vascular resistance and increases peripheral vasodilation Dosage: PO 12.5 mg BID, increased incrementally to maximum 100 mg BID	Used to lower blood pressure (decreases peripheral resistance and peripheral vasodilation) Side effects: flushing, headache, nausea, vomiting, tachycardia, palpitations, lupus syndrome, and leukopenia	Monitor blood pressure and pulse rate Observe for orthostatic hypotension, tachycardia, palpitations, headache, dizziness, nausea, vomiting Give drug with meals to increase absorption
Magnesium sulfate Depressive effects on central nervous system; decreases acetylcholine release → neuromuscular transmission of impulses in smooth, skeletal and cardiac muscle Produces peripheral vasodilation Given IV in preeclampsia and eclampsia; dosage varies Loading dose 4 g in 250 mL 5% D/W at 5 mL/30 sec (approximately 20 min) or in continuous infusion; then 1–3 g/hr until contractions stop or therapeutic levels are maintained	Used to prevent convulsions in preeclampsia and eclampsia. Also tocolytic to treat preterm labor and uterine tetany Side effects: *Maternal:* extreme thirst, hypotension, flaccidity, circulatory collapse, depression of CNS and cardiac system. *Fetal:* crosses placenta, lethargy, hypotonia Antidote: calcium gluconate 10%. Keep 10-mL vial available at bedside	Observe carefully for signs of magnesium toxicity: extreme thirst, feeling hot all over; loss of patellar reflex, muscle weakness Monitor respirations (> 12/min), BP (hypotension), and P closely in order to assess effect of drug. Never leave patient alone Patellar reflex should be checked frequently Check urine output continuously (> 30 mL/hr)

Appendix 14-3. *(Continued)*

Name of Drug and Action	Uses and Side Effects	Nursing Implications
Ritodrine (Yutopar) Analog of beta-adrenergic agonist Alters calcium balance in cells and decreases contractility of smooth muscles, suppresses uterine contractions Usual initial dose is 0.1 mg/min using microdrip at the recommended dilution Effective dose usually between 0.15 and 0.35 mg/min continued for 12 hours after uterine contractions cease Phase in PO dose	Treatment of premature labor or during labor when contractions are unusually frequent and not coordinated; most effective when given in early latent phase of labor; rarely stops active labor Side effects: nausea, vomiting, dizziness, transient hypotension, and tachycardia Hydrate woman prior to infusion with IV solution of 1000 mL normal saline Continuous monitoring (Swan–Ganz) of mother and infant important as mother and infant deaths have occurred	Take blood pressure and pulse every 5 min until stable Cardiac monitoring for IV route; notify physician if pulse over 120 Discontinue drug 6 hours before birth Arrhythmias: maintain bedrest—quiet environment Fowler's or side-lying position Monitor uterine activity and FHT Check for toxicity; CNS symptoms, dyspnea, cardiac irregularities; pulmonary edema Screen with ECG prior to beginning therapy Monitor hydration status carefully—limit fluids to 3000 mL/day
Terbutaline (Brethine) B_2 adrenergic agonist; stimulates B_2 receptors, relaxes smooth muscle of uterus and bronchus 0.25–0.5 mg sub q every 1–4 hrs until contractions stop; 5 mg PO maintenance dose	Relaxes uterus in preterm labor Also used for fetal distress to increase placental flow Side effects: tachycardia, palpitations, sweating, tremors, restlessness, lethargy, drowsiness, headache, nausea, vomiting	In addition to above, screen baseline glucose status and follow levels; follow urinary ketones; check for hypertension, muscle cramps, CNS symptoms indicating toxicity
Nifedipine Classification: calcium channel blocker Reduces the flow of extracellular calcium ions into the intracellular space of the myometrial smooth muscle cells, thereby inhibiting contractile activity Usual dose: PO immediate release 10 mg TID; increase in 10-mg increments q 4–6 h, not to exceed 180 mg/24 hours Well absorbed either orally or sublingually	Used as a tocolytic Side effects: hypotension, tachycardia, facial flushing, headache, and pulmonary edema	Monitor blood pressure, pulse, and respiratory status Encourage client to change position slowly Instruct to notify nurse of dyspnea, edema of extremities, or nausea/vomiting

✦ Appendix 14-4. NUTRITIONAL GUIDELINES FOR PREGNANCY

A. Influences on dietary habits and nutrition.
1. Food—many emotional connotations originating in infancy.
2. Eating habits influenced by:
    a. Emotional factors.
    b. Cultural factors.
    c. Religious beliefs.
    d. Nutritional information.
    e. Age—especially adolescent and aged.
    f. Physical health.
    g. Personal preferences.

B. Nutritional needs in pregnancy.
1. Influenced by above factors.
2. Must supply caloric and nutritional needs of mother as well as promote optimum fetal growth.
3. May be complicated by:
    a. Poor maternal nutrition before pregnancy.
    b. Medical complications prior to pregnancy (diabetes, anemia).
    c. Complications resulting from pregnancy (toxemia, anemia).
    d. Pica (cravings).

C. Weight gain in pregnancy.
1. Recommendations based on pre-pregnancy weight for height:
    Normal: 11.5–16 kg (25.3–35.2#).
    Underweight: 12.5–18 kg (27.5–39.6#).
    Overweight: 7–11.5 kg (15.4–25.3#).
✦ 2. Weight gain during 2nd and 3rd trimesters.
    Normal: 0.4 kg/week (0.88#).
    Underweight: 0.5 kg/week (1.1#).
    Overweight: 0.3 kg/week (0.66#).
3. Weight gain accounted by:
    a. Product of conception.

Fetus—average size	7–8 pounds
Placenta	2–2.5
Amniotic fluid	2
Uterus	2
Breasts	1–4
Extracellular fluid	3–5
Blood volume	4–5
	21–30.5 pounds

    b. Rest of weight gain deposited as fat stores or fluid representing energy stored for lactation.

D. Revised daily food guide.
1. This revised daily guide meets RDA standards for daily nutrients except for:
    a. Iron and folacin—cannot be ingested in sufficient quantities by dietary means. Must be supplemented during pregnancy.
✦ b. 300 additional calories needed to meet recommended allowances.
2. Protein intake includes both animal and vegetable protein.
    a. Vegetable protein may be omitted in those whose income will allow by increasing animal servings to three 3-oz. servings.
    b. One serving at least should be red meat.
3. Whole-grain items are better choices than leavened breads and cereals. They contain more magnesium, zinc, folacin, and vitamin B_6.
4. At least two tablespoons of fat or oils should be consumed daily for vitamin E and essential fatty acids.

E. Special diets.
✦ 1. Adolescents.
    a. Have high proportion of low-birth-weight infants.
    b. Dietary habits often poor. Plan menu to include necessary items around foods they like.
    c. Stress balanced diet—avoid empty calories.
2. Low sodium.
    a. Presently sodium restriction is *deemphasized*.
    b. Sodium essential in maintaining increased body fluids needed for adequate placental flow, increased tissue requirements, and renal blood flow.
    c. If moderate salt intake is necessitated, avoid highly salted foods such as canned soups, potato chips, soda pop.
3. Weight control.
    a. Presently, weight loss in pregnancy is discouraged.
    b. Even obese patient should gain 15–25 pounds to ensure adequate nutrition for fetal growth.
    c. Strict dieting may lead to ketosis, which has proven harmful to fetal brain development.
    d. Stress careful dietary planning to include essential nutrients and avoid empty calories.
    e. Weight reduction program should begin *after* lactation only.
✦ 4. Vegetarians.
    a. Sound nutritional planning to include those combinations of foods which, when combined, include all essential amino acids. May require iron and zinc.
    b. May require B-complex supplement, especially vitamin B_{12}, which comes only from animal sources.

MATERNAL/NEWBORN AND GYNECOLOGICAL NURSING QUESTIONS

1. A nurse in her first trimester of pregnancy is working in the hospital. The nurse knows that she should avoid

   1. Any patient with an infection.
   2. A 3-month-old infant with a generalized rash.
   3. A child with a fever and upper respiratory disorder.
   4. A patient who has just been diagnosed with lupus erythematosus.

2. Following a saline-induced therapeutic abortion, a patient has developed disseminated intravascular coagulation (DIC). The most critical nursing intervention for this patient is to

   1. Administer ordered medications.
   2. Allay anxiety—provide emotional support.
   3. Administer ordered oxygen at 6 L/min.
   4. Encourage fluid intake.

3. A patient's laboratory results indicate a creatinine level of 7 mg/dL. This finding would lead the nurse to place the highest priority on monitoring the patient's

   1. Temperature.
   2. Intake and output.
   3. Capillary refill.
   4. Pupillary reflex.

4. After a normal labor and delivery, the infant weighs only 5 pounds and is considered premature. One of the most important interventions to provide nutrition for this preterm infant is to

   1. Use a regular nipple with a large hole.
   2. Feed every 4–6 hours.
   3. Use a preemie nipple for bottle feeding.
   4. Use milk high in fat for the formula.

5. A common test used to determine fetal status in the presence of preeclampsia is the nonstress test (NST). If this test is "reactive," the nurse knows that it means

   1. The test was normal, showing an increased fetal heart rate (FHR) with fetal movement.
   2. The test was normal, showing no change in FHR with fetal movement.

3. The test was abnormal, indicating a need for an immediate oxytocin challenge test (OCT).
   4. Ultrasound is indicated to determine fetal habitat and placental placement.

6. A diabetic patient who is pregnant asks about breast-feeding. The most accurate response regarding breast-feeding by diabetic mothers is that it is

   1. Contraindicated because insulin is passed to the infant through the milk.
   2. Not contraindicated; however, the diabetic's milk production and mechanism may be faulty.
   3. Contraindicated because it puts too much stress on the mother's body.
   4. Not contraindicated but encouraged.

7. A new mother is concerned because her physician said that her baby had jaundice. The nurse understands that it is a(an)

   1. Normal condition that appears at 2–3 days of life.
   2. Normal condition that appears 8–24 hours after birth.
   3. Abnormal condition that appears within the first 24 hours of life.
   4. Abnormal condition that appears at 2–3 days of life.

8. A newly pregnant patient who is slightly overweight asks how much weight she should gain during her pregnancy. The most appropriate answer is

   1. "For your size, a little heavy, about 15 pounds would be best."
   2. "It really doesn't matter exactly how much weight you gain, as long as your diet is healthy."
   3. "A gain of about 25 pounds is best for mother and baby."
   4. "Because you are a little overweight, it would be best for you not to gain too much weight."

9. Which of the following statements is usually true about cervical changes in primiparas?

   1. Effacement precedes dilation.
   2. Effacement and dilation occur simultaneously.
   3. Dilation precedes effacement.
   4. Effacement is not necessary.

10. A patient is 3 days postpartum. Her vital signs are stable; her fundus is 3 fingerbreadths below the umbilicus, and her lochia rubra is moderate. Her breasts are hard and warm to the touch. The nurse would evaluate that the patient

   1. Is showing early signs of breast infection.
   2. Is normal for 3 days postpartum.
   3. Needs ice packs applied to her breasts.
   4. Should remove her nursing bra to reduce discomfort.

11. The first day postpartum for a new mother, the nurse observes that she appears frightened and says, "The baby has been breathing funny: fast and slow, off and on." The most appropriate nursing response would be

   1. "That's normal when the baby breast-feeds."
   2. "There's nothing to worry about. I'm going to take the baby back to the nursery now."
   3. "I'll watch the baby for a while to see if there is something wrong."
   4. "Don't be frightened. It's a normal breathing pattern. I'll sit here while you finish feeding him."

12. An amniocentesis is performed for genetic cell analysis. The nurse counsels the patient that this test cannot be performed until 14 weeks' gestation because

   1. This is when the heartbeat is first heard.
   2. The fetus is not mature enough until this time.
   3. There is not enough amniotic fluid until this time.
   4. The genetic results will not be accurate until this time.

13. A serology test for syphilis is given to a pregnant woman. The nurse explains to the patient that the reason this test is given is that

   1. Latent syphilis becomes highly active during pregnancy due to hormonal changes.
   2. Syphilis may be passed to the fetus after 4 months of pregnancy.
   3. Syphilis is no longer a problem, but the law still requires the serology test.
   4. Syphilis may be passed to the infant during delivery.

14. Nursing care of a pregnant patient who received regional anesthesia would include

   1. Walking the patient to ensure medication is evenly distributed.
   2. Asking the patient to turn from side to side every 15 minutes.

   3. Monitoring blood pressure every 3–5 minutes until stabilized.
   4. Giving the patient sips of water to swallow during the procedure.

15. Assessing a patient with eclampsia, the nurse knows that a cardinal symptom is

   1. Weight gain of 1 pound a week.
   2. Concentrated urine.
   3. Hypertension.
   4. Feeling of lassitude and fatigue.

16. The nurse would anticipate a possible complication in infants delivered by cesarean section. The nurse would assess for

   1. Respiratory distress.
   2. Renal impairment.
   3. ABO incompatibility.
   4. Kernicterus.

17. If a patient experiences a ruptured ectopic pregnancy, an expected sign or symptom would be

   1. Elevated blood glucose levels.
   2. Sudden excruciating pain in lower abdomen.
   3. Sudden hypertension.
   4. Extensive external bleeding.

18. A patient, 34 weeks pregnant, has just been admitted to the labor room in the first stage of labor. Which of the following clinical manifestations would be considered abnormal and would be reported to the physician immediately?

   1. Expulsion of a blood-tinged mucous plug.
   2. Continuous contraction of 2 minutes' duration.
   3. Feeling of pressure on perineum causing her to bear down.
   4. Expulsion of clear fluid from the vagina.

19. An eclamptic patient has been receiving magnesium sulfate IV 2 g/hour. What symptom would indicate that the current dose be continued?

   1. Absence of deep tendon reflexes.
   2. A respiratory rate of 16 per minute.
   3. Urine output of 50 mL over the last 4 hours.
   4. Heart skipping a beat.

20. An 11-lb. 6-oz. baby girl was delivered by cesarean section to a diabetic mother. Priority data collection of the infant of a diabetic mother would be for

   1. Hypoglycemia.
   2. Sepsis.
   3. Hyperglycemia.
   4. Hypercalcemia.

21. Of the following conditions, which one is *not* a result of metabolic error in the fetus?

    1. Phenylketonuria.
    2. Maple syrup urine disease.
    3. Glutamicacidemia.
    4. Pyloric stenosis.

22. A patient has given birth to a stillborn with congenital deformities. She knows this but says she wants to see her baby. What is the nurse's best approach?

    1. "That's your right. I'll bring the baby to you."
    2. "It would be better to let your husband see the baby; then he can tell you."
    3. "Are you really sure you want to? You might regret it later."
    4. "Let's talk about it first. Tell me what you expect."

23. Of the following conditions, the one recognized as a known teratogen is

    1. Scarlet fever.
    2. Rubella.
    3. Coronary heart disease.
    4. Dental x-rays.

24. A patient is gravida 3 para 2 and is in a labor room. After a vaginal exam, it is determined that the presenting head is at station +3. The appropriate nursing action is to

    1. Continue to observe the patient's contractions.
    2. Check the fetal heart rate for a prolapsed cord.
    3. Prepare for delivery of the baby.
    4. Check with the physician to see if an oxytocin drip is warranted.

25. Pelvic inflammatory disease (PID) is an inflammatory condition of the pelvic cavity and may involve the ovaries, tubes, vascular system, or pelvic peritoneum. The nurse explains to the patient that the most common cause of PID is

    1. Tuberculosis bacilli.
    2. *Streptococcus*.
    3. *Staphylococcus*.
    4. Gonorrhea.

26. Normal menstrual cycles and ovarian function are regulated by the hormones

    1. FSH and LH.
    2. LH and progesterone.
    3. FSH and progesterone.
    4. Estrogen and progesterone.

27. As the nurse walks into the newborn nursery, she sees a baby in respiratory distress from apparent mucus. The first nursing action is to

    1. Carefully slap the infant's back.
    2. Thump the chest and start cardiopulmonary resuscitation.
    3. Pick the baby up by the feet, keeping the head lower.
    4. Call the code team.

28. A patient, 18 weeks pregnant, is concerned because she had a fever and rash about 2½ weeks ago. The nurse's best response is

    1. "It's best to talk with the physician about that."
    2. "It's unlikely the fetus would have been affected as the first trimester is the most important time."
    3. "What do you think the problems are with that?"
    4. "Are you thinking you may have to terminate the pregnancy?"

29. A 14-year-old girl came to the clinic for a birth control method. She sat through the class that describes the methods available to her. After class, she asked the nurse, "Which method is best for me to use?" The best response is

    1. "You are so young, are you sure you are ready for the responsibilities of a sexual relationship?"
    2. "Because of your age, we need your parents' consent before you can be examined and then we'll talk."
    3. "Before I can help you with that question, I need to know more about your sexual activity."
    4. "The physician can best help you with that after your physical examination."

30. Assessing a newborn infant, the nurse knows that postmature infants may exhibit

    1. Heavy vernix, little lanugo.
    2. Large size for gestational age.
    3. Increased subcutaneous fat, absent creases on feet.
    4. Small size for gestational age.

31. A primigravida, age 36, delivered an 8-lb. 6-oz. baby girl by cesarean section. Which of the following nursing actions would *not* be included in the patient's immediate postoperative care?

    1. Taking vital signs q 15 min for 2–3 hours.
    2. Checking lochia for amount and color q 15 min for 2–3 hours.
    3. Assisting the patient to turn, cough, and deep breathe.
    4. Offering oral fluids q 15 min for 2–3 hours.

32. Counseling a patient who is starting to use oral contraception, the nurse explains that birth control pills work by the mechanism of

    1. Inhibiting chorionic gonadotropin production.
    2. Inhibiting follicle-stimulating hormone production.
    3. Inhibiting progesterone and estrogen production.
    4. Stimulating luteinizing hormone production.

33. A new mother of a 3-week-old infant comes to the clinic complaining of feeling down, sad, having no energy and wanting to cry. The priority intervention is to

    1. Notify the family that the mother needs more support.
    2. Spend extra time talking to the mother to help her express her feelings.
    3. Notify the physician for medication.
    4. Identify postpartum depression so that appropriate interventions may be made.

34. An appropriate nursing intervention to help a nursing mother care for cracked nipples would be

    1. Applying benzoin to toughen the nipples.
    2. Keeping the nipples covered with warm, moist packs.
    3. Offering to give the baby a bottle.
    4. Rub hindmilk on the nipples.

35. A patient is very concerned because her 1-day-old son, who was very alert at birth, is now sleeping most of the time. The appropriate nursing response would be

    1. "Most infants are alert at birth and then require 24 to 48 hours of deep sleep to recover from the birth experience."
    2. "Your son's behavior is slightly abnormal and bears careful observation."
    3. "Would you like the pediatrician to check him to ease your mind?"
    4. "Your son's behavior is definitely abnormal, and we should keep him in the nursery."

36. During a physical exam of an infant with congenital hip dysplasia, the nurse would observe for which of the following characteristics?

    1. Symmetrical gluteal folds.
    2. Limited adduction of the affected leg.
    3. Palpable femoral pulse when the hip is flexed and the leg is abducted.
    4. Limited abduction of the affected leg.

37. A neonatal nurse would be aware that small-for-gestational-age (SGA) infants are more likely to develop which of the following neonatal conditions?

    1. Hyperthermia.
    2. Hyperglycemia.
    3. Respiratory distress.
    4. Hypothermia.

38. If RhoGAM is given to a mother after giving birth to a healthy baby, the condition that must be present for the globulin to be effective is that the

    1. Mother is Rh positive.
    2. Baby is Rh negative.
    3. Mother has no titer in her blood.
    4. Mother has some titer in her blood.

39. A patient delivered a 34-week, 1550-g female infant. The infant demonstrates nasal flaring, intercostal retraction, expiratory grunt, and slight cyanosis. The rationale for placing the baby in a heated isolette is

    1. The infant has a small body surface for her weight.
    2. Heat increases flow of oxygen to extremities.
    3. Her temperature control mechanism is immature.
    4. Heat within the isolette facilitates drainage of mucus.

40. A 28-year-old patient has just learned that her pregnancy test is positive. The nurse will reinforce nutritional counseling by telling the patient that her diet should

    1. Maintain iron intake and increase calorie intake by 500 calories.
    2. Increase iron and folic acid and increase calorie intake by 300 calories.
    3. Increase iron and multivitamins but maintain calorie intake.
    4. Decrease iron but increase calorie intake by 200–300 calories.

41. In the delivery room, a patient has just delivered a healthy 7-pound baby boy. The physician instructs the nurse to suction the baby. The nursing intervention is to

    1. Suction the nose first.
    2. Suction the mouth first.
    3. Suction neither the nose nor mouth until the physician gives further instructions.
    4. Turn the baby on his side so mucus will drain out before suctioning.

42. The nurse is doing data collection on a postpartum patient. Suspecting infection, the nurse would assess for

    1. Dark red lochia.
    2. Bradycardia.
    3. Discomfort and tenderness of the abdomen.
    4. Generalized rash.

43. A 24-year-old patient who has just learned she is pregnant tells the nurse that she smokes one pack of cigarettes a day. In counseling, the nurse encourages her to stop smoking because newborns of mothers who smoke are often

    1. Premature and have respiratory distress syndrome.
    2. Small for gestational age.
    3. Large for gestational age.
    4. Born with congenital abnormalities.

44. A patient, 36 weeks pregnant, is having a contraction stress test (oxytocin challenge test). After 35 minutes, her uterus begins to contract, and the nurse observes three 40-second-long contractions in a 10-minute period. She has two contractions within 5 minutes, and her uterus remains contracted after the second contraction. The first nursing action is to

    1. Turn off the oxytocin.
    2. Administer oxygen by mask.
    3. Turn her on her left side.
    4. Assess the fetal heart rate.

45. Oxygen and humidity are part of the treatment for premature infants. Of the following, the statement that best describes the purpose of this treatment is that it

    1. Is necessary because premature infants have a depressed Moro reflex.
    2. Facilitates perfusion of the kidney to clear blood wastes more quickly.
    3. Helps the infant adjust better to the early transition of extrauterine life.
    4. Assists the immature respiratory system with systemic oxygenation.

46. Following a cesarean section, paralytic ileus may be a complication. According to the physician's orders, an important assessment would be to

    1. Administer PO fluids only.
    2. Insert a nasogastric tube.
    3. Listen for bowel sounds.
    4. Insert a rectal tube.

47. A patient's physician has suggested that a lecithin/sphingomyelin (L/S) ratio be done. The patient is 34 weeks pregnant. She is very nervous and asks the nurse why this test must be done. The best response is that this test

    1. Will indicate the sex of the baby.
    2. Determines the maturity of the baby's lungs.
    3. Has diagnostic capability to ascertain if anything is wrong.
    4. Detects neural tube defect.

48. A nurse working in a prenatal clinic recognizes that the physician should immediately see any patient who presents with

    1. Heartburn.
    2. Diastolic blood pressure over 85.
    3. Ankle edema.
    4. Blurred vision.

49. A nursing mother has developed mastitis and has symptoms of chills, 103°F temperature, and elevated pulse. The nurse, making a home visit, should include instructions to

    1. Leave the breast free of support or binding brassiere.
    2. Apply heat to the breast.
    3. Continue to breast-feed as necessary.
    4. Empty the breast every 4 hours regardless of infant's feeding schedule.

50. A nurse is in the situation of an emergency delivery and, as the baby's head is born, observes the cord draped around the baby's neck. The nursing action is to

    1. Wait until the placenta is delivered to prevent damage.
    2. Gently push the baby's head back in to release pressure.
    3. Cut the cord to prevent damage to the baby.
    4. Slip the cord over the baby's head to prevent circulatory impairment.

MATERNAL/NEWBORN AND GYNECOLOGICAL NURSING

Answers with Rationale

1. (2) It is very possible that the child has German measles. German measles or rubella, if contracted in the first trimester of pregnancy, may result in a child with congenital malformations of the heart, eye, and ear, as well as mental retardation.

   NP:P; CN:H; CL:C

2. (1) In DIC, the patient begins to hemorrhage after the initial hypercoagulability uses up the clotting factors in the blood. Administering heparin, therefore, is a critical nursing intervention. Heparin prevents clot formation and increases available fibrinogen, coagulation factors, and platelets. The other actions have lesser priority. Oxygen would be administered at 2–3 L/min.

   NP:I; CN:PH; CL:AN

3. (2) This elevated creatinine suggests impaired renal function. Monitoring intake and output will provide data related to renal function. The other findings would not be indicative of renal function.

   NP:D; CN:PH; CL:A

4. (3) A regular nipple is too hard and will make it difficult for the infant to suck, causing unnecessary fatigue. A preemie soft nipple should be used because it is very important that the infant receive nutrition without tiring.

   NP:P; CN:PH; CL:A

5. (1) Reactive = good outcome. Increased FHR with movement indicates normal reaction and adequate CNS integration. Ultrasound is not indicated.

   NP:D; CN:PH; CL:C

6. (4) Insulin does not cross into the milk. The mother's calorie intake needs to be adjusted with increased protein intake. Insulin must be adjusted and care must be exercised during weaning. Breast-feeding may actually have an antidiabetogenic effect and this requires less insulin.

   NP:I; CN:PH; CL:A

7. (1) Jaundice (icterus neonatorum) is a normal newborn condition that appears 48–72 hours after birth and begins to subside on the sixth to seventh day. If the levels go above 13 mg/100 mL, it is considered to be beyond the "safe" physiologic limit. The condition is caused by the breakdown of excess fetal red blood cells after birth.

   NP:P; CN:PH; CL:C

8. (3) The optimum weight gain for both mother's and baby's health is 24–25 pounds. Dieting is contraindicated. There is a lower incidence of prematurity, stillbirths, and low-birth-weight infants with a weight gain of at least 25 pounds.

   NP:I; CN:H; CL:A

9. (1) Primiparas normally go through effacement before dilation of the cervix. Multiparas tend to dilate and efface simultaneously.

   NP:P; CN:H; CL:K

10. (2) From the assessment findings of the lochia and fundus, the new mother is progressing normally during the postpartum period. The breast signs indicate normal engorgement, which occurs about 3 days after birth. With stable vital signs, infection is not likely to be a problem. Applying warm packs and wearing a nursing bra will reduce discomfort.

    NP:D; CN:H; CL:A

11. (4) An infant's normal breathing pattern is irregular. Staying with the patient helps give her support, and the nurse can reassure her that the infant is all right.

    NP:I; CN:PH; CL:A

Coding for Questions/Answers Abbreviations: **Nursing Process: NP,** Data Collection: D, Planning: P, Implementation: I, Evaluation: E, **Client Needs: CN,** Safe, Effective Care Environment: S, Health Promotion and Maintenance: H, Psychosocial Integrity: PS, Physiological Integrity: PH, **Clinical Area: CA,** Medical Nursing: M, Surgical Nursing: S, Maternal/Newborn Nursing: MA, Pediatric Nursing: P, Psychiatric Nursing: PS, **Cognitive Level: CL,** Knowledge: K, Comprehension: C, Application: A, Analysis: AN

12. (3) Amniocentesis cannot be done until adequate amniotic fluid is available, which is at about 14 weeks' gestation. It usually is done for genetic counseling purposes before 18 weeks, as the test result requires 2–4 weeks, and elective abortion after 22 weeks is contraindicated. Chorionic villus sampling (CVS) may replace this test as diagnostic information is available from 8–12 weeks.

NP:P; CN:H; CL:C

13. (2) The venereal disease syphilis is again becoming increasingly prevalent. It may cause abortion early in pregnancy and may be passed to the fetus after the fourth month of pregnancy, causing congenital syphilis in the infant. Gonorrhea and herpesvirus II may be passed to the infant during delivery, but syphilis is usually passed to the infant in utero.

NP:I; CN:H; CL:C

14. (3) Regional anesthesia, such as an epidural–spinal combined or epidural, may result in vasodilatation by causing blood to pool in the extremities. This may lead to maternal hypotension so the BP should be monitored. Immediate treatment is to elevate both legs for a few minutes in order to return the blood to the central circulation and then turn the patient on her side to reduce pressure on the veins and arteries in the pelvic area.

NP:P; CN:PH; CL:A

15. (3) High blood pressure is one of the cardinal symptoms of toxemia or eclampsia, along with excessive weight gain, edema, and albumin in the urine.

NP:D; CN:H; CL:A

16. (1) During a normal birth, the fetus passes through the birth canal, and pressure on the chest helps rid the fetus of amniotic fluid that has accumulated in the lungs. The baby delivered by cesarean section does not go through this process, and thus, may develop respiratory problems. The other conditions are not related to c-section.

NP:E; CN:H; CL:A

17. (2) In a ruptured ectopic pregnancy, there may be signs of shock, excruciating pain, and minimal bleeding. There should be no effect on blood glucose levels or blood pressure initially (1).

NP:D; CN:PH; CL:C

18. (2) A uterus that is contracted for more than 1 full minute is a sign of tetany, which could lead to uterine rupture. This symptom must be reported to the physician immediately so interventions can be initiated. The other answers are all normal conditions that occur with labor. The patient should be cautioned against bearing down this early, as it is not effective and can cause edema of the cervix.

NP:I; CN:H; CL:AN

19. (2) The respiratory rate must be maintained at a rate of at least 12 per minute as a precaution against excessive depression of impulses at the myoneural junction. When deep tendon reflexes are absent (1) and the urine output is decreased (3), the medication should be held to prevent complications of depression of the CNS. If the patient is complaining of irregular heartbeats (4), she is experiencing a sign of magnesium toxicity.

NP:E; CN:H; CL:AN

20. (1) Infants of diabetic mothers are prone to develop hypoglycemia, respiratory distress, and hypocalcemia. The infant of a diabetic mother may develop sepsis (2), but usually from a cause unrelated to the diabetes itself. Hyperbilirubinemia is also fairly common in these infants.

NP:D; CN:H; CL:A

21. (4) This is an example of a congenital abnormality and does not fall into the category of a metabolic or biochemical disorder. Phenylketonuria (1) is an inability to metabolize the amino acid phenylalanine; maple syrup urine disease (2) is defective metabolism of branched-chain keto-acids; glutamicacidemia (3) is an increase in total amino nitrogen.

NP:E; CN:H; CL:K

22. (4) The mother has a right to see her infant, but must have some anticipatory guidance. Finding out what the mother's expectations are will help the nurse better prepare the mother to see her dead child.

NP:I; CN:PS; CL:A

23. (2) *Teratogen* is a term denoting "monster-former," and rubella in the first trimester is known to produce monster babies. X-rays are also considered teratogens. Dental x-rays (4) would not have high roentgens; thus, they have little chance of being dangerous.

NP:P; CN:PH; CL:K

24. (3) If the head is +3, it is just about crowning, and because the patient is a multipara, it would be reasonable to assume delivery is imminent. Answers (1) and (4) are not appropriate nursing actions and answer (2) is wrong because there is no data suggesting a prolapsed cord.

NP:I; CN:H; CL:A

25. (4)   Gonorrhea accounts for 65–75 percent of all cases of PID. *Streptococcus* (2), *Staphylococcus* (3), and TB bacilli (1) are less frequent causes.

    NP:I; CN:H; CL:C

26. (1)   Normal menstrual cycles and ovarian function are regulated by FSH and LH, which are produced in the hypothalamus.

    NP:P; CN:H; CL:K

27. (3)   The airway must be cleared before anything else can help. Of the choices, (3) is the best for clearing the airway by creating a gravity or postural drainage situation.

    NP:I; CN:PH; CL:A

28. (3)   Although the first trimester is the danger period with German measles, the nurse should first ascertain the patient's concerns before she gives any direction. Answer (4) is putting words in the patient's mouth.

    NP:I; CN:H; CL:A

29. (3)   Consultation with a patient on the best form of birth control for her is dependent on the frequency of intercourse, number of partners, and her own motivation and reliability. The other responses cut off the patient and do not form a therapeutic relationship.

    NP:I; CN:H; CL:A

30. (4)   Babies that are postmature often look as though they have lost weight. They exhibit long nails, little subcutaneous fat, and the skin is very dry. Often, meconium is stained green or yellow.

    NP:D; CN:H; CL:C

31. (4)   Oral fluids are usually withheld after surgery until normal conscious levels are reached and bowel sounds are heard. Giving oral fluids before normal consciousness returns can lead to vomiting and aspiration. A c-section is also considered a surgical procedure, and normal postop as well as postpartum care should be given.

    NP:P; CN:H; CL:C

32. (2)   Birth control pills are small doses of estrogen and progesterone that maintain sufficient levels in the body to inhibit the pituitary from producing the follicle-stimulating hormone.

    NP:I; CN:H; CL:C

33. (4)   This answer is more comprehensive than any of the others because it includes them. It is very im-

portant to identify postpartum depression to prevent possible injury or suicide. The mother may or may not require medication, but it is necessary to intervene now. (The majority of postpartum depression conditions appear around the 4th postpartum week.)

    NP:I; CN:H; CL:AN

34. (4)   Keeping the nipples moist and soft is the best treatment. Hindmilk (released after initial letdown or release of milk) has a high fat concentration and will help to keep nipples moist. Never use harsh agents such as benzoin or alcohol. Teach the mother to use general hygiene practices—wash the breasts once daily; do not use soap as it removes natural oils. To prevent further problems with engorgement, bottles should not be offered.

    NP:P; CN:H; CL:A

35. (1)   Normally, most newborns are alert at birth and then require deep sleep to recover from the birth experience. This should be explained first, and then if the patient is still concerned, the nurse could offer to have the pediatrician talk to her.

    NP:I; CN:H; CL:A

36. (4)   Abduction is limited in the affected leg. The nurse would also find asymmetrical gluteal folds and an absent femoral pulse when the affected leg is abducted.

    NP:D; CN:H; CL:A

37. (4)   A large proportion of body surface to body weight increases susceptibility to hypothermia. These infants are also more prone to hypoglycemia. Postmature infants are most likely to develop respiratory distress.

    NP:E; CN:H; CL:K

38. (3)   RhoGAM will not work if there is any titer in the blood; thus, it is important to administer it within 72 hours after delivery or abortion if the mother shows no evidence of antibody production. The mother would be Rh negative and the baby Rh positive for RhoGAM to be needed.

    NP:D; CN:H; CL:AN

39. (3)   The premature infant has poor body control of temperature and needs immediate attention to keep from losing heat. Reasons for heat loss include little subcutaneous fat and poor insulation, large body surface for weight, immaturity of temperature control, and lack of activity.

    NP:P; CN:H; CL:C

40. (2) During pregnancy, iron supplements and folic acid must be added to the diet because studies have found that pregnant women cannot assimilate enough from their regular diet. Calories are increased by 300 to be certain that the mother-to-be and fetus have enough nutritional intake.

    NP:I; CN:H; CL:K

41. (2) It is important to suction the mouth first. If the nose were to be suctioned first, stimulation of the delicate receptors in the nose could cause the infant to aspirate mucus from the mouth.

    NP:I; CN:H; CL:A

42. (3) The major symptoms of infection would be rapid pulse, foul-smelling lochia or discharge, and discomfort and tenderness of the abdomen. A generalized rash (4) would not be a sign of postpartum infection but would indicate a viral infection, such as measles, or an allergic reaction to a medication or food. A rash should never be ignored; rather, it should be charted and its cause investigated.

    NP:D; CH:H; CL:A

43. (2) Women who smoke have almost twice the chance of delivering a low-birth-weight infant (< 2500 g) than nonsmokers.

    NP:I; CN:H; CL:K

44. (1) The first action is to turn the Pitocin off. If the fetal heart rate has dropped in response to the prolonged contraction, turning the mother on her side (3) and administering oxygen (2) may be necessary.

    NP:I; CN:H; CL:A

45. (4) The premature infant's poorly developed ability to control respirations is a frequent problem. Additional respiratory support with oxygen will decrease potential hypoxemia. The oxygen will also help oxygenate the systemic circulation if the infant has a tendency for hypoventilation.

    NP:P; CN:H; CL:C

46. (3) Following a c-section the patient will not be fed until bowel sounds are present, abdominal distention relieved, and flatus is passed. Answer (3) would be the first action, followed by (2) and (4) if necessary.

    NP:D; CN:H; CL:A

47. (2) This test examines amniotic fluid for the presence of surfactant to determine fetal lung maturity. When lecithin is two or more times greater than sphingomyelin, the infant is unlikely to develop respiratory distress syndrome. This ratio usually occurs at the 35th week of pregnancy. An amniocentesis test will determine the sex of the baby (1) and whether there is a problem (3) such as Down syndrome.

    NP:E; CN:H; CL:C

48. (4) Blurred vision is an advanced indicator of pregnancy-induced hypertension (PIH) and the physician should see the patient immediately.

    NP:P; CN:H; CL:A

49. (2) The most effective nursing action is local application of heat to the breast. Other treatment will include antibiotics and analgesics for pain. This mother needs a snug-fitting, supportive brassiere. Breast-feeding may or may not be continued; if not, the breast should be emptied every 4 hours to prevent engorgement.

    NP:I; CN:H; CL:A

50. (4) The nursing action is to gently slip the cord (which is fairly elastic) over the baby's head. The nurse would never wait until the placenta is delivered (1), as the infant could become hypoxic. The nurse could not push the baby's head back in (2). The cord should not be cut (3) at this time to prevent hypoxia.

    NP:I; CN:H; CL:A

Pediatric Nursing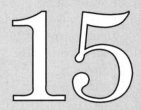

GROWTH AND DEVELOPMENT*

Maturation

A. The process of maturation.
   1. Process of attaining maximum growth and development.
   2. Process of the unfolding of inherited tendencies, independent of any special practice or training.
◆ B. Major principles of growth and development.
   ◆ 1. Occurs in an orderly sequence.
   2. Continuous, but continuity may be interrupted by spurts of growth and periods of no growth.
   ◆ 3. Progresses at individualized rates.
   4. Different ages vary for specific body structures.
   5. Each individual has an inherent growth pattern.
   6. Increases in structure (growth) are accompanied by increases in function (development).
C. Major influences on growth and development.
   1. Genetic factors.
   2. Environmental variations.

Profiles of Growth and Development

A. Physical development.
   1. Growth rate.
      a. Rapid during infancy.
      b. Slow and steady during childhood.
      c. Spurt during puberty.
      d. Decreases: maximum height attained during adolescence.
   ◆ 2. Height.
      a. Average length is 20 inches at birth.
      b. Increases 10 inches in the first year.
      c. Increases 5 inches in the second year.
      d. Increases 3 inches per year from the third to the sixth year.
      e. Increases by about 2 inches per year after sixth year.
      f. Peak reached by boys at about 14 years of age.
      g. Peak reached by girls at about 13 years of age.
   ◆ 3. Weight.
      a. Average weight is 7½ pounds at birth.
      b. Doubles by the end of the fifth month, and triples by the end of first year.
      c. Increases by about 5 pounds per year until puberty, and then increases rapidly.
      d. Levels off with only little gain after puberty.
   4. Body proportions.
      a. Striking changes from birth to maturity.

      b. At birth, head is one-fourth of the total body length; the adult head is only about one-eighth of the total body length.
   ◆ 5. Bone formation.
      a. What will later be bone begins as connective tissue, which gradually becomes cartilage, and finally, through the process of ossification, becomes bone.
      b. Bone formation complete in girls at about 17 years of age.
      c. Bone formation is complete in boys at about 19 years of age.
   6. Teeth formation.
      a. First two lower central incisors appear between the fifth and seventh month followed by about one new tooth per month.
      b. The set of 20 deciduous teeth should be complete by the age of 2½ years. (For chart of Dental Development, *see* Appendix 15-9.)
◆ B. Motor development.
   1. Includes learning, controlling, and integrating muscular responses.
   2. Occurs in an orderly sequence, and is related to the maturation of the nervous system.
   3. Begins at the head, moves downward, and proceeds from the center of the body toward the extremities.
   4. Effective use of the hands for seizing and grasping objects (prehension) begins between the second and third month.
   5. Ability to walk alone (locomotion) is attained gradually and begins with holding up the head; most infants have learned to walk alone between the ages of 12 and 14 months.
◆ C. Intellectual development.
   1. Intelligence is the ability to think, to reason, to remember, and to imagine.
   2. Intelligence develops gradually and continuously.
D. Emotional development.
   1. Emotions begin to develop early.
   2. Few individuals react to the same emotion in the same way.
   3. Emotions of fear, excitement, anger, and joy are recognizable at 1 year of age.
   4. Emotions are expressed by facial expressions, vocalization, and body movements.

HOSPITALIZATION

Stages of Separation Anxiety

◆ A. Protest.
   1. Characteristics: cries loudly, throws tantrums.
   2. Nursing behaviors: stay close to the child to provide warmth and support.

* For Growth and Development Milestones by age group, *see* Chapter 3.

✦ B.   Despair.
1.   Characteristics: withdraws, shows no interest in eating, playing or interacting; typical during extended hospitalization.
2.   Nursing behaviors: recognize the anxiety and establish a relationship with the child; attempt to engage and involve the child in an activity.

✦ C.   Denial.
1.   Characteristics: exhibits behavior that is often mistaken for happy adjustment; ignores mother and may regress.
2.   Nursing behaviors: reassure the mother, develop a relationship with the child, and provide warmth and support to the child during long hospitalization.

Hospitalization of the Infant

✦ **Psychological Implications**
A.   Separation from the parent is threatening.
B.   Decrease in sensory stimuli.
C.   Causes of breakdown in mother–infant relationship.
1.   Maternal guilt.
2.   Hostile, cold hospital environment.
3.   Lessened opportunity for mothering role; mother may feel inadequate.
4.   Subordination of the parents by the staff.

Implementation
A.   Take positive nursing action to prevent the detrimental effects of hospitalization.
B.   Provide a prehospitalization nursing interview with the parents and give a tour of the pediatric unit.
1.   Explain procedures, regulations, and the rationale behind the rules; arrange for parents to meet the staff.
2.   Encourage parents to visit frequently and/or to possibly room in.
C.   Counsel the parents regarding the infant's illness.
1.   Elicit their understanding of the disease as well as its likely progressive course.
2.   Correct any misconceptions and, if appropriate, reassure them that they are not the cause of the illness.
✦ D.   Encourage the parents to participate in the infant's care if they show an interest in doing so.
1.   Teach the parents procedures they are capable of doing.
2.   Show respect for superior knowledge of their infant in respect to likes, dislikes, and habits.
✦ E.   Assume role of the absent mother.
1.   Limit, initially, the number of people handling the infant; allow one person to become familiar with the infant and gradually introduce others.

2.   Provide closeness and warmth by cuddling.
3.   Avoid isolating the infant from sensory stimulation.
a.   Provide stimulation during feeding.
b.   Hang brightly colored mobiles within the infant's sight.
4.   Play with the infant.

Hospitalization of the Toddler and Preschool Child

Psychological Implications
A.   Hospitalization is a very threatening experience for a child.
1.   Unfamiliar situations and procedures are experienced.
2.   Growing sense of identity and independence may be disrupted.
✦ B.   Experiences separation anxiety; child mourns the absence of the mother through protest, despair and denial.
✦ C.   The loss of "body integrity" is feared.
1.   Does not realistically perceive how the body functions.
2.   May overreact to a simple procedure; some toddlers believe that drawing blood will leave a hole and that the rest of their blood will leak out.
✦ D.   Disruption of normal rituals and routines are resented; toddlers are often very rigid about those procedures that allow them a sense of security and control over otherwise frightening circumstances.
E.   Loss of mobility is frustrating to a child.
F.   Most recent acquired behaviors are frequently abandoned, and toddler reverts to safer, less mature patterns (regression).

Implementation
A.   Introduce the child to hospital surroundings, preferably prior to hospitalization.
B.   Explain all the procedures in simple terms and allow for further discussion, if desired.
C.   Encourage parents to room in or to visit frequently once the child is hospitalized.
✦ D.   Suggest that the mother leave an object that the child associates with her for the child to "care for" until she can return. This procedure assures the child that his mother will return.
✦ E.   Encourage the parents to be honest about when they are going and coming. Do not tell the child they will stay all night and then leave when the child is asleep.
F.   Paste family pictures to the crib.
✦ G.   Use puppet play to explain procedures and to gain an understanding of the child's perception of his hospitalization. Use puppets to work out anxiety, anger, and frustration.

✦ H. When recording developmental history elicit exact routines and rituals that the child uses; attempt to modify hospital routine to continue these rituals.

I. Provide stretchers, wheelchairs, and carts for immobilized children.

J. Do not punish the child for reverting to less mature behavior patterns; explain the reasons for its occurrence to the parents.

Hospitalization of the School-Age Child

Psychological Implications

✦ A. School-age child needs to understand why things are happening as they are.

✦ B. Child has heightened concern for privacy and needs to protect body image.

C. Child is modest and fears disgrace.

D. Hospitalization interrupts busy school life, and child fears he or she will be replaced or forgotten by peer group.

E. Absence from peer group means a disruption of close friendships.

Implementation

A. Inform the child about his or her illness; take the opportunity to explain how the body functions.

B. Explain all procedures completely; allow the child to see special rooms (i.e., intensive care, cardiac catheter lab) prior to being sent to them for treatments.

C. Provide opportunities for the child to socialize with his or her peer group at meals and through team tournaments of cards, chess, and checkers.

D. Allow telephone privileges for calls to his or her home and friends.

E. Provide outlets (e.g., dart board and a boxing bag) for anger and frustration.

F. Give the child opportunity to make choices and exert independence.

G. Protect the child's privacy.

H. Provide tutors to prevent disruption of education.

I. Provide the opportunity to master developmental tasks of age group.

Hospitalization of the Adolescent

Psychological Implications

✦ A. Concern with disruption of social system and peer group.

✦ B. Fear of alteration of body image.

✦ C. Fear of loss of independence.

D. Fear of change in future plans.

E. Concern with interruption in development of heterosexual relationships.

F. Resentment of loss of privacy.

G. The degree to which the young adult is affected depends on several factors.

1. Whether the illness is chronic or acute.

2. Whether the final prognosis necessitates a change in the young adult's future aspirations.

3. The number of changes that he or she must accept.

Implementation

✦ A. Adolescents should be placed in rooms with their peers.

B. Allow telephone privileges with some limitations of time.

✦ C. Enhance the adolescent's feeling of self-worth, and encourage as much independence as possible.

D. Allow reasonable heterosexual relationships to develop.

E. Provide for privacy.

F. Assist adolescent in role model identification.

G. Realistically discuss problems of the illness with the adolescent.

H. Always provide honest information.

I. Encourage the adolescent, if able, to accept reasonable responsibility for unit decorum.

General Assessment—Infant to Adolescent

General Principles

A. Maturational ability of the child to cooperate with the examiner is of major importance to adequate physical assessment.

✦ B. When planning physical assessment of the child, the following points should be considered.

1. Establish a relationship with the child prior to the examination.
    a. Determine child's maturational level.
    b. Allow the child an opportunity to become more accustomed to the examiner.

2. Explain in terms appropriate to the child's level of understanding the extent and purpose of the examination.

3. Realize that the physical examination may be a stressful experience for the child, who is helpless and depends on others for protection.

4. Limit the physical examination to what is essential in determining an adequate nursing diagnosis.

5. Proceed from the least to the most intrusive procedures.

6. Allow active participation of the child whenever possible.

7. Consider cultural influences and practices—incorporate appropriately into exam.

The Infant

A. Accomplish as much of the examination as possible while the infant is sleeping or resting undisturbed.

B. Assess general condition.

1. Symmetry and location of body parts.

2. Color and condition of the skin.
3. State of restlessness and sleeplessness.
4. Adjustment to feeding regimen.
5. Quality of cry.

✦ C. Congenital anomaly appraisal.
 1. Neurological system.
    a. Reflexes: absent or asymmetrical (*see* Appendix 15-2).
    b. Head circumference: microcephaly, hydrocephaly.
       (1) Average newborn 33–35.5 cm at birth.
       (2) 40 cm at 3 months.
       (3) 45 cm at 9 months.
       (4) At birth, the head size is 2 cm larger than the chest. Equals or exceeds chest size until 2 years of age.
    c. Fontanelles: closed, bulging.
       (1) Anterior measures 3.5 cm by 3.5 cm and closes by 18 months.
       (2) Posterior measures 1 cm by 1 cm and closes at 6–8 weeks.
    d. Eyes: cataracts, lid folds, spots on iris.
 2. Respiratory system.
    a. Breath sounds: signs of aspiration, asymmetry of lung expansion, retractions, grunting.
    b. Apnea.
 3. Cardiovascular system.
    a. Color: cyanosis.
    b. Rate and rhythm: murmurs, tachycardia, bradycardia.
    c. Energy level: cannot suck for 15 minutes without exhaustion or cyanosis.
 4. Gastrointestinal tract.
    a. History of polyhydramnios.
    b. Patency: mucus, spitting, cyanosis, cannot pass nasogastric tube to stomach.
    c. Mouth: palate or lip not intact.
    d. Anus: not patent.
 5. Genitourinary.
    a. Umbilical vessels: missing normal two arteries and one vein.
    b. Urine: abnormal stream.
    c. Masses: abdominal (Wilms' tumor).
    d. Boys: undescended testicles, hernia, urethra not opening at the end of the penis.
    e. Girls: labial adhesions.
 6. Skeletal system.
    a. Fractured clavicle.
    b. Dislocated hip: asymmetric major gluteal folds, hip click.
    c. Legs and feet: clubbing, without straight tibial line.
    d. Spine: curved, inflexible, open.

✦ D. Common problems.
 1. Ear infections.
    a. Increased temperature, irritability.
    b. Rubbing or pulling ear.
    c. Change in eating habits.
 2. Upper respiratory infections.
    a. Duration of symptoms, severity.
    b. Wheezing, barking cough, anxiety, restlessness, use of accessory muscles.
    c. If throat is sore, check white patches on tonsils.
 3. Rashes.
    a. Onset, duration, description, location.
    b. Any event such as new food, exposure to animals.
 4. Contact dermatitis.
    a. Allergic problems.
    b. Diaper area rash: use of soap, lotions, powders; method of cleaning cloth diapers.
 5. Hernias.
    a. Inguinal: lump in groin, with or without pain.
    b. Umbilical: can it be pushed back without difficulty or pain.
 6. Scalp—cradle cap.
    a. Scalp scaling, crusted; method of washing hair.
    b. Application of any lotions or balms to hair.
 7. Birthmarks.
    a. Change in size, color, shape.
    b. Any bleeding or irritation.
 8. Eye symmetry.
    a. Frequency of a problem with eye alignment (time of day eyes wander).
    b. Light reflex symmetrical in both eyes.

E. Screening procedures.
 1. Developmental landmarks—DDST (Denver Developmental Screening Test).
 2. Vision.
 3. Hearing.
 4. Growth charts: head circumference, weight, length.

F. Nursing guidance areas.
 1. Growth and development changes.
 2. Stranger anxiety.
 3. Separation anxiety.
 4. Transitional objects.
 5. Accident prevention.

Toddler and the Preschool Child

A. General considerations.
✦ 1. Remember that separation anxiety is most acute at toddler age and body integrity fears most acute at preschool age.
 2. Involve the parent in examination as much as possible.
 3. Restrain child as much as necessary to protect the child from injury.

a. Car seat restraints must be in rear seats only (if car has airbags).

b. Restraints in car seats must have upper anchorage devices and locking clips or Universal Child Safety Seat System (UCSSS).

4. Give careful explanation of each portion of the exam.

5. Allow the child to handle the equipment and try out on doll.

✦ B. Common problems.

1. Feeding and eating.

a. Review food ingested in last 48 hours.

b. Types of foods, adequate source of vitamins, minerals.

2. Temper tantrums.

a. Frequency, duration, precipitating event.

b. Response of caretaker.

3. Toilet training.

a. Check ability to ambulate (indicating neuromuscular maturity).

b. Bothered by wet diapers. Interested in toileting.

4. Respiratory infections: *see* Infant section.

5. Communicable diseases.

a. Onset of symptoms, progression of disease, treatment of symptoms.

b. Observation of complications.

6. Gastrointestinal.

a. Onset, duration, intake and output.

b. Signs of dehydration.

C. Screening procedures (same as Infant).

School-Age Child

A. General considerations.

1. Modesty important.

2. Explain all procedures.

3. Direct questions to child.

✦ B. Common problems.

1. School.

a. Signs of school phobias, vomits before school, delays going.

b. Increase in physical complaints.

2. Nervous habits (stuttering, twitching, etc.).

a. Onset, duration, precipitating event.

b. Anxiety of child and parent over problem.

3. Injury prevention.

a. Booster seat in car until child is 60 lb. or 8 years old (dictated by individual state laws).

b. Ride in back seat only until 12 years old.

c. Seat belts.

d. Bicycle/skateboard safety (local/state helmet laws); water safety (swimming lessons).

4. Safety rules in home: ensure guns are locked and unloaded; ensure child has supervision before and after school; teach a family "password" to protect from strangers.

5. Accidental trauma.

a. Understanding of accident.

b. Prevention, physical limitations/sports.

6. Respiratory infections: *See* Infant section.

7. Gastrointestinal infections: *See* Preschooler section.

C. Screening procedures.

1. Snellen vision testing.

2. Sweep check audiometry.

3. Height and weight measurement. Monitor for obesity.

4. Inspection of skin and teeth.

D. Nursing guidance areas.

1. Need for autonomy.

2. Toilet training.

3. Imaginary friends.

4. Fear of dark.

5. Rituals and routines.

6. Encourage regular activity/exercise.

Adolescent

A. General considerations.

1. Examine child alone if he wishes (privacy important).

2. Note signs of puberty.

3. Ascertain feelings about body image.

✦ B. Common problems.

1. Acne.

a. Existing skin care program.

b. Personal hygiene.

2. Dysmenorrhea.

a. Degree of pain, missed school.

b. Use of analgesics.

c. Amount of exercise.

3. Obesity.

a. Eating patterns.

b. Family concern.

c. Amount of exercise.

C. Screening procedures (same as School Age).

D. Nursing guidance areas.

1. Hazards of cigarette smoking and alcohol.

2. Transmission and symptoms of venereal disease.

3. Review sex education.

4. Accident prevention—particularly automobile.

5. Principles of nutrition.

PEDIATRIC DIAGNOSTIC PROCEDURES

Neurological Diagnostic Procedures

Lumbar Puncture

A. Withdrawal of cerebral spinal fluid by insertion of a hollow needle between lumbar vertebrae

(L_3 and L_4 or L_4 and L_5) into subarachnoid space to identify intracranial pressure, signs of infection, or hemorrhage.

B. Nursing responsibilities prior to procedure.
    1. Maintain base line record of vital signs.
    2. Explain to the parents and child exactly what will happen.
C. Nursing responsibilities during procedure.
    1. Place child on side in knee–chest position with head flexed on chest.
    2. Help child remain steady in this position and reassure child throughout procedure.
D. Nursing responsibilities following procedure.
    1. Keep child flat in bed.
    2. Encourage fluid intake.
    3. If headache occurs when sitting up, return child to flat position and give analgesic.
    4. Observe neurological status for signs of deterioration.

✦ **CT (Computed Tomography) Scan**

A. Provides visualization of neuroanatomy; differentiates tissue density compared to water.
B. Visualizes brain along vertical or horizontal plane from any axis.
C. Can distinguish hemorrhage, tumors, congenital abnormalities, and inflammatory or hypoxic processes.
D. May use contrast medium for enhanced views.
E. Nursing considerations.
    1. Patient/family education about what to expect. Machine may provoke claustrophobia.
    2. Patient required to lie still during procedure. May require restraints or sedation.
    3. Assess carefully for allergy of anaphylaxis to contrast (iodine based). Observe IV site carefully to avoid extravasation.

✦ **MRI (Magnetic Resonance Imaging)**

A. Allows high-quality imaging of morphology of structures.
B. Distinguishes structures by response to radio frequency pulses in a magnetic field.
C. Tissue differentiation superior to other techniques.
D. Requires immobilization throughout procedure (sedation and respiratory monitoring *required* for young patients).
E. Nursing considerations.
    1. Education of patient/family about procedure and what to expect. Reassure older children.
    2. Reinforce medical information as needed.
    3. Follow sedation protocol.
    4. Careful monitoring of vital signs, SaO_2, and respiratory status during procedure.
    5. Observe carefully for reaction to contrast medium.

Electroencephalogram (EEG)

A. Provides information about electrical activity of cerebral cortex.
B. Used to assess neuronal functioning and to diagnose seizure activity; shows characteristic abnormalities for seizures.
C. Also may be used in part to determine brain death.
D. May be combined with simultaneous video recording.
✦ E. Nursing responsibilities.
    1. Explain procedure and sensations to expect.
    2. Activities during procedure may include hyperventilation, sleep deprivation, and anti-seizure drug withdrawal.
    3. Shampoo head afterward to remove all glue and gel.
    4. Clarify any misconceptions (patient does not receive shocks via leads, etc.).

Electromyelogram

A. Visualization of the spinal subarachnoid space to define it and to evaluate lesions involving neural elements.
B. Nursing responsibilities prior to procedure.
    1. Ensure child is NPO 6–8 hours before procedure.
    2. Maintain baseline record of vital signs and neurological status.
    3. Administer sedative as ordered.
C. Nursing responsibilities following procedure.
    1. Frequently observe neurological signs and vital signs and compare to baseline.
    2. Ensure adequate hydration—check for adequate voiding.
    3. Keep flat for 24 hours and promote rest.
    4. Watch for signs of infection.
    5. Slightly elevate head (30 degrees) for 8 hours if some contrast media is retained.

✦ **Angiogram**

A. Radiopaque substance is injected into cerebral vasculature or its extracranial sources to evaluate vascular anomalies, lesions, or tumors.
B. Nursing responsibilities prior to procedure.
    1. Prep area where cannulization is to be made (usually femoral or brachial).
    2. Ensure child has no solid food for 6–8 hours prior to procedure.
    3. Keep baseline record of neurological and vital signs.
    4. Frequently a sedative is administered to relax child.
C. Nursing responsibilities following procedure.
    1. Observe for changes in level of consciousness, transient hemiplegia, seizures, sensory or

motor deterioration, or elevation of blood pressure with widening pulse pressure.

2. Encourage fluid intake.
3. Check extremity for adequate peripheral pulses, color, temperature.

Cardiovascular Diagnostic Procedures

✦ Cardiac Catheterization

A. A procedure in which a catheter is passed into the heart and its major vessels for examination of blood flow, pressures in all chambers and vessels, and oxygen content and saturation. The catheter may be passed through the arterial system into the left side of the heart or through the venous system into the right side of the heart.

B. Nursing responsibilities before procedure.
1. Prepare patient and/or parents and child for procedure by showing equipment, procedures, table.
2. Establish vital sign base line.
3. Promote good physical condition prior to test.

C. Nursing responsibilities during procedure.
1. Carefully observe vital signs.
2. Observe for cyanosis or pallor, bradycardia, and apnea.
3. Assist in restraining and comforting the child.
4. Follow sedation protocol.

D. Nursing responsibilities following procedure.
1. Check for peripheral pulses, distal to the site in the extremity used for catheter.
2. Take and record vital signs every 15 minutes; observe for subnormal temperature.
3. Observe for thrombosis: warmth of extremities, weak arterial pulses, cyanosis, blanching of extremity, skin color.
4. Check for progressive return to normal.
5. Observe for hypotension (internal bleeding) and signs of infection.
6. Check incision site for bleeding or hematoma; maintain pressure dressing as ordered.
7. Observe for reactions to dye used in procedure.

✦ Echocardiography

A. A noninvasive cardiac procedure that records high frequency sound vibrations and reflects mechanical cardiac activity.

B. Usually used to diagnose valvular and other structural anomalies, thickness of septum and ventricular walls.

C. Nursing responsibilities.
1. Before procedure, assure child that procedure is painless, and prepare child for procedure to help ensure cooperation.
2. After procedure, provide general reassurance (no specific care is indicated).

✦ Electrocardiography

A. 12-lead ECG used to diagnose arrhythmias (as in adults).

B. May need to time test with nap for small children unable to stay still.

Gastrointestinal Diagnostic Procedures

For additional GI tests, *see* Chapter 7.

✦ Barium Enema

A. A procedure in which a barium mixture is placed in the large intestine via a rectal catheter for x-ray visualization of the entire large intestine.

B. Nursing responsibilities prior to procedure.
1. Cleanse the bowel through enemas.
2. Restrict diet (clear fluids for 24 hours).

C. Nursing responsibilities following procedure.
1. Avoid impaction from barium.
   a. Provide child with large fluid intake.
   b. Administer laxative or cleansing enemas.
2. Advise parents and child that stools will be white for 24–72 hours following procedure.

Renal Diagnostic Procedures

Evaluation of Blood

A. CBC with differential.
B. Blood Urea Nitrogen (BUN).
C. Creatinine.
D. Uric acid.

Evaluation of Urine

A. pH.
B. Protein.
C. Specific gravity.
D. Presence of glucose and ketones.

✦ Cystoscopy

A. Direct visualization of bladder and urethra done under general anesthesia.

B. Nursing responsibilities.
1. Prior to procedure—NPO 6–8 hours.
2. Following procedure—check I&O, observe for urinary retention and hematuria.

✦ Intravenous Pyelogram (IVP)

A. A radiographic study of kidneys, bladder, and other structures via contrast media injection.

B. Nursing responsibilities.
1. Prior to IVP—NPO 6–8 hours; bowel cleaned with cathartic; have child void.
2. Following procedure—evaluate for dye reaction; assess child's alertness and gag reflex; check for signs of perforation (intense pain in stomach).

Additional Procedures

A. Renal/Bladder Ultrasound.
B. Urodynamic evaluation.

C. CT/MRI.

D. Renal biopsy.

NEUROLOGICAL SYSTEM

Traumatic Brain Injury

Definition: Any trauma to the scalp, skull, meninges, or brain caused by mechanical force or penetration.

Characteristics

✦ A. Types of injuries.
   1. Most injuries are caused by physical forces that impact on the head through acceleration and deceleration.
   2. Concussion is most common—violent jarring of the brain within the skull.
   3. Contusion and laceration.
   4. Closed or open head injuries.

✦ B. Complications.
   1. Epidural hemorrhage—bleeding usually arterial and brain compression develops quickly.
   2. Subdural hemorrhage—bleeding between dura and cerebrum. Bleeding usually venous and develops gradually—more common than epidurals.

Assessment

✦ A. Assess level of consciousness—changes appear earlier than in vital signs.

✦ B. Observe for pupillary changes—pupil dilates on ipsilateral side of injury.

C. Nausea and vomiting.

D. Changes in vital signs reflecting increased intracranial pressure.

E. Seizure activity, nuchal rigidity.

F. Observe any unusual behavior in children—fussiness, restlessness, irritability.

✦ Implementation

A. Continually check for signs of increasing intracranial pressure: level of consciousness, vital signs, restless, irritable behavior.

B. Maintain adequate respiratory exchange—increased CO_2 levels increase cerebral edema.

C. Protect from injury—bedrest and siderails up and padded.

D. Position head to promote fluid drainage—elevated 15–30 degrees.

E. Prevent infection if drainage from ear or nose—maintain strict asepsis.

F. Provide adequate nutrition (clear liquids) and hydration (measure I&O and monitor IV, if in place).

Hydrocephalus

✦ *Definition:*   Abnormal accumulation of spinal fluid within the brain causing an increase in intracranial pressure. Accumulation may be due either to blockage of the flow of spinal fluid or to the lack of proper absorption of the spinal fluid. May occur as congenital defect or as a result of trauma, infection, or surgery.

Assessment

A. Gradual increase in size and shape of head.

B. Suture lines separated with bulging fontanelles.

C. Dilated scalp veins.

D. Strabismus and nystagmus.

E. "Sunset" eyes (sclera visible above the iris).

F. Projectile vomiting and anorexia.

G. Irritability, lethargy, and high-pitched cry.

H. Poor neck control.

Treatment and Implementation

✦ A. Preoperative care.
   1. Feed small amounts with care to prevent vomiting.
   2. Change position frequently to prevent pneumonia and pressure sores on the head.
   3. Support the infant's head when turning or moving.
   4. Prevent infection.
   5. Carefully observe vital signs.
   6. Observe for signs of increased intracranial pressure.
   7. Provide emotional support for both parents and infant.

✦ B. Surgical procedure: ventriculovenous shunt performed to reduce the volume of spinal fluid within the ventricles.

✦ C. Postoperative care.
   1. Maintain open airway.
   2. Carefully observe vital signs.
   3. Measure head circumference and look for signs of increased intracranial pressure indicating shunt malfunction.
   4. Give nothing by mouth for 4–6 hours after surgery.
   5. Carefully begin to feed clear fluids.
   6. Meet the needs of the normal newborn.
   7. Position the head opposite the side of the shunt; protect operative site.
   8. Support the head when turning or changing the position. Use gel form or protective device.
   9. Observe for infection—increased temperature, pulse, and irritability.
   10. Administer antibiotics as ordered.
   11. Give emotional support to infant and parents.

Neural Tube Defects (NTD)

Definition: Defect in the spinal column caused either by failure of the posterior part of the laminae of the vertebrae to fuse or by absence of part of the laminae.

The defect usually occurs in the lumbosacral area, but it may occur at any level of the spine.

✦ **Types of Spina Bifida**

A. *Spina bifida occulta:* Bony defect in the spine that may have a visible dimple or a small tuft of hair in the area; usually not visible externally. Generally requires no treatment.

B. *Meningocele:* Protrusion of meninges and cerebrospinal fluid through the opening in the spine, which may be covered only by a thin membranous sac. Usually causes no paralysis; treatment involves closure of sac.

C. *Myelomeningocele:* Protrusion of meninges, cerebrospinal fluid, spinal cord, and nerves through the defect in the spine; there may be paralysis below the level of the defect.

Assessment

A. May be detected prenatally by elevated concentrations of alphafeto proteins and prenatal ultrasonography.

B. Presence of hydrocephalus a frequent complication.

C. Neurological involvement.

D. Urological involvement.
   1. Frequent bladder infections.
   2. Potential for progressive renal damage.

E. Orthopedic involvement.

F. Bowel function.

G. Special considerations.
   1. Children with NTDs are especially prone to developing latex allergies. Exposure to latex should be limited or avoided in infants and throughout all treatment.
   2. Use of folic acid supplements in pregnancy has shown to decrease incidence of NTDs.

Treatment and Implementation

✦ A. Preoperative care.
   1. Prevent infection.
   2. Observe movement of the extremities.
   3. Observe bowel and bladder function.
   4. Provide normal newborn care.

✦ B. Surgical procedure.
   1. Ileal conduit surgery is frequently required.
   2. Removal of the protrusion.
   3. Closure of the defect.

C. Postoperative care.
   1. Observe for signs of CNS infection (meningitis).
      a. Increased temperature.
      b. Foul smelling urine; cloudy urine.
   2. Credé method of managing urinary retention involves systematic "milking" of the bladder at periodic intervals. May need to teach parents procedure.
   3. Provide range-of-motion exercises to lower extremities.
      a. Prevent contractures.
      b. Use foot brace to prevent footdrop.
   4. Provide good skin care.
   5. Give emotional support to infant and parents.

Seizure Disorders

Definition: A series of seizures that result from focal or diffuse paroxysmal discharges in cortical neurons—symptoms of abnormal brain function. May be congenital or acquired.

Etiology

A. Seizure disorders are idiopathic—cause unknown or acquired—result of brain injury caused by trauma, hypoxia, infection, toxins, or other acquired factors.

B. Seizures more common during first 2 years than any other period.

C. Most common cause by age group.
   1. Young infants—birth injury, hemorrhage, anoxia, and congenital defects of the brain.
   2. Late infancy and early childhood—infections frequent cause; infrequent in middle childhood.
   3. Children older than 3 years—idiopathic epilepsy most common.

Assessment

✦ A. Simple partial seizure.
   1. Localized (confined to a specific area) motor symptoms, accompanied by autonomic or somatosensory symptoms.
   2. Manifestations.
      a. Aversive seizure—most common motor seizure in children. Eye(s) turn away from focus side.
      b. Sylvan seizures—most common during sleep. Tonic–clonic movements involving face.
      c. Jacksonian march—rare in children. Sequential clonic movements.
   3. Complex partial (psychomotor) seizure.
      a. Area of brain most involved is temporal lobe (thus, this type of seizure is called psychomotor).
      b. Most common in children from 3 years to adolescence.
      c. Characterized by complex sensory phenomena, a period of altered behavior and amnesia (child is not aware of behavior).
      d. May perform such mannerisms as lip smacking, chewing, picking at clothes, etc.
      e. May appear dazed, but loses consciousness for only a few seconds.

◆B. Generalized seizures.
  ◆ 1.   Tonic–clonic seizures, traditionally known as "grand mal."
      a. May begin with an aura, then a tonic phase (lasting 10–20 seconds)—stiffening or rigidity of muscles, particularly arms and legs; eyes roll up; followed by loss of consciousness; may be apneic and become cyanotic.
      b. Clonic phase follows (lasts about 30 seconds, but may last as long as 30 minutes)—hyperventilation with rhythmic, violent jerking of all extremities; may foam at the mouth and become incontinent; full recovery may take several hours.
      c. Status epilepticus—a series of seizures that run together and do not allow the child to regain consciousness between attacks.
         (1) A neurological emergency with generalized tonic–clonic seizures.
         (2) State can lead to exhaustion, respiratory failure, and death.
         (3) Usually treated with IV diazepam or Lorazepam. Respiratory monitoring is *essential* after administration of benzodiazepines.
  ◆ 2.   Absence seizures, formerly "petit mal."
      a. Brief duration, often just 5–10 seconds; brief loss of consciousness; almost no change in muscle tone.
      b. May occur 20–30 times/day.
      c. Common in children; may appear to be "daydreaming," or inattentive.
    3. Myoclonic seizure.
      a. Characterized by a brief, generalized jerking or stiffening of the extremities.
      b. Seizure may throw person to the floor; no loss of consciousness.
    4. Atonic or akinetic seizures, also called "drop attacks."
      a. Onset between 2 and 5 years of age.
      b. Characterized by sudden, brief loss of muscle tone.
      c. Person may fall to ground, momentary loss of consciousness.
    5. Infantile spasms.
      a. Most common in first 6–8 months of age; more common in males; usually low intelligence later in life.
      b. Characterized by sudden, brief, symmetrical contractions; head flexed, legs drawn up, arms extended.
      c. May experience numerous attacks during the day without postictal drowsiness.

Implementation

◆ A. Prevent injury during seizure.
    1. Remove any objects that may cause harm.
    2. Remain with child during seizure and provide privacy if possible.
    3. Do not force jaws open during seizure.
    4. Tongue depressor used only with physician's orders and only prior to seizure beginning.
    5. Do not restrict limbs or restrain.
    6. Loosen restrictive clothing.
    7. Check that airway is open. Do not initiate artificial ventilation during a tonic–clonic seizure.
    8. Following seizure, turn head to side to prevent aspiration and allow secretions to drain.
  B. Observe and document seizure pattern.
    1. Note time, level of consciousness, and presence of aura before seizure.
    2. Record type, character, progression of movements.
    3. Note duration of seizure and child's condition throughout.
    4. Observe and record postictal state.
  C. Administer and monitor medications—complete control achieved in 50–70 percent of epileptic children.
  ◆ 1. Drugs prescribed for partial or generalized seizures—carbamazepine (Tegretol), phenytoin (Dilantin), and valproic acid.
    2. Drug of choice for absence seizures is ethosuximide (Zarontin).
    3. Administer dose accurately.
    4. Keep medication out of reach of children.
◆ D. Observe for drug side effects.
    1. Dilantin can cause hypertrophy of gums and stomatitis.
    2. Zarontin can provoke blood dyscrasia.
    3. Observe for signs of toxicity.
◆ E. Administer postseizure procedures—will influence speed of recovery.
    1. Reduce stimuli—noise, lights, conversation.
      a. Place sources of light behind child.
      b. Keep away from fluorescent lights.
    2. Remain with child after consciousness returns.
      a. Speak and move slowly.
      b. Use simple phrases—give child time to respond.
    3. Encourage rest following a seizure (child will be exhausted) and maintain privacy.
◆ F. Provide seizure precautions in the hospital.
    1. Keep bed rails raised and padded.
    2. Have suction and oxygen available.
  G. Emotional factors.
    1. Assist family to understand the disease.

2. Explain how to help child have as normal a life as possible.
3. Prevent overprotection.

Cerebral Palsy

Definition: Nonprogressive paralysis resulting from either developmental brain defects, birth trauma, or anoxia to the brain. Premature birth appears to be the most important determinant.

Assessment

✦ A. Poor motor development; slow at walking and in other movements.
B. Involuntary movements of extremities and head.
C. Weakness of the extremities.
✦ D. Spasticity of the extremities.
   1. Voluntary muscles lose normal smooth movements.
   2. Increased deep tendon reflexes and contractures of antigravity muscles.
E. One or all of the extremities may be involved.
F. Seizures may occur.
G. Vision disturbance (20 percent).

Implementation

A. Care should be individualized to the needs of the specific child.
B. Prevention of contractures of the joints.
C. Good nutrition.
D. Good dental care.
E. Encourage activities of daily living.
F. Encourage normal growth and development.

Poliomyelitis

✦ *Definition:*   An acute viral infection that affects the spinal cord and brain stem; may lead to paralysis or death. Polio is no longer a threat in the western hemisphere.

Characteristics

A. A contagious disease caused by three viruses—types 1, 2, and 3.
B. Incubation period is usually 7–14 days with range of 5–35 days.
C. Communicable—throat holds virus for about 1 week, feces 4–6 weeks.
✦ D. Manifests in three forms—abortive, nonparalytic (most common), and paralytic.

Assessment

✦ A. Assess symptoms of different types.
   1. Abortive—fever, sore throat, headache, anorexia, vomiting, abdominal pain. May last few hours to days.
   2. Nonparalytic—same as above but more severe with stiff neck, back, and legs.

   3. Paralytic (spinal and bulbar types)—similar course as nonparalytic; apparent recovery followed by paralysis.
✦ B. Assess if polio vaccine (OPV) was given and if full course was received.

Implementation

A. Preventive—education of public to fully immunize children with IPV series. (*See* Appendix 15-3.)
B. Maintain complete bedrest during acute period of infection.
C. Provide respiratory support (mechanical ventilation) if respiratory paralysis occurs.
D. Assist with physiotherapy (most important factor in recovery) following acute stage.
E. Evaluate for potential complications.

Meningitis

Definition: An acute inflammation of the meninges.

Characteristics

A. May be caused by viral or bacterial agents.
B. Diagnosis based on symptoms and culture of CSF.

✦ Assessment

A. Symptoms of nuchal–spinal rigidity: headache, irritability, nausea, vomiting, fever.
B. Positive Kernig's and Brudzinski's signs.
C. Increased ICP.

Implementation

✦ A. Isolate child until the causative agent is identified.
B. Administer antibiotics on time if bacterial cause.
C. Manage fluids: prevent dehydration and over-hydration (causes an increase in cerebral edema).
D. Monitor neurological signs carefully.
✦ E. Maintain bedrest and position child comfortably; most children prefer a side-lying or flat position; sitting up increases pain. May elevate head of bed with increased ICP.
F. Maintain patent airway; administer oxygen if ordered.
G. Provide quiet activities that are age appropriate.

Reye's Syndrome

✦ *Definition:*   Acute encephalopathy with fatty degeneration resulting in marked cerebral edema and enlargement of the liver with marked fatty infiltration.

Characteristics

A. Children from 2 months to adolescence contract illness; ages 6 and 11 years most often affected.
B. Usually follows a viral infection, especially varicella and influenza B.

✦ STAGES OF SYNDROME

- Stage 1: vomiting, lethargy, and drowsiness.
- Stage 2: CNS changes, disorientation, delirium, aggressiveness and combativeness, central neurologic hyperventilation, hyperactive reflexes and stupor.
- Stage 3: comatose, hyperventilation, decorticate posturing.
- Stage 4: increasing comatose state, loss of ocular reflexes, fixed, dilated pupils.
- Stage 5: seizures, loss of deep tendon reflexes, flaccidity, and respiratory arrest.

✦ C. Aspirin is now contraindicated with influenza—use Tylenol. (Incidence of Reye's is down since change from aspirin to Tylenol.)

Assessment

A. Prodromal symptoms: malaise, cough, rhinorrhea, sore throat.
B. Changes in level of consciousness.
C. Temperature changes.
D. Check laboratory findings.
   1. Associated with liver dysfunction—SGOT, SGPT, and LDH; decreased prothrombin; bilirubin and alkaline phosphate unchanged.
   2. Associated with renal dysfunction—reduced blood sugar levels to below 50 mg/100 mL, reduced insulin levels and decreased glucagon.

Implementation

✦ A. Most important nursing intervention—monitor for signs of increased intracranial pressure.
   1. Major effort is toward recognizing and reducing cerebral edema, as this may lead to death.
   ✦ 2. Monitor IV mannitol when administered to reduce blood osmolarity while increasing urine output, thus reducing cerebral edema.
B. Prepare for tracheal intubation and controlled ventilation (to decrease ICP).
C. Monitor vital signs frequently and decrease temperature as needed.
D. Monitor closely for signs of seizure activity and utilize seizure precautions.
E. Provide nursing care appropriate for semiconscious child.
   1. Maintain head elevation at 30 degrees.
   2. Monitor reflexes as indicative of clinical stage of syndrome.
F. Provide adequate fluid balance.
   1. Ensure adequate urinary output of at least 1 mL/1 kg body weight/hr.
   2. Provide and monitor intravenous fluids.
   3. Observe closely for cerebral edema or dehydration.

G. Provide respiratory care; suctioning, ventilation, and oxygen as ordered.
H. Provide emotional and supportive care.

CARDIOVASCULAR SYSTEM

Congenital Heart Defects

✦ *Definition:*   A structural defect of the heart or great vessels. The defects are present at birth. *Cyanotic* (with cyanosis) defects allow unoxygenated blood to circulate throughout the body. *Acyanotic* (without cyanosis) defects shunt blood previously oxygenated back to the lungs and allow oxygenated blood to go to the body.

Fetal Circulation

✦ A. Major structures of fetal circulation.
   1. Ductus venosus—a structure that shunts blood past the portal circulation.
   2. Foramen ovale—an opening between the right and left atria of the heart that shunts blood past the lungs.
   3. Ductus arteriosus—a structure between the aorta and the pulmonary artery that shunts blood past the lungs in uterine development.
✦ B. Normal changes in circulation at birth.
   1. The umbilical arteries and vein and the ductus venosus become nonfunctional.
   2. The lungs expand, reducing resistance, and greater amounts of blood enter the pulmonary circulation.
   3. Increased blood in the pulmonary circulation increases the return of blood to the left atrium, which initiates the closure of the flap of tissue covering the foramen ovale.
   4. The ductus arteriosus contracts and the blood flow decreases; eventually, the duct closes.
✦ C. Indications of heart disease in newborns.
   1. Congestive heart failure.
      a. Begins before 1 year of age in majority of infants.
      b. Cyanosis—persistent with administration of 100 percent oxygen.
   2. Arrhythmias.
   3. Nonductal murmur.

Coarctation of Aorta

Definition: Stenosis or narrowing of the aorta.

✦ **Assessment**

A. Increased blood pressure in the arms.
B. Decreased blood pressure in the thighs; may have no femoral pulses that are palpable.

C. Headache and nose bleeds.

D. May have no audible murmurs.

Treatment and Implementation

A. Resection of the aorta or insertion of a graft.

B. Surgery delayed as long as possible, depending on the condition of the vessel.

Patent Ductus Arteriosus

Definition: Failure of the ductus arteriosus to close after birth.

✦ Assessment

A. Dyspnea on exertion.

B. Growth failure; poor feeding habits.

C. Loud, machinerylike murmur.

D. Low diastolic-type blood pressure.

Treatment and Implementation

A. Closing of ductus.

B. Surgery usually performed at 2 or 3 years of age.

Atrial Septal and Ventricular Septal Defects (ASD/VSD)

Definition: Failure of the septum in either the atrium or the ventricle to completely develop. The extent of severity of the defect is dependent on the size and location of the opening.

✦ Assessment

A. Frequent upper respiratory infections.

B. Cyanosis on exertion.

C. Loud murmurs.

D. Signs of congestive heart failure (not always present —depends on size of defect and amount of shunting).

Treatment and Implementation

A. Surgical closure to repair defect.

B. Surgery delayed as long as possible to allow child to grow.

Tetralogy of Fallot

Definition: Combination of four heart defects—ventricular septal defect, pulmonary stenosis, overriding of aorta, and hypertrophy of the right ventricle.

✦ Assessment

A. Cyanosis.

B. Growth failure.

C. Polycythemia.

D. Fatigue with exercise.

E. Hypoxic episodes with potential for convulsions.

F. The child normally assumes a squatting position to facilitate breathing.

Treatment and Implementation

A. Surgical closure.

B. Surgery delayed as long as possible.

Transposition of the Great Vessels

Definition: Reversal of the position of the aorta and the pulmonary artery, not compatible with survival unless a large defect is present in the septum.

✦ Assessment

A. Profound cyanosis.

B. Dyspnea.

C. Tachycardia.

D. Signs of heart failure.

Treatment and Implementation

A. Preoperative care.
1. Prevent infection.
2. Encourage rest.
3. Observe vital signs with care.
4. Provide emotional support for the child and family.
5. Prepare for surgery with the usual preoperative teaching of breathing exercises (e.g., cough and deep breathing; blow bottles).

✦ B. Surgical procedure.
1. In infancy a shunt is usually necessary to get more oxygenated blood to the body.
2. Palliative surgery: creation of a patent ductus arteriosus or pulmonary artery banding to decrease blood flow through lungs.
3. Corrective surgery: arterial switch procedure.

✦ C. Postoperative care.
1. Maintain pulmonary function with suctioning, oxygen, deep breathing, and/or care of the chest tubes.
2. Observe vital signs, intake and output, and color.
3. Provide good skin care.
4. Provide adequate rest periods.
5. Maintain child comfort with medications and necessary positioning.
6. Provide emotional support for the child and the family.

Implementation—Congenital Heart Disease in Children

✦ A. Monitor regular analysis of oxygen concentration in isolette to ensure appropriate levels.

✦ B. Obtain vital signs at least every 4 hours or more frequently if warranted.

✦ C. Check for signs of impending heart failure.
1. Increase in weight, edema.
2. Increased pulse, respirations.

✦ **Table 15-1. CONGENITAL HEART DEFECTS**

Cyanotic Defects	Acyanotic Defects
Conditions that allow unoxygenated blood into the systemic circulation or conditions that result in obstruction of pulmonary blood flow. A.　Signs and symptoms 　　1.　Cyanosis. 　　2.　Retarded growth and failure to thrive 　　3.　Lack of energy 　　4.　Frequent respiratory infections. 　　5.　Polycythemia. 　　6.　Clubbing of fingers and toes. 　　7.　Squattting. 　　8.　Cerebral changes—fainting, confusion, CVAs. B.　Diseases in the cyanotic category. 　　1.　Complete transposition of the great vessels. 　　2.　Tetralogy of Fallot. 　　3.　Truncus arteriosus. 　　4.　Tricuspid atresia. 　　5.　Total anomalous pulmonary venous connection. 　　6.　Hypoplastic left heart syndrome.	Conditions that interfere with normal blood flow through the heart either by slowing it down, or by shunting blood from left to the right side of the heart. A.　Signs and symptoms. 　　1.　Audible murmur 　　2.　Discrepancies in pulse pressure in the upper and lower extremities. 　　3.　Tendency of develop respiratory infections. 　　4.　May develop heart failure with little stress. B.　Diseases in the acyanotic category. 　　1.　Patent ductus arteriosus. 　　2.　Atrial septal defect. 　　3.　Coarctation of the aorta. 　　4.　Pulmonic stenosis. 　　5.　Aortic stenosis. 　　6.　Atrioventricular canal (endocardial cushion defects).

　　3.　Presence of adventitious breath sounds, respiratory distress.
　　4.　Increase in cyanosis.
　　5.　Liver margin palpable for more than 1–2 cm below costal margin.
✦ D.　Monitor strict I&O and daily weights for changes that may indicate alterations in the infant's fluid status.
✦ E.　Note laboratory values for oxygen saturation and signs of polycythemia.
　　1.　Oxygen saturation of arterial blood that is less than 92 percent is considered a sign of cyanotic heart disease.
　　2.　Hematocrit higher than 52 percent may be a sign of polycythemia.
　F.　Position infant in the knee–chest position during hypercyanotic episodes. The toddler assumes the squatting position by himself.
　G.　Feed the child by nipple or nasogastric tube. Formula should contain appropriate caloric concentration and fluid volume.
　H.　General principles.
　　1.　Encourage normal growth and development.
　　2.　Counsel parents to avoid overprotection.
　　3.　Deal with parents' concerns and anxieties.
　　4.　Educate parents about conditions, tests, planned treatments, medications.
　　5.　Assist parents in developing ability to assess child's physical status.
　I.　Organize care and feedings to provide sufficient periods of rest.

HEART CONDITIONS

Rheumatic Fever

✦ *Definition:*　General systemic disease with damage to the connective tissue (collagen disease) caused by an antigen–antibody reaction to the beta-hemolytic *Streptococcus*.

✦ **Assessment**

A.　Migratory or polyarthritis.
B.　Abdominal pain.
C.　Low-grade fever.
D.　Weight loss and anorexia.
E.　Myocarditis with a murmur.
F.　Increased C-reactive protein in the blood; elevated erythrocyte sedimentation rate.
G.　Evaluate supporting evidence.
　　1.　Recent scarlet fever.
　　2.　Positive throat culture for group A *streptococci*.

Implementation

✦ A.　Maintain complete bedrest until the symptoms subside.
✦ B.　Monitor medications—antibiotics (penicillin is drug of choice) and salicylates for inflammation.
C.　Position legs in good body alignment, and make child comfortable.
D.　Provide diversional activities that do not require strenuous effort.
E.　Observe vital signs, especially the pulse, with care.

F.   Track weight.

G.   Provide emotional support.

Congestive Heart Failure

Definition: The heart is unable to meet the metabolic demands of the body; it is unable to pump the blood it contains out to the body. The most common cause of CHF in children is related to congenital anomalies.

Assessment

✦ A.   Observe for the following signs of pulmonary and venous congestion.

   1.   Tachycardia.

   2.   Tachypnea, progressing to respiratory distress.

   3.   Intercostal, supraclavicular, substernal retractions.

   4.   Fluid retention (weight gain).

   5.   Rales, wheezing, or rhonchi.

   6.   Hepatic engorgement.

✦ B.   Infant signs and symptoms: increased respiratory rate and infections; rales; enlarged liver and spleen, generally no edema, may see periorbital edema; babies do not display distended jugular veins but fontanelles may be full or bulging.

Implementation

A.   Promote rest.

   1.   Provide outlets such as drawing, doll play, and reading for the child who may be frustrated by restricted activity.

   2.   Organize care to limit time spent disturbing child's rest.

✦ B.   Increase oxygen supply and reduce oxygen demands.

   1.   Ensure child has a secure airway.

   2.   Administer oxygen via most appropriate route.

C.   Diet supervision.

   1.   Provide small frequent feedings.

   2.   Make high-calorie diet more palatable through imaginative play and an attractive food arrangement.

   3.   Educate parents about diet and its purpose.

D.   Medication supervision.

   1.   Afterload reducing medications (ACE inhibitors, e.g., Captopril and Enalapril). Monitor I&O, heart rate, blood pressure (hypotension).

✦   2.   Digoxin.

     a.   Monitor vital signs every hour during digitalization. If pulse under 90–100, notify RN or physician (may hold medication).

     b.   Observe for digoxin toxicity.

       (1)   Nausea, vomiting, diarrhea.

       (2)   Anorexia.

       (3)   Dizziness and headaches.

       (4)   Arrhythmias.

       (5)   Muscle weakness.

     c.   Always check pulse prior to giving digoxin.

✦   3.   Diuretics (Lasix and Diuril).

     a.   Observe for electrolyte abnormalities.

     b.   Weigh the child daily.

E.   Emotional support to avoid anxiety and stress.

Kawasaki Disease

✦ *Definition:*   A children's disease, most frequently seen in boys under age 2 of Asian ancestry. It responds like a viral disease of lymph nodes; cause is suspected to be infection with organism or toxin.

Assessment

A.   Age, sex, and ancestry to determine if child fits usual profile.

✦ B.   Symptoms: acute phase—fever, rash, swollen hands and feet, redness of the eyes, swollen lymph glands in the neck, inflammation of mouth, lips, and throat.

C.   Subacute phase: fissures on lips and skin, joint pain, cardiac disease and thrombocytosis.

D.   Lab findings: elevated ESR, elevated liver enzymes, anemia, or leukocytosis, elevated platelet count and elevated C-reactive protein level.

Treatment

A.   Since cause is unknown, no specific treatment is ordered. Immune globulin (IVIG) therapy often is initiated.

B.   Monitor high doses of aspirin to reduce fever, pain, and inflammation.

   1.   Dose: 80–100 mg/kg/day given when fever is high.

   2.   Given until platelet count is normal (to prevent thrombocytosis).

C.   Intravenous immune globulin given to prevent coronary artery disease if administered early.

   1.   Commonly given initially in high doses for its anti-inflammatory effect.

   2.   Later given in low doses for its antiaggregation platelet action.

Cardiac Surgery

Preoperative Implementation

✦ A.   Extensively prepare the child and the parents for the experience—demonstrate tubes and bandages and describe the scar that will be present after the operation.

✦ B.   Teach coughing and deep breathing to the child.

C.   Conduct the child and the parents on a tour of the intensive care unit and introduce them to the staff.

D. Observe the child for signs of infection.

E. Make sure all laboratory tests are completed.

Postoperative Implementation

✦ A. Maintain adequate pulmonary function.
1. Keep airway patent.
2. Patient should deep breathe and cough. Encourage use of incentive spirometry.
3. Suction if necessary.
4. Oxygen.
5. Chest suction for refilling lungs.
6. Check rate and depth of respirations.
7. Check water-seal chest drainage.

B. Maintain adequate circulatory functioning.
1. Check vital signs.
2. Replace blood when necessary, as ordered.
3. Check intake and output every hour.

C. Provide for rest through organized care.

D. Establish adequate hydration and nutrition.

✦ E. Take measures to prevent postoperative complications.
1. Antibiotic therapy.
2. Turn patient frequently.
3. Skin care.
4. Check extremities for occlusions of major vessels with blood clots: cyanosis, paleness of extremity, or coldness to the touch.
5. Passive range of motion.
6. Check dressing for signs of hemorrhage.

RESPIRATORY SYSTEM

Bronchiolitis

Definition: Inflammation of the bronchioles caused by thick mucus that traps air in the alveoli, which leads to poor air exchange. Bronchiolitis usually occurs before 18 months of age.

✦ **Assessment**

A. Abrupt onset of increased respiratory rate.

B. Harsh, nonproductive cough with expiratory wheeze and grunt.

C. Nasal discharge.

D. Tachycardia.

E. Cyanosis.

F. Dehydration (sunken fontanelle, poor skin tugor, decreased urinary output).

G. Irritability.

Treatment and Implementation

✦ A. Maintain patent airway; place upright to facilitate breathing.

B. Give nothing by mouth until dyspnea is improved.

C. Maintain intravenous feedings as ordered.

✦ D. Observe for dehydration: sunken fontanelle, decreased urinary output, poor skin tugor.

E. Provide cool humidity and oxygen as necessary.

F. Conserve energy—allow to rest.

G. Monitor cardiac, respiratory, and oxygen saturation.

H. Medications include: aerosolized ribavirin, RespiGam, Synagis.

Croup–Laryngotracheobronchitis

✦ *Definition:* Group of symptoms resulting from a variety of inflammatory conditions of the upper airway. The condition occurs in children 3–5 years of age.

Assessment

✦ A. Gradual onset, then hoarseness and barking cough.

✦ B. Inspiratory stridor, usually for 3–7 days (worse at night).

C. Mild elevation of temperature (102°F).

D. Hypoxemia.

E. If sudden onset, with inspiratory stridor, plan for hospital care.

✦ **Treatment and Implementation**

A. Observe vital signs with care, every 1–2 hours; check temperature if in cool mist tent.

B. Check oxygen saturation to keep above 93 percent.

C. Provide emotional support for the child and family.

D. Set up cool mist tent if severe dyspnea experienced. (May teach parents to use steam from shower if child is not hospitalized.)

E. Monitor hydration status; give clear liquids as tolerated.
1. Supplemental IV if needed.
2. Monitor urinary output, specific gravity to maintain fluid balance.

Bronchitis

✦ *Definition:* Inflammation of the large airways, usually associated with a URI.

✦ **Assessment**

A. Fever, usually preceded by an upper respiratory infection.

B. Hacking, moderately productive cough.

C. Crackles and wheezes.

D. Monitor for acute respiratory distress with acute symptoms.

Implementation

✦ A. Provide humidified air.

B. Urge fluids.

C. Provide postural drainage.

D. Observe vital signs with care.

E. Administer cough suppressants and expectorant as ordered.

Pneumonia

✦ *Definition:* Inflammation of the lung tissue caused primarily by bacteria or viruses.

✦ **Assessment**
   A. Cough that is usually nonproductive.
   B. Increased pulse and respirations.
   C. High fever (low-grade with viral pneumonia).
   D. Dyspnea and cyanosis.
   E. Convulsions.
   F. Increased white blood count.

Treatment and Implementation
   A. Maintain isolation if ordered.
✦ B. Treat symptoms.
      1. Control fever with antipyretic drugs, cool mattress, or sponge baths.
      2. Position to aid breathing; monitor oxygen therapy.
   C. Urge fluids; monitor I&O and fluid balance.
   D. Observe vital signs with care.
   E. Provide rest.
   F. Monitor medications—antibiotics.

Epiglottitis

✦ *Definition:* An acute bacterial infection of the epiglottis; may occasionally be of viral origin. Usually caused by *Hemophilus influenzae* type B or *Streptococcus pneumoniae*. May produce severe upper airway obstruction.

Assessment
   A. Illness occurs most frequently in young children, 3–7 years of age.
   B. May be preceded by URI—rapid onset.
✦ C. Inspiratory stridor and retractions, cough, muffled voice.
   D. High temperature (100°–104°F).
   E. May have acute respiratory distress.
   F. Difficulty swallowing with excessive drooling.

Implementation
✦ A. Keep child upright and in "sniffing" position —supine may cause occlusion of the airway.
✦ B. Never use restraints or a tongue blade or elicit gag reflex—all may cause occlusion of the airway.
✦ C. Provide cool mist therapy.
✦ D. Keep tracheostomy set/intubation at bedside at all times.
   E. Monitor vital signs with special emphasis on respirations.
   F. Monitor temperature every 2 hours—acetaminophen and ibuprofen given for temperature over 100°F, as ordered.
   G. Isolate child for 24 hours after starting antibiotics.
   H. Monitor endotracheal tube patency if intubated.

Tonsillitis and Adenoiditis

Definition: Infection and inflammation of the palatine tonsils and adenoids. Primary causes are Group A betahemolytic *Streptococcus* and viruses.

✦ **Assessment**
   A. Assess for difficulty swallowing or breathing.
   B. With adenoiditis, child is unable to breathe through nose and must mouth breathe (may be noisy, snoring at night).
   C. Observe for fever, sore throat, and anorexia.
   D. Assess for general malaise and dehydration.
   E. Assess for pain in ear and recurring otitis media.
   F. Observe for signs of respiratory distress.

Implementation
PREOPERATIVE INTERVENTIONS

✦ A. Provide emotional support and preop teaching for the child.
   B. Provide routine preoperative care.

POSTOPERATIVE INTERVENTIONS

✦ A. Maintain in prone or Sims' position until fully awake to facilitate drainage of secretions and prevent aspiration. Then change to semi-Fowler's.
✦ B. Avoid suctioning and coughing to prevent hemorrhage.
✦ C. Observe for signs of postop bleeding and shock.
      1. Restlessness.
      2. Alterations in vital signs (increased pulse, decreased blood pressure, increased respiration).
      3. Frequent swallowing.
      4. Excessive thirst.
      5. Vomiting of blood.
      6. Pallor.
   D. Maintain calm, quiet environment to prevent anxiety, which can lead to shock.
✦ E. Provide ice collar.
   F. Encourage fluids.
      1. Encourage cold fluids, popsicles, ice chips, or any food or liquid child will take; no red color foods/fluids.
      2. Do not use straws.
   G. Administer analgesics for pain as ordered.
   H. Complete discharge teaching.

Asthma

✦ *Definition:* A pulmonary disorder in which physical or chemical irritants cause the release of histamine and other substances that cause edema of the bronchial walls, excess secretion of mucus by the bronchial glands, and constriction of the bronchi.

✦ Table 15-2. SYMPTOMS OF UPPER AND LOWER RESPIRATORY OBSTRUCTIVE CONDITIONS	
Upper Respiratory Obstructive Conditions (Inspiration Problems—Croup, Epiglottitis)	Lower Respiratory Obstructive Conditions (Expiration Problems—Bronchitis, Bronchiolitis, Pneumonia)
1. Toxicity	1. Toxicity
2. Fatigue	2. Fatigue
3. Air hunger	3. Air hunger
4. Marked inspiratory stridor with hoarseness	4. Increasingly severe dyspnea
5. Increasing dyspnea	5. Intercostal retractions
6. Severe sternal reactions	6. Prolonged expiratory phase
7. Prolonged inspiratory phase	7. Increased respiratory rate
8. Increased respiratory rate	8. Increased cardiac rate
9. Increased cardiac rate	9. Harsh cough
10. Barking cough	10. Expiratory wheeze and grunt
	11. Moist rales

Characteristics

A. An attack may be provoked by exposure to certain foods, infections, vigorous activity, or emotional excitement.

B. Bronchiolar musculature goes into spasm.

C. Thick, tenacious mucus accumulates and causes obstruction of air passages.

D. Trapping of air occurs causing obstructive emphysema.

E. Symptoms include wheezing and crackles.

F. Attack may occur slowly or quickly.

G. Child usually coughs continually.

H. Cyanosis may occur, especially in lips and nailbeds.

I. Child appears anxious and upset.

J. Symptoms may become rapidly worse with acute respiratory failure with cyanosis and acidosis.

Implementation

A. Relieve bronchospasm.

B. Identification and removal of suspected allergen or "trigger," or treat underlying infection.

✦ C. Medication supervision.

   1. Beta-2 agonists: Albuterol, terbutaline—given in aerosolized form.

   2. Corticosteroids—reduces inflammation, which relieves airway obstruction.

   3. Cromolyn—used prophylactically, prevents allergic responses.

   4. Newer medications: Leukotrine modulators (Zafirlukast—Accolyte® and Montelukast—Singulair®). Most used for severe persistent asthma.

   5. Teach child to use peak expiratory flow meter before and after using medications.

D. Removal and control of secretions.

   1. Large fluid intake to liquefy secretions and maintain electrolyte balance.

   2. Mist tent.

   3. Chest physiotherapy and postural drainage.

E. Emotional support for parents and child to reduce anxiety.

F. Child educated to live optimally with chronic problem.

Cystic Fibrosis

Definition: Generalized dysfunction of the exocrine glands, which produce excessive mucus and abnormal secretion of sweat. The changes in secretions eventually cause dysfunction of the pancreas and the lungs. The disorder is hereditary and is inherited as a recessive trait.

Assessment

✦ A. Pancreas involvement consists of copious, foul-smelling stools with large amount of fat but no trypsin. The infant has a good appetite but fails to gain weight.

✦ B. Lung involvement consists of chronic cough and recurrent upper respiratory infections.

✦ C. Sweat gland involvement consists of an increased sweat chloride test of over 60 mEq/liter.

D. An associated problem is the poor absorption of fat-soluble vitamin D; this may lead to osteoporosis.

E. Infants with meconium ileus—often the first sign.

Implementation

✦ A. Provide special nutritive foods; 130 percent more than normal daily requirements.

   1. Pancreatic enzymes (Viokase and Cotazym) with meals and snacks.

   2. Water-soluble vitamins and fat-soluble vitamins (A, D, and E) and mineral supplements daily.

   3. A moderately low-fat, high-calorie and protein diet; additional salt during summer.

✦ B. Monitor drugs.

   1. A new drug, dornase alfa (Pulmozyme®), improves lung function.

   2. Antibiotics, inhaled (Tobramycin) and IV, and corticosteroids to treat infection.

C. Prevent respiratory infection.
1. Keep the lungs clear of mucus.
2. Provide mist tent at night to liquefy secretions.
3. Provide aerosol Mucomyst therapy and postural drainage.
4. Promote postural drainage and breathing exercises.
D. Provide good skin care to prevent irritation.
E. Educate the parents or interested others in proper care.
1. Teach at least two people the special procedures that are necessary for the infant's care.
2. Teach the proper care of the equipment, especially the cleaning process.
3. Encourage the responsible persons to participate in the infant's care while still hospitalized.
4. New drugs: most target gene therapy. Many clinical trials underway in 2003.
5. Refer the parents to the Cystic Fibrosis Foundation (www.cff.org) for additional help.
6. Refer parents to other community agencies if requested.
F. Give emotional support to child and family— median age of survival now approximately 35 years.

Otitis Media

Definition: Inflammation of the middle ear resulting from an infection-producing organism. Incidence greatest from 6 months to 2 years.

Assessment
A. Pain in the ears; child will pull or rub ear.
B. Fever; associated with URI.
C. Crying, irritability.
D. Restlessness and lethargy.

Treatment and Implementation
A. Monitor use of antibiotics and analgesics.
B. Myringotomy—incision that opens up the tympanic membrane or insertion of tubes.
C. Observe vital signs.
D. Take measures to reduce fever if present.
E. Provide good skin care; maintain cleanliness of the ear canal.
F. Advise parents to never put child in bed with a bottle and to feed child in upright position.

GASTROINTESTINAL SYSTEM

Cleft Lip

Definition: A congenital defect that involves a fissure or split in the upper lip resulting from failure of the two sides of the face to unite properly.

Treatment and Implementation
A. Preoperative care.
1. Use a large-holed, soft nipple with crosscut or "gravity flow" nipple for feedings.
2. Prevent infections.
3. Place nipple on side opposite defect.
4. Bubble frequently.
B. Surgical procedure.
1. Closure of lip.
2. Performed at 6–12 weeks of age or when infant is 10 pounds.
C. Postoperative care.
1. Observe for respiratory distress and swelling of tongue, nostrils, and mouth.
2. Avoid circumstances that will cause crying.
3. Watch for hemorrhage.
4. Use elbow restraints and provide supervised rest periods to exercise arms.
5. Feed with rubber-tipped medicine dropper on the side opposite the repaired cleft for 3 weeks.
6. After feeding, clean suture line with half-strength hydrogen peroxide.
7. Prevent crust formation on suture line by frequent cleansing and application of ointment.
8. Lay infant on side or back with support to prevent rolling over on the abdomen.
9. Prevent infections.
10. Support family and repare for discharge needs.

Cleft Palate

Definition: A birth defect in which a fissure or split in the roof of mouth (palate) results from failure of two sides of the face to unite. There may be involvement of both the hard and soft palate.

Assessment
A. Poor sucking reflex so infant unable to form a vacuum in the mouth.
B. If able to talk, there may be a speech impediment.
C. Increased incidence of upper respiratory infections.

Treatment and Implementation
A. Preoperative care.
1. Prevent infections.
2. Give nothing by mouth.
B. Surgical procedure.
1. May be performed in stages if the defect is bilateral.
2. The repair is usually made after 18 months of age.
C. Postoperative care.
1. Place child on abdomen to prevent aspiration.
2. Observe for signs of airway obstruction.

3. Apply hand restraints to prevent damage to the mouth.
4. Provide good oral hygiene.
5. Prevent infections.
6. Provide safe toys with no small parts.
7. Sedate and attempt to keep infant content.
✦ 8. Feed liquids using a cup or spoon—introduce method before surgery.

Hypertrophic Pyloric Stenosis (HPS)

✦ *Definition:*   Severe narrowing in the opening between the stomach and the intestine resulting from enlargement (hypertrophy) of the pyloric muscle. The condition is more common in the male infant and usually is diagnosed between 4 and 6 weeks of age.

Assessment

✦ A. Projectile vomiting soon after or during a feeding.
   1. Vomiting usually begins 30–60 minutes after feedings.
   2. Progressively increases in frequency and force; usually begins at about 1 week of age.
   3. Vomitus contains no bile.
   4. Formula appears to be almost the same as when ingested.
   5. May progress to complete obstruction.
B. Weight loss and dehydration; crying and fussy (constant hunger).
✦ C. Peristaltic waves passing left to right during or after feeding.
✦ D. Palpate epigastrium just to the right of umbilical area for classic "olive"-shaped mass.

Treatment and Implementation

✦ A. Preoperative care.
   1. Elevate head of bed 30 degrees.
   2. Give nothing by mouth.
   3. Maintain intravenous feedings as ordered to prevent dehydration and correct electrolytes.
   4. Adjust nasogastric tube to low suction.
✦ B. Surgical procedure.
   1. Pyloromyotomy—the incision of pylorus muscles.
   2. Fredet–Ramstedt procedure.
✦ C. Postoperative care.
   1. Maintain patent airway.
   2. Check position of NG tube. Adjust nasogastric tube to low suction for a few hours.
   3. Maintain intravenous fluids.
   4. Elevate head of bed 30 degrees.
   5. Check dressing for bleeding; observe for shock.
   6. Feed small amounts of clear liquids frequently, and increase them as tolerated; begin feedings 4 to 6 hours after surgery and progress slowly.
   7. Do not handle infant excessively after feeding.

Esophageal Atresia with Tracheoesophageal Fistula (TEF)

✦ *Definition:*   Closure of the esophagus during embryonic development; usually ends in a blind pouch. TEF is an abnormal connection between the trachea and esophagus (occurs in 1 in 3000 births).

Assessment

A. Excessive amounts of saliva with drooling.
✦ B. Early recognition important to prevent aspiration.
C. Respiratory distress with each feeding.
   1. Check to see if food is expelled through nose following feeding.
   2. Assess for severe coughing and choking.
   ✦ 3. Three C's of TEF—coughing, choking, and cyanosis when fed.
D. Abdominal distention caused by inspired air going into stomach.

Treatment and Implementation

✦ A. Preoperative care.
   1. Observe carefully.
   2. Maintain patent airway; suction if necessary.
   3. Elevate head of bed 30 degrees to decrease chance of aspiration.
   4. Give nothing by mouth; monitor IV fluids.
   5. Allow sucking with pacifier.
B. Surgical procedure.
   1. Repair the esophagus.
   2. Gastrostomy tube for feeding access (decompresses stomach and prevents aspiration of gastric contents from fistula).
C. Postoperative care.
   1. Maintain patent airway; suction; administer oxygen.
   2. Monitor IV fluids—record I&O; record specific gravity.
   3. Prevent infection—meticulous care of operative site.
   4. Feed through gastrostomy tube (usually after third postoperative day).
      a. Continue until infant tolerates oral feedings (10–14 days).
      b. Monitor gradual increase in feedings.
   5. Provide rest with infrequent handling.
   6. Elevate head of bed 30 degrees.
   7. Meet sucking needs with pacifier.

Obstruction of the Bowel

Definition: Impairment of the forward flow of intestinal contents by partial or complete blockage. May be caused by congenital intestinal obstruction—could be life threatening; or mechanical or muscular obstruction.

◆ **Assessment**

A. Absent or abnormal stools.

B. Presence of vomiting—may be projectile.

◆ C. Distended abdomen.

   1. Presence of slightly protuberant abdomen is normal.

   2. If abdomen is distended or excessively hard, evaluate for possible obstruction.

   3. Monitor respiratory status carefully as abdominal distention impinges on ability to expand diaphragm.

◆ D. Hyperactive bowel sounds above level of obstruction; hypoactive or absent below.

Implementation

◆ A. Check on passage of meconium which should occur during first 3 days after birth.

   1. If not, assess the child for abdominal distention.

   2. If more than 20 mL of gastric contents is aspirated through nasogastric tube, assess for lower intestinal obstruction.

B. Attempt to pass a nasogastric tube into stomach and aspirate contents as ordered.

C. Evaluate for excessive mucus and choking.

D. Observe for presence of cyanosis and choking on first feeding.

◆ E. Check for projectile vomiting following feedings.

   1. Evaluate infant's diet. (Overfeeding can cause projectile vomiting.)

   2. If vomiting occurs, evaluate for signs of infection or increased intracranial pressure.

   3. If these conditions are not present, vomiting may be a sign of an obstruction.

F. Document evidence of abdominal pain.

G. Evaluate for absent or abnormal stools.

Intussusception

Definition: Invagination or telescoping of one part of the bowel into another part below it. The condition occurs most frequently in boys between the ages of 3 and 12 months.

Assessment

◆ A. Sudden onset—severe colic-like pain in the abdomen; if child pulls knees to chest, this is an indication of pain.

B. Progressive vomiting.

◆ C. Bloody stools (like currant jelly).

D. Shock.

Treatment and Implementation

◆ A. Barium enema, which may be effective in reducing the bowel; if successful, makes surgery unnecessary.

◆ B. Preoperative care if surgery necessary.

   1. Adjust nasogastric tube to low suction.

   2. Give nothing by mouth.

   3. Maintain intravenous liquids.

   4. Provide emotional support.

◆ C. Surgical procedure.

   1. May only need to manipulate the bowel back to its normal position.

   2. A resection may be required, depending on when the diagnosis was made.

   3. Excision of involved area with end-to-end anastomosis.

D. Postoperative care.

   1. Maintain intravenous fluids.

   2. Adjust nasogastric tube to low suction.

   3. Begin oral feeding of clear fluids.

   4. Observe vital signs.

   5. Check dressing for bleeding.

Hirschsprung's Disease (Congenital Megacolon)

◆ *Definition:* Lack of normal nerve ganglia in the distal end of the colon. Length of colon involved varies with each individual. Condition is more common in males.

Assessment

◆ A. Newborn may or may not pass meconium.

◆ B. Progressive abdominal distention.

C. Reluctance to feed.

D. Occasional vomiting, bile stained.

E. Constipation is progressive as diet increases.

F. In older child, symptoms may be constipation, foul odor, and ribbonlike stools.

Treatment and Implementation

◆ A. Prior to surgery, monitor oral antibiotics, liquid diet, and saline colonic irrigation.

◆ B. Surgical procedure—colostomy.

C. Postoperative: maintain optimal nutrition and maintain skin care of colostomy.

Acute Diarrhea

Definition: Frequent, watery bowel movements (3–30/day) that result from an increased wavelike movement in the intestines.

◆ **Types of Diarrhea**

A. Infectious—caused by either bacterial or viral organism (most common).

B. Noninfectious—caused by an irritant in the intestinal tract, e.g., foods, drugs, laxatives, or other irritants.

C. Diarrhea may be a separate disease or a symptom of another disease.

Assessment

A. May be mild to severe.

B. Increased rate of peristalsis.

✦ C. Frequent stools, usually foul smelling, greenish in color, watery, and expelled with force.

D. Abdominal distention.

E. Irritability.

F. Weight loss and dehydration (*see* Dehydration below).

✦ G. Lab tests: stool culture if blood present; ova and parasite stool tests if culture negative.

✦ **Treatment and Implementation**

A. Replace electrolytes with oral rehydration solutions if possible.

✦ B. With severe diarrhea and dehydration, monitor IV—admission to the hospital may be necessary.
1. Measure intake and output.
2. Weigh infant daily.

C. Give antibiotics if caused by an organism and/or to prevent secondary infection.

D. Give nothing by mouth—rest for GI tract (24–48 hours). Desire for food will increase as stools decrease.

E. Isolate infant to prevent spread of diarrhea throughout the nursery.

F. Give good skin care.

Dehydration

Definition: Loss of water with resulting sodium excess. (Fluid volume deficit is when water and sodium losses are proportional.)

Assessment

✦ A. Increased heart rate and respirations.

B. Increased irritability and fussiness.

C. Dry skin with loss of normal elasticity; dry mucous membranes.

D. Depressed fontanelles, and eyes that appear sunken.

E. Decreased urine.
1. Urine may be dark in color (concentrated).
2. Increase in urine specific gravity.
3. Acidosis is a common result.

✦ **Implementation**

A. Administer oral rehydration therapy (ORT)—according to protocol.

B. Maintain strict recording of intake and output.

C. Supervise IV therapy if ordered.
1. Monitor electrolyte laboratory results and urine specific gravity.
2. IV treatment is guided by serum sodium levels.

D. Maintain skin care; monitor for diaper rash.

E. Family teaching (handwashing, avoiding high-sugar containing fluids to rehydrate, avoid BRAT diet).

Celiac Disease (Gluten-Induced Enteropathy)

Definition: A chronic disease of intestinal malabsorption precipitated by ingestion of gluten or protein portions of wheat or rye flour.

Characteristics

✦ A. A major cause of malabsorption in children, second only to cystic fibrosis.

B. Highest incidence occurs in Caucasians.

C. Major problem is an intolerance to gluten, a protein found in most grains.

✦ D. Basic defect is believed to be an inborn error of metabolism or an autoimmune response.

E. Inadequate fat absorption; as disease progresses it affects absorption of all ingested elements.

F. Long-term effects can be anemia, poor blood coagulation, osteoporosis, and lymphoma.

G. Usually occurs when child begins to ingest grains. It may begin as early as 6 months and continue until fifth year.

Assessment

✦ A. Diarrhea or loose stools: bulky, foul smelling, pale, and frothy.

B. Failure to gain weight after a bout of diarrhea.

C. Abdominal distention.

D. Anorexia.

E. Irritability and restlessness.

F. Celiac crisis.
1. Vomiting and diarrhea.
2. Acidosis and dehydration.
3. May be precipitated by respiratory infection, fluid and electrolyte imbalance, or emotional upset.
4. Excessive perspiration.
5. Cold extremities.

Implementation

A. Monitor appropriate diet.
✦ 1. Wheat and rye gluten as well as barley and oats are eliminated.
✦ 2. Low fat.
3. Slow feedings, small amounts at a time.
4. Strict intake and output.
5. Strict calorie control.
6. Supplemental vitamins and iron.

B. Give parental support.

C. Teach parents to recognize impending celiac crisis.

Inflammatory Bowel Disease (Ulcerative Colitis and Crohn's Disease)

✦ *Definition:* Inflammation of the colon and the rectum in which the mucous membrane becomes hyperemic, bleeds easily, and tends to ulcerate.

Etiology

A. Unknown, although the increased incidence within families has given rise to the hypothesis that suggests a hereditary predisposition or an emotional and/or environmental causation.

B. Incidence is highest in young adults and middle-age groups.

✦ Assessment

A. Diarrhea.

B. Weight loss—moderate to severe.

C. Rectal bleeding.

D. Abdominal pain, nausea, and vomiting.

E. Anemia.

F. Fever and dehydration.

G. Adolescents tend to be passive, pessimistic, fearful, and strongly, though ambivalently, attached to a parent.

H. Assist with diagnostic procedures.
   1. Barium enema.
   2. Mucosal biopsy.
   3. Stool examination and blood tests.

Implementation

✦ A. Control inflammation.
   1. Supervise medication regime (Sulfasalazine, corticosteroids, cyclosporine, ASA, and Azothioprine.).
   2. Provide adequate hydration with intravenous therapy and oral fluids as indicated.

✦ B. Provide for rest of intestinal tract.
   1. Observe for type and amount of bowel activity, symptoms of bleeding, and hyperactive peristalsis.
   2. Administer sedatives sparingly and observe for side effects.

✦ C. Maintain diet therapy.
   1. Encourage well-balanced, high-protein, high-caloric diet and vitamin therapy.
   2. May require special formulas, continuous NG feedings at night, or TPN to rest bowel.
   3. Record I&O.
   4. Avoid presenting cold foods because they increase gastric motility.
   5. Avoid gas-forming foods, sharp cheeses, highly spiced foods, smoked or salted meats, fried foods, raw fruits, and vegetables.
   6. Arrange for attractive environment with opportunities for socialization at mealtimes.

D. Provide counseling.
   1. Educate patient about diet, medication, and symptoms of bleeding.
   2. Observe for signs of psychological problems; initiate referral if necessary.

E. Colectomy may be needed in severe cases; is curative in Crohn's disease

Obesity

Definition: Excessive accumulation of body fat, which is over 10 percent of that normal for a young adult with regard to age, height, and body build. May be defined as body weight over 120 percent ideal weight.

Characteristics

A. The impact of childhood obesity becomes most obvious at adolescence when body image and peer approval become important.

B. Occasionally, obesity is a sign that the child may be missing other kinds of satisfaction.

C. Sometimes food is the only source of pleasure a child can find.

D. Eating may relieve anxiety for some children.

E. The child is often the victim of nagging and begins to associate overweight with feelings of worthlessness.

F. Usually, a strong familial tendency toward obesity exists.

Assessment

A. Height and weight according to standard growth and development scale.

B. Possible genetic factors related to the child.

C. Eating patterns and habits and food types.

D. Length of time child has been obese.

E. Child's and family's feelings and attitudes about obesity.

F. Consider cultural implications of body size and usual diet.

Implementation

A. Provide a balanced diet with limited calories.

B. Set up a routine of daily exercise; frequently, groups for after-school exercise programs can be organized by school nurses.

C. Help the young person work through underlying problems causing or caused by obesity.

D. Provide family counseling.
   1. Examine the eating patterns of the family. Some cultures have a high proportion of starches; others associate large meals with prosperity.
   2. Suggest the use of positive reinforcement for the adolescent rather than shaming the child.
   3. Have family support child by removing high-calorie food from their meals.

INTESTINAL PARASITES AND POISONING

Definition: Worms affect the gastrointestinal system as well as other systems and, as parasites, feed off the host body.

Roundworms

✦ Characteristics

A. Eggs are laid by the worm in the gastrointestinal tract of any host animal and passed out in feces.

B. After the worms have been ingested, egg batches are laid.

C. Larvae in the host invade lymphatics and venules of the mesentery and migrate to the liver, the lungs, and the heart.

D. Larvae from lungs reach the host's epiglottis and are swallowed; once in the gastrointestinal tract, the cycle is repeated—larvae mature and mate, and the female lays eggs.

Assessment

A. Atypical pneumonia.

✦ B. Gastrointestinal symptoms—nausea, vomiting, anorexia, weight loss, and stooling patterns.

C. Insomnia.

D. Irritability.

E. Signs of intestinal obstruction, vomiting and dehydration.

Treatment and Implementation

✦ A. Treatment—piperazine citrate or mebendazole (Vermox).

B. Nursing management.
  1. Prevention of infection through the use of a sanitary toilet.
  2. Hygiene education of the family.
  3. Careful disposal of infected stools.

Pinworms (Oxyuriasis)

Characteristics

A. Life cycle.
  1. Eggs ingested.
  2. Eggs mature in cecum, then migrate to anus.
  ✦ 3. Worms exit at night and lay eggs on host's skin.

B. Itching and reingestion occur.

Assessment

A. Acute or subacute appendicitis.

B. Eczematous areas of skin.

C. Irritability.

D. Loss of weight and anorexia.

E. Insomnia.

✦ F. Diagnosis by tape test—place transparent adhesive tape over anus and examine tape for evidence of worms.

Treatment and Implementation

A. Treatment.
  ✦ 1. Drug of choice is mebendazole. One dose of pyruinium pamoate (Povan) 5 mg/kg of body weight; repeat dose after 2 weeks to prevent reinfection.
  2. All infected persons living communally must be treated simultaneously.

B. Nursing management.
  1. During treatment, maintain meticulous cleansing of the skin, particularly in the anal region, and the hands and the nails.
  2. Bed linens and clothing must be boiled.
  3. Use ointment to relieve itching.
  4. Teach careful hygiene as a preventative measure.

Hookworms

Characteristics

✦ A. Life cycle.
  1. Eggs of the worm are evacuated from the human bowel in feces and left in the soil.
  2. Once the larvae are infective (in 5–10 days), they invade the host when in contact with the skin—which occurs either by handling the soil or by walking barefoot.

B. The worms live in the upper gastrointestinal tract of the host or suck blood from the intestinal wall for nourishment.

Assessment

A. Disturbed digestion.

B. Unformed stools containing undigested food.

C. Tarry stool with decomposed blood.

D. Blood loss.
  1. Pallor.
  2. Dull hair.
  3. Anemia.
  4. Increased pulse.
  5. Mental apathy.

Treatment and Implementation

A. Treatment.
  ✦ 1. Drug of choice is mebendazole or tetrachloroethylene.
  2. Possibly blood transfusions.

✦ B. Nursing management.
  1. NPO the evening preceding the treatment.
  2. Avoid fats, oils, and alcohol for 12 hours following medication.
  3. Prevention of infection.
    a. Hygiene instruction.
    b. Use of shoes in hookworm areas.
  4. Careful disposal of stools.

Giardiasis

✦ *Definition:* The most common intestinal parasite pathogen in the United States, this condition is caused by the protozoan, *Giardia lamblia*.

Characteristics

A. Often occurs in children in day care centers (estimates are 9–38 percent).

✦ B. Major mode of transmission is person-to-person, water (especially potentially contaminated mountain lakes and streams), food, and animals.

C. Adults may be asymptomatic, but children usually manifest symptoms.

Assessment

✦ A. Infants and young children.
   1. Diarrhea.
   2. Vomiting and anorexia.
   3. Failure to thrive.

✦ B. Children over 5 years of age.
   1. Abdominal cramps.
   2. Loose stools—may be intermittent.
   3. Stools may be watery, pale, and smelly.

C. Assess condition through stool specimens—may need 6 or more over several weeks.

Implementation

A. The most important nursing measure is to teach prevention—meticulous sanitary practices during diaper changes and cleaning of children.
   1. Inform parents of importance of handwashing.
   2. Drink water that is purified, especially when out in the open.

✦ B. Administer drugs available for treatment: quinacrine, furazolidone (drug of choice), and metronidazole.
   ✦ 1. If cost is a factor, quinacrine is usually given: administer with or after meals and crush tablets into jam or syrup.
   2. Quinacrine has most side effects: nausea and vomiting.

Poisoning

Definition: Ingestion of toxic substances, which may result in death or severe illness.

Characteristics

✦ A. The most common age group affected is 2 year olds because of the exploration of the environment through tasting.

✦ B. The major cause of poisoning is improper storage of toxic agents.
   1. Legislation has mandated childproof tops on prescription drugs, but many children can still remove the tops.
   2. Some new forms of drugs, such as transdermal patches or lozenges, are packaged so that they present a danger.

✦ C. General principles of care for poisoning.

   1. Identify the toxic substance and retrieve the poison.
   2. Notify the local poison control center and inform them of the toxic substance.
   3. Reverse the effect of the poison.
      ✦ a. Induce vomiting with syrup of ipecac or apomorphine.
         (1) Families of small children should keep this substance in the house in case of accidental poisoning.
         (2) Dose is 15 mL for children and 30 mL for young adults; follow with tap water.
         (3) Child should vomit within 30 minutes—important to bring up the syrup of ipecac to avoid cardiac complications.
      ✦ b. Activated charcoal may be used to carry toxic substance out of the body.
   ✦ 4. Vomiting is contraindicated with some substances.
      a. If child or person is in a coma, in shock, convulsing, or exhibits no gag reflex.
      b. If person has ingested low-viscosity hydrocarbons or corrosive substances (acid or alkaloid).

Types of Poisoning

✦ A. Acetaminophen poisoning.
   1. Toxic at 150 mg/kg body weight.
   2. Symptoms: diaphoresis; nausea and vomiting; lethargy; weakness; slow, weak pulse; depressed respirations; decreased urine; coma; liver failure.
   3. Intervention: induce vomiting with syrup of ipecac; lavage; antidote—acetylcysteine (Mucomyst) binds with acetaminophen.

✦ B. Salicylate poisoning.
   1. Toxic dose is 4–7 g/kg body weight.
   2. Symptoms: hyperventilation (from severe acidosis); diaphoresis; nausea and vomiting; diarrhea; delirium; dizziness; confusion; bleeding.
   3. Intervention: induce vomiting; lavage; activated charcoal; IV fluids; dialysis in severe cases; vitamin K if bleeding present.

✦ C. Chemical poisoning.
   1. Toxic dose: any corrosive chemical is toxic.
   2. Symptoms: respiratory problems, burns.
   3. Interventions: avoid emesis, which could cause further damage; dilute with water if ordered; maintain patent airway; give steroids if ordered.

Lead Poisoning

Definition: Poisoning from ingestion of paint or other lead-based materials.

Incidence

✦ A. Occurrence usually between 12 and 36 months of age.
 B. Death results in 25 percent of the cases of lead encephalopathy.
 C. Many neurologic residual problems in survivors.

Assessment

✦ A. Gastrointestinal symptoms.
   1. Unexplained, repeated vomiting.
   2. Vague, chronic abdominal pain.
✦ B. Central nervous system symptoms.
   1. Irritability.
   2. Drowsiness.
   3. Ataxia.
   4. Convulsive seizures.

Prevention and Treatment

 A. Education.
   ✦ 1. Inspection of buildings 25 years old or older that have lead-based paint on walls.
   2. Education of parents regarding danger of old paint or old lead pipes.
 B. Treatment.
   ✦ 1. IV calcium disodium edetate (EDTA) in several treatments to chelate lead from body.
   2. IM EDTA given but is very painful.
   ✦ 3. Observe for signs of hypocalcemia or tetany from chelation treatments.
   ✦ 4. Provide for seizure precautions.
   5. Check intake and output to evaluate kidney response to chelation.

RENAL SYSTEM

Acute Glomerulonephritis (AGN)

✦ *Definition:* Inflammation of the glomeruli that may be due to an antigen–antibody response to the beta-hemolytic *Streptococcus*, which causes changes in the glomerular filtering system. Most common in children 4–7 years of age.

Assessment

 A. Onset usually 2–3 weeks following an infection in site other than kidney.
 B. Edema of the face (periorbital and worse in mornings).
 C. Grossly bloody urine (cola-colored).
 D. Headache and vomiting.
 E. Oliguria and anuria.
 F. Fatigue; anorexia; irritability; lethargy.
 G. Anemia and malnutrition.
 H. Hypertension and slowed pulse.
 I. Encephalopathy and heart failure.

Treatment and Implementation

✦ A. Administer antibiotics if bacterial culture is positive.
✦ B. Maintain bedrest.
 C. Restrict salt and fluid in diet as necessary.
 D. Administer antihypertensive drugs as necessary (reserpine, magnesium sulfate).
 E. Observe vital signs.
 F. Observe intake and output; weigh daily.
✦ G. Monitor diet: elevated BUN and oliguria—restrict protein moderately; acute renal failure—restrict protein severely.
 H. Prevent infections.

Nephrotic Syndrome

Definition: Degenerative, noninflammatory disease of the renal tubules with an increase in permeability of the glomerular membrane and necrotic lesions of the tubules.

Assessment

 A. Gradual development of generalized edema. Periorbital and facial edema my be severe.
 B. Malnutrition due to loss of appetite.
 C. Anemia.
 D. Marked proteinuria.
 E. Nephrotic crisis indicated by abdominal pain, fever, and skin eruptions; will subside in a few days with a diuretic.
✦ F. Abnormal laboratory tests.
   1. Urine.
     a. Increased albuminuria.
     b. Increased casts and white blood cells.
     c. Increased lipid granules.
   2. Blood.
     a. Decreased total protein to < 4 g/100 mL.
     b. Decreased albumin and gamma globulin.
     c. Increased blood lipids and cholesterol.
     d. Increased sedimentation rate.

Treatment and Implementation

✦ A. Isolate child to prevent infections from increased susceptibility.
✦ B. In treatment of edema, provide good skin care, change position frequently, observe intake and output, track weight accurately, and measure abdominal girth at umbilicus.
 C. Prepare for the side effects of medications (prednisone) and be accurate with the dosage.
 D. Provide diet high in protein, possibly low in sodium, and high in calories.

Enuresis

✦ *Definition:* Involuntary urination in a child who is of age to have bladder control or previously had control —occurs most often in boys 4–5 years old.

Assessment

 A. Obtain accurate history (toilet training, prior habits).

B. Assess for UTI or diabetes.

C. Signs of infections or child abuse.

D. Developmental milestones.

E. Family response to enuresis.

Implementation

A. Prepare child for diagnostic procedures.

✦ B. Administer medications—antibiotics if infection, possible anticholinergics.

C. Assist with emotional care—increasing self-esteem, teaching.

Extrophy of the Bladder

Definition: A rare defect in which the bladder wall fails to close during development and a portion of the bladder wall extrudes through the abdominal wall; the upper urinary tract is normal.

Assessment

A. A mass of bright red tissue in the lower abdomen where the abdominal wall has not closed.

B. Assess for continual leaking from an open urethra.

Treatment and Implementation

A. Surgical reconstruction in several stages; the initial stage is completed shortly after birth.

B. Some children require permanent urinary diversion because it is impossible to reconstruct a functional bladder.

C. Nursing management.

   1. Position infant side-lying to promote drainage and help reduce risk of infection.

   2. Prevent trauma to exposed bladder; avoid abduction of the legs.

   3. Clean exposed area daily using meticulous skin care to protect from urine leakage and infection.

   4. Observe for obstruction in drainage tubes (decreased urine output, blood drainage from urethra, bladder spasms).

   5. Complete discharge teaching.

      a. Dressing change protocol.

      b. Prevention of infection.

      c. Observe for changes in urinary function.

BLOOD CELL DISORDERS

Sickle Cell Anemia

✦ *Definition:* Tendency of red blood cells to be crescent shaped when under low oxygen tension. The disorder results from the presence of an abnormal type of hemoglobin and is transmitted as a recessive dominant trait, particularly among blacks.

Assessment

✦ A. In noncrisis state the infant experiences the following symptoms.

   1. Severe chronic anemia.

   2. Periodic crises with abdominal and joint pain.

   3. Enlarged spleen from increased activity.

   4. Jaundice from excessive red blood cell destruction.

   5. Widening of the marrow spaces of the bones.

   6. Renal dysfunction.

✦ B. In crisis state the infant experiences episodes with the following characteristics.

   1. Thrombotic crisis is the most frequent type and is caused by occlusion of the small blood vessels, which produces distal ischemia and infarction.

      a. Swelling of hands and feet.

      b. Large joints and surrounding areas may become painful and swollen.

      c. Severe abdominal pains.

   2. Sequestration crisis is less frequent and occurs only in young children; it is caused by pooling of blood in spleen.

      a. Enlargement of the spleen.

      b. Circulatory collapse.

Treatment and Implementation

A. Alleviate pain with analgesics.

✦ B. Prevent dehydration with intravenous infusion if necessary and increased fluid intake.

C. Supplemental oxygen.

D. Keep child warm.

E. Offer parents genetic counseling.

F. Counsel the family on physiology and prognosis of disease.

G. Teaching: emphasize signs of crises, preventing crises, safe activities, Medic-Alert® bracelet.

Thalassemias

✦ *Definition:* An inherited group of hemolytic anemias caused by too few hemoglobin polypeptide chains. A chronic condition. Most often seen in individuals of Mediterranean descent.

✦ ### Assessment

A. Assess for skin breakdown, especially leg ulcers.

B. Observe for jaundice and elevated serum bilirubin.

C. Check for intolerance to fatty foods and abdominal discomfort.

D. Check blood studies, fetal hemoglobin as high as 90 percent.

Implementation

A. Supportive: rest, decreased activity, heat lamp to open wounds, excellent skin care.

✦ B. Monitor packed red cells or chelating agents (DTPH, Deferoxamine with vitamin C; folic acid may be given).

C. Prepare for splenectomy if transfused cells are rapidly destroyed by spleen.

Hemophilia

✦ *Definition:*   A sex-linked disorder in which certain factors necessary for coagulation of the blood are missing. Sex-linked traits are passed from unaffected carrier females to affected males along the X chromosome.

✦ **Characteristics**

A. Hemophilia A—Factor VIII deficiency: treated with monoclonal factor VIII concentrate.

B. Hemophilia B—Factor IX deficiency (Christmas disease): treated with purified, concentrated factor IX.

Assessment

✦ A. Type A or B—symptoms.
1. Possible bleeding tendency in neonatal period because factors are not passed through the placenta.
2. Excessive bruising.
3. Large hematomas from minor trauma.
4. Persistent bleeding from minor injuries.
5. Hemarthrosis with joint pain, swelling, and limited movement.
6. Possible progressive degenerative changes with osteoporosis, muscle atrophy, and fixed joints.
7. Abnormalities in clotting studies (PT, PTT, fibrinogen).

B. Type C—symptoms.
1. Usually appears as a mild bleeding disorder.
2. Autosomal dominant trait with both sexes affected.

Implementation

A. Prevent bleeding.
✦ 1. Protect child from environment by padding crib and playpen.
2. Supervise child carefully when child is learning to walk.

B. Observe for signs of blood transfusion reaction.

✦ C. Treatment if bleeding occurs.
1. Apply cold compresses and pressure.
2. Hemarthrosis (effusion of blood into joint).
a. Immobilize joint initially.
b. Initiate passive range of motion within 48 hours to prevent stiffness.
3. Immobilize site of bleeding.

D. Administer needed factors or blood products.

E. Monitor HIV status appropriately. (Many were inadvertently infected before blood was routinely screened.)

Anemia

Definition: A deficit of red blood cells or hemoglobin caused by impairment of red blood cell production or increased erythrocyte destruction.

Assessment

✦ A. Assess for early changes in behavior: listlessness, fatigue, sluggishness, and anorexia.

✦ B. Assess for late symptoms: pallor, weakness, tachycardia; signs of shock.

C. Observe for sources of blood loss (GI tract).

D. Check with RN to determine if nutritional deficiency is present: iron, folic acid, vitamin B_6 or B_{12}.

E. Consider racial/ethnic background.

✦ **Implementation**

A. Decrease oxygen demand—rest and quiet activities.

B. Prepare child for multiple blood draws.

C. Prevent infection by maintaining nutritious diet with vitamin and iron supplements, excellent hygiene, and avoidance of exposure to infections.

D. Teach parents that stools will be dark with iron supplements and that vomiting and diarrhea can occur.

E. Monitor blood transfusions and observe for signs of transfusion reactions.

F. Administer iron injections as ordered by special method (Z-track if severe iron deficiency is present) and take special precautions.

Infectious Mononucleosis

✦ *Definition:*   An acute, self-limited infectious disease, believed to be viral in origin (primarily the Epstein–Barr virus), that causes an increase in the mononuclear elements of the blood. Most common in individuals younger than age 25.

Assessment

A. Incubation period is around 11 days.

B. Blood test ("monospot") used to make diagnosis, in combination with clinical signs.

✦ C. Symptoms.
1. Malaise.
2. Sore throat with pharyngitis (may be severe).
3. Prolonged fever (2 weeks).
4. Enlargement of the lymph nodes.
5. Splenomegaly (enlargement of the spleen).
6. About 10–20 percent of the cases exhibit skin rashes that appear between days 4 and 10. The rash is usually the macular type, occurring primarily on the trunk.

Implementation

A. Symptomatic and supportive. No specific treatment.

1. Maintain bedrest initially. Promote rest.
2. Increase activity gradually.
3. Administer acetaminophen for fever, chills, and muscle pain as ordered.
4. Prevent secondary infections by limiting contacts while acutely ill.
5. Acyclovir may be given to patients who are immunosuppressed.

B. No isolation procedures are required.

Blood Transfusions

Assessment

✦ A. Identify type of blood therapy—whole blood, packed red cells, platelets.
✦ B. Check type and crossmatch.
  C. Baseline vital signs.
  D. Review institution policy about blood products.

Implementation

✦ A. Check identification of child with blood slip and Identaband.
  B. Ensure proper IV tubing and filter is used for blood administration (per institution policy).
✦ C. Hang blood only with normal saline—never with dextrose and water.
✦ D. Observe for transfusion reaction or allergic reaction—if either occurs, STOP transfusion immediately and notify RN or physician.
✦ E. Do not use blood that is discolored, cloudy, or that has been unrefrigerated for more than 30 minutes.

MUSCULOSKELETAL SYSTEM

Juvenile Rheumatoid Arthritis

Definition: Systemic disease with multiple manifestations, arthritis being the most characteristic; etiology unknown. Incidence 1 in 2000 children—more in Caucasians. Onset generally seen between 2 and 16 years of age.

Pathology

  A. Inflammation of joints.
  B. Edema and congestion of synovial tissues.
✦ C. As the disease progresses, synovial fluid fills the joint space and causes narrowing, fibrous ankylosis, and bony fusion.
  D. Growth centers adjacent to affected joints may undergo either premature closure or accelerated epiphyseal growth.

Assessment

✦ A. Involvement of joints.
  1. Arthritis may start slowly with gradual development of joint stiffness, swelling, and loss of motion.
  2. Affects knees, ankles, feet, wrists, and fingers most frequently, although any joint may be involved.
  3. Affected joints are swollen, warm, painful, and stiff.
  4. Young children appear irritable and anxious, guarding their joints.
  5. Weakness and atrophy of muscles appear around affected joints.
  6. Chronically affected joints may become deformed, dislocated, or fused.

  B. Systemic involvement.
  1. Frequent occurrence.
  2. Irritability, anorexia, and malaise.
  3. Fever.
  4. Intermittent macular rash on occasion.
  5. Enlarged liver and spleen (hepatosplenomegaly) and generalized lymphadenopathy in 20 percent of the patients.
  6. Anemia is common in active cases of the disease.
  7. Inflammation of eyes with redness, pain, photophobia, decreased visual acuity, and nonreactive pupil.

Treatment and Implementation

✦ A. Although there is no specific cure, care can be given to prevent joint destruction, maintain joint mobility and function.
  1. Exercise joints.
  2. Provide night splints.
  3. Educate parents in how adolescent should perform exercises, and impress upon them the adolescent's need for physical therapy and night splints.

  B. Provide emotional support to the chronically ill adolescent and his family.
✦ C. Administer medications; major goal is to relieve pain.
  1. Nonsteroidal anti-inflammatories (NSAIDs).
     a. Monitor levels carefully.
     b. Observe for gastric irritation—give with meals.
  2. Slower-acting antirheumatic drugs (SAARDs).
     a. Injectable gold given in weekly injections.
     b. Observe for side effects: dermatitis, stomatitis, thrombocytopenia.
  3. Cytotoxic drugs—may be given when child is not responding to NSAIDs or SAARDs.
  4. Corticosteroids—reduce inflammation and prevent joint damage; given in low doses and every other day to reduce side effects.
     a. Observe for side effects and toxicity.
        (1) Masked infection.
        (2) Hypertension.
        (3) Vascular disorders.
        (4) Mental disturbances.

(5) Edema with weight gain.

(6) Increased appetite.

(7) Peptic ulcer.

b. Observe vital signs regularly.

5. Immunologic modulators—to decrease inflammation and alter the immune response (example: etanercept).

◆ D. Maintain joint function—exercise joints, apply heat and night splints.

E. Prevent eye damage—report any sign of eye problems.

Scoliosis

◆ *Definition:*   Lateral curvature of the spine that occurs during the growth spurt at puberty.

Assessment

A. One leg shorter in length than the other.

B. One hip or one shoulder higher than the other hip or shoulder.

◆ C. A marked curve in upper part of spine.

1. Size of curve—20–50 degrees treated nonsurgically; more than 50 degrees treated surgically.

2. Pattern of curve—when main curve is thoracic, more likely deformity will occur.

◆ D. Types.

1. Kyphosis: flexion deformity usually at thoracic spine.

2. Lordosis: fixed extension deformity usually occurring to compensate for other abnormalities.

3. Scoliosis: lateral curvature of the spine.

a. Nonstructural: caused by changes outside the spine treated with exercises.

b. Structural: the spine itself has rotated, treated by bracing, exercise, insertion of the Harrington Rod or Luque procedure.

Treatment and Implementation

◆ A. Nonsurgical correction of curvature.

1. Exercise.

2. Plastic braces (orthoses).

◆ 3. TLSO (thoracolumbosacral) or Boston brace (usually when curve is 20–25 degrees)—worn 16–23 hours per day.

4. Halo traction.

5. Casting.

◆ B. Surgical correction options.

◆ 1. Considerations: any patient with a curve of 40 degrees is considered to be a candidate for surgery—after growth stops, a lateral curve can continue to progress at about 1 degree a year.

2. Spinal fusion: prevents progression of scoliosis and is done by inserting bone chips to achieve fusion of the vertebrae.

◆ 3. Harrington instrumentation: straightens the spine, acts as a splint to allow solid fusion of bony parts. Steel rods are placed along the spine and attached by wires at the cephalo and caudal ends of the spine.

◆ 4. Dwyer and Zielke instrumentation: anterior spinal fusion and instrumentation; used as first part of two-part surgery with Harrington instrumentation (posterior).

◆ 5. Luque Segmental Spinal instrumentation: rigid internal fixation of the spine; a method of internal segmental spinal instrumentation by wiring each vertebra to steel rods.

6. Vaneda and CD fixation systems: use surgically placed hooks, rods, and screws to correct curvature.

7. USS Hardware: screws and rods are surgically placed to create a frame to correct.

8. Video-assisted thoracoscopy is currently being performed for anterior fusion and stabilization with promising results.

◆ C. Instruct on use of Milwaukee brace.

1. Teach adolescent to wear the brace correctly and remove it only to bathe or as prescribed by the physician.

2. Explain necessity for good skin care where brace touches.

3. Assist adolescent to understand the need for the brace, and help the patient deal with the altered body image.

◆ D. Provide care when child undergoes surgery.

◆ 1. Harrington instrumentation.

a. Decortication of the bone over the laminas and spinous processes.

b. Bone grafts from iliac crest are inserted to achieve fusion of the vertebrae.

c. Rods are inserted along the vertebrae and attached by Harrington hooks and wires to achieve tension along the spine.

d. Casting is required postoperatively to protect the spinal fusion and to add stability.

◆ 2. Luque procedure.

a. Placement of wire loops under the lamina at each vertebral level.

b. Steel rods aligned along the curvatures of the spine are fixated to the spine by the wires.

◆ E. Preoperative care.

1. Evaluate child's level of understanding regarding condition and development progression.

2. Check preop labwork to assure all values are within normal limits.

3. Assist child with pulmonary function tests. Teach child to do tri-flows, cough, and deep

breathe. Explain the importance of doing this postoperatively.

4. Evaluate child's and parents' understanding of surgical procedure. Explain to their level of understanding. Discuss postoperative course with child and parents to help them know what to expect. Answer questions they may have.

5. Visit the ICU with family and child to familiarize them with the surroundings.

✦ F. Postoperative care.

1. Check vital signs every 15 minutes until stable, then every hour.

2. Watch for signs and symptoms of hypovolemia, tachycardia, BP. (Blood loss in the OR is considerable.)

3. Assess respiratory function—BS, RR, chest excursion, color, GFR (grunting, flaring, retractions); check ABGs. (Continual assessment of respiration function with vital signs is essential; pneumothorax or punctured lung is a risk after surgery.)

4. Maintain strict I&O; monitor urine output after 1 hour. Urine output must be adequate; if low, may indicate hypovolemia.

5. Check specific gravity to assess hydration status.

6. Start tri-flows as soon as awake after 1 hour. Encourage to cough and deep breathe between use of tri-flows.

✦ 7. Check CMS (circulation–color, movement, sensation) of lower extremities and feet q 1 h × 8 hours, q 2 h × 24 hours, then q 4 h.

✦ 8. Turn after 1 or 2 hours by logrolling only. Maintain alignment of spine.

9. Medicate child prior to turning or doing procedures (per orders).
   a. It is important to keep child comfortable, but watch for signs of respiratory depression with large doses of narcotics.
   b. Observe vital sign changes as indicative of pain.

10. Maintain NPO until child has positive bowel sounds, is passing flatus, or has had a stool.

11. Start diet with ice chips only. (Paralytic ileus is a common side effect.)

12. Check skin and dressing every 2 hours to assess for skin breakdown and bleeding.

13. Instruct child to flex feet to improve circulation and maintain muscle tone.

G. Rehabilitation.

1. Harrington instrumentation.
   a. Most children are casted after recovery from surgery; they can get up 1–2 weeks after the cast has been applied.
   b. Cast stays on 6 months.

   c. Once cast is removed, a Milwaukee brace or thoracolumbar support is worn approximately 3 months—removed only at night.

2. Luque CD and thoracoscopic procedures.
   a. After the wound is stable and child recovered from anesthesia, child may sit at the side of the bed.
   b. Progresses to ambulation. No postop immobilization is required.

Legg–Calvé–Perthes Disease

✦ *Definition:* A self-limiting disease in which aseptic necrosis of the femoral head produces hip deformation and dysfunction. Usually affects children 3–12 years of age, most common in males age 4–8.

Assessment

✦ A. Pain in hip or knee, most evident on rising or at end of the day.

B. Limp or joint dysfunction on the affected side.

C. Stiffness and tenderness over hip capsule.

Treatment and Implementation

✦ A. Goal of treatment is to keep head of the femur contained in the acetabulum.
   ✦ 1. Reduce inflammation and restore motion—active motion is encouraged during this phase.
   ✦ 2. Containment may be done by using non–weight-bearing devices (casts, abduction brace, or leather sling).

✦ B. Conservative treatment may be continued for 2–4 years—early treatment essential to avoid permanent damage.

C. Most care is outpatient so nursing emphasis is on teaching.
   1. Teach family use of corrective devices.
   2. Support normal growth and development and school progress.

Congenital Clubfoot (Talipes Equinovarus)

✦ *Definition:* Congenital deformity in which the foot is twisted out of its normal position. The deformity is described according to the position of the foot and ankle. The most common type is talipes equinovarus (95 percent), in which the foot is pointed downward and inward.

Assessment

A. Assess whether foot deformity is accompanied by other problems such as neurological defects or spina bifida.

B. General health status of infant in preparation for treatment.

C. Determine aspects of treatment: occurs in three stages and includes exercises, manipulation, casting, and splinting.

Implementation

✦ A. Treatment consists of correction, maintenance, and follow-up.
1. Manipulation followed by serial casting (right after birth).
2. Casts changed every few days, as needed due to rapid growth of infant.
3. More severe forms may require surgery.
4. Splinting may also be used.

✦ B. Assist in passive exercises (manipulation) of the foot following a demonstration by RN or physician: hold position to count of 10 and continue for 10 minutes several times a day.

C. Instruct parents in cast and/or splint care.

INTEGUMENTARY SYSTEM

Eczema (Atopic Dermatitis)

Definition: Inflammation of the skin that can occur on any area of the body. Generally seen in children with allergic tendencies.

Assessment

A. Local redness of the skin (erythema).
B. Papules and vesicles apparent on face, neck, and body folds.
C. Rash characterized by itching, crusting, scaling, and oozing.
D. Question when symptoms appear—may be when new foods are introduced (eggs, cow's milk, etc.); stress can exacerbate outbreaks.

Treatment and Implementation

A. Treat the symptoms. Aim of treatment is to reduce inflammation, pruritis, and hydrate the skin.
B. Provide sedation.
C. Keep infant comfortable.
D. Prevent scratching and secondary infections.
E. Provide emotional support.
F. Eliminate the source of allergic sensitivity, if known (ex., dust-carrying objects such as stuffed animals, molds, cigarettes).

Impetigo

✦ *Definition:* A skin infection caused by *Streptococcus* or *Staphylococcus*. Usually begins as a scratch or scrape that becomes infected.

Assessment

✦ A. Assess for multiple macular–papular rash seen at various stages of healing.

B. Check rupture of papules, which produce serous exudate and form a crust.
C. Assess location: usually found on face, head, and neck.

Implementation

✦ A. Monitor topical and/or systemic antibiotic therapy (penicillins or cephalosporins).
B. For older child and adult, administer frequent cleansing with soap or Burow's solution and remove crusts.
C. Monitor antibiotic therapy—topical and/or systemic.
D. Cut nails to avoid scratching.
E. Provide isolation protection for newborn; emphasize thorough handwashing and overall good hygiene.
F. Prevent secondary infections.

Burns

Definition: Destruction of body tissue caused by heat. It is the most frequent accidental injury occurring to infants and children.

✦ Degree of Burns

A. First-degree—superficial—involves only the epidermis with redness, swelling, and pain.
B. Second-degree—partial thickness—involves superficial skin layers with redness, blisters, and pain; scarring may occur.
C. Third-degree—full thickness—involves the epidermis and some of the dermis, with charring and destruction of the nerve endings, sweat glands, and hair follicles.

Treatment and Implementation

A. Exposed method (reverse isolation).
B. Pressure dressings.
C. Wet dressings (sterile).
D. Skin grafts.
E. Prevent infection.
F. Maintain optimum circulating volume; observe intake and output.
G. Align body carefully to prevent contractures.
H. Provide a well-balanced diet.
1. Give twice normal amount of calories.
2. Give 3 to 4 times normal requirement of protein.

See interventions for Burns in Chapter 10.

ENDOCRINE SYSTEM

Diabetes Mellitus

Definition: A total or partial deficiency of insulin—the most common childhood endocrine disorder. Incidence peaks in adolescence.

Characteristics

A. Type I: An absolute deficiency of insulin and patients are insulin deficient.
   1. Often diagnosed in early childhood or adolescence.
   2. Requires replacement of insulin.
B. Type II: The body fails to use insulin properly and may also have deficient insulin levels.
C. Type II diabetes has increased dramatically in children.
D. Prognosis: degenerative changes associated with diabetes mellitus begin in young adults who have had the disease for 10–20 years.
   1. Arteriosclerosis with hypertension.
   2. Retinal changes and cataracts.
   3. Nephropathy.

✦ Assessment

A. As with adults, random blood glucose levels >200 mg/dL or fasting glucose >130 mg/dL.
B. Clinical signs.
   1. Loss of weight.
   2. Increased thirst and appetite, polydipsia, polyphagia, polyuria, and nocturia, decreased attention span.
   ✦ 3. Onset frequently associated with ketoacidosis —an acute, life-threatening condition.
      a. Drowsiness.
      b. Dryness of skin.
      c. Flushed cheeks.
      d. Acetone breath.
      e. Hyperpnea.
      f. Nausea, vomiting, and abdominal pains.

Treatment and Implementation

✦ A. Monitor blood glucose and administration of insulin via injection or pump.* (Oral hypoglycemic agents generally do not produce satisfactory results because they require some pancreatic function to be effective.)
   1. Side effects: hypoglycemia with hunger, irritability, nervousness, headaches, and slurred speech.
   2. Combine insulin treatment with controlled diet.
✦ B. Monitor diet.
   1. Diet should be adequate for normal growth and development and regulated according to diabetic needs.
   2. The type of diet prescribed is influenced by the philosophy of the physician.
   3. Diets vary from free diets to strict dietary control.
C. Provide family and patient education.

* *See* Insulin chart in Chapter 10.

   1. Signs and symptoms of disease, including acidosis and hypoglycemia.
   2. Instruction in insulin injection or pump, sterile technique, and blood glucose monitoring.
   3. Diet control as prescribed by the physician.
   4. Prevention of infections through adequate skin and foot care.
   5. Knowledge of the effects of increased physical activity and stress on food needs.
   6. Patient's responsibility for administering insulin and managing diet.
   7. Normal activity and life style appropriate.
D. Provide special counseling because of adolescent's heightened sensitivity to being different and their frequently unusual dietary habits.

Hypothyroidism

✦ *Definition:*   Deficiency in secretions of thyroid hormones resulting from a rudimentary thyroid gland, which is either hypoactive or absent. The condition is recognizable when the child is 2–3 months old.

✦ Assessment

A. Body growth is retarded.
B. Eyes are puffy.
C. Tongue protrudes and is thick and large.
D. Hands and feet are short and square.
E. Skin is very dry, pale, and coarse.
F. Hair is very dry and coarse.
G. Frequently, there is an umbilical hernia.
H. Feeding difficulties include choking, lack of interest in food, and sluggishness.
I. Respiratory difficulties include apneic episodes, noisy respirations, and nasal obstructions.

✦ Treatment and Implementation

A. Medication must be started immediately in infants to avoid mental deficiency.
   1. Infants given thyroid hormone—Synthroid is drug of choice.
   2. Cytomel is used when rapid response needed.
B. Dosage based on age, weight, and response to treatment.
C. 50 percent of the children treated before the age of 6 months will achieve an IQ of 90 or more.

PEDIATRIC ONCOLOGY

Characteristics

A. Signs and symptoms of pediatric malignancy may be subtle and not easily recognized.
B. Causal factors associated with cancer in children are not clearly defined.
C. Current treatment focuses on chemotherapy, radiation, a combination of the two, and surgical intervention.

✦ **Cardinal Symptoms**
  A. Unusual mass or swelling.
  B. Unexplained paleness or weakness.
  C. Tendency to bruise.
  D. Persistent pain or limp.
  E. Prolonged, unexplained fever.
  F. Headaches, often with vomiting.
  G. Sudden eye or vision changes.
  H. Excessive, rapid weight loss.

Wilms' Tumor (Nephroblastoma)

✦ *Definition:*   Rapidly developing, malignant solid tumor of the kidneys containing embryonal elements. The incidence is 1 in 10,000 and peak age of occurrence is 3 years. Multimodal therapy can give 90 percent cure in localized tumors (Stage I or II).

Assessment

✦ A. Presence of a mass on either side of the abdomen with possible pain. (The mass itself should initiate a diagnostic workup.)
  B. Fever and hypertension.
  C. Possible weight loss and anemia.
  D. Diagnostic tests: ultrasound, CT scan, blood studies, venogram.

Treatment and Implementation

  A. Preoperative care.
  ✦ 1. Avoid palpation of the tumor to prevent spreading. If a mass is present, defer palpation of abdomen to physicians **only.**
     2. Provide emotional support for the family.
     3. Observe intake and output with care.
  B. Surgical procedure, chemotherapy, and possible radiation.
     1. Tumor can be shrunk with chemotherapy before surgery.
     2. Nephrectomy if the nonaffected kidney is functioning.
  C. Postoperative care.
     1. Observe for toxic reactions to chemotherapy, such as mouth lesions.
     2. If radiation therapy is given, provide good skin care.

Brain Tumor

Definition: The second most common childhood cancer. Benign or malignant brain mass. In children, the tumor is usually located in the cerebellum or the midbrain.

Characteristics

  A. Seventy-five percent of childhood brain tumors are impossible to remove or are so situated as to cause damage if completely removed.
  B. Incidence—occurs most frequently in the 5–7 age group.
  C. Location—most occur in the posterior fossa.
✦ D. Types most frequently seen in children.
     1. Astrocytoma.
        a. Located in the cerebellum.
        b. Insidious onset and slowly progressive course.
        c. Surgical removal usually possible.
     2. Medulloblastoma.
        a. Located in the cerebellum.
        b. Highly malignant.
        c. Prognosis poor.
     3. Ependymoma.
        a. Usually, there is ventricular blockage, leading to signs of increased intracranial pressure.
        b. Treated with incomplete internal compression and radiation therapy.
     4. Brain stem gliomas.
        a. Seventy-five percent of childhood brain tumors.
        b. Develops slowly with initial symptoms of cranial nerve palsies.
     5. Neuroblastoma.
        a. Malignant solid tumor found in infants and young children.
        b. Generally arises in the adrenal gland.

Assessment

  A. Variety of symptoms depending on location of tumor.
✦ B. Increased intracranial pressure.
     1. Vomiting without nausea; anorexia.
     2. Headache.
     3. Diplopia.
✦ C. Enlargement of the head in children under 4 years old.
  D. Mental change: lethargy, irritability, drowsiness, and stupor.
  E. Unsteady gait and muscular uncoordination (ataxia).
  F. Vital sign disturbances.

Implementation

  A. Control and relief of symptoms.
✦ B. Seizure precautions.
✦ C. Postoperative care for surgical removal.
     1. Maintain child flat in bed on unaffected side.
     2. Logroll for change of position.
     3. Control fever with hypothermia mattress.
     4. Frequently observe vital signs until stable, every 15–30 minutes.
     5. Reinforce dressing, if wet, with sterile gauze.
     6. Notify RN of increased wetness in dressing— possible cerebrospinal fluid leakage.
  D. Minimize increases in ICP: prevent vomiting, coughing, straining with stool; keep lights dim and noise down.

E. Provide emotional support for family and child.

F. Monitor radiation therapy.

BONE TUMORS

Osteogenic Sarcoma

✦ *Definition:* A malignant tumor originating from osteoblasts (bone-forming cells). The most common malignant bone tumor in children.

Characteristics

✦ A. Tumor usually located at the end of the long bones (metaphysis).

B. Most frequently seen at the distal end of the femur or the proximal end of the tibia.

Assessment

✦ A. Primary symptoms are pain at site, swelling, and limitation of movement.

B. Lungs most common site of metastasis.

C. Occurs twice as frequently in boys as in girls.

Treatment and Implementation

A. Therapy aimed at saving the limb whenever possible.

B. Provide care for amputation followed by chemotherapy.

✦ C. Administer drugs and monitor for side effects.
1. Antimetabolities—high-dose methotrexate.
2. Synthetic agents—cisplatin.
3. Antibiotics—Doxarubicin, Bleomycin.
4. Alkylating agents—Ifosfamide, Cyclophosphamide.
5. Plant alkaloids—Vincristine.

D. Provide supportive emotional care.

Ewing's Sarcoma

Definition: A malignant tumor of the bone originating from myeloblasts with early metastases to lungs, lymph nodes, and other bones.

Assessment

✦ A. Tumor usually located on the shaft of the long bones; femur, tibia, and humerus common sites.

✦ B. Primary symptoms.
1. Pain at site.
2. Swollen area with tenderness.
3. Fever.

C. Swollen area and tenderness.

D. Occurs twice as frequently in boys as in girls.

✦ #### Treatment and Implementation

A. Usually radiation, sometimes followed by amputation; monitor for side effects.

B. Chemotherapy to treat tumor and prevent metastases.

C. Administer drugs and monitor for side effects—chemotherapeutic agents same as "C" in Osteogenic Sarcoma above.

D. Encourage inclusion of patient in discussions of treatment, options, risks, and prognosis.

E. Listen to parents, child, and siblings as they work through denial, anger, acceptance—allow them their grieving process.

F. Promote age appropriate activities and group discussions with peers.

G. Assist parents in avoiding overprotection.

H. Treat the side effects of chemotherapy and radiation.

BLOOD AND LYMPH CANCER

Leukemia

Definition: Unrestrained growth of abnormal, immature white blood cells, which causes destruction of the red blood cells. Leukemia is the most common cancer in children. Annual incidence is around 4–5 per 100,00 in Caucasian children younger than 15 years old and less in black children under age 15.

Assessment

✦ A. Increased number of white blood cells that are immature and do not function normally.

✦ B. Anorexia, nausea, and vomiting.

✦ C. Weight loss, fatigue, and weakness.

D. Abdominal pain, joint pain.

E. Fever.

F. Petechiae and bruising.

G. Enlarged liver and spleen.

H. Anemia.

I. Onset is usually rapid.

Treatment and Implementation

A. Support child and family during diagnostic procedures: LP, MRI, biopsy, bone marrow aspiration.

✦ B. Administer antimetabolite drugs (methotrexate); observe for side effects and signs of toxicity.

✦ C. Prevent infection.
1. Avoid contact with communicable diseases.
2. Do not give regular immunizations while in treatment.
3. Provide oral hygiene; avoid toothbrushes.
4. Prevent and/or treat candida oral infections.
5. Change intravenous tubing daily, as institutional protocol.
6. If WBC very low, reverse isolation.

D. Handle child gently.

E. Encourage good nutrition.

1. Administer antiemetic 30 minutes before eating.
2. Offer cold liquids high in calories to supplement diet.
F. Prevent hemorrhage.
   1. Handle infant carefully.
   2. Pad sides of bed.
   3. Follow platelet count closely.
G. Provide emotional support for the child and the family during therapy.

Hodgkin's Disease*

✦ *Definition:*   Malignancy of the lymph system characterized by a large, primitive, reticulumlike, malignant cell. Peak occurrence is adolescent boys. Long-term survival rate is 80–90 percent in early stages.

Assessment
A. Enlarged, painless lymph nodes. Nodes are firm and movable.
B. Lessened sensitivity to specified antigens (anergy).
C. Frequent infections.
D. Prognosis is guarded for advanced stages (overall 5-year survival rate appears to be about 30 percent).

✦ Stages
A. Stage I.
   1. Disease restricted to single anatomic site or localized in a group of lymph nodes.
   2. Asymptomatic.
B. Stage II.
   1. Stage II: two or three adjacent lymph nodes in the area on the same side of the diaphragm are affected.
   2. Stage IIE: as above and disease within extra-lymphatic organ.
C. Stage III: Disease of lymph on both sides of diaphragm.
D. Stage IV: as above and disease within extralymphatic organ. Disease is widely disseminated into the lymph areas and organs.

Treatment and Implementation
✦ A. Provide for symptomatic relief for the side effects of radiation (used for Stages I, II, and III in an effort to eradicate the disease) and chemotherapy (used in combination is usual treatment of choice).
B. Combination chemotherapy most frequently used is ABVD regimen (doxorubin, bleomycin, vinblastine and decarbazine). (MOPP was used).
C. Radiation is primary treatment for early stage Hodgkin's; in later stages, it is combined with chemotherapy.

* For non-Hodgkin's Lymphoma, *see* Medical-Surgical chapter (10).

D. Counseling.
   1. Assist the family and the adolescent to accept the process of treatment.
   2. Encourage independence where possible.
E. Observe for complications.
   1. Pressure from enlargement of the lymph glands on vital organs.
   2. Respiratory problems from the compression of the airway.

CANCER TREATMENT

Chemotherapy

Basic Principles
A. Chemotherapeutic agents work on rapidly dividing cells.
B. Tumor's location and cell type affect choice of drugs.
✦ C. Most antineoplastic drugs are metabolized in the liver and excreted by the kidneys so these organs must be in functioning order to prevent toxicity.

Assessment
A. Assess if more than one chemotherapeutic agent is being administered.
B. Identify potential side effects of medications.
   1. GI disturbance.
   2. Loss of hair.
   3. Bone marrow suppression.
C. Assess for fluid and electrolyte imbalances associated with drug therapy.
D. Assess for adequate urine output.
E. Monitor laboratory values.
F. Assess oral cavity for irritation and bleeding gums.

Implementation
A. Establish baseline data.
   1. Nutritional status.
   2. Oral condition.
   3. Skin condition.
   4. Degree of mobility.
   5. Psychological status.
   6. Neurological condition.
B. Observe for side effects of cell breakdown.
   1. BUN on rise.
   2. Stone formation in urinary tract.
✦ C. Observe for side effects of rapidly dividing cells.
   1. Gastrointestinal mucosa—diarrhea, nausea, vomiting.
      a. Administer antiemetics.
      b. Provide mouth care with hydrogen peroxide every 4 hours. No toothbrush or glycerin.
      c. Administer anesthetic spray to mouth prior to meals.

d. Provide frequent cold, high-calorie beverages.

2. Hair follicles—loss of hair.
   a. Prepare patient for loss—suggest wig, scarf.
   b. Reassure that it will return in 6 weeks.
   c. Apply tourniquet around scalp during chemotherapy plus 2–3 hours following to lessen amount of hair lost.

Common Chemotherapy Drugs

✦ A. Corticosteroids—prednisone used most frequently.
   1. Side effects.
      a. Ravenous appetite.
      b. Change in fat distribution.
      c. Retention of fluid.
      d. Hirsutism.
      e. Occasional hypertension.
      f. Psychological disturbance.
   2. Nursing management—watch blood sugar and tapering of medication.

✦ B. 6-Mercaptopurine (6MP).
   1. Interrupts the synthesis of purines essential to the structure and function of nucleic acids.
   2. Side effects.
      a. Produces very little toxicity in children.
      b. Increases amount of uric acid that the kidneys must excrete.
   3. Nursing management.
      a. Observe kidney function.
      b. Increase fluid intake.

✦ C. Methotrexate.
   1. A folic acid antagonist (antimetabolite) that suppresses the growth of abnormal cells enough to permit regeneration of normal cells.
   2. Side effects.
      a. Ulceration of oral mucosa.
      b. Nausea, vomiting, diarrhea, and abdominal pain.
   3. Nursing management.
      a. Observe for ulcerations—drug must be temporarily discontinued at the appearance of ulcers.
      b. Observe renal function—primary route of drug excretion.

✦ D. Cytoxan, Ifosfamide, Cyclophosphamide.
   1. Alkylating agent suppresses cellular proliferation; it has greater effect on abnormal than normal cells.
   2. Side effects—hemorrhagic cystitis.
   3. Nursing management—provide large quantities of fluids preceding and immediately following drug administration to prevent side effects.

✦ E. Vincristine.
   1. Plant alkaloid.
   2. Side effects.
      a. Insomnia.
      b. Severe constipation.
      c. Peripheral neuritis or palsies.
   3. Frequently used to induce remissions rapidly, after which the patient is maintained on another, less toxic drug.

Radiation

✦ Basic Principles

A. Radiation affects all cells but is particularly lethal to rapidly developing cells.

B. Radiation can be utilized in conjunction with chemotherapy.

C. Radiation may be used to eradicate the tumor or to relieve pressure.

✦ Assessment

A. Assess for fatigue.

B. Assess fluid and electrolyte imbalances due to vomiting, diarrhea, and urinary frequency associated with radiation therapy.

C. Monitor hemoglobin and hematocrit.

D. Assess skin condition in radiated area.

E. Assess for dental caries and gum disease.

F. Assess condition of hair.

✦ Implementation

✦ A. Treatment of radiation sickness.
   1. Symptoms—nausea, vomiting, malaise.
   2. Offer frequent high caloric feedings (milk shakes with extra protein and vitamins).
   3. Make food trays attractive, palatable.

✦ B. Observe side effects of cell breakdown.
   1. Rising potassium, phosphate, creatinine, BUN.
   2. Accumulation of uric acid.
   3. Stone formation in urinary tract.

✦ C. Treat side effects of cell breakdown.
   1. Increase fluid intake.
   2. Monitor intake and output.

✦ D. Treat skin breakdown.
   1. Check patient regularly for any redness or irritation at radiation site.
   2. Immediately notify physician.
   3. Usual treatment—apply lotion to area, cover loosely with sterile gauze.
   4. Avoid any irritation to area from clothing, soap, or weather extremes.

✦ E. Treat bone marrow depression.
   1. Carefully watch lab values.
   2. Isolate (low leukocytes) patient if WBC dangerously low.
   3. Avoid injections (low platelets).

4. Antibiotics.
5. Meticulous handwashing—limit contacts, especially people who are sick.

SPECIAL TOPICS IN PEDIATRICS

Failure to Thrive

Definition: A syndrome characterized by an infant's failure to grow and develop with or without characteristic posturing or "body language." Etiology is nonspecific. May be organic or nonorganic.

Assessment

◆ A. History of infant includes feeding problems, vomiting, sleep disturbance, irritability, sucking ability, aversion to formula, and irregularity in daily activities.

◆ B. Abnormal nutritional intake may be related to deficient intake, malabsorption, or poor assimilation.
1. Number of calories, quality of calories, and feeding patterns.
2. Weigh daily and observe reaction to nutritional program.

C. Nature of mother–child relationship.
1. Relationship patterns.
2. Ability of mother to perceive infant's needs.

Implementation

◆ A. Priority—provide sufficient nutrients so that infant will grow.
1. Develop a structured feeding routine.
2. Weigh daily to assess weight gain.

◆ B. Provide nurturing to infant.
1. Ensure a warm, loving environment through holding, cuddling, and physical contact.
2. Spend time talking to infant and building a trusting relationship.
3. Maintain as much eye-to-eye contact as possible.

C. Provide a positive, quiet, nonstimulating environment to promote psychosocial growth.

D. Assist mother to develop a positive relationship with infant.

E. Document feeding behaviors and monitor infant progress.

The Child with Cognitive Impairment (Mental Retardation)

Definition: Impairment of intelligence that results in a limited capacity to adapt to the environment and to achieve skills necessary for progress on the developmental continuum.

General Concepts

◆ A. Cognitive impairment is defined as significantly below average intelligence that occurs in association with developmental delays (motor, language, and adaptive behavior).

◆ B. May result from genetic, familial, birth-related factors, or acquired conditions.
1. Genetic conditions: inborn errors of metabolism, chromosomal abnormalities (Down syndrome).
2. Fetal or birth-related factors: fetal alcohol syndrome, maternal infections, asphyxia, prematurity, hyperbilirubinemia.
3. Familial factors: low parental intelligence or environmental deprivation.
4. Acquired conditions: meningitis, lead poisoning.

Classifications of Cognitive Impairment

◆ A. Mild (educable).
1. Child can acquire simple basic learning skills.
2. IQ between 50 and 75.
3. Social and sensorimotor skills can be developed.
4. Child can learn self-support skills.

◆ B. Moderate (trainable).
1. Child can acquire simple social skills.
   a. Communication.
   b. Minimal social interaction skills.
2. IQ between 35–50 and 55.
3. Minimal learning ability; delays in motor development.
4. Can be independent with supervision.

◆ C. Severe (minimally trainable).
1. Can benefit from habit training.
2. IQ between 20–35 and 40.
3. Requires supervision.
4. Poor communicative, social, and sensorimotor skills.
5. Marked delay in motor development.

◆ D. Profound—custodial.
1. Minimal capacity to function.
2. IQ below 20–25.
3. Requires constant supervision (custodial care).
4. Gross retardation.

Incidence

A. Approximately 3 percent of the general population is considered to be mentally retarded.

B. Cognitive impairment occurs in all races and both sexes; there is no differentiation as to socioeconomic status.

C. Incidence of mental retardation according to classification.
1. Educable—75 percent.
2. Trainable—23 percent.
3. Custodial—2 percent.

Implementation

✦ A. Treat the child according to developmental age rather than chronological age.
   1. Respond to the child on a level he or she can understand. If the developmental age is 2 years and chronological age is 10, respond to and deal with child as if a 2 year old.
   2. Assessment is often vague and inaccurate so expectations at the developmental age should not be rigid.
✦ B. Provide the child with as much stimulation and love as a normal child.
   C. Watch for infections and disease; retarded children are frequently more susceptible.
   D. Challenge with behavioral modification, as it frequently works well with these children.
   E. Empathize with parents' reaction to the birth of a mentally retarded child.
      1. Birth presents a threat to the parents' marital relationship and family dynamics.
   ✦ 2. Stages of parental reaction.
      a. Denial: initial reaction of defense, which protects the parents from admitting that this child, this extension of themselves, is not normal.
      b. Initial recognition: aware of difference between their child and other children.
      c. Active recognition: the parents begin to search for information on their child's problem and are ready to seek professional advice.
   F. Work with staff to formulate a plan for dealing with the mentally retarded child if child is to live at home with parents.

Down Syndrome

✦ *Definition:* Physical malformation and degree of mental retardation resulting from a chromosomal defect, usually number 21.

Assessment

✦ A. Face characterized by rounded shape, flattened nose, thickened tongue, almond-shaped eyes, and flattened occiput.
✦ B. Muscles flaccid; motor development will be slow.
   C. Extremities characterized by short, fat hands with simian crease on the palms and little finger curved inward.
   D. Mental capacity varies from mild to severe retardation. These children are usually very happy.

✦ Implementation

   A. Individualize according to needs of the infant and the family.
   B. Give assistance in contacting community agencies that can assist the family with the infant's needs.

C. Encourage developmental activities initiated at the proper time.
D. Observe for other anomalies in the infant.
E. Alert the family of the necessity to take precautions against infection.
F. Refer the family to a geneticist.

Attention Deficit/Hyperactivity Disorder

✦ *Definition:* A developmental disorder that involves a group of behavioral symptoms such as hyperactivity, hyperkinesis, or overactivity. Incidence may be as low as 1 percent or as high as 20 percent in school-age children.

Assessment

✦ A. Identify child by assessing presence of diagnostic criteria (DSM-III).
   1. Inattention.
   2. Impulsive.
   3. Hyperactivity.
   B. Additional traits that may be present: negativistic, emotional liability, easily frustrated, and learning disabilities.

Implementation

   A. Coordinate treatment plan with family and physician and educational counselor.
   B. Provide safe environment with minimal stimulation—short contact times.
✦ C. Monitor diet—limit sugar, additives, artificial colors.
   D. Administer medication if ordered—Ritalin (now very controversial).

Phenylketonuria (PKU)

✦ *Definition:* Failure of the body to normally metabolize the amino acid phenylalanine. The condition is genetically transmitted.

Characteristics

✦ A. High levels of this amino acid in the blood are toxic and can cause mental retardation.
✦ B. Brain development arrested by 4 months of age if left untreated.
   C. Moderate to severe retardation by 1 year of age if left untreated. Retardation level correlates with high PKU levels and this condition is irreversible.

Assessment

✦ A. Observe for signs.
   1. Lethargy.
   2. Anorexia.
   3. Anemia.
   4. Skin rashes.
   5. Diarrhea.

B. Check results of early PKU test and determine if later test was done or needs to be done (takes several days of protein in formula to reveal metabolism error).

Treatment and Implementation

✦ A. Most state health departments mandate PKU testing (Guthrie blood test) either before the infant's discharge if infant has feeding source (protein) in the hospital or with a return visit within 2 weeks.

✦ B. Restrict phenylalanine in the diet until about 5 years of age—Lofenalac formula.

✦ C. Eliminate foods high in protein, e.g., meat, poultry, fish, eggs, nuts, legumes, and milk products.

D. Suggest genetic counseling to the parents.

E. Gently remind parents to have all future children born to them screened for PKU.

Child Abuse

Definition: Physical maltreatment or negligence (not including accidental mishaps) of children that results from an absence of reasonable standards of protection and care by the parents or the child's caretaker.

Epidemiology

✦ A. Incidence.
   1. An estimated 879,000 cases of child abuse or battered children occurred in 2000.
   2. Of all injuries in children under 5 years of age, as seen in hospital emergency departments, about 10 percent are actually caused by parents or are the result of negligence.
   3. Children less than 1 year old accounted for 44% of child maltreatment fatalities.
   4. Neglect is the most common form of maltreatment—physical abuse occurred in 28% of reported cases.

✦ B. Distribution.
   1. 50 percent are 7 years or younger.
   2. 25 percent are less than 4 years old.
   3. 25 percent are 12–18 years old.

✦ C. Psychological factors.
   1. Abused child usually has demanding behaviors.
   2. Abuse usually occurs close in time to a crisis or stressful event.
   3. Abuse usually occurs after the parent is provoked to anger.
   4. Majority of perpetrators (75 percent) are parents, 10 percent are relatives, and only 2 percent caregivers.

D. Victims.
   1. Shaken baby syndrome has been documented in children up to 5 years old.

   2. In 2000, 60% of perpetrators were female.
   3. Risk of becoming a battered child is three times greater for children born prematurely than for those born full-term.
   4. Stepchildren have a higher abuse risk than do nonstepchildren.

Clinical Indications of Abuse

✦ A. Account of the injury/ies.
   1. Cause given for the injury is implausible.
   2. Cause given for the injury is punishment, which is inappropriate considering the age of the child.
   3. Discrepancies in the initial account as presented by neighbors or other family members.
   4. Delay in seeking medical help for the child.

✦ B. Indications for diagnosis of abuse.
   1. Physical examination.
      a. Bruises, welts, and scars in various stages of healing.
      b. Finger-mark pattern of bruises on the body.
      c. Bite, rope, or choke marks in evidence.
      d. Cigarette and/or hot water burns are visible.
      e. Eye damage, subdural hematoma, and/or intra-abdominal injuries.
      f. Radiographic findings of multiple bone injuries at different stages of healing.
   2. Other observations.
      a. Child perceived as passive, noncommunicative and/or withdrawn.
      b. Child perceived as failing to thrive.

✦ C. Characteristics of abusers—parents, caretakers, relatives.
   1. Abusers usually abused as children.
   2. Abusers unable to utilize outside help when angry with their children.
   3. Abusers usually are isolated and lonely individuals under age 40.
   4. Frequently, spouse of abuser does not know how to prevent abuse.
   5. Frequently, abusive parents make unreasonable demands of their children.
   6. Abusing parents often exhibit certain personality problems such as dependency, low self-esteem, immaturity, and inability to cope with feelings.

D. Legal responsibilities of health team members.
   ✦ 1. Both nurses and doctors have a legal responsibility to report incidences of children who are suspected of being abused to the proper authorities.
   2. Designated community authorities have the responsibility to determine further placement of the abused child.

Accidental Injuries

Incidence

✦ A. Accidents are the leading cause of deaths from 1 to 44 years of age.

B. The majority of accidents occur in or near the home.

✦ C. Most common types of fatal accidents by age.
1. Infant under 12 months—congenital anomalies and prematurity.
2. Accidents eighth leading cause of death < 1 year.
3. 1–4 years.
   a. Motor vehicle accidents.
   b. Drowning.
   c. Fires or burns.
   d. Suffocation.
   e. Falls.
4. 5–9 years.
   a. Motor vehicle accidents.
   b. Drowning.
   c. Fires/burns.
   d. Overland transport (bicycles, skateboards).
5. 10–24 years. Motor vehicle accidents are major cause of death.

Treatment and Implementation

A. If accidental poisoning occurs, contact local poison control center for pertinent information. Keep the poison container if available.

B. Take children to the nearest emergency room for proper treatment of any type of injuries.

C. Accident prevention is very important; educate both the child and the parents.

Sudden Infant Death Syndrome (SIDS)

Definition: The sudden, unexplained death of an infant during sleep.

Characteristics

✦ A. Largest single cause of death after neonatal period—third leading cause of death in infants.

✦ B. Peak incidence 2–4 months; rare after 6 months.

✦ C. Higher incidence in winter months, in low-income groups, and in low-birth-weight infants.

D. Most deaths are unobserved and occur during sleep.

E. On autopsy, inflammation of upper respiratory tract is found.

F. Etiology unknown and controversial. Many theories involving carbon dioxide sensitivity, poor response to stimulus, vitamin or mineral deficiency, allergic reaction, strep B from the mother.

Treatment

✦ A. Recent research suggests that there is a correlation between SIDS and infants sleeping on their abdomen.
1. New research indicates that an infant should be placed on back only for sleep (even sleeping on their side is considered potentially dangerous).
✦ 2. Incidence of SIDS decreased by more than 40 percent since "back-to-sleep" program started in 1994.

B. If apneic episode is discovered (infant responds when stimulated, called near-miss SIDS), physician should be notified for further workup and treatment.

Appendix 15-1. NUTRITION

Nutrition for the Infant

✦ A. Caloric requirements
1. Birth to 6 months: 100–108 Kcal/kg/day.
2. Protein: 2.2g/kg/day.

✦ B. Fluids.
1. First 6 months—120–150 mL/kg/24 hours.
2. Requirements increase in hot weather.

✦ C. Number of feedings per 24 hours.
1. First week—6–10 per day.
2. 1 week to 1 month—6–8 per day.
3. 1–3 months—5–6 per day.
4. 3–6 months—4–5 per day.
5. 6–12 months—3 per day.

✦ D. Vitamins.
1. Breast-fed infants—supplement with vitamins C, D, and A.
2. Formula-fed infants—vitamin supplements depend on type of formula and which vitamins are already included in it.
3. Mixing cereal with vitamin C-containing juices will aid iron absorption.
4. Vitamin supplements may be added at 3–6 mo. if advised by health care provider.

✦ E. Solid foods—recent trends indicate introduction of solid foods at 4–6 months of age.
1. Cereal—infants are least allergic to rice.
2. Fruits and vegetables.
   a. New foods should be introduced once a day in small amounts until the infant becomes accustomed to them.
   b. Introduce only one new food per week.
   c. Bananas and applesauce are well tolerated.
   d. Orange juice is usually not well tolerated, initially. It can be introduced, diluted with water, when the infant is two or three months old.
   e. Green and yellow vegetables can be introduced at about 4 months of age.
3. Eggs.
   a. Introduce after infant is 6 months old.
   b. Usually yolks are well tolerated, but sometimes there are allergic reactions to egg whites—should not be introduced until 12 months.
4. Meat.
   a. May be introduced at 4 months.
   b. Usually more palatable if mixed with fruits or vegetables.
5. Starchy foods.
   a. May be introduced after the infant is 6 months old.
   b. Should not be substituted for green vegetables or fruit.
   c. Chief value is caloric.
   d. Zwieback and other crackers are good for the gumming infant.
6. Whole milk should not be given until after 1 year of age.

F. Diarrhea (temporary).
1. Usually caused by contaminated food, or viral infection.
2. Review feeding preparation and storage of formula with caretaker.
3. Usually corrected by oral rehydration therapy (ORT). *See* page 531.
4. BRAT (bananas, rice, applesauce, and toast) diet is NOT recommended.

G. Constipation.
1. Increase fluid intake.
2. In infant 3 months old or older, increase cereal, fruit, and vegetable intake.
3. On occasion, prune juice (half an ounce) may be given.

H. Avoid honey until at least 1 year old (risk of infantile botulism).

Nutrition for the Second Year

A. Rate of growth is slowing down; thus, there is a decreased caloric need.
B. Self-selection—children usually select a balanced diet over a period of several days.
C. Child should be feeding self, with some assistance.

Nutrition for the Preschooler

A. Child begins to imitate family's likes and dislikes.
B. Finger foods are popular.
C. Single foods are preferable to a combination of foods.
D. Do not let child drink sweet liquids from a "sippy cup" all day—ruins their teeth.

Nutrition for the School-Age Child

A. Patterns of good eating habits are established at this time.
B. Provide fruits as snacks.

Adolescent Eating Patterns

A. Adolescents often gain weight easily and then resort to fad diets.
B. Girls adapt themselves to fashionable weight goals, some of which may be unhealthy.
C. Eating of nonnutritious foods in a social setting.

Malnutrition

A. Kwashiorkor—caused by a lack of protein.
B. Rickets—caused by a lack of vitamin D.
C. Scurvy—caused by a lack of vitamin C.

✦ Appendix 15-2. REFLEXES IN THE NEWBORN

Palmar Grasp

A. Automatic reflex of full-term newborns; eliciting by placing finger in infant's palm.

B. Present at birth.

C. Disappears at 4 months.

Asymmetrical Tonic Neck Reflex

A. Infant assumes fencer's position—when head is turned to one side, arm on that side is extended, and opposite arm is flexed.

B. Present at birth.

C. Disappears at 4 months.

Moro's Reflex (Startle Reflex)

A. When infant is suddenly jarred or hears a loud noise, the body stiffens, the legs are drawn up, and the arms are brought up, out, and then in front in an embracing position.

B. Present at birth.

C. Disappears at 4 months.

Reciprocal Kicking

A. Movements of newborns are jerky and usually alternate in the legs.

B. Evolving at birth.

C. Disappears at 9 months.

Rooting

A. When infant's cheek is brushed, the head will turn to that side.

B. Present at birth.

C. Rooting while awake disappears at 3–4 months.

D. Rooting while asleep disappears at 7–8 months.

Sucking

A. Infants make sucking movements when anything touches their lips.

B. Present at birth.

C. Involuntary sucking disappears at or about 9 months.

Neck Righting Reflex

A. When the head is turned to one side, the opposite shoulder and trunk will follow.

B. Evolving at 4 months.

C. Involuntary movement disappears at 9–12 months.

Babinski's Sign

A. Extension of the great toe on stroking the sole of the foot.

B. Present at birth.

C. Disappears after 2 years.

◆ **Appendix 15-3. IMMUNIZATION SCHEDULE**

Recommended Childhood and Adolescent Immunization Schedule, United States, 2005
Vaccines are listed under routinely recommended ages for administration. *Bars* indicate recommended age range. *Ovals* indicate age for vaccines to be administered if previously recommended doses were missed or given earlier than the recommended minimum age.

						Age					
Vaccine	Birth	1 month	2 months	4 months	6 months	12 months	15 months	18 months	4–6 years	11–12 years	14–16 years
Hepatitis B	Hepatitis B-1*		Hepatitis B-2		Hepatitis B-3					Hep B	
Diphtheria, tetanus, toxoids and acellular pertussis			DTaP	DTaP	DTaP		DTaP		DTaP	Td	
Hemophilus influenzae type b			Hib	Hib	Hib	Hib					
Inactivated Polio[a]			IPV	IPV	IPV				IPV		
Pneumococcal			PCV	PCV	PCV	PCV			PCV		
Measles, mumps, and rubella						MMR-1			MMR-2	MMR	
Varicella						Var			Var		

■ Range of acceptable ages for vaccination	⬭ "Catch-up" vaccination

HepB 1 only if mother HBsAG(⁻)

[a] OPV (trivalent oral polio vaccine) is no longer recommended. IPV eliminates risk of vaccine-associated paralytic polio.

Approved by Advisory Committee on Immunization Practices (ACIP), the American Academy of Pediatrics (AAP), and the American Academy of Family Physicians (AAFP).

Note: this schedule is reviewed and subject to change every 6 months. To be up-to-date, check current schedule on CDC or ACIP website.

Immunizations

A. Refer to schedule above.
B. Current schedule recommends children receive 20 injections by age 6 years old—combination vaccines are coming into practice (Pediatrix and Rixensart®).
C. Providers need to adjust administration when combination vaccine (combine DTaP, IVP and Hep B) series are begun, but not completed.
D. Generally vaccines are interchangeable, but care must be taken to assure series is completed, and record keeping accurate.
E. Educating parents.
    1. Need for immunizations.
    2. Minimizing pain and psychological trauma—most well child visits at 12 scheduled dates will still include at least 3 injections (or as many as 5, if no combination vaccines are used).
    3. Independent studies have refuted claims that MMR causes autism.
    4. Multiple immunizations given simultaneously do NOT overwhelm immune system—thought to use about 0.1% of immune system capacity.
    5. If extra doses of vaccines are given if switched to combination vaccines, no harm has been demonstrated.
    6. Educate parents about possible side effects (fever, fussiness, local reaction) to immunizations—and management (acetaminophen/ibuprofen to manage fever and pain, massage and warm compresses to local reactions).

✦ Appendix 15-4. CALCULATION OF MAINTENANCE FLUID REQUIREMENTS IN CHILDREN

Body Weight	Fluid Requirement
0–10 kg	100 mL/kg/24 hr
11–20 kg	1000 cc + 50 mL/kg/24 hr
21–40 kg	1500 cc + 20 mL/kg/24 hr

Divide total fluid requirement by 24 to obtain hourly fluid rate.

Appendix 15-5. ORAL REHYDRATION THERAPY (ORT) FOR MILD–MODERATE DEHYDRATION

A. Fluids available: Pedialyte®, Infalyte®, and Rehydrate®.
B. Dehydration: 40–50 mL/kg of rehydration fluids over 4 hours, containing 75–90 mEq of sodium per liter.
C. Maintenance: Fluids should contain 40–60 mEq/L sodium (breast milk, lactose-free formula or half-strength lactose fluids).
D. Approximately 10 mL/kg replacement with rehydrating solution should be used for each diarrheal stool after rehydration therapy is complete.

Appendix 15-6. DRUG ADMINISTRATION FOR CHILDREN

A. Clark's weight rule for pediatric dosage.

$$\frac{\text{Child's weight in pounds}}{150} \times \text{Adult dose} = \text{Approximate dose for children}$$

B. Intravenous microdrip usually has 60 drops/mL.
C. Conversion of administration units.
  1 tsp = 5 mL
  1 tbl = 15 mL
  1 mL = 16 minims
  1 grain = 60 mg
  1 g = 1000 mg
  1 oz = 30 mL
  1 dram = 4 mL

✦ Appendix 15-7. PEDIATRIC COMMUNICABLE DISEASES

Disease	Characteristics	Transmission	Nursing Care
Varicella (Chickenpox)	Acute viral disease; onset is sudden with high fever; maculopapular rash and vesicular scabs in multiple stages of healing. Incubation is 10–21 days	Spread by droplet or airborne secretions; scabs not infectious	Isolate Treat symptoms: Acetaminophen, fluids for fever Prevent scratching Observe for complications—could be fatal
Erythema Infectiosum (Fifth disease)	Rash in 3 stages: I—Facial Erythema ("slapped cheek" appearance) Lasts 1–4 days II—Symmetrically distributed maculopapular red spots on upper and lower extremities Progresses from proximal to distal locations, may last >7 days III—Rash subsides but *can* reappear Caused by human parvovirus B19 (HPV) Incubation: Usually 4–14 days, can be up to 21 days	Unknown Possibly respiratory secretions and/or blood	Standard precautions Isolation of hospitalized child only necessary if immunosuppressed or if in aplastic crisis May precipitate aplastic crisis in patients with chronic hemolytic disorders
Lyme Disease	1st sign generally a ring-shaped rash (erythema migrans), fever, headache, red eyes, arthralgia, lymph anenopathy and general malaise Complications: meningitis, facial palsy, pericarditis	Caused by *Borrelia burgdorferi,* transmitted by infected ticks	Oral antibiotic administration (tetracycline) in early localized infection—educate parents Promote rest and fluid intake Anticipatory guidance to families in areas known to have ticks (bug repellant use, clothing covering legs)
Mumps	Acute viral disease, characterized by fever, swelling, and tenderness of one or more salivary glands. Potential complications, including meningoencephalitis	Spread by droplet and direct and indirect contact with saliva of infected person. Most infectious 48 hours prior to swelling	Prevent by vaccination (MMR) Isolate—respiratory precautions Treat symptoms: ice pack to neck and force fluids Watch for symptoms of neurological involvement: fever headache vomiting stiff neck
Rubeola (Measles)	Acute viral disease, characterized by conjunctivitis, bronchitis, Koplik's spots on buccal mucosa, dusky red and splotchy rash 3–4 days, and usually photophobia. Complications can be severe in respiratory tract, eye, ear, and nervous system. Incubation is 10–12 days.	Spread by droplet or direct contact	Symptomatic: rest until cough and fever subside, cool mist humidifier, force fluids, dim lights in room, tepid baths, lotion to relieve itching.
Rubella (German measles)	Viral infection, slight fever, mild coryza, and headache. Discrete pink-red maculopapules that last about three days. Incubation 14–21 days. Basically a benign disease	Spread by direct and indirect contact with droplets. Fetus may contract measles in utero if mother has the disease	Highly associated with congenital anomalies in fetus Symptomatic: bedrest until fever subsides Preventable by vaccine (MMR)

✦ **Appendix 15-7. PEDIATRIC COMMUNICABLE DISEASES** *(Continued)*

Disease	Characteristics	Transmission	Nursing Care
Diphtheria	Local and systemic manifestations: malaise, fever, cough with stridor. Toxin has affinity for renal, nerve, and cardiac tissue. Incubation 2–6 days or longer	Spread by droplets from respiratory tract or carrier	Antitoxin and antibiotic therapy to kill toxin. Strict bedrest to prevent exertion. Liquid or soft diet. Observe for respiratory obstruction/ depression—suctioning, humidified oxygen, and emergency tracheotomy may be necessary
Scarlet Fever	Usually seen in children 6–12 y.o. Incubation 1–7 days Manifested by sore throat, headache, abrupt, high fever, vomiting, then "beefy red" tonsils and "strawberry tongue." Sandpaper-like erythematous rash, spreads from chest and arms to abdomen, groin and buttocks. Complications: sinusitis, arthritis, glomerulonephritis, retropharyngeal or peritonsillar abscess	Caused by *Streptococcus* pyogenes (**Group A** β-hemolytic streptococci—GAS) Transmitted by droplets, direct contact with infected person or indirectly by contact with contaminated articles or food	Treat fever, sore throat Administer antibiotics (penicillin) Respiratory precautions until 24 hrs of antibiotics completed Encourage fluids
Tetanus (lockjaw)	Acute or gradual onset. Muscle rigidity and spasms, headache, fever, and convulsions. Death may result from aspiration, pneumonia, or exhaustion. Incubation 3–21 days	Organisms in soil that enter body through wound. Not communicable man to man.	Toxins must be neutralized. Bedrest during illness in quiet, darkened room. Avoid stimulation that can cause spasms. Observe for complications of laryngospasm and respiratory failure
Pertussis (whooping cough)	Dry cough occurring in paroxysms Dyspnea and fever may be present Lymphocytosis Incubation 5–21 days	Direct contact or droplet from infected person Infants at risk DPt series is complete	Symptomatic—keep warm, humidified air, bedrest Maintain nutritional status, encourage fluids Protect from secondary infections

✦ **Appendix 15-8. VITAL SIGNS FOR CHILDREN AT DIFFERENT AGES**

Vital Sign Chart

Age	Range of Normal Pulse	(Average)	Average Blood Pressure	Average Respiration
Newborn	100–180	140	90/60	30–50
1 year	80–150	120	96/65	20–40
2 years	80–130	110	99/65	20–30
4 years	80–120	100	99/65	20–25
6 years	75–115	100	100/56	20–25
8 years	70–110	90	105/56	15–20
10 years	70–110	90	110/58	15–20

Pulse

A. Increased rate is significant if maintained during sleep.

B. Body temperature elevation causes an increase of 8–10 pulse beats for each degree of elevation.

◆ Appendix 15-9. DENTAL DEVELOPMENT

Deciduous Teeth

	Age at Eruption		Age at Shedding	
	Maxillary	**Mandibular**	**Maxillary**	**Mandibular**
Central incisors	6–8 months	5–7 months	7–8 years	6–7 years
Lateral incisors	8–11	7–10	8–9	7–8
Cuspids	16–20	16–20	11–12	9–11
First molars	10–16	10–16	10–11	10–12
Second molars	20–30	20–30	10–12	11–13

Permanent Teeth

	Age at Eruption	
	Maxillary	**Mandibular**
Central incisors	7–8 years	6–7 years
Lateral incisors	8–9	7–8
Cuspids	11–12	9–11
First molars	6–7	6–7
Second molars	12–13	12–13
First premolars	10–11	10–11
Second premolars	10–12	11–13
Third molars	17–22	17–22

PEDIATRIC NURSING QUESTIONS

1. In assessing an infant with pyloric stenosis, which of the following clinical manifestations would be present?

   1. Palpable olive-size mass in the upper right quadrant.
   2. Visible peristaltic waves passing right to left during and after feeding.
   3. Severe projectile vomiting 1 hour after each feeding.
   4. Fluid overload, demonstrated by bulging fontanelles, widely separated cranial sutures, and urine specific gravity of 1.002.

2. When a child is admitted with the diagnosis of croup, why are cool mist vaporizers better to use than hot steam vaporizers?

   1. The temperature of the mist is irrelevant because the child needs humidity.
   2. More moisture can be delivered in cool mist than with hot steam.
   3. Small children are more resistant to anything that is hot.
   4. The cool mist relieves swelling in the airways and makes breathing easier.

3. A 4-year-old child with celiac disease is admitted to the hospital with abdominal pain, distention and vomiting. Intussusception is the suspected diagnosis. The nurse, in completing data collection, will ask the parents if the symptoms

   1. Occurred suddenly.
   2. Developed over the last few days.
   3. Were mild, but bothersome.
   4. Were preceded by the ingestion of certain foods.

4. When a toddler is hospitalized, the nurse knows that separation anxiety can be reduced by

   1. Having parents absent when painful procedures are performed.
   2. Not telling the toddler about upcoming painful experiences.
   3. Setting limits and routines for parental visits.
   4. Having parents present as much as possible, preparing for separations, and use of transitional objects ("Loveys").

5. The nurse will provide teaching to the parents of infants with gastroesophageal reflux. Included in these instructions will be directions to

   1. Feed the baby only when the baby is hungry.
   2. Maintain the desired positioning and adhere to a frequent feeding schedule.
   3. Allow the baby to complete the feeding before attempting to burp the baby.
   4. Place the baby in a supine position with the head of the bed elevated at least 45 degrees.

6. Which of the following characteristics of acute glomerulonephritis is it essential for the nurse to know in order to deliver comprehensive care to a 5-year-old child?

   1. Polyuria (increased urine output) is a clinical manifestation of this disorder.
   2. Acute glomerulonephritis is usually preceded by a streptococcal infection of the upper respiratory tract or skin.
   3. It is necessary to monitor for hypotension and tachycardia.
   4. Weight loss is a common clinical manifestation.

7. The most accurate area to check the pulse of an infant is at the

   1. Carotid artery.
   2. Apex of the heart.
   3. Brachial artery.
   4. Temporal artery.

8. An 8-year-old child with an acute asthma attack is admitted to the hospital. A priority assessment of the child will be

   1. Noisy, hoarse inspirations.
   2. Wheezing on expiration.
   3. Labored abdominal breathing.
   4. Flail chest with inspiratory wheeze.

9. A medication order for a child is for one fluid dram of liquid. The medication cup is measured in mLs. How many mLs will be administered?

   1. 1 mL.
   2. 4 mL.
   3. 8 mL.
   4. 30 mL.

10. The nurse is monitoring a child with hydrocephalus who has a ventriculoperitoneal (VP) shunt. What clinical manifestations will the nurse be most concerned about?

1. Growth spurt, increased appetite, and thirst.
2. Upper respiratory infection with coughing, a recent growth spurt, and a palpable shunt catheter.
3. Growth spurt, fever, and irritability changing to lethargy.
4. Diarrhea, recent weight loss, and a soft, round abdomen.

11. When providing diversional activities for a child in isolation, the nurse will remember that

   1. Any articles brought into the unit should be washable.
   2. These children are always on bedrest.
   3. The room is usually darkened to protect the child's eyes.
   4. Most children are satisfied with books.

12. In children, the period of negativism begins when the child

   1. Learns he can manipulate his or her parents.
   2. Copies negative behavior of siblings.
   3. Is struggling between dependence and independence.
   4. Is learning manual skills.

13. A 12-month-old child is admitted to the pediatric unit with suspected bronchiolitis. The priority assessment is

   1. Retractions and inspiratory stridor.
   2. Flaring nostrils and expiratory stridor with wheezing.
   3. Rapid, shallow respirations with subcostal retractions.
   4. Elevated temperature and expiratory stridor.

14. A child has been admitted to the pediatric unit with the diagnosis of congestive heart failure (CHF). The nurse will assess for *early* symptoms of CHF which include

   1. Arrhythmias and conduction blocks.
   2. Hypotension, decreased urine output, and weak pedal pulses.
   3. Cyanosis, peripheral edema, and bradycardia.
   4. Hepatomegaly, bulging fontanelles, and tachypnea.

15. Considering a 17-month-old child's developmental level, the most effective technique to reestablish nutritional status after the immediate postoperative period would be

   1. Semisoft foods QID.
   2. Finger foods at frequent intervals.

3. Regular diet put into a blender and given in liquid state.
4. A high-roughage diet.

16. A 2-year-old toddler was diagnosed with iron-deficiency anemia. Which of the following statements best describes the anemias of childhood?

   1. The clinical manifestations of anemia are directly related to the decrease in oxygen-carrying capacity of the blood.
   2. Significant deficiencies of all vitamins will result in reduced production of red blood cells.
   3. A 2-year-old child with a hemoglobin of 5 g/100 mL will not manifest signs and symptoms of the disorder.
   4. All anemias in childhood are potentially terminal.

17. The nurse has just completed data collection for a 4-year-old child. Which of the following findings is most characteristic of thrombocytopenia?

   1. Petechiae, hematuria, purpura.
   2. Urticaria, epistaxis, hypertension.
   3. Purpura, tachycardia, hypotension.
   4. Vertigo, petechiae, bradycardia.

18. When determining if a child has Down syndrome characteristics, which of the following would *not* be present?

   1. Abnormal palmar creases.
   2. Protruding tongue.
   3. Low-set ears.
   4. Loose joints and flaccid muscles.

19. When assessing clinical indicators of adequate cardiac output in children, which of the following signs are *most* important?

   1. Blood pressure, skin temperature, and capillary refill.
   2. Pedal pulses, blood pressure, and skin temperature.
   3. Pedal pulses, skin temperature, and capillary refill.
   4. Blood pressure, urine output, and skin temperature.

20. A mother with a 4-month-old infant comes to the clinic for a well-baby examination. The nurse advises the mother to change the formula she is feeding the baby to one that contains iron. The nurse explains that the reason for this is

   1. Iron is required by the infant's eyes as they begin to focus and develop.
   2. The infant requires extra iron to grow.

3. The infant's iron source from the mother is depleted.

4. The infant requires more iron for the breakdown of bilirubin.

21. Which of the following symptoms is the priority assessment because it is suggestive of a complication of a central nervous system infection?

    1. Separation of cranial sutures.
    2. Depressed anterior fontanelle.
    3. Oliguria.
    4. Photophobia.

22. A child with the diagnosis of Guillain–Barré syndrome would have which of the following nursing diagnoses included on the care plan?

    1. Fluid Volume Deficit; Impaired Gas Exchange; and Altered Nutrition.
    2. Ineffective Breathing Pattern; Pain; and Urinary Incontinence.
    3. Urinary Incontinence; Risk for Impaired Skin Integrity; and Ineffective Airway Clearance.
    4. Impaired Gas Exchange; Anticipatory Grieving; and Pain.

23. An obese 14 year old is admitted to the adolescent unit with a tentative diagnosis of type 1 diabetes mellitus. Adolescent diabetics frequently have more difficulty than diabetics in other age groups because

    1. The disease is usually more severe in adolescents than in younger children.
    2. Adolescents as a group have poor eating habits.
    3. Adolescents have a difficult time with long-acting insulin.
    4. Adolescents have difficulty regulating their insulin.

24. A first-grader was sent to the school nurse by her teacher because the teacher feared the child had lice in her hair. The most effective way of recognizing lice instead of dandruff is to know that

    1. Prepubescent children rarely have dandruff.
    2. There will be an area of alopecia on the nape of her neck.
    3. The child is scratching her head almost incessantly.
    4. Lice would not fall off the hair shaft when the hair is moved.

25. What anatomical condition must be present in order for an infant with complete transposition of the great vessels to survive at birth?

    1. Coarctation of the aorta.
    2. Large septal defect.

3. Pulmonic stenosis.
4. Mitral stenosis.

26. When taking the history from the mother of a baby who has pyloric stenosis, the nurse would expect her to say that the baby vomits

    1. Continuously.
    2. Immediately after feedings.
    3. Between feedings.
    4. When new foods are introduced.

27. A child with hemophilia A has experienced an episode of hemarthrosis. The first intervention is to

    1. Teach the parents to offer aspirin for comfort.
    2. Apply an ice pack.
    3. Encourage ambulation.
    4. Apply pressure for at least 5 minutes.

28. A child is admitted to the pediatric unit with a diagnosis of dehydration. The child weights 10 kg. Oral rehydration therapy is ordered, 40 mL/kg over 4 hours. The child will receive how many milliliters per hour?

    1. 100 mL/hour.
    2. 400 mL/hour.
    3. 200 mL/hour.
    4. 50 mL/hour.

29. Assessing a child with a possible cardiac condition, the nurse knows that a child with a large patent ductus arteriosus would exhibit which of the following symptoms?

    1. Often assumes a squatting position.
    2. Becomes cyanotic on exertion.
    3. Is acyanotic but has difficulty breathing after physical activity.
    4. Has breathing difficulty and is cyanotic with slight activity.

30. The correct position for a nurse to place an infant with extrophy of the bladder is

    1. Prone.
    2. Supine, flat.
    3. Side-lying.
    4. Trendelenburg's.

31. A young patient with cystic fibrosis is receiving dornase alfa (Pulmozyme). To check for the desired therapeutic effect, the nurse would monitor the patient's

    1. Weight.
    2. Lung sounds.
    3. Cardiac rhythm.
    4. Serum chloride.

32. Which one of the following therapeutic approaches would be appropriate in the nursing/ medical management of a 12 year old with juvenile rheumatoid arthritis?

    1. Encourage prolonged periods of complete joint immobilization.
    2. Apply warm compresses and night splints to the affected joint.
    3. Discourage the child's active participation in his care in the initial phases of the disease.
    4. Allow unlimited salicylates as necessary for control of pain.

33. A patient gave birth to a baby who weighed only 5 pounds and is considered premature. The infant will be on formula. One of the most important principles in providing nutrition is to use a

    1. Regular nipple with a large hole.
    2. Regular nipple.
    3. Preemie nipple for bottle feeding.
    4. Pacifier between feedings.

34. A mother calls the emergency hotline and asks how she should cope with a 7 year old who was just diagnosed with mumps. She has 3 other children at home and none have been vaccinated. What precautions should the nurse tell her about?

    1. No precautions; just symptomatic care for the child.
    2. Isolation precautions, especially respiratory.
    3. Airborne precautions.
    4. Indirect precautions.

35. To obtain an apical pulse on an infant, the diaphragm of the stethoscope is placed at the apex of the heart. When placing the diaphragm on the infant's chest, the nurse would locate it

    1. At the left nipple, where the heart's point of maximum impulse is located.
    2. To the left of the midclavicular line, at the third to fourth intercostal space.
    3. At the left edge of the sternum and fifth intercostal space.
    4. At the left midclavicular line and fifth intercostal space.

36. A 10-year-old child in respiratory difficulty is admitted to the emergency room and given a β-adrenergic drug with nebulized albuterol. The nurse observes that he is short of breath with circumoral cyanosis and sweating. The nursing action will be to

    1. Notify the physician immediately.
    2. Encourage the child to lie down and administer oxygen.
    3. Reassure the child that the medication will begin working soon.
    4. Encourage the child to sit upright and reassure the child to reduce fear and stress.

37. Once a child has had one poison ingestion, statistically he is nine times more likely to have another poisoning episode within the year. To prevent further poisoning incidents, the most important information the nurse should give to the child's mother is to

    1. Keep purses out of the child's reach.
    2. Never give medications to others in front of the child.
    3. Keep all cabinets locked at all times.
    4. Keep medicine only in high cupboards.

38. An infant radiant warmer is used in the newborn nursery to ensure maintenance of adequate body temperature. The major safety factor involved with the use of the warmer is for the nurse to

    1. Ensure the warmer is on manual control.
    2. Tape the thermometer skin probe in place.
    3. Inspect the skin under the temperature probe at routine intervals.
    4. Adjust temperature of the warmer each day to ensure it is set at 102°F.

39. Working with children who have acyanotic heart defects, the nurse is aware that

    1. Occurrence of cardiac failure is rare after the age of 6 months.
    2. Bacterial endocarditis is not a complication of acyanotic congenital heart disease.
    3. An infant or young child with acyanotic heart disease requires alteration in their activity level by their parents.
    4. Children with congenital heart disease are usually asymptomatic.

40. The nurse explains to the mother of a 1 year old that the child is more likely to have otitis media than her 13-year-old brother because

    1. Her hands are often contaminated when she crawls on the floor.
    2. She is still "cutting" new teeth.
    3. The angle of the child's eustachian tube is straighter than her brother's.
    4. She is not old enough to have learned how to "clear" her nasal passages.

41. With a diagnosis of hemophilia B, part of the teaching plan for a child's parents will include treatment measures to control minor bleeding episodes. These will include

1. Topical coagulants, cold packs, and constant pressure to affected areas.
2. Elevation of the affected area, oral anticoagulants, and warm compresses.
3. Gentian violet, ice packs, and pressure dressings.
4. Bedrest, topical coagulants, and cold compresses.

42. A mother of a 3-month-old infant asks the nurse if her baby can eat solid food now so she can sleep through the night. The appropriate response is to say

   1. "Infants obtain all the nutrients they need from the formula and they really can't digest foods well at that early age."
   2. "Infants at age 3 months do not usually sleep through the night, so solid food probably will not help this problem."
   3. "Rather than giving her solid food, it would be best to give the baby her bath at night to relax her and then she might sleep through the night."
   4. "It sounds like she's not getting enough food to satisfy her, so it is probably a good idea to start introducing solid food."

43. A 1 year old is hospitalized with bronchitis; she is receiving care for the respiratory condition. An appropriate toy for her would be a

   1. Book with pop-up pages.
   2. Set of blocks.
   3. Mobile hanging from the crib.
   4. Terry cloth teddy bear.

44. A 2-year-old boy has been admitted to the pediatric unit for a diagnostic workup. When his mother left, the child cried, screamed, and threw toys out of his bed. The nurse will recognize this behavior as

   1. A spoiled child.
   2. A sign of mental retardation.
   3. Separation anxiety.
   4. Normal.

45. An appropriate nursing intervention when caring for an infant with an acute upper respiratory infection and elevated temperature would be to

   1. Give frequent cold sponge baths to decrease the fever.
   2. Push solid food intake to maintain caloric needs.
   3. Give small amounts of clear liquids frequently to prevent dehydration.
   4. Dress the child warmly to prevent chilling.

46. The nurse is caring for a hospitalized toddler who was toilet trained at home. He wets his pants. The best response to this situation is to say

   1. "It's okay; try not to wet your pants next time."
   2. "That's okay; now let's get you cleaned up."
   3. "I know you understand how to use the toilet; what happened?"
   4. "Your mom told me you don't wet anymore; what's wrong?"

47. The nurse is completing a general assessment on a neonate. The nurse will suspect Hirschsprung's disease when the neonate

   1. Has foul smelling, ribbonlike stools and is anemic.
   2. Fails to pass meconium within 24–48 hours after birth and is reluctant to ingest fluids.
   3. Is continuously hungry and fails to gain weight.
   4. Has 7–8 watery, bile-containing stools in the first 24–48 hours after birth.

48. A mother calls the pediatric hotline and tells the nurse that her 3 year old has a virus and a fever. She asks how much aspirin she should give the child. The best response is

   1. "You'll have to call your physician."
   2. "Give her no more than 3 baby aspirin every 4 hours."
   3. "Give her Tylenol, not aspirin."
   4. "Follow directions on the aspirin bottle for her age and weight."

49. An infant was born with spina bifida and has remained on the pediatric unit for observation. The most important assessment would be to

   1. Measure head circumference daily.
   2. Monitor for contractures.
   3. Observe for signs of infection.
   4. Measure intake and output.

50. Important discharge instructions the nurse will give the parents of a child with frequent otitis media would include

   1. Proper administration of antibiotics, pain control, and reporting irritability that deteriorates to lethargy.
   2. Stopping the antibiotics when the acute pain is diminished to prevent developing resistance to the common antibiotics.
   3. Children should be kept away from school and other children and their activity restricted until the full course of medication is completed.
   4. Avoiding any additional dental work because of the likelihood of recurrence of otitis media.

PEDIATRIC NURSING

Answers with Rationale

1. (1) A small mass may be found in the upper right quadrant. Peristaltic waves pass left to right with this condition. Pyloric stenosis presents in early infancy with projectile vomiting right after feeding. Dehydration and electrolyte imbalances are possible complications if therapy is not performed; thus, fluid overload is not a symptom.

   NP:D; CN:PH; CL:A

2. (4) Swollen, irritated tissues will vasoconstrict, and swelling is reduced in response to cold and humidity. Humidity also helps loosen secretions. While amounts of moisture delivered may vary, the vasoconstriction offered by cold mist is most beneficial.

   NP:P; CN:PH; CL:C

3. (1) When intussusception is suspected, the nurse would validate the sudden onset of symptoms because this completes the classical picture of this condition. This is one of the most frequent causes of bowel obstruction in children, especially those with celiac or cystic fibrosis disease.

   NP:D; CN:PH; CL:A

4. (4) Parents and transitional objects have been shown in research to decrease anxiety. Having parents present as much as possible, especially for painful procedures, helps decrease anxiety. Explaining upcoming procedures in language the toddler can understand will also help decrease their anxiety.

   NP:P; CN:H; CL:C

5. (2) Positioning will decrease the amount of reflux and consistent feeding schedules will decrease the tendency to overfeed if the child is very hungry. Small meals tend to cause less reflux.

   NP:I; CN:PH; CL:A

6. (2) This is important to understand because antibiotics are one of the primary aspects of care if the disorder was preceded by an infection of group A beta-hemolytic streptococci. Answer (1) is wrong because there is decreased urine output with edema formation. Answer (3) is a complication.

   NP:P; CN:PH; CL:C

7. (2) The apical pulse at the apex of the heart, using a stethoscope, is the most reliable way to take an infant's pulse. The brachial artery can be used in checking the pulse of an infant, but it is difficult to locate. The carotid arteries (1) are difficult to locate in an infant.

   NP:P; CN:PH; CL:K

8. (2) The hallmark of asthma is wheezing. Wheezing is an expiratory sound. There is no vocal cord involvement so "hoarseness" (1) is unlikely. Abdominal breathing (3) does not occur with asthma. Flail chest, an unstable chest wall, is not present with asthma (4).

   NP:D; CN:PH; CL:A

9. (2) The answer is 4 mL because 4 mL is equal to one dram of fluid.

   NP:P; CN:PH; CL:A

10. (3) The major complications of VP shunts are infection and malfunction. Children can "outgrow" shunts or distal ends can dislodge after growth spurts. Fever can be a sign of an infected shunt, and irritability deteriorating to lethargy could be due to increased intracranial pressure (ICP) from a blocked shunt. Appetite usually decreases with increasing ICP; respiratory infections should not change shunt patency.

    NP:D; CN:PH; CL:AN

11. (1) Things that go into the room will have to be disinfected before they are removed, so they should be washable. The children are not always on

---

Coding for Questions/Answers Abbreviations: **Nursing Process: NP,** Data Collection: D, Planning: P, Implementation: I, Evaluation: E, **Client Needs: CN,** Safe, Effective Care Environment: S, Health Promotion and Maintenance: H, Psychosocial Integrity: PS, Physiological Integrity: PH, **Clinical Area: CA,** Medical Nursing: M, Surgical Nursing: S, Maternal/Newborn Nursing: MA, Pediatric Nursing: P, Psychiatric Nursing: PS, **Cognitive Level: CL,** Knowledge: K, Comprehension: C, Application: A, Analysis: AN

bedrest (2), nor does the room necessarily have to be dark (3).

NP:P; CN:H; CL:A

12. (3) Negativism begins as the child learns to do some things independently and then becomes frustrated by things he or she cannot do. This period begins at about 2 years and is normal for this stage of development. This behavior occurs naturally and does not depend on siblings, learning skills, or learning he/she can manipulate parents.

NP:P; CN:H; CL:C

13. (2) Low obstructive respiratory syndrome has expiratory stridor with a characteristic wheeze and grunt. The respirations are rapid and shallow because of severe long distention, but retractions are mild. Increased temperature is most likely in high obstructive respiratory conditions.

NP:A; CN:PH; CL:A

14. (4) A child's liver becomes engorged early in the disease process of CHF and hepatomegaly is easily palpated. Bulging fontanelles and tachypnea are signs of fluid overload. Arrhythmias and conduction changes (1) may occur later in response to hypoxia; cyanosis (3), hypotension, and decreased urine output (2) are *late* signs.

NP:D; CN:PH; CL:A

15. (2) The developmental period is the autonomy stage. The child wants to do things for himself and will respond well to finger foods offered frequently. If the child will eat a variety of nutritious finger foods, the nutritional status will be reestablished more effectively. Semisoft or blended food will not be as appealing to a 17 month old. High roughage is not appropriate during the post-operative period.

NP:P; CN:PH; CL:A

16. (1) Clinical manifestations of fatigability, anorexia, weakness, and tachycardia are a result of vitamin B_{12} and folic acid deficiency. This results in reduced production of red blood cells, and a 2-year-old child will manifest symptoms of this disorder.

NP:P; CN:PH; CL:C

17. (1) Thrombocytopenia (a platelet count 50,000 or below) is characterized by petechiae, purpura, and, on occasion, spontaneous hematuria. The lower the platelet count, the greater the risk of spontaneous bleeding.

NP:D; CN:PH; CL:C

18. (3) Although low-set ears are a sign of congenital defects, they are usually associated with some kidney problem. The other characteristics will be present with Down syndrome.

NP:D; CN:PH; CL:A

19. (3) Children can maintain normal blood pressure when experiencing serious hemodynamic deficits. Signs of peripheral perfusion change early in assessing decreased cardiac output and are reliable clinical indicators. Urine output is a late sign.

NP:D; CN:PH; CL:A

20. (3) Between 3 and 5 months, the infant has used the iron provided by the mother and requires further supplementation if bottle feeding. Options (1) and (4) are not accurate and while iron is important for growth, extra iron is not advised.

NP:I; CN:PH; CL:C

21. (1) Meningitis is a common CNS infection of infancy and early childhood. Increased intracranial pressure, which can accompany meningitis, accounts for separation of the cranial sutures, bulging not depressed (2) fontanelles, and/or projectile vomiting. Oliguria (3) and photophobia (4) are not symptoms common to CNS infection.

NP:E; CN:PH; CL:AN

22. (3) As paralysis progresses, urinary incontinence becomes a problem; skin can break down without frequent positioning changes and exercises. Airway problems are of major concern with ascending paralysis. Pain is generally not a problem, nor is gas exchange unless the airway is compromised and lung function affected by chest paralysis.

NP:P; CN:PH; CL:C

23. (2) As young adults start spending more time with their peer group, they frequently adopt eating habits of this group, which are often not appropriate for diabetics.

NP:E; CN:PS; CL:C

24. (4) Lice secrete a cementlike substance that allows them to hold tenaciously onto the hair shaft. Dandruff will easily brush off. Alopecia (2), loss of hair, will not occur. Often lice do not cause itching.

NP:D; CN:H; CL:C

25. (2) Because complete transposition results in two closed blood systems, the child can survive only if a large septal defect is present.

NP:D; CN:PH; CL:K

26. (2) Stenosis of the pyloric sphincter impedes gastric emptying; therefore, feedings are vomited immediately after feedings when the stomach is full.

NP:D; CN:PH; CL:C

27. (2) Ice will produce vasoconstriction to help control bleeding into the joint and promote comfort. Aspirin and ambulation will provoke further bleeding. Pressure to the joints is ineffective in controlling internal bleeding.

NP:I; CN:PH; CL:A

28. (1) Dehydration formula is usually 40–50 mL/kg over 4 hours. In this case the child would receive 400 mL every 4 hours or 100 mL/hour.

NP:AN; CN:S; CL:A

29. (3) PDA is acyanotic. Options (2) and (4) are cyanotic. If the ductus is large and much blood is shunted into the pulmonary circulation, there may be growth retardation and limitation of physical activity. Squatting (1) occurs with cyanotic disorders.

NP:D; CN:PH; CL:C

30. (3) Placing an infant in a side-lying position will promote the drainage of urine from the bladder and help reduce the risk of urinary tract infection.

NP:I; CN:PH; CL:A

31. (2) Dornase alfa reduces the viscosity of the sputum in patients with cystic fibrosis. Pulmonary function is improved and the incidence of respiratory tract infections is lessened. Lung sounds reflect the presence or absence of lung congestion, which may indicate infection and are, therefore, monitored closely as an indicator of the therapeutic effect of this drug.

NP:E; CN:PH; CL:A

32. (2) Warm compresses will help to relieve the pain and night splints are important. During an exacerbation of this childhood disorder, hospitalization is usually required; however, affected joints should *not* be immobilized for extended periods of time (1) as residual effects (joint atrophy) will ensue. Active participation in care (3) should be encouraged in all stages of the disease. Unlimited salicylates (4) could be dangerous to the child.

NP:P; CN:PH; CL:C

33. (3) A regular nipple is too hard, even one with a large hole in it, and will make it difficult for the infant to suck, causing unnecessary fatigue. Use a preemie soft nipple.

NP:I; CN:H; CL:K

34. (2) The child should be isolated from the other children because mumps is spread by droplet, direct and indirect contact via the respiratory tract as well as saliva. Options (3) and (4) are incomplete.

NP:I; CN:S; CL:A

35. (2) This is the appropriate location on an infant's chest for an apical pulse. Over age 7, the apical pulse is found at the location described in answer (4).

NP:I; CN:PH; CL:C

36. (4) The child's immediate situation needs to be addressed before calling the physician. The nebulized albuterol and medication are usually effective immediately. Breathing is more effective in an upright position; and reassuring the child will help to improve breathing.

NP:I; CN:PH; CL:AN

37. (3) The other answers are also necessary information, but keeping cabinets locked is critical. It is not enough to keep only medicine in high cupboards (4) because other products, such as cleaning materials, can be poison. The child's mother should also be given the telephone number of a poison control center.

NP:I; CN:H; CL:A

38. (3) The probe can cause irritation. If this occurs, the probe is placed in a different location. An infant's skin is very delicate and becomes irritated easily. The warmer should be on automatic, not manual. The thermometer is not taped in place and the temperature should not exceed 102° F.

NP:P; CN:S; CL:A

39. (1) Cardiac failure rarely occurs after the age of 6 months. If the child has gone 6 months without failure, then either the cardiac problem is not severe or the child is compensating successfully. Bacterial endocarditis is a possible complication (2), and usually a child sets his own pace of activity (3).

NP:P; CN:PH; CL:C

40. (3) It is easier for infectious agents to travel from the nasopharyngeal area to the middle ear in younger than in older children because the eustachian tube is straighter when they are younger.

NP:I; CN:PH; CL:C

41. (1) Local measures that sometimes help control minor bleeding episodes are topical coagulants, constant pressure, and cold packs (which cause vasoconstriction) to the bleeding areas. The other

options will not help to control minor bleeding episodes.

NP:I; CN:H; CL:A

42. (1) Studies have indicated that breast milk or formula will provide sufficient nutrition to infants up to 6 months and even 1 year. Many pediatricians begin introducing solid food about 6 months of age, because infants cannot easily digest food before this time. Sleeping patterns for infants vary on an individual basis and the introduction of solid food does not ensure a full night's sleep.

NP:I; CN:H; CL:A

43. (4) Because the child is in a mist tent, she will need a toy that can get wet, then dry out. A book (1) might not last in this misty environment. The blocks (2) would be difficult to play with and the mobile (3) is for a younger child.

NP:P; CN:H; CL:AN

44. (3) This is the protest (first) stage of separation anxiety. Because this is an expected reaction to hospitalization at this age, it may also be considered normal, but this is not as specific an answer as (3).

NP:E; CN:H; CL:C

45. (3) Small amounts of liquid are tolerated better, preventing gastric distention and impingement on the diaphragm causing further distress. Large amounts of fluids are lost through the respiratory tract with increased rate and effort, so fluid must be replaced; solids (2) are often not tolerated. Tepid sponge baths are helpful; cold baths (1) are not appropriate.

NP:I; CN:PH; CL:A

46. (2) The nurse knows that children tend to regress when under the stress of hospitalization, so it is important not to make a judgment or imply that the child should know better. The best approach: be matter-of-fact, not blaming.

NP:I; CN:H; CL:A

47. (2) These are signs of decreased autonomic innervation to the colon—classic Hirschsprung's disease. The other answers indicate other intestinal disorders.

NP:D; CN:PH; CL:C

48. (3) Children from 2 months to adolescence are advised not to take aspirin with a viral infection due to the connection to Reye's syndrome, and acute encephalopathy condition. Tylenol is the treatment of choice for any virus infection. This is a nurse's area of knowledge and they physician does not need to be contacted.

NP:I; CN:PH; CL:C

49. (1) While all of the assessments would be done, the most important is to measure head circumference daily. An increase in size would indicate a neurological condition developing (hydrocephalus is a frequent complication). Infection (3) might occur in the urinary tract; I&O (4) is also related to the possible urological complications. Contractures (2) could be prevented through proper positioning.

NP:D; CN:PH; CL:A

50. (1) A full course of antibiotics is necessary to destroy the causative organism. Any change in neurological status could be a developing CNS infection (e.g., meningitis). Children usually feel able to return to school after 24–48 hours of antibiotics, and will self-limit their own activity. Avoiding dental hygiene (4) is not advised nor helpful in preventing otitis media.

NP:I; CN:P; CL:CH

Mental Health Nursing 16

MENTAL HEALTH CONTINUUM

Mental Illness

Definition: Mental illness is the general term that is used for a variety of behavioral reactions to life stresses that range from severe personality disorganization to the milder forms of temporary inability to cope with daily stress. Mental health, according to the World Health Organization, is "the presence of physical and emotional well-being."

Characteristics

◆ A.   Mental illness is a major health problem in the United States. One out of three individuals experiences some form of mental illness during a period of his or her life.
   B.   There has been an ever-increasing number of patients admitted to mental hospitals or special units in private hospitals.
   C.   The criteria of mental illness might be said to be the extent to which problems are not dealt with through rational decisions.
   D.   *See* Table 16-1, Mental Assessment Summary.

Community Mental Health Movement

A.   National Mental Health Act placed emphasis on the quality of care hospitalized mentally ill patients received.
B.   It also emphasized the level of skills necessary to deliver higher-quality care and lower rate of chronic hospitalized patients.
C.   Object of act was to alter the state hospital model, which was linked to chronicity and severity of disease.
D.   Primary objectives were stated as preventing mental illness, coping with symptoms of illness, and returning the patient to community as soon as possible.

Anxiety

◆ *Definition:*   Anxiety is an affective state that is subjectively experienced as a response to an internal or external threat, real or imagined. It is experienced as a painful, vague uneasiness; tension; or diffuse apprehension. It is a form of energy whose presence is inferred from its effect on attention, behavior, learning, and perception.

Table 16-1. MENTAL ASSESSMENT SUMMARY

General appearance, manner, and attitude
Assess *physical appearance.*
Note *grooming,* mode of dress, and *personal hygiene.*
Note *posture.*
Note speed, pressure, pace, quantity, volume, and diction of *speech.*
Note relevance, content, and organization of *responses.*

Expressive aspects of behavior
Note *general motor* activity.
Assess *purposeful movements* and *gestures.*
Assess style of *gait.*

Consciousness
Assess *level of consciousness.*

Thought processes and perception
Assess coherency, logic, and relevance of *thought processes.*
Assess *reality orientation:* time, place, and person.
Assess *perceptions* and reactions to stimuli.
Assess mutism; ability to respond.

Thought content and mental trend
Ask questions to determine general themes that identify *degree of anxiety.*
Assess ideation and concentration.

Mood or affect
Assess prevailing or variability in mood by observing behavior and asking questions such as "How are you feeling right now?" Check for presence of abnormal *euphoria.*
If you suspect *depression,* continue questioning to determine depth.

Memory
Assess *past and present memory* and *retention* (ability to listen).
Assess *recall* (recent and remote).

Judgment
Assess *judgment* and interpretations.

Insight
Assess *insight,* the ability to understand.

Intelligence and fund of information
Assess *intelligence.*
Assess *fund of information.*

Sensory ability
Assess the five *senses.*

Developmental level
Assess patient's *developmental level.*

Addictive patterns
Identify *addictive patterns.*

Coping devices and defense mechanisms
Identify *defense-coping mechanisms* and their effect.

Characteristics

✦ A. Anxiety is subjectively perceived by the conscious portion of the personality.

B. It can occur as a result of conflicts between the personality and the environment or between different aspects within the personality.

C. It may be a reaction to threats of deprivation of something vital to the person, biologically or emotionally.

D. The individual may be unaware of the conflicts.

E. The degree of anxiety is in relation to its effect on the individual.

F. Level of anxiety is influenced by:
  1. The extent to which the self feels threatened.
  2. The extent to which behavior reduces anxiety.

G. Varying levels of anxiety are common to all individuals at one time or another.

H. Anxiety can be transmitted from individual to individual.

I. Realistic anxiety can be constructive.

✦ J. Anxiety may be placed on a continuum of degrees.
  1. Absent (ataraxia).
    a. Uncommon or under influence of drugs.
    b. Apparent in the person who takes drugs.
    c. Indicator of a low level of motivation.
  2. Mild.
    a. Senses are alert.
    b. Attentiveness is heightened.
    c. Motivation is increased.
  3. Moderate.
    a. Selective inattention because it narrows perception.
    b. Point at which it becomes pathological depends on individual.
    c. May be seen as behaviors that are complaining, arguing, teasing.
    d. Can convert to physical symptoms, such as headache, low back pain, nausea, diarrhea.
  4. Severe.
    a. All senses gravely affected—extremely painful psychologically.
    b. Nursing intervention always indicated.
    c. Cannot be used constructively by patient.
    d. Defense mechanisms may be used to control severe levels of anxiety.
    e. Behavior becomes automatic.
  5. Panic.
    a. Individual is overwhelmed.
    b. Personality may disintegrate.
    c. Condition is now pathological.
    d. Anxiety cannot be tolerated very long.
    e. Individual cannot control his or her behavior—feels helpless.
    f. Behavior wild and desperate, causing possible bodily harm to self and others.
    g. Needs immediate intervention.
      (1) Constant presence of attendant.
      (2) Medication.
      (3) Nonstimulating environment.

K. Anxiety is always present in emotional disorders.

L. Physiological reactions to anxiety.
  1. Increased heart rate.
  2. Increased or decreased appetite.
  3. Increased blood supply to skeletal muscles.
  4. Tendency to void.
  5. Dry mouth.
  6. "Butterflies" in stomach, nausea, vomiting, cramps, diarrhea.
  7. "Fight or flight" response.

Implementation

A. Intervene when patient is unable to cope with anxiety or is ineffective in reducing it.

B. Be aware of own anxiety—may escalate patient's anxiety.

C. Maintain positive attitude toward patient.
  1. Acceptance.
  2. Matter-of-fact approach.
  3. Willingness to listen and help.
  4. Calmness and support.

D. Recognize anxiety-produced behavior.

E. Provide activities that decrease anxiety and provide a physical outlet for energy.

F. Establish nurse–patient relationship.
  1. Allow patient to express feelings.
  2. Proceed at patient's pace.
  3. Avoid forcing patient to express feelings.
  4. Assist patient in identifying anxiety.
  5. Assist patient in learning new ways of dealing with anxiety.

G. Provide appropriate physical environment.
  1. Nonstimulating.
  2. Structured.
  3. Arrange to prevent physical exhaustion or self-harm.

H. Administer medication as directed and, after assessment, as needed.

ANXIETY DISORDERS

Definition: A mild to moderately severe psychological disorder that affects thought and feeling processes. The individual suppresses and represses unpleasant thoughts and/or feelings to alleviate the discomfort of the resulting anxiety. The consequent conflicts are handled by means of anxiety reaction, phobias, obsessive–compulsive reaction, dissociation, hypochondriasis, and neurasthenia.

Characteristics

A. No apparent physiologic basis for symptoms.

B. Threats to ego cause anxiety, and ego protects the person by developing defenses.

C. A neurosis is an attempt to deal with anxiety.

D. Behavior is affected by anxiety.
   1. Individuals have little difficulty talking, but conversation may be vague and unrevealing.
   2. Individual is generally unaware of his or her behavior patterns.
   3. Behavior becomes stereotyped and rigid.
   4. Individual becomes more dependent as time goes on.

E. Secondary gains from anxiety become associated problems.
   1. These are the fringe benefits that patient receives from symptoms.
   2. Secondary gains reinforce maladaptive behavior.

F. Common defense mechanisms include repression and projection.

G. Evidence of low self-esteem is observable.

H. No gross distortion of reality (as is seen in schizophrenia).

I. Personality is not grossly disorganized.

J. The martyr syndrome is common.

Implementation

✦ A. Remain with extremely anxious patient.

B. Nurse needs to understand and recognize own feelings and attitudes in dealing with anxiety.

C. Convey an attitude of acceptance and understanding of patient's symptoms because patient relies on them to control anxiety.

✦ D. Plan nonthreatening activities that will reduce anxiety and enhance self-esteem.

E. Do not make unreasonable demands on the patient.

F. Avoid using labels for patient's behaviors.

✦ G. Provide a safe, supportive environment.

H. Be alert to the specific needs of patient as demonstrated by his or her behavior.

Generalized Anxiety Disorder (GAD)

A. Anxiety is diffuse (free-floating).

B. Anxiety cannot be controlled by means of defense mechanisms.

✦ C. Psychological symptoms.
   1. Cannot concentrate on work.
   2. Feels depressed and guilty.
   3. Harbors fears of sudden death or insanity.
   4. Dreads being alone.
   5. Confused.
   6. Tense.
   7. Agitated and restless.

✦ D. Physiological symptoms.
   1. Tremors.
   2. Dyspnea.
   3. Palpitations.
   4. Tachycardia.
   5. Numbness of extremities.

E. Specific nursing approaches.
   1. Calm, serene approach with recognition of own anxiety.
   2. Nonverbal reassurance.
   3. Listen.
   4. Provide physical outlet for anxiety.
   5. Remain with patient.
   6. Decrease environmental stimuli.

Phobic and Panic Disorders

A. By means of displacement, anxiety is transferred from the original source to a symbolic idea or situation.

B. Phobic disorders are classified into types.
   ✦ 1. Agoraphobia—most common form.
      a. Marked fear of and avoidance of being alone or in public places where escape might be difficult or help not available in case of sudden incapacitation.
      b. Increasing constriction of normal activities until fear dominates the individual's life.
   2. Acrophobia—fear of high places.
   ✦ 3. Social phobia.
      a. A persistent irrational fear and compelling desire to avoid a situation in which the individual is exposed to scrutiny by others.
      b. Fear of acting in a way that may be humiliating or embarrassing.
      c. Distress about disturbance and feelings.
   4. Simple phobia.
      a. A persistent irrational fear and compelling desire to avoid simple objects or situations.
      b. Distress about symptoms.

✦ C. Panic attacks.
   1. Characterized by recurrent attacks of severe anxiety lasting minutes to hours.
   2. Symptoms: palpitations, sweating, shaking, dyspnea, fear of losing control, fear of dying.
   3. Attacks appear suddenly with no warning—may become associated with specific situations.

✦ D. Specific nursing approaches.
   1. Slowly develop a trusting relationship with the patient.
   2. Do not force patient into feared situations.
   3. Divert patient's attention from the phobia.
   4. Direct patient's focus to awareness of self.
   5. Encourage but do not force patient to discuss fears and feelings.
   6. Support patient during program of phobic desensitization.
      a. Programs for fear of flying or elevators are examples of desensitization.

b. Virtual reality software programs are helping patients to desensitize from phobias.

Obsessive–Compulsive Disorder

✦ A. Anxiety is associated with the persistence of undesired ideas, impulses, or images; repetitive ritualistic actions alleviate anxiety.
   B. Specific nursing approaches.
   ✦ 1. Avoid punishment or criticism for compulsive repetition of acts.
      2. Set limits to protect patient from harmful acts.
      3. Provide climate of acceptance and understanding.
      4. Orient nursing care around patient's need to perform rituals.
      5. Provide for patient's physical needs.

Post-Traumatic Stress Disorder

✦ *Definition:* Condition follows a traumatic event that is outside the range of common experience (military combat, rape, assault, etc.).

Characteristics
   A. Traumatic event is consistently reexperienced in dream state, as flashbacks, connected to events that trigger memory.
   B. As event is reexperienced, patient suffers behavioral and emotional symptoms (difficulty sleeping, irritability).
   C. Individual is not able to adjust to the event.
   D. Persistent avoidance of stimuli associated with trauma occurs.

Assessment
   A. Symptoms of anxiety and depression.
   B. Nightmares, difficulty falling/staying asleep.
   C. Angry outbursts.
   D. Feelings of detachment, guilt.
   E. Flat affect, emotionally labile.

Implementation
✦ A. Implement treatment protocol for anxiety disorders.
   B. Assist patient to go through recovery process.
      1. Deal with conscious awareness of traumatic experience.
      2. Adjust to acceptance of experience.
   C. Protect patient from self-destructive behaviors or acting-out behaviors.

Defense Mechanisms

✦ *Definition:* Defense mechanisms are automatic, psychological methods that are used by an individual to relieve or decrease anxieties caused by internal or external dangers or stressors (*see* Table 16-2).

Characteristics
✦ A. The purpose of adjustive techniques is to attempt reduction of anxiety and reestablishment of equilibrium.
   B. An individual's adjustment depends on the ability to vary responses so that anxiety is decreased.
   C. Individuals use essentially the same techniques, which may vary in form.
   D. The exercise of a defense mechanism may be a conscious process, but it is usually generated at the unconscious level.
   E. Defense mechanisms are compromise solutions (*see* Table 16-2) that include many forms.
   F. Healthy adjustment to life forces.
      1. A healthy adjustment is characterized by:
         a. Infrequent need to use unconscious adjustive techniques.
         b. Ability to form new responses.
         c. Ability to change external environment.
         d. Ability to modify one's own needs.
   ✦ 2. Healthy adjustment mechanisms may include rationalization, sublimation, compensation, and suppression.
✦ G. Unhealthy adjustment to life forces.
      1. An unhealthy adjustment is characterized by:
         a. The inability or loss of ability to vary responses.
         b. The individual's retreat from the problem or from reality.
         c. Continual use, which may interfere with maintenance of self-image.
      2. Unhealthy defense mechanisms may include regression, repression, denial, projection, and isolation.

Implementation
   A. Be aware of your own behavior and the use of defense mechanisms.
   B. Avoid criticizing the patient's behavior.
   C. Assist the patient in learning new or alternative techniques for healthier adaptation.
   D. Use techniques to help alleviate the patient's anxiety.
   E. Do not attempt to arbitrarily eliminate defense mechanisms without replacement—they serve a purpose for the patient.

MOOD (AFFECTIVE) DISORDERS

Manic Episode of Bipolar Disorder

✦ *Definition:* One manifestation of an affective disorder that involves mood swings of elation, euphoria, and grandiose behavior with or without a history of depression.

✦ Table 16-2. DEFENSE MECHANISMS

Compensation	Covering up a lack or weakness by emphasizing a desirable trait, or making up for a frustration in one area by overemphasis in another area. Learned early in childhood and may be recognized in adult behavior; for example, the physically handicapped individual who is an outstanding scholar.
Denial	Refusal to face reality. The ego protects itself from unpleasant pain or conflict by rejecting obvious facts or truth. Example: A person's not seeing a doctor because he does not want to know the truth. Individual who avoids reality by becoming ill.
Displacement	Discharging pent-up feelings from one object to a less dangerous object. Example: Your supervisor yells at you and you yell at your husband.
Dissociation	Emotional conflict is handled by altering consciousness, identity, memory or perception. Example is amnesia for an event that was traumatic.
Fantasy	Gratification by imaginary achievements and wishful thinking. Example: Children's play.
Fixation	Persistence into later life of interests and behavior patterns appropriate to an earlier age.
Identification	Assumption of desirable personality attributes of one admired. Satisfaction can be derived from assuming the success or the experience of others. Example: Nurse who feels sick watching a traumatic procedure on her patient.
Insulation	Passive withdrawal. Inaccessible to avoid further threatening circumstances. Sometimes the person appears cold and indifferent to his surroundings. Insulation is usually harmless, but can become very serious if it prevents interaction with others.
Isolation	Walling off of certain ideas, attitudes, or feelings. Isolation is separating the feelings from the intellect, by putting our emotions concerning a specific traumatic event into an isolated compartment. Example: An individual talks about a significant situation such as an accident or death without a display of feelings. This pattern can be positive if used temporarily to keep the ego from being overwhelmed.
Projection	Attribution of one's own undesirable traits to someone else. Example: The child who says to a parent, "You hate me," after the parent has spanked the child. In an adult, this technique may be a predominant indicator of paranoia. The paranoid patient projects hate for others by saying that others are out to get him or her.
Rationalization	The attempt that is almost universally employed to prove or justify behavior. It is face saving to give a reason that is acceptable rather than the real reason, as in remarks such as, "It wasn't worth it anyway" and "It's all for the best." This mechanism relieves anxiety temporarily and helps the person avoid facing reality.
Reaction-Formation	Prevention of dangerous feelings and desires from being expressed by exaggerating the opposite attitude—a kind of denial. The overly neat, polite, conscientious individual may have an unconscious desire to be untidy and carefree. The behavior becomes pathological when it interferes with tasks or produces anxiety and frustration.
Regression	Resorting to an earlier developmental level in order to deal with reality. Regression is an immature way of responding, and is frequently seen during a physical illness. It is sometimes used to an extreme degree by the mentally ill, who may regress all the way back to infancy.
Repression	The unconscious process in which undesirable and unacceptable thoughts are kept from entering the conscious. This repressed material may be the motivation for some of our behavior. The superego is largely responsible for repression; the stronger, more punitive the superego, the more emotion will be repressed. The child who is frustrated and downtrodden by a parent may rebel in later life against authority.
Sublimation	The mechanism by which a primitive or unacceptable tendency is redirected into socially constructive channels. This adjustment pattern is at least partly responsible for many artistic and cultural achievements, such as painting and poetry.
Suppression	The act of keeping unpleasant feelings and experiences from awareness.
Symbolization	An idea or object used by the conscious mind to represent an actual event or object. Sometimes the meaning is not clear because the symbol may be representative of something unconscious. Children use symbolization in this way and have to learn to distinguish between the symbol and the thing being symbolized. Examples include obsessive thoughts or behavior (handwashing, cleansing) and the incoherent speech of the schizophrenic (by the time the painful thoughts reach the surface, they are so jumbled that they lose their painfulness).
Undoing	A specific action is performed that is considered to be the opposite of a previously unacceptable action. This action is felt to neutralize or "undo" the original action. Example: Lady MacBeth rubbing and washing her hands.

Characteristics

A. Specific etiology is unknown. May be related to a genetic predisposition to illness or to increased levels of dopamine in the brain. Attempts are now being made to discover why lithium is therapeutic in hopes of solving the mystery of manic illness.

B. Women experience this illness slightly more frequently than men. The lifetime risk of developing this illness is 1 to 2 percent of the population.

C. The first manic episode usually occurs before age 30 and, interestingly, is more common in the higher socioeconomic group.

✦ D. Mania refers to a pronounced, elated, high mood that is evidenced by a high level of activity and general demeanor of cheerfulness. (*See* Table 16-3.)

✦ E. Cyclothymic disorder is the second category of bipolar disorder and refers to a milder form of the same illness.
   1. No severe manic or depressive episodes.
   2. Diagnosis is after patient has experienced chronic mood swings from hypomanic to depressive episodes for 2 years.

F. Hypomanic disorder—a less extreme form of mania.
   1. Mood swings not severe enough to require hospitalization.
   2. Mild elation, euphoria, "high."
   3. Therapeutic intervention and medication usually not necessary.

G. Mixed episode.
   1. Both manic and depressive episodes are experienced almost every day.
   2. Episodes are severe and require hospitalization.

✦ Assessment

A. Mood is one of euphoria, which can lead to grandiose behavior and delusions.

✦ B. Individual overresponds to stimuli.
   1. Rapid talk, with play on words and *flight of ideas.*
   2. Increased motor activity.
   3. Increased thought processes.

C. Individual exercises poor judgment, i.e., spends money foolishly, runs up charge accounts, erratically gives away belongings, etc.

D. Individual's attitude is narcissistic and will not tolerate guidance or criticism.

E. Individual gives little attention to physical health.
   1. Poor sleep habits with no apparent fatigue.
   2. Poor nutrition.
   3. Poor, or even bizarre, habits of grooming.

F. Behavior varies from delightful and playful to restless, irritable, sarcastic, and even antagonistic and combative.

✦ **Table 16-3. AFFECTIVE ILLNESS**

Depression Type	Distinguishing Feature
Bipolar	
Manic–depressive	History of elation episodes disorder with depression
Cyclothymic	Same history—milder disorder symptoms
Mixed episodes	Both features
Unipolar	
Manic episode	History of mania, without history of depression
Major depressive	History of depression without disorder any history of elation
Depression with psychotic features	
Hypomania	Less extreme form of mania
Dysthymic disorder	
Depressive neurosis	Symptoms of depression fluctuate but are less severe

G. If behavior is not controlled, the individual will become incoherent, overtly aggressive, and hostile.

✦ H. With no intervention, condition may progress to delirium, a dangerous state of excitement and exhaustion.

Implementation

✦ A. Maintain safe environment.
   1. Reduce external stimuli such as noise, people, and motion.
   2. Eliminate patient's participation in competitive activities.
   3. Redirect patient's energy into brief but useful activities.

✦ B. Establish a nurse–patient relationship.
   1. Maintain an accepting and nonjudgmental attitude.
   2. Create conditions favorable to the development of mutual trust.
   3. Avoid entering into patient's playful, joking activity if it appears to be a manic reaction.
   4. Allow the patient to verbalize his or her feelings, especially hostility.

✦ C. Set realistic limits on behavior.
   1. Set scope and limitations to behavior to provide for a sense of security.
   2. Restrain destructive behavior.
   3. Be firm and consistent.

✦ D. Give attention to physical needs.
   1. Provide a diet that is high in calories, vitamins, and fluids.
   2. Ensure adequate rest and sleep.
   3. Protect patient from inadvertent self-harm.

Major Depressive Episode/Disorder

Definition: A condition in which the feeling state of the individual is abnormal and manifests itself by a complex of symptoms. The symptoms may be mild and only slightly debilitating or pathological, implying overwhelming intensity and long duration.

Characteristics

✦ A. The most common of all psychiatric illnesses, depression is a symptom probably experienced by 15 out of 100 adults in our society. The most common age for adult onset is between 25 and 44 years.

B. One cause is now thought to involve a genetic link; other possible causes are personality traits such as low self-esteem, neurochemical imbalances, and other biological factors.

C. Most acute depressive episodes are self-limiting and last from a few weeks (with treatment) to a few months.

D. More than half of those persons who experience a first episode go on to suffer a recurrence.

E. About 20 to 25 percent never return to their pre-morbid state of mental health.

F. May be a single episode or recurrent (2 or more) episodes.

Assessment

✦ A. The distinguishing quality of depression is mood; affect is one of sadness or gloom.

✦ B. Behavior is slowed down, with purposeful movement nearly diminished.

✦ C. Personal appearance is neglected.

D. Thought processes are slowed down until there is paucity of thinking.

✦ E. Attitudes are pessimistic and self-denigrating, and focus is on the problems and uselessness of life. The individual lacks inner resources and strengths to cope effectively.

F. Physical symptoms usually reflect a preoccupation with body and poor health. Weight loss, insomnia, and general malaise are typically in evidence.

G. Social interaction is reduced and inappropriate. The depressed patient feels isolated but cannot resolve that condition because he or she cannot contribute to a relationship.

H. A common outcome of depression is possible suicide (refer to section on Suicide).

Major Depressive Subtypes

✦ **Dysthymic Disorder**

✦ A. Characterized by a chronic depressive syndrome (mild to moderate in degree) that is present for most of the day.

   1. Mild symptoms are present for at least 2 years.

   2. Depression may be episodic or constant.

B. Psychosis is not present.

C. Several of the following symptoms are usually present with this diagnosis.

   1. Low energy level.

   2. Loss of interest in pleasurable activities.

   3. Pessimistic attitude toward the future; thoughts of suicide.

   4. Tearful, crying demeanor.

   5. Feelings of low self-esteem.

   6. Decreased ability to concentrate.

Seasonal Affective Disorder (SAD)

A. Change in mood or depression influenced by lack of natural light at a particular time of the year.

   1. Relationship between sunlight, biological rhythm and depressed mood.

   2. Condition occurs mostly in winter months when natural (sun) light is decreased—disappears in spring and summer.

B. Application of full-spectrum light through special light bulbs or lamps appears to alleviate or lessen disorder.

Implementation

✦ A. Provide a safe milieu, and protect the patient from self-injury (prevent suicide).

✦ B. Provide a structured environment to mobilize the patient.

   1. Encourage daily activities, and allow time for them.

   2. Provide stimulation for occupational and recreational activity.

   3. Reactivate interests outside of the patient's present concerns.

   4. Motivate patient for treatment.

   5. Encourage psychotherapy and occupational therapy activities.

C. Build trust through nurse–patient relationship.

   1. Employ a supportive and unchallenging approach.

   2. Project behaviors and attitudes that are accepting and nonjudgmental.

   3. Show interest. Listen and give positive reinforcement.

   4. Redirect the patient's monologue away from painful and depressing thoughts.

   5. Focus on the patient's underlying anger, and encourage its expression.

D. Help build the self-esteem of the patient.

   1. Encourage simple tasks that invite successful experiences.

   2. Limit decision making with the severely depressed.

   3. Support use of defenses to alleviate suffering.

E. Be attentive to the patient's physical needs: provide adequate nutrition and opportunity for sleep and exercise.

Suicide

Definition: The act of killing oneself intentionally.

Characteristics

✦ A. Suicide is the seventh most common cause of death in the United States today.

B. Suicide statistics.
1. Suicide ranks fourth as the cause of death in the 15 to 40 age group.
2. For every successful suicide, it is believed that there are 5 to 10 attempted suicides.
3. Women make more suicide attempts than men.
4. Suicide is more common in the elderly age group.
5. Adolescent suicide is increasing.
6. Suicides are incurred by means of auto accidents; because they are not reported as such, statistics remain low.

✦ C. Causes of suicide attempts.
1. Depression is the primary cause.
2. The secondary cause is alcohol.
3. Inability to cope with problems in living.
4. Attempts to control others.

✦ D. Depressed individuals, when severely ill, rarely commit suicide.
1. They do not have the drive and energy to make a plan and follow it through when severely depressed.
2. Danger period is when depression begins to lift.

✦ E. Eight out of 10 known suicide cases give warnings or messages through direct or indirect means.

F. Danger symptoms range from depression, disorientation, and defiance to intense dependence on another.

✦ Assessment

✦ A. Recognize level of depression and potential for suicide (when depression begins to lift).

✦ B. Determine presence of suicide ideation.

C. Observe behavior closely as clues to potential suicide.

D. Listen to verbalization to determine what is meaningful for patient.

E. Observe physical status so you can intervene if necessary (if patient is not eating, sleeping, etc.).

F. Recognize ambivalence when patient is considering suicide.

Implementation

✦ A. Provide safe environment to protect patient from self-destruction.

✦ B. Observe closely at all times, especially when depression is lifting.

C. Establish supportive relationship, letting the patient know you are concerned for his welfare.

D. Encourage expression of feelings, especially anger.

✦ E. Determine patient's capacity to entertain suicide ideas.
1. Ask questions such as, "Are you thinking of suicide?" "Did you think you might do something about it?" "What?" "Have you taken any steps to prepare?" "What are they?"
2. Important to recognize a continued desire to commit suicide.

F. Determine the lethality of a suicide plan (details of the plan, lethality of proposed method—gun versus pills—and availability of means).

G. Focus on strengths and successful experiences that can enhance self-esteem.

✦ H. Follow a structured schedule, and involve the patient in activities with others.

I. Work out a plan for coping when patient next experiences ideas of suicide.

J. Help the patient plan for continued professional support after discharge.

SOMATOFORM DISORDERS

✦ *Definition:*   Somatoform disorders (also called *psychosomatic disorders*) are physical symptoms that may involve any organ system, and whose etiologies are, in part, precipitated by psychological factors.

Characteristics

A. An individual must adapt and adjust to stresses in life.
1. The way a person adapts depends on individual characteristics and extent of one's inner stability.
2. Emotional stress may exacerbate or precipitate an illness.

B. Psychosocial stress or anxiety is an important factor in symptom formation.
1. If stress or anxiety cannot be expressed through verbalization, it may find expression through particular organ symptoms.
2. Exact relationship between stress and illness is unknown.
3. Illness provides focus for individual away from original anxiety, thereby providing secondary gains of sympathy and attention from others.

✦ C. Structural changes in body systems may occur and pose a life-threatening situation.
1. Individual not faking illness; it is real and requires direct medical attention.
2. Correcting physical illness may not alter the underlying cause of anxiety.

D. There can be synergistic reaction from repressed feelings and overexcited organs.

✦ E. Psychosomatic illness provides individual with coping mechanisms.
1. Means to handle anxiety and stress.
2. Ways to gain socially acceptable attention.
3. Rationalization for failures.
4. Means for adjusting to dependency needs.
5. Ways to handle anger and aggression.
6. Ways to punish self and others.
F. Kinds of defense mechanisms used in this condition.
1. Repression.
2. Denial.
3. Projection.
4. Conversion.
G. A psychosomatic disorder may involve any body system and be related to any disease process.

Assessment

✦ A. Observe closely and assess patient's condition.
1. Collect data about the physical illness, psychosocial adjustment, life situations, natural stresses, strengths, etc.
2. Report the kinds of things that aggravate or release the symptom.
B. Assess the whole person, physically and emotionally, not just the symptoms.

Implementation

A. Develop nurse–patient relationship.
1. Respect the patient and acknowledge his or her problems.
2. Assist the patient to express his or her feelings.
3. Help the patient to release anxiety and explore new coping mechanisms.
4. Allow the patient to meet dependency needs.
5. Allow the patient to feel in control of his or her life.
B. Reduce demands on the patient.
C. Encourage the patient to work through problems and to learn new methods of responding to stress.
D. Provide safe and nonthreatening environment.
1. Balance therapy and recreation.
2. Decrease distracting stimuli.
3. Provide activities that can deemphasize or help to alleviate the patient's physical symptoms.

Conversion Disorder

✦ A. Conversion disorder is the development of a physical symptom (blindness, paralysis, deafness) with no physical etiology identified.
1. The symptom is real, in that the patient actually cannot see, walk, hear, etc.
2. Anxiety that results from an unconscious conflict is converted into the physical symptom for which there is no physiologic explanation.

✦ B. Understand that patient's lack of concern or indifferent attitude is at the same time a symptom of the illness.
✦ C. Recognize that illness is frequently used for primary gains, i.e., solving conflict by not solving it and removing the source of anxiety. Illness used for *secondary gain* provides patient with sympathy and attention to physical handicap.
D. Specific nursing approaches.
1. Do not confront the patient with his or her illness.
2. Divert patient's attention from symptoms.
3. Do not respond to patient's secondary gains.
4. Reduce pressure or demands on patient.
5. Create positive relationship.
6. Use a matter-of-fact approach.
7. Provide patient with recreational and socializing activities.
8. Teach necessities of daily living, and give assistance as needed, i.e., if patient is blind, teach patient how to feed self—do not feed patient, for this behavior is feeding into secondary gains (attention).

Hypochondriasis

✦ A. A severe, morbid preoccupation with one's own body; abnormal anxiety about one's health.
✦ B. Preoccupation with an imagined illness for which no observable symptoms or organic changes exist.
✦ C. Differentiate from *malingering*—deliberately making up an illness to prolong hospitalization.
D. Specific nursing approaches.
1. Accept the patient and his or her complaints; anticipate demands to break demanding cycle.
2. Provide diversional activities in which the patient can succeed and raise self-esteem.
3. Use friendly, supportive approach.
4. Provide for patient's physical needs.
5. Assist patient to refocus interest.

EATING DISORDERS

✦ Anorexia Nervosa

Definition: A potentially life-threatening (results in death 10 percent of the time) syndrome of self-starvation with underlying emotional disturbance characterized by an intense fear of gaining weight or becoming fat. The psychological aversion to food results in emaciation and physical problems.

Characteristics

✦ A. Almost exclusively female—90 to 95 percent.
B. Most common in adolescent girls and young adults (age 12 to mid-30s).

C. Often unnoticed in early stages; female "goes on diet to lose weight."

D. Dynamics of disorder.
1. History of a "model child"; extreme perfectionism.
2. Intense fear of obesity leads anorectic to report feeling fat.
✦ 3. Not a disturbance in appetite but distorted body image perceptions: related to disturbance in sense of self, identity, and autonomy.
4. Hormones altered—are they cause or effect of disorder?
5. Anorectics do not want treatment. Potentially lethal disease: mortality 5 to 18 percent.
6. Many anorectics have a single episode, then recover. Factors associated with positive prognosis include onset of problem before age 15 and weight gain within 2 years.

Assessment

✦ A. Loss of weight: refusal to maintain body weight or profound weight loss of 15 percent or more.
✦ B. No menstrual period for 3 months.
C. Physical symptoms.
1. Malnutrition.
2. Fractures—calcium leaked from bones.
3. Teeth enamel eroded and poor gums.
4. Hypotension, hypothermia.
5. Anemia and reduced white blood cells.
6. Hypoproteinemia.
D. Monitor for potential complications.
1. Severe electrolyte imbalance (decreased potassium, kidney failure).
2. Heart failure and coma, and possible death.

Implementation

A. Actions to improve nutritional status (to stabilize medical condition).
✦ 1. Diet.
a. High protein, high carbohydrate, especially amino acids.
b. Identify foods patient prefers.
c. Small, nutritious, attractive feedings.
2. Nasogastric feedings: if patient refuses to eat, administer tube feedings as ordered.
B. Psychological care.
✦ 1. Care plan.
a. Formulate plan that all staff agree on. Do not allow manipulation. Do not engage in power struggle.
b. Do not focus on food, taste, recipes, etc.
c. Remain with patient when eating or monitor when patient eats with others.
d. Do not accept excuses to leave eating area (to vomit).

e. Set limits on amount patient must eat. Reward when patient adheres to plan.
f. Ensure that weight is taken same time every day with patient dressed in only a hospital gown.
g. Be warm and caring in approach to patient both verbally and physically.
2. Therapy.
✦ a. Medications.
(1) Antidepressants—treats lack of caring about weight loss.
(2) SSRIs for depression.
b. Focused on behavior therapy.
(1) Set limits with positive and negative reinforcement.
(2) Establish contract that specifies weight gain/loss correlated with privileges, restrictions.
c. Insight-oriented therapy: correcting patient's body perceptions and misconceptions about feelings, needs, self-worth, autonomy.
d. Family therapy important focus as issues of control and autonomy are connected to eating.

Bulimia

✦ *Definition:* Eating disorder characterized by loss of control during binge eating, frequently followed by self-induced vomiting.

Characteristics

A. Etiology is unknown but this disorder is often accompanied by an underlying psychopathology.
B. More common in women than men.
C. Begins in adolescence or early adulthood and often follows a chronic course over many years.
D. Generally aware that eating patterns are abnormal (in contrast to anorectics).
E. Typically evidences impaired impulse control, low self-esteem, and depression.

Assessment

A. Degree of disruption in life caused by eating disorder.
B. Degree of depression: often due to guilt over eating binges. (Studies suggest link between bulimia and affective disorder.)
C. Weight fluctuation and potential danger of weight loss.

Implementation

✦ A. Patient is usually not hospitalized but does require therapy.
B. Behavior modification and insight-oriented therapy used with limited success.

C. Care plan is similar to anorexia nervosa with focus on interrupting binge/purge cycle and altering attitudes toward food and self.

SLEEP DISORDERS

Definition: Sleep disorders or sleep pattern disturbance can be categorized into 4 different groups: primary sleep disorders (dyssomnias and parasomnias), sleep disorders related to mental conditions, a medical condition, or substance-induced disorder.

Assessment

A. Dyssomnias.
   1. Prmary insomnia.
      a. Difficulty falling asleep or continuing sleep.
      b. Problems with nonrestorative sleep.
   2. Primary hypersomnia.
      a. Prolonged sleep and excessive sleepiness which interferes with daily functioning.
      b. Excessive sleepiness is not caused by insomnia and is not accounted for by inadequate sleep.
   3. Breathing-related sleep disorders.
      a. Sleep apnea, obstructive type (upper airway partially collapses and opening it involves at least partial arousal).
      b. Predisposing factors: obese, middle-aged men with a history of snoring.
   4. Narcolepsy.
      a. A pattern of brief episodes of deep sleep, occurring daily.
      b. May be accompanied by cataplexy (sudden collapse of muscle tone or recurrent episodes of rapid eye movement).
   5. Circadian rhythm sleep disorders.
      a. A recurrent pattern of sleep disruption due to mismatched sleep-wake schedules.
         (1) Disturbance causes stress or impairment of functioning.
         (2) Disturbance is not connected to other sleep disorders or a substance abuse.
      b. Specific types: delayed sleep phase, jet lag, shift work phase or unspecified.
B. Parasomnias.
   1. Somnambulism—sleep walking, nightmares, sleep terrors.
   2. Bruxism—teeth grinding.
   3. Enuresis—bed-wetting.

Implementation

A. Intervention is based on thorough identification of the type of sleep disturbance.
   1. Diagnostic sleep tests (polysomnography) assists in confirming the diagnosis.
   2. Treatment is based on subjective analysis unless specific symptoms suggest other disorders.
B. Interventions may include principles of sleep hygiene, coping mechanisms, medication, reduction or removal of an obstruction (sleep apnea), CPAP by nasal mask; in general, treatment is specific to each individual's problem.

ATTENTION DEFICIT-HYPERACTIVITY DISORDER (ADHD)

Definition: Emotional disorder characterized by a persistent pattern of hyperactivity–impulsivity.

Characteristics

A. More common in males—18 percent of boys and 8 percent of girls.
B. Children with this disorder represent 40–50 percent of child disorders as inpatients and even a higher percentage as outpatients.

Assessment

✦ A. Assess for symptoms of inattention that are maladaptive.
   1. Makes careless mistakes.
   2. Difficulty sustaining attention in tasks or play.
   3. Does not listen when spoken to directly.
   4. Has difficulty organizing tasks.
   5. Easily distracted.
   6. Forgetful in daily activities.
✦ B. Assess for symptoms of hyperactivity–impulsivity.
   1. Fidgets with hands or feet.
   2. Leaves seat when expected to stay seated.
   3. Runs/climbs excessively.
   4. Has difficulty playing quietly.
   5. Constantly "on the go."
   6. Talks excessively.
✦ C. Assess symptoms of impulsivity.
   1. Blurts out answers before question is completed.
   2. Has difficulty waiting for turn.
   3. Intrudes/interrupts others' conversations and games.
D. Assess for symptoms of conduct disorder, i.e., persistent disregard for rights of others (aggression, destruction of property, etc.).

Implementation

A. Develop therapeutic relationship with child.
B. Refer to special education programs for attention difficulties.
C. Conduct relationship therapy and play therapy with child for emotional problems related to disorder.

Table 16-4. PROFILE DIFFERENTIATION	
Schizophrenic	**Anxiety Disorder**
Major ego impairment. Includes faulty reality testing, delusions, hallucinations (especially auditory).	No grave impairment of reality testing. No hallucinations or delusions.
Serious impairment of patient's life, including social, vocational, and sexual.	Difficulty in relating, but interaction with others not prevented. Personality usually remains organized.
Little insight into problems and behavior. Patient generally does not recognize he or she is ill.	Some awareness into problems. Keenly feels subjective suffering. Often unconsciously fights any changes in status (getting well).
Severe personality disorganization, e.g., judgment, memory, and perceptions.	Less severe disorganization. Can function but with decreased efficiency.
May be caused by both physiological or psychological factors.	Always a functional disorder; not organic in origin.
Usually requires hospitalization and long-term treatment.	Usually does not require hospitalization. May require long-term treatment.
Maladaptive adjustment mechanisms used in rigid, fixed way. May be seen as severe regression.	Suppression and repression used to handle internal conflicts; defenses are largely symbolic.
No secondary gain received.	Symptoms generally exploited for secondary gain.

D. Work with parents to set up home environment that promotes successful completion of developmental tasks.

SCHIZOPHRENIC DISORDERS

✦ *Definition:*   A syndrome that carries with it varied etiology, psychodynamics, and psychopathology. The clinical course of the illness varies from patient to patient, so the nurse should view the disease as a syndrome with varying clinical entities. It is characterized by disturbances in thought, communication, relationships, behavior, and perception.

Characteristics
A.   Schizophrenia may be the result of many variables: genetic constellation, individual adaptive patterns, poor family relationships, lack of ego strength, earlier traumatic experiences, or distorted cognition.
✦ B.   Regression and repression are regarded as the primary mechanisms of schizophrenia.
C.   Major maladaptive disturbances: impaired interpersonal relationships, ineffective mental and emotional processes, and disturbances in overt behavior patterns.
D.   Individuals generally demonstrate personality disorganization with a break from reality as opposed to anxiety disorders. (*See* Table 16-4.)
E.   Schizophrenic reactions may become acute and/or chronic.

Primary Disturbances
A.   Thoughts are confused and disorganized so that ability to communicate clearly is limited.

B.   Feelings (affect) may be expressed in an inappropriate manner.
C.   Behavior may be bizarre or lack purposeful direction.
D.   Close and trusting interpersonal relationships are difficult to establish.

Positive Symptoms

A.   *Delusions*—fixed misinterpretation of reality; false beliefs maintained despite evidence to the contrary (somatic delusions are false beliefs that something is wrong with the body).
B.   *Hallucinations*—unwilled sensory perceptions with no basis in reality; auditory, visual, olfactory, tactile, gustatory.
C.   *Disordered speech and behavior.*
1.   Disordered speech includes frequent derailment or incoherence.
2.   Behavior is disorganized—catatonic or random, purposeless.
D.   Terms associated with disordered speech or behavior.
1.   *Withdrawal*—behavior that signifies the patient's desire to regress into more satisfying world of own making (autism).
2.   *Depersonalization*—feelings of estrangement or unconnectedness of body parts from self.
3.   *Echolalia*—a condition in which the individual consistently repeats what is heard.
4.   *Echopraxia*—a condition in which the individual mimics what is done.
5.   *Neologism*—term that refers to the coining of a new word.
6.   *Word salad*—communication characterized by jumbled words with no coherent message.

**SUMMARY OF SCHIZOPHRENIA
CLASSIFICATIONS (DSM-IV-TR)**

Positive symptoms
* Hallucinations
* Delusions
* Disordered speech
* Loose associations—when one thought does not connect to another or does not make any logical sense
* Bizarre or disordered behavior

Negative symptoms
* Poverty of speech, alogia
* Affective blunting
* Social withdrawal
* Apathy
* Lack of volition, avolition
* Poor grooming, anhedonia
* Attentional impairment

Negative Symptoms

A. *Flat affect*—feelings or emotions minimal (i.e., flat, blunted, or inappropriate).

B. *Alogia or poverty of speech*—answers questions with one word which may signify lack of thoughts.

C. *Avolition*—when the patient is unable to follow goal-directed behavior; this is not the same as laziness.

D. *Anhedonia*—the inability to experience joy or pleasure in any aspect of life.

E. *Note:* The above 4 symptoms can be remembered by the "four As": Affect flattened, Alogia, Avolition, and Anhedonia.

Implementation

A. General nursing approaches.
   ✦ 1. Establish nurse–patient relationship.
      a. Develop positive and trusting relationship.
      b. Provide a safe and secure environment.
   ✦ 2. Stress situational reality.
      a. Help patient to reality-test and come out of fantasy world.
      b. Involve the patient in reality-oriented activities.
      c. Help the patient to find satisfaction in the external environment.
   3. Accept the patient as he or she is.
      a. Do not invalidate disturbed thoughts or fantasies.
      b. Do not invalidate the patient's sense of self by your inappropriate responses.
   4. Use only therapeutic communication techniques.
      a. Encourage patient to express negative and/or positive emotions.
      b. Encourage patient to express thoughts, fears, and problems.
      c. Match your nonverbal with your verbal communications.
      d. Communicate clearly with the patient.
   5. Do not foster a dependency relationship.
   6. Avoid stressful situations that can increase the patient's anxiety (i.e., moving the patient into group therapy too soon).

B. Approaches to specific behaviors.
   ✦ 1. Working with delusions.
      a. Help the patient to recognize distorted views of reality.
      b. Focus on patient's strengths.
      c. Provide a safe, nonthreatening milieu.
      d. Divert focus from delusional material to reality.
      e. Provide situations that can create successful experiences for the patient.
      f. Specific nursing responses.
         (1) Avoid confirming or feeding into delusion.
         (2) Stress reality by denying you believe the patient's delusion.
         (3) Respond to patient's feelings, i.e., validate his or her feelings by saying, "I sense you are afraid. Is this true?"
   ✦ 2. Working with hallucinations.
      a. Provide a safe, structured environment with routine activities.
      b. Protect patient from self-injury or hurting others prompted by "voices."
      c. Initiate short, frequent interactions.
         (1) Respond verbally to anything real that patient talks about.
         (2) Avoid denying or arguing with patient about the hallucinations he or she is experiencing.
         (3) Involve the patient in reality-based tasks or activities (i.e., a person cannot sing and hallucinate at the same time).
         (4) Increase patient's social interaction gradually from interaction with one person to interaction with small groups as tolerated.
   ✦ 3. Working with withdrawn behavior.
      a. Assist patient in developing a satisfying relationship with you.
         (1) Initiate interaction.
         (2) Show sincerity for a trusting relationship by being consistent in keeping appointments, in attitudes, and in nursing practice.
         (3) Be honest and direct in what you say and do.

(4) Deal with your feelings incurred by patient's hostility or rejection.
b. Help patient to modify self-perception.
  (1) Structure situations in which patient will succeed.
  (2) Focus on patient's assets or strengths to enhance self-esteem.
  (3) Relieve patient from making choices until able to make decisions.
c. Teach patient how to restore social skills.
  (1) Gradually increase opportunities for social contacts with staff and other patients.
  (2) Increase opportunities for social contact with significant others (family) as appropriate.
d. Focus on reality situations.
  (1) Use nonthreatening approach.
  (2) Provide safe nonthreatening milieu.
e. Attend to physical needs of nutrition, sleep, exercise, occupational therapy.

Schizophrenic Subtypes

✦ A. *Catatonic type:* underactivity results in bizarre posturing *(waxy flexibility)* and overactivity leads to agitation. Catatonic excitement is the opposite of mute, withdrawn behavior normally seen in catatonia.
✦ B. *Disorganized type:* inappropriate affect: giggling and silly laughter (formerly labeled hebephrenia).
✦ C. *Undifferentiated type:* characterized by a combination of symptoms, none of which discriminates a specific type of disorder.
D. *Residual type:* refers to a patient who has had episodes of schizophrenia but now has no positive symptoms—negative symptoms remain present.
E. Follow general approaches—nursing guidelines for schizophrenia—for the above subtypes.
✦ F. *Paranoid type:* a reaction that manifests delusions of persecution and other maladaptive behavior.
  ✦ 1. Clinical signs and symptoms.
    a. Extreme suspiciousness and mistrust of others.
    b. Hostility toward others.
    c. Delusions of persecution or grandeur.
    d. Chronic insecurity, inadequate self-concept, low self-esteem.
    e. Chronic high anxiety level.
    f. Patient denies delusional role.
    g. Hypochondriasis.
  ✦ 2. Nursing care.
    a. Establish a trusting relationship.
      (1) Be consistent and friendly despite patient's hostility.
      (2) Avoid talking and laughing when the patient can see but not hear you.

(3) If patient is very suspicious, relate one to one and not in a group situation.
(4) Involve the patient in the treatment plan.
(5) Give nonpunitive support.
b. Reduce anxiety associated with interpersonal interactions.
  (1) Avoid power struggles, i.e., do not argue with the patient because it increases anxiety and hostility.
  (2) Proceed with nursing therapy slowly because a paranoid patient is suspicious and often mistrustful of others.
  (3) Show consistency and honesty.

Schizoaffective Disorder

✦ *Definition:* Condition that does not directly fit either schizophrenia or a mood disorder and, thus, is a mixture of symptoms.

Characteristics

✦ A. Illness characterized by episodes of depression, mania, or both, concurrent with symptoms of schizophrenia.
  1. Thought processes similar to schizophrenic disorder.
  2. Bizarre behavior and mood disorders range from depression to elation (bipolar disorder).
✦ B. Patients treated according to symptoms manifested—schizophrenic and/or mood disorder.
C. Drug therapy may be either antipsychotic (usually prescribed) or antidepressant drugs.
D. Check implementation sections for both Schizophrenic and Mood Disorders.

Paranoid Personality Disorder

Definition: Diagnosis of paranoid disorder is made when paranoid features dominate the personality. Other symptoms of maladaptive or schizophrenic behavior may be absent.

Characteristics

✦ A. Paranoia is characterized by extreme suspiciousness and withdrawal from all emotional contact with others.
B. Onset is usually gradual.
C. Onset of paranoid reactions may be precipitated by certain stressful events in patient's life.
✦ D. More common paranoid psychosis is manifested by delusional thoughts.
  1. Most common delusions are of persecution (people are out to harm, injure, or destroy).
  2. Other delusions may center around grandeur, somatic complaints, or delusions of jealousy.
E. Implementation principles similar to paranoid schizophrenic disorder.

DISSOCIATIVE DISORDERS

✦ *Definition:*   A sudden temporary alteration in the integrative functions of consciousness, identity, or motor behavior.

Characteristics

✦ A.   Patient attempts to deal with anxiety through various disturbances or by blocking certain areas of the mind from conscious awareness.

B.   Patient has a psychological retreat from reality.

C.   Repression is used to block awareness of traumatic event.

D.   Dissociative identity disorder (DID) dominated by two or more personalities, each of which controls the behavior while in the consciousness.

Assessment

A.   Amnesia: circumscribed, selective, generalized and continuous.

✦ B.   *Fugue* or transient disorientation—patient is unaware that he or she has traveled to another location.

C.   Interference in lifestyle and interpersonal relationships.

D.   Accompanying symptoms such as depression, suicide ideation, etc.

✦ E.   Depersonalization—sense of detachment from self.

Implementation

A.   Support therapeutic modality as established by treatment team.

B.   Reduce anxiety-producing stimuli.

C.   Redirect patient's attention away from self.

D.   Avoid sympathizing with patient.

E.   Increase socialization activities.

PERSONALITY DISORDERS

Definition: An individual with a personality disorder adjusts to life situations with difficulty and interacts with others in an unsatisfactory manner. Behavioral problems rather than symptoms are exhibited. This individual is known as a psychopathic or sociopathic personality.

Characteristics

A.   Three major categories referred to as clusters: odd-eccentric, dramatic-emotional, and fearful-anxious.

B.   Several traits are common to all 3 clusters.

1.   Lacks understanding of how their behavior affects others; lacks insight.

2.   Cannot take responsibility for own behavior.

3.   When threatened cannot change own behavior, but attempts to change environment.

C.   Other general traits common to personality disorders:

✦ 1.   Exhibits inflexible and maladaptive responses to stress, which produce dysfunctional behavioral problems.

✦ 2.   Experiences difficulty in developing warm interpersonal relationships.

a.   Affective responses are shallow.

b.   Relationships tend to be superficial.

✦ 3.   Responds poorly to intellectual and emotional demands made of them.

4.   Aggressive and sexual impulses are expressed overtly.

5.   Tolerance for anxiety is low so that the person will go to any length to avoid situations that provoke anxiety; inability to tolerate frustration.

a.   The attempts to gain relief from anxiety produce inappropriate behavior.

b.   Individual is unaware that behavior is contrary to social expectations.

6.   Exhibits poor impulse control and poor judgment; rejects all authority.

✦ 7.   Social assets include intelligence and charm; skilled in manipulation.

8.   Behavior often perceived as direct or indirect attack on laws and mores of society.

✦ D.   Personality profiles.

1.   *Antisocial personality.*

a.   Lies, cheats, and steals (a pathologic diagnosis common in prisons).

b.   Patient shows evidence of emotional immaturity.

c.   Indicates little or no capacity for good judgment.

d.   Rationalizes behavior so that it appears justified; lacks a moral conscience.

e.   Is the typical "con artist."

2.   *Inadequate personality.*

a.   Responds to intellectual and emotional demands ineffectively.

b.   Does not learn from experience or punishment, indicating poor judgment.

c.   Is socially unstable.

d.   Lacks ability to adapt.

3.   *"Social deviate"* personality types.

a.   Sadist—inflicts pain on another.

b.   Masochist—inflicts pain on self.

c.   Voyeur—enjoys "Peeping Tom" behavior.

d.   Exhibitionist—exposes own body for pleasure.

4.   *Addictive personality* (*see* section on Substance Dependence).

5.   *Schizoid personality.*

a.   Lacks close interpersonal relationships.

b.   Is shy, and behavior is withdrawn.

c. Projects eccentric behavior patterns.

d. Unable to express hostility; affect is flat.

6. *Paranoid personality*.

   a. Suspects intentions of others.

   b. Unable to sustain interpersonal relationships because of inability to trust.

   c. Experiences jealousy and envy in relating to others.

Implementation

A. Participate in planning a therapeutic nurse–patient relationship that focuses on reinforcement of positive behavior.

1. Accept the patient for what and where he or she is (in terms of abilities).

   a. Set realistic expectations.

   b. Assess capabilities realistically so that excessive expectations will not reinforce failure.

✦ 2. Maintain control, and protect other patients from antisocial behavior.

3. Allow patient to express frustration and hostility.

4. Assist patient to tolerate frustration and postpone satisfaction.

5. Explore new alternatives for patient's living patterns that are socially acceptable.

6. Be aware of your own negative attitudes that may arise in working with these patients.

✦ B. Set limitations firmly and with consistency.

1. Avoid falling into the patient's charming and manipulative ways.

2. Understand that the patient's anxiety will increase if manipulative behavior is ineffective.

C. Recognize that punishment does not resolve problems or change behavior.

1. Confront behavior but do not demean the patient.

2. Plan a supportive environment.

   a. Provide the patient with a sense of security.

   b. Provide opportunities for patient to learn how to cope with impulses.

D. Help patient to formulate realistic future plans.

E. Low self-esteem, which may lead to self-destructive behavior, requires planned interventions.

1. Work with patient to see assets and strengths and positive attributes—group feedback is useful for this intervention.

2. Use of cognitive behavior techniques (stopping negative thoughts) is useful.

3. Self-destructive behavior may necessitate a stable, safe, secure environment with clear expectations of behavior, firm limits and strict consequences.

F. Set specific guidelines for working with sociopathic behavior.

1. Attempt to develop a trusting relationship; it is difficult because the patient usually does not want help.

2. Follow the total care plan as determined by the physician. This is important because therapy is oriented toward reconstruction of personality.

3. Focus on reality, and do not allow patient to manipulate.

4. Give approval only for acceptable behavior.

Nursing Approaches to Maladaptive Behavior

Aggressive or Combative Behavior

A. Observe sharply for clues that the patient is getting out of control.

1. Note rising anger from patient's verbal and nonverbal behavior.

2. Note erratic or unpredictable responses to staff or other patients.

B. Intervene immediately when you become aware that patient's loss of control is imminent.

C. Approach the patient in a nonthreatening manner.

D. Set firm limits on unacceptable behavior.

E. Maintain calm demeanor, and do not show fear.

F. Avoid engaging in an argument or provoking the patient.

G. Summon assistance only when indicated: sudden involvement of many people will increase the patient's agitation.

H. Remove the patient from a threatening situation as soon as possible.

I. Use seclusion and/or restraints only if necessary.

J. Attempt to calm the patient so that control can be regained.

K. Be supportive and remain with the patient.

L. Use a problem-solving focus following outburst of aggressive or combative behavior.

1. Encourage discussion of feelings surrounding incident.

2. Attempt to discuss causal factors of the behavior.

3. Examine the patient's initial response to stimulus, and explore alternative responses.

4. Point out consequences of aggressive behavior.

5. Discuss the patient's role in taking responsibility for aggressive behavior.

Verbally Abusive Behavior

A. Do not respond in kind to abusive comments.

B. Try not to take abuse personally.

C. Interact with the patient on a therapeutic basis.

1. Help the patient examine own feelings.

2. Do not reject the patient.

3. Give patient feedback concerning your reactions to abusive comments.

4. Teach alternative ways to express feelings.

D. Maintain a calm, accepting approach to patient.

Demanding Behavior

A. Do not ignore demands; they will only increase in intensity.

B. Attempt to determine causal factors of behavior, e.g., high anxiety level.

C. Set limits to your own response patterns when patient is demanding.

D. Control own feelings of anger and irritation.

E. Teach alternative means for getting needs met.

F. Plan nursing care to include frequent contacts that are initiated by the nurse.

G. Alert the staff to try to give patient needed reassurance.

Rape Trauma Syndrome

Definition: Rape is a nonconsensual sexual assault on a person that is basically an act of violence; only secondarily considered a sex act.

Characteristics

◆ A. Recognize that the assault of rape is a humiliating and violent experience, and that the victim is experiencing severe psychological trauma.

B. 93% of victims are female and 90% of perpetrators are male.

C. Accept the fact that the victim was indeed raped and that the victim is to be supported, not treated as the "accused."

D. Before assessment, inform victim of her rights: privacy rights, notification of private physician, notification of a rape crisis advocate, confidentiality and consent to all tests.

E. Understand that the victim's behavior might vary from hysterical crying and/or laughing to very calm and controlled.

◆ F. Crisis response.

1. Acute phase: shock, crying, high anxiety, hysterical, incoherent, agitated, fearful, volatile, poor problem-solving ability.

2. Reconstitution phase: denial, appears calm and controlled, withdrawn, fearful, begins to talk about feelings, expresses anger, makes decisions.

3. Resolution phase: realistic attitudes, able to express feelings, controlled anger, acceptance of facts.

Implementation

A. Treatment focus.

◆ 1. Emotional—crisis counseling and call Women Against Rape or rape advocate.

a. Degree of emotional trauma.

b. Presence of symptoms.

◆ 2. Encourage victim to report rape to the authorities.

◆ 3. Medical—immediate medical care: assess assault and degree of trauma.

a. Assist with a complete physical examination.

b. Carefully assess and document all physical damage: injuries; signs of physical entry.

4. Legal—do not bathe, douche, or change clothes; gather evidence.

◆ B. Interventions.

◆ 1. Provide immediate privacy for examination.

◆ 2. Choose a staff member of the same sex to be with the victim.

◆ 3. Remain with the victim.

4. Administer physical care.

◆ a. Do not allow patient to wash genital area or void before examination; these actions will remove any existing evidence such as semen.

b. Keep patient warm.

c. Prepare patient for complete physical examination to be completed by physician (same sex as patient if possible).

◆ d. Physical exam includes:

(1) Head-to-toe exam.

(2) Pap smear.

(3) Saline suspension to test for presence of sperm.

(4) Acid-phosphatase to determine recency of attack.

e. Physical treatment may include:

(1) Prophylactic antibiotics.

(2) Tranquilizers.

5. Provide emotional support.

◆ a. Demonstrate a nonjudgmental and supportive attitude.

b. Express warmth, support, and empathy in relating to the victim.

c. Listen to what the victim says, and document all information.

d. Encourage the victim to relate what happened, having her tell you in her own words if it appears that she would like to talk about the experience.

e. Do not insist if patient chooses not to talk; allow the victim to cope in her own way.

f. During the interview, continue to be sensitive to the victim's feelings and degree of control. If, in relating the attack, she becomes hysterical, do not continue questioning at this time.

6. Termination of crisis relationship.
   a. Counsel patient to receive repeat test for sexually transmitted diseases in 3 weeks or sooner if symptoms appear.
   b. Help reestablish contact with significant people.
   c. Refer to appropriate community resource for follow-up care—many cities have a "hot line" that offers crisis counseling to victims.
   d. Keep accurate records, as they may be important in future legal proceedings.

COGNITIVE DISORDER (ORGANIC BRAIN SYNDROME)

✦ *Definition:* Cognitive disorders are psychiatric disorders with organic etiology that may be reversible (delirium) or irreversible (dementia) and include clinically significant deficits in cognition or memory that result in significant changes in a patient's level of functioning.

Characteristics
✦ A. Delirium.
   1. Disturbance of consciousness that develops over a short period of time.
   2. Approximately 10 percent of all hospitalized elderly have delirium.
   3. Global intellectual impairment with rapid onset.
   4. Condition may last hours or weeks—usually resolves in a few days.
✦ B. Dementia, Alzheimer's type (DAT). *See* Dementia section in Chapter 13.
   C. Dementia due to HIV disease.
   1. Dementia is present as a direct consequence of HIV infection.
   2. Involves diffuse, multifocal destruction of white matter and subcortical structures.
   3. Characterized by forgetfulness, slowness, poor concentration, difficulty with problem solving, and hallucinations.

Assessment
A. Assess onset, which may be slow or fast, and level of deterioration.
✦ B. Assess for degree of cognitive impairment.
   1. Memory loss and loss of capacity to learn.
   2. Judgment impairment.
   3. Disorientation, perceptual disturbance.
   4. Decreased attention span.
   5. Decreased motivation and self-concern.
   6. Labile mood, irritability, and depression.
   7. Behavioral impairment.
      a. Ritualistic, stereotyped behavior.
      b. Possible combativeness and inappropriate responses.
      c. Regressive behavior.

Implementation
✦ A. Nursing interventions are the same for any cognitive disorder, including delirium, dementia, and Alzheimer's disease.
   B. Monitor medications for dementia management.
   1. Acetylcholinesterase inhibitors.
      a. Inhibits the enzyme acetylcholinesterase which slows the breakdown of acetylcholine, thereby allowing more information to be transmitted from one cell to another.
      b. Memory and general cognitive activity increases, thus slowing the progression of dementia, especially early in the process of the disease.
      c. Common drugs in the category are donepezil (Aricept), revastigmine (Exelon), and galantamine (Reminyl).
      d. These drugs have both positive and negative results and must be individualized.
   2. Depressive symptoms for dementia.
      a. SSRIs appear to be more efficacious (Celexa, Prozac, Paxil and Zoloft).
      b. Evidence less side effects than other antidepressants.
   3. Psychosis and dementia.
      a. If psychotic thoughts are a problem, drugs are required.
      b. When psychosis is associated with violence or dangerous behavior, Haldol (.5 mg or more) is indicated.
      c. For chronic aggressive behavior, Risperdal (2–6 mg) is effective.
      d. Seroquel is also effective and does not worsen cognition.
   4. Anger and aggression.
      a. For an acute episode, Haldol may be recommended.
      b. For gradually evolving tendencies, Depakote (125 mg BID increasing to 1500 mg daily) may be administered.
   C. Refer to pages 399–400 in Chapter 13 for more information on dementia.

SUBSTANCE RELATED DISORDERS

Definition: Substance dependence includes any process by which an individual ingests any mind-altering, nonprescribed chemical that produces physiological and/or psychological dependence. Withdrawal symptoms are usually manifest when substance is not taken.

Characteristics

◆ A. *Psychological dependence*—emotional dependence, desire, or compulsion to continue taking the substance or drug to experience "normal" functioning.

◆ B. *Tolerance*—the need for greatly increased amounts of the substance to obtain the desired effect.

◆ C. *Physiological dependence*—physical need for the substance manifested by appearance of withdrawal symptoms when substance is withheld.

D. Withdrawal from substance causes substance specific syndrome—leads to impairment.

Alcohol Abuse

Definition: The abuse of any alcoholic substance combined with physical and psychological addiction.

Characteristics

A. Alcohol consumption is permitted by law and supported by most people in our society as a recreational activity.

B. A fine line exists between the social drinker and the addicted or problem drinker.

◆ C. The greatest difference involves the degree of compulsion to drink and the inability to survive the trials of everyday living without the ingestion of alcohol.

D. Alcoholism, the third largest health problem in the United States (heart disease and cancer rank first and second), affects 15 million people.

E. Alcoholism is involved in about 30,000 deaths and one-half million injuries (auto accidents) every year.

F. Alcoholism decreases life span 10 to 12 years.

G. Loss to industry caused by alcoholism is estimated at $15 billion a year (affecting primarily the 35 to 55 age group).

H. Major U.S. social concern is the dramatic rise in teenage alcoholism (estimated to affect 3 million adolescents).

I. The legal definition of intoxication in most states is 0.10% or more blood alcohol level.

Dynamics of Alcoholism

◆ A. Alcoholic disease implies the consumption of alcohol to such a degree that it interferes with the individual's physical, emotional, and social functioning.
   1. The syndrome consists of two phases: problem drinking and alcohol addiction.
   2. Dependence on other drugs is very common.

B. Genetic or familial predisposition to dependence may exist.

C. Alcohol blocks synaptic transmission, depresses the central nervous system (CNS), and releases inhibitions. It acts initially as a stimulant but is actually a depressant.
   1. Chronic excessive use can lead to brain damage (sedative effect on CNS).
   2. High blood levels may cause malfunctions in cardiovascular and respiratory systems.

D. Psychological effects of alcohol appear to be the gratification of oral impulses and the reduction of superego forces; abuse leads to shame and guilt and impaired ego function.

E. Alcohol may be said to be a defense against overwhelming psychological needs and conflicts; therefore, the patient needs to work on problems causing his or her distress.

◆ F. Illnesses associated with chronic alcoholism.
   1. Korsakoff's syndrome (related to thiamine deficiency).
   2. Delirium tremens (DTs).
   3. Chronic gastritis.
   4. Malnutrition resulting in beriberi, pellagra, cerebellar degeneration, and anemia.
   5. Laënnec's cirrhosis, hepatitis and fatty liver.
   6. Peripheral neuropathy (related to vitamin B deficiency).
   7. Osteoporosis.
   8. Individual is prone to infection, blood dyscrasias, and sexual dysfunction.

G. Alcohol withdrawal.
   1. Hangover: mild alcohol withdrawal; symptoms include headache, nausea, vomiting.
   2. General withdrawal symptoms.
      a. Nausea and vomiting.
      b. Insomnia.
      c. Anorexia.
      d. Anxiety, restlessness.
      e. Tremors, sweating.

Characteristics of an Alcoholic

A. Dependent personality but resents authority.

B. Sets high self-expectations but has a low tolerance for frustration.

C. Inclined toward patterns of failure.

D. Uses alcohol to gain a false sense of success, power, confidence, and self-worth.

E. Uses alcohol to ease suffering, reduce anxiety, and to help cope with life stresses.

F. Functions with less intellectual, emotional, and social ability as need for alcohol increases.

G. Risk-taking propensity.

Implementation

◆ A. Help reestablish the patient's healthy physical condition.
   1. Provide adequate nutrition with fluids and a high-vitamin (especially vitamin B_6 and

B complex), high-calorie, and high-protein diet.

2. Promote adequate rest and sleep.

✦ B. Observe patient for symptoms of impending delirium tremens—an acute condition usually occurring within 24–72 hours after the last ingestion of alcohol. May appear 7–10 days after drinking periods when little or no food is ingested.

   1. Major symptoms of DTs: tremors, hallucinations, paranoia, disorientation, seizures, illusions, severe agitation.

   2. Death from DTs may occur (10–15 percent die from cardiac failure).

✦ C. Maintain a controlled and structured environment until the patient is able to manage his or her own circumstances.

   1. Set behavior limits, and confront the manipulative patient.

   2. Suggest group interaction for lonely patients.

   3. Remember that the patient needs support, firmness, and a reality-oriented approach.

✦ D. Treatment techniques.

   1. Patient must first go through detoxification —intensive care to prevent the toxic state and then the return to a nonalcoholic state.

   2. Stress need for a change in attitudes.

     a. To accept fact that alcoholism is an illness.

     b. To accept fact that life must be managed without the support of alcohol.

   3. Promote psychotherapy techniques of group and family therapy; establish positive nurse–patient relationship therapy.

     a. Therapy goals.

       (1) Focus on the underlying emotional problems.

       (2) Offer assistance in handling anxiety.

       (3) Focus on relief of inferiority feelings and low self-esteem.

     b. Advantages of group therapy.

       (1) Patient receives support from peers.

       (2) Patient can receive negative feedback from peers without feeling threatened.

       (3) Patient can be supported in efforts to change by nonprofessional groups (AA), but change will not occur unless patient wants to be helped.

   4. Encourage rehabilitation or long-term supportive care.

     a. Continued psychotherapy on an outpatient basis.

     b. Referral to Alcoholics Anonymous.

✦   c. Medication such as *Antabuse* (alcohol-sensitizing drug that causes vomiting

and cardiovascular symptoms if the patient drinks after taking drug).

     d. Referral to social or vocational rehabilitation community program.

E. Nursing attitudes.

✦   1. Maintain a nonjudgmental attitude toward the alcoholic.

✦   2. Approach patient with firmness and consistency.

   3. Accept the individual but not his or her deviant behavior.

   4. Support patient's attempts to change life patterns.

   5. Assist patient to develop a support system— AA, church, etc.

Substance Dependence

Definition: Substance dependence is the dependency on drugs other than alcohol or tobacco that alter perception and/or mood.

Characteristics of Opioid (Narcotic) Addiction

A. The most common narcotics are heroin and morphine.

✦ B. Emotional dependence on the drug (to alter mood) is followed by physiological dependence on the drug.

✦ C. Narcotics have a sedative effect on the CNS.

✦ D. As tolerance level increases, greater amounts of the drug are necessary to produce pleasurable effects.

E. Addiction tends to be chronic; the rate of relapse is high.

✦ F. Withdrawal symptoms occur when substance is withdrawn.

   1. Anxiety.

   2. Nausea and vomiting.

   3. Sneezing, yawning, and watery eyes.

   4. Tremor and profuse perspiration.

   5. Stomach cramps and dehydration.

   6. Convulsions and coma.

G. Characteristics of the narcotic addict personality.

   1. Emotionally immature with feelings of inadequacy and inferiority.

   2. Difficulty in establishing interpersonal relationships; untruthful and insecure.

   3. Poor judgment and inability to tolerate frustration.

Characteristics of Sedative–Hypnotic Addiction

✦ A. The most common barbiturates are Seconal and Amytal Sodium; other commonly abused drugs are Valium, Quaalude, and Nembutal.

B. Barbiturates have a sedative effect on the CNS— sudden withdrawal may cause seizures or death.

C. Danger of death from overdose.

D. Emotional dependence on the drug is followed by physiological dependence on the drug.

E. Originally may have been taken to relieve pain or sleeplessness.

F. Addicts usually have emotional problems and an anxious temperament.

Characteristics of Other Common Addictions

✦ A. Amphetamines and methamphetamines.

1. The most common amphetamines are Desoxyn and Dexedrine.

2. They are CNS stimulants so that overuse may result in brain damage.

3. They have the effect of producing a "high."

4. Large doses produce a hyperactive and agitated state.

5. They produce an emotional addiction, especially for persons who feel insecure and inadequate.

6. They reduce appetite and awareness of bodily needs so that the person's physical condition suffers.

B. LSD—"acid."

1. A hallucinogenic drug that mimics hallucinations seen in psychoses.

2. Produces changes in perception and logical thought processes.

3. Not considered addictive per se, but individual may become emotionally dependent on the drug.

4. Experiences following LSD ingestion range from ecstasy to terror; the consequences are unpredictable.

C. Marijuana.

1. There is psychological dependence, but the abuse potential is lessened because it produces neither tolerance nor physical dependence.

2. Produces "dreamy" state and feelings of euphoria, hilarity, and well-being.

3. Moods vary according to environmental stimuli.

4. Changes in perception of space and time seem to distort and extend.

5. High dosage may produce hallucinations and delusions.

✦ D. Cocaine.

1. Classified as a stimulant.

2. Usually sniffed, smoked, or used intravenously.

3. Strong psychological dependence may occur.

4. Does not develop a physiological dependence or tolerance.

5. Chronic users often abuse or are dependent on a narcotic, alcohol, or an antianxiety drug to lessen withdrawal symptoms of cocaine.

E. PCP—"crystal," "elephant tranquilizer," angel dust.

1. Usually smoked with marijuana. May also be sniffed, ingested, or injected.

2. Reactions vary from sense of well-being to total disorientation and hallucinations.

3. Considered an extremely dangerous street drug.

4. Psychological dependence may occur.

5. Cerebral cellular destruction and atrophy may occur with even small amounts.

6. Overdoses or "bad trips" are characterized by erratic and unpredictable behavior, withdrawal, disorientation, self-mutilation, and self-destructive behaviors.

7. Overdoses are treated with sedatives, with a decrease of environmental stimuli, and with protection of the patient from self-harm and harm of others.

Implementation

A. General nursing approaches and attitudes are similar to those enumerated for alcoholism.

B. Special approaches to drug addiction.

1. First step is withdrawal treatment; accomplished abruptly ("cold turkey") or gradually over a period of days.

2. The substitute drug methadone is used to reduce the physical reaction to withdrawal.

3. Extended medical and psychiatric treatment for physical and emotional deterioration must be part of convalescence.

4. Resocialization process of patient needs supportive treatment from professional and/or community resources.

5. Rehabilitation programs must be directed toward helping the person reenter the mainstream of society.

a. Many organizations operated by former addicts offer help in rehabilitation.

b. Therapeutic communities and group therapy programs also assist with rehabilitation.

6. Specific guidelines.

a. Provide a structured environment, and set consistent and strict limits.

b. Identify patient's attempts to manipulate; maintain control.

c. When patient distorts reality, affirm the situational facts.

d. Give equal concern to patient's physical, social, and emotional needs.

MEDICATION THERAPY

Psychotropic Drugs

Definition: Psychotropic drugs are those used in psychiatry in conjunction with other forms of therapy to temporarily modify behavior. They con-

Table 16-5. DRUG CLASSIFICATION CHART

Trade Name	Daily Dose	Trade Name	Daily Dose
Antipsychotics		**Antidepressants (Mood Elevators)**	
Thorazine	20–1500 mg	*MAO Inhibitors*	
Mellaril	100–800 mg	Nardil	15–90 mg
Serentil	30–400 mg	Parnate	10–30 mg
Trilafon	6–64 mg	*Tricyclics*	
Prolixin Decanoate	12.5–25 mg	Pamelor	50–100 mg
Prolixin, Permitil	0.5–20 mg	Tofranil	75–300 mg
Stelazine	2–50 mg	Elavil	75–300 mg
Taractan	30–600 mg	Norpramin	75–300 mg
Navane	6–60 mg	Aventyl	40–200 mg
Haldol	2–40 mg	Vivactil	20–60 mg
Haldol Decanoate	50 mg/mL	Sinequan	75–300 mg
Loxitane	20–250 mg	Ludiomil	100–225 mg
Clozaril	300–900 mg	Wellbutrin	100–300 mg
		Selective Serotonin Reuptake Inhibitors (SSRIs)	
"Atypical" Antipsychotics			
Risperdal	1–4 mg	Paxil	10–40 mg
Seroquel	150–750 mg	Zoloft	25–150 mg
Zyprexa	5–10 mg	Prozac	10–40 mg
		Celexa	20–40 mg
Antianxiety Drugs		Lexapro	10 mg
Atarax	200–400 mg		
Vistaril	200–400 mg	**Antimanic Drugs**	
	50–100 mg	Depakote	125–500 mg
Librium, Librax	10–100 mg	Lithium carbonate	300–1800 mg
Valium	4–30 mg	(Lithane, Lithonate)	
Serax	30–160 mg	Tegretol	200–1200 mg
Centrax	20 mg		
Xanax	0.25–0.5 mg	**Antipanic Agents**	
Ativan	2–16 mg	Klonopin	.5–20 mg
Restoril	15–30 mg	Paxil	10–40 mg
BuSpar	15–130 mg	Xanax	.25–1 mg
Klonopin	0.5–20 mg	Zoloft	25–100 mg
		Antiparkinson Drugs	
		Cogentin	1–6 mg
		Artane	1–15 mg
		Akineton	2–10 mg
		Kemadrin	5–30 mg
		Symmetrel	100–200 mg
		Benadryl	30–60 mg

trol symptoms but do not cure disorder. (*See* Table 16-5.)

Characteristics

✦ A. Psychotropic drugs affect both the central and autonomic nervous systems.

B. These drugs affect behavior indirectly by chemically interacting with other chemicals, enzymes, or enzyme substrates.
  1. Changes in cellular, tissue, and organ functions occur.
  2. Drug effects vary from cellular activity to psychosocial interaction.

Antipsychotic Drugs

A. These drugs are also known as ataractics, neuroleptics, or major tranquilizers.

B. Introduced about 1953.

✦ C. Most common drugs are phenothiazine derivatives (Thorazine, Stelazine, Trilafon, and the long-acting Prolixin).

✦ D. A new class of drugs are "atypical" antipsychotics —Risperdal, Seroquel, and Zyprexa.
  1. These drugs have few or no extrapyramidal symptoms.
  2. Target both positive and negative symptoms.

◆ E. Another common antipsychotic drug is derived from butyrophenone (Haldol).
1. These drugs are less sedative than phenothiazines.
2. High incidence of severe extrapyramidal reactions.
3. Side effects include leukocytosis, blurred vision, dry mouth, urinary retention.
4. Avoid alcohol.

◆ F. Clozapine (Clozaril), Loxitane, and loxapine are new drugs for management of psychotic symptoms in patients who do not respond to other antipsychotics.
1. Side effects—similar to other antipsychotics: be aware of blood dyscrasias (leukopenia, neutropenia, agranulocytosis, eosinophilia).
2. Monitor monthly bilirubin, CBC, liver function studies, and weekly WBC—if WBC is less than 2000 µL, drug is discontinued.

G. Other classes of drugs are thioxanthenes (Taractan and Navane).

H. Formerly called "atypical" antipsychotics—Risperal, Seroquel, Zyprexa and Geodan—these drugs target positive and negative symptoms and have few or no extrapyramidal effects.

I. Antipsychotic drugs control hallucinations, delusions, and bizarre behavior and can calm an excited patient without producing a marked impairment of motor function or sleep.

◆ J. Side effects.
◆ 1. Blood dyscrasias.
a. Agranulocytosis occurs in first 3 to 5 weeks of treatment. *Symptoms:* fever, sore throat.
b. Leukopenia, preceded by altered white blood count.
◆ 2. Extrapyramidal effects occur in 30 percent of patients, affecting voluntary movements and skeletal muscles.
a. Parkinsonism—symptoms occur in 1–4 weeks; signs are similar to classic parkinsonism: rigidity, shuffling gait, pill-rolling hand movement, tremors, dyskinesia, and masklike face.
b. Akathisia—very common; occurs in 1–6 weeks; uncontrolled motor restlessness, foot tapping, agitation, pacing.
c. Dystonia—occurs early, 1–2 days; limb and neck spasms; uncoordinated, jerky movements; difficulty in speaking and swallowing, rigidity and spasms of muscles.
d. Tardive dyskinesia—develops late in treatment; estimated to occur in up to 50 percent of chronic schizophrenics.
(1) Antiparkinson drugs are of no help in decreasing symptoms.

(2) This is a permanent side effect; symptoms are shuffling gait, drooling, and general dystonic symptoms.
◆ 3. Hypotension—orthostatic hypotension may occur. Monitor closely when patient is elderly. Keep patient supine for 1 hour and advise to change positions slowly.
◆ 4. Anticholinergic effects—dry mouth, blurred vision, tachycardia, nasal congestion, and constipation. Treat symptomatically.
5. Drugs potentiate CNS depression, especially with alcohol.
6. Antacids reduce absorption.
◆ 7. *Neuroleptic malignant syndrome*—a rare complication caused by antipsychotics—a medical emergency (20 percent mortality rate) and must be recognized and treated immediately.
a. Signs and symptoms: irregular vital signs, hyperpyrexia, altered mental status, elevated CPK.
b. Treatment: discontinue drug, administer dopamine-enhancing drug and/or Dantrium.

Antiparkinson Drugs

A. The term *extrapyramidal disease* refers to motor disorders often associated with pathologic dysfunction in the basal ganglia.
1. Clinical symptoms of the disease include abnormal involuntary movement, changes in tone of the skeletal muscles, and a reduction of automatic associated movements.
2. Reversible extrapyramidal reactions may follow the use of certain drugs.
3. The most common drugs are the phenothiazine derivatives.

◆ B. Antiparkinson drugs act on the extrapyramidal system to reduce disturbing symptoms caused by antipsychotic drugs.
1. They are usually given in conjunction with antipsychotic drugs.
◆ 2. Two of the most common drugs are Artane and Cogentin.
3. Side effects are dizziness, gastrointestinal disturbance, headaches, urinary hesitancy, and memory impairment.

C. Benadryl, an antihistamine, is often given in place of Artane or Cogentin.
1. Controls the extrapyramidal side effects of phenothiazines.
2. Preferred because it does not cause as many untoward side effects as other antiparkinson drugs.

Anxiolytic (Antianxiety) Drugs

✦ A. These drugs induce sedation, relax muscles, and inhibit convulsions; major use to reduce anxiety.

B. These drugs are the most frequently prescribed drugs in medicine; demand is great for relief from anxiety, and they are safer than sedative–hypnotics.

✦ C. They potentiate drug abuse. Greatest harm occurs when combined with alcohol and other CNS depressants.

D. They are prescribed in neuroses, psychosomatic disorders, or functional psychiatric disorders, but do not modify psychotic behavior.

E. Drugs from two major classes. Benzodiazepines: safer and more common (Librium, Valium, Ativan, Restoril, Centrax, Versed, Serax, and Xanax—being tested for use in depression, panic, and obsessive–compulsive disorders). Nonbenzodiazepines: BuSpar, Sonata, Ambien, Equanil.

F. New benzodiazepines have shorter onset and half-lives (triazolam, Doral) and Klonopin with usual onset and half-life.

✦ G. Side effects.
  1. Drowsiness (avoid driving or working around equipment).
  2. Blurred vision, constipation, dermatitis, mental confusion, anorexia, polyuria, menstrual irregularities, and edema.
  3. Habituation and increased tolerance.
  4. Pancytopenia, thrombocytopenia, and granulocytopenia.

Antidepressant Drugs

✦ A. The tricyclics, the most commonly used antidepressants, include Elavil, Norpramin, Tofranil, Aventyl, Vivactil, and Pamelor.
  ✦ 1. Anticholinergic: take 1 to 6 weeks to be effective. Produces antagonism of the parasympathetic system.
  ✦ 2. Blocks uptake of norepinephrine and serotonin.
  3. Patients with morbid fantasies do not respond well to these drugs.
  ✦ 4. Side effects.
    a. Anticholinergic effects: dry mouth, blurred vision, constipation, postural hypotension.
    b. CNS effects: tremor, agitation, angry states, mania, and seizures.
    c. Cardiovascular and cardiotoxic effects: changes in the electrical conduction; with history of cardiac disease, have an ECG.
    d. Sedation.
    e. Most side effects appear in first 1–2 weeks and diminish over the next few weeks.

5. If patient is switched from a tricyclic drug to an MAO inhibitor, a period of 1–3 weeks must elapse between drugs.

✦ B. The MAO inhibitors include Marplan, Nardil, and Parnate.
  1. MAO inhibitors are toxic, potent, and produce many side effects.
  2. They should not be the first antidepressant drug used; effect is at best equal to a tricyclic and side effects more dangerous.
  ✦ 3. Side effects.
    a. Most dangerous is hypertensive crisis.
    b. Drug interactions can cause severe hypertension, hypotension, or CNS depression.
    c. Postural hypotension, headaches, constipation, anorexia, diarrhea, and chills.
    d. Tachycardia, edema, impotence, dizziness, insomnia, and restlessness.
    e. Manic episodes and anxiety.
  ✦ 4. All patients must be warned not to eat foods with high tyramine content (aged cheese, wine, beer, chicken liver, yeast), certain combination foods such as pizza, drink alcohol, or take other drugs, especially sympathomimetic drugs (amphetamines, L-Dopa, epinephrine).
  5. MAO inhibitors must not be used in combination with tricyclics due to elevated tyramine levels.

✦ C. Hypertensive crisis.
  1. Severe symptoms: throbbing occipital headache, confusion, drowsiness, vomiting, stiff neck, chills, and chest pain.
  2. Monitor for potential complications: encephalopathy, heart failure.
  3. Treatment.
    a. Drug of choice: Regitine, IV 5 mg (or Thorazine) with close monitoring; antihypertensive.
    b. Monitor vital signs, ECG, and neurological signs; BP q 5 minutes.
    c. Norepinephrine is administered for severe hypotension.

✦ D. A new class of drugs, introduced in 1988 with Prozac, are chemically and pharmacologically distinct from other antidepressant drugs.
  1. Selective inhibitors of the uptake of serotonin (SSRIs).
    ✦ a. Studies suggest that increased serotonin in critical areas of the brain modifies certain affective behavior. Results in the increased concentration of active serotonin in critical synaptic areas in the brain.
    b. A number of neurochemical pathways can be affected by existing antidepressants—

drugs are highly selective for the serotonin pathway and exert little or no effect on the uptake of other neurotransmitters or receptor sites.

◆ c. Examples are Prozac, Zoloft, Paxil, Wellbutrin, Celexa and Lexapro.

2. Exhibit fewer side effects than other antidepressant drugs.

a. Anticholinergic side effects such as dry mouth and constipation are fewer with these drugs.

b. Side effects observed are nausea (the most common), anxiety/nervousness, insomnia, drowsiness, and headache.

c. Coadministration of alcohol is not recommended.

E. A later class of drugs are now being used as antidepressants with few to no side effects.

1. Trazodone HCL (Desyrel) inhibits uptake of serotonin.

2. Nefazodone (Serzone) and venlafaxine (Effexor) block uptake of both norepinephrine and serotonin.

3. Useful to treat severely depressed and melancholic patients.

4. Some patients experience anxiety, nausea, vomiting, and dizziness.

Mood-Stabilizing (Antimanic) Drugs

A. These drugs control mood disorders, especially the manic phase, and elevate mood when patient is depressed.

B. Before lithium therapy is begun, baseline studies of renal, cardiac, and thyroid status obtained.

C. Most common form of drug is lithium carbonate, a naturally occurring metallic salt.

◆ D. Drug must reach certain blood level before it is effective.

1. Stabilizing concentration occurs in 5–7 days; therapeutic effects 7–28 days.

2. Serum level can be simply and reliably measured in mEq/L of blood.

◆ E. Lithium is metabolized by the kidney.

1. Deficiency of sodium results in more lithium being reabsorbed, thus increasing risk of toxicity.

2. Excessive sodium causes more lithium to be excreted and may lower level to a nontherapeutic range.

3. Normal dietary intake of sodium and adequate fluids to prevent dehydration are important guidelines with lithium.

4. Serum levels measured 2–3 times weekly (12 hours after last dose) in beginning of therapy; for long-term maintenance therapy, every 2–3 months.

◆ F. Drug concentration and side effects.

1. Therapeutic range of serum levels is 0.6–1.2 mEq/L; for acute manic state, 1.0–1.5 mEq/L.

2. Side effects occur at upper ranges, usually above 1.5 mEq/L.

3. Gastrointestinal disturbances, metallic taste in mouth, muscle weakness, fatigue, thirst, polyuria, and fine hand tremors.

4. Hypothyroidism is a long-term effect of lithium therapy.

◆ G. Lithium toxicity.

1. Appears when blood level exceeds 1.5–2.0 mEq/L. Many appear sooner depending on individual patient.

2. Central nervous system is the chief target.

3. Initial symptoms include nausea, vomiting, drowsiness, tremors, slurred speech, blurred vision, muscle twitches, and oliguria.

4. If drug is continued, coma, convulsions, and death may result.

5. Treatment for toxicity: gastric lavage, correction of fluid balance, drug (mannitol) to increase urine excretion.

6. For patients who cannot take lithium, seizure medications may be prescribed (Depakote).

Drug Administration in a Psychiatric Setting

A. Give correct *drug* and *dose* at correct time to correct *patient* according to physician's orders.

B. Learn the specific actions and uses of drugs.

C. Become familiar with the side effects and precautions associated with major drug groups.

D. Observe patient carefully for side effects.

E. Be familiar with the drug groups that are not compatible—know half-life of drugs and drug interactions.

F. Refer to psychotropic drug classification chart in Table 16-5.

OTHER FORMS OF THERAPY

Crisis Intervention

◆ *Definition:* Crisis intervention is the form of therapy aimed at immediate intervention into an acute episode or crisis that the individual is unable to cope with alone.

Profile of a Crisis Situation

A. The individual is typically in a state of equilibrium (homeostatic balance).

1. State is maintained by behavioral patterns that govern interchange between the individual and the environment.

2. The individual uses learned coping techniques to deal with simple problems as they arise.

B. Crisis situation develops when a problem (triggering event) becomes too complex to be handled by previously learned coping techniques.

1. Functioning modes become grossly disorganized.
◆ 2. Individual is more amenable to intervention in circumstances of inability to resolve crisis.
3. Potential for problem resolution as a result of intervention is positive.

C. Precipitant factors of a crisis.

1. Threat to one's sense of security.
   a. Situational crisis: may include an actual or potential loss of job, friend, or mate.
   b. Developmental crisis: may include any change in role as occurs in marriage or birth of a child.
   c. Concurrence of two or more severe problems.
2. Precipitants typically occur within 2 weeks of onset of disorganization.

Characteristics

◆ A. Crisis is self-limiting, acute, and lasts 1–6 weeks.
◆ B. Crisis is initiated by a triggering event (death, loss, etc.); usual coping mechanisms are inadequate for the situation.
C. Situation is dangerous to the person; he or she may harm self or others.
◆ D. Individual will return to a state that is better, worse, or the same as before the crisis; therefore, intervention by the therapist is important.
E. Person is totally involved—hurts all over.
F. At this time, the individual is most open for intervention; therefore, major changes can take place.

Stages of Crisis Development

A. Initial perception and comprehension of scope of problem.
B. Rise in tension and anxiety, which instigates the usual coping mechanisms.
C. Consultation with the usual supportive contacts.
D. Familiar methods prove unsuccessful, and tension increases.
E. Seeks new problem-solving methods; if unsuccessful, the problem remains and interferes with individual's life.
1. Functioning becomes disorganized.
2. Extreme anxiety is likely to be experienced.
3. Perception is narrowed.
4. Coping ability is further impaired.
5. Situation may cause self-harm or harm to others.
6. Individual totally involved with crisis situation.

F. Resolution will occur within 6 weeks with or without intervention.

Principles of Crisis Intervention

◆ A. Goal is the return of patient to precrisis level and maintenance of functioning.
◆ B. Intervene immediately because it is important that intervention occur within the 6-week time limit.
C. Assess problem accurately and keep focus on this problem with reality-oriented therapy ("here and now" focus).
D. Set limits.
E. Remain with patient or have significant person available as necessary.
F. Explore coping mechanisms available to patient.
1. Develop strengths and capitalize on them.
2. Do not focus on weakness or pathology.
3. Help explore the available situational supports.
G. Help the patient to understand the problem and to integrate the events in his or her life.
H. Determine if continuing therapy with a professional may be needed for future support.

Domestic Violence

Definition: In a domestic or family setting, the abuser becomes destructive and abusive; threatens or attacks the victim.

Characteristics

A. The abuser (the majority are males) makes demands and threats against the victim, who attempts to appease the abuser.
B. The abuser loses control and hurts the victim and then tries to make up for this behavior by becoming loving and apologetic.
C. Most often other family members or outsiders do not know what is happening inside the family.
D. Often the victim hides the abuse and will not seek help from their family or the outside.
E. Abusers evidence certain characteristics similar to sociopathic personalities.
1. Poor self-esteem.
2. Suspicious and dependent.
3. History of sexual abuse or violent abuse during childhood.
F. Victims also have low self-esteem, are dependent and often depressed; they feel helpless and without power to change the situation.

Assessment

A. Recognize and assess for abuse in the victim (bruises, cuts, broken bones, etc.).
B. Assess the family situation.
C. Report suspected cases of domestic abuse.

Implementation

A. Assure privacy for the victim during examination; remind victim that information is confidential to allay fears.
B. Establish a nurse–patient relationship to provide climate for the victim to feel safe in discussing family situation.
C. Encourage therapy for both victim and abuser; suggest group therapy, family counseling and support groups.
D. Suggest therapy for the victim that focuses on building self-esteem, self-protective abilities and problem-solving ability.

Electroconvulsive Therapy (ECT)

◆ *Definition:*   Use of electrically induced seizures for the safe and effective treatment of severe depression, psychotic depression and mania.
A. Electric current passed through the brain induces seizures; breaks up behavior patterns by causing temporary amnesia.
◆ B. Advantages.
  1. Works more quickly than antidepressants.
  2. Safer for elderly with history of cardiac illness than antidepressant medication therapy.
  3. Major depressive episode with vegetative aspects has improvement rate of 80 percent.
C. Administration.
  ◆ 1. Three types of medication administered: anticholinergic (*atropine, Robinul*), to block vagal stimulation so secretions are reduced; short-acting, *general anesthesia* administered IV to make the patient more comfortable; and a *muscle relaxant (Anectine)*, to reduce complications from the convulsion itself.
  ◆ 2. Preparation: informed consent, medical history, and physical exam; lab workup and education of patient.
◆ D. Side effects: memory loss for recent events and difficulty learning new information—effects resolve in 6–9 months; headaches, muscle aches, weight gain, hypertension, and, occasionally, cardiac arrhythmias.
◆ E. In several weeks, as memory returns, most of the self-deprecation and sadness will have dissipated.
◆ F. Nursing considerations.
  1. Keep NPO for at least 4 hours.
  2. Have patient void and remove dentures prior to treatment.
  3. Check that consent form is signed.
  4. Provide support by listening to the patient's expression of fear concerning the procedure.
  5. Assure patient that she or he will not be alone during or after treatment.
  6. Assist physician during treatment.
  7. Reorient patient following procedure, and explain feelings of confusion.
  8. Observe and record patient's response to treatments.

Socialization or Motivational Therapy

A. Intended to motivate and get patient moving again.
◆ B. Patient can socialize and be motivated by means of group therapy, occupational therapy, environmental therapy.
C. Encourage patient's participation in therapy.
D. Support patient's efforts to share feelings.

Energetic Psychotherapies

A. New emerging therapies are dealing with issues that traditional therapies took years to resolve.
B. Several forms of new style therapies are being used.
  1. EMDR: Eye Movement Desensitization and Reprocessing is the most popular and well known.
  2. TFT: Thought Field Therapy.
  3. EFT: Emotional Freedom Technique.
  4. WHEE: Wholistic Hybrid EMDR, a combination of EFT and EMDR.
C. Treatment of psychological problems has been accomplished with algorithms of sequences focusing on eye movements (EMDR) and tapping on energy meridians in precise order (TFT or EFT and WHEE).
D. Types of populations treated with energetic therapies.
  1. Post-traumatic stress syndrome (especially combat veterans).
  2. Phobias and panic disorders.
  3. Crime victims.
  4. Excessive grief.
  5. Children with traumas of assault or natural disaster.
  6. Sexual assault or sexual dysfunction.
  7. Dissociative disorders.
  8. Chemical dependence.
E. Advantages of these therapies.
  1. Remarkable results for resolution of problems (high efficacy). Almost 1 million people treated with these techniques.
  2. Takes only a few sessions; previously, it could take years to resolve these problems.
  3. Results show:
    a. Decrease in subjective distress (traumatic memories).
    b. Significant increase in confidence and positive beliefs.
    c. Increase in insight and cognitive changes.

Appendix 16-1. GLOSSARY

Acting out Expression of unconscious emotional conflicts of hostility or love in actions that the person does not consciously know are related to such conflicts of feelings.

Affect Generalized feeling, tone, or mood.

Aggression Any verbal/nonverbal activity that may be forceful abuse of self, another person, or thing.

Ambivalence The simultaneous existence of contradictory and contrasting emotions toward a person or object at the same time, that is, love and hate.

Amnesia A condition where the individual experiences a loss of memory because of physical or emotional trauma.

Anxiety A persistent feeling of tension and apprehension arising from within the individual. Response to vague, unspecific danger that may be real or imagined.

Apathy Pathological indifference.

Autism Detachment from reality when self-preoccupation and involvement predominate.

Compulsion An irresistible urge to repeat an act that must be carried out to avoid anxiety.

Conflict A struggle between two or more opposing forces.

Covert Hidden, below the surface.

Cyclothymia Alterations in mood from high to low.

Defense mechanism Originally identified by Anna Freud, an activity of the ego that defends itself by not allowing unacceptable thoughts or feelings to come into awareness to cause anxiety.

Delusion A false belief maintained in spite of facts or evidence to the contrary.

Depression An unshakable feeling of sadness accompanied by feelings of hopelessness, worthlessness, and the feeling of a bleak future.

Disorientation A condition in which the individual manifests loss of ability to recognize or locate himself in respect to time, place, or other persons.

Echolalia A condition in which the individual constantly repeats what is heard.

Echopraxia A condition in which the individual mimics what is done.

Ego A Freudian term denoting the aspect of the psyche that is conscious and most in touch with external reality; the "I" part of the person. Also, that part of the personality that makes decisions, is conscious, and represents the thinking–feeling part of a person.

Electroconvulsive shock (ECT) A medical procedure of applying electric current to certain areas in the brain. Used in the treatment of certain psychiatric disorders (especially depression).

Etiology The cause or causes of disease.

Euphoria A feeling of elation or joy.

Fear Response to an actual person or situation of external danger.

Fixation A stage in development when there is an abnormal attachment; inability to move on to later developmental tasks.

Frustration A feeling that may contain elements of anger, hopelessness, or defeat, which results when goals set by perceived needs are blocked.

Fugue A condition experienced as a transient disorientation—patient is unaware that he or she has physically escaped or run to another place.

Functional Used in psychiatry to denote mental illness existing without known physical causes or structural changes.

Hypochondriasis A state of morbid concern about one's body or health for which there is no physical evidence.

Hysteric Involves elements of both conscious and unconscious exaggerated reaction, often in a dramatic manner, to a specific situation.

Id A Freudian term denoting a division of the psyche from which come blind, instinctual impulses that lead to immediate gratification of primitive needs, dominated by the pleasure principle.

Ideas of reference A distortion of reality wherein a person believes that activities of others have a personal reference to one's self.

Illusion Distorted perceptual experience in which the individual misinterprets actual data from the environment. Examples: a mirage on the desert; seeing a lake when it is only light refraction.

Insight An individual's understanding of the origin and mechanisms of his or her attitudes and behavior.

Interpersonal Existing between two or more persons.

Intrapersonal Existing within one person.

Labile Refers to rapid shifts in emotions from high to low.

Manipulation The process by which one individual influences another individual to function in accordance with his needs without regard to the other's needs or goals.

Mental retardation A term for mental deficiency or lack of normal development of intelligence.

Milieu The total environment, emotional as well as physical.

Narcissistic Loving one's self excessively in a childish or an infantile fashion.

Negativism A strong resistance to suggestions coming from others.

Neologism A term that refers to the coining of a new word, as seen in schizophrenia.

Obsession A persistent repetitive and unwanted thought.

Organic Based on structural alterations, gross or microscopic.

Overt Discernible; out in the open.

Parataxic A term coined by Sullivan to mean distorted perception.

Phobia The dread of an object, an act, or a situation that is not realistically dangerous but that has come to represent a danger.

Premorbid personality The status of an individual's personality (conflicts, defenses, strengths, weaknesses) before the onset of clinical illness.

Psyche A term meaning the mind or the mental and emotional "self."

Psychogenic Originating within the psyche or mind. Sometimes used to describe physical disorders that are believed to stem from the emotions.

Rapport A component of a relationship in which one feels harmony or empathy with another.

Continues

Appendix 16-1. GLOSSARY *(Continued)*

Regression Reverting to types of behavior characteristic of an earlier level of development.

Resistance A mechanism an individual employs to avoid certain ideas or feelings coming into consciousness.

Schizoid A term used to describe a form of personality disorder characterized by an unsocial, withdrawn, shy type of personality.

Seclusive A term describing persons who are unsociable, reserved, secretive, and adverse to interacting with people.

Soma A term meaning body.

Superego A Freudian term referring to a system within the total psyche that is developed by incorporating parental standards such as moral values; the two components of superego are conscience and ego ideal.

Unconscious A term coined by Freud to refer to that part of the mind where mental activity is always going on, but not on a conscious level.

Undoing A defense mechanism aimed at the removal of a painful memory.

Waxy flexibility A condition associated with catatonic schizophrenia, in which a posture is maintained for long periods of time.

MENTAL HEALTH NURSING QUESTIONS

1. A depressed patient refuses to get out of bed, go to activities, or participate in any of the unit's programs. The most appropriate nursing action is to

   1. Tell her the rules of the unit are that no patient can remain in bed.
   2. Suggest she should get out of bed or she will go hungry later.
   3. Tell her that the nurse will assist her out of bed and help her to dress.
   4. Allow her to remain in bed until she feels ready to join the other patients.

2. A young adult is admitted to the hospital for a diagnostic workup. She has recently lost weight and has not had a menstrual period for 3 months. While collecting data, the nurse will focus on a(n)

   1. Interpersonal relationship.
   2. Eating disorder.
   3. Hormone irregularity.
   4. Diet consultation.

3. When encouraged to join an activity, a depressed patient on the psychiatric unit refuses and says, "What's the use?" The approach by the nurse that would be most effective is to

   1. Sit down beside her and ask her how she is feeling.
   2. Tell her it is time for the activity, help her out of the chair, and go with her to the activity.
   3. Convince her how helpful it will be to engage in the activity.
   4. Tell her that this is a self-defeating attitude and it will only make her feel worse.

4. When a depressed patient becomes more active and there is evidence that her mood has lifted, an appropriate goal to add to the nursing care plan is to

   1. Encourage her to go home for the weekend.
   2. Move her to a room with three other patients.
   3. Monitor her whereabouts at all times.
   4. Begin to explore the reasons she became depressed.

5. A client with a history of alcohol abuse is admitted to the emergency room with delirium tremens (DTs). The physician orders Valium 10 mg, IV with vitamin B_6, vital signs every 30 minutes, regular diet, and an environment with no stimuli. Which intervention will the nurse implement first?

   1. Vital signs.
   2. Valium 10 mg.
   3. IV with vitamin B_6.
   4. Quiet environment.

6. When a patient's hallucinations become more insistent, demanding, and difficult to ignore, the nurse assesses his mental status as

   1. Improving.
   2. Deteriorating.
   3. Remaining the same.
   4. Showing more evidence of paranoia.

7. During the last 15 years, suicide has increased dramatically in the age group of

   1. Menopausal women.
   2. Adolescents.
   3. Elderly men.
   4. Children under age 12.

8. Group therapy has been an accepted method of treatment for psychiatric patients for several years. The best rationale for this form of treatment is

   1. It is the most economical—one staff member can treat many patients.
   2. The format of the therapy is realistic and does not deal with unconscious material.
   3. It enables patients to become aware that others have problems and that they are not alone in their suffering.
   4. It provides a social milieu similar to society in general, where the patient can relate to others and validate perceptions in a realistic setting.

9. A 60-year-old male patient has been admitted to the psychiatric unit, with symptoms ranging from fatigue, an inability to concentrate, and an inability to complete everyday tasks, to refusal to care for himself and preferring to sleep all day. One of the first interventions should be aimed at

   1. Developing a good nursing care plan.
   2. Talking to his wife for cues to help him.
   3. Encouraging him to join activities on the unit.
   4. Developing a structured routine for him to follow.

10. A patient becomes very dejected and states that life isn't worth living and no one really cares what happens to him. The best response from the nurse would be

1. "Of course, people care. Your wife comes to visit every day."
2. "Let's not talk about sad things. Why don't we play Ping-Pong?"
3. "I care about you, and I am concerned that you feel so down."
4. "Tell me, who doesn't care about you?"

11. A female patient on a psychiatric unit has just told the nurse that she is thinking of committing suicide. The appropriate intervention would be to

1. Notify the charge nurse.
2. Ask the patient if she has a plan.
3. Request special one-to-one observation.
4. Administer the PRN ordered medication.

12. A nurse observes a patient sitting alone in her room crying. As the nurse approaches her, the patient states, "I'm feeling sad. I don't want to talk now." The nurse's best response would be

1. "It will help you feel better if you talk about it."
2. "I'll come back when you feel like talking."
3. "I'll stay with you a few minutes."
4. "Sometimes it helps to talk."

13. A client with the diagnosis of manic episode is racing around the psychiatric unit trying to organize games with the patients. An appropriate nursing intervention is to

1. Have the patients play Ping-Pong.
2. Suggest video exercises with the other patients.
3. Take the client outside for a walk.
4. Do nothing, as organizing a game is considered therapeutic.

14. When assessing a patient for possible suicide, an important clue would be if the patient

1. Is hostile and sarcastic to the staff.
2. Identifies with problems expressed by other patients.
3. Seems satisfied and detached.
4. Begins to talk about leaving the hospital.

15. A male patient on the psychiatric unit becomes upset when a visitor does not show up, and in a rage, breaks a chair. The first nursing intervention should be to

1. Stay with the patient during the stressful time.
2. Ask direct questions about the patient's behavior.
3. Set limits and restrict the patient's behavior.
4. Plan with the client for how he can better handle frustration.

16. A patient with a diagnosis of obsessive–compulsive disorder constantly does repetitive cleaning. The nurse knows that this behavior is probably most basically an attempt to

1. Decrease the anxiety to a tolerable level.
2. Focus attention on nonthreatening tasks.
3. Control others.
4. Decrease the time available for interaction with people.

17. A patient has been admitted with a diagnosis of DTs. The nurse knows that the primary reason the patient is so fearful and apprehensive is that

1. He has a serious mental illness.
2. He may die, as 15 percent of the people with DTs do die.
3. His illusions and hallucinations are very real to him.
4. He has to give up alcohol until the symptoms recede.

18. A patient is experiencing a high degree of anxiety. It is important to recognize if additional help is required because

1. If the patient is out of control, another person will help to decrease his anxiety level.
2. Being alone with an anxious patient is dangerous.
3. It will take another person to direct the patient into activities to relieve anxiety.
4. Hospital protocol for handling anxious patients requires at least two people.

19. A 56-year-old patient is tentatively diagnosed as having Korsakoff's syndrome. In developing a strategy to care for this patient, the nurse knows that this condition is a(n)

1. Neurological condition common with alcohol poisoning.
2. Neurological degeneration caused by vitamin deficiency.
3. Organic brain lesion brought on by repeated hepatitis attacks.
4. State resulting from severe, long-term psychosis.

20. Three days after admission for depression, a 54-year-old female patient approaches the nurse and says, "I know I have cancer of the uterus. Can't you let me stay in bed and have some peace before I die?" In responding, the nurse must keep in mind that

1. The patient must be postmenopausal.
2. Thoughts of disease are common in depressed patients.

3. Patients suffering from depression can be demanding, making many requests of the nurse.
4. Antidepressant medications frequently cause vaginal spotting.

21. As a depressed patient begins to participate in her treatment program, an indication that she is ready for discharge will be when she has

   1. Formulated a plan to return home and continue therapy.
   2. Talked to her boss about returning to work.
   3. Identified her weak areas and is working on them.
   4. Asked the staff for advice about her future.

22. A patient with Alzheimer's disease is talking to the tree in the corner of the room as if it were a person. An appropriate intervention would be to

   1. Tell the patient that he is talking to a tree.
   2. Ignore the incident.
   3. Write the incident in the chart.
   4. Begin a conversation with the patient.

23. The nurse observes a patient's daughter, who is visiting her mother, sitting alone and crying. When approached, the daughter states, "I'm really concerned about Mom." The nurse's best response would be

   1. "Are you concerned about her hospitalization?"
   2. "Tell me what's concerning you."
   3. "Would you like to talk with the social worker?"
   4. "Would you like to talk to her physician?"

24. Of the following approaches to a patient with organic brain syndrome, the most therapeutic would be to

   1. Use short, concrete, specific interactions.
   2. Give complete explanations to the patient about his problems.
   3. Provide a flexible therapy schedule.
   4. Confront the patient whenever he loses contact with reality.

25. In assisting in the treatment of a person on a "bad trip" from LSD ingestion, the nurse would

   1. Stay with the patient.
   2. Ask him what help he would like to have.
   3. Encourage verbalization of feelings and perceptions.
   4. Provide ongoing orientation.

26. A schizophrenic patient is admitted to the psychiatric unit. As the nurse approaches the patient with medication, he refuses it, accusing the nurse

of trying to kill him. The nurse's best strategy would be to tell him that

   1. "It is not poison and you must take the medication."
   2. "I will give you an injection if necessary."
   3. "You may decide if you want to take the medication by mouth or injection, but you must take it."
   4. "It's all right if you don't take the medication right now."

27. An elderly, depressed patient has orders for electro-convulsive therapy (ECT). Of the medications administered, the primary purpose of a muscle relaxant is to

   1. Decrease anxiety before ECT.
   2. Reduce complications from the procedure.
   3. Reduce tension in the patient's muscles.
   4. Block vagal stimulation.

28. A patient with the diagnosis of organic brain syndrome, dementia type, confabulates when talking with the nurse. The nurse's best response and the rationale for it is to

   1. Tell him she knows he is distorting the situation and not telling the truth because she knows alcoholics need to have moral values reinforced.
   2. Sit him down and repeatedly give him the correct version of his activity until he remembers it, because one way of learning is to have something repeatedly stressed.
   3. Constantly reiterate the correct story each time he confabulates because a realistic goal with this patient is to correct memory distortion.
   4. Accept his stories without challenge as he is unable, because of organic damage, to recall accurately.

29. A 50-year-old patient has just been admitted to the psychiatric unit with a diagnosis of depression. The nurse can best approach her by saying

   1. "You have just been admitted, and I'd like to show you the unit."
   2. "Would you like to come with me to occupational therapy and see if you can find a project you would enjoy?"
   3. "My name is Mary. I will introduce you to all of the other patients."
   4. "My name is Mary. I am a nurse on this floor and I will be spending some time with you."

30. A patient has been in the hospital for 3 weeks. His diagnosis is paranoid ideation. The nurse will know that the patient's condition is improving when he

1. Stops talking about the paranoid ideas.
2. Says that he wants to go home.
3. Asks the nurse if his ideas are real.
4. Describes his paranoid ideas to the nurse in great detail.

31. An antisocial patient refuses to participate in unit activities, staying in his room reading until late at night. When he is on the unit, he makes fun of the other patients, calling them "nuts" or "stupid." Considering his diagnosis and behavior, the nursing plan that would be most effective for the staff to follow is to

   1. Let the patient know the rules on the unit.
   2. Allow the patient to isolate himself so that he does not upset the other patients.
   3. Confer with the patient, the staff, and his psychiatrist about his lack of participation on the unit.
   4. Require the patient's participation in activities.

32. A patient with a diagnosis of schizophrenia who threatened a neighbor with a knife was placed on a 72-hour hold by the courts and the psychiatrist. The hold is up, and the psychiatrist and court must determine if the patient is

   1. Gravely disabled and unable to take care of himself.
   2. A danger to himself and others.
   3. Able to pay for his hospitalization and treatment.
   4. Willing to remain in treatment if he is discharged.

33. A patient tells the nurse that she is having a great deal of difficulty talking to her husband. She says, "He treats me like a child. Nothing I say seems to matter to him." The best response is

   1. "Tell me more about how you and your husband communicate."
   2. "How do you feel about his reactions to you?"
   3. "He sounds very childish himself."
   4. "Why do you think he treats you like a child?"

34. As a male nurse is coming on duty, one of the patients meets him in the elevator and says, "You look like a wreck today." The best response would be

   1. "You don't look so good yourself."
   2. "If you can't say anything nice, perhaps you shouldn't say anything at all."
   3. "I don't understand what you mean by that."
   4. "I was a little rushed this morning."

35. The nurse is in the dayroom with a group of patients when a patient who has been quietly watching TV suddenly jumps up screaming and runs out of the room. The nurse's priority intervention would be to

   1. Turn off the TV, and ask the group what they think about the patient's behavior.
   2. Follow after the patient to see what has happened.
   3. Ignore the incident because these outbursts are frequent.
   4. Send another patient out of the room to check on the agitated patient.

36. A patient's deafness has been diagnosed as conversion disorder. Nursing interventions should be guided by which of the following?

   1. The patient will probably express much anxiety about her deafness and require much reassurance.
   2. The patient will have little or no awareness of the psychogenic cause of her deafness.
   3. The patient's need for the symptom should be respected; thus, secondary gains should be allowed.
   4. The defense mechanisms of suppression and rationalization are involved in creating the symptom.

37. A nursing student failed her psychology final exam and spent the entire evening berating the teacher and the course. This behavior would be an example of

   1. Reaction-formation.
   2. Compensation.
   3. Projection.
   4. Acting out.

38. In planning nursing care for the individual with a somatoform or psychosomatic illness, the nurse needs to consider which of the following general concepts?

   1. The nurse must incorporate concepts of adaptation, stress, body image, and anxiety.
   2. The area of symptom formation may be symbolic to the patient.
   3. Psychosomatic illnesses may be life threatening.
   4. All of the above concepts are important.

39. The most effective nursing intervention for a severely anxious patient who is pacing vigorously would be to

   1. Instruct her to sit down and quit pacing.
   2. Place her in bed to reduce stimuli and allow rest.

3. Allow her to walk until she becomes physically tired.
4. Give her PRN medication and walk with her at a gradually slowing pace.

40. A patient has been in the hospital for 4 weeks. He is dying of terminal cancer. During this time, he has never mentioned his condition or the fact that he is dying. The nurse's knowledge of the dying process leads to the conclusion that the patient is

1. In the grieving process and does not wish to talk.
2. Still in the denial phase.
3. Depending on his family for support and talks to them.
4. Afraid that by talking about dying it will become reality.

41. A new staff nurse is on an orientation tour with the head nurse. A patient approaches her and says, "I don't belong here. Please try to get me out." The staff nurse's best response would be

1. "What would you do if you were out of the hospital?"
2. "I am a new staff member, and I'm on a tour. I'll come back and talk with you later."
3. "I think you should talk with the head nurse about that."
4. "I can't do anything about that."

42. A patient on the psychiatric unit frequently gets out of control and is inappropriately aggressive. A plan to teach this patient how to cope would include

1. A problem-solving focus involving alternative responses.
2. Confronting the patient about this behavior.
3. Informing the patient of the consequences of his behavior (i.e., restraints).
4. Frequent times in seclusion as a part of a behavior modification program.

43. A patient is admitted with the diagnosis of alcoholism. The initial goal of the treatment program would be to

1. Set limits on the patient's behavior.
2. Reestablish a healthy physical condition.
3. Determine what circumstances led to the condition.
4. Use group psychotherapy as the primary method of treatment.

44. A patient in the hospital asks the nurse what the drug Prozac is used for. The best response would be

1. "You had better ask your physician."

2. "It is given for depression. Why do you ask?"
3. "It is an antidepressant medication that has fewer side effects than other drugs."
4. "Why are you asking about Prozac?"

45. A patient is admitted to the hospital with the diagnosis of narcotic addiction–heroin. In collecting data on the patient, the nurse knows that the effect of this drug on the patient is

1. Sedative.
2. Stimulating.
3. Hallucinogenic.
4. A sense of well-being.

46. Nursing responsibility working on a psychiatric unit includes being able to recognize indications or signals of impending violent or assaultive behavior. This behavior could be

1. Foul language.
2. Hallucinations that are threatening, new, and commanding in nature.
3. Sudden withdrawal and refusal to speak.
4. Increased tendency to approach people and make physical contact, such as touching faces.

47. A patient has been given the diagnosis of compulsive disorder. As part of her treatment plan, the patient will join a daily group therapy session at 10:30 in the morning. The rationale for choosing this time of day is

1. Anxious patients are more relaxed in the morning.
2. Mornings are better for group therapy because clients have the rest of the day to work through problems that come up during the sessions.
3. Most groups are planned for the morning when physicians are on the unit.
4. The patient will have just completed her ritualistic activity.

48. A 75-year-old patient has the diagnosis of organic brain syndrome (OBS). In planning the daily schedule, it is important for the nurse to understand that the patient

1. May have moderate-to-severe memory impairment and short periods of concentration.
2. Will be more comfortable with a rigid daily schedule.
3. Is more likely to be able to remember current experiences than past ones.
4. Can usually be trusted to be responsible for her daily care needs.

49. A patient was admitted with the diagnosis of antisocial behavior. He had beat up his girlfriend and was brought to the hospital for a court-ordered evaluation. During the nurse's interaction with the patient he asked where she lives, whom she dates, and other personal information. He said, "I just want to get to know you better. I like you. You're the only one I can really talk to." The best nursing response would be

1. "You're getting too involved with me. Maybe another nurse would be more appropriate for you."
2. "Let's talk about my purpose in working with you and your feelings about it."
3. "Why are you focusing on me all the time?"
4. "I think you're trying to avoid talking about you and your problems."

50. The nurse finds a manipulative patient in the TV room at midnight watching an old movie. The nurse reminds him that the TV set is to be shut off at 12:30 AM. He ignores her. When the nurse returns 30 minutes later, he tells her not to turn off the TV because he is just starting another movie and he intends to watch it. The best nursing response is

1. "Ok, but that's it after this one!"
2. "No one else is allowed to watch TV this late."
3. "Apparently there is some confusion about the rules."
4. "You are aware of the TV rule and I'm turning off the TV now."

MENTAL HEALTH NURSING

Answers with Rationale

1. (3)   Be positive, definite, and specific about expectations. Do not give depressed patients a choice or try to convince them to get out of bed. Physically assist the patient to get up and dressed to mobilize her.

   NP:I; CH:PS; CA:PS; CL:A

2. (2)   Weight loss and no menstrual period for 3 months are symptoms of anorexia nervosa, so an eating disorder should be assessed. This could be the cause of hormone irregularity (3). Diet consultation (4) would be part of the treatment plan.

   NP:D; CN:H; CA:PS; CL:A

3. (2)   The nursing intervention is directed toward mobilizing the patient without asking her to make a decision or trying to convince her to go. The nurse must be direct, specific, and not take no for an answer.

   NP:P; CN:PS; CA:PS; CL:C

4. (3)   The goal is to implement suicide precautions because the danger of suicide is when the depression lifts and the patient has the energy to formulate a plan. The nurse would not encourage her to go home (1) where she could not be observed constantly. She could be moved into a room with other patients (2), but this is not the priority concern.

   NP:P; CN:S; CA:PS; CL:A

5. (3)   The most important order to implement first is fluids (IV) with B_6 supplement. The main cause of an alcoholic's going into DTs is lack of nutrients, especially vitamin B_6. This patient also requires the glucose supplement from the IV fluids. The other orders would then be implemented.

   NP:I; CN:PS; CA:PS; CL:AN

6. (2)   The more demanding and absorbing hallucinations (hearing voices) become, the more the patient's condition may be deteriorating. Secondarily, this may indicate increased paranoia (4). Paranoid schizophrenia is only one form of this condition, and hallucinations occur in all types of schizophrenia.

   NP:D; CN:PS; CA:PS; CL:A

7. (2)   The number of suicides has increased dramatically in the adolescent age group in the last 15 years. As more elderly are living longer, the number of suicides has also increased, but it is proportional.

   NP:D; CN:PH; CA:PS; CL:K

8. (4)   Because many people's problems occur in an interpersonal framework, the group setting is a way to correct faulty perceptions, as well as to work on more effective ways of relating to others.

   NP:P; CN:PS; CA:PS; CL:C

9. (4)   While a good nursing care plan is important, the priority would be to get the patient mobilized. Even without a specific diagnosis, the nurse will realize that part of what is happening with the patient is a depressed mood. Providing a structured plan of activities for the patient to follow will help his mood to lift and provide a focus so that he will not be centered on internal suffering.

   NP:I; CN:PS; CA:PS; CL:A

10. (3)   A depressed person needs to experience that someone is concerned for his welfare and that there is a person he can relate to during his hospitalization. Answers (1) and (2) negate the patient's feelings and answer (4) may focus on uncomfortable thoughts that will deepen the depression.

    NP:I; CN:PS; CA:PS; CL:A

11. (2)   The most appropriate intervention is to follow through with the patient and ask if she has a plan. The patient may tell the nurse her plan, which would assist in formulating the treatment options. After this, the nurse would notify the charge nurse and request suicide observation.

    NP:I; CN:PS; CA:PS; CL:A

Coding for Questions/Answers Abbreviations: **Nursing Process: NP,** Data Collection: D, Planning: P, Implementation: I, Evaluation: E, **Client Needs: CN,** Safe, Effective Care Environment: S, Health Promotion and Maintenance: H, Psychosocial Integrity: PS, Physiological Integrity: PH, **Clinical Area: CA,** Medical Nursing: M, Surgical Nursing: S, Maternal/Newborn Nursing: MA, Pediatric Nursing: P, Psychiatric Nursing: PS, **Cognitive Level: CL,** Knowledge: K, Comprehension: C, Application: A, Analysis: AN

12. (3) Simply offering comfort by staying with the patient and being open for communication is the most therapeutic. The other responses place an additional burden on the patient if she does not wish to talk.

NP:I; CN:PS; CA:PS; CL:C

13. (3) Engaging the patient in a large-muscle activity, like walking with the nurse, will direct the patient's energy but not be too stimulating, as would a competitive game such as Ping-Pong.

NP:I; CN:PS; CA:PS; CL:A

14. (3) Most suggestible of suicide is the sudden sense of satisfaction or relief (perhaps from finally making the decision to commit suicide) and detachment. Hostility (1), identifying with others (2), or thinking of the future (4) do not as clearly suggest suicidal thinking.

NP:E; CN:PS; CA:PS; CL:AN

15. (3) The first intervention is to set firm, clear limits on his behavior. The nurse would also remain with the patient until he calms down (1) and then encourage him to discuss his feelings rather than act out.

NP:I; CN:PS; CA:PS; CL:A

16. (1) The primary reason for the compulsive activity is to decrease the anxiety caused by obsessive thoughts. The patient is not trying to focus her attention on tasks (2), control others (3), or lessen interaction with others (4).

NP:P; CN:PS; CA:PS; CL:C

17. (3) A patient experiencing DTs may have illusions and/or hallucinations. These are very frightening to him because they seem real and the patient does not recognize that they are part of his illness.

NP:E; CN:PS; CA:PS; CL:C

18. (1) If the patient and/or the situation gets out of control, anxiety will only increase. Additional help may prevent this from occurring.

NP:P; CN:PS; CA:PS; CL:AN

19. (2) Korsakoff's syndrome (also called polyneuritic psychosis) is a form of organic brain syndrome that is associated with long-term alcohol abuse and a deficiency of vitamin B complex, especially thiamine. Answer (2) is more specific than answer (1). This condition is not caused from a lesion, hepatitis (3), or psychosis (4).

NP:P; CN:PS; CA:PS; CL:K

20. (2) Concern with having a life-threatening disease is a common issue with depressed patients. While demanding behavior (3) may be a symptom, it is not the issue here. Whether or not the patient is postmenopausal (1) is not relevant.

NP:P; CN:PS; CA:PS; CL:C

21. (1) A plan to return home and continue therapy shows that the patient has begun to realistically and responsibly deal with her problems. Talking to her boss (2) is positive but not as comprehensive as (1). Identifying and working on weak areas (3) usually are intermediate steps toward discharge. In asking the staff for advice (4), the patient is not ready or willing to accept responsibility for herself.

NP:E; CN:PS; CA:PS; CL:AN

22. (4) The goal is to keep the patient in reality as much as possible, so beginning a real conversation is the best intervention. The nurse would also write the incident on the patient's chart (3) because it is an indication of his condition.

NP:I; CN:PS; CA:PS; CL:A

23. (2) The nurse should offer on-the-spot support to visiting family members. They are important components of the therapeutic process and need assistance in dealing with their thoughts and feelings about the patient.

NP:I; CN:PS; CA:PS; CL:A

24. (1) Organic brain syndrome patients need specific, concrete instructions and a safe, consistent environment with reality orientation. Confrontation (4) and environmental instability (3) further confuse the patient by increasing his anxiety level. Giving too much information (2) is confusing.

NP:P; CN:PS; CA:PS; CL:A

25. (1) The patient needs to have external stimuli decreased but does not need to be isolated. It is much less traumatic if the nurse remains with the patient. Encouraging verbalization (3) or answering questions during this period would not be therapeutic.

NP:I; CN:PS; CA:PS; CL:C

26. (3) Giving the patient a choice of how he would like to take his medication, while being firm that he must take it, gives the patient a sense of control and helps to reduce the power struggle. Telling the patient that the medication is not poison (1) will do little to persuade him to comply. Answer (2) would represent a punishment. The patient must take his medication; therefore, answer (4) is not appropriate.

NP:I; CN:PS; CA:PS; CL:AN

27. (2) The purpose of a muscle relaxant is to reduce complications from convulsions that occur with ECT. This medication would reduce muscle tension (3), but this answer is not as specific. Atropine is given to block vagal stimulation (4).

NP:E; CN:PS; CA:PS; CL:K

28. (4) Confabulation is filling in memory gaps caused by organic deterioration of brain cells. Attempts to correct stories (2), reeducate (3), or refute (1) may increase anxiety, thus being unproductive and/or detrimental. It would also lower the patient's self-esteem.

NP:I; CN:PS; CA:PS; CL:A

29. (4) Acknowledge the patient by introducing yourself and start a one-to-one relationship by spending time with her. Let the patient know that the nurse cares about her by staying with her.

NP:I; CN:PS; CA:PS; CL:A

30. (3) When the patient is able to question his ideas or ask if they are real, it is a sign of improvement. Wanting to go home (2) or stopping talking about the paranoid ideas (1) is not necessarily an indication of improvement.

NP:E; CN:PS; CA:PS; CL:C

31. (3) In dealing with manipulative behavior, it is important that all members of the team and the patient are clear about expectations. Answer (1) is nontherapeutic as it pits the nurse against the patient. Answer (2) is not a reasonable choice because the patient is not involved in treatment. Answer (4) is nontherapeutic.

NP:P; CN:PS; CA:PS; CL:AN

32. (2) The staff and court must determine if the patient is a danger to self and others. Answer (1) may be a correct answer, but the patient was admitted to the hospital for threatening a neighbor. Answers (3) and (4) are not pertinent to the decision.

NP:E; CN:PS; CA:PS; CL:K

33. (2) The patient needs to recognize her feelings, and this response will assist her to do so. Answer (1) keeps the conversation on the cognitive level and does not deal with her feelings. Answer (3) is making a judgment. Answer (4) is asking for an intellectual analysis, which may or may not help the patient, and which may cause her to feel she must justify herself.

NP:I; CN:PS; CA:PS; CL:A

34. (3) Asking for clarification of such a statement might reveal more feelings than implied by the casual comment. This type of statement may be indicative of anger or projected feelings. Answer (1) is sarcastic, and (2) and (4) cut off further exploration of what the patient may really be saying. It would not be appropriate to continue with a personal explanation of why the nurse looks bad.

NP:I; CN:PS; CA:PS; CL:A

35. (2) The immediate priority is to find the patient and assess what further intervention may be needed. Whether or not the behavior has happened frequently in the past (3) is irrelevant, because the behavior exhibited now is significant and should be followed up. Sending another patient (4) is inappropriate as an immediate intervention may be necessary.

NP:I; CN:PS; CA:PS; CL:A

36. (2) This disorder has an unconscious mechanism in place; thus, there is a relative lack of distress or anxiety regarding the symptom. The patient is likely to demonstrate "la belle indifference," an unconcerned, indifferent attitude toward the loss of function with no awareness of the psychogenic cause. Answer (3) is incorrect as secondary gains should be minimized. Answer (4) is incorrect as repression and displacement are the operating mechanisms.

NP:P; CN:PS; CA:PS; CL:C

37. (3) The patient is placing blame on others and not taking responsibility for her own behavior. Reaction-formation (1) is preventing "dangerous" feelings from being expressed by exaggerating the opposite attitude. Compensation (2) is covering up a weakness by emphasizing a desirable trait. Acting out (4) is not a defense mechanism.

NP:D; CN:PS; CA:PS; CL:C

38. (4) Psychosomatic illnesses involve the "holism" of the individual; thus, all three of the concepts are important. If the nurse considers all of these concepts in planning nursing care, interventions will be therapeutic.

NP:P; CN:PS; CA:PS; CL:C

39. (4) This patient is in severe anxiety heading for a panic level. She requires immediate medication, constant attention, and a gradual lessening of activity according to her expressed level of energy. With moderate anxiety, directed activity helps to reduce the level.

NP:I; CN:PS; CA:PS; CL:A

40. (2) The fact that he has not talked about dying in a month, or even about his illness, leads the nurse to suspect denial. In this situation, the nurse would not confront him with reality but wait until he is ready to talk.

    NP:E; CN:PS; CA:PS; CL:C

41. (2) As a new staff member, the nurse should clarify who she is and why she is there. She also should acknowledge the patient's attempt to initiate interaction by offering to talk at a more appropriate time. Answer (1) might be used in a later interaction, but is not appropriate at this time.

    NP:I; CN:PS; CA:PS; CL:A

42. (1) The most effective method is problem solving, allowing the patient to explore his feelings, responses, consequences, and try out new, alternative responses. Confrontation (2) may only increase the maladaptive behavior. Threatening the patient with restraints (3) or putting him in seclusion (4) is punitive, not creating a climate where he would learn new behavior.

    NP:P; CN:PS; CA:PS; CL:AN

43. (2) The first step in the treatment plan would be to focus on the physical condition of the patient—to provide a healthy diet with vitamin supplements (these patients are usually low in vitamin B), and adequate rest and sleep. Setting limits (1), providing structure (3), and group psychotherapy (4) would be implemented later.

    NP:P; CN:PS; CA:PS; CL:C

44. (2) It is therapeutic to answer the question, then make an open-ended response to encourage the patient to talk. Answers (1) and (3) close off communication, and (4) does not answer the question.

    NP:I; CN:PS; CA:PS; CL:K

45. (1) Narcotics like heroin or morphine have a sedative effect on the central nervous system. Cocaine is a stimulant (2) and LSD is hallucinogenic (3). Marijuana gives one a sense of well-being (4).

    NP:D; CN:PS; CA:PS; CL:K

46. (2) Violent behavior often occurs as a response to a real or imagined threat. Hallucinations can be threatening in nature. Foul language may or may not be an indication of impending violence. Threatening hallucinations are more predictive of possible acting out behavior.

    NP:D; CN:PS; CA:PS; CL:C

47. (4) It is best to plan any activity, particularly therapy, to follow the compulsive activity because anxiety is lowest at this time.

    NP:P; CN:PS; CA:PS; CL:AN

48. (1) It is important to remember that OBS patients usually have some memory and concentration impairment. The degree depends on the individual and is influenced by the basic personality structure and the cause of the problem.

    NP:P; CN:PS; CA:PS; CL:A

49. (2) The nurse is structuring the relationship and giving the patient an opening to talk about his feelings. She is also refocusing the communication. Answer (1) is incorrect because the nurse is avoiding the issue of the patient's feelings. Answer (2) is incorrect because it asks him to analyze and give a reason for his behavior. The focus needs to be on his feelings and behaviors. Answer (4) is incorrect because it is a judgmental statement and may put the patient on the defensive.

    NP:I; CN:PS; CA:PS; CL:A

50. (4) The nurse is setting clear limits on the patient's behavior. He is testing her to see if she will follow through on what she said she would do. Answer (1) is incorrect. She is allowing the patient to manipulate her, which will reinforce his noncompliance. Answers (2) and (3) are also incorrect. The nurse is not addressing the real issue and she is opening up the subject for negotiation rather than setting clear limits.

    NP:I; CN:PS; CA:PS; CL:A

Simulated NCLEX-PN CAT Tests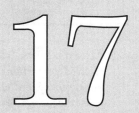

COMPREHENSIVE TEST 1 QUESTIONS

1. After discharge from the hospital, a patient is being treated with chemotherapy and radiation therapy at an outpatient clinic. Before radiation therapy begins, discharge teaching should include

   1. Radiation therapy can cause pneumonitis.
   2. Radiation ionizes atoms in the chemical system of the cells and causes side effects.
   3. Radiodermatitis may occur in the course of therapy.
   4. Radiation therapy causes cell damage that may result in gastrointestinal side effects.

2. You are assigned to care for a patient on an ECG monitor. You observe the tracing shown below. You recognize this strips shows

   1. A normal sinus rhythm.
   2. Multifocal PVCs.
   3. Ventricular tachycardia.
   4. Third-degree heart block.

   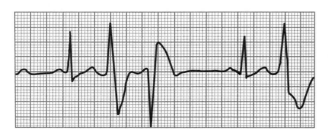

3. To facilitate the breathing of a 1-year-old child who has croup, the nurse should position the child in

   1. Prone position.
   2. Semi-Fowler's position.
   3. Supine position.
   4. Low-Fowler's position.

4. Immediately following a normal, spontaneous birth, the newborn infant is dried thoroughly and banded, and erythromycin is placed in both eyes. The mother asks the nurse, "Why are you putting medicine in my baby's eyes?" The nurse's reply should be based on an understanding that erythromycin is administered optically to infants to prevent

   1. Gonorrheal infection.
   2. Retrolental fibroplasia.
   3. Blindness.
   4. Transferral of human immunodeficiency virus (HIV).

5. What is the major assessment that will enable the nurse to identify hypoglycemia in a newborn?

   1. Restlessness and a whining cry.
   2. Stuporlike behavior with no cry.
   3. A shrill, intermittent cry.
   4. A weak, soft cry.

6. The nurse is providing care for a patient who just learned that she has terminal cancer. The patient says to the nurse, "I don't know why you are all so concerned; I'm not that sick." The defense mechanism she is using is

   1. Denial.
   2. Rationalization.
   3. Projection.
   4. Regression.

7. The nurse should understand that vitamin K is administered to infants in the newborn nursery to

   1. Help conjugate bilirubin in the infant.
   2. Prevent Rh sensitization in the infant.
   3. Reduce the possibility of hemorrhage in the infant.
   4. Increase the infant's resistance to infection.

8. Following a normal, spontaneous birth by a diabetic mother, the infant is admitted to the newborn nursery. After a first feeding of sterile water, the infant is given glucose water. The next nursing action should be to

   1. Observe the infant for hyperbilirubinemia.
   2. Administer formula or, preferably, breast milk to the infant.
   3. Monitor the infant's respiratory status.
   4. Monitor the infant's glucose levels using Dextrostix.

9. When providing nursing care for a patient who is receiving oxygen, what is the primary characteristic of oxygen that is dangerous?

   1. Oxygen supports combustion.
   2. Oxygen burns rapidly.
   3. Oxygen is explosive.
   4. Oxygen is present in higher concentrations than normal air.

10. A depressed patient refuses to join group activities and sits in a corner all day. The therapeutic intervention is to

    1. Assign the patient to clean the unit kitchen.
    2. Insist that the patient join group therapy.
    3. Formulate a structured schedule of daily activities for the patient.
    4. Allow the patient to not participate until medication is effective.

11. A 23-year-old male patient is admitted to an emergency room with first-degree (superficial, partial thickness) burns of his entire right arm and second- (partial thickness) and third-degree (full thickness) burns of his neck, abdomen, and back. Assessing the burns according to the Rule of Nines, the nurse should calculate that the burns affect

    1. 1–18 percent of his body.
    2. 19–33 percent of his body.
    3. 34–49 percent of his body.
    4. Over 50 percent of his body.

12. A patient develops jaundice after a Sengstaken tube is removed. The physician orders lactulose 30 mL via nasogastric tube. The therapeutic effect of this drug is to

    1. Increase prothrombin production.
    2. Decrease the blood ammonia concentration.
    3. Decrease potassium levels.
    4. Increase the albumin levels.

13. The nurse would evaluate that the drug lactulose is working when the patient has

    1. Watery diarrhea.
    2. Two or three stools per day.
    3. Constipation.
    4. Blood in the stool.

14. After the first week of hospitalization for a severely burned patient, the nurse will check that his diet includes foods that are

    1. High protein, low sodium, and low carbohydrate.
    2. Low fat, low sodium, and high calorie.
    3. High protein and high carbohydrate.
    4. High protein, high vitamin B-complex, and low-sodium.

15. List the patient characteristics that would influence his or her adaptation to the hospital (include all the numbers that apply): _____

    1. Age.
    2. Sense of humor.
    3. Level of consciousness.
    4. English language ability.
    5. Nationality.
    6. Disease state.

16. A patient who is receiving radiation therapy comes to the clinic for a scheduled treatment. The nurse notices that the patient's skin appears wet and weeping. The nursing action is to

    1. Not give the treatment and tell the patient to avoid bathing the skin until the weeping has stopped.
    2. Give the treatment and make a note on the patient's record concerning the skin condition.
    3. Not give the treatment and notify the charge nurse of the patient's skin condition.
    4. Give the treatment and instruct the patient to use antibiotic lotion on the lesions.

17. Which of the following nursing diagnoses would be *most* appropriate for the patient with decreased thyroid function?

    1. Altered growth and development related to increased growth hormone production.
    2. Altered thought processes related to decreased neurologic function.
    3. Fluid volume deficit related to polyuria.
    4. Hypothermia related to decreased metabolic rate.

18. A 7 month old has received a tentative diagnosis of mental retardation. The parents have come to the hospital for further assessment and counseling. During the nursing assessment, an observation that will help confirm the diagnosis of mental retardation is that the child

    1. Is unable to sit unsupported for brief periods.
    2. Is able to approach a toy and grasp it.
    3. Frequently rolls from back to stomach.
    4. Can grasp a spoon and bring it to her mouth.

19. When working with parents of a newly diagnosed retarded child, the nurse should formulate a nursing plan that

    1. Is based on a careful family assessment, including the parents' grief reaction.
    2. Will help the parents make decisions about long-term plans for the child.
    3. Will interpret the parents' feelings about their child and the grief process they are experiencing.
    4. Presents information about institutional placement for the child.

20. A 50-year-old patient was admitted to a hospital for a breast biopsy. Following the biopsy, the patient

was scheduled for surgery. After a radical mastectomy, the nurse would position the patient

1. On the patient's operative side.
2. On the patient's unoperative side.
3. In semi-Fowler's, with the patient's affected arm flat on the bed.
4. In semi-Fowler's, with the patient's affected arm elevated.

21. The physician prescribes a soft diet for an adult patient who has a diagnosis of congestive heart failure. She complains to the nurse about the diet. The nurse should explain that the purpose of this diet is to

1. Minimize the effort of mastication and digestion.
2. Increase elimination.
3. Prevent an increased workload on the heart.
4. Reduce the caloric intake.

22. A pregnant patient who has a history of mild diabetes that is controlled by insulin asks the nurse what will happen to her insulin requirements during her pregnancy. Which of the following responses would be best for the nurse to make?

1. "Because your case is so mild, you are not likely to need much insulin during your pregnancy."
2. "It's likely that, as the pregnancy progresses to term, you will need increased insulin."
3. "Every case is individual, so there's really no way to say."
4. "If you follow the diet well and don't gain too much weight, your insulin needs should stay about the same."

23. When reviewing the urinalysis report of a patient with the diagnosis of cystitis, the nurse would be surprised to find that it shows

1. Red blood cells present in the urine.
2. Negative glucose.
3. Specific gravity, 1.015.
4. No white or red blood cells in the urine.

24. Prior to surgery, a patient must give informed consent. This implies that the patient must

1. Be fully informed regarding the surgery.
2. Be allowed to read his records.
3. Must understand the intended outcome.
4. Understand that he may rescind his consent.

25. A 56-year-old male patient is admitted to a hospital with a diagnosis of fever of unknown origin. He is an alcoholic who has recently resumed heavy drinking. One day, when approached by the nurse, he says, "I'm really no good. I drink and don't take care of my family, and I'm a rotten father." Which of the following responses to this statement would be most therapeutic?

1. "But now you are doing something about your problem."
2. "It sounds as though you are feeling pretty guilty about drinking."
3. "I'm sure that you are a good father."
4. "What makes you think you are no good?"

26. When assessing the developmental level of a 3-month-old infant at a well-baby clinic, the nurse would expect the infant to

1. See objects only as shapes and shadows.
2. Focus her eyes only momentarily.
3. Distinguish between light and dark only.
4. Focus her eyes on objects and people.

27. Select the location (1–5) at which you would place your stethoscope as you start auscultating breath sounds:

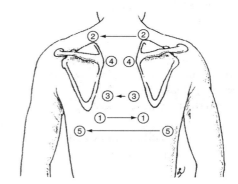

28. Part of the discharge teaching for a patient who is taking nitroglycerin is to instruct him to store this medication

1. In the refrigerator.
2. In a clear, tightly closed glass jar.
3. In a dark, tightly closed glass jar.
4. Not more than 3 months.

29. A 30-year-old patient was admitted to the hospital with a diagnosis of bipolar disorder, manic episode. She manifests an excess of energy and cannot sit still. The most useful activity that the nurse might suggest for this patient would be to

1. Play volleyball outside.
2. Engage in group exercises.
3. Play table tennis in the day room.
4. Go outside for a walk with the nurse.

30. Following total hip replacement surgery, one of the goals is to prevent thrombus formation from venous stasis. A nursing action to achieve this goal is to

    1. Help the patient to perform total range-of-motion exercises every 2 hours.
    2. Get the patient up in a wheelchair as soon as possible.
    3. Put antiembolic stockings on the patient.
    4. Elevate the foot of the patient's bed.

31. When teaching a woman about adequate nutrition that is essential during early pregnancy for optimal fetal development, the nurse should recommend a balanced, nutritious daily diet that is supplemented by

    1. Iron and folacin.
    2. Vitamin C.
    3. Additional minerals.
    4. Vitamin B complex.

32. A patient was returned to the unit following exploratory abdominal surgery. A nasogastric tube is in place. Understanding possible early complications of abdominal surgery, the nurse should assess the patient for

    1. Constipation.
    2. Clay-colored stools.
    3. Infection.
    4. Hemorrhage.

33. Prior to administering a dose of digoxin to a 5-year-old child, the nurse observes that the child's temperature is 37.7°C (99.8°F) and her pulse rate is 100. The appropriate nursing action would be to

    1. Notify the charge nurse.
    2. Recognize that these are signs of digoxin toxicity and withhold the dose.
    3. Administer the medication.
    4. Administer the medication, but tell the charge nurse that the child's pulse rate is higher than normal.

34. After a normal labor and delivery, the infant weighs 2400 g (5 lb) and is considered premature. Which of the following actions should the nurse consider most important for providing adequate nutrition for the infant who will not breast-feed?

    1. Feed the infant formula with a regular nipple with a large hole.
    2. Offer a full-strength formula feeding every 2–4 hours.
    3. Use a preemie nipple and dilute formula.
    4. Feed the infant glucose water for the first 2 days.

35. The mother of a premature infant visits her every day. During a visit, the nurse asks the mother if she would like to feed the infant. She says, "Oh, no; you do it so well. I want my baby to be well cared for." The most appropriate response is to say

    1. "I'll feed her today. Maybe tomorrow you can try it."
    2. "It's not difficult at all. She is just like a normal baby, only smaller."
    3. "You can learn to feed her as well as I can; I wasn't good when I first fed a premature infant either."
    4. "It's frightening sometimes to feed an infant this small, but I'll stay with you to help."

36. After a nasogastric tube is inserted for tube feedings, the test to confirm placement is

    1. Regular intermittent bubbling when the end of the tube is submerged in water.
    2. Hearing a rush of air in the stomach when 1 mL of air is injected into the tube.
    3. X-ray confirmation.
    4. No coughing or choking when the tube was inserted.

37. The nurse should assess for which of the following clinical manifestations in the patient with Cushing's syndrome?

    1. Hypertension, diaphoresis, nausea, and vomiting.
    2. Tetany, irritability, dry skin, and seizures.
    3. Unexplained weight gain, energy loss, and cold intolerance.
    4. Water retention, moon faced, hirsutism, and purple striae.

38. The patient with hyperparathyroidism should have extremities handled gently because

    1. Decreased calcium bone deposits can lead to pathologic fractures.
    2. Edema causes stretched tissue to tear easily.
    3. Hypertension can lead to a stroke with residual paralysis.
    4. Polyuria leads to dry skin and mucous membranes that can break down.

39. Bethanechol chloride (Urecholine) is prescribed PRN for a patient following a transurethral resection (TUR). The nurse will administer the medication when the patient

    1. Complains of bladder spasms.
    2. Complains of severe pain.
    3. Is unable to void.
    4. Has frequent episodes of painful urination.

40. The nurse should understand that the period when it is most difficult to control a pregnant woman's diabetes is

   1. Early in the pregnancy.
   2. Early in the postpartum period.
   3. During the delivery process.
   4. During labor.

41. A 73-year-old patient has a history of chronic obstructive pulmonary disease (COPD). Upon admission to the hospital with a diagnosis of angina, the nurse would question which one of the following orders?

   1. A 4-g sodium diet.
   2. Oxygen at 5–7 L/min via nasal cannula.
   3. IV fluids of 5 percent dextrose in 0.45 percent NaCl at 80 mL/hr.
   4. Nitroglycerin gr 1/150 sublingual PRN for angina.

42. A 57-year-old patient has been admitted with a diagnosis of pneumococcal pneumonia. She has a temperature of 38.9°C (102°F), and complains of nausea and lethargy. When providing care for the patient, the nurse will remember that one of the most important goals in the treatment of pneumonia is to

   1. Keep the environment free of allergens.
   2. Administer limited fluids.
   3. Conserve the patient's energy.
   4. Encourage the patient to frequently turn and cough.

43. The nurse must carefully handle nasal and bronchial secretions from a patient with the diagnosis of pneumonia because

   1. Bloody sputum will be present.
   2. These secretions may spread the disease.
   3. The sight may be upsetting to the other patients.
   4. Standard Precautions must be observed for all patients with pneumonia.

44. A 1-month-old infant is brought by her mother to a well-baby clinic for a checkup and to receive her first immunization. The mother is concerned because the baby sleeps so much of the day. The nurse should tell the mother that infants

   1. Sleep all day and stay awake most of the night until they get on a regular routine.
   2. Should now be having only one nap during the day.
   3. Need at least 12 hours of sleep out of every 24 hours.
   4. Usually sleep about 20 hours out of every 24 hours.

45. A patient who has a diagnosis of esophageal varices has had a Sengstaken–Blakemore tube inserted to control the bleeding. The most important safety intervention for this patient is

   1. Providing good mouth care.
   2. Monitoring IV fluid intake.
   3. Keeping scissors at the bedside.
   4. Deflating the balloon on a regular basis.

46. An infant weighs 2880 g (6 lb) at birth. By 6 months of age, the normal infant should weigh about

   1. 19.6 kg (21 lb).
   2. 3840 g (8 lb).
   3. 5760 g (12 lb).
   4. 11.8 kg (26 lb).

47. An elderly patient has had an open reduction of the hip, with fixation by a nail. Postoperatively, the primary nursing intervention is to

   1. Keep her affected hip in acute flexion.
   2. Elevate her affected leg to avoid edema.
   3. Keep her affected hip in abduction.
   4. Keep the head of the bed flat.

48. Following a patient's hip replacement surgery, a Hemovac is put in place to assist with drainage. During the first postoperative hours, the nurse should observe for

   1. Infection at the incision site.
   2. Hemorrhage.
   3. Color of the drainage.
   4. Edema at the incision site.

49. A female patient's disruptive behavior on the psychiatric unit has been extremely annoying to the other patients. One approach the nurse may find effective is to

   1. Tell the patient that she is bothering others and confine her to her room.
   2. Ignore the patient's behavior, realizing that it is consistent with her illness.
   3. Set consistent limits on the patient's behavior.
   4. Make a definite, structured plan that the patient will have to follow.

50. A 32-year-old female is in her 37th week of pregnancy and is showing signs of preeclampsia. When assessing the patient, the nurse should observe for the most common early signs of preeclampsia, which are

   1. Increased blood pressure, proteinuria, and edema.

2. Decreased blood pressure, proteinuria, and edema.

3. Increased blood pressure, glucose in the urine, and weight gain.

4. Hypertension, hyperreflexia, and edema.

51. In a preoperative assessment, the nurse will document all of the following database parameters. Which one is more important for a diabetic patient rather than other surgical patients?

1. Blood sugar level.
2. White blood cell count.
3. Vital signs.
4. Skin condition.

52. An adult patient who was diagnosed as having cholelithiasis has had several episodes of gallbladder attacks over the past year. Which of the following symptoms should the nurse recognize as the one that would most likely cause the patient to go to a physician?

1. Chronic pain in the lower right abdomen.
2. Chronic pain in the lower left abdomen.
3. Fatty food intolerance while eating.
4. Fatty food intolerance several hours after eating.

53. The nursing action that will provide the best source of relief for a woman in early labor with back pain would be to

1. Direct her attention to the television or talk to her.
2. Help her to walk around.
3. Administer a prescribed narcotic analgesic to her.
4. Apply counterpressure to her sacrum.

54. When assessing a patient who is taking lithium carbonate for a manic-type disorder, the nurse should be alert for the expected side effect of

1. Dehydration.
2. Muscle weakness.
3. Drowsiness.
4. Anuria.

55. A teenage girl comes to a prenatal clinic where it is determined that she is 12 weeks pregnant. During counseling the nurse is helping the patient select the best protein foods from the school cafeteria. Of the following choices, the nurse should suggest that she choose

1. A slice of pizza.
2. Pasta with tomato sauce.
3. A peanut butter sandwich.
4. Tomato soup and crackers.

56. The nurse should teach a mother-to-be that energy requirements of pregnancy increase the daily calorie requirement. The nurse will know the mother-to-be understands when she says that her daily calories should be increased by _____ calories.

57. The most effective nursing measure to maintain optimal positioning and function for a patient who has had a cerebrovascular accident (CVA) is to

1. Place the patient in a prone position for 15 to 30 minutes, three times a day.
2. Change the patient's position every 4 hours.
3. Maintain the patient on the affected side as much of the time as possible.
4. Change the patient's position from the affected to the unaffected side every 2 hours.

58. A 45-year-old patient is brought to the hospital by her husband because she refuses to get dressed or go out, cries most of the time, and says life is not worth living. A major depressive episode is the admitting diagnosis. A priority goal of this patient's nursing care plan would be to

1. Provide a safe environment.
2. Build up the patient's self-esteem.
3. Pay attention to the patient's physical needs.
4. Establish a nurse–patient relationship.

59. The most important developmental task for the nurse to encourage a mother to teach her child prior to surgery for cleft palate repair would be

1. Drinking with a straw.
2. Using a spoon.
3. Using a soft nipple.
4. Drinking from a cup.

60. A mother is unable to breast-feed her sick infant, who has a gastrostomy tube in place. An appropriate nursing action is to encourage the mother to

1. Accept the fact that the infant will need formula while in the hospital.
2. Discontinue the idea of breast-feeding.
3. Pump her breasts and bring the milk to the hospital.
4. Wait until the infant leaves the hospital and then resume breast-feeding.

61. Tranylcypromine sulfate (Parnate), an MAO inhibitor, is prescribed for a depressed patient about to be discharged. The nurse should include in the discharge instructions the information that

1. Parnate takes 2–3 weeks to become effective.

2. Drowsiness and blurred vision can be dangerous side effects of Parnate.
3. Parnate potentiates the action of other drugs.
4. Parnate should not be taken with foods that are aged or that contain tyramine.

62. A patient on a sodium-restricted diet using salt substitute should be counseled about the risk for developing

    1. Hypercalcemia.
    2. Hyperkalemia.
    3. Hyponatremia.
    4. Hypovolemia.

63. When caring for a patient following abdominal surgery, the most important nursing intervention to prevent pulmonary complications would be to

    1. Administer oxygen to the patient as prescribed.
    2. Instruct the patient to turn, cough, and deep breathe every 2 hours.
    3. Encourage the patient to hyperventilate every hour.
    4. Assist the patient out of bed to a chair on the second postoperative day.

64. When discussing family planning methods with a couple, the nurse should

    1. Include only the female in the discussion.
    2. Ensure that the couple have a thorough understanding of the method they choose.
    3. Choose the method that would best suit the couple.
    4. Point out that most methods are 99.9 percent effective, so it makes no difference which method they choose.

65. When a patient returns to the unit following a cardiac catheterization, the nursing activity that should immediately follow taking vital signs is

    1. Placing the patient in a warm bed and encouraging sleep.
    2. Providing the patient with fluids.
    3. Assessing the patient's peripheral pulses.
    4. Reapplying the patient's dressing where the dye was injected.

66. A 4-month-old infant was brought to the emergency room after rolling off the couch and hitting his head. Which one of the following assessments by the nurse could indicate increased intracranial pressure?

    1. Apical pulse of 108.
    2. Bulging fontanelle when calm.
    3. Crying and reaching for the parents.
    4. Pupils equal and reactive to light.

67. A 23-year-old woman is admitted to a hospital at 8:00 PM with a tentative diagnosis of appendicitis. On admission, the patient states that she has been experiencing pain all day. During the initial assessment, the nurse should be especially alert for

    1. High fever.
    2. Nausea and vomiting unrelated to eating.
    3. Tenderness in the upper right abdominal quadrant.
    4. Lethargy.

68. Following the completion of laboratory studies, a patient is scheduled for an appendectomy. Nursing interventions during the preoperative period will include keeping the patient

    1. Lying flat in bed, with no heat or ice application to the affected area.
    2. In bed in semi-Fowler's position, with ice to the affected area.
    3. In any position, with a heating pad on the tender area.
    4. In any position, with an ice bag on the tender area.

69. The orders are to give warfarin (Coumadin) 12.5 mg. On hand are 5 mg tablets. The nurse would give the patient _____ tablet(s).

70. A teenage girl comes to a clinic and tells the nurse that she is sexually active and would like some form of birth control. After discussing the various methods of contraception, she decides she would like to use an oral contraceptive. The nurse should tell her that the physician will need to know

    1. The names of her sexual contacts.
    2. A complete history of her sexual experiences.
    3. If she has a history of thrombophlebitis or migraine headaches.
    4. If her parents approve and will sign a written consent.

71. When preparing a 5-year-old child for an intrusive diagnostic test, the nurse should consider the fact that children at this age

    1. Are too young to fear intrusive procedures.
    2. Respond poorly to verbal directions.
    3. Understand simple directions.
    4. Are quiet, shy, and withdrawn.

72. An 81-year-old patient has right side heart failure and is confined to bed. Which of the following assessments by the nurse would indicate a deterioration in his condition?

1. Clear lung sounds.
2. Pitting edema of the sacral area.
3. Stating, "I don't want breakfast today."
4. Weight loss.

73. The nurse is assigned a patient whose orders include heparin therapy. The substance that the nurse will keep at the bedside as the antidote is

1. Magnesium sulfate.
2. Vitamin K.
3. Protamine sulfate.
4. Calcium gluconate.

74. A 24-year-old woman is brought into an emergency room by her roommate. She appears to be unconscious, is unresponsive, and her friend can give no information about the cause of her condition. The period of time allowed for checking the patient's level of unresponsiveness would be

1. 30 minutes to 1 hour.
2. A few seconds.
3. 1 minute.
4. Several minutes.

75. The nurse should recognize that the most appropriate method of ordering low-sodium meals for a 6-year-old child would be to

1. Help the child fill out the menu.
2. Have one of the child's parents fill out the menu after learning about the diet.
3. Fill out the menu for the child.
4. Ask the dietitian to order the meals.

76. Which nursing behavior is correct when applying a topical transdermal medication patch?

1. Wipe the planned site of application with alcohol.
2. Apply the patch to an area that will be covered by clothing.
3. Gently rub the patch on the skin before taping it down.
4. Remove the old patch before applying a new one.

77. A female patient is extremely anxious while waiting for the results of her breast biopsy. She is hyperventilating and complaining of numbness in her fingers and toes. Her arterial blood gas (ABG) results show an elevated blood pH and decreased carbon dioxide level. Based on the data, the nurse recognizes that the patient's condition is

1. Metabolic acidosis.
2. Metabolic alkalosis.
3. Respiratory acidosis.
4. Respiratory alkalosis.

78. A 60-year-old woman is admitted to a hospital for treatment and rehabilitation after suffering a cerebrovascular accident (CVA). The patient has some residual expressive aphasia. In dealing with this problem, the most therapeutic nursing action would be to

1. Anticipate all of the patient's needs and requests.
2. Encourage patient communication by writing or using an alphabet board.
3. Encourage every attempt to communicate without correcting words or usage.
4. Encourage the patient to use pantomime as a way of communicating.

79. When a patient has visual loss in the right half of each visual field, the most effective nursing approach to assist the patient to compensate for this loss would be to

1. Place the items that are frequently used on the unaffected side.
2. Position the patient so that the unaffected side is toward the activity in the room.
3. Frequently encourage the patient to position and turn her head to scan the environment on her affected side.
4. Approach the patient on her unaffected side.

80. A 26-year-old woman is admitted to a hospital at 40 weeks' gestation in active labor. Initial assessment indicates that her cervix is 4 cm dilated, and she is having strong contractions every 4 minutes, lasting 40 seconds. She complains of back discomfort and an urge to bear down. The nurse should suspect that the

1. Patient's cervix is fully dilated.
2. Fetus is in a posterior position.
3. Patient requires analgesic medication.
4. Patient needs to get up and walk around.

81. Of the following patients, the one who is at the *greatest* risk for developing fluid volume deficit is a(n)

1. 23-year-old man exercising vigorously.
2. 34-year-old woman on diuretic therapy.
3. 71-year-old man unconscious and on tube feeding.
4. 82-year-old woman in uncompensated heart failure.

82. You are assigned a patient who is to be treated with a cobalt implant for intracavity irradiation for cervical CA. Her treatment will be completed in 72 hours. Which protective measures are indicated for personnel and visitors? List the numbers that apply: _____.

1. Place "Radiation Treatment" sign on door to patient's room and on front of patient's chart.
2. All nurses and visitors wear a protective shield. (Keep lead shield at patient's doorway.)
3. Complete care of the patient as fast as possible and leave the room quickly.
4. Do not allow pregnant women to visit or to be assigned as staff for this patient, but children under age 18 may visit.
5. Visitors limit exposure to 1 hour/day and keep a distance from the patient.

83. To decrease the risk of compromised venous return when a patient is in hypovolemic shock, the most appropriate position would be

1. Supine with feet slightly elevated.
2. Low-Fowler's.
3. Feet elevated and head lowered.
4. Head and feet slightly elevated.

84. A 16-year-old boy has fractured his right tibia during the high school football game. A long leg cast was applied, and he was admitted to the hospital for observation. He starts to complain of severe pain in his right leg. The *best* course of action by the nurse would be to

1. Administer the ordered analgesic.
2. Elevate the right leg.
3. Notify the physician.
4. Perform a neurovascular check.

85. Which of the following laboratory values should the nurse recognize as the normal serum potassium level?

1. 1.010–1.030.
2. 3.5–5.5 mEq/L.
3. 135–145 mg.
4. 22 kg.

COMPREHENSIVE TEST 1

Answers with Rationale

1. (4) All of the information is accurate regarding radiation; however, the patient's initial symptoms usually are related to GI function. The patient should not be told about pneumonitis but could be told to report any unusual symptoms. Answer (2) is technical and not necessary for patient understanding of the disease process.

NP:I; CN:S; CA:M; CL:A

2. (2) The rhythm strip is showing *multifocal PVCs*. It is important to recognize because the patient could be hypoxic or in acidosis (with a diagnosis of COPD or diabetes mellitus). Lidocaine may be administered to decrease automaticity and increase electrical stimulation threshold of the ventricles.

NP:D; CN:PH; CA:M; CL:AN

3. (2) Semi-Fowler's position is the most appropriate to facilitate breathing. Some children prefer being on their abdomen, which is also acceptable.

NP:I; CN:PH; CA:P; CL:C

4. (3) Every newborn receives silver nitrate 1 percent, or more commonly, a broad-spectrum antibiotic such as erythromycin in the eyes. The purpose of this is to prevent blindness caused by the mother having a sexually transmitted disease, such as chlamydia or gonorrhea.

NP:I; CN:H; CA:MA; CL:K

5. (3) Infants with signs and symptoms of hypoglycemia usually have a high-pitched or shrill cry that may be intermittent. A drug-addicted infant may also have a high-pitched cry, but it will be persistent.

NP:D; CN:H; CA:MA; CL:C

6. (1) The answer is denial. The patient is simply refusing to accept her terminal illness to protect herself from the unpleasant reality of possible death. Denial is a stage of the grief process.

NP:E; CN:PS; CA:PS; CL:C

7. (3) Vitamin K is necessary for blood coagulation. The newborn has a transitory deficiency in the clotting ability of the blood. Bacteria are necessary for the production of vitamin K in the intestines, and bacteria are not present in sufficient numbers in the newborn until several days after birth.

NP:P; CN:H; CA:MA; CL:K

8. (4) Dextrostix results yield data about the blood glucose level; this is essential data for monitoring hypoglycemia in the infant of a diabetic mother. Glucose water is not given as a first feeding because if the infant aspirates, lung tissue would be damaged.

NP:I; CN:PH; CA:M; CL:AN

9. (1) Oxygen itself does not burn, but, if present in large amounts, it will allow a small fire to spread rapidly.

NP:P; CN:S; CA:M; CL:K

10. (3) An important goal for depressed patients is to keep them busy with a structured schedule. It may be too early for the patient to join a group, and cleaning the kitchen may not increase self-esteem.

NP:I; CN:PS; CA:P; CL:A

11. (3) According to the Rule of Nines, the patient's right arm would be considered as 9 percent; his abdomen, 9 percent; and his back, 18 percent, for a total of 36 percent. Burn degree is not taken into account.

NP:D; CN:PH; CA:M; CL:A

12. (2) Lactulose reduces blood ammonia. It acidifies colon contents resulting in retention of the ammonium ion and decreased ammonia absorption.

NP:E; CN:PH; CA:M; CL:C

13. (2) Several stools per day would indicate that the drug is working and ammonia is being eliminated. Diarrhea indicates drug overdose.

NP:E; CN:PH; CA:M; CL:A

Coding for Questions/Answers Abbreviations: **Nursing Process: NP,** Data Collection: D, Planning: P, Implementation: I, Evaluation: E, **Client Needs: CN,** Safe, Effective Care Environment: S, Health Promotion and Maintenance: H, Psychosocial Integrity: PS, Physiological Integrity: PH, **Clinical Area: CA,** Medical Nursing: M, Surgical Nursing: S, Maternal/Newborn Nursing: MA, Pediatric Nursing: P, Psychiatric Nursing: PS, **Cognitive Level: CL,** Knowledge: K, Comprehension: C, Application: A, Analysis: AN

14. (3) A diet high in protein and carbohydrates is essential so that the protein is available for tissue-cell rebuilding and repair. Sodium is not a factor for burn diets.

NP:I; CN:S; CA:M; CL:A

15. The answers are 1, 3, 4, and 6. While sense of humor may help adaptation, it is not a major influence. Nationality is also not important; rather, it is the ability to communicate with personnel that influences how a patient adapts.

NP:P; CN:H; CA:M; CL:A

16. (3) During the time the reaction occurs, patients are taken off radiation therapy and instructed to use antibiotic lotion and steroid cream to prevent infection.

NP:I; CN:PH; CA:M; CL:A

17. (4) Because the thyroid gland regulates the metabolic rate, a decrease in thyroid function would result in a decreased metabolic rate. Growth and development and altered thought processes are not affected by the thyroid gland.

NP:P; CN:PH; CA:M; CL:C

18. (1) At 6 months, a child should be sitting with minimal support. Often, with retarded children, their flaccid muscles and loose joints prevent the attainment of simple developmental milestones. The ability to sit is one of the most important milestones.

NP:D; CN:PS; CA:PS; CL:A

19. (1) Parents cannot be expected to make decisions and long-term plans for the child while they are still experiencing grief. The focus of nursing should be on accepting parents' feelings and promoting communication.

NP:P; CN:PS; CA:PS; CL:A

20. (4) Semi-Fowler's position with the patient's arm elevated will enhance lymphatic and venous drainage of fluid in the affected arm. The other positions are not therapeutic.

NP:I; CN:PH; CA:S; CL:A

21. (3) A soft diet decreases bulk and promotes elimination of solid wastes. Ease in defecation prevents straining and an increased workload for the heart.

NP:I; CN:PH; CA:M; CL:AN

22. (2) Because of the diabetes and normal changes caused by pregnancy, there is usually an increased need for insulin in the second and third trimesters.

NP:I; CN:PH; CA:MA; CL:A

23. (4) White blood cells and red blood cells are usually present in urine samples from patients with cystitis. White blood cells are a response to the inflammation; the irritation of the mucosa and irritation of the urethra cause bleeding.

NP:E; CN:PH; CA:M; CL:C

24. (1) The consent to receive health services includes informed consent, which means that prior to granting a consent, the patient must be fully informed regarding treatment, tests, surgery, etc. The patient must also understand the intended outcome (3) and the potentially harmful results.

NP:P; CN:S; CA:S; CL:A

25. (2) The nurse paraphrases the patient's comments to give feedback, to show an understanding of what was said, and to encourage the patient to continue expressing feelings without making a judgment about the drinking.

NP:I; CN:PS; CA:PS; CL:A

26. (4) At 3 months, an infant is able to focus on objects or people. The other characteristics occur earlier in development.

NP:D; CN:H; CA:P; CL:K

27. The answer is 2; as you start auscultating breath sounds, you start at the top (labeled 2 in the question) of the back and move down according to the numbers (to the fifth position).

NP:I; CN:PH; CA:M; CL:A

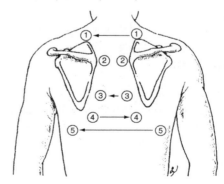

28. (3) Nitroglycerin should be kept in a dark, tightly closed jar. The potency is 6 months, not 3.

NP:I; CN:PH; CA:M; CL:C

29. (4) This activity would channel her energy because it would involve large-muscle activity, but would not increase external stimuli as group or competitive activities would.

NP:I; CN:PS; CA:PS; CL:A

30. (3)   Antiembolic stockings and leg exercises (flexing feet and ankles) are the best means of preventing thrombus formation. Total ROM (1) is not appropriate, as the hip must remain in abduction and flexion must be prevented. The patient should be up in a walker by the second postoperative day.

NP:I; CN:PH; CA:S; CL:A

31. (1)   Iron and folacin cannot be ingested in sufficient quantities by dietary means; thus, they must be supplemented during pregnancy. Additional vitamins (C and B complex) (2, 4) and minerals (3) may be appropriate, but they are not critical daily supplements as they can be obtained through food.

NP:I; CN:PH; CA:MA; CL:C

32. (4)   Because an incision has been made into the abdomen, hemorrhage can be a complication of abdominal surgery. Infection (3) would be a later complication.

NP:D; CN:PH; CA:S; CL:A

33. (3)   A normal pulse rate for a 5-year-old child is 100; elevated temperature is not a sign of digoxin toxicity.

NP:I; CN:PH; CA:P; CL:AN

34. (3)   A regular nipple is too hard and will make it too difficult for the infant to suck, causing unnecessary fatigue. A soft preemie nipple should be used. Formula should be diluted at first, progressing to full strength. The first feeding will be sterile water, then glucose water, and then formula.

NP:I; CN:PH; CA:MA; CL:A

35. (4)   The nurse, while recognizing and accepting this mother's apprehension, assures her that she will have assistance.

NP:I; CN:PS; CA:MA; CL:A

36. (3)   When a tube feeding is ordered, x-ray confirmation of tube placement must be done for safety. Otherwise, the test would be to aspirate stomach contents and check the pH. Answer (1) is no longer considered safe nursing practice for NG placement. Answer (2) can be done as the initial test for placement but must be followed by checking pH.

NP:E; CN:PH; CA:M; CL:A

37. (4)   Clinical manifestations of Cushing's syndrome include water retention, moon face, hirsutism, and purple striae.

NP:D; CN:PH; CA:M; CL:C

38. (1)   The parathyroid glands regulate calcium in the body. Excessive activity results in calcium leaving the bones and teeth to enter the bloodstream. This makes the bones more brittle and susceptible to fracture.

NP:P; CN:PH; CA:M; CL:A

39. (3)   Bethanechol chloride (Urecholine) stimulates the parasympathetic nervous system. It increases the tone and motility of the smooth muscles of the urinary tract. This drug is used frequently following a transurethral resection (TUR) when the patient has a lack of muscle tone and is unable to void. Bladder spasms (1) can be relieved with belladonna or opium suppositories.

NP:E; CN:PH; CA:S; CL:A

40. (2)   Early postpartum is a crucial period, for the placenta contains the hormone insulinase, which blocks the use of insulin during pregnancy.

NP:P; CN:H; CA:MA; CL:C

41. (2)   High levels of oxygen in patients with COPD will knock out the carbon dioxide center and lead to respiratory arrest.

NP:E; CN:PH; CA:M; CL:AN

42. (3)   The patient's energy should be conserved to enable the body to use all of its resources for fighting the disease. Fluid intake should be at least 3000 mL/day.

NP:P; CN:PH; CA:M; CL:A

43. (2)   Pneumonia may be caused by a virus, bacteria, or fungi, which would be present in the secretions and thus, if not handled carefully, would spread the disease. Standard Precautions are always good nursing care, but this is not as specific an answer.

NP:I; CN:S; CA:M; CL:A

44. (4)   Most newborns are awake for eating and care only. The mother should not worry if the infant sleeps most of the time because this is normal.

NP:I; CN:H; CA:P; CL:K

45. (3)   The respiratory system can become occluded if the balloon slips and moves up the esophagus, putting pressure on the trachea. This would result in respiratory distress. Scissors should be kept at the bedside so that the tube can be cut if distress occurs.

NP:P; CN:S; CA:M; CL:A

46. (3)   Healthy infants should double their birth weight by 5–6 months of age.

NP:E; CN:H; CA:P; CL:K

47. (3) The hip should be kept in abduction to prevent flexion. The hip must not be in acute flexion. If the affected leg is elevated, flexion of the hip occurs and this could cause dislocation of the hip. Position should be changed frequently and can be done by raising or lowering head of the bed.

    NP:I; CN:PH; CA:S; CL:A

48. (2) The nurse will observe for hemorrhage during the first few hours. Later, the nurse will observe for infection. It is also important to check for patency of the Hemovac.

    NP:D; CN:PH; CA:S; CL:A

49. (3) Setting limits is important to decrease the disruptive behavior and prevent the patient from being rejected by others—with subsequent lowering of self-esteem.

    NP:I; CN:PS; CA:PS; CL:A

50. (1) Classical manifestations of mild preeclampsia (also called pregnancy-induced hypertension or PIH) are elevated blood pressure, proteinuria, and edema.

    NP:D; CN:H; CA:MA; CL:C

51. (1) The diabetic patient preparing for surgery must have the blood sugar level closely monitored so that the correct amount of insulin can be administered. Balancing of blood glucose will result in fewer complications.

    NP:I; CN:PH; CA:S; CL:AN

52. (4) Pain is due to contraction of the gallbladder, which has stones present. The gallbladder empties when fat is present in the stomach. The gallbladder is located in the upper right side of the abdomen along the side of the liver.

    NP:E; CN:PH; CA:M; CL:C

53. (4) Counterpressure provides significant pain relief by supporting the sacrum as the fetus's head is driven down by the contractions. The knee–chest position also may provide pain relief. If it is early labor, it is too early for any analgesics.

    NP:I; CN:H; CA:MA; CL:A

54. (2) Muscle weakness is an expected side effect and one that the patient may have to learn to live with while on the medication. Dehydration (1) is not a side effect that should be evaluated; drowsiness (3) is a toxic side effect. A usual side effect is polyuria, not anuria (4).

    NP:D; CN:PH; CA:PS; CL:C

55. (3) A peanut butter sandwich has 12 g of protein, more than the other foods. A normal teenager requires 78 g of protein a day.

    NP:I; CN:H; CA:MA; CL:A

56. The answer is *300*. The increased energy and nutritional demands of pregnancy require approximately 300 additional calories a day.

    NP:E; CN:H; CA:MA; CL:C

57. (1) Changing the patient's position to prone three times a day will encourage optimal functioning. The position protocol is 2 hours on the unaffected side, 20 minutes on the affected side, and 30 minutes prone TID. Prolonged pressure on the affected side contributes to contractures, deformities, and pressure ulcers due to loss of motor tone and circulation.

    NP:I; CN:PH; CA:M; CL:A

58. (1) The highest priority with a depressed patient is to protect the patient from self-injury by providing a safe milieu to prevent suicide. The other goals are also important, but have lower priority.

    NP:P; CN:PS; CA:PS; CL:A

59. (4) It is imperative that the child know how to drink from a cup, because this is the only way the child can effectively drink following this surgery. The child will not be able to drink from a bottle or straw.

    NP:P; CN:PH; CA:S; CL:A

60. (3) While the gastrostomy tube is in place, the mother cannot breast-feed. It is important, however, to continue the flow of breast milk so that when the baby is ready, breast-feeding can be resumed.

    NP:I; CN:PH; CA:P; CL:C

61. (4) Parnate is an MAO inhibitor and cannot be taken with foods high in tyramine, such as cheese, wine, and chocolate. Answers (1) and (2) refer to tricyclic medications. MAO medications should never be taken with alcohol or other medications.

    NP:I; CN:PH; CA:PS; CL:A

62. (2) Because many salt substitutes contain potassium, use of salt substitutes can lead to elevated blood potassium levels.

    NP:P; CN:PH; CA:M; CL:C

63. (2) The most effective method of preventing pulmonary complications is to instruct the patient to turn, cough, and deep breathe frequently.

    NP:I; CN:PH; CA:S; CL:A

64. (2) Contraceptive methods must be thoroughly understood if they are to be used properly and prevent pregnancy. Both partners should be informed.

NP:I; CN:H; CA:MA; CL:C

65. (3) The nurse must ensure that the peripheral circulation is intact. The other activities are completed but are not considered priority.

NP:E; CN:PH; CA:S; CL:AN

66. (2) Indications of increased intracranial pressure include decreased pulse and respirations, decreased level of consciousness, and decreased pupillary response to light. An apical pulse of 108 (1) is within normal range for an infant. A bulging fontanelle unrelated to crying can be seen in the infant prior to the closure of the anterior fontanel by the age of 18 months.

NP:E; CN:PH; CA:P; CL:A

67. (2) Patients with appendicitis will have a low-grade fever, tenderness in the lower right quadrant, and nausea and vomiting unrelated to eating. Pain is primarily in the lower right quadrant.

NP:D; CN:PH; CA:S; CL:C

68. (2) Semi-Fowler's position relieves abdominal pain and tension. Ice is used to decrease pain. Heat (3) is never used because it could cause the appendix to rupture, thus causing peritonitis.

NP:I; CN:PH; CA:S; CL:A

69. The answer is *2.5 tablets*. This computation can be done using the formula D (dose desired) ÷ H (dose on hand) × Q (quantity of dose on hand). 12.5 ÷ 5 × 1 = 2.5 tablets.

NP:P; CN:PH; CA:M; CL:A

70. (3) Since one of the suspected side effects of the pill is thrombophlebitis, it is important to know the patient's history. If the history indicates a predisposition, the pill would not be the contraceptive method of choice. Regardless of her age, she may obtain contraceptive counseling. Names of sexual contacts (1) are important only for tracing sexually transmitted diseases.

NP:D; CN:H; CA:MA; CL:C

71. (3) A preschooler can understand simple directions and may be fearful of such tests. Although a 5-year-old child may be quiet and shy (4), these qualities are not applicable to this situation.

NP:P; CN:PS; CA:P; CL:C

72. (2) Right side heart failure manifests systemic symptoms rather than respiratory involvement. Symptoms include weight gain and edema of the dependent parts of the body. Although anorexia can be a symptom, skipping one meal does not indicate anorexia.

NP:E; CN:PH; CA:M; CL:AN

73. (3) Protamine sulfate is the antagonist for heparin. Answer (2), vitamin K, is the antagonist for Coumadin. Answer (4) is the antagonist for magnesium sulfate.

NP:E; CN:PH; CA:M; CL:A

74. (2) The nurse should take a few seconds (4–10) to check unresponsiveness in a patient who appears to be unconscious. It is important to give the patient a chance to awaken and respond before initiating other interventions, but not to wait too long.

NP:D; CN:PH; CA:M; CL:AN

75. (1) Ordering meals in this manner allows the child some independence and control, while providing an excellent teaching opportunity.

NP:P; CN:PH; CA:P; CL:C

76. (4) By first removing the old patch, the risk of overdosing the patient is minimized. The skin should not be wiped with alcohol and the patch should be applied without rubbing. Patches may be placed under clothing or on exposed skin.

NP:I; CN:PH; CA:M; CL:A

77. (4) Because the patient is breathing rapidly, she is exhaling excessive amounts of carbon dioxide. This loss of carbon dioxide decreases the H^+ ion concentration, causing the blood pH to increase, resulting in respiratory alkalosis.

NP:D; CN:PH; CA:S; CL:AN

78. (3) Recovery of language is related to frequent attempts to communicate with a responsive listener. Allowing the patient to use her own form of communication to express needs encourages further attempts to communicate. Pantomime (4) is useful but should not replace verbal communication.

NP:I; CN:PH; CA:M; CL:A

79. (3) Homonymous hemianopsia is a common visual deficiency associated with hemiplegia. Loss of the visual field must be compensated for by the patient's increased conscious awareness of hazards to personal safety.

NP:P; CN:PH; CA:M; CL:A

80. (2) A posterior fetal position often causes severe back pain and a bearing-down sensation during contractions.

    NP:P; CN:H; CA:MA; CL:C

81. (3) The unconscious patient cannot ask for fluids and will only receive ordered fluids via the feeding tube. Although individuals who exercise vigorously or are on diuretic therapy could develop fluid volume deficit, these individuals can compensate for the loss of fluids by taking oral fluids. The patient with uncompensated heart failure is more likely to develop fluid volume excess.

    NP:E; CN:PH; CA:M; CL:AN

82. The answers are 1, 2, and 5. Completing care as soon as possible is not the point—limiting exposure to 15 minutes/day is what is advised. It is true that pregnant women cannot be exposed; anyone under 18 also cannot be admitted.

    NP:I; CN:S; CA:M; CL:A

83. (4) Supine position with head on a pillow and legs elevated is the best position to decrease risk of compromised venous return. Trendelenburg's position compromises ventilation and baroreceptor mechanisms. If respirations are compromised, the bed can be raised 30–45 degrees.

    NP:I; CN:PH; CA:M; CL:A

84. (4) Because the pain may be a result of neurovascular impairment, the nurse should assess the neurovascular status of the extremity. If the status is within normal limits, then the analgesic can be administered (1). If the status is not within normal limits, the physician should be notified (3). Elevating the leg (2) will improve venous return, but not necessarily decrease the pain.

    NP:I; CN:PH; CA:S; CL:AN

85. (2) Electrolytes (potassium) are measured in milliequivalents per liter, and 3.5–5.5 mEq/L is the normal serum potassium level.

    NP:D; CN:PH; CA:M; CL:C

COMPREHENSIVE TEST 2 QUESTIONS

1. An adult patient has come to the clinic complaining of pain in her joints. A review of the record shows a diagnosis of osteoarthritis. The nurse could suggest comfort measures for this patient that would include

   1. Applying warm, moist packs to the joints.
   2. Undertaking exercises that stress the muscles.
   3. Wearing a copper bracelet to lessen the pain.
   4. Sleeping on a soft mattress to ease the pain.

2. A patient's physician has placed him on a low potassium diet. List the numbers of the following foods that he should avoid because they are high in potassium. The numbers that apply are

   _____ .

   1. Butter.
   2. Shellfish.
   3. Milk.
   4. Frozen vegetables.
   5. Orange juice.
   6. Dried dates.

3. An adult patient is scheduled to undergo arthroplasty of the hip. A priority postoperative nursing intervention is to

   1. Turn the patient to the operated side.
   2. Maintain abduction of the affected hip.
   3. Maintain acute flexion of the hip.
   4. Maintain adduction of the hip.

4. On the second morning following arthroplasty of the hip, the patient is allowed out of bed. To accomplish this, the first intervention would be to assist the patient to

   1. Dangle legs at the bedside.
   2. Transfer from the bed to a chair.
   3. Transfer from the bed to a walker.
   4. Transfer from the bed to crutches for support.

5. In assessing the respiratory status of a 1 year old with a suspected diagnosis of bronchiolitis. What is the priority assessment indicating the need for oxygen?

   1. Flaring nostrils.
   2. Cyanosis.
   3. Bradycardia.
   4. Deep, shallow breathing.

6. If a pregnant woman does not know her LMP date, the sign most useful to calculate her EDC would be the

   1. Appearance of the linea nigra.
   2. Fetal size detected by ultrasound.
   3. Estriol level at 12 weeks.
   4. Detection of Goodell's sign.

7. Before a patient goes to surgery, an operative permit must be signed. The most appropriate sequence for having the permit signed is to

   1. Have the patient sign the permit and have it witnessed as soon as she is admitted, so she knows what surgery she will be having.
   2. Prepare the patient for surgery, give the preoperative narcotics, and have her sign the permit before she goes to sleep.
   3. Ensure that the surgeon has explained the surgery to the patient, answer her questions, have her sign the permit, and then complete the final preparations for surgery.
   4. Have the patient sign the operative permit and then notify the physician.

8. The charge nurse asks the LVN to give a pregnant patient diet counseling. The patient says she does not want to gain too much weight because her husband likes her thin. Which of the following responses would be the best?

   1. "It's best for the baby if you don't try to stay too thin."
   2. "If you are careful about the foods you eat, especially those high in calories, you will not gain too much."
   3. "Let's talk about the importance of good nutrition and weight gain in pregnancy."
   4. "Why don't you have your husband come to the clinic next time, and we can all talk about nutrition."

9. A 70-year-old male patient is admitted to a skilled nursing facility (SNF) with the diagnosis of organic brain syndrome. The history shows that the patient is often disoriented. The nurse knows that the time to watch for this behavior is

   1. When he first gets out of bed in the morning.
   2. After he has been up and ambulating.
   3. After his family visits.
   4. When he awakens, especially at night.

10. A 62-year-old patient is admitted to the hospital with a diagnosis of congestive heart failure. She has had angina for many years, and recently her symptoms have been getting worse as a result of arteriosclerosis. In establishing a patient care plan, a primary goal of treatment is to

   1. Reduce the workload of the heart.
   2. Promote rest for the heart.
   3. Reduce fluid retention.
   4. Reduce circulating blood volume.

11. A 6-month-old infant is admitted to the pediatric unit with a diagnosis of severe diarrhea. The most important nursing objective is to

   1. Make constant assessment of the infant's dehydration level.
   2. Accurately record the number of the infant's stools.
   3. Dispose of the infant's stools in proper containers.
   4. Monitor the infant's electrolyte lab results.

12. The most effective means of controlling external bleeding of an extremity is

   1. Direct pressure.
   2. Pressure points.
   3. Tourniquets.
   4. Elevation.

13. A depressed 50-year-old patient is admitted to the psychiatric hospital. For the nurse assigned to work with the patient and orient her to the unit, one of the first goals would be to

   1. Show the patient where she will be sleeping.
   2. Introduce the patient to the other patients.
   3. Allow the patient to move at her own pace in getting used to the unit.
   4. Establish a nurse–patient relationship.

14. A 35-year-old patient is brought to the hospital by her husband. She has been hearing voices, acting bizarre, and singing her sentences instead of talking. A tentative diagnosis of schizophrenic disorder is made. The patient begins to take chlorpromazine (Thorazine) 200 mg TID, and by the second day, she is having limb spasms and jerky movements. The nurse should assess this behavior as

   1. Dystonic movements.
   2. Tardive dyskinesia.
   3. Parkinsonism.
   4. Extrapyramidal movements.

15. The physician orders a medication to counteract the adverse effects of chlorpromazine (Thorazine). The nurse expects that this medication will be

   1. Haloperidol (Haldol).
   2. Trifluoperazine hydrochloride (Stelazine).
   3. Benztropine mesylate (Cogentin).
   4. Levodopa (L-Dopa).

16. A premature infant is placed in an isolette. The rationale for humidifying the air in the isolette is to

   1. Improve respiratory capacity.
   2. Prevent hyperbilirubinemia.
   3. Increase the infant's temperature.
   4. Prevent drying of bronchial secretions.

17. A patient gives birth to a normal, premature, female infant. The infant's physician diagnoses respiratory distress syndrome (RDS). The concentration of oxygen that the infant receives will be regulated based on her PO_2 and PCO_2 levels. The nurse understands that critical monitoring is necessary because high levels of oxygen

   1. Produce kernicterus.
   2. Cause retinal spasms leading to the development of retrolental fibroplasia.
   3. Cause peripheral circulatory collapse.
   4. May cause respiratory damage.

18. An adult patient has just returned from the recovery room following lower bowel surgery for an obstruction. She is unable to void and her physician orders a Foley catheter. The nurse will perform the catheterization implementing

   1. Surgical asepsis.
   2. Clean technique using Standard Precautions.
   3. The physician's instructions.
   4. Medical asepsis.

19. A 63-year-old patient was recently diagnosed with cervical cancer and has received a radium needle implant. When working with the charge nurse to prepare the patient for discharge, what is the most important discharge teaching?

   1. No adverse symptoms will occur.
   2. Radioactive symptoms will occur for at least 6 weeks.
   3. Report vaginal or rectal bleeding immediately to the physician.
   4. Persistent nausea and vomiting may occur for a while after discharge, but these symptoms are not dangerous.

20. An adult patient who sustained a head injury when he fell off a ladder is admitted to a neurological unit. The nurse will assess for increased intracranial pressure. What is the earliest sign of intracranial pressure the nurse will look for?

1. Vomiting.
2. Increased blood pressure.
3. Agitation.
4. Lethargy.

21. The day before scheduled abdominal surgery, the results of a patient's laboratory tests indicate a white blood cell count of 9800/mm^3. The most appropriate intervention is to

    1. Check the chart for a physician's order for antibiotics.
    2. Notify the surgeon immediately.
    3. Take no action because it is a normal value.
    4. Call the laboratory and have the test repeated.

22. When a patient is scheduled for surgery, nursing responsibilities for the preoperative period would include notifying the charge nurse if the patient's

    1. Erythrocyte count is 6 million/mm^3.
    2. Oral temperature is 99.6°F.
    3. Hemoglobin is 14 g/100 mL.
    4. Urinalysis indicates ketonuria.

23. An adult patient whose diagnosis is personality disorder, borderline, is committed for 14 days on a locked psychiatric unit. When confronted with inappropriate behavior of talking another patient into leaving the unit without permission, the borderline patient responds, "Well, if it wasn't me, someone else would have talked her into leaving." This response is a typical example of

    1. Denial.
    2. Rationalization.
    3. Suppression.
    4. Reaction formation.

24. An adult patient with a diagnosis of epilepsy is being admitted to the hospital for a general workup and medication management. As the nurse enters the patient's room, he is just beginning to have a seizure. The first nursing action would be to

    1. Push the patient's emergency help buzzer.
    2. Protect the patient's head and body from damage.
    3. Hold the patient down.
    4. Place a tongue blade between the patient's teeth.

25. A hospitalized 24-year-old man is constantly trying to manipulate the staff as a way of getting his needs met. Which response to the patient would indicate that the nurse understands how to therapeutically respond to manipulation?

    1. "I won't allow you to manipulate me."

    2. "I won't do as you ask, but I will stay with you and talk."
    3. "If this behavior doesn't stop, I shall have to tell your doctor."
    4. "Let's focus on your anxiety so we can deal with all this manipulation."

26. Calculate the following drug dosage: If you were to give a patient one-half of a grain ¼ tablet, the patient would receive _____ grain(s) of medication.

27. When establishing discharge goals for a 9 year old with cystic fibrosis, a major component of the child's care at home will be to

    1. Avoid catching a cold.
    2. Continue breathing exercises.
    3. Control fat intake.
    4. Continue an antibiotic regimen.

28. For patients with peptic ulcer disease, nursing assessment should include observations for possible complications including

    1. Pain with defecation.
    2. Mucus in the stool.
    3. Bright-red bloody stools.
    4. Tarry stools.

29. Cimetidine (Tagamet) is ordered for a patient with peptic ulcer disease. The nurse will know that the drug has been effective when the patient no longer

    1. Tells the nurse she is nauseated after eating.
    2. Complains of intermittent pain.
    3. Complains of pain when her stomach is empty.
    4. Tells the nurse she can eat only small, bland meals.

30. A 14-year-old patient who is admitted to the hospital will most likely experience fears of

    1. Being displaced.
    2. Separation.
    3. Loss of independence.
    4. The unknown.

31. A 14-year-old patient has been admitted to the adolescent unit with a diagnosis of Type 1 diabetes mellitus. Symptoms that the patient will exhibit when the insulin injection is delayed would include

    1. Thirst, polyuria, and decreased appetite.
    2. Flushed cheeks, acetone breath, and increased thirst.
    3. Nausea, vomiting, and diarrhea.
    4. Weight gain, acetone breath, and thirst.

32. When teaching a 14-year-old patient about regulating his diabetes at home, what is the most important information to include?

   1. Limiting vigorous exercise.
   2. Eliminating sugar from his diet.
   3. Testing his blood for sugar at regular intervals.
   4. Limiting carbohydrates in his diet.

33. An adult patient is admitted to the hospital with a diagnosis of acute glomerulonephritis. His symptoms have been mild, consisting of fatigue, anorexia, and mild hypertension. One of the primary goals of the patient's treatment would be to

   1. Restore fluid and electrolyte balance.
   2. Encourage bedrest during the acute phase of illness.
   3. Give a high-protein diet to restore nutritional status.
   4. Assist patient to choose foods high in potassium.

34. A nursing action that will lessen the severity of a patient's orthostatic hypotension is to

   1. Turn him from side to side every 2 hours.
   2. Limit times he will have to get in and out of bed.
   3. Change his position routinely, especially from horizontal to vertical.
   4. Encourage him to move very slowly.

35. When caring for a patient whose physician has ordered furosemide (Lasix), the nurse should recognize that the medication is having the desired effect when

   1. The patient becomes very thirsty.
   2. The patient passes stones in the urine.
   3. Infection is decreased.
   4. Production of urine is increased.

36. An adult female patient, admitted to a psychiatric unit 2 days ago with a diagnosis of acute depression, attempts suicide. The staff intervenes in time to prevent the patient from harming herself. The most important rationale for having the staff discuss the suicide attempt is that they must

   1. Reenact the attempt so the staff can understand exactly what happened.
   2. File an accident report so the hospital administration is kept informed.
   3. Discuss the patient's behavior prior to the attempt to identify cues that might have warned them.
   4. Prevent a second suicide attempt because there is high probability that the patient will try again in the immediate future.

37. A curarelike medication and a barbiturate are given to patients before electroconvulsive therapy (ECT). The nurse understands that these medications will reduce the potential side effects of

   1. Cardiac arrest and loss of memory.
   2. Convulsions and fractures.
   3. Fractures and anxiety.
   4. Anxiety and loss of memory.

38. A 4-week-old infant is brought to the hospital by her mother, who is concerned about her weight loss and frequent crying. Pyloric stenosis is the suspected diagnosis. The nurse assessing the infant should know that the most obvious sign or symptom of this condition is

   1. Constant hunger and fussiness.
   2. Peristaltic waves passing left to right after a feeding.
   3. Frequent diarrhea.
   4. Spitting up after a feeding.

39. The most important nursing goal prior to surgery for correction of pyloric stenosis would be to

   1. Prevent dehydration.
   2. Educate the parents about the procedure.
   3. Provide sensory stimuli for the infant.
   4. Prevent development of a negative attitude toward feeding.

40. An infant is usually placed in a heated crib immediately after birth to

   1. Prevent loss of body heat.
   2. Increase oxygen intake.
   3. Facilitate drainage of mucus.
   4. Provide an environment similar to the uterus.

41. A 38-year-old patient with right upper quadrant tenderness and jaundice is admitted to the hospital. Infectious hepatitis is suspected. Before the diagnosis is confirmed, the priority nursing objective is to

   1. Observe enteric precautions.
   2. Institute isolation techniques.
   3. Use only needle precautions.
   4. Use standard precautions.

42. Which of the following symptoms would indicate possible thrombophlebitis?

   1. Pain along a vein.
   2. Severe cramping.
   3. Edema.
   4. Area surrounding a vein is warm to touch.

43. The LVN has a full workload and must reassign some of her patients to the nursing assistant. The most appropriate to reassign is a(n)

    1. Patient just returning from the recovery room following colostomy surgery.
    2. CVA patient who has been hospitalized for 2 days.
    3. Oncology patient who is in severe pain controlled by epidural analgesia.
    4. Newly admitted patient with suspected pancreatitis.

44. A 72-year-old patient in a long-term care facility has a diagnosis of Alzheimer's disease. The patient shuffles up to the station, crying and screaming, "Nobody cares if I live or die! You all hate me! All hate me!" The response by the nurse that would be most therapeutic is

    1. "What makes you think we hate you?"
    2. "You are always saying that, and you know we all love you."
    3. "Here is a cigarette. Now go in the dayroom and watch TV."
    4. "You seem very upset. Let's take a walk and talk about it."

45. A 7-year-old patient received a diagnosis of sickle cell anemia. When her parents are given genetic counseling, they will be told that if only one parent has the sickle cell trait, the number of children who will get the disease is

    1. None.
    2. All of their children.
    3. Half of their children.
    4. Twenty-five percent of their children.

46. The group of signs and symptoms that best describe a patient who is experiencing heatstroke would be

    1. Pale, moist skin; rapid pulse; and slow, deep respirations.
    2. Hot, dry skin; rapid pulse; and slow, deep respirations.
    3. Hot, dry skin; normal pulse; and normal respirations.
    4. Pale, moist skin; weak pulse; and rapid respirations.

47. In planning the daily schedule of a patient who has Alzheimer's disease, it is important for the nurse to understand that this patient

    1. May have moderate to severe memory impairment and short periods of concentration.
    2. Will respond to a rigid daily schedule, which will help him be more comfortable.

    3. Is more likely to be able to remember current experiences than past ones.
    4. Can usually be trusted to be responsible for his daily care needs.

48. Transmission-based respiratory precautions indicate that when the disease is airborne, the precaution that must be used is

    1. A mask.
    2. A gown.
    3. Eye shield
    4. Shoe covers.

49. An adult patient was admitted to the hospital with a diagnosis of carcinoma of the left lung. Following a left lobectomy, the patient is returned to the unit with a chest tube in place. The chest tube is inserted to

    1. Supply oxygen to the thoracic cavity.
    2. Remove fluid from the alveolar sacs.
    3. Provide a means of instilling medication into the thoracic cavity.
    4. Provide for removal of air and fluid from the pleural space.

50. When a chest tube is inserted, it is connected to a water-seal suction. The purpose of the water is to

    1. Provide humidity for the oxygen.
    2. Maintain a closed system so air cannot enter the pleural space.
    3. Provide a sterile environment for drainage.
    4. Provide an accurate means to measure drainage.

51. An important preoperative nursing procedure for a patient who is scheduled for a craniotomy would be to

    1. Shampoo the hair.
    2. Administer a cleansing enema.
    3. Give a complete bath.
    4. Shave the head.

52. Following a craniotomy, postoperative nursing care for the patient will include

    1. Placing the patient in Trendelenburg's position.
    2. Administering morphine sulfate for pain.
    3. Placing the patient in a belt restraint and soft wrist restraints.
    4. Recording rectal temperatures frequently.

53. A 45-year-old patient is scheduled to have an abdominal hysterectomy. While the nurse is orienting the patient to her surroundings, she states that she is afraid of what will happen the next day. The most appropriate nursing response is to

1. Assure the patient that the surgery is very safe and that problems are rare.
2. Let the patient talk about her fears as much as she wishes.
3. Explain that the patient has an excellent physician and that she has nothing to worry about.
4. Explain that anxiety has been proven to prolong length of hospitalization.

54. When caring for a patient who has undergone an abdominal hysterectomy, which of the following nursing measures would best prevent atelectasis?

   1. Have the patient turn, cough, and deep breathe every 2 hours.
   2. Put pillows under the patient's knees to decrease pressure on the incision, thereby increasing her willingness to take deep breaths.
   3. Apply a scultetus binder as soon as the patient is fully awake to assist with deep breathing.
   4. Closely observe the patient's intake of fluids to liquefy secretions.

55. A 40-year-old patient is scheduled to have an amniocentesis. This procedure would be primarily performed to detect

   1. The presence of twins.
   2. Down syndrome.
   3. Tay–Sachs disease.
   4. The sex of the fetus.

56. A 35-year-old patient was admitted to the nursing unit 4 hours ago with a diagnosis of asthmatic reaction. The nurse will assess for a characteristic symptom of asthma, which is

   1. Flushed skin.
   2. Wheezing type of respiration.
   3. Hemoptysis.
   4. Chest pain.

57. The team leader overhears the nurse assigning the nursing assistant (NA) to check on a patient who has just returned from surgery following a transurethral prostatic resection (TURP). He has a 3-way Foley catheter inserted. The nurse has asked the NA to see if the catheter is draining. The team leader's intervention would be to

   1. Remind the nurse to chart the drainage from the catheter because the physician will want to know.
   2. Do nothing because this assignment is appropriate for the NA.
   3. Instruct the nurse that this is not an appropriate assignment for the NA.
   4. Tell the nurse that she, the team leader, will check on the patient herself and report.

58. A patient who is experiencing dyspnea appears anxious. The best nursing approach is to

   1. Ignore the anxiety, understanding it will decrease when his breathing improves.
   2. Stay with the patient and be supportive.
   3. Tell the patient his breathing will soon improve.
   4. Notify the physician.

59. When planning for a safe environment for a senile elderly patient, which of the following should be considered necessary for comfort and safety?

   1. Handrails in halls.
   2. A portable walker.
   3. Floors with wall-to-wall carpeting.
   4. Handrails by the toilets.

60. A pregnant mother of a 10-year-old son says that he has begun to ask questions about the pregnancy. She is afraid he's going to ask her "where the baby comes from" and asks the nurse what to say. The nurse's best response would be

   1. "Ignore it and gently change the subject."
   2. "Ask a male family member to discuss it with the boy."
   3. "Give him a simple explanation of the facts of reproduction."
   4. "Redirect the question to him to find out what he specifically wants to know."

61. When caring for a patient who has renal failure, the nurse should be concerned about a change in

   1. Blood pressure.
   2. Pulse.
   3. Proteinuria.
   4. Respirations.

62. After a normal delivery, a newborn appears jaundiced. The physician has ordered a continuous bili light and forced fluids between feedings. An important nursing action when an infant has phototherapy is to

   1. Cover the eyes with eye patches to prevent retinal damage.
   2. Dress the infant to prevent chilling.
   3. Isolate the infant to prevent cross-contamination.
   4. Avoid handling the infant so as not to interfere with the treatment.

63. When caring for a newborn infant, the nurse should know that physiologic jaundice in a newborn usually appears

   1. Within the first 24 hours and disappears after 3 days.
   2. Within the first 24 hours and lasts 6–7 days.

3. On the second or third day and lasts 48 hours.
4. On the second or third day and begins to decrease on the sixth or seventh day.

64. Confabulation is a symptom frequently seen in dementia. Confabulation can be best defined as

1. Amnesia of recent events.
2. A defense mechanism to control anxiety.
3. The falsifying of facts to fill in memory gaps.
4. A mechanism to lower self-esteem.

65. When preparing a patient for an intravenous pyelogram (IVP), nursing care will include

1. An NPO regimen.
2. Forced fluids.
3. Enemas until clear.
4. A 24-hour urine collection.

66. A 36-year-old male patient comes to the emergency room with complaints of severe right flank pain radiating to the inguinal and testicular area. He is pale, diaphoretic, and nauseated. The physician orders an analgesic, a routine urinalysis, and admission to the hospital. The nurse should reinforce these orders by instructing the patient to

1. Save his urine for measurement and straining.
2. Drink as much fluid as possible.
3. Notify the nursing staff of the amount of his voidings.
4. Refrain from eating and not drink until further notice.

67. The charge nurse asks the LVN to check on any allergies a patient who is scheduled for an immediate intravenous pyelogram (IVP) may have. The reason for obtaining this data is

1. The intravenous dye contains iodine.
2. It is routine information and should be charted.
3. The patient will require antibiotic therapy.
4. The patient's symptoms may suggest an allergic reaction.

68. A patient is experiencing dyspnea associated with congestive heart failure. A nursing measure that would relieve the dyspnea would be to place the patient in

1. Supine position.
2. High-Fowler's position.
3. Reverse Trendelenburg's position.
4. Semi-Fowler's position.

69. When monitoring a patient who is receiving a blood transfusion, the nurse should recognize that the

signs and symptoms most characteristic of an allergic reaction to blood are

1. Decreasing blood pressure, distention of neck veins, and rash.
2. Backache, increased temperature, and chills.
3. Wheezing, hives, and laryngeal edema.
4. Tachycardia, hives, and flushed skin.

70. If an allergic reaction to a blood transfusion occurs, the first nursing action should be to

1. Notify the physician.
2. Call the charge nurse.
3. Slow the rate of infusion.
4. Shut off the transfusion.

71. You are tabulating a patient's intake and output record for your shift.

INTAKE
IV   = 1000 mL normal saline
Coffee   = 1 cup
Water   = 6 ounces
Soup   = 1 cup
Jello   = 3 ounces
Ice Cream   = 3 ounces

How many milliliters will you document as the patient's intake? _____

72. For a patient with pulmonary tuberculosis, the most important nursing intervention is to

1. Maintain secretion precautions.
2. Force fluids to a total of 2500 mL or more per day.
3. Maintain bedrest during first 2 weeks.
4. Administer chemotherapy medication on time.

73. A patient who has undergone a thyroidectomy will be maintained in semi-Fowler's position postoperatively to

1. Assist the patient to be more comfortable.
2. Prevent respiratory distress.
3. Avoid strain on the suture line.
4. Prevent bleeding.

74. A terminally ill patient says to the nurse, "Well, I've given up all hope. I know I'm going to die soon." The most therapeutic response to this statement is

1. "One should never give up all hope. We are finding new cures every day."
2. "Would you like to talk about dying?"
3. "You've given up all hope?"
4. "You know, your physician will be here soon. Why don't you talk to him about your feelings and giving up all hope?"

75. The condition of a patient who has been on an on-cology unit for 2 months becomes critical. Of the following tasks, the one with the highest priority is to

   1. Attend to the patient's physical needs and assess her condition for changes.
   2. Support the family and give them needed encouragement.
   3. Encourage the patient to express and talk about her fears of dying.
   4. Contact the patient's lawyer so she can tie up loose ends.

76. A patient's physician has ordered that he be fed via hyperalimentation. This procedure is a method of

   1. Providing the necessary fluids and electrolytes to the body.
   2. Providing complete nutrition by the intravenous route.
   3. Tube feeding that provides necessary nutrients to the body.
   4. Blood transfusion.

77. An important nursing goal in planning care for a patient with chronic organic brain syndrome (OBS) is to

   1. Encourage the patient to function dependently.
   2. Continually orient the patient to reality.
   3. Provide an unstructured environment with appropriate recreational activities.
   4. Plan a daily schedule that is varied and interesting.

78. Regression is a defense mechanism used by psychiatric patients. The best description of this mechanism is that it

   1. Is an immature way of responding.
   2. Works most effectively to eliminate anxiety.
   3. Fosters dependence.
   4. Provides security through childlike behavior.

79. The nurse should expect that the dietary requirements of a patient who has been admitted with jaundice will

   1. Limit carbohydrates.
   2. Restrict fatty foods.
   3. Avoid all juices.
   4. Include parenteral fluids.

80. When two types of insulin are being administered, the intermediate acting insulin is drawn into the syringe _____ the regular insulin.

   1. Before.
   2. After.

81. A 55-year-old female was brought to the hospital by ambulance after telling her husband that she had intense chest pain, anxiety, and nausea. Her admitting diagnosis is suspected myocardial infarction. When providing care for the patient in the emergency department, the nurse should understand that myocardial infarction results from a

   1. Critical reduction in blood supply to the myocardium.
   2. Marked increase in cardiac output.
   3. Sudden irregularity of cardiac contraction.
   4. Marked decrease in cardiac output.

82. An elderly patient develops arrhythmias while she is being admitted to the hospital. Which of the following medications should the nurse expect to be administered first?

   1. Morphine sulfate, U.S.P.
   2. Lidocaine hydrochloride, U.S.P.
   3. Nitroglycerin (Nitrostat).
   4. Meperidine hydrochloride (Demerol).

83. An infant, 3 days old, is admitted to the pediatric unit from the nursery. His diagnosis is esophageal atresia, type III. The infant's mother says to the nurse, "I feel as though I've done something wrong to make my baby sick." Which of the following responses would be most appropriate?

   1. "Your baby was born with this. You've done the best you can."
   2. "It does no good to feel that way. Your baby is sick and needs you."
   3. "A lot of mothers feel guilty when their babies are sick."
   4. "I can understand your feelings, but remember that this is a congenital defect that you did not cause."

84. An infant returns from surgery for esophageal atresia with fistula with a gastrostomy tube in place. On the second postoperative day, the intervention for tube placement is to

   1. Return the tube to gravity drainage.
   2. Secure the tube above the level of the stomach.
   3. Leave the tube as it is.
   4. Plug the tube.

85. Anticoagulants are prescribed for an adult patient. The nurse should understand that the action of this medication will

   1. Relieve pain from myocardial damage.
   2. Prevent extension of a coronary thrombus.
   3. Improve coronary circulation.
   4. Improve cardiac output.

COMPREHENSIVE TEST 2

Answers with Rationale

1. (1) Heat increases circulation to the area. There is no scientific evidence that stressing muscles with exercise (2) or wearing a copper bracelet (3) helps arthritis in any way. A soft mattress (4) would cause greater strain on joints.

   NP:I; CN:PH; CA:M; CL:C

2. The answers are 3, 5, 6—milk (*3*), orange juice (*5*), and dried dates (*6*). All are high in potassium. The other 3 foods are high in sodium.

   NP:P; CN:H; CA:M; CL:A

3. (2) Abduction, not adduction, of the hip should be maintained and acute flexion avoided. The patient may be turned to the affected side only with physician's orders.

   NP:I; CN:PH; CA:S; CL:A

4. (3) The intervention should avoid flexion of the hip, so do not dangle the patient's legs (1) or move the patient to a chair (2). The correct action is to use a walker to provide support for walking. Crutches (4) will not provide enough support.

   NP:I; CN:PH; CA:S; CL:A

5. (1) Early signs of respiratory distress and the need for oxygen include nasal flaring, increased respiratory rate, retractions, and tachycardia. Cyanosis (2) and bradycardia (3) are later signs.

   NP:D; CN:PH; CA:P; CL:A

6. (2) Fetal size is usually detected by ultrasound. Another gestational age determinant is quickening, which is first perceived movement of the baby between 17 and 19 weeks' gestation.

   NP:D; CN:H; CA:MA; CL:C

7. (3) Informed consent by a patient who is mentally competent is required in order to have an operative permit signed. This means the physician must talk to the patient, and the patient must not be under the influence of narcotics. The operative permit does not have to be witnessed.

   NP:P; CN:S; CA:S; CL:A

8. (3) Adequate nutrition and weight gain in pregnancy are directly related to decreased mortality and morbidity in the newborn. Helping the patient understand the role of nutrition and weight gain will help her to explore the best way to talk with her husband about his concerns.

   NP:I; CN:PS; CA:PS; CL:A

9. (4) Because of an elderly person's slowness in adapting to dim light, the patient is most likely to be disoriented if he awakens in the dark.

   NP:D; CN:PS; CA:PS; CL:A

10. (1) Congestive heart failure results when the heart is unable to pump adequate amounts of blood. The cardiac workload and activity should be reduced to allow the heart to rest.

    NP:P; CN:PH; CA:M; CL:C

11. (1) While all the objectives listed in the answers are important, assessment of dehydration level and acidosis are the most crucial, for this condition can be life threatening.

    NP:P; CN:PH; CA:P; CL:C

12. (1) Direct pressure is the most effective way of controlling bleeding. It can be augmented by elevating the wound above the level of the heart. Pressure points (2) only slow bleeding, as collateral circulation is almost always present. Tourniquets (3) are seldom needed and are used as a last resort.

    NP:I; CN:PH; CA:M; CL:K

Coding for Questions/Answers Abbreviations: **Nursing Process: NP,** Data Collection: D, Planning: P, Implementation: I, Evaluation: E, **Client Needs: CN,** Safe, Effective Care Environment: S, Health Promotion and Maintenance: H, Psychosocial Integrity: PS, Physiological Integrity: PH, **Clinical Area: CA,** Medical Nursing: M, Surgical Nursing: S, Maternal/Newborn Nursing: MA, Pediatric Nursing: P, Psychiatric Nursing: PS, **Cognitive Level: CL,** Knowledge: K, Comprehension: C, Application: A, Analysis: AN

13. (4) With a psychiatric patient, establishing a relationship in which she can begin to trust another person is a primary goal and should begin during orientation. During this process, the nurse will also accomplish answers (1) and (2).

NP:P; CN:PS; CA:PS; CL:A

14. (1) Although these side effects are Parkinson-like (3) and are extrapyramidal (4), the more specific answer is dystonia, the form that occurs in the first 1 or 2 days.

NP:D; CN:PS; CA:PS; CL:AN

15. (3) The drugs of choice to counteract the extrapyramidal side effects are Cogentin or Artane. Haldol (1) and Stelazine (2) may be used instead of Thorazine to control behavior; L-Dopa (4) is used in Parkinson's disease, not for Parkinson-like side effects.

NP:P; CN:PS; CA:PS; CL:C

16. (4) The infant will have a weak cough and gag reflex and have difficulty removing mucus. Should the bronchial secretions become dry, they become tenacious and almost impossible for the infant to cough up, as well as difficult to remove by suctioning. Oxygen is very drying to the mucous membranes and should always be humidified while being administered, whether to an infant or adult.

NP:P; CN:H; CA:MA; CL:C

17. (2) High blood levels of oxygen cause spasms of the retinal vessels, and the destruction of these vessels can cause retrolental fibroplasia, which leads to blindness.

NP:E; CN:PH; CA:MA; CL:C

18. (1) Nurses observe surgical asepsis while performing catheterizations because of the sterility of the system being entered. Physicians' instructions do not include outlining the steps of the procedure for catheterization.

NP:I; CN:S; CA:S; CL:A

19. (3) Any sign of vaginal or rectal bleeding after a radium implant should be reported immediately to the physician, as it would indicate that complications have developed.

NP:I; CN:S; CA:M; CL:AN

20. (4) Lethargy is the earliest sign of increased intracranial pressure. It is due to compression of the brain from edema or hemorrhage (or both).

NP:D; CN:PH; CA:M; CL:A

21. (3) The normal WBC is 5000 to 10,000/mm^3. If the results were abnormally high, the surgeon would have to be notified, and the surgery may be canceled. Also, if the white count is high, antibiotics may be ordered. Tests with abnormal results are not routinely repeated unless the results are grossly abnormal.

NP:I; CN:PH; CA:S; CL:AN

22. (4) All the other reports are within normal range. The ketonuria indicates a probable diabetic complication or other metabolic condition.

NP:E; CN:PH; CA:S; CL:AN

23. (2) Rationalization is the most common defense mechanism used by borderline individuals. They usually do not feel guilt.

NP:E; CN:PS; CA:PS; CL:C

24. (2) The primary nursing goal during a seizure is to protect the patient from physical injury and, if possible, to maintain a patent airway. After a seizure has begun, the nurse would not use a tongue blade (4) because it can cause damage. The nurse would never hold the patient down (3).

NP:I; CN:PH; CA:M; CL:A

25. (2) It is important to set limits but not to reinforce low self-esteem, so staying with the patient would be therapeutic.

NP:I; CN:PS; CA:PS; CL:AN

26. When you take one-half of a ¼ grain tablet, you are left with ⅛ grain, the correct dosage.

NP:P; CN:PH; CA:M; CL:A

27. (2) The major objective is to keep lungs clear of mucus. Because these children tend to have shallow breathing, breathing exercises are an important activity to achieve this goal.

NP:P; CN:PH; CA:P; CL:C

28. (4) A bleeding peptic ulcer would cause tarry stools. Bright-red bloody stools (3) indicate a bleeding problem low in the gastrointestinal tract.

NP:D; CN:PH; CA:M; CL:A

29. (3) Tagamet blocks gastric acid secretion, so the patient will no longer experience pain when her stomach is empty. Nausea (1) is not an expected side effect of the drug.

NP:E; CN:PH; CA:M; CL:C

30. (3) Having recently achieved some measure of independence, adolescents have a fear of losing it.

NP:E; CN:H; CA:P; CL:K

31. (2) All the other choices have one wrong answer. Decreased appetite (1), diarrhea (3), and weight gain (4), are symptoms not usually associated with this condition.

NP:E; CN:PH; CA:P; CL:C

32. (3) Regular testing for sugar via finger-sticks is important as a guide to dietary and insulin control. If a patient is in good health and understands the increased glucose needs of the body following exercise, there is no reason to restrict activities (1). All sugar is usually not eliminated (2) if correct ADA exchanges are used and carbohydrates make up 60 percent of the diet.

NP:I; CN:PH; CA:P; CL:A

33. (2) Bedrest would protect the poorly functioning kidneys (activity may increase urinary abnormalities), as well as facilitate diuresis. Protein is usually restricted if oliguria is present, but a high-protein diet (3) would not be implemented. Fluids may be restricted, as well as potassium and sodium.

NP:P; CN:PH; CA:M; CL:A

34. (3) Orthostatic hypotension occurs when the body position is changed infrequently; it can be lessened by routinely altering the patient's position from horizontal to upright. Moving slowly (4) may help, but would not be as useful.

NP:I; CN:PH; CA:M; CL:C

35. (4) Furosemide (Lasix) actually increases blood flow to the kidney, thereby increasing the production of urine. The patient may become thirsty, but answer (4) is more specific. The patient may or may not have kidney stones, and Lasix is not given for this diagnosis. Answer (3) is wrong because Lasix is not antimicrobial.

NP:E; CN:PH; CA:M; CL:A

36. (3) Even though all of the reasons are important and should not be ignored, the most important task is that the staff learn to assess the patient's behavior correctly and to identify cues that might indicate an impending suicide attempt.

NP:E; CN:PS; CA:PS; CL:AN

37. (3) The curarelike drug lessens strong muscular contractions during the convulsion that can cause fractures, and the barbiturate is given to reduce anxiety by putting the patient to sleep for 5 to 10 minutes.

NP:E; CN:PH; CA:PS; CL:C

38. (2) Observing peristaltic waves is one of the most distinctive signs of pyloric stenosis. The infant is also probably suffering from hunger, but crying and being fussy (1) is a more nonspecific sign.

NP:D; CN:PH; CA:P; CL:A

39. (1) Dehydration from persistent vomiting is the most frequent complication of pyloric stenosis.

NP:P; CN:PH; CA:P; CL:C

40. (1) The infant is wet and delivery rooms are usually cool, resulting in heat loss from the infant through conduction, convection, and radiation. Placing the infant in a heated crib decreases heat loss. Trendelenburg's position is used to facilitate drainage, not the heated crib itself.

NP:P; CN:H; CA:MA; CL:C

41. (1) Recognizing that these symptoms may represent infectious hepatitis, which is communicable by excreta, the nurse will protect patients and personnel by observing enteric precaution isolation until the diagnosis is confirmed. After the diagnosis is confirmed, the patient will be infectious for 1 week (3 weeks prior to and 1 week after developing jaundice).

NP:D; CN:PH; CA:M; CL:A

42. (4) The area surrounding a vein would be warm to touch and red, indicating an inflammatory response. Pain may be present, but it would not be along a vein. Neither cramping nor edema is significant for a thrombus.

NP:D; CN:PH; CA:M; CL:C

43. (2) The most appropriate patient would be the one with the CVA diagnosis. This patient would have been in the hospital for 2 days, so the initial assessment would have been completed. This condition does not demand immediate assessment or intervention, as does the colostomy patient (1) assessing for hemorrhage, vital signs, etc.; the oncology patient (3) to determine the effectiveness of the pain protocol; and the new patient with suspected pancreatitis (4) who needs a complete assessment.

NP:P; CN:S; CA:M; CL:AN

44. (4) The nurse acknowledges the patient and his feelings without focusing directly on them. Answer (1) asks for an analysis of feelings; (2) is making

light of the patient's feelings; (3) is ignoring the problem.

NP:I; CN:PS; CA:PS; CL:A

45. (1) No children will get sickle cell anemia. Both parents must have the recessive gene to have a child with the disease. One parent can pass the gene on so that the children may be carriers.

NP:I; CN:H; CA:M; CL:C

46. (2) A person experiencing heatstroke will most likely have hot, dry skin; a rapid pulse; and slow, deep respirations.

NP:D; CN:PH; CA:M; CL:C

47. (1) It is important to remember that these patients usually have some memory and concentration impairment. The degree depends on the individual and is influenced by the basic personality structure and the cause of the problem. Past experiences are more likely to be remembered. This patient cannot be responsible for his daily needs.

NP:P; CN:PS; CA:PS; CL:A

48. (1) A mask must be used for respiratory precautions when the disease is airborne; for droplet precautions, a mask is indicated when working within 3 feet of the patient. Contact precautions do not indicate a mask, but require gloves.

NP:P; CN:S; CA:M; CL:A

49. (4) Air enters the chest cavity when it is opened, and fluid collects during surgery. A tube is placed in the pleural space to drain this collection of fluid and to allow for the reexpansion of the lung.

NP:P; CN:PH; CA:S; CL:K

50. (2) The end of the drainage tube is kept under water; this water seals the tube so air cannot enter and be drawn back into the pleural space.

NP:P; CN:PH; CA:S; CL:K

51. (1) While a complete bath is usually given, the most important preoperative procedure is the shampoo. A cleansing enema is usually not given because of the potential increase in intracranial pressure. The physician will shave the patient's head.

NP:I; CN:PH; CA:S; CL:A

52. (4) Hyperthermia is a complication of brain surgery, and since the patient probably is not fully oriented, a rectal temperature should be taken. Trendelenburg's position increases intracranial pressure; morphine may depress respirations. Re-

straints are not routinely used; however, siderails are used for safety.

NP:P; CN:PH; CA:S; CL:A

53. (2) Allowing the patient to express her fears results in a decrease in anxiety and a more realistic and knowledgeable reaction to the situation.

NP:I; CN:PS; CA:S; CL:A

54. (1) Atelectasis is collapse of alveoli caused by mucus plugs in the small bronchioles due to inadequate ventilation. Turning, coughing, and deep breathing improve ventilation and help prevent the collapse. Liquefying secretions (4) is important, but answer (1) is more critical.

NP:I; CN:PH; CA:S; CL:A

55. (2) Amniocentesis is done primarily to determine fetal trisomy 21 (Down syndrome) in pregnant women over 35 years of age. Carrying twins (1) is not relevant to performing this test. Ashkenazic Jews (3) have a high incidence of Tay–Sachs disease, and for a person with this ethnic background, the test might be performed; it is not related to age. While this test does reveal the sex of the fetus (4), it is not the primary purpose.

NP:P; CN:H; CA:MA; CL:C

56. (2) Asthma is defined as recurrent paroxysms of dyspnea with a characteristic wheezing. Flushed skin and hemoptysis are not present. Rales may be present, but chest pain is not.

NP:D; CN:PH; CA:M; CL:A

57. (3) This situation involves management skills and teaching because the team leader should instruct the nurse that the NA cannot complete the necessary assessment needed for safe patient care. The Foley is inserted if considerable bleeding is expected; therefore, an RN or LVN should evaluate the drainage. If the Foley is not draining sufficiently, a complication of hemorrhage, displacement of the catheter, or perforation of the bladder during surgery might have occurred and the physician should be notified immediately. For the team leader to do the assignment herself is not appropriate because the nurse needs guidance.

NP:I; CN:S; CA:PS; CL:AN

58. (2) The dyspneic patient may be very anxious and will look to the nurse for support and reassurance. The best way to provide this is to remain with him. Do not ignore the anxiety (1); it is a symptom of the condition. Telling him his breathing will improve

(3) is giving him false reassurance.

NP:I; CN:PS; CA:M; CL:A

59. (4) The patient should be encouraged to use toilet rails for support. Hall handrails (1) are useful but not as important as rails by the toilet. The patient is not yet ready for a walker (2). Carpeting (3) has been found to hold unpleasant odors and is difficult to clean.

NP:P; CN:S; CA:M; CL:C

60. (4) Always clarify with children what it is they want to know before giving them facts; then give them simple, direct answers. Ignoring the question (1) may only postpone the answer or, worse, give the child the idea that it is an unspeakable subject.

NP:I; CN:PS; CA:MA; CL:AN

61. (1) While pulse (2) and respirations (4) may change, hypertension is the major concern. Patients in early stages of renal failure become hypertensive due to poor kidney perfusion and function, probably caused by renal ischemia.

NP:E; CN:PH; CA:M; CL:AN

62. (1) The infant's eyes are covered with patches during treatment because of the possibility of damage to the retina. The light is warm, so the baby will not be fully dressed. This condition is not contagious, so isolation (3) is not indicated.

NP:I; CN:PH; CA:MA; CL:A

63. (4) Physiologic jaundice occurs as the bilirubin level in the blood rises. As liver function increases, bilirubin is excreted and blood levels of bilirubin go down.

NP:E; CN:PH; CA:MA; CL:K

64. (3) As the patient experiences memory gaps, he fills them in with stories unsubstantiated by facts. This allows him to preserve his self-esteem, not lower it (4).

NP:P; CN:PS; CA:PS; CL:K

65. (1) Realizing that the patient could require surgical removal of an existing stone, the nurse will monitor the NPO status as a precautionary measure.

NP:P; CN:PH; CA:M; CL:A

66. (1) The patient's urine should be measured and strained for stones. If surgery is anticipated, the patient will be maintained NPO regardless of the status of his nausea.

NP:I; CN:PH; CA:M; CL:A

67. (1) Anaphylactic reactions have occurred in patients with hypersensitivity to iodine derivatives from the intravenous dye used for the pyelogram. If the patient is allergic to shellfish, which contains iodine, he may well be allergic to the dye.

NP:P; CN:PH; CA:M; CL:C

68. (2) High-Fowler's position allows for good lung expansion, as well as decreasing venous return from the lower extremities.

NP:I; CN:PH; CA:M; CL:A

69. (3) These are classic symptoms of an allergic reaction. Answer (2) lists symptoms of a hemolytic reaction. All other symptoms listed are a combination of transfusion reactions.

NP:D; CN:PH; CA:M; CL:A

70. (4) If the nurse suspects an allergic reaction, the blood should be shut off immediately, and then the charge nurse and the physician should be notified.

NP:I; CN:PH; CA:M; CL:A

71. The total intake is 1720 mL. The nurse would change the containers and ounces to mL and add: 1000 mL IV; 1 cup coffee = 180 mL; 6 ounces water = 180 mL; 1 cup soup = 180 mL; 3 ounces Jello = 90 mL; and 3 ounces ice cream = 90 mL.

NP:P; CN:PH; CA:M; CL:A

72. (1) It is important to maintain respiratory precautions until 2–3 weeks after chemotherapy has begun to prevent spread of the disease. Patients should drink fluids, but they don't have to be forced (2). Bedrest (3) is not necessarily advocated, and drugs should be given in a single daily dose to be most effective.

NP:I; CN:PH; CA:M; CL:A

73. (3) The nurse will want to avoid strain on the sutures, which could cause bleeding. This position will not prevent respiratory distress, but will help relieve it.

NP:E; CN:PH; CA:S; CL:C

74. (3) This reflective response will open communication and enable the patient to express whatever concerns or feelings she has without confining her to a discussion of dying (2).

NP:I; CN:PS; CA:M; CL:A

75. (1) The highest priority is observing for changes in physical status and then giving the patient emotional support. Supporting the family (2) is part of

the role as a nurse, but contacting the lawyer (4) is not a responsibility.

NP:P; CN:PH; CA:M; CL:A

76. (2) This is a method that involves infusion of a solution of protein, glucose, electrolytes, vitamins, and minerals—complete nutrition by the intravenous route.

NP:P; CN:PH; CA:M; CL:C

77. (2) OBS patients require frequent orientation to reality because they forget recent events. They should be encouraged to function independently in a safe, structured environment. The daily schedule should be planned and predictable.

NP:P; CN:PS; CA:PS; CL:C

78. (2) Regression is a way to reduce anxiety and cope with different situations by going back to a time when the patient felt more safe, secure, and comfortable.

NP:P; CN:PS; CA:PS; CL:K

79. (2) Gallbladder and liver function are stimulated by ingestion of fats, so they will be restricted. Juices (3) and carbohydrates (1) will be included in the diet.

NP:P; CN:PH; CA:M; CL:C

80. (2) The answer is after. You would first draw the regular insulin into the syringe to prevent inadvertent injection of intermediate-acting insulin into the Regular insulin bottle, which would inactivate its rapid action.

NP:P; CN:S; CA:M; CL:A

81. (1) Critical reduction of blood supply to the myocardium for a prolonged period results in sustained oxygen deprivation. As a result, cardiac muscle is destroyed.

NP:P; CN:PH; CA:M; CL:K

82. (2) Death-producing arrhythmias must be treated immediately with lidocaine or another antiarrhythmic medication. Although a narcotic analgesic (1, 4) will also be given to decrease pain and a nitroglycerin IV drip (3) will probably be started, these medications are not the priority.

NP:P; CN:PH; CA:M; CL:C

83. (4) The nurse recognizes the mother's feelings, but tries to show that they are not based on fact.

NP:I; CN:PH; CA:M; CL:C

84. (1) The gastrostomy tube is returned to gravity drainage until the infant can tolerate feedings. After the second or third day, the gastrostomy tube is pinned to the infant's shirt, above the level of the stomach. This allows gastric secretions to pass to the duodenum.

NP:I; CN:PH; CA:S; CL:A

85. (2) Anticoagulants are administered to decrease the occurrence of venous thrombosis and emboli, as well as to prevent the extension of a clot that has already formed.

NP:E; CN:PH; CA:M; CL:K

APPENDIX—DIRECTORY OF BOARDS OF NURSING

Alabama Board of Nursing
770 Washington Ave.
RSA Plaza, Suite 250
Montgomery, Alabama 36130-3900
(334) 242-4060

Alaska Board of Nursing
3601 C Street, Suite 722
Anchorage, Alaska 99503
(907) 269-8161

Health Services Regulatory Board
LBJ Tropical Medical Center
Pago Pago, American Samoa 96799
(685) 633-1222

Arizona State Board of Nursing
1651 E. Morten, Suite 150
Phoenix, Arizona 85020
(602) 331-8111

Arkansas State Board of Nursing
1123 South University, Suite 800
Little Rock, Arkansas 72204
(501) 686-2700

California Board of Vocational Nursing
2535 Capitol Oaks Drive, Suite 205
Sacramento, California 95833
(916) 263-7800

Colorado State Board of Nursing
1560 Broadway, Suite 880
Denver, Colorado 80202
(303) 894-2430

Connecticut Board of Examiners for Nursing
410 Capitol Avenue
Hartford, Connecticut 06134
(860) 509-7624

Delaware Board of Nursing
861 Silver Lake Blvd.
Dover, Delaware 19904
(302) 739-4522

District of Columbia Board of Nursing
825 N Capitol Street, NE, 2nd Floor
Washington, DC 20002
(202) 442-4778

Florida State Board of Nursing
4080 Woodcock Drive, Suite 202
Jacksonville, Florida 32207
(904) 858-6940

Georgia Board of Nursing
237 Coliseum Drive
Macon, Georgia 31217
(478) 207-1640

Guam Board of Nurse Examiners
PO Box 2816
Agana, Guam 96910
(671) 734-7295

Hawaii Board of Nursing
Box 3469
Honolulu, Hawaii 96801
(808) 586-3000

Idaho State Board of Nursing
280 N 8th Street, Suite 210
Boise, Idaho 83720
(208) 334-3110

Illinois Dept. of Professional Regulations
100 West Randolph, Suite 9-300
Chicago, Illinois 60601
(312) 814-2715

Indiana State Board of Nursing
402 W. Washington Street
Indianapolis, Indiana 46204
(317) 232-2960

Iowa Board of Nursing
400 SW 8th Street
Des Moines, Iowa 50309
(515) 281-3255

Kansas State Board of Nursing
900 SW Jackson Street, Suite 551S
Topeka, Kansas 66612
(785) 296-4929

Kentucky Board of Nursing
312 Whittington Parkway, Suite 300
Louisville, Kentucky 40222
(502) 329-7011

Louisiana State Board of Nursing
3510 N Causeway Blvd., Suite 501
Metairie, Louisiana 70003
(504) 838-5332

Maine State Board of Nursing
158 State House Station
Augusta, Maine 04333
(207) 287-1133

Maryland Board of Nursing
4140 Patterson Avenue
Baltimore, Maryland 21215
(410) 585-1900

Massachusetts Board of Registration in Nursing
239 Causeway Street
Boston, Massachusetts 02114
(617) 727-9961

Michigan Board of Nursing
CIS/Office of Health Services
611 West Ottawa
Lansing, Michigan 48933
(517) 373-9102

Minnesota Board of Nursing
2829 University Avenue, SE, Suite 500
St. Paul, Minnesota 55414
(612) 617-2270

Mississippi Board of Nursing
1935 Lakeland Drive, Suite B
Jackson, Mississippi 39216
(601) 987-4188

Missouri State Board of Nursing
3605 Missouri Boulevard
Jefferson City, Missouri 65102
(573) 751-0681

Montana State Board of Nursing
301 South Park
Helena, Montana 59620
(406) 444-2071

Nebraska Health and Human Services System
Department of Licensure-Nursing
301 Centennial Mall South
Lincoln, Nebraska 68509
(402) 471-4376

Nevada State Board of Nursing
4330 South Valley View Blvd.
Las Vegas, Nevada 89103
(702) 486-5800

New Hampshire Board of Nursing
78 Regional Drive, Bldg. B
Concord, New Hampshire 03302
(603) 271-2323

New Jersey Board of Nursing
124 Halsey Street, 6th Floor
Newark, New Jersey 07101
(973) 504-6586

New Mexico Board of Nursing
4206 Louisiana Blvd., NE, Suite A
Albuquerque, New Mexico 87109
(505) 841-8340

New York State Board of Nursing
89 Washington Avenue
2nd Floor, West Wing
Albany, New York 12234
(518) 474-3817

North Carolina Board of Nursing
3724 National Drive, Suite 201
Raleigh, North Carolina 27612
(919) 782-3211

North Dakota Board of Nursing
919 S 7th Street, Suite 504
Bismarck, North Dakota 58504
(701) 328-9777

Ohio Board of Nursing
17 South High Street, Suite 400
Columbus, Ohio 43215
(614) 466-3947

Oklahoma Board of Nursing
2915 N. Classen Boulevard, Suite 524
Oklahoma City, Oklahoma 73106
(405) 962-1800

Oregon State Board of Nursing
800 NE Oregon Street, Suite 465
Portland, Oregon 97232
(503) 731-4745

Pennsylvania State Board of Nursing
124 Pine Street
Harrisburg, Pennsylvania 17101
(717) 783-7142

Council on Higher Education of PR
P.O. Box 23305, University Station
Rio Piedras, Puerto Rico 00931
(809) 758-3350

Rhode Island Board of Nursing
105 Cannon Building
Three Capitol Hill
Providence, Rhode Island 02908
(401) 222-5700

South Carolina Board of Nursing
110 Centerview Drive, Suite 202
Columbia, South Carolina 29210
(803) 896-4550

South Dakota Board of Nursing
4300 South Louise Ave., Suite C-1
Sioux Falls, South Dakota 57106
(605) 362-2760

Tennessee Board of Nursing
426 Fifth Avenue North
Nashville, Tennessee 37247
(615) 532-5166

Texas Board of Nurse Examiners
333 Guadalupe, Suite 3-460
Austin, Texas 78701
(512) 305-7400

Utah State Board of Nursing
160 East 300 South
Salt Lake City, Utah 84111
(801) 530-6628

Vermont State Board of Nursing
109 State Street
Montpelier, Vermont 05609
(802) 828-2396

Virgin Islands Board of Nurse Licensure
P.O. Box 4247
St. Thomas, Virgin Islands 00803
(340) 776-7397

Virginia State Board of Nursing
6606 W Broad Street, 4th Floor
Richmond, Virginia 23230
(804) 662-9909

Washington State Nursing Care
Quality Assurance Commission
1300 Quince Street, SE
Olympia, Washington 98504
(360) 236-4740

West Virginia Board of Examiners
for Registered Nurses
101 Dee Drive
Charleston, West Virginia 25311
(304) 558-3596

Wisconsin Department of Regulation & Licensing
1400 E Washington Avenue
Madison, Wisconsin 53708
(608) 266-0145

Wyoming State Board of Nursing
2020 Carey Avenue, Suite 110
Cheyenne, Wyoming 82002
(307) 777-7601

BIBLIOGRAPHY

CHAPTER 1

Bloom, BS. (Ed.). (1956). *Taxonomy of educational objectives: the classification of educational goals, Handbook I*. New York: David Mckay.

Hertz, J, Yocum, C, Gawel, S. (2000). *1999 Practice analysis of newly licensed registered nurses in the US*. Chicago: National Council of State Boards of Nursing.

National Council of State Boards of Nursing. (1998). Model Nursing Practice Act. Chicago: Author.

National Council of State Boards of Nursing. (Effective 2005). *Test plan for the national council licensure examination for practical nurses*. Chicago: Author.

Smith, JE, Crawford, LH, Gawel, SH. (2000). *Linking the NCLEX-PN national licensure examination to practice: 2000 practice analysis of newly licensed practical/vocational nurses in the US*. Chicago: National Council of State Boards of Nursing, Inc.

CHAPTER 2

American Hospital Association. (2001). *A patient's bill of rights*. Chicago: AHA.

American Nurses' Association. (2001). *Code of ethics for nurses with interpretive statements*. Washington, DC: ANA.

American Nurses' Association. (1997). *Unlicensed assistive personnel legislation*. Washington, DC: ANA.

American Nurses' Association. (1998). *Standards of clincial nursing practice* (2nd ed.). Washington, DC: ANA.

Bernzweig, E. (1996). *The nurse's liability for malpractice*. (6th ed.). St. Louis: Mosby.

Boucher, MA. (1998, February). Delegation alert. *American Journal of Nursing, 98*(2), 26–32.

Brent, N. (2000). *Nurses and the law: a guide to principles and applications* (2nd ed.). Philadelphia: Saunders.

California Board of Registered Nursing. (1997). *Nursing practice act: rules and regulations*. Sacramento, CA.

Canavan, K. (1997, May). Combating dangerous delegation. *American Journal of Nursing, 97*(5), 57–58.

Gerber-Zimmerman. (1997, May). Delegating to unlicensed assistive personnel. *Nursing 97, 27*(5), 71.

Guido, G. (1998). *Legal issues in nursing: a source book for practice* (2nd ed.). Norwalk, CT: Appleton & Lange.

Kany, K. (1999, October). Working with UAPs. *American Journal of Nursing, 99*(10), 71.

LeMone, P, Burke, K. (2004). *Medical surgical nursing: Critical thinking in client care* (3rd ed.). Upper Saddle River, NJ: Prentice Hall Health.

Parkman, C, Calfee, B. (1997, April). Advance directives: honoring your patient's end-of-life wishes. *Nursing 97, 98*(4), 48–53.

Sheehan, J. (2001, November). Delegating to UAPs. *RN Magazine, 64*(11), 65–66.

Smith, S. (1998, July). RNs and UAPs: not much difference? *RN Magazine, 62*(7), 37–38.

Smith, S, Duell, D, Martin, B. (2004). *Clinical nursing skills* (6th ed.). Upper Saddle River, NJ: Prentice Hall Health.

Ventura, M. (1999, February). Staffing issues. *RN Magazine, 62*(2), 26–30.

Ventura, M. (1996, September). Workload, UAPs and you. *RN Magazine, 59*(9), 41–45.

CHAPTER 3

American Psychiatric Association. (2000). *Diagnostic and statistical manual of mental disorders* (text revision—4th ed.). Washington, DC: Author.

Ball, J, Bindler, R. (2003). *Pediatric nursing* (3rd ed.). Norwalk, CT: Appleton & Lange.

Bandura, A. (1986). *Social foundations of thought and action: a social cognitive theory*. Upper Saddle River, NJ: Prentice Hall Health.

Engle, G. (1964). Grief and grieving, *American Journal of Nursing, 64*(9).

Erickson, E. (1963). *Childhood and society* (2nd ed.). New York: Norton.

Fogel, C, Lauver, D. (1990). *Sexual health promotion*. Philadelphia: Saunders.

Furman, J. (2001, April). Living with dying: how to help the family caregiver. *Nursing 2001, 31*(4), p. 36.

Kübler-Ross, E. (1993). *Death and dying*. New York: Macmillan.

Lark, S. (2002). *The estrogen decision*. Berkeley, CA: Celestial Arts.

Piaget, J. (1973). *Origins of intelligence in children*. New York: Norton.

Selye, H. (1976). *The stress of life*. New York: McGraw-Hill.

Selye, H. (1974). *Stress without distress*. New York: Signet Books.

Stuart, G, Laraia, M, Sundeen, S. (2002). *Principles and practice of psychiatric nursing* (7th ed.). St. Louis: Mosby.

CHAPTER 4

Blais, K, Hayes, J, Kozier, B, Erb, G. (2001). *Professional nursing practice: concepts and perspectives* (4th ed.). Upper Saddle River, NJ: Prentice Hall Health.

Board of Registered Nursing. (2003). *Pain assessment: the fifth vital sign.* State of California.

Guiliamo, K, (1997, May). Organ transplants. *Nursing 97, 27*(5), 34–39.

Heffernan, L. (1998, February). Organ donation: the legal aspects. *RN Magazine, 61*(2), 51–52.

McCaffery, M, Pasero, C. (2001, July). Assessment and treatment of patients with mental illness: implementing the JCAHO pain management standards. *American Journal of Nursing, 101*(7), 69.

McCaffrey, M. (2001, April). Overcoming barriers to pain management. *Nursing 2001, 31*(4), 18.

McCaffrey, M. (1999, July). Assessing pain in a confused, nonverbal patient. *Nursing 99, 29*(7), 18.

McCaffery, M, Pasero, C. (2000, September). Pain control. *Nurseweek,* Sunnyvale, CA.

Metules, TJ, Unkle, DW. (2000, April). Spinal cord injury falls into two categories. *RN Magazine, 63*(4), 85.

Pagana, K, Pagana, T. (2002). *Mosby's manual of diagnostic and laboratory tests* (2nd ed.). St. Louis: Mosby.

Taylor, C, Lillis, C, LeMone, P. (2001). *Fundamentals of nursing: the art and science of nusring care* (4th ed.). Philadelphia: Lippincott.

Wong-Baker. (2000). *Choosing a FACES pain scale,* Revised. www.painsourcebook.ca/pdfs/pps92.

CHAPTER 5

Abrams, AC. (2000). *Clinical drug therapy: rationales for nursing practice* (6th ed.). Philadelphia: Lippincott.

Boyer, MJ. (2002). *Math for nurses: a pocket guide to dosage calculations and drug preparations* (5th ed.). Philadelphia: Lippincott.

Chase, S. (1997, March). Pharmacology in practice. *RN Magazine, 60*(3), 22–24.

Craven, R, Hirmle, C. (2000). *Fundamentals of nursing: human health and function* (3rd ed.). Philadelphia: Lippincott.

Cobb, M.D. (1990, March). Dealing fairly with medication errors. *Nursing 90, 20*(3), 42–43.

Deglin, J, Vallerand, A. (2003). *Davis's drug guide for nurses* (7th ed.). Philadelphia: Davis.

Grajeda-Higley, L. (2000). *Pharmacology: a physiology approach.* Upper Saddle River, NJ: Prentice Hall Health.

Hodgen, B. (2002). *Saunders nursing drug handbook.* Philadelphia: Saunders.

Karch, A, Karch, F. (2001). Take part in the solution: how to report medication errors. *American Journal of Nursing, 101*(10), 25.

Kuhn, M. (1998). *Pharmacotherapeutics: a nursing process approach.* Philadelphia: Davis.

Leahy, J, Kizilay, P. (1998). *Foundations of nursing practice: a nursing process approach.* Philadelphia: Saunders.

Malseed, R, Goldstein, F, Baldon, N. (1995). *Pharmacology: drug therapy and nursing considerations* (4th ed.). Philadelphia: Lippincott.

Phillips, L. (1997). *Manual of IV therapeutics* (2nd ed.). Philadelphia: Davis.

Physicians' desk reference to pharmaceutical specialties and biologicals (55th ed.). (2003). Montvale, NJ: Medical Economics.

Wilburn, S. (2000, February). Preventing needlesticks in your facility. *American Journal of Nursing, 100*(2), 96.

Wilson, B, Shannon, M, Stang, C. (2000). *Nurses drug guide.* Upper Saddle River, NJ: Prentice Hall Health.

Wilson, B, Shannon, M. (2001). *Dosage calculation* (4th ed.). Upper Saddle River, NJ: Prentice Hall Health.

CHAPTER 6

Brown, J. (2002). *Nutrition now* (3rd ed.). Belmont, CA: Wadsworth Group.

Eisenberg, P. (1994, November). Gastrostomy and jejunostomy tubes. *RN Magazine, 57*(11), 54–59.

Loan, T, Magnuson, B, Williams, S. (1998, August). Debunking six myths about enteral feeding. *Nursing 98, 28*(8), 43–48.

Metheny, W, Wiersema, M, Clark, J. (1998, January). pH, color and feeding tubes. *RN Magazine, 61*(1), 25–27.

US Department of Agriculture and US Department of Health and Human Services. (1992). *Food guide pyramid—A guide to daily food choices.* Washington, DC: USDA/HNIS.

Whitney, E, Cataldo, C, Rolfes, S. (2002). *Understanding normal and clinical nutrition* (6th ed.). St. Paul, MN: West Publishing.

Williams, SR. (2001). *Basic nutrition & diet therapy* (11th ed.). St. Louis: Mosby.

Williams, M. (2002). *Nutrition for health, fitness, and sport.* Boston: McGraw-Hill.

CHAPTER 7

Carroll, P. (1997, November). Analyzing the Chem 7. *RN Magazine, 60*(11), 32–36.

Carroll, P. (1997, September). Clarifying the CBC. *RN Magazine, 60*(9), 47–50.

Chernecky, C, Berger, B. (2001). *Laboratory tests and diagnostic procedures* (3rd ed.). Philadelphia: Saunders.

Corbett, J. (2000). *Laboratory tests and diagnostic procedures* (5th ed.). Upper Saddle River: Prentice Hall Health.

Fischbach, F. (2000). *Manual of laboratory and diagnostic tests* (6th ed.). Philadelphia: Lippincott Williams & Wilkins.

Frizzell, J. (1998, February). Avoiding lab test pitfalls. *American Journal of Nursing, 98*(2), 34–37.

Gaedeke, MK. (2000). *Laboratory and diagnostic handbook.* Menlo Park: Addison-Wesley.

Gibbar Clements, T, et al. (1997, July). PT and APTT: seeing beyond the numbers. *Nursing 97, 27*(7), 49–51.

Kee, J. (2002). *Laboratory and diagnostic tests* (6th ed.). Upper Saddle River: Prentice Hall Health.

Pagana, K, Pagana, T. (2002). *Diagnostic testing and nursing implications* (6th ed.). St. Louis: Mosby.

Tasota, F, Wesmiller, S. (1998, December). Keeping blood pH in equilibrium. *Nursing 98, 28*(12), 35–40.

CHAPTER 8

Abrutyn, E, Goldman, DA, Scheckler, WE, Biello, L. (2001). *Saunders infection control reference service.* Philadelphia: Saunders.

Beezhold, T, et al. (1996). Latex allergy can induce clinical reaction to specific foods. *Clinical and experimental allergy, 26,* 416–422.

Black, J, Matassarin-Jacobs, E. (2001). *Medical–surgical nursing: clinical management for continuity of care* (6th ed.). Philadelphia: Saunders.

Borton, D. (1996, September). Gloves: on or off? *Nursing 96, 26*(9), 46–47.

Borton, D. (1997, January). Isolated precautions. *Nursing 97, 27*(1) 49–51.

Calianno, C. (1996, May). Nosocomial pneumonia. *Nursing 96, 26*(5), 34–39.

Carroll, P. (1998, June). Preventing nosocomial pneumonia. *RN Magazine, 68*(6), 44–47.

Centers for Disease Control. (2002). Recommendations for prevention of HIV transmission in healthcare settings. *MMWR, 36*(suppl 25).

Decennial International Conference on Nosocomial and Healthcare Associated Infections.

Doenges, M, Moorhouse, M. (2002). *Nurse's pocket guide: diagnosis, interventions, and rationales* (7th ed.). Philadelphia: Davis.

Emerging Infectious Diseases. (1998). Using nurse hotline calls for disease surveillance. www.cdc.gov/nicdod/eid/vol4no2/rodman.htm.

Friedman, M. (2000, February). Improving infection control in home care: from ritual to science-based practice. *Home Healthcare Nurse, 18*(2), 99.

Gritter, M. (1998, September). The latex threat. *American Journal of Nursing, 98*(9), 26–32.

Larson, E. (1995). APIC guideline for handwashing and hand anasepsis in health care settings. *American Journal of Infection Control, 23,* 251–269.

Sheff, B. (1999, February). Minimizing the threat of C. difficile. *Nursing 99, 29*(5), 33–38.

Smeltzer, S, Bare, B. (2000). *Brunner & Suddarth's textbook of medical–surgical nursing.* Philadelphia: Lippincott.

CHAPTER 9

Armstrong, J. (2002, April). Chemical warfare. *RN Magazine, 65*(4), 32–39.

Fell-Carlson, D. (2003, January). Terrorist Danger. *Nurseweek California,* Sunnyvale, CA.

Fell-Carlson, D. (2003, January). The nurse's role in managing threat. *Nurseweek California,* Sunnyvale, CA.

Henderson, D. (1999, February). The looming threat of bioterrorism. *American Association for Advancement of Science, 283*(5406). 1279–1282.

Hoffman, R, Norton, J. (2000, December). Lessons learned from a full-scale bioterrorism exercise. *Emerging Infectious Diseases, 6*(6), 652–653.

Kilpatrick, J. (2002, May). Nuclear attacks. *Nurseweek California,* Sunnyvale, CA, 47–51.

Maniscalco, P, Christem, H. (2002). *Understanding terrorism and managing the consequences.* Upper Saddle River, NJ: Pearson Education.

Nicolson, G. (2001, December). Protection from biological warfare agents. *Townsend letter for doctors & patients.* Port Townsend, WA: 62–67.

Salvucci, A. (2002, October). Bioterrorism safeguards. *Bottom Line,* Stamford, CT: Boardroom.

Steinhauer, R. (2002, May). Bioterrorism, *RN Magazine, 65*(3), 48–54.

Steinhauer, R. (2002, June). The emergency management plan. *RN Magazine, 72*(6).

References Found on the Internet

American College of Emergency Physicians (2002). NBC Task Force; Office of Emergency Preparedness, Final Report: Resources for Dealing with Stress Brought on by Recent Terrorist Attacks. www.acep.org/Government & Advocacy.

American Hospital Association (2002). Chemical & Biological Terrorism Preparedness Checklist; Policy Forum, Hospital Preparedness for Mass Casualties. www.hospitalconnect.com/ahapolicyforum/resources /disaster.

Association for Professionalism Infection Control and Epidemiology, Inc., Mass Casualty Disaster Plan Checklist: A Template for Healthcare Facilities. www.apic.org/bioterror/checklist.doc.

Army Regulation 40-13 Medical Services. (1985). Medical Support—Nuclear, Chemical Accidents & Incidents. www.cdc.gov/nuclear.

Centers for Disease Control and Prevention (2000). Biological & Chemical Terrorism: Strategic Plan for Preparedness and Response. www.cdc.gov/mmwr/preview/mmwrht/rr4901 al.htm.

Centers for Disease Control and Prevention. Emerging Infectious Diseases (2002, September). Preparing at the Local Level for Events Involving Weapons of Mass Destruction. www.cdc.gov/nicdod/EID/vol8no9/01-0520.htm.

Centers for Disease Control and Prevention. Interim Recommendations for the Selection & Use of Protective Clothing and Respirators Against Biological Agents. cdc.gov/niosh/unp-intrecppe.html.

Centers for Disease Control and Prevention. Issues in Healthcare Settings, Part II. Recommendations for Isolation Precautions in Hospitals. cdc.gov/nicdod/hip/isolat/isopart2.htm.

Centers for Disease Control and Prevention. National Center for Infectious Diseases. www.cdc.gov/ncidod/publicat.htm.

Centers for Disease Control and Prevention. National Institute for Occupational Safety and Health. Chemical protective clothing. www.cdc.gov/niosh/npptl/chemprcloth.html.

Centers for Disease Control and Prevention. Office of Communication. CDC Radiation Studies, Nuclear Terrorism & Health Effects. www.cdc.gov/od/oc/media/9-11 pk.html.

Centers for Disease Control and Prevention. Public Health Emergency Preparedness & Response FAQS about Anthrax. www.cdc.gov/documentsapp/faqanthrax.asp#Qr001.

Centers for Disease Control and Prevention. Strategic Planning Workgroup. (2002). Biological & Chemical Terrorism: Strategic Plan for Preparedness Response. www.cdc.gov/mmwr/preview/mmwrhtml/rr 4904al.htm.

Centers for Disease Control and Prevention. Trends. www.cdcnac.org/geneva98/trends/trends_6.htm.

Center for Strategic and International Studies. Combating chemical, biological, radiological, and nuclear terrorism. www.cis.org/home/and/reports contactchembiorad.

Centers for Disease Control and Prevention (2000). Biological & Chemical Terrorism: Strategic Plan for Preparedness and Response. www.cdc.gov/mmwr/rpeview/mmwrht/rr 4901 al.htm.

Centers for Disease Control and Prevention. Emerging Infectious Diseases (2002, September). Preparing at the Local Level for Events Involving Weapons of Mass Destruction. www.cdc.gov/nicdod/EID/vol8no9/01-0520.htm.

Centers for Disease Control and Prevention. Interim Recommendations for the Selection & Use of Protective Clothing & Respirators Against Biological Agents. cdc.gov/niosh/unp-intrecppe. html.

Centers for Disease Control and Prevention. Issues in Healthcare Settings, Recommendations for Isolation Precautions in Hospitals. cdc.gov/nicdod/hip/isolat/isopart2.htm.

Centers for Disease Control and Prevention. National Center for Community Emergency Response Team (CERT). Training: Participant handbook. www.cert-la.com/manuals/tc & intro.pwf.

Electronic Journal of Biotechnology. (1999). Biological Warfare, bioterrorism, biodefence and the biological antitoxin weapons convention. www.ejb.org/content/vol2/issue 3/full//.

Emergency Weapons of Mass Destruction Responses. (2001). Emergency decontamination triage and treatment. www.2.sbccom.army.mil/hid.

Emerging Infectious Diseases. (1998). Using Nurse Hotline Calls for Disease Surveillance. www.cdc.gov/nicdod/eid/vol4o2/rodman.htm.

Federal Emergency Management Agency. (FEMA). 2001. Federal Response Plan-ESF#8. www.fema.gov/rrr/frpesf8.shtm.

Guidance for Radiation Accident Management. (2002). Managing radiation emergencies. www.orau.gove/reacts/dyndrome.htm.

Guidance for Radiation Accident Management. (2002). Oak Ridge Associated Universities Basics of Radiation Safety Around Radiation Sources. www.orau.gov/reacts/guidance.htm.

JCAHO Standards, Security Management Plan. Occupational Safety & Health Administration. (1999, April). Technical information—rubber latex gloves & other natural rubber products. www.osha.gov/as/opa/fol9/TIB 19990412-html.

Recommendations for Chemical Protective Clothing Database. www.cdc.gov/niosh/nepc/ncpc2.html.

Smallpox and Smallpox Vaccines: Adverse Reactions—Thinktwice, Smallpox. www.thinktwice.com/smallpox.htm.

Weapons of mass destruction, information for EMS first responders. www.oswegocountyems.org/WMD%20sheet%2ohtml.html.

CHAPTER 10

Acello, B. (2000, March). Meeting JCAHO standards for pain control. *Nursing 2000, 30*(3), 52–54.

American Nurses Association. (1996, March). Standards of clinical practice. *Nursing 96, 26*(3), 32f–j.

Amsterdam, E, et al. (1997, March 15). Chest pain with normal coronary arteries. *Patient Care,* p. 43.

Arnolds, S. (1997). What you should know about cardiac stress testing. *Nursing 97, 37*(1), 58–61.

Back, J, (1999, January). Clinical practice guidelines for chronic nonmalignant pain syndrome. *Musculoskeletal Rehabilitation, 13,* 47–58.

Barker, E. (1999, May). Brain attack!: a call to action. *RN Magazine, 62*(5), 54.

Barker, E. (1998, February). The xenon CT: a new neuro tool. *RN Magazine, 61*(2), 22–26.

Bates, B. (2002). *Guide to physical examination and history taking* (8th ed.). Philadelphia: Lippincott Williams & Wilkins.

Beare, P, Myers, J. (1998). *Adult health nursing* (3rd ed.). St. Louis: Mosby.

Beers, M, Berkow, R. (1999). *The Merck manual of diagnosis and therapy.* Whitehouse Station, NJ: Merck Research Laboratories.

Beezhold, T, et al. (1996). Latex allergy can induce clinical reaction to specific foods. *Clinical and Experimental Allergy, 26,* 416–422.

Black, J, Hawkes, J, Keene, A. (2001). *Medical-surgical nursing: clinical management of positive outcomes* (6th ed.). Philadelphia: Saunders.

Bozinko, C, Lowe, K, Reigart, C. (1998, November). A new option for burn victims. *RN Magazine, 61*(11), 37–39.

Burrell, L, Gerlach, M, Pless, B. (2001). *Foundations of contemporary nursing practice* (3rd ed.). Upper Saddle River, NJ: Prentice Hall Health.

Cantwell-Gab, K. (1996). Identifying chronic peripheral arterial disease. *American Journal of Nursing, 96*(7), 40–46.

Carroll, P. (1999, January). Chest injuries. *RN Magazine, 62*(1), 36–40.

Carroll, P. (1998, May). Closing in on safer suctioning. *RN Magazine, 61*(5), 22–26.

Chettie, C. (2002, October). West Nile Virus, *Nurseweek,* 24–25.

Chiocca, E. (1997, September). Actionstat. *Nursing 97, 27*(9), 33.

Chulay, M, Guzzetta, C, Dossey, B. (1997). *AACN handbook of critical care nursing.* Stamford, CT: Appleton & Lange.

Cooper, C. (2000). Reducing the use of physical restraints in nursing homes. *Postgradutae Medicine, 107*(2).

Corbett, J. (2000). *Laboratory tests and diagnostic procedures* (5th ed.). Stamford, CT: Appleton & Lange.

Crumlish, C, et al. (2000). When time is muscle. *American Journal of Nursing, 100*(1), 26–31.

Cutler, J, et al. (1998, February 28). Preventing hypertension. *Patient Care, 32*(4), 64–77.

Deedwania, P, LaRosa, J, Superko, H. (1999, Spring). Managing dyslipidemia. *Patient Care.*

Deglin, J, Vallerand, A. (2003). *Davis's drug guide for nurses* (7th ed.). Philadelphia: Davis.

Dibartolo, V. (1998, December). 9 steps to effective restraint use. *RN Magazine, 61*(12), 23–26.

Doenges, M, Moorhouse, M, Geissler-Murr, A. (2002). *Nurse's pocket guide: diagnosis, interventions, and rationales* (8th ed.). Philadelphia: Davis.

Finkelman, A. (2001, January). *Managed Care: a nursing perspective.* Upper Saddle River, NJ: Prentice Hall Health.

Fischbach, F. (2001). *Nurses' quick reference to common laboratory and diagnostic tests* (3rd ed.). Philadelphia: Lippincott Williams & Wilkins.

Garza, A, Forshner, H. (1997, December). Hepatitis update. *RN Magazine, 60*(12), 39.

Gorski, L. (2001, January). TPN update: making each visit count. *Home Healthcare Nurse, 19*(1), 15.

Gritter, M. (1998, September). The latex threat. *American Journal of Nursing, 98*(9), 26–32.

Guyton, AC. (2000). *Textbook of medical physiology* (10th ed.). Philadelphia: Saunders.

Habel, M, Strong, MA. (1997, January). Providing excellent care for patients with post-polio syndrome. *Nurseweek,* pp. 10–11.

Hayes, D. (1997). Mitral valve prolapse revisited. *Nursing 97, 27*(10), 34–39.

Heffernan, L. (1998, February). Organ donation: the legal aspects. *RN Magazine, 61*(2), 51–52.

Heslin, J. (1997, January). Peptic ulcer disease. *Nursing 97, 27*(1), 34–36.

Hickey, JV. (2002). *Clinical Practice of Neurological and Neurosurgical Nursing* (5th ed.). Lippincott Williams & Wilkins.

Hilton, G. (2001, September). Acute head injury: distinguishing subdural from epidural hematoma. *American Journal of Nursing, 101*(9), 51.

Hudak, C, Gallo, B, Morton, P. (2001). *Critical care nursing: a holistic approach* (8th ed.). Philadelphia: Lippincott.

Hurley, M. (1998). New hypertension guidelines. *RN Magazine, 61*(3), 25–28.

Hutcherson, C. (1998, May). What five regulatory trends mean to you. *Nursing 98, 28*(5), 54–57.

Ignatavicius, D, Workman, L, Mishler, M. (2003). *Medical–surgical nursing across the health care continuum* (4th ed.). Philadelphia: Saunders.

Iomko, J. (2000). Demystifying cardiac markers. *American Journal of Nursing, 100*(1), 36–40.

Joint Commission for the Accreditation of Hospitals. (2002, February). *Comprehensive accreditation manual for hospitals: the official handbook.* Sentinel Events. Chicago: JCAHO.

Joint Commission on Accreditation of Healthcare Organization (JCAHO). (2002). *Comprehensive accreditation manual for hospitals.* Oakbrook Terrace, IL: JCAHO.

Kuhn, M. (2002). *Pharmacotherapeutics* (5th ed.). Philadelphia: Davis.

LeMone, P, Burke, K. (2004). *Medical–surgical nursing: critical thinking in client care* (3rd ed.). Upper Saddle River, NJ: Prentice Hall Health.

Lewis, A. (1999, October). Neurologic emergency. *Nursing 99, 29*(10), 33, 54–55.

Lewis, S, Heitkemper, M, Dirksen, S. (2004). *Medical–surgical nursing* (6th ed.). St. Louis: Mosby.

Little, C. (2000). Renovascular hypertension. *American Journal of Nursing, 100*(2), 46–51.

Mancini, M, Kaye, W. (1999). AEDs: changing the way you respond to cardiac arrest. *American Journal of Nursing, 99*(5), 26–30.

Marthalwe, M, Keresztes, P, Tazbir, J. (2003, August). SARS—What have we learned? *RN Magazine, 66*(8), 58–62.

McCaffrey, M. (1999, July). Assessing pain in a confused, nonverbal patient. *Nursing 99, 29*(7), 18.

McCaffery, M, Pasero, C. (2000, September). Pain control. *Nurseweek,* Sunnyvale, CA.

McCance, K, Huether, S. (2002). *Pathophysiology* (4th ed.). St. Louis: Mosby.

McConnell, EA. (1999, January). Myths and facts . . . about fractures. *Nursing 99, 29*(1), 17.

McGrath, D. (1997). Mitral valve prolapse. *American Journal of Nursing, 97*(5), 40.

McKee, R. (1999, May). Clarifying advance directives. *Nursing 99, 29*(5), 52–53.

Meissner, J. (1997, October). Caring for patients with pancreatitis. *Nursing 97, 27*(10), 50–51.

Metules, TJ. (2002, April). Stroke prevention depends on skilled assessment. *RN Magazine, 65*(4), 66.

Miller, C, Holden, P. (1999, June). Women and asthma; facts about the disease. *Nurseweek,* pp. 14–15.

O'Donnell, L. (1996). Complications of MI. *American Journal of Nursing, 96*(9), 24–30.

Oertel, L. (1999, November). Monitoring warfarin therapy. *Nursing 99, 29*(11), 41–44.

Packer, M, Cohn, J. (1999, January 21). Consensus recommendations for the management of chronic heart failure. *American Journal of Cardiology.*

Pettinicchi, T. (1998, March). Trouble shooting chest tubes. *RN Magazine, 28*(3), 58–60.

Phillips, J. (1998). Abdominal aortic aneurysm: confronting a compound problem. *Nursing 98, 28*(5), 34–39.

Phipps, W, Sands, J, Marek, J. (2004). *Medical–surgical nursing: concepts and clinical practice* (7th ed.). St. Louis: Mosby.

Porth, C. (2002). *Pathophysiology: concepts of altered health states* (6th ed.). Philadelphia: Lippincott.

Rice, K. (1998). Peripheral arterial occlusive disease, Part I. *Nursing 98, 28*(2), 33–38.

Riley, M. (1997). Elective cardioversion. *RN Magazine, 60*(5), 27–29.

Rockett, J. (1999). Endothelial dysfunction and the promise of ACE inhibitors. *American Journal of Nursing, 99*(10), 44–45.

Shelton, B. (1998, December). Mounting an offense against lobar pneumonia. *Nursing 98, 28*(12), 42–46.

Smeltzer, S, Bare, B. (2000). *Brunner & Suddarth's textbook of medical–surgical nursing* (9th ed.). Philadelphia: Lippincott.

Smith, S, Duell, D, Martin, B. (2004). *Clinical nursing skills* (6th ed.). Upper Saddle River: Prentice Hall Health.

Stockert, P. (1999, March). Getting UTI patients back on track. *RN Magazine, 62*(3), 49–51.

Taber's cyclopedic medical dictionary (9th ed.). Philadelphia: Davis.

Taylor, E. (2002). *Spiritual care.* Upper Saddle River, NJ: Prentice Hall Health.

Thelan, L, Urden, L, Lough, M, Stacy, K. (2002). *Critical care nursing: diagnosis and management* (4th ed.). St. Louis: Mosby.

Tierney, L, McPhee, S, Papadakis, M. (2004). *Current medical diagnosis and treatment* (43rd ed.). New York: Lange Medical Books/McGraw-Hall.

US Department of Health and Human Services, Public Health Service. (1992, February). *Acute pain management: operative or medical procedures and trauma.* USDHHS, Pub. No. 920032.

Urben, L, Lough, M, Stacy, K. (1996). *Priorities in critical care nursing* (2nd ed.). St. Louis: Mosby.

Walsh, E. (1998). Peripheral arterial occlusive disease, Part II. *Nursing 98, 28*(2), 39–44.

Warmkessel, J. (1997, June). Caring for patients with non-Hodgkin's lymphoma. *Nursing 97, 27*(6), 48–49.

Warren, C. (1999). What is homocysteine? *American Journal of Nursing, 99*(10), 39–41.

CHAPTER 11

American Medical Association. (1990). *Handbook of first-aid and emergency care.* New York: Random House.

Asselin, M, Cullen, H. (2001, March). New guidelines for BLS and ACLS. *Nursing 2001, 31*(3), 48–50.

Black, J, Matassarin-Jacob, E. (2001). *Medical–surgical nursing* (6th ed.). Philadelphia: Saunders.

Bailey, M. (1996, March). Emergencies handbook. *Nursing 96, 26*(3), 61–64.

Harwood, S. (1997, February). Anaphylaxis. *Nursing 97, 27*(2), 33.

Laskowski-Jones, L. (1997, September). Managing hemorrhage. *Nursing 97, 27*(9), 36–41.

Lewis, A. (1999, January). Pediatric emergencies. *Nursing 99, 29*(1), 33–39.

Phipps, W, Sands, J, Marek, J. (2003). *Medical–surgical nursing: concepts and clinical practice* (7th ed.). St. Louis: Mosby.

Porth, C. (2002). *Pathophysiology: concepts of altered health states* (6th ed.). Philadelphia: Lippincott.

Sloan, A. (1996, August) DNR—Do not resuscitate, lose your job? *RN Magazine, 59*(8), 51–54.

Smeltzer, S, Bare, B. (2000). *Brunner & Suddarth's textbook of medical–surgical nursing* (9th ed.). Philadelphia: Lippincott.

Smith, S, Duell, D, Martin, B. (2004). *Clinical nursing skills* (6th ed.). Upper Saddle River, NJ: Prentice Hall Health.

Tierney, L, McPhee, S, Papadakis, M. (2004). *Current medical diagnosis and treatment* (43rd ed.). New York: Lange Medical Books/McGraw-Hill.

CHAPTER 12

Barker, E. (1998, June). Beyond conventional radiation. *RN Magazine, 61*(6), 34–36.

Campbell, M, Pruett, J. (1996, January). Radiation therapy. *RN Magazine, 59*(1), 46–47.

Greifzu, S. (1996, July). Chemo quick guide—Taxol and other agents. *RN Magazine, 59*(7), 938–939.

Greifzu, S. (1996, June). Plant alkaloids. *RN Magazine, 59*(6), 36–37.

Greifzu, S. (1996, May). Hormonal agents. *RN Magazine, 59*(5), 41–42.

Greifzu, S. (1996, March). Antimetabolites. *RN Magazine, 59*(3), 32–33.

Held-Warmkessel, J. (1998, April). Chemotherapy complications. *Nursing 98, 28*(4), 41–45.

Navarro, T. (1998, November). Chemotherapy extravasation. *American Journal of Nursing, 98*(11), 38.

Oncology update. (1997, October). *Nursing 97, 27*(10), 44–45.

Wakeling, K. (1999, July). The latest weapon in the war against cancer. *RN Magazine, 62*(7), 58–60.

Bence, Sharlene A. (2000, April). Stop cervical cancer in its tracks. *Nursing 2000, 30*(4).

Brown, CG, Yoder, LH. (2002, April). Stomatitis: an overview. *American Journal of Nursing, 102*(4).

Brown, K, Esper, P, et al. (Eds.). (2001). *Chemotherapy and biotherapy guidelines and recommendations for practice.* Pittsburgh: Oncology Nursing Press.

Carr, B, Burke, C. (April, 2001). Outpatient chemotherapy: hypersensitivity and anaphylaxis. *American Journal of Nursing, 101*(4).

——— (US Preventive Services Task Force). (May, 2003). Chemoprevention of breast cancer: recommendations and rationale. *American Journal of Nursing, 103*(5).

Connor, TH. (2002). *Occupational Hazards Related to Antineoplastic Agents.* The University of Texas-Houston Health Science Center www.uth.tmc.edu/schools/sph/an_agents/index.htm

Del Gaudio, D, Menonna-Quinn, D. (1998, November). Chemotherapy: potential occupational hazards. *American Journal of Nursing, 98*(11), 59.

Engstrom, PF. (2000, May). Cancer Prevention: from Concept to Practice. *Career.*

Held-Warmkessel, J. (1998, April). Chemotherapy complications. *Nursing 98, 28*(4), 41–45.

Hinson-Smith, V. (2000). Breast cancer survivors: learning from the faces of hope. *Nursing* 2000.

Kazda, R. (2001, April). Coming out on top: one woman coping with chemotherapy-induced alopecia finds strength in humor. *American Journal of Nursing, 101*(4).

Lewis, S, Heitkemper, M., Dirksen, S. (2000). *Medical surgical nursing assessment and management of clinical problems.* St. Louis: Mosby.

——— Low- versus high-dose radiation therapy. (2002, December). (Horizons). *Journal of Neuroscience Nursing.*

Machia, J, Napoli, M. (2001, April). Breast cancer: risk, prevention, and tamoxifen. *American Journal of Nursing, 101*(4).

Mosby's Medical, Nursing, & Allied Health Dictionary (1998). (5th ed.). St. Louis: Mosby.

Myers, J. (2000, April). Chemotherapy-induced hypersensitivity reaction. *American Journal of Nursing, 100*(4).

Napoli, M. (April, 2000). The lingo of chemo: how language misleads patients with cancer. *American Journal of Nursing, 100*(4).

National Cancer Institute http://cis.nci.nih.gov/fact/5_9.htm

National Institutes of Health, Division of Safety, Clinical Center Pharmacy Department and Cancer Nursing Service. *Recommendations for the safe handling of cytotoxic drugs.* (2002, January). www.nih.gov/od/ors/ds/pubs/cyto/index.htm

Navarro, T. (1998, November). Chemotherapy extravasation. *American Journal of Nursing, 98*(11).

Nielsen, E, Brant, J. (2002, April). Chemotherapy-induced neurotoxicity: assessment and interventions for patients at risk. *American Journal of Nursing, 102*(4).

Occupational Safety & Health Administration. (1999). *Controlling occupational exposure to hazardous drugs.* OSHA technical manual. www.osha-slc.gov/dts/osta/otm/otm_vi/otm_vi_2.html (31 Jan. 2002).

Oncology Nursing Society, www.ons.org

Sitton, E. (2000, August). Beaming in on radiation therapy. *Nursing 2000, 30*(8).

——— Support for preventive mastectomies. (2001, October) *Nursing 2000, 31*(10).

Wakeling, K. (1999, July). The latest weapon in the war against cancer. *RN Magazine, 62*(7), 58–60.

Welch, J, Silveira, J. (Eds.). (1997). *Safe handling of cytotoxic drugs: an independent study module* (2nd ed.). Pittsburgh: Oncology Nursing Press.

CHAPTER 13

Adresen, G. (1998, March). Assessing the older patient. *RN Magazine, 61*(3), 47–53.

American's life expectancy reaches record high. (2003, June). *RN Magazine, 66*(6), 98.

Anderson, M. (1995). *Caring for the elderly client.* Philadelphia: Davis.

Bauer, J. (2003, June). "Silent" strokes increase elderly patients' risk of developing dementia. *RN Magazine, 66*(6), 23.

Carneveli, D, Patrick, M. (1997). *Nursing management for the elderly* (4th ed.). Philadelphia: Lippincott.

Centers for Disease Control and Prevention. (2003). Deaths: preliminary data for 2001. National Vital Statistics Report, 51(5). www.cdc.gov/nchs/data/nvsr/nvsr51/nvsr51_05.Pdf (26 Mar. 2003).

Dibartolo, V. (1998, December). 9 steps to effective restraint use. *RN Magazine, 61*(12), 23–24.

Ebersole, P, Hess, P. (1998). *Toward healthy aging* (5th ed.). St. Louis: Mosby.

Eliopolis, C. (1997). *Gerontological nursing* (4th ed.). Philadelphia: Lippincott Williams & Wilkins.

Finch, M. (2003, April). Assessment of skin in older people. *Nursing Older People, 15*(2), 29.

Gallagher, B. (2001, August). Managing pain in elderly patients at home. *Nursing 2001, 31*(8), 18.

Garrison, J. (2003, May). Heart failure and older people. *Nursing Older People, 15*(3), 38.

Gray-Vickery, P. (1999, September). Elder abuse. *Nursing 99, 29*(9), 52–53.

Haban, S. (2000, November). Elder abuse and neglect. *American Journal of Nursing, 100*(11), 49.

Higginbotham, E. (2003, March). The misuse of psychotropics in the elderly. *RN Magazine, 66*(3), 67–68.

Ignatavicius, D. (2000, January). Do you help staff rise to the fall-prevention challenge? *Nursing Management, 31*(1), 27.

Jubeck, M. (1994, May). Teaching the elderly: a common sense approach. *Nursing 94, 24*(5), 70–71.

Lewis, SM, Heitkemper, MM, Dirksen, SR. (2000). *Medical surgical nursing. Assessment and management of clinical problems.* St. Louis: Mosby.

Lueckenotte, AG. (1998). *Pocket guide to gerontologic assessment* (3rd ed.). St. Louis: Mosby.

Miller, C. (1999). *Nursing care of older adults* (3rd ed.). Philadelphia: Lippincott.

Morris, R. (1998, August). Elder abuse: what the law requires. *RN Magazine, 61*(8), 52–53.

Shuster, J. (1997, November). Adverse drug reactions. *Nursing 97, 27*(11), 34–39.

Stanly, M, Beare, PG. (1999). *Gerontological nursing* (2nd ed.). Philadelphia: Davis.

Venaree, E. (2003, June). Help reduce adverse drug events in elderly outpatients. *RN Magazine, 66*(6), 95.

Whetstone, G, Boswell, S. (2002, September). The geriatric heart: nurses need to be aware of how aging and disease affect the myocardium. *American Journal of Nursing, 102*(9), 22.

Wold, G. (1993). *Basic geriatric nursing.* St. Louis: Mosby.

Zhan, C. (2002, March). One in five elderly is prescribed inappropriate medications: safety is a major concern. *American Journal of Nursing, 102*(3), 18.

CHAPTER 14

American Academy of Pediatrics, American Heart Association (2000). *Neonatal resuscitation textbook* (4th ed.).

Bernstein, J. (1995). Ectopic pregnancy: a nursing approach to excess risk among minority women. *JOGNN 24*(9), 803–10.

Bougere, M. (1998). Abruptio placentae. *Nursing 98, 28*(2), 47.

Carr, D, Gabbe, S. (1998). Gestational diabetes: detection, management, and implications. *Clinical Diabetes* [Online] 16(1), 4. Available: www.diabetes.org.clinicaldiabetes/v16n1j-f98/pg4.htm

Gilbert, E, Harmon, J. (1998). *Manual of high-risk pregnancy and delivery* (2nd ed.). St. Louis: Mosby.

Hockenberry, MJ, Wilson, D, Winkelstein, ML, Kline, NE. (2003). *Wong's nursing care of infants and children* (7th ed.). St. Louis: Mosby.

Letko, M. (1996). Understanding the Apgar score. *JOGNN, 25*(4), 299–303.

Lowdermilk, DL, Perry, SE, Bobak, IM. (2004). *Maternity and women's health care nursing* (8th ed.). St. Louis: Mosby.

Lowe, N, Reiss, R. (1996). Parturition and fetal adaptation. *JOGNN, 25*(4), 339–49.

Lucas, L, Jordan, E. (1997). Phenytoin as an alternative treatment for preeclampsia. *JOGNN, 26*(3), 263–69.

Mandeville, L, Troiano, N. (1998). *High-risk and critical care intrapartum nursing.* Philadelphia: Lippincott Williams & Wilkins.

Olds, S, London, M, Ladewig, P. (2004). *Maternal-newborn nursing: a family and community-based approach* (7th ed.). Upper Saddle River, NJ: Prentice Hall.

Oliveto, TM. (1997). Emergency! Severe preeclampsia. *American Journal of Nursing, 97*(7), 47.

Orlando, S. (1995). The immunologic significance of breast milk. *JOGNN, 24*(7), 678–83.

Persson, B, Hanson, U. (1998). Neonatal morbidities in gestational diabetes mellitus. *Diabetes Care* [On-line] 21(2). Available: www.diabetes.org/diabetescare/supplement298/b79.htm

Schnare, S, Matsoda, K. (1997). today's contraceptive choices. *RN Magazine, 60*(12), 30–37.

Tomlinson, P, Bryan, A. (1996). Family centered intrapartum care: revisiting an old concept. *JOGNN, 25*(4), 331–337.

CHAPTER 15

American Academy of Pediatrics. (2003). Recommended childhood immunization schedule—United States, January–December 2003. Available from AAP Web site: www.aap.org.

American Academy of Pediatrics Car Safety Seats. (2003). *A guide for families.*

Ball, J, Bindler, R. (2003). *Pediatric nursing* (3rd ed.). Upper Saddle River, NJ: Prentice Hall Health.

Bates, B. (1995). *A guide to physical examination history taking* (6th ed.). Philadelphia: Lippincott.

Bazinski, M. (1999). *Manual of pediatric critical care.* St. Louis: Mosby.

Betz, C, Hunsburger, M, Wright, S. (Eds.). (1994). *Family-centered nursing care of children* (2nd ed.). Philadelphia: Saunders.

Buck, M. (2001). Pediatric vaccine update. *Pediatric Pharmacotherapy* 7(3).

Centers for Disease Control and Prevention. (2000). *Attention deficit / hyperactivity disorder.* Division of Birth Defects, Child Development and Disability and Health, Development Disabilities Branch. Available from CDC Web site: www.cdc.gov.

Centers for Disease Control and Prevention. (2003, May). *Childhood injury fact sheet.* National Center for Injury Prevention and Control. Available from CDC Web site: www.cdc.gov.

Centers for Disease Control and Prevention. (2003, May). *10 Leading causes of death, United States, 2000, all races, both sexes.* National Center for Injury Prevention and Control. Available from CDC Web site: www.cdc.gov.

Curley, M, Smith, J, Moloney-Harmon, P. (1996). *Critical care nursing of infants and children.* Philadelphia: Saunders.

Estrada, B. (2000, May). Pediatric bulletin: what's new in varicella vaccine? *Infections in Medicine*, 17(3). Available from Infections in Medicine®.

Fretz, A, Eldridge, T, Shega, C. (1998). *The Skidmore-Roth outline series: pediatric nursing* (2nd ed.). Englewood, CO: Skidmore-Roth.

Garfunkel, L, Kaszorous, J, Christy, C. (2003). *Mosby's pediatric clinical advisor.* St. Louis: Mosby Yearbook.

Gern, J. (1999). *Pediatric asthma: risk factors and clinical implications.* Proceedings from the American Lung Association/American Thoracic Society International Conference, Day 1, April 25, 1999. As published on Medscape®.

Gern, J. (1999). *Diagnosis and treatment of childhood asthma: geographic and socioeconomic variables.* Proceedings from the American Lung Association/ American Thoracic Society International Conference, Day 1, April 25, 1999. As published on Medscape®.

Gibson, E, Dembofsky, CA, Rubin, S, Greenspan, JS. (2000, May). Infant sleep practices two years into the "Back to Sleep" campaign. *Clinical Pediatrics*, 39(5), 285–289.

Green, M. (ed). (1994). *Bright futures, guidelines of health supervision of infants, children and adolescents.* Arlington, VA: National Center of Education in Maternal and Child Health.

Lewis, D, Shala, A. (1999, April). Syncope in the pediatric patient, the cardiologist's perspective. *Pediatric Clinics of North America, 46*(2), 205–219.

Melish, M. (1996, May). Kawasaki syndrome. *Pediatrics in Review, 17*(5), 153–162.

Morris, C. (2000, May). Pediatric iron poisonings in the United States. *South Med Journal, 93*(4), 351–358.

National Center for Injury Prevention and Control. (2003). *Child maltreatment.* http://www.cdc-gov/

Patel, SR, Benjamin, RS. (2000, May). *Sarcomas of soft tissue and bone.* Harrison's Online, The McGraw-Hill Company, 2000. Available from Medscape®.

Shiminski-Maher, T, Shields, M. (1995, October). Pediatric brain tumors: diagnosis and management. *Journal of Pediatric Oncology Nursing, 12*(4), 188–198.

Siegler, R. (1995, December). The hemolytic uremic syndrome. *Pediatric Clinics of North America, 42*(6), 1505–1522.

Tumiston, S. (2003). *A practical guide to using the new combination vaccines.* Contemporary Pediatrics, 20*(2),* 36–53.

US Department of Health and Human Services. (2002). *Child maltreatment 2000: reports from the states to the national child abuse and neglect data system.* Washington, DC: US Government Printing Office.

Veasy, G, et al. (1987, February). Resurgence of acute rheumatic fever in the intermountain area of the United States. *New England Journal of Medicine, 316,* 421–427.

Velasco-Whetsell, M, et al. (2001). *Pediatric nursing.* New York: McGraw-Hill Nursing Care Services.

Welch, M. (1999). *Pediatric asthma: new options for young children.* Proceedings from the American Lung Association/American Thoracic Society International Conference Day 1, April 25, 1999. As published on Medscape®.

Wong, D. (2001). *Whaley & Wong's essentials of pediatric nursing* (6th ed.). St. Louis: Mosby.

Wubbel, DO, McCracken, G. (1998, March). Management of bacterial meningitis: 1998. *Pediatrics in Review, 19*(3), 78–84.

Chapter 16

American Psychiatric Association (2000). *Diagnostic and statistical manual of mental disorders* (4th ed.). Washington, DC: Author.

Aguilera, DC. (1998). *Crisis intervention and methodology* (8th ed.). St. Louis: Mosby.

Geldmucher, D. M. (2004). *Alzheimer's dementia (contemporary diagnosis and management).* Newtown, PA: Handbooks in Health Care.

Haber, J, Krainovich-Miller, B, McMahon, AL, and Price-Hoskins, P. (1997). *Comprehensive psychiatric nursing* (5th ed.). St. Louis: Mosby.

Kneisl, C, Wilson, H, Trigoboff, E. (2004). *Contemporary psychiatric-mental health nursing.* Upper Saddle River, NJ: Pearson Education Inc.

Physicians desk reference (2003). Montvale, NY: Medical Economics Company.

Stuart, G, Laraia, M. (2002). *Principles and practice of psychiatric nursing* (7th ed.). St. Louis: Mosby.

Sundeen, S, et al. (1998). *Nurse-client interaction: implementing the nursing approach* (6th ed.). St Louis: Mosby.

Varcarolis, EM. (1998). *Foundations of psychiatric mental health nursing.* Philadelphia: Saunders.

INDEX

LICENSE AGREEMENT AND LIMITED WARRANTY

CD-ROM OPERATING INSTRUCTIONS

The enclosed CD-ROM contains review questions and practice tests. Each time you wish to access this material, you will insert the CD into your CD drive and run the software directly from the CD. The program will not be installed on your computer's hard drive.

FOR WINDOWS PLATFORMS

1. Insert CD into computer
2. Go to *My Computer*
3. Click on the folder in your CD drive
4. Double click on the *NNRPNTest* icon

FOR MACINTOSH PLATFORMS

1. Insert CD into computer
2. Go to *Desktop*
3. Click on the folder to your CD drive
4. Double click on the *NNRPNTest* icon

If you are having technical issues related to any part of the CD-ROM, please visit our technical support web site at http://www.jbpub.com/support.